SCAI

Interventional Cardiology Review

THIRD EDITION

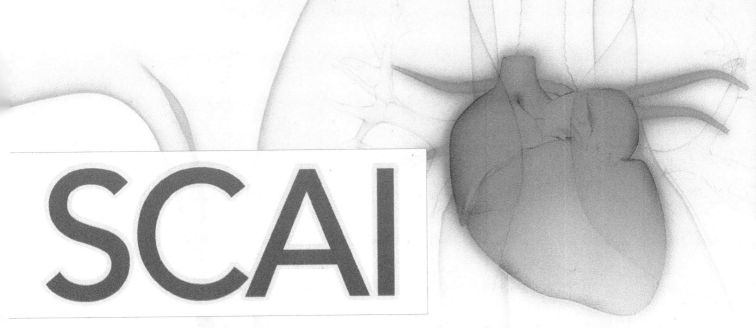

SCAI
Interventional Cardiology Review

THIRD EDITION

Morton J. Kern, MD, MSCAI, FAHA, FACC

Professor of Medicine
University California Irvine
Chief of Medicine
Long Beach Veterans Administration Health Care System
Long Beach, California
Associate Chief, Cardiology
University California Irvine
Orange, California

Arnold H. Seto, MD, MPA, FSCAI, FACC

Associate Professor of Medicine
University California Irvine
Chief, Cardiology
Long Beach Veterans Administration Health Care System
Long Beach, California

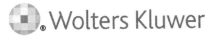. Wolters Kluwer

Philadelphia • Baltimore • New York • London
Buenos Aires • Hong Kong • Sydney • Tokyo

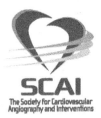

SCAI
The Society for Cardiovascular
Angiography and Interventions

Acquisitions Editor: Sharon Zinner
Developmental Editor: Ashley Fischer
Editorial Coordinator: Maria M. McAvey and Lindsay Ries
Production Project Manager: Marian Bellus
Design Coordinator: Stephen Druding
Manufacturing Coordinator: Beth Welsh
Marketing Manager: Rachel Mante Leung
Prepress Vendor: S4Carlisle Publishing Services

Third Edition

Library of Congress Cataloging-in-Publication Data

Names: Kern, Morton J., editor. | Seto, Arnold, H., editor. | Society of
  Cardiac Angiography and Intervention.
Title: SCAI interventional cardiology review / [edited by] Morton J. Kern,
  Arnold H. Seto.
Other titles: SCAI interventional cardiology board review book. |
  Interventional cardiology review | Society of Cardiac Angiography and
  Intervention interventional cardiology review
Description: 3rd edition. | Philadelphia: Wolters Kluwer Health, 2018. |
  Preceded by SCAI interventional cardiology board review / edited by Morton
  J. Kern. 2nd edition. 2014.
Identifiers: LCCN 2017052635 | ISBN 9781496360557 (hardback)
Subjects: | MESH: Cardiovascular Surgical Procedures | Catheterization |
  Diagnostic Techniques, Cardiovascular | Heart Diseases—surgery
Classification: LCC RC669.2 | NLM WG 168 | DDC 616.1/20076—dc23 LC record available at https://lccn.loc.gov/2017052635

DEDICATION

*To Margaret and Anna Rose, who provide unwavering
support without measure.*

—Morton J. Kern

*To Lily for her inexhaustible understanding, and to
Dr. Kern for opening so many doors
for me for the past decade.*

—Arnold H. Seto

ACKNOWLEDGMENT

*We thank the SCAI leadership and membership for their support and
the opportunity to further their educational mission through this book.*

—Morton J. Kern and Arnold H. Seto

CONTRIBUTORS

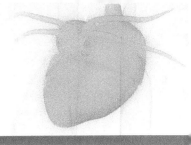

Mazen Abu-Fadel, MD, FACC, FSCAI
Associate Professor of Medicine
Vice Chief, Section of Cardiovascular Medicine
Director, Interventional Cardiology & Cardiac Cath Lab
Program Director, Interventional Cardiology Fellowship
University of Oklahoma Health Sciences Center
Oklahoma City, Oklahoma

Robert J. Applegate, MD, FACC, FAHA, MSCAI
Professor of Internal Medicine and Cardiovascular Medicine
Section of Cardiovascular Medicine
Wake Forest School of Medicine
Winston-Salem, North Carolina

Ehrin J. Armstrong, MD, MSc, MAS, FACC, FSCAI, FSVM
Director, Interventional Cardiology
Director, Vascular Laboratory
VA Eastern Colorado Healthcare System
Division of Cardiology
Associate Professor of Medicine
University of Colorado School of Medicine
Aurora, Colorado

Alaa S. Ayyoub, MD
Interventional Cardiology Fellow
Department of Cardiovascular Medicine
Lahey Hospital and Medical Center
Burlington, Massachusetts

Subhash Banerjee, MD, FSCAI, FACC, FAHA
Chief of Cardiology
VA North Texas Healthcare System
University of Texas Southwestern
Medical Center
Dallas, Texas

P. Matthew Belford, MD, FACC, FSCAI
Wake Forest School of Medicine
Winston-Salem, North Carolina

Ryan A. Berg, MD, FSCAI, FACC
VA Central California Healthcare System
Associate Professor of Medicine
University of California, San Francisco Fresno
Fresno, California

Emmanouil S. Brilakis, MD, PhD, FSCAI, FACC, FESC, FAHA
Director, Center for Advanced Coronary Interventions
Minneapolis Heart Institute
Minneapolis, Minnesota

M. Nicholas Burke, MD, FSCAI, FACC
Senior Consulting Cardiologist
Director, CV Emergency Programs, CV Lab, and
CTO Program at Minneapolis Heart Institute at Abbott
Northwestern Hospital
Minneapolis, Minnesota

John D. Carroll, MD, FSCAI, FACC
Professor of Medicine and Cardiology
Director of Interventional Cardiology
University of Colorado School of Medicine
Denver, Colorado

Jeffrey Cavendish, MD, FSCAI
Kaiser Permanente San Diego Hospital
San Diego, California

Charles E. Chambers, MD, MSCAI
Professor of Medicine and Radiology
Penn State University College of Medicine
Hershey, Pennsylvania

Adnan K. Chhatriwalla, MD, FACC, FSCAI
Medical Director, Structural Intervention
Saint Luke's Mid America Heart Institute
Assistant Professor
University of Missouri-Kansas City School of Medicine
Kansas City, Missouri

Creighton W. Don, MD, MS, PhD, FSCAI
Associate Professor of Medicine
University of Washington Medical Center
Seattle, Washington

Douglas E. Drachman, MD, FACC, FSCAI
Director, Cardiovascular Fellowship Program
Director, Interventional Cardiology Fellowship Program
Interventional Cardiology Associates
Boston, Massachusetts

Ted Feldman, MD, MSCAI, FACC, FESC
NorthShore University Health System
Evanston, Illinois

José Luis Ferreiro, MD, PhD
Heart Diseases Institute
Bellvitge University Hospital-IDIBELL
University of Barcelona
L'Hospitalet de Llobregat
Barcelona, Spain

Francesco Franchi, MD
Assistant Professor
University of Florida College of Medicine-Jacksonville
Jacksonville, Florida

Mario Gössl, MD, FSCAI
Minneapolis Heart Institute
Minneapolis, Minnesota

Mayra Guerrero, MD, FACC, FSCAI
NorthShore University HealthSystem
Evanston, Illinois

Sartaj Hans, MD, FACC
The John Ochsner Heart and Vascular Institute
University of Queensland
Ochsner Medical Center
University of Queensland Ochsner Medical Center
New Orleans, Louisiana

Robert A. Harrington, MD, FSCAI, FACC
Arthur L. Bloomfield Professor of Medicine
Chairman of the Department of Medicine
Stanford University
Stanford, California

Beau M. Hawkins, MD, FACC, FSCAI
Director, Heart, Lung and Vascular Clinic
Assistant Professor of Medicine
University of Oklahoma Health Sciences Center
Oklahoma City, Oklahoma

Khalil Ibrahim, MD
Johns Hopkins Hospital
Baltimore, Maryland

Ignacio Inglessis, MD
Medical Director Structural Heart Disease Program
Massachusetts General Hospital
Assistant Professor
Harvard Medical School
Boston, Massachusetts

Farouc A. Jaffer, MD, PhD, FSCAI, FACC
Cardiovascular Research Center
Director of Coronary Intervention and CTO-PCI Program
Massachusetts General Hospital
Associate Professor
Harvard Medical School
Boston, Massachusetts

Navin K. Kapur, MD
Director, Acute Mechanical Circulatory Support Program
Director, Interventional Cardiology Research Laboratories
Director, Cardiac Biology Research Center within the
Molecular Cardiology Research Institute (MCRI)
Associate Professor, Tufts University School of Medicine
Boston, Massachusetts

Morton J. Kern, MD, MSCAI, FAHA, FACC
Professor of Medicine and Associate Chief of Cardiology
University California Irvine
Chief of Medicine
Long Beach Veterans Administration Health Care System
Long Beach, California

Ajay J. Kirtane, MD, SM, FSCAI, FACC
Chief Academic Officer, CIVT
Director, NYP/Columbia Cardiac Catheterization Laboratories
Columbia University Medical Center / New York-Presbyterian Hospital
New York, New York

Sandeep Krishnan, MD, RPVI
Interventional Cardiology Fellow
University of Washington Medical Center
Seattle, Washington

Zoran Lasic, MD, FSCAI, FACC
Northwell Health Physician Partners
New York, New York
Assistant Professor
Donald and Barbara Zucker School of Medicine at Hofstra/Northwell
New York, New York

Carl J. Lavie, MD, FACC
The John Ochsner Heart and Vascular Institute
University of Queensland Ochsner Clinical School
University of Queensland School of Medicine
New Orleans, Louisiana

Michael S. Lee, MD, MPH, FSCAI, FACC
Associate Professor
University of California, Los Angeles
Los Angeles, California

Justin P. Levisay, MD, FACC, FSCAI
NorthShore University HealthSystem
Evanston, Illinois

Michael S. Levy, MD, MPH
Lahey Hospital
Burlington, Massachusetts

Michael Lim, MD, FSCAI, FACC
Jack Ford Shelby Endowed Professor in Cardiology
Co-Director, Center for Comprehensive Cardiovascular Care
Director, Division of Cardiology
St Louis University
Saint Louis, Missouri

Amir S. Lofti, MD
Baystate Cardiology
Springfield, Massachusetts
Associate Professor of Medicine
Tufts University School of Medicine
Boston, Massachusetts

Gopi Manthripragada, MD
Assistant Clinical Professor
University of California
Los Angeles, California

Ronan Margey, MD, MRCPI, FSCAI, FACC
Heart & Vascular Centre
Mater Private Hospital
Citygate, Mahon, Cork

Richard V. Milani, MD, FACC
The John Ochsner Heart and Vascular Institute
University of Queensland Ochsner Clinical School
New Orleans, Louisiana

Julie M. Miller, MD, FSCAI, FACC, FAHA
Associate Professor of Medicine
Director, Vascular Cardiology Program
Johns Hopkins Hospital
Baltimore, Maryland

Keshav Nayak, MD, FSCAI, FACC
Associate Professor
Uniformed Services University of the Health Sciences
Naval Medical Center San Diego
San Diego, California

Vivian G. Ng, MD
Columbia University Medical Center
New York, New York

Eric A. Osborn, MD, PhD, FSCAI, FACC
Instructor
Harvard Medical School
Beth Israel Deaconess Medical Center
Boston, Massachusetts

Pranav M. Patel, MD, FSCAI, FACC
Chief of Cardiology
University of California, Irvine
Orange, California

Jayendrakumar S. Patel, MD
Fellow, Heart and Vascular Institute
Cleveland Clinic
Cleveland, Ohio

Karen S. Pieper, MS
Associate Director Clinical Trials Statistical Operations
Duke Clinical Research Institute
Duke University Medical Center
Durham, North Carolina

Matthew J. Price, MD, FSCAI, FACC
Director of the Cardiac Catheterization Laboratory
Assistant Professor, Scripps Translational Science Institute
Scripps Clinic
La Jolla, California

Sunil V. Rao, MD, FSCAI, FACC
Chief of Cardiology
Durham VA Medical Center
Associate Professor of Medicine
Duke University Medical Center
Durham, North Carolina

Jeremy D. Rier, DO
Interventional Cardiology Fellow
Penn State Hershey Medical Center
Hershey, Pennsylvania
Durham, North Carolina

F. David Russo, MD
Duke University Medical Center
Durham, North Carolina

Abdulfattah Saidi, MD
University of Utah School of Medicine
Vernal, Utah

Michael H. Salinger, MD, FSCAI, FACC
Clinical Assistant Professor
University of Chicago Pritzker School of Medicine
NorthShore University HealthSystem
Evanston, Illinois

Sonia R. Samtani, MD
Interventional Cardiology Fellow
University of California, Irvine
Orange, California

Arnold H. Seto, MD, MPA, FSCAI, FACC
Associate Professor of Medicine
University California Irvine
Chief, Cardiology
Long Beach Veterans Administration Health Care System
Long Beach, California

Binita Shah, MD, MS, FSCAI, FACC
VA New York Harbor Health Care System (Manhattan Campus)
Assistant Professor of Medicine and Associate Director of Research
NYU School of Medicine
New York, New York

Mehdi H. Shishehbor, DO, MPH, PhD, FSCAI
Director, Cardiovascular Interventional Center
Heart and Vascular Institute
Cleveland Clinic
Cleveland, Ohio

Vikas Singh, MD
Structural Heart Disease Fellow
Massachusetts General Hospital
Harvard Medical School
Boston, Massachusetts

Paul Sorajja, MD, FSCAI, FACC, FAHA
Director, Center of Valve and Structural Heart Disease
Minneapolis Heart Institute
Minneapolis, Minnesota

Daniel H. Steinberg, MD, FSCAI
Associate Professor
Medical University of South Carolina
Charleston, South Carolina

Sasha Still, MD
Baylor University Medical Center
Dallas, Texas

William Suh, MD, FSCAI
Interventional Cardiologist
Associate Professor
University of California, Los Angeles
Los Angeles, California

Molly Szerlip, MD, FSCAI, FACC, FACP
The Heart Hospital Baylor Plano
Plano, Texas

Jose D. Tafur Soto, MD
The John Ochsner Heart and Vascular Institute
University of Queensland Ochsner Clinical School
New Orleans, Louisiana

Mladen I. Vidovich, MD, FSCAI, FACC
Chief, Section of Cardiology
Jesse Brown VA Medical Center
Associate Professor of Medicine
University of Illinois at Chicago
Chicago, Illinois

Frederick G.P. Welt, MD, FSCAI, FACC
Associate Chief of Cardiovascular Medicine
University of Utah School of Medicine
Director of the Cardiac Catheterization Laboratory
Vernal, Utah

Christopher J. White, MD, MSCAI, FACC
The John Ochsner Heart and Vascular Institute
University of Queensland Ochsner Clinical School
New Orleans, Louisiana

Dominik M. Wiktor, MD
Assistant Professor
University of Colorado School of Medicine
Cardiac & Vascular Center—Anschutz
Aurora, Colorado

Katherine Yu, MD
Cardiology Fellow
University of California, Irvine
Orange, California

Gilbert Zoghbi, MD, FSCAI, FACC
Gilbert Stern Cardiovascular Foundation
South Haven, Mississippi

PREFACE

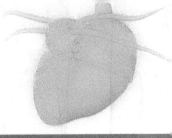

Interventional cardiology is among the most dynamic and rapidly changing specialties in medical practice. There have been 18 annual ABIM board certification examinations for interventional cardiology since its inception in 1999. New procedures and new data are generated yearly. Certifying examinations continue to include many areas of updated knowledge. For this reason, a concise yet comprehensive review of the pertinent material is important. We believe that this contribution to continuing education meets one of the major missions of the SCAI. The SCAI Interventional Cardiology Board review book is designed to assist fellows-in-training, students, residents, and those physicians wishing to renew their cognitive and procedural knowledge base and pass the test to maintain certification in this specialty.

Coronary interventions are the mainstay of the field and occupy a major part of testable material. New and emerging percutaneous structural heart disease interventions will certainly take their place alongside the coronary knowledge base. To fulfill the cognitive basis for current and future practitioners of interventional cardiology, well-known studies are used to support modern pharmacologic therapies, pathophysiologic mechanisms directing interventional modalities, and current practice guidelines likely to be included by the examiners.

As in the prior edition, we have attempted to cover all the major topics as outlined by the ABIM certifying examination materials. Notable in this new edition is sections on structural heart interventions focusing on transcatheter aortic valve replacement, percutaneous mitral valve repair (MitraClip), closure of atrial septal defects, and left atrial appendage occluder indications. The sections on basic science deal with the fundamentals of atherosclerosis, including endothelial function and restenosis; the pharmacology of interventional practice; and the important principles of imaging, anatomy, and coronary physiology for application in PCI. Specific commonly encountered coronary interventional patient subsets, critical aspects of patient management, peripheral vascular disease, and finally, guidelines are reviewed.

From basic to clinical science, each of the expert contributors discusses what are considered the most important aspects of their topics. Of course, as with any review text, it is impossible to include all aspects of every topic of a complex medical field. Each expert has provided several questions and answers, which the reader will find useful in their study for the examination. Study questions have been included in the online supplement.

I want to acknowledge the continued and highly supportive role that the Society of Cardiac Angiography and Intervention plays in the education of interventional cardiologists. The mission of SCAI is to be the leading society for interventional cardiologists in education, representation, and advocacy. I believe this book exemplifies that mission. It is our hope that the SCAI Interventional Cardiology Review will benefit all those interested in interventional cardiology, especially those preparing for their Board Exam, ultimately providing interventional cardiologists with high-quality education for the advancement of patient care.

On a personal note, I thank my co-editor, Dr. Arnold Seto and my colleagues, who contributed their knowledge and precious time. Many of the contributors are members of the SCAI Early Career Interventional Committee or Early Leadership Mentor Award recipients. Their contributions further reflect their competence and commitment.

I remain indebted to my friends in the SCAI. The SCAI plays a unique role in the life of a cardiologist. As evidenced by the growing membership, now more than 4,000 members strong, the SCAI fills a vital need in our professional community and the cardiologist's professional life. The SCAI has been and, I believe, will continue to be a stable, strong resource for communication, education, and professional support.

Morton J. Kern, MD, MSCAI, FAHA, FACC
Long Beach Veterans Administration Health Care System, Long Beach, California and University California Irvine, Orange, California

---

In this age of advanced information technology, you are more likely to consult the latest journal article from a smartphone than to pick up a physical book. Based on typical printing timelines and the rapidity of advances in the field, by the time any book is published, it may already seem out-of-date. Yet there remains a role for a board review text such as this, with expert summaries of a wide breadth of material that simply cannot be found with an internet search, and certainly not as efficiently. The board exam by design tests established facts and practices that are at least 2 years old, making the contents of this book as contemporaneous as you will need.

I thank all of the contributors to this endeavor for their hard work, and hope you make the most of the collective knowledge and experience contained in this book.

Arnold H. Seto, MD, MPA, FSCAI, FACC
Long Beach Veterans Administration Health Care System, Long Beach, California and University California Irvine, Orange, California

CONTENTS

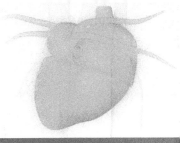

SECTION I. Basic Science and Pharmacology

Chapter 1: Arterial Disease—Atherosclerosis 1
Abdulfattah Saidi and Frederick G. P. Welt

Chapter 2: Restenosis 11
Abdulfattah Saidi and Frederick G. P. Welt

Chapter 3: Platelet—Inhibitor Agents 27
José Luis Ferreiro and Francesco Franchi

Chapter 4: Anticoagulant and Fibrinolytic Agents for NSTE-ACS, PCI, and STEMI 38
Vivian G. Ng and Ajay J. Kirtane

Chapter 5: Vasoactive and Antiarrhythmic Drugs in the Catheterization Laboratory 53
Gilbert Zoghbi

SECTION II. Fundamentals of Interventions

Chapter 6: Fundamentals of X-ray Imaging, Radiation Safety, and Contrast Media 62
Jeremy D. Rier and Charles E. Chambers

Chapter 7: Coronary Hemodynamics: Pressure and Flow 79
Morton J. Kern, Amir S. Lofti, and Arnold H. Seto

Chapter 8: Intravascular Ultrasound, Optical Coherence Tomography, and Near-Infrared Spectroscopy 93
Sonia R. Samtani and Arnold H. Seto

Chapter 9: Vulnerable Plaque Imaging 105
Eric A. Osborn and Farouc A. Jaffer

Chapter 10: Hemodynamics for Interventional Cardiologists 116
Morton J. Kern and Arnold H. Seto

Chapter 11: Coronary Angiography for PCI 143
Morton J. Kern and Arnold H. Seto

Chapter 12: Introduction to Statistics in Clinical Research for Interventional Cardiology 156
Robert A. Harrington and Karen S. Pieper

SECTION III. Equipment

Chapter 13: Equipment Selection for Coronary Interventions 164
Keshav Nayak, Arnold H. Seto, Jeffrey Cavendish, and Morton J. Kern

Chapter 14: Niche Devices: Atherectomy, Cutting and Scoring Balloons, and Laser 175
P. Matthew Belford and Robert J. Applegate

SECTION IV. Stable and Acute Coronary Syndrome PCI

Chapter 15: Coronary Stents 187
F. David Russo and Sunil V. Rao

Chapter 16: Elective Percutaneous Coronary Intervention for Stable Coronary Artery Disease and Silent Myocardial Ischemia 196
Ronan Margey, Douglas E. Drachman and Katherine Yu

Chapter 17: Acute Coronary Syndromes 215
Arnold H. Seto

Chapter 18: STEMI Intervention: *Emphasis on Guidelines* 224
Khalil Ibrahim and Julie M. Miller

Chapter 19: High-Risk Percutaneous Coronary Intervention, Cardiogenic Shock, and Acute Mechanical Circulatory Support Devices 249
Daniel H. Steinberg and Navin K. Kapur

SECTION V. Higher-Risk PCI and Complex Angiographic Subsets

Chapter 20: Multivessel Percutaneous Coronary Interventions 258
Creighton W. Don and Sandeep Krishnan

Chapter 21: Bifurcation Lesions and Intervention 272
Alaa S. Ayyoub and Michael S. Levy

Chapter 22: Small Vessel and Diffuse Disease 281
Mladen I. Vidovich

Chapter 23: Left Mainstem Intervention 292
Michael S. Lee and Gopi Manthripragada

Chapter 24: Bypass Graft Intervention and Embolic Protection 299
Emmanouil S. Brilakis, Mario Gössl, Paul Sarojja, and Subhash Banerjee

Chapter 25: Complications of Coronary Intervention . . 306
Ryan A. Berg and Michael Lim

Chapter 26: Chronic Total Occlusion Percutaneous Coronary Intervention 313
Emmanouil S. Brilakis, M. Nicholas Burke, and Subhash Banerjee

SECTION VI. Vascular Access and Hemostasis

Chapter 27: Vascular Access: Radial and Femoral Approaches 323
Beau M. Hawkins and Mazen S. Abu-Fadel

Chapter 28: Vascular Access Site Management
(Closure Devices and Complications) 330
Robert J. Applegate

SECTION VII. Women, Prevention, and Guidelines

Chapter 29: Women and Percutaneous Interventions. . 339
Binita Shah, Sasha Still, and Molly Szerlip

Chapter 30: Primary and Secondary
Coronary Prevention 349
Carl J. Lavie and Richard V. Milani

Chapter 31: PCI Guidelines for Interventional
Cardiology Boards 354
Zoran Lasic

SECTION VIII. Peripheral Vascular Disease and Interventions

Chapter 32: Thoracic Aortic, Abdominal Aortic,
and Lower Extremity Interventions 364
Ehrin J. Armstrong and Douglas E. Drachman

Chapter 33: Carotid and Cerebrovascular/
Acute Stroke Intervention 373
Jose D. Tafur Soto, Sartaj Hans, and Christopher J. White

Chapter 34: Atherosclerotic Renal Artery Disease 391
Pranav M. Patel

Chapter 35: Deep Venous Thrombosis 400
Jayendrakumar S. Patel and Mehdi H. Shishehbor

SECTION IX. Structural Heart Disease and Interventions

Chapter 36: Imaging for Structural Heart Disease 406
Mazen Abu-Fadel

Chapter 37: Atrial Septal Defect and Patent
Foramen Ovale 417
Dominik M. Wiktor and John D. Carroll

Chapter 38: Left Atrial Appendage Closure 424
Matthew J. Price

Chapter 39: Mitral Valvuloplasty and Percutaneous
Mitral Valve Repair 430
Ted Feldman, Mayra Guerrero, Michael H. Salinger,
and Justin P. Levisay

Chapter 40: Transcatheter Aortic Valve Replacement. . 442
William Suh

Chapter 41: Hypertrophic Cardiomyopathy 451
Paul Sorajja

Chapter 42: Paravalvular Leaks 458
Adnan K. Chhatriwalla and Paul Sorajja

Chapter 43: Pericardial Disease Interventions 464
Paul Sorajja

Chapter 44: Interventional Procedures in Adult
Congenital Heart Disease 469
Vikas Singh and Ignacio Inglessis

Index   477

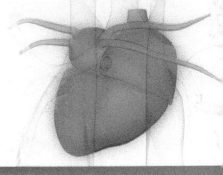

1 Arterial Disease—Atherosclerosis

Abdulfattah Saidi, MD and Frederick G. P. Welt, MD,

FSCAI, FACC

Atherosclerosis

There is increasing understanding of the molecular and cellular pathophysiology of the vascular responses to injury leading to atherosclerosis. A common thread that links these events is an inflammatory response to injury. The inflammatory process not only initiates these lesions, but often dictates their clinical presentation. A fundamental knowledge of these processes is necessary to understand the natural history of atherosclerosis, as well as therapies employed during coronary intervention. This chapter will review the pathophysiology of atherosclerosis and the conversion of stable atherosclerotic plaques to ones that cause acute coronary syndromes.

Atherosclerosis: A Response to Injury

Atherosclerosis is a chronic inflammatory disease initiated and sustained by injury to the vascular wall (1). Largely through extensive epidemiologic studies, several injurious processes have been identified (Table 1.1). These include metabolic conditions such as sustained exposure to low-density lipoprotein (LDL), hyperglycemia associated with diabetes, and hyper-homocysteinemia. Other factors, including physical (hypertensive changes in shear stress), environmental (tobacco smoke), and possibly infectious (Chlamydia Pneumoniae) processes, have also been implicated. The common thread of injury to the vessel wall is an inflammatory response that involves a complex and incompletely understood sequence of interactions among endothelial and smooth muscle cells (SMCs), leukocytes, and platelets. These cells and their secreted growth factors and cytokines combine with lipids and components of the vessel wall to eventually form the mature atherosclerotic plaque. The central role of inflammation in the pathogenesis of atherosclerosis is evidenced by numerous epidemiologic studies that demonstrate a correlation between circulating markers of inflammation (e.g., fibrinogen,

C-reactive protein [CRP], serum amyloid protein, myeloperoxidase) and subsequent risk of coronary events (2,3).

Atherosclerosis: Pathogenesis

There are several key biologic events involved in atherogenesis; extracellular lipid accumulation, leukocyte recruitment, foam cell formation, neointimal growth (as a result of SMC migration and proliferation and extracellular matrix deposition), as well as vessel remodeling (Fig. 1.1).

EXTRA- AND INTRACELLULAR LIPID ACCUMULATION

The key event in the creation of the incipient atherosclerotic lesion is the accumulation of lipoproteins within the intima. These lipoproteins may subsequently be modified by processes such as oxidation, and glycation in the presence of aging and hyperglycemia. The modification of these lipoproteins helps to elicit a cascade of molecular and cellular events, including stimulation of growth factor and cytokine production from endothelial and SMCs. These early events lead to recruitment of leukocytes and eventually to SMC proliferation and migration, all of which act to form the mature atherosclerotic plaque.

Of pivotal importance is the understanding that hyperlipidemia is an inflammatory state. The interaction between inflammation and hyperlipidemia is evident in the presence of foam cells, the hallmark of the fatty streak, which is the initial lesion of atherosclerosis. The foam cell is a macrophage named for the abundance of lipids within the cell. Macrophages bind and internalize modified lipoprotein particles via a number of "scavenger receptors," including scavenger receptor-A family members, CD36, and macrosialin. Foam cells are able to further modify lipoproteins. In addition, lipoproteins can prove toxic to macrophages, leading to necrotic debris and free cholesterol clefts and ester within the lesion. This necrotic debris along with expression of the tissue factor and other molecules, leads to a very prothrombotic environment within the plaque and is a serious threat to local blood flow in the setting of loss of integrity of the barrier between plaque and blood stream.

LEUKOCYTE RECRUITMENT

Leukocytes, especially macrophages, play pivotal roles in atherosclerosis through their release of critical cytokines and growth factors that influence not only atherogenesis, but also influence processes of plaque rupture and thrombosis. The process of leukocyte recruitment, attachment, and migration into the plaque is under the influence of a variety of molecules. As a response to injury, such as the accumulation of lipoproteins, endothelial cells express certain adhesion molecules, such as E-selectin, which interact with ligands on the surface of circulating leukocytes to begin a process of loose association and rolling along the surface of the vessel (4). Subsequent tight binding mediated by the integrin class of adhesion molecules stops the leukocyte prior to the process of diapedesis. Although their pathologic role is uncertain, soluble forms of cell adhesion molecules

TABLE 1.1 Causes of Vascular Injury

Metabolic
- Hyperlipidemia
- Hyperglycemia
- Hyperhomocysteinemia

Physical
- Shear forces (hypertension)
- Laminar versus nonlaminar flow (i.e., bifurcations)

Environmental
- Tobacco smoke

Infectious
- Chlamydia
- Herpes simplex
- Cytomegalovirus

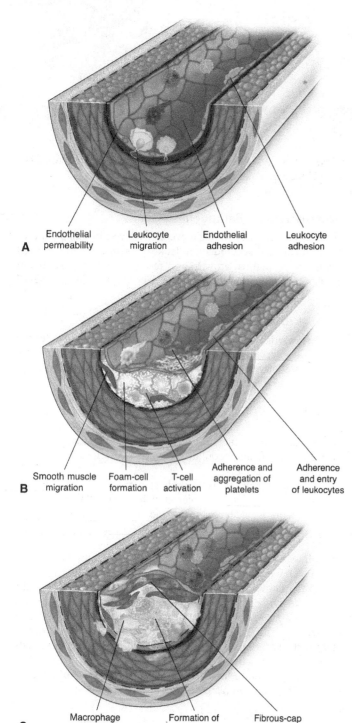

A Endothelial permeability | Leukocyte migration | Endothelial adhesion | Leukocyte adhesion

B Smooth muscle migration | Foam-cell formation | T-cell activation | Adherence and aggregation of platelets | Adherence and entry of leukocytes

C Macrophage accumulation | Formation of necrotic core | Fibrous-cap formation

FIGURE 1.1 Stages of atherosclerotic plaque growth. **A:** Initial stage of atherosclerosis involves injury to the vessel wall, with subsequent expression of inflammatory adhesion molecules, which leads to leukocyte recruitment. **B:** Intermediate lesions involve macrophages imbibing oxidized LDL, leading to foam cell formation. There is continued leukocyte recruitment, formation of an early lipid core, and SMC proliferation and migration. **C:** The advanced or mature atherosclerotic plaque consists of a necrotic lipid core with foam cells, necrotic debris, and free cholesterol esters. In addition, there is a fibrous cap consisting of SMCs and extracellular matrix. LDL, low-density lipoprotein; SMC, smooth muscle cell. (From: Ross R. Atherosclerosis—An inflammatory disease. *N Engl J Med.* 1999;340:115–126, with permission.)

(CAMs) can be found in plasma. Human studies have demonstrated that plasma levels of intracellular cell adhesion molecules (ICAM-1) and E-selectin correlate with clinical manifestations of coronary atherosclerosis (5).

Also central to the recruitment of leukocytes to areas of vascular injury, chemokines are a group of chemoattractant cytokines produced by a variety of somatic cells that include SMCs, endothelial cells, and leukocytes. One important chemokine of the C-C class, monocyte chemoattractant protein-1 (MCP-1), participates in the recruitment of monocytes in particular (6). Also critical is the C-X-C chemokine, interleukin-8 (IL-8), which participates in the recruitment of leukocytes to areas of vascular injury. IL-8 has been extensively documented in the recruitment of neutrophils (7), and more recent evidence suggests that the murine analogue of IL-8, KC, also plays a critical role in the recruitment of monocytes to injured areas (8).

As lesions mature, there tends to be excess accumulation of leukocytes at the "shoulder" regions of plaques where the eccentric plaque merges with the more normal architecture of the vessel. This clustering is thought to make these "shoulder" regions more vulnerable to the consequences of atherosclerosis (9). In addition, it has long been observed that atherosclerotic lesions develop preferentially at areas of bifurcations within the coronary tree. This likely is related to disturbances in flow patterns and resultant areas of flow separation and altered shear stress, leading to preferential areas of upregulation of adhesion molecules and increased leukocyte recruitment (10). In addition, monocytes may contribute to vascular calcification in response to two cytokines: monocyte colony stimulating factor and receptor activator of NF-κB (RANKL) (11). Emerging evidence indicates that atherosclerotic plaque calcification is positively correlated with vulnerability. Several inflammatory mediators have been shown to modulate arterial calcification, thus increasing the risk of plaque rupture. Among these factors, RANKL/OPG axis might be of particular interest as a promising biomarker of plaque vulnerability in subjects with diffuse coronary calcification (12).

INNATE VERSUS ADAPTIVE IMMUNITY

There are two major branches of the immune system: the innate or nonspecific arm, and the adaptive or specific arm (13). There are several key differences that distinguish these two arms. The innate arm relies predominantly on phagocytic cells, such as neutrophils and monocyte/macrophages, the cells most classically associated with atherosclerosis. The innate arm is not antigen-dependent and exhibits immediate response to foreign material. On the other hand, the adaptive arm is characterized by a specific antigen dependent response that has the characteristic of conferring memory against the pathogen. Unlike, the immediate response of the innate arm, the adaptive arm involves a lag time between exposure to the pathogen and response. The primary effector cells of this arm are lymphocytes. These two arms work in concert with dendritic cells of the innate immune system, representing a link between innate and adaptive immunity because they are phagocytic cells, which then present antigens to cells of the adaptive system (14).

INNATE IMMUNE RESPONSE IN ATHEROSCLEROSIS

The monocyte is thought to be the first leukocyte recruited to the incipient atheroma after encountering complex signals that include soluble factors affecting general monocyte function in circulation. In addition, local factors affect the cells upon monocytes' adhesion to the endothelium and their migration into the tissue. The defining cell of the fatty streak is the foam cell, a macrophage named for the abundance of lipids within the cell. Macrophages bind and internalize oxidized lipoprotein particles via a number of "scavenger receptors," including scavenger receptor-A family members, CD36, and macrosialin. Foam cells can also further modify lipoproteins, making them more inflammatory. Lipoproteins can also lead to toxicity of macrophages, resulting in cell death and eventually leaving necrotic debris and free cholesterol clefts and ester within the lesion. Two main directions of monocyte-to-macrophage differentiation are recognized: type 1, induced by inflammatory stimuli like IFN-γ or LPS and type 2, induced by IL-4, IL-13 and other anti-inflammatory cytokines. Type 1 macrophages (M1) produce high amounts of reactive oxygen species and inflammatory cytokines like tumor necrosis factor (TNF) or IL-1β. Type 2 macrophages show a high expression of scavenger receptors that produce extracellular matrix components and remodeling enzymes and secrete anti-inflammatory cytokines IL-1ra, CCL18, and IL-10, and express typical surface markers (15–17). The phenotype of plaque-associated macrophages (PAMs) seems to be mixed, because infiltrating monocytes/macrophages are described to express markers of both M1 (TNF) and M2 (STAB1, CD163) (18). Macrophages amplify the inflammatory response through the secretion of cytokines such as TNF-α and IL-1-β (13). Other cells of the innate immune response that have been implicated in atherosclerosis include mast cells, natural killer cells, and neutrophils (19).

ADAPTIVE IMMUNE RESPONSE IN ATHERSOCLEROSIS

In contrast to the monocyte, the CD4$^+$ T-cell is the primary cell of the adaptive arm of the immune response present at atherosclerotic sites. It is believed that these T-cells and their secreted cytokines influence progression and vulnerability of plaques (19). As an example, interferon (IFN)-γ appears to inhibit the growth of SMC and promote apoptosis (programmed cell death) of these cells, leading to plaque vulnerability. In addition, IFN γ appears to limit production of structural proteins (collagen and elastins) that SMCs (smooth muscle cells) secrete, and may lead to a plaque more prone to rupture (20). CD4$^+$ T-cells also express a CD40 ligand on their surface, which is subsequently released as a soluble factor. Among its effects, the soluble CD40 ligand appears to influence a variety of cell types to produce the highly procoagulant substance called tissue factor. There are subsets of CD4$^+$ T-cells that have been identified by cellular receptors and the typical cytokines released from these cells. CD4$^+$ T$_H$1 T-cells are the predominant types at atherosclerotic lesions and are believed to promote atherosclerosis. CD4$^+$ T$_H$2 T-cells, on the other hand, are likely anti-atherogenic. In addition, regulatory T-cells are present, which seem to suppress activation of other T-cells acting as an anti-atherogenic mechanism.

Lastly, B-cells can also be identified within an atherosclerotic lesion. Antibodies to oxidized LDL can be identified in human and animal models (19) and it is thought that this humoral immune response acts as a protectant against atherosclerosis, possibly by intercepting and neutralizing antigens prior to their reaching sites of atherosclerosis. There is other evidence to suggest that infection with agents such as chlamydia pneumonia or perhaps viruses can create antibodies with auto-immune features that promote atherogenesis (21).

SMOOTH MUSCLE MIGRATION, PROLIFERATION, AND EXTRACELLULAR MATRIX DEPOSITION

SMCs and their products are responsible for giving structure to the mature atherosclerotic plaque, which is initially little more than a collection of lipids and foam cells. Under the influence of growth factors and chemoattractants, such as platelet-derived growth factors and thrombin, SMCs migrate out from the media into the neointima where they begin to proliferate. In addition, SMCs produce extracellular matrix constituents, including collagen, proteoglycans, elastin, fibrinogen, fibronectin, and vitronectin. These proteins often account for a substantial volume of the plaque and are important in determining the structural integrity of the fibrous cap. Giachelli et al. have shown evidence that these cells express bone matrix proteins that have been subsequently corroborated by other investigators (22–24). This highlights the role of VSMC in vascular calcification. In some patients, an additional process of mineralization of the atherosclerotic plaque will occur with deposition of calcium and osteopontin. Mineralization does not equate to a stable plaque, and has been associated with higher risk, especially in the elderly (25).

PLAQUE ANGIOGENESIS AND HYPOXIA

A newly emerging area of interest is the potential role of angiogenesis in plaque growth and in the pathogenesis of atherosclerotic complications. New vasculature under the influence of angiogenic growth factors, such as hypoxia inducible factor (HIF)/vascular endothelial growth factor (VEGF) (26), may grow from the vaso vasorum within the adventitia into the plaque. These vessels may be disrupted and cause plaque hemorrhage independent of plaque rupture. The extravasated erythrocytes provide a local depot of cholesterol-rich red cell membranes and heme, a source of iron that is a stimulant for oxidative stress, which promotes further growth.

In addition, analogous to tumor growth, these vessels may stimulate plaque growth. There is experimental evidence demonstrating inhibition of plaque growth by angiogenic inhibitors in a mouse model of atherosclerosis (27,28). Furthermore, neo vessel density is higher in nonstenotic segments and stenotic noncalcified plaques than in normal segments or calcified lesions (29).

Hypoxemia not only promotes angiogenesis but also contributes to proteolysis through the promotion of matrix metalloproteinases (MMPs), a family of interstitial collagenases that weaken the fibrous cap and gellatinases capable of catabolizing nonfibrillar collagen, to which endothelial cells adhere (30–32). Proteolysis would ultimately lead to dissolution of the plaque extracellular matrix and plaque vulnerability. Hypoxemia promotes the formation of proinflammatory cytokines and leukotrienes and activates Akt and betacatenin pathways with subsequent macrophage activation (31,33). In addition, conditions resulting in lipids accumulation in macrophages are amplified with accumulation of triglyceride containing cytosolic lipid droplets and adipose differentiation protein (ADRP) expression, even in the absence of exogenous lipids. The lipid accumulation is a result of increased triglyceride biosynthesis, reduced [beta]-oxidation of fatty acids and increased expression of stearoyl-coenzyme A desaturase (SCD-1), an important enzyme in the synthesis of fatty acids (33–35).

THE MATURE ATHEROSCLEROTIC PLAQUE

The mature atherosclerotic plaque is therefore composed of several components, including a fibrous cap consisting of SMCs and extracellular matrix proteins overlying a necrotic lipid core consisting of free cholesterol esters, foam cells, other leukocytes (such as T-cells), and necrotic debris of dead foam cells (Fig. 1.1). These plaques commonly are eccentric in nature and there is heterogeneity in terms of the thickness of the cap, as well as in the distribution of leukocytes that tend to cluster in shoulder regions. Both of these features have potential import in terms of the propensity of plaques to cause acute coronary syndromes.

VASCULAR REMODELING

While angiography remains the mainstay of diagnosis in coronary artery disease, its major limitation is that it provides information only on the luminal encroachment of lesions and not on the architecture of the vessel wall. Use of intravascular ultrasound has provided a much broader understanding of the nature of atherosclerosis by allowing systematic investigation of plaque architecture not only at sites of flow-obstructing lesions but throughout the vessel. Although the interventional cardiologist is most concerned with focal obstructive lesions in proximal portions of the vessel, it is important to realize that it is now recognized that atherosclerosis is almost always universally present throughout the coronary tree. The amount of impingement of the plaque on the lumen is controlled not only by the growth of plaque volume but also on vascular remodeling. Vascular remodeling involves the restructuring of cellular or noncellular components of the wall, and can occur under a variety of stimuli (36). For example, under situations of hypertension, muscle mass of the vessel wall can increase in order to normalize wall stress. In atherosclerosis, remodeling may consist of compensatory enlargement of the vessel to preserve luminal area (**Fig. 1.2**). Central to the process of vascular remodeling are the MMPs, a family of zinc-dependent proteases that have been demonstrated to be upregulated in areas of vessel wall remodeling and are thought to play a central role also in plaque rupture (37).

Clinical Sequelae of Atherosclerosis

A convenient way of thinking about coronary artery disease is as a spectrum of syndromes from stable angina at one end (associated with exertional angina) and relatively benign outcomes to stent thrombosis (ST) segment elevation myocardial infarction (MI) at the other end (associated with sudden complete thrombotic occlusion of an epicardial blood vessel and high rates of morbidity and mortality). The intermediate syndromes of unstable angina and non-Q-wave myocardial infarction exist between these two extremes. Unstable angina, non-Q-wave MI, and ST-segment elevation MI are collectively termed as the acute coronary syndromes due to their similar pathophysiology and worse prognosis compared to stable angina. This is explained by the fact that complications from atherosclerosis can result from two related but distinct mechanisms: (a) simple luminal narrowing can lead to an imbalance between supply and demand for blood, typically resulting in stable exertional angina, or (b) atheromatous plaques may rupture, resulting in a thrombus with varying degrees of occlusion (38). Critical to the understanding of coronary disease is the knowledge that the propensity for thrombotic complications depends on a variety of vascular biologic factors, not just the degree of stenosis. Equally as important, the atherosclerotic

process fundamentally alters the normal vasomotor functions of the endothelium necessary to autoregulate blood flow in accordance with the demands of hemodynamics, a condition termed *endothelial dysfunction*.

PROGRESSIVE LUMEN ENCROACHMENT AND STABLE ANGINA

As atherosclerotic lesions grow in size, depending on the amount of compensatory vascular remodeling that occurs, they may gradually encroach upon the lumen of the vessel (Fig. 1.2). As a response to reduction in flow, there is vasodilation of the distal micro-circulation to increase flow. This reduces coronary vascular reserve or the ability of the coronary circulation to increase blood flow in response to demand, which typically leads to exertional angina, something that is short in duration and relieved by rest. At what point luminal encroachment causes symptoms depends on many factors, including the severity of the lesion, the demand of the distal cardiac bed, and the oxygen carrying capacity of the blood stream. In general, however, lesions begin to produce symptoms when they reach approximately 60% to 70% in diameter stenosis. Modern techniques of interrogating intracoronary hemodynamics with flow and pressure wires have taught the interventional cardiologist that lesions with the same degree of angiographic stenosis may have very different hemodynamic consequences (39). See Chapter 7 Coronary Hemodynamics (40,41).

PLAQUE RUPTURE, THROMBOSIS, AND THE ACUTE CORONARY SYNDROMES

James Herrick published his findings of thrombus as the predominant cause of sudden coronary obstruction in 1912 (42). DeWood, in his landmark 1980 paper (43), demonstrated that ST segment elevation was associated with angiographic occlusion of epicardial vessels (**Fig. 1.3**) and that thrombosis was present at the time of infarct, a finding confirmed by autopsy studies (**Fig. 1.4**) and by angioscopy. Visible thrombus is associated with both unstable angina and acute myocardial infarction.

Insights into acute coronary syndromes come from studies with mandated angiography after randomization to either placebo or thrombolytic therapy. The angiograms revealed an unexpected finding, namely that the majority of lesions responsible for myocardial infarction were <50% in diameter stenosis (44). In addition, similar angiographic studies also showed that mild and moderate stenoses may progress to produce myocardial infarction in a matter of weeks to months. In analysis of four serial angiographic studies, only •15%

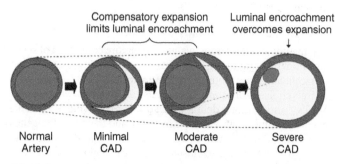

FIGURE 1.2   Schematic of vascular remodeling. As the atherosclerotic lesions progress, initial enlargement of the entire vessel allows preservation of the luminal area. As atherosclerosis becomes severe, enlargement is overcome by progression of the atherosclerotic plaque and the luminal area is compromised. CAD, coronary artery disease. (Adapted from: Glagov S, Weisenberg E, Zarins CK. Compensatory enlargement of human coronary arteries. *N Engl J Med.* 1987;316:1371–1375.)

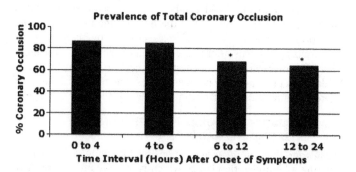

FIGURE 1.3   Percent of vessels totally occluded in patients presenting after acute myocardial infarction as a function of time after onset of symptoms. (Adapted from: DeWood MA, et al. Prevalence of total coronary occlusion during the early hours of transmural myocardial infarction. *N Engl J Med.* 1980;303:897–902, with permission.)

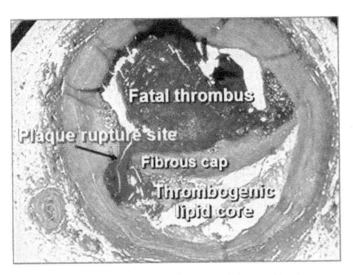

FIGURE 1.4 Histologic example of a ruptured plaque with subsequent thrombosis, leading to a fatal myocardial infarction. (From: Constantinides P. Plaque hemorrhages, their genesis and their role in supra-plaque thrombosis and atherogenesis. In: Glagov S, Newman WP III, Schaffer SA, eds. *Pathology of the Human Atherosclerotic Plaque*. New York, NY: Springer-Verlag; 1990:393–411, with permission.)

of acute myocardial infarctions were found to arise from lesions with degrees of stenosis >60% on an antecedent angiogram (45) (Fig. 1.5). The implication of these data is that the vascular biologic state of the lesion is responsible for its propensity to cause an infarct, not the severity of stenosis. These data should not be misinterpreted to suggest that lesion severity is correlated with danger of infarction. Rather, noncritical lesions represent a larger population than critical lesions. In addition, as described earlier, compensatory enlargement of the vessel often accompanies atherosclerosis. Therefore, even mildly stenotic lesions may represent large plaques by volume. In summary, thrombosis, often on a noncritical stenosis, caused by lesion disruption causes the majority of myocardial infarctions.

The proximate event leading to thrombosis at a lesion is plaque rupture (or less commonly endothelial denudation) leading to exposure of blood to highly thrombotic sub-endothelial components

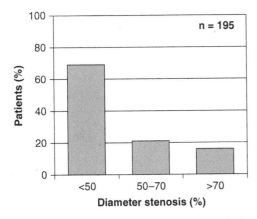

FIGURE 1.5 Compiled data from four thrombolytic trials showing that the majority of underlying lesions responsible for acute myocardial infarction are less than 50% diameter stenosis. (From: Smith SC. Risk-reduction therapy: the challenge to change. Paper presented at the 68th scientific session of the American Heart Association, November 13, 1995, Anaheim, California. *Circulation*. 1996;93:2205–2211, with permission.)

of the plaque. Histologic studies have identified several features that appear to be associated with plaques more vulnerable to rupture. These include a thin fibrous cap, a large lipid core, and an abundance of inflammatory cells largely concentrated at the shoulder regions of the plaque (Fig. 1.6) (9). It is thought that inflammation is the key regulator of the structural integrity of the plaque. One of the largest trials to date to examine the natural history of atherosclerosis is the Providing Regional Observations to Study Predictors of Events in the Coronary Tree (PROSPECT) study (46). In this trial, 697 patients with acute coronary syndrome undergoing percutaneous intervention had interrogation of all major epicardial arteries with gray scale and radiofrequency intravascular ultrasound. Patients were followed over 2 years. One hundred and six nonculprit lesions were subsequently associated with adverse cardiac events. Correlates that predicted a subsequent event had a plaque burden greater than 70%, the presence of a thin-capped fibroatheroma, and a minimal luminal area less than 4.0 mm^2.

The structural integrity of the plaque is dependent on a balance between two components: SMC mass and extracellular matrix content. In turn, SMC mass is a balance between migration of cells from the media and subsequent proliferation in the neointima on the one hand, and cell death on the other. There is evidence to suggest that cytokines released from inflammatory cells control apoptosis, or programmed cell death (47). Extracellular matrix content is a balance between production from SMCs and degradation by a variety of proteases (Fig. 1.7). Production of extracellular matrix content is dependent on both the number of cells present and their activity. Activated T-cells in the plaque secrete interferon-γ (IFN-γ), an inhibitor of SMC collagen synthesis. Inflammatory cells in atherosclerotic plaques also produce enzymes, such as MMP and cathepsins, which are capable of degrading important constituents of the extracellular matrix (i.e., collagens, elastin) (9). Therefore, inflammatory cells can contribute to plaque weakening by decreasing SMC mass, decreasing extracellular matrix content, and by increasing extracellular matrix degradation.

How and why plaques rupture when they do is a subject of increasing study. The variability of plaque rupture involves a number of postulated mechanisms, including circadian variation (48), stress events (49) and the abrupt release of cortisol and adrenaline, as well as high-circumferential biomechanical forces acting at the shoulder regions of plaques (50).

Therefore, there is an interesting combination of both biochemical and biophysical characteristics that make plaques rupture.

While frank plaque rupture is the major antecedent cause of thrombotic complications of the acute coronary syndromes, other processes may also be responsible. Local superficial denudation of endothelial cells (perhaps secondary to apoptosis) may expose the internal elastic membrane representing an important thrombotic substrate. There is some evidence that these endothelial erosions occur more frequently in women and in diabetics. The frequency of superficial erosion has increased concomitant with increased medical therapy, making vulnerable plaque a decreasing proximate cause for acute coronary syndromes (51). The evidence for this notion comes from both intravascular imaging studies (52) and studies supporting a temporal shift in acute coronary syndrome presentation from ST-segment elevation myocardial infarction (STEMI) to non-STEMI (NSTEMI) (53). The hypothesis put forward is that increasing therapy largely with statins has decreased plaque LDL cholesterol and inflammation shifting plaques more toward a stable phenotype, making plaque erosion a more dominant form of plaque thrombosis. This may have implications for therapy not only due to the lack of ruptured plaque but also because of the different nature

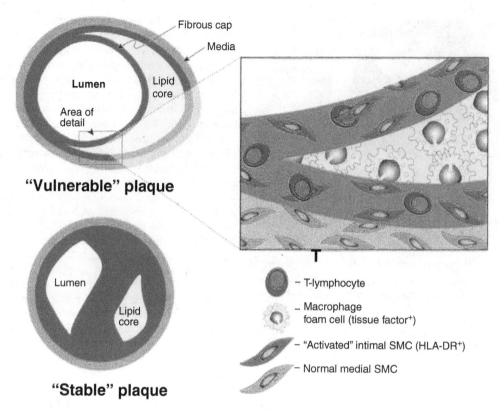

"Vulnerable" plaque

"Stable" plaque

– T-lymphocyte

– Macrophage
foam cell (tissue factor+)

– "Activated" intimal SMC (HLA-DR+)

– Normal medial SMC

FIGURE 1.6   Characteristics of stable versus vulnerable plaques. Vulnerable plaques have thinner fibrous caps and larger, more inflammatory, cell-rich lipid cores. SMC, smooth muscular cell. (From: Libby P. Molecular bases of the acute coronary syndromes. *Circulation.* 1995;91:2844–2850, with permission.)

of the adherent thrombus, which in the case of plaque erosion may be more platelet-based (**Fig. 1.8**). Mechanical injury during percutaneous coronary intervention is also another source of local plaque disruption that may lead to thrombotic complications.

The final pathway through which either plaque rupture or endothelial denudation leads to alterations in flow is through thrombosis. Exposure of blood to the lipid core is a potent stimulus for thrombus formation, largely on the basis of exposure to tissue factors associated with lipid-laden and necrotic macrophages. There is a balance between procoagulant–anticoagulant and fibrinolytic–antifibrinolytic factors

in the blood stream, which likely predetermines the consequence of any given plaque disruption. In the presence of an intact and robust fibrinolytic system, a mural thrombus might undergo rapid lysis, limiting its clinical consequences to unstable angina or non-Q-wave myocardial infarction. Similarly, patients on antiplatelet agents, such as aspirin, obviously are protected to some degree. In the presence of prothrombotic factors, such as elevated levels of fibrinogen or plasminogen activator inhibitor-1 (PAI-1), growth of a thrombus to occlusion may occur more frequently. A nonocclusive mural thrombus may be incorporated into the plaque during the process of healing, providing a mechanism for plaque growth.

There are numerous trials of anti-platelet therapy that corroborate the thrombotic paradigm of the acute coronary syndromes. Trials of lipid-lowering therapy have similarly demonstrated an interesting corroboration of theories of plaque vulnerability. These trials have demonstrated marked reductions in subsequent coronary events associated with lipid lowering, with essentially no change in lesion severity (45). As stated earlier, the hypothesis is that lipids within the plaque provide the critical initiating and sustaining inflammatory stimulus for plaque growth and rupture, and the beneficial actions of "statin" lipid-lowering agents may derive in part from the reduction of inflammation leading to stabilization of the fibrous cap and reduced thrombogenicity of the inner core. There is increasing evidence to support lipid-lowering therapy as a vital adjunct to acute as well as chronic therapy for patients presenting with acute coronary syndromes.

Endothelial Dysfunction

In 1986, Ludmer and colleagues reported that in patients with atherosclerosis, a paradoxical reaction occurred when acetylcholine

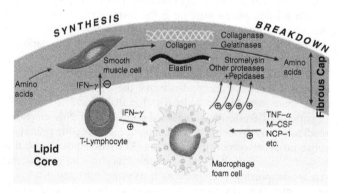

FIGURE 1.7   Thickness of the fibrous cap is a balance between synthesis of extracellular matrix proteins by smooth muscle cells and the breakdown of these products by degradative enzymes. These processes are largely under the influence of inflammatory cells. CSF, cerebrospinal fluid; IFN-γ, interferon γ; TNF-α, tumor necrosis factor α. (From: Libby P. Molecular bases of the acute coronary syndromes. *Circulation.* 1995;91:2844–2850, with permission.)

Coronary Artery Cross Sections

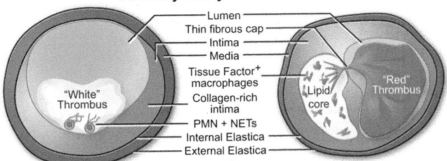

Thrombosis due to Erosion	Thrombosis due to Rupture
Fibrous cap thick & intact	Thin fibrous cap with fissure
"White" platelet-rich thrombus	"Red" fibrin-rich thrombus
Collagen trigger	Tissue Factor trigger
Smooth muscle cells prominent	Macrophages prominent
Often sessile, non-occlusive Thrombus	Often occlusive thrombus
Usually less remodelled outward	Usually expansively remodelled
Neutrophil extracellular traps (NETs) involved	Less NET involvement?
More frequent in Non-STEMI?	More frequently cause STEMI?

FIGURE 1.8 Illustration of differences between plaque erosion and plaque rupture as causes of presentation with acute coronary syndrome. Non-STEMI, non-ST-segment elevation myocardial infarction; STEMI, ST-segment elevation myocardial infarction. (From: Libby P. Superficial erosion and the precision management of acute coronary syndromes: not one-size-fits-all. *Eur Heart J.* 2017;38(11):801–803, permission needed.)

was administered via an intracoronary route (54). Normally, acetylcholine leads to vasodilation of the epicardial coronary arteries; however, it was found that in patients with atherosclerosis it led to vasoconstriction even in territories without significant lumen encroachment. Acetylcholine had previously been identified as working through an endothelial-dependent mechanism (55) and hence, the concept of clinical endothelial dysfunction was born.

The endothelium is a monolayer of cells derived from the embryonic mesoderm that form a continuous layer on the intimal surface of the entire cardiovascular system, including the arteries, veins, and chambers of the heart (endocardium); the capillary walls consist solely of endothelial cells. The endothelial cell has a variety of functions that play important roles in the maintenance of vascular integrity, including the regulation of vascular tone, vascular permeability, vessel wall inflammation, and thromboresistance through expression of anticoagulants such as heparin sulfate and enzymes that destroy them (56,57). Given these properties, it is important for the endothelium to undergo rapid repair when damaged, and for apoptotic cells to be quickly replaced by circulating endothelial progenitor cells (EPCs), which are also central to angiogenesis throughout our lifespan (58).

Vascular tone is regulated by numerous factors whose counterbalance maintains normal vascular tone and responds to various physiologic stimuli. Nitric oxide (NO), generated from L-arginine by the action of endothelial NO synthase (eNOS) in the presence of cofactors such as tetrahydrobiopterin, diffuses to the vascular smooth muscle cells (VSMCs) and activates guanylate cyclase, which results in cGMP-dependent vasodilation (59). The endothelium also mediates the hyperpolarization of VSMCs via a NO-independent pathway, which increases K$^+$ conductance and subsequently propagates the depolarization of VSMCs, maintaining vascular tone through the production of endothelium-derived hyperpolarizing factors (EDHFs)

(60). While Some vasoconstrictive molecules such as endothelin 1, through activation of ETA receptors, lead to vasoconstriction and proliferation. Additional peptides (such as endothelin 2 and endothelin 3) have been recently discovered (61,62). Endothelin 1 has also been expressed in the active plaque (63,64). Thromboxane A$_2$, serotonin, and angiotensin II also play similar roles. Vascular permeability and cell-to-cell communication is controlled by endothelial proteins such as vascular endothelial cadherin (65). All of these factors act in a complex interactive fashion to maintain vascular tone in a variety of physiologic states.

Atherogenic stimuli activate cell signaling and therefore modulate cellular function in endothelial cells. The interaction between endothelial cells and immune cells is augmented in response to atherogenic stimuli by an upregulated expression of adhesion molecules. Vascular smooth muscle function is also modified through the altered production of vasoactive substances by endothelial cells (66). A dysfunctional endothelium is an early marker of the development of atherosclerotic changes and can also contribute to cardiovascular events (67). Vascular reactivity tests represent the most widely used methods of clinical assessment of endothelial function, given the limited ability to visualize vessels <500 μm in diameter. The aim of these tests is to activate or block endothelial cell function while measuring consequent changes in vascular tone in selected vascular districts and are thus functional assessments of the microcirculation (68). These methods include coronary flow reserve (CFR) and coronary blood flow (CBF). It is also important to note that there are also noninvasive methods for evaluating endothelial dysfunction, although a thorough discussion of these is beyond the scope of this chapter.

CFR is defined as the ratio of near maximal to basal myocardial flow in response to maximal hyperemia. It is an amalgamated measure of CBF through both epicardial coronary arteries and the coronary microcirculation. A decrease in CFR could be attributed to both, and thus in the absence of epicardial vessel obstruction, it reflects solely on the microcirculation (69,70).

Acetyl choline produces primarily a vasodilator response in patients with normal coronaries. In contrast, in patients with coronary artery disease or endothelial dysfunction, acetylcholine causes dose-dependent vasoconstriction (71). Adenosine acts predominantly on vessels less than 150 μm in diameter via stimulation of adenosine A_2 receptors on the SMCs and thus reflects changes in resistance as reflected in changes in flow (72,73). These are two distinct mechanisms, of which the former is endothelial dependent and the latter is endothelial independent. An increase ≥50% increase in CBF above baseline in response to acetyl choline and CFR ratio of >2.5 in response to adenosine is considered normal (72). An abnormal response to both acetyl choline and adenosine indicates dysfunction in epicardial and resistance vessels involving endothelium-dependent and endothelium-independent mechanisms. An abnormal response to adenosine with normal response to acetyl choline indicates endothelial-independent dysfunction, while an abnormal response to acetyl choline suggests an endothelial-dependent dysfunction (72).

Endothelial dysfunction has been associated with stable angina, as well as unstable angina and MI. Marks et al. followed patients with chest pain/ischemic cardiac disease and normal coronary angiograms over a mean period of 8.5 years and noted a nearly threefold higher mortality for those patients with an abnormal CFR (20% vs. 7%; p = 0.016) (74). Britten et al., who followed patients with angiographically normal or minimally diseased coronary arteries over an average of 6.5 years, noted a more than threefold higher cardiovascular event rate in patients in the lowest tertile compared with the highest tertile of CFR (18% vs. 5%, p = 0.019) with 36% of all events related to acute coronary syndrome (75). An interesting study was conducted at the Mayo Clinic by Rubinshtein et al. to evaluate the relation between the Framingham risk score (FRS) and the presence of coronary risk factors to coronary microcirculatory vasodilator function in patients with early coronary atherosclerosis. The authors evaluated 1,063 patients (age: 50 ± 12 years, 676 (64%) females) without significant narrowing (<30%) on coronary angiography who underwent invasive assessment of coronary endothelial function. CBF in response to the endothelium-dependent vasodilator acetylcholine was evaluated, as well as the microvascular (endothelium-independent) CFR in response to intracoronary adenosine. CBF and CFR were analyzed in relation to the FRS and the presence of traditional and novel risk factors. The estimated 10 years risk in this group was 5.4 ± 5.2%. Higher FRS was associated with lower CBF in men (p = 0.008) and was a univariate predictor of lower CFR (p = 0.012) in all patients. Multivariable analysis identified a higher FRS (p < 0.001), female sex (p < 0.001) and a positive family history of coronary disease (p = 0.043) as independent predictors of reduced CFR.

Other associations with endothelium-dependent microvascular dysfunction included age, elevated body mass index (BMI), diabetes mellitus, impaired glucose metabolism (high plasma glucose level and glycosylated hemoglobulin), hypercholesteremia, and elevated L-arginine, while high-sensitivity CRP had no association. Would change this to "This was one of the largest studies evaluating the risk of endothelial dysfunction. The authors concluded that in patients without obstructive coronary disease, higher FRS was anin dependent predictor of reduced CFR (76)."

The main treatment of endothelial dysfunction is through the modification of risk factors, although the search for targets is the subject of ongoing research. Current management focuses on lifestyle modification and cardiac rehabilitation (77), lipid-lowering agents

TABLE 1–2 Endothelium independent and dependent vasodilators

Endothelium Independent
- Direct NO donors
  - NO Gas
  - Na Nitroprusside
  - Na Trioxodinitrate
- NO donors requiring metabolism
  - Nitroglycerine
  - Isosorbide dinitrate
  - Amyl Nitrate
  - Nicorandil
- Smooth muscle cell relaxers
  - Ca-Channel Blockers

Endothelium Dependent
- Acetylcholine
- 5-Hydroxytryptamine
- Bradykinine

that could improve dysfunction through their anti-inflammatory and anti-oxidant properties, and the ability to restore vascular NO availability (67), angiotensin-converting enzyme inhibitors and angiotensin rennin blockers (78), β-blockers (79), L-arginine (80), ranolazine (81), xanthine derivatives (82), and enhanced external counterpulsation (83). Calcium channel blockers are effective in Prinzmetal's angina, but ineffective in endothelial dysfunction (84). The agents used routinely as coronary vasodilators in the cath lab can be classified as endothelial dependent or independent in their mechanisms and are included in **Table 1.2**.

Medical Therapy of Atherosclerosis and the Inflammatory Link

Medical therapy of atherosclerosis centers around the control of risk factors with a special emphasis on lipid lowering. As mentioned earlier, a central link in the development and consequences of atherosclerosis revolves around inflammation. Many have postulated that the profound impact of statin therapy on reduction of coronary events has to do with the anti-inflammatory effects of LDL lowering, as well as the possible pleiotropic effects of statins that confer benefits beyond lowering the lesion levels of cholesterol. The clearest link between inflammation and statins comes from the JUPITER trial (85). This trial tested the hypothesis that in patients with relatively normal levels of cholesterol (LDL-C < 130 mg/dL), patients with higher levels of inflammation as measured by high sensitivity CRP (>2.0 mg/dL) would benefit from statin therapy. In patients randomized to Rosuvastatin, there was a 44% reduction in the primary endpoint, a composite of cardiovascular death, nonfatal MI, nonfatal stroke, hospitalization for unstable angina, or arterial revascularization. Whether newer lipid-lowering agents such as the novel PCSK9 inhibitors will have the same reduction in inflammation and cardiovascular events is as yet unknown.

Furthermore, whether targeting inflammation alone can reduce cardiovascular events, a central test of the inflammation hypothesis, is not yet known. The Cardiovascular Inflammation Reduction Trial will test this hypothesis. In this trial, 7,000 patients with prior myocardial infarction and either type 2 diabetes or the metabolic syndrome will be randomized to low-dose methotrexate (an anti-inflammatory agent without a lipid-lowering effect) or a placebo over an average follow-up period of 3 to 5 years. The primary endpoint is a composite of nonfatal MI, nonfatal stroke, and cardiovascular death (86).

Conclusions

Over the past decades, the molecular and cellular pathophysiology of atherosclerosis and related arteriopathies has been extensively studied. A more thorough knowledge of these processes has led to increasingly effective therapies for the treatment of atherosclerosis and acute coronary syndromes. Much remains to be determined, however, regarding the molecular mechanisms of atherosclerosis and the identification of plaques prone to cause acute coronary syndrome.

Key Points

■ The molecular and cellular pathophysiology of atherosclerosis and related arteriopathies has revealed the role of inflammatory cells on lipid metabolism in the vessel wall.

■ The treatment of atherosclerosis and acute coronary syndrome relies on therapies directed at endothelial cell stabilization and the suppression of links between vessel surface and thrombosis.

■ The identification of plaques prone to rupture, and of more effective and economical methods to treat restenosis focus on processes of lipid accumulation, fibrous cap degradation, and vascular smooth muscle proliferation.

References

1. Ross R. The pathogenesis of atherosclerosis–an update. N Engl J Med. 1986;314(8):488–500.
2. Ridker PM, et al. Comparison of C-reactive protein and low-density lipoprotein cholesterol levels in the prediction of first cardiovascular events. N Engl J Med. 2002;347(20):1557–1565.
3. Brennan ML, et al. Prognostic value of myeloperoxidase in patients with chest pain. N Engl J Med. 2003;349(17):1595–1604.
4. Cybulsky MI, Gimbrone MA Jr. Endothelial expression of a mononuclear leukocyte adhesion molecule during atherogenesis. Science. 1991;251(4995):788–791.
5. Ridker PM. Intercellular adhesion molecule (ICAM-1) and the risks of developing atherosclerotic disease. Eur Heart J. 1998;19(8):1119–1121.
6. Rollins BJ. Chemokines. Blood. 1997;90(3):909–928.
7. Webb LM, et al. Binding to heparan sulfate or heparin enhances neutrophil responses to interleukin 8. Proc Natl Acad Sci USA. 1993;90(15):7158–7162.
8. Huo Y, et al. The chemokine KC, but not monocyte chemoattractant protein-1, triggers monocyte arrest on early atherosclerotic endothelium. J Clin Invest. 2001;108(9):1307–1314.
9. Libby P. Molecular bases of the acute coronary syndromes. Circulation. 1995;91(11):2844–2850.
10. Walpola PL, et al. Expression of ICAM-1 and VCAM-1 and monocyte adherence in arteries exposed to altered shear stress. Arterioscler Thromb Vasc Biol. 1995;15(1):2–10.
11. Matsuzaki K, et al. Osteoclast differentiation factor (ODF) induces osteoclast-like cell formation in human peripheral blood mononuclear cell cultures. Biochem Biophys Res Commun. 1998;246(1):199–204.
12. Quercioli A, et al. Coronary artery calcification and cardiovascular risk: the role of RANKL/OPG signalling. Eur J Clin Invest. 2010;40(7):645–654.
13. Hansson GK, et al. Innate and adaptive immunity in the pathogenesis of atherosclerosis. Circ Res. 2002;91(4):281–291.
14. Bobryshev YV. Dendritic cells in atherosclerosis: current status of the problem and clinical relevance. Eur Heart J. 2005;26(17):1700–1704.
15. Gratchev A, et al. Alternatively activated macrophages differentially express fibronectin and its splice variants and the extracellular matrix protein betaIG-H3. Scand J Immunol. 2001;53(4):386–392.
16. Gratchev A, et al. Alternatively activated antigen-presenting cells: molecular repertoire, immune regulation, and healing. Skin Pharmacol Appl Skin Physiol. 2001;14(5):272–279.
17. Gratchev A, et al. Interleukin-4 and dexamethasone counterregulate extracellular matrix remodelling and phagocytosis in type-2 macrophages. Scand J Immunol. 2005;61(1):10–17.
18. Brocheriou I, et al. Antagonistic regulation of macrophage phenotype by M-CSF and GM-CSF: implication in atherosclerosis. Atherosclerosis. 2011;214(2):316–324.
19. Packard RR, Lichtman AH, Libby P. Innate and adaptive immunity in atherosclerosis. Semin Immunopathol. 2009;31(1):5–22.
20. Amento EP, et al. Cytokines and growth factors positively and negatively regulate interstitial collagen gene expression in human vascular smooth muscle cells. Arterioscler Thromb. 1991;11(5):1223–1230.
21. Perschinka H, et al. Cross-reactive B-cell epitopes of microbial and human heat shock protein 60/65 in atherosclerosis. Arterioscler Thromb Vasc Biol. 2003;23(6):1060–1065.
22. Giachelli C, et al. Molecular cloning and characterization of 2B7, a rat mRNA which distinguishes smooth muscle cell phenotypes in vitro and is identical to osteopontin (secreted phosphoprotein I, 2aR). Biochem Biophys Res Commun. 1991;177(2):867–873.
23. Bostrom K, et al. Bone morphogenetic protein expression in human atherosclerotic lesions. J Clin Invest. 1993;91(4):1800–1809.
24. Shanahan CM, et al. High expression of genes for calcification-regulating proteins in human atherosclerotic plaques. J Clin Invest. 1994;93(6):2393–2402.
25. Vliegenthart R, et al. Coronary calcification improves cardiovascular risk prediction in the elderly. Circulation. 2005;112(4):572–577.
26. Libby P, Folco E. Tension in the plaque: hypoxia modulates metabolism in atheroma. Circ Res. 2011;109(10):1100–1102.
27. Moulton KS. Plaque angiogenesis and atherosclerosis. Curr Atheroscler Rep. 2001;3(3):225–233.
28. Moulton KS, et al. Angiogenesis inhibitors endostatin or TNP-470 reduce intimal neovascularization and plaque growth in apolipoprotein E-deficient mice. Circulation. 1999;99(13):1726–1732.
29. Gossl M, et al. Segmental heterogeneity of vasa vasorum neovascularization in human coronary atherosclerosis. JACC Cardiovasc Imaging. 2010;3(1):32–40.
30. Kolev K, et al. Matrix metalloproteinase-9 expression in post-hypoxic human brain capillary endothelial cells: H_2O_2 as a trigger and NF-kappaB as a signal transducer. Thromb Haemost. 2003;90(3).528–537.
31. Deguchi JO, et al. Chronic hypoxia activates the Akt and beta-catenin pathways in human macrophages. Arterioscler Thromb Vasc Biol. 2009;29(10):1664–1670.
32. Burke B, et al. Hypoxia-induced gene expression in human macrophages: implications for ischemic tissues and hypoxia-regulated gene therapy. Am J Pathol. 2003;163(4):1233–1243.
33. Hulten LM, Levin M. The role of hypoxia in atherosclerosis. Curr Opin Lipidol. 2009;20(5):409–414.
34. Parathath S, et al. Hypoxia is present in murine atherosclerotic plaques and has multiple adverse effects on macrophage lipid metabolism. Circ Res. 2011;109(10):1141–1152.
35. Bostrom P, et al. Hypoxia converts human macrophages into triglyceride-loaded foam cells. Arterioscler Thromb Vasc Biol. 2006;26(8):1871–1876.
36. Gibbons GH, Dzau VJ. The emerging concept of vascular remodeling. N Engl J Med. 1994;330(20):1431–1438.
37. Galis ZS, Khatri JJ. Matrix metalloproteinases in vascular remodeling and atherogenesis: the good, the bad, and the ugly. Circ Res. 2002;90(3):251–262.
38. Fuster V, et al. The pathogenesis of coronary artery disease and the acute coronary syndromes (1). N Engl J Med. 1992;326(4):242–250.
39. Kern MJ. Coronary physiology revisited: practical insights from the cardiac catheterization laboratory. Circulation. 2000;101(11):1344–1351.
40. Tonino PA, et al. Angiographic versus functional severity of coronary artery stenoses in the FAME study fractional flow reserve versus angiography in multivessel evaluation. J Am Coll Cardiol. 2010;55(25):2816–2821.
41. Tonino PA, et al. Fractional flow reserve versus angiography for guiding percutaneous coronary intervention. N Engl J Med. 2009;360(3):213–224.

42. Herrick JB. Landmark article (JAMA 1912). Clinical features of sudden obstruction of the coronary arteries. *JAMA.* 1983;250(13):1757–1765.

43. DeWood MA, et al. Prevalence of total coronary occlusion during the early hours of transmural myocardial infarction. *N Engl J Med.* 1980;303(16):897–902.

44. Ambrose JA, et al. Coronary angiographic morphology in myocardial infarction: a link between the pathogenesis of unstable angina and myocardial infarction. *J Am Coll Cardiol.* 1985;6(6):1233–1238.

45. Smith SC Jr. Risk-reduction therapy: the challenge to change. Paper presented at the 68th scientific session of the American Heart Association, November 13, 1995, Anaheim, California. *Circulation.* 1996;93(12):2205–2211.

46. Stone GW, et al. A prospective natural-history study of coronary atherosclerosis. *N Engl J Med.* 2011;364(3):226–235.

47. Seshiah PN, et al. Activated monocytes induce smooth muscle cell death: role of macrophage colony-stimulating factor and cell contact. *Circulation.* 2002;105(2):174–180.

48. Muller JE, et al. Circadian variation in the frequency of onset of acute myocardial infarction. *N Engl J Med.* 1985;313(21):1315–1322.

49. Leor J, Kloner RA. The Northridge earthquake as a trigger for acute myocardial infarction. *Am J Cardiol.* 1996;77(14):1230–1232.

50. Lee RT, et al. Circumferential stress and matrix metalloproteinase 1 in human coronary atherosclerosis. Implications for plaque rupture. *Arterioscler Thromb Vasc Biol.* 1996;16(8):1070–1073.

51. Libby P. Superficial erosion and the precision management of acute coronary syndromes: not one-size-fits-all. *Eur Heart J.* 2017;38(11):801–803.

52. Saia F, et al. Eroded versus ruptured plaques at the culprit site of STEMI: in vivo pathophysiological features and response to primary PCI. *JACC Cardiovasc Imaging.* 2015;8(5):566–575.

53. Katz JN, et al. Evolution of the coronary care unit: clinical characteristics and temporal trends in healthcare delivery and outcomes. *Crit Care Med.* 2010;38(2):375–381.

54. Ludmer PL, et al. Paradoxical vasoconstriction induced by acetylcholine in atherosclerotic coronary arteries. *N Engl J Med.* 1986;315(17):1046–1051.

55. Furchgott RF, Zawadzki JV. The obligatory role of endothelial cells in the relaxation of arterial smooth muscle by acetylcholine. *Nature.* 1980;288(5789):373–376.

56. de Agostini AI, et al. Localization of anticoagulantly active heparan sulfate proteoglycans in vascular endothelium: antithrombin binding on cultured endothelial cells and perfused rat aorta. *J Cell Biol.* 1990;111(3):1293–1304.

57. Marcus AJ, et al. The endothelial cell ecto-ADPase responsible for inhibition of platelet function is CD39. *J Clin Invest.* 1997;99(6):1351–1360.

58. Urbich C, Dimmeler S. Endothelial progenitor cells: characterization and role in vascular biology. *Circ Res.* 2004;95(4):343–353.

59. Forstermann U, Munzel T. Endothelial nitric oxide synthase in vascular disease: from marvel to menace. *Circulation.* 2006;113(13):1708–1714.

60. Busse R, et al. EDHF: bringing the concepts together. *Trends Pharmacol Sci.* 2002;23(8):374–380.

61. Yanagisawa M, et al. A novel peptide vasoconstrictor, endothelin, is produced by vascular endothelium and modulates smooth muscle Ca^{2+} channels. *J Hypertens Suppl.* 1988;6(4):S188–S191.

62. Barton M, Yanagisawa M. Endothelin: 20 years from discovery to therapy. *Can J Physiol Pharmacol.* 2008;86(8):485–498.

63. Kinlay S, et al. Role of endothelin-1 in the active constriction of human atherosclerotic coronary arteries. *Circulation.* 2001;104(10):1114–1118.

64. Hasdai D, et al. Mechanical pressure and stretch release endothelin-1 from human atherosclerotic coronary arteries in vivo. *Circulation.* 1997;95(2):357–362.

65. Dejana E, Tournier-Lasserve E, Weinstein BM. The control of vascular integrity by endothelial cell junctions: molecular basis and pathological implications. *Dev Cell.* 2009;16(2):209–221.

66. Hirase T, Node K. Endothelial dysfunction as a cellular mechanism for vascular failure. *Am J Physiol Heart Circ Physiol.* 2012;302(3):H499–H505.

67. Bonetti PO, Lerman LO, Lerman A. Endothelial dysfunction: a marker of atherosclerotic risk. *Arterioscler Thromb Vasc Biol.* 2003;23(2):168–175.

68. Virdis A, Taddei S. How to evaluate microvascular organ damage in hypertension: assessment of endothelial function. *High Blood Press Cardiovasc Prev.* 2011;18(4):163–167.

69. Gould KL, Lipscomb K, Hamilton GW. Physiologic basis for assessing critical coronary stenosis. Instantaneous flow response and regional distribution during coronary hyperemia as measures of coronary flow reserve. *Am J Cardiol.* 1974;33(1):87–94.

70. Uren NG, et al. Relation between myocardial blood flow and the severity of coronary-artery stenosis. *N Engl J Med.* 1994;330(25):1782–1788.

71. Vrints CJ, et al. Impaired endothelium-dependent cholinergic coronary vasodilation in patients with angina and normal coronary arteriograms. *J Am Coll Cardiol.* 1992;19(1):21–31.

72. Hasdai D, et al. Evaluation of patients with minimally obstructive coronary artery disease and angina. *Int J Cardiol.* 1996;53(3):203–208.

73. Hori M, Kitakaze M. Adenosine, the heart, and coronary circulation. *Hypertension.* 1991;18(5):565–574.

74. Marks DS, et al. Mortality in patients with microvascular disease. *J Clin Hypertens (Greenwich).* 2004;6(6):304–309.

75. Britten MB, Zeiher AM, Schachinger V. Microvascular dysfunction in angiographically normal or mildly diseased coronary arteries predicts adverse cardiovascular long-term outcome. *Coron Artery Dis.* 2004;15(5):259–264.

76. Rubinshtein R, et al. Coronary microcirculatory vasodilator function in relation to risk factors among patients without obstructive coronary disease and low to intermediate Framingham score. *Eur Heart J.* 2010;31(8):936–942.

77. Eriksson BE, et al. Physical training in Syndrome X: physical training counteracts deconditioning and pain in Syndrome X. *J Am Coll Cardiol.* 2000;36(5):1619–1625.

78. Tiefenbacher CP, et al. ACE inhibitors and statins acutely improve endothelial dysfunction of human coronary arterioles. *Am J Physiol Heart Circ Physiol.* 2004;286(4):H1425–H1432.

79. Kaski JC, et al. Cardiac syndrome X: clinical characteristics and left ventricular function. Long-term follow-up study. *J Am Coll Cardiol.* 1995;25(4):807–814.

80. Palloshi A, et al. Effect of oral L-arginine on blood pressure and symptoms and endothelial function in patients with systemic hypertension, positive exercise tests, and normal coronary arteries. *Am J Cardiol.* 2004;93(7):933–935.

81. Deshmukh SH, et al. Ranolazine improves endothelial function in patients with stable coronary artery disease. *Coron Artery Dis.* 2009;20(5):343–347.

82. Emdin M, et al. Improved exercise capacity with acute aminophylline administration in patients with syndrome X. *J Am Coll Cardiol.* 1989;14(6):1450–1453.

83. Kronhaus KD, Lawson WE. Enhanced external counterpulsation is an effective treatment for Syndrome X. *Int J Cardiol.* 2009;135(2):256–257.

84. Lanza GA, et al. Atenolol versus amlodipine versus isosorbide-5-mononitrate on anginal symptoms in syndrome X. *Am J Cardiol.* 1999;84(7):854–856, A8.

85. Ridker PM, et al. Rosuvastatin to prevent vascular events in men and women with elevated C-reactive protein. *N Engl J Med.* 2008;359(21):2195–2207.

86. Everett BM, et al. Rationale and design of the cardiovascular inflammation reduction trial: a test of the inflammatory hypothesis of atherothrombosis. *Am Heart J.* 2013;166(2):199–207 e15.

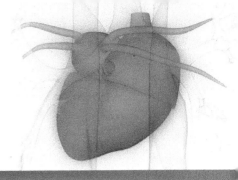

Restenosis

Abdulfattah Saidi, MD and Frederick G. P. Welt, MD,

FSCAI, FACC

Despite the advent of effective interventional vascular therapies, post-intervention restenosis remains an important limitation of the technique regardless of the type of intervention (1,2). Compared to balloon angioplasty, bare-metal stents (BMSs) decreased the in-stent restenosis (ISR) rate to approximately 30% (3). Drug-eluting stents (DESs) reduced the restenosis rates to 5% to 18% depending on the population (4–7). The aim of this chapter is to understand the pathogenesis, the clinical indicators and biochemical markers associated with increased post-procedure restenosis.

Definitions and Clinical Sequelae of Restenosis

For most clinical trials, restenosis is defined by the binary endpoint of a reduction of 50% of the luminal diameter compared to the reference vessel (8). This arbitrary definition endeavors to separate clinically important lesions from those without sequelae. Restenosis can also be described in continuous terms, which is helpful in understanding the pathophysiology of the process. For example, late lumen loss (LLL) is defined as the continuous angiographic measure of lumen deterioration and is calculated by subtracting minimal lumen diameter (MLD) at immediate follow-up from late-post-procedural MLD. This parameter has been used as a surrogate marker for the effects of different anti-restenotic therapies and to determine BMS and DES outcomes (9,10). Importantly, when viewing restenosis as a continuous variable, it can be noted that virtually all patients suffer some degree of restenosis in a typical Gaussian distribution (Fig. 2.1). However, it is only the few patients who have severe *symptomatic* ISR (usually with a lesion severity of >70%).

The average amount of LLL is 0.8 to 1.0 mm after implantation of a BMS, regardless of the size of the original vessel lumen. This is of critical significance, especially for smaller vessels. A 4-mm-diameter vessel would lose 44% of lumen area, with a loss of 1 mm in diameter. If a vessel with a 2-mm diameter experiences the same 1 mm of late loss (LL), there is a 75% loss of lumen area and angiographic restenosis. Therefore, LL and angiographic restenosis are related to the diameter of the reference vessel (11). One of the most important concepts to understand is that restenosis rates vary greatly, depending on the particular definition used in any given study.

Discordance between LL and binary restenosis is multifactorial and a topic of debate. While LL has been very useful as a surrogate marker for the effectiveness of a given drug to prevent clinical restenosis, the relationship between LL and binary restenosis is nonlinear and is characterized by a curvilinear function (Fig. 2.2) (12), suggesting that there is a threshold for clinical significance below which a given amount of LL and the degree of tissue growth is immaterial, and thus does not reflect a worse clinical restenosis rate.

The clinical sequelae of angiographic ISR are not always in concordance with the degree of restenosis. In a meta analysis of all patients with angiographic ISR from the BENESTENT I, BENESTENT II pilot, BENESTENT II, MUSIC, WEST 1, DUET, FINESS 2, FLARE, SOPHOS, and ROSE studies that recruited 2,690 patients who underwent percutaneous revascularization, restenosis (≥50% diameter stenosis) occurred in 607 patients and was clinically silent in almost half those patients. Multiple factors play a role in how patients present, including reference diameter and lesion severity in follow-up (13).

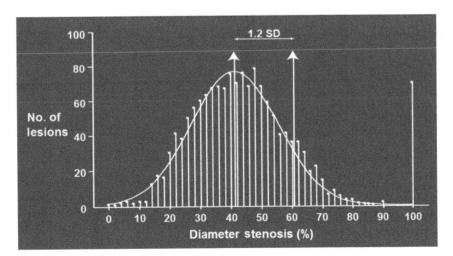

FIGURE 2.1 Histogram of percent diameter stenosis at follow-up angiography of 1,445 lesions treated with percutaneous intervention. The superimposed curve represents the theoretic Gaussian distribution. SD, standard deviation. (From: Rensing BJ, Hermans WR, Deckers JW, et al. Lumen narrowing after percutaneous transluminal coronary balloon angioplasty follows a near Gaussian distribution: a quantitative angiographic study in 1,445 successfully dilated lesions. *J Am Coll Cardiol.* 1992;19:939–945.)

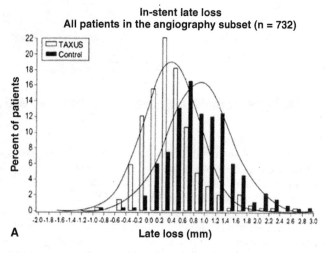
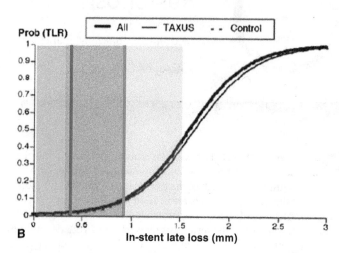

FIGURE 2.2   Data from the TAXUS IV trial shows the in-stent late loss (LL) for the Taxus and control bare-metal stent (BMS) in panel **(A)**. Panel **(B)** shows the probability of target lesion revascularization (TLR) as a function of in-stent LL, revealing a curvilinear distribution. Superimposed are the mean and standard deviations for the Taxus stent LL (*red*) and the control BMS (*blue*). The distribution of the Taxus stent LL falls along the relatively flat portion of the curve, whereas the distribution for the BMS falls along the steeper portion of the curve where there is greater correlation between LL and TLR. (From: Ellis SG, Popma JJ, Lasala JM, et al. Relationship between angiographic LL and TLR after coronary stent implantation: analysis from the TAXUS-IV trial. *J Am Coll Cardiol.* 2005;45:1193–1200.)

Traditionally, restenosis had been viewed as a largely benign condition, presenting most commonly with stable angina. There is substantial evidence to the contrary, however. Bare-metal ISR has shown variability in presentation. While many patients present with stable exertional symptoms, unstable angina is a frequent presentation (26%–53%) and acute myocardial infarction (MI) has been described in 3.5% to 20% of patients (14,15). DESs have similar presentations. In one series, the rates of unstable angina and MI were comparable between the two groups 18% and 2%, respectively (16).

Restenosis of left main stenting carries severe adverse consequences. Despite such concerns, multiple case series from Rotterdam and Milan show promising results with left main stenting in comparison to coronary artery bypass surgery. The safety of the LM stenting has also been well-documented in randomized trials. Routine follow-up angiography is no longer recommended (17–19).

Multiple studies have confirmed that restenosis following balloon angioplasty or stent implantation is a relatively accelerated process compared to atherosclerosis. With balloon angioplasty, clinically important restenosis is almost always apparent by 6 months (20,21). Similarly, with stents, the average time at which ISR is apparent is at 5.5 months, with some evidence that there is a shorter interval if presentation was with an acute MI (22).

Risk Factors for Restenosis

Risk factors can be loosely identified as both biologic in nature and mechanical, although there is considerable interplay between the two. The three most important clinical risk factors for restenosis are increased stent length, smaller MLD, and the presence of diabetes (23).

Biologic Associations—Diabetes Mellitus

Data from the Swedish Coronary Angiography and Angioplasty Registry (SCAAR) involving >35,000 patients implanted with four different types of DES (Endeavor, SES, Taxus Express, and Liberte)

in real-world practice at 2-year follow-up showed DES restenosis rates were significantly higher in patients with diabetes (24).

In another study of 954 patients undergoing percutaneous coronary intervention (PCI), target lesion revascularization (TLR) was required in 28% of patients with insulin-dependent diabetes, compared with 16.3% in individuals without diabetes (25). The high risk for restenosis among patients with diabetes may be associated with metabolic alterations that promote endothelial dysfunction, accelerate intimal hyperplasia, and increase platelet aggregability and thrombogenicity (26).

Genetic Abnormalities

Evidence also suggests that some patients may be genetically predisposed to restenosis. Genetic abnormalities associated with high risk for restenosis include polymorphisms in genes coding for angiotensin-converting enzyme (ACE) inhibitor (27), glycoprotein receptor IIIa PLA1/2, haptoglobin 2/2.25, and IL-8 (28). Resistance to antiproliferative drugs due to polymorphisms in the genes that encode the intracellular receptor mammalian target of rapamycin (mTOR) or proteins involved in paclitaxel or sirolimus metabolism have been shown to confer drug resistance both in vitro and in vivo (29,30). Decreased binding of sirolimus to mTOR because of mutations in FK binding protein-12 (FKBP-12) and mTOR and mutations of downstream effector molecules of mTOR may all cause resistance to sirolimus (30).

Inflammation

Attempts have been made to identify markers of inflammation and thrombosis that correlate with an increased risk of ISR. A strong correlation between the number of macrophages in tissue samples obtained at the time of directional atherectomy and the propensity for restenosis was noted (31). Because obtaining pathologic specimens is neither feasible nor practical, however, investigators have pursued local and systemic biomarkers that could assist in determining ISR risk. Neumann et al. determined the expression of neutrophil adhesion molecule L selectin and CD11b from blood proximal and distal to the angioplasty site in patients. They found upregulation of markers following balloon angioplasty (32). Mickelson used systemic venous blood sampling for measurement of CD11b and found similar results with a propensity toward adverse clinical events (33). Monocyte chemoattractant protein-1 (MCP-1) is a potent chemokine for monocytes. Plasma levels of MCP-1 were measured before and 1, 5, 15, and 180 days after percutaneous transluminal coronary angioplasty (PTCA) in 50 patients who underwent PTCA and who had repeated angiograms at 6-month follow-up. Restenosis occurred in 14 (28%) patients. The MCP-1 level was no different at baseline between patients with or without restenosis. However, after the procedure, restenotic patients, compared with non-restenotic patients, had statistically significant (p < 0.0001) elevated levels of MCP-1. In contrast, plasma levels of other chemokines, such as RANTES and interleukin-8 (IL-8), did not differ between the two groups after PTCA (34).

The plasma level of C-reactive protein (CRP) is considered a risk predictor for cardiovascular (CV) diseases. Nevertheless, the relationship between CRP and ISR has been controversial. Studies have supported the notion that increased inflammation following PCI is higher with BMS compared to DES, as conferred by lower periprocedural CRP levels with DES (35,36). When the goal of the study was to investigate if CRP was linked to restenosis, the results were mixed (37–39).

Circulating matrix metalloproteinases (MMPs) have recently been identified as being potentially useful in identifying patients at greater risk of developing ISR following DES implantation. MMP-2 and MMP-9 are known to play fundamental roles in the migration of vascular smooth muscle cells (VSMCs), and also in matrix remodeling during wound healing, and are produced by VSMCs, endothelial cells, macrophages, lymphocytes, and mast cells in response to mechanical injury. Significant elevations in MMP-9 levels at baseline and MMP-2 and MMP-9 levels 24 hours post-PCI have proven to be strongly associated with the development of ISR following DES implantation.

Conversely, low and near-normal MMP-2 and MMP-9 levels were associated with a lack of a significant restenotic response (40).

Mechanical Associations—Stent Expansion and Apposition

Stent underexpansion and malapposition predispose to stent thrombosis more than to increased restenosis. Some studies suggested that incomplete expansion also impacts drug delivery and subsequently enhances neointimal hyperplasia (NIH) (41,42). In the era of drug-eluting stents, the concept of geographical miss was introduced, referring to an area of the treated segment that was exposed to balloon injury but not covered with stent struts and thus did not receive adequate suppressive therapy.

A less common mechanical association is stent fracture, defined as complete or partial separation of a stent at follow-up that was contiguous after the original stent implantation (43). The incidence of stent fracture with DES has been reported as 1% to 8% (44–46). With stent fracture, the scaffolding is impaired, and subsequent drug delivery may be impacted (47).

Patterns of In-Stent Restenosis

Mehran et al. developed an angiographic classification of ISR according to the geographic distribution of intimal hyperplasia in reference to the implanted stent (Fig. 2.3) (48). Four classes were defined as the following:

Class I: Focal ISR group. Lesions are ≤10 mm in length and are positioned at the unscaffolded segment (i.e., articulation or gap), the body of the stent, the proximal or distal margin (but not both), or a combination of these sites (multifocal ISR).

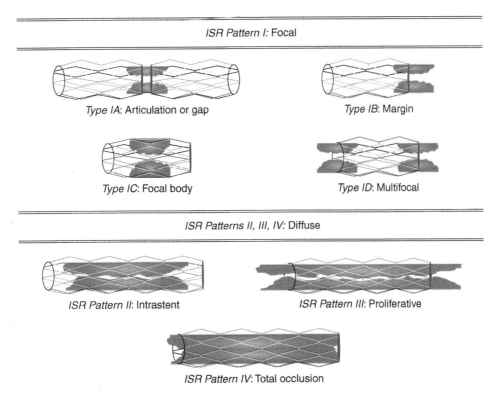

FIGURE 2.3 Common patterns of in-stent restenosis. (From: Mehran R, Dangas G, Abizaid AS, et al. Angiographic patterns of in-stent restenosis: classification and implications for long-term outcome. *Circulation.* 1999;100(18):1872–1878.)

Class II: "Diffuse intrastent" ISR. Lesions are >10 mm in length and are confined to the stent(s), without extending outside the margins of the stent(s).
Class III: "Diffuse proliferative" ISR. Lesions are >10 mm in length and extend beyond the margin(s) of the stent(s).
Class IV: ISR with "total occlusion." Lesions have a thrombolysis in myocardial infarction (TIMI) flow grade of 0.

The pattern of ISR is different between BMS and DES, with a diffuse pattern more likely with the DES and a more focal pattern seen with BMS. Of interest, patients presenting with MI are likely to present with a diffuse pattern when compared to a non-MI presentation (16,22).

Pathogenesis of Restenosis

The pathogenesis of restenosis is significantly different than atherogenesis with respect to both the content of the lesion and the time required for development. Restenosis develops much more rapidly than atherosclerosis and is sometimes referred to as an accelerated arteriopathy. Forrester proposed a paradigm for restenosis and suggested three phases; (1) the inflammatory phase, (2) a granulation or cellular proliferation phase, and (3) a remodeling phase involving extracellular matrix (ECM) protein synthesis (49). More recently, Park et al. have suggested the occurrence of in-stent neoatherosclerosis, although the prevalence of these histologic findings is uncertain (50) (see section titled Neoatherosclerosis).

Differences between Post-Balloon Angioplasty and In-Stent Restenosis

Prior to discussing the molecular and cellular mechanisms of restenosis, it is worth elucidating the important differences that exist between restenosis following balloon angioplasty when performed alone and in stents.

Balloon Angioplasty

Detailed IVUS studies have demonstrated that restenosis is caused both by neointimal proliferation and shrinkage (and recoil) of the artery. Elastic recoil is an acute process that is observed within a few minutes after balloon deflation, resulting in an inward collapse of the vessel wall. More stretching leads to an increased inward recoil force upon balloon inflation. The recoil force can result in up to a 50% loss of cross-sectional area and a 33% loss in luminal diameter (51). However, negative remodeling recognized as contraction of the external elastic laminae is a process that typically presents weeks to months after injury. Neointimal proliferation is considered to be an inflammatory response at the site of injury, coupled to smooth muscle cell proliferation and migration and excessive ECM production. These last two processes contribute to neointima (NI) formation (52,53). In terms of their relative contribution, acute and chronic negative remodeling play a larger role in balloon-injury-associated restenosis.

In-Stent Restenosis

Angiographic analysis of the pivotal stent studies (the Stent Restenosis Study [STRESS] and Belgian Netherlands Stent Study [BENESTENT]) revealed major quantitative and qualitative differences between

angioplasty-induced injury and injuries associated with stent placement. The initial luminal gain with stents is greater due to scaffolding (less or no recoil) of the vessel. In addition, late negative remodeling is abrogated by the presence of the rigid frame of the stent. However, the LLL is greater with stented vessels due to greater neointimal growth (54,55). Hoffman et al. compared stented and nonstented lesions using serial IVUS studies, confirming the observation that the main mechanism of ISR is due to NIH rather than negative remodeling (56). Therefore, stents reduce restenosis because they are able to achieve a larger initial lumen and prevent late remodeling despite inducing more LL (Fig. 2.4).

The neointimal formation of ISR is similar to that following balloon angioplasty. The exaggerated NI response seen with stenting is likely due to differences in vessel injury and a more potent inflammatory response. Kornowski et al., using a porcine model, demonstrated that an increase in vessel injury or vascular inflammation results in an increase in neointimal formation. Pigs in which the stent struts perforated the internal elastic lamina and external elastic lamina had greater histologic evidence of inflammatory response and subsequently a larger volume of neointimal formation (57).

Other contributing factors to an increased inflammatory response include increased balloon pressure required to place the stent and contact metal allergy. Contact allergy to metals including nickel and molybdenum may account for the elevated inflammatory response in some patients. BMS slowly elute metal ions that may stimulate a delayed-type hypersensitivity response within the stented vessel (58). A study was conducted in Germany on 131 patients after stent implantation who had cutaneous patch testing to investigate the relation between nickel and molybdenum hypersensitivity and ISR. All 10 patients with a positive test result had restenosis (p = 0.03), requiring target vessel revascularization (TVR) (58).

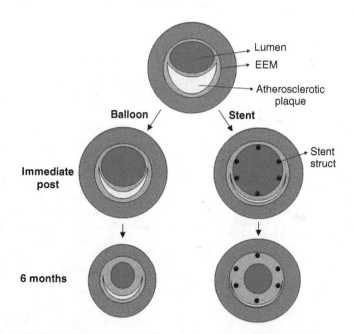

FIGURE 2.4 Illustration of differences in mechanisms of restenosis between plain balloon angioplasty and stenting. In balloon angioplastied vessels, restenosis is caused by a combination of neointimal growth and negative remodeling. Stented arteries have lower rates of restenosis despite incurring greater neointimal growth due to their ability to achieve a larger initial lumen size, and the elimination of negative remodeling. EEM, external elastic membrane.

Inflammation Mechanisms of Leukocyte Recruitment and Infiltration

Expansion of a balloon or stent causes injury with vessel wall dissection, crush injury of SMCs and de-endothelialization. In response to vessel injury, leukocyte recruitment and infiltration occur where platelets and fibrin have been deposited. Within areas of injury such as atherosclerotic and postangioplasty restenotic lesions, and in areas of ischemia-reperfusion injury, in vivo studies have shown that leukocytes and platelets are deposited together. For the inflammatory response after angioplasty, this interaction between platelets and leukocytes appears to be important (59).

This interaction has been explained by Diacovo et al. who have put forth a paradigm of leukocyte attachment to surface-adherent platelets followed by transmigration (60). As with atherosclerosis, the initial loose association of leukocytes is mediated through the selectin class of adhesion molecules, particularly by platelet P-selectin followed by their firm adhesion and trans-platelet migration, processes that are dependent on the integrin class of adhesion molecules (60,61). The β_2 integrin molecule Mac-1 (CD11b/CD18) is present on both neutrophils and monocytes and appears to be of central importance in leukocyte recruitment following vascular injury. In addition to promoting the accumulation of leukocytes at sites of vascular injury, the binding of platelets to neutrophils amplifies the inflammatory response by inducing neutrophil activation, upregulating cell adhesion molecule expression, and generating signals that promote integrin activation and chemokine synthesis. These processes of activation may be mediated through the release of soluble CD40 ligand, a pro-inflammatory molecule stored most abundantly in platelets. Bolstering this data, both neutrophil–platelet and monocyte–platelet aggregates have been identified in the peripheral blood of patients with coronary artery disease, and may be markers of disease activity and prognosis (62,63).

Evidence for the Role of Inflammation in Restenosis

In most cases, ISR does not appear to be a case of accelerated atherosclerosis but rather a distinct temporal and pathophysiologic process, knowing that inflammation is an important common link between atherogenesis and restenosis. Farb et al. investigated stented arteries from pathologic samples of 116 stents from 87 patients greater than 90 days postprocedure. They found a statistically significant association between extent of medial damage, inflammation, and restenosis (64). Also linking leukocytes and restenosis is data by Moreno et al., in tissue retrieved from directional atherectomy at the time of angioplasty showing a strong positive correlation between the number of macrophages in the tissue and subsequent risk of restenosis (31).

Systemic markers of inflammation following angioplasty have also provided insight into the mechanisms of restenosis mentioned earlier (65–68).

In several experimental animal models, cell adhesion molecules critical for leukocyte recruitment have been found to be upregulated by an atherogenic diet (69–71), induction of diabetes (72), and increased shear stress (73). After balloon endothelial denudation in a rabbit model, vascular cell adhesion molecule-1, intracellular cell adhesion molecule-1, and MHC class II antigens, all have been shown to be upregulated in a sustained fashion (74). A particularly potent inflammatory stimulus appears to be the implantation of a chronic indwelling endovascular stent, leading to a brisk early inflammatory response with abundant surface-adherent leukocytes of both monocyte and granulocyte lineage (75,76). Days and weeks later, macrophages invade the forming NI and are observed clustering around stent struts often forming giant cells.

Evidence of the importance of monocytes comes from studies in which blockading early monocyte recruitment with anti-inflammatory agents resulted in reduced late neointimal thickening (76–78). Activated macrophages may influence vascular repair through various mechanisms, including production of a variety of mediators, such as members of the interleukin family, tumor necrosis factors (TNFs), monocyte chemoattractant protein-1, and growth factors such as platelet-derived growth factors, basic fibroblast growth factors, and heparin-binding epidermal growth factors (79).

Several studies have also shown infiltration of neutrophils within the arterial wall following vascular injury (80–82). As with macrophages, a concomitant reduction in neutrophil number and smooth muscle proliferation can be seen with administration of anti-inflammatory agents, resulting in less neointimal growth (75). The mechanisms by which neutrophils may affect vascular repair are not as fully understood as with monocytes/macrophages. While neutrophils are not typically thought to secrete growth factors, they can contribute to tissue injury through the release of reactive oxygen species and proteases (79). In addition, it has been reported that rabbit vascular smooth cells are stimulated to proliferate when co-cultured with neutrophils or neutrophil-conditioned media (83). Neutrophils are also known to secrete cytokines, including IL-1, TNF-α, and IL-6 (84).

Differences between Balloon and Stent Injury

Systematic investigation in both human and animal studies suggests important differences between vascular biologic responses to balloon- and stent-induced injury. Inoue et al. used flow cytometry to measure CD11b (a member of the integrin family of adhesion molecules) expression on neutrophils following PCI and found substantially higher levels on neutrophils from patients undergoing stent implantation, as compared to balloon angioplasty alone. This increased inflammatory response may help explain the larger neointimal growth seen in stented arteries (85).

Animal studies have also demonstrated differences in response to vascular injury between balloon-angioplastied and stented arteries. Heparin, an archetypal modulator of vascular repair in animal models, has long been known to reduce neointimal growth following vascular injury (86,87). Heparin is equally effective at reducing NIH following balloon injury or stent implantation (88,89). Studies have shown that heparin maximally inhibits NIH in stented rabbit iliac arteries only when given in a prolonged fashion (14 days), whereas maximal inhibition of balloon-injured arteries requires only transient early heparin therapy (3 days) (88). An explanation of this difference is suggested by immunohistologic and molecular studies. Data demonstrate that there is a distinct pattern of leukocyte infiltration that distinguishes the superficial injury associated with simple balloon-induced de-endothelialization from the deep chronic injury associated with stent implantation. In a rabbit iliac artery model, balloon injury is associated with early and transient infiltration of neutrophils without monocyte accumulation, while stent implantation is associated with an early influx of neutrophils, followed by sustained recruitment of monocytes over days to weeks. These differences are mirrored by molecular studies in which mRNA levels of the monocyte chemokine MCP-1 and the neutrophil chemokine IL-8 at sites of vascular injury were determined utilizing semi-quantitative reverse transcriptase polymerase chain reactions. In balloon injury, there is only transient (hours) expression of MCP-1 and IL-8. In contrast, in stented arteries, there was sustained expression of IL-8 and, more prominently, MCP-1 as late as 14 days (90).

Intracellular Molecular Basis of VSMC Proliferation

Because vascular smooth muscle cell (VSMC) proliferation and migration are so central to the development of restenosis and effective therapies, it is important to understand the basics of the intracellular signaling pathways that propagate these processes. The two major cascades that regulate the function of VSMC are the tyrosine kinase cascade and the cyclic-adenosine monophosphate (AMP) pathway. Growth factors bind to the receptors and activate tyrosine kinase that leads to a phosphorylation cascade, eventually activating *ras* proteins. This stimulates *raf* proteins to activate mitogen-activated protein kinase kinase (MAPKK), resulting in intranuclear activation of transcription factors that induce proliferation and migration of VSMC. The cyclic-AMP pathway leads to the activation of protein kinase A (PKA), which phosphorylates and activates the transcription factor cAMP responsive element binding protein (CREB). In addition, PKA phosphorylates *raf*, inhibiting the other major pathway involved in the activation of VSMC (91). In vitro and in vivo studies demonstrate that the inactivation of *ras* and the activation of the cyclic-AMP pathway leads to a >50% reduction in neointimal formation at 14 days postballoon injury in rat carotid arteries. A similar effect on NI formation is observed with inhibiting MAPKK by the dominant inhibitor mutant gene (92–94).

Downstream from these events, other molecular processes regulate the progression of the cell through the cell cycle. The progression from the G_0 to G_1 phase is regulated by cyclin-dependent kinases (CDK), particularly cyclin D-CDK and cyclin E-CDK-2. Endogenous inhibitors of CDK (CKI) such as p21[cip1], p27[kip1], and INK4 families regulate the process of entering G_1 and keep VSMC in the G_0 phase. Vascular inflammation and injury decreases the level of p27[kip1] thereby promoting cell division. On the contrary, activation of cAMP leads to an increase in p27[kip1], promoting the proliferating cells to enter a quiescent phase (91). This matrix of balanced events and intracellular signals leads to the conversion of VSMC to myofibroblasts and migration to the site of injury. Histologic analysis in the porcine model demonstrates that these actin (+) cells colonize the residual thrombus, which forms a cap across the thrombus and proliferates toward the tunica media. The myofibroblasts then degrade the thrombus and replace it with ECM, leading to the formation of the neointimal mass (95). The amount of NI produced is determined by the degree of inflammation generated during vascular injury (96).

Negative Remodeling

Remodeling is a change in arterial size following vascular injury (97). This process is primarily responsible for luminal loss after angioplasty and atherectomy (98). The process of negative remodeling may be observed 1 to 6 months after balloon angioplasty and accounts for about 60% to 65% of luminal loss observed by IVUS (97,99). The adventitia plays a crucial role in both the proliferation and concentric compression of the external elastic lamina (negative remodeling) (100). Three days after balloon injury in animals, a large number of proliferating cells were located in the adventitia, with significantly

fewer positive cells found in the media and lumen. Seven days after injury, proliferating cells were found primarily in the NI, extending along the luminal surface. In situ hybridization for PDGF A-chain and β-receptor mRNAs revealed that the expression of these two genes was closely correlated with the sites of proliferation at each time point (100,101). Upon vessel injury, inflammatory cells stimulate conversion of adventitial fibroblasts to myofibroblasts that express α-smooth muscle actin and secrete ECM, leading to constriction of the vessel and the formation of a fibrotic scar within the adventitia surrounding the site of injury. Wilcox used antibodies against α-smooth muscle actin, myosin, and desmin to demonstrate the proliferation of myofibroblasts in the NI and the adventitia (101). Other studies demonstrated that using intra-coronary radiation was effective in slowing the process when directed toward the adventitia, suggesting that the adventitia is not a passive player in restenosis.

An Integrated View of the Pathophysiology of Restenosis

When a balloon and stent injure a mature atherosclerotic plaque, a series of events are initiated (**Fig. 2.5**). The initial injury immediately following stent placement is de-endothelialization, with dissection into the tunica media and occasionally the adventitia, resulting in stretching of the entire artery. A layer of platelets and fibrin are deposited at the injured site. Activated platelets on the surface expressing adhesion molecules, such as P-selectin and GP Ibα, attach to circulating leukocytes via platelet receptors such as P-selectin glycoprotein ligand (PSGL-1) and begin a process of rolling along the injured surface. Leukocytes then bind tightly to the surface and stop rolling (mediated through the leukocyte integrin [i.e., Mac-1] class of adhesion molecules) via direct attachment to platelet receptors such as GP Ibα and through cross linking with fibrinogen to the GP IIb/IIIa receptor. Migration of leukocytes across the platelet–fibrin layer and diapedesis into the tissue is driven by chemical gradients of cytokines released from smooth muscle cells and resident inflammatory cells.

The next event is granulation or cellular proliferation. Growth factors are subsequently released from platelets, leukocytes, and smooth muscle cells, which stimulate the proliferation and migration of smooth muscle cells from the media into the NI. The resultant NI consists of smooth muscle cells, extracellular matrices, and macrophages recruited over several weeks. Over time, the artery remodels, with involvement of ECM protein degradation and resynthesis. Accompanying this phase is a shift to less cellular elements and greater production of ECM. After balloon injury, the shift to more ECM leads to shrinkage of the entire artery and negative remodeling. In the stented artery, this phase has less impact due to the rigid scaffolding of the stent, which prevents negative remodeling. In both balloon angioplastied and stented arteries, there is eventual re-endothelialization of at least part of the injured vessel surface.

Neoatherosclerosis

It has recently been recognized from pathologic examinations that, in a subset of patients, a lesion will develop within the stented segment that more closely resembles a native atherosclerotic plaque (102). This has been termed neoatherosclerosis (**Fig. 2.6**). Histologically, in-stent neoatherosclerosis is manifested by the accumulation of lipid-laden foamy macrophages, which start in the peri-strut area or adjacent to the luminal surface and then progress to a typical

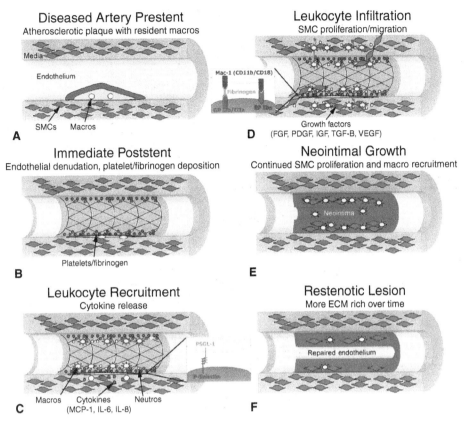

Diseased Artery Prestent
Atherosclerotic plaque with resident macros

Immediate Poststent
Endothelial denudation, platelet/fibrinogen deposition

Leukocyte Recruitment
Cytokine release

Leukocyte Infiltration
SMC proliferation/migration

Neointimal Growth
Continued SMC proliferation and macro recruitment

Restenotic Lesion
More ECM rich over time

FIGURE 2.5 Panel **(A)** illustrates a mature atherosclerotic plaque prior to intervention. Panel **(B)** illustrates the immediate result of stent placement with endothelial denudation and platelet/fibrinogen deposition. Panel **(C)** and **(D)** illustrate leukocyte recruitment, infiltration, and smooth muscle cell (SMC) proliferation and migration in the days following injury. Panel **(E)** demonstrates neointimal thickening in the weeks following injury, with continued SMC proliferation and monocyte recruitment. Panel **(F)** illustrates the long-term (weeks to months) change from a predominantly cellular to a less cellular and more ECM-rich plaque. ECM, extracellular matrix; MCP-1, monocyte chemoattractant protein-1; IL-6, IL-8, interleukin-6; interleukin-8; VEGF, vascular endothelial growth factor. (From: Welt FG, Rogers C. Inflammation and restenosis in the stent era. *Arterioscler Thromb Vasc Biol.* 2002;22:1769–1776.)

appearing fibroatheroma. This process may be associated with necrotic core formation and calcification (102).

The mechanism of neoatherosclerosis is still poorly understood but may include delayed endothelial coverage of the stented segments. Furthermore, antiproliferative effects of the eluted drugs in DES are likely to not only delay coverage but also lead to reduced production of nitric oxide and anti-thrombotic molecules (103–105). This process appears to occur faster (months to years) in neoatherosclerosis compared to atherosclerosis in native coronary arteries (decades) (103,106).

In-stent neoatherosclerosis occurs more frequently in DES than BMS, possibly due to polymer coating-induced inflammation, with an infiltration of macrophages, lymphocytes, and giant cells (107). An autopsy study published by Nakazawa and others (102) showed that the prevalence of neoatherosclerosis is significantly higher in lesions with first-generation DES compared to BMS (31% vs. 16%, respectively). Otsuka et al. (106) demonstrated no significant difference in the prevalence of neoatherosclerosis in CoCr-everolimus-eluting stent (EES) and first-generation SES and paclitaxel-eluting stent (PES) with implant durations of 30 days to 3 years. An autopsy stent registry of 384 cases and 614 stented lesions (266 lesions with BMS, 285 with first-generation DES, and 63 with second-generation DES) were analyzed histologically for neoatherosclerosis (108). The prevalence of neoatherosclerosis for implant duration ≤1 year

was similar in the first- and second-generation DES (13% vs. 17%, respectively) but higher than BMS (0%). Similar results were found when the lesions were assessed for the duration of implant >1 year and ≤3 years (51% for first-generation DES, 48% for second-generation DES, and 6% for BMS). For a duration of implant >3 years, only data from first-generation DES and BMS were available (65% vs. 38%, respectively).

Therapy

There have been multiple agents identified in preclinical studies that have shown efficacy against restenosis in animal models but failed when tested in large-scale clinical trials. It was not until agents directed against smooth muscle cell proliferation were married with local delivery techniques that significant reduction in restenosis was observed.

Mechanical Strategies

Mechanical strategies have been applied to reduce the frequency of ISR, which include: (i) IVUS-guided, high-pressure deployment to achieve larger mean luminal diameter (MLD), (ii) prior debulking therapy, and (iii) avoidance of predilation with "direct" stenting.

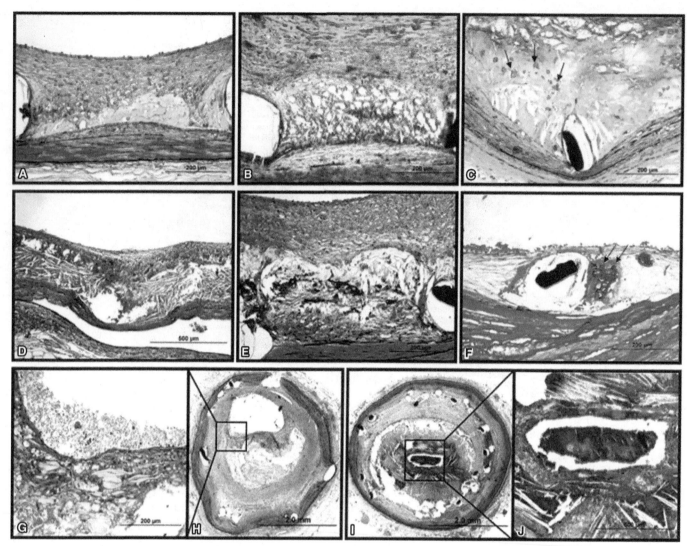

FIGURE 2.6 Representative images of various stages of newly formed atherosclerotic changes within neointima after stent implantation. **A:** Foamy macrophage clusters in the peristrut region of sirolimus-eluting stents (SESs) implanted for 13 months antemortem is seen. **B:** Fibroatheroma with foamy macrophage-rich lesion and early necrotic core formation in SES of 13 months' duration. **C:** Fibroatheroma with peristrut early necrotic core, cholesterol clefts, surface foamy macrophages, and early calcification (*arrows*) in SES at 13 months. **D:** Peristrut late necrotic core in the neointima, characterized by large aggregate of cholesterol cleft in SES at 17 months. **E:** Fibroatheroma with calcification in the necrotic core in SES of 10 months' duration. **F:** A peristrut calcification (*arrows*) with fibrin in SES of 7 months' duration. **G** and **H:** A low-power magnification image (**H**) of a severely narrowed bare-metal stent (BMS) implanted 61 months, with a thin-cap fibroatheroma. Note macrophage infiltration and a discontinuous thin fibrous cap in a high-power magnification image (**G**). **I:** A low-power magnification image shows a plaque rupture with an acute thrombus that has totally occluded the lumen in BMS implanted for 61 months antemortem. **J:** A high-power magnification image shows a discontinuous thin-cap with occlusive luminal thrombus. (From: Nakazawa G, Otsuka F, Nakano M, et al. The pathology of neoatherosclerosis in human coronary implants bare-metal and drug-eluting stents. *J Am Coll Cardiol.* 2011;57:1314–1322.)

These strategies may achieve some reduction in restenosis rates in certain cases; however, large randomized controlled trials failed to support this notion (109–111).

Bare-Metal Stents

Bare-metal stents were developed as a mechanical scaffolding of the arterial wall for the primary reduction of restenosis. The BENESTENT study was the earliest randomized controlled study that assessed long-term outcomes after BMS implantation. The study was conducted in 520 patients with stable coronary disease who were randomly assigned to a Palmaz–Schatz stent versus balloon angioplasty. There was a 30% reduction of primary endpoint between the two groups in

favor of the BMS. The primary clinical endpoints included death, MI, cerebrovascular events, the need for coronary artery bypass grafting (CABG), or a second PCI involving the previously treated lesion. The primary angiographic end-point was the minimal luminal diameter at follow-up. The clinical and angiographic outcomes were statistically better in the stent group in comparison to the angioplasty group, mainly with respect to restenosis rates (22% vs. 32%, respectively) (3).

Pharmacologic Therapies

Therapies directed toward the various pathways implicated in the restenosis have been attempted in both animal and human studies and include antiplatelet, anti-inflammatory, and antiproliferative agents.

Anticoagulant Therapy

The Antiplatelet Trialist Collaboration Investigators demonstrated a reduction of 25% of platelet aggregation in patients undergoing angioplasty but with no impact on restenosis. The addition of Ticlopidine to aspirin was more effective in reducing thrombosis compared to aspirin or aspirin plus warfarin, but had no impact on restenosis (112). Dipyridamole, another agent which stimulates prostacyclin synthesis and potentiates the action of prostacyclin and blocks the uptake of adenosine (a potent vasodilator) and inhibits phosphodiesterase, which increases platelet cyclic AMP levels leading to platelet inhibition, has yet failed to show difference in the rate restenosis (113). Other antiplatelet agents, thromboxane inhibitors, and prostacyclin analogues have showed similar disappointing results (114). The addition of aspirin and sulotroban in another study showed no reduction in the rates of restenosis either (115).

Glycoprotein IIb with IIIa form the platelet fibrinogen receptor, the final step in the cascade of platelet aggregation. Leucocytes bind through adhesion molecules indirectly through cross-linking of fibrinogen and glycoprotein IIb/IIIa. This is one of the links that allows leucocyte migration into the tissue, contributing to inflammation and, finally, neointimal formation (116). The direct effect of abciximab on inhibition of human coronary smooth muscle cells (hcSMCs), proliferation, migration, and invasion was tested ex vivo (117). The chemotactic and invasive potential of hcSMC was significantly inhibited when Abciximab was administered 24 hours prior and during migration, and there was a modest dose-dependent effect on proliferation. However, trials of the use of glycoprotein IIb/IIIa antagonist molecules were conducted for efficacy in patients undergoing PCI in acute coronary syndromes, and the rates of restenosis were evaluated in some of these studies. These studies collectively showed no effect on restenosis.

Similarly, oral antiplatelet agents have also been studied. Cilostazol, an antiplatelet agent, was approved by the US Food and Drug Administration (FDA) in 1998 for the treatment of intermittent claudication, and has been in use in other countries since 1988 for related indications. The pharmacologic effects of cilostazol are largely a result of selective inhibition of phosphodiesterase-3 (PDE3). In PDE3-rich cells, such as platelets and VSMCs, inhibition of PDE3 increases intracellular levels of cyclic-AMP, which activates PKA and ultimately results in phosphorylation of PKA substrates. These substrates mediate the potent antiplatelet effect of cilostazol, increase VSMCs relaxation and cardiac contractility, and inhibit VSMC proliferation (118). Initial nonrandomized studies showed evidence that cilostazol affects restenosis in both patients who underwent either balloon angioplasty or stenting (119).

Cilostazol for Restenosis (CREST) trial was a modern-era randomized study that sought to test the efficacy of cilostazol in preventing restenosis after stent implantation in a native coronary artery (120). The study enrolled 705 patients undergoing stenting at 19 sites who were randomized to therapy with cilostazol 200 mg/day (n = 354) or placebo (n = 351). All patients received aspirin before the procedure; a 300-mg loading dose of clopidogrel was given to those patients who were not already receiving clopidogrel. Both aspirin and cilostazol were continued for 6 months; clopidogrel was discontinued after 1 month. The primary end-point of the study was the MLD in the first lesion stented, as measured by quantitative coronary angiography at 6 months. Secondary endpoints were mean percentage diameter stenosis per stented lesion and rate of restenosis, defined as 50% luminal narrowing. Incidence of death, rate of TLR, and major adverse

cardiovascular events (MACE) were also monitored. At 6 months, cilostazol demonstrated a significant reduction in MLD compared to a placebo. In-segment restenosis was observed in 22.01% of patients receiving cilostazol and in 34.46% of those receiving a placebo (p = 0.002). Similarly, ISR was observed in significantly fewer patients in the cilostazol group (20.8%) than in the placebo group (31.4%). Consistent with the results of previous studies, reductions in the rates of ISRs were particularly large in patients with diabetes (17.7% vs. 37.7%, for cilostazol and placebo, respectively; p = 0.01). In summary, there is data supporting the use of cilostazol for reduction of ISR, particularly in diabetic patients who are at high risk of restenosis. Recent meta-analysis of 10 randomized studies continued to support the use of cilostazol for the reduction of restenosis (121).

Heparin has been the archetypal modulator of vascular repair in animal models and has been shown to reduce neointimal proliferation and restenosis following vascular injury (86,87). However, the maximum inhibition of NIH is noted with continued infusion for the duration of the experiment rather than intermittent use (88). This effect was also witnessed in the SHARP (Subcutaneous Heparin and Angioplasty Restenosis Prevention) trial, which randomized 339 patients to subcutaneous therapy versus no therapy. The 4-month follow-up showed no difference in outcome or restenosis (122). Low-molecular-weight heparin has been evaluated in multiple studies and demonstrated no reduction in restenosis (123,124). Hirudin, a small molecule that is a direct thrombin inhibitor, has shown promising results in animal femoral arteries with reductions in restenosis rates; however, subsequent clinical randomized studies showed no difference in restenosis when compared to heparin (125–127).

Agents that Prevent Inflammation and Cell Proliferation

Cell proliferation plays a key role in restenosis and, as described earlier, is driven primarily by inflammation. Therefore, there has been great interest in anti-inflammatory and anti-proliferative agents as therapies to prevent restenosis. Broadly speaking, the classic anti-inflammatory agents such as corticosteroids and colchine, a metaphase inhibitor, have shown little to no benefit in clinical trials (128,129).

Prevention of Vascular Recoil and Remodeling

The Coronary Angioplasty Study Amlodipine Restenosis (CAPARES) randomized 635 patients to Amlodipine versus placebo in patients undergoing coronary intervention. The treatment was started 2 weeks prior to the procedure and continued for 4 months. There was no difference in minimum lumen diameter measured by quantitative angiography, but the incidence of repeat PTCA and the composite major adverse clinical events were significantly reduced during the 4-month follow-up period after PTCA with amlodipine, as compared with a placebo (130).

Individual trials using Nifedipine, Verapamil, and Diltiazem were not able to demonstrate an effect either (131–133). Although meta analysis data demonstrated that patients treated with calcium channel blockers had a 32% reduction in angiographic restenosis compared to controls, the practice of routine use of these agents was never solidified, mostly due to concerns about increased incidence of ischemic events following MI (134).

Some authors have suggested that the rate of restenosis may be modified by the gene deletion/insertion (D/I) polymorphism of the ACE gene. Patients being treated with ACE inhibitors or angiotensin receptor blockers (ARB) with DD homozygotes with two deletion alleles had a higher rate of restenosis. This finding may be attributed to patient selection bias, given that patients with diabetes have higher rates of restenosis and are likely to be on an ACE or ARB. However, it was not found to be an independent predictor of restenosis, and there is no reason to test prior to interventions (135).

Drug-Eluting Stents

Local drug delivery has several important advantages in the treatment of restenosis. Most importantly, potentially toxic drugs can be delivered in sufficiently high doses locally to have an effect without systemic toxicity. Some of the unique features of restenosis as a target are that the exact site and time of the onset of disease are well-known, given that implantation of the stent is the inciting event. DESs that allow a predictable elution of a high dose locally of a therapeutic agent have been shown to be very effective in preventing ISR. The ability of the stent to deliver an agent locally reduces proliferation of VSMC with essentially undetectable levels in peripheral blood and lack of any systemic toxicity (136).

Local drug delivery is a complex process governed by the dose and rate of release of the agent, tissue retention, and the inherent properties of the drug. Low doses may be ineffective, while higher doses can lead to tissue death and fibrin deposition, leading to increased rates of thrombosis with delayed healing (137,138). In summary, release rates must be targeted to match the biologic process being modified. Interestingly, with sirolimus as opposed to paclitaxel, fast release is just as effective in comparison to slow release in reduction of late luminal loss (139). The drug can be delivered by the stent through a variety of media that play a role in the rate of restenosis. Some drugs can be linked to the stent directly through processes of quaternary binding. However, most drugs require a polymer to harbor the drug and allow timed release. In this process, non-erodable polymers had to be developed with minimal inflammatory stimuli. Polymer release kinetics plays a critical role in the prevention of restenosis. The Paclitaxel In-Stent Controlled Elution Study (PISCES) trial 3 demonstrated this principle, involving the use of the Conor stent with six different polymer-drug release formulations. The duration of the drug release had a far greater impact on the inhibition of NIH than the dose of drug delivered. For example, 10 μg of paclitaxel released over 10 days following DES implantation appeared to have little effect on NIH formation, whereas the same dosage of drug released over a 30-day period led to a profound reduction in NIH, with more than half (57%) the reduction of the LLL, while 30 μg of the same drug released over a 10-day period also was less effective (140). Molecular biology studies have suggested that the genes responsible for the proliferative response potentially remain active for a period up to 21 days after vessel injury. These clinical findings therefore support the concept of a certain threshold of drug, delivered over a biologically appropriate period of time, to inhibit the inflammatory and subsequent NIH response (141).

Sirolimus

Sirolimus (rapamycin) is a natural macro-cyclic lactone with potent immunosuppressive and antimitotic action produced by a fungus, *Streptomyces hygroscopicus*. The agent binds intracellularly to the FKBP-12 forming the immunosuppressive complex that inhibits the mTOR, a key regulatory kinase. That leads to an increase in the levels of p27^{kip1}, which inhibits the cyclin-CDK complex, blocking the G_1-S transition and thereby restricting proliferation of VSMC (142).

There have been four pivotal trials conducted with sirolimus-eluting stents (SESs) that led to FDA approval in April 2003. After initial impressive results from the First in Man (FIM) (139) experience, a double-blind, randomized, controlled trial was launched. The Randomized Study with the Sirolimus-Eluting Velocity Balloon-Expandable Stent (RAVEL) randomized 238 patients to either a single SES or the same single BMS (143). The SES was prepared for release similar to the slow-release method from the FIM study. One-half of the patients presented with unstable angina. All patients received heparin during PCI, clopidogrel, or ticlopidine for 8 weeks after the procedure, and aspirin (100 mg or more/day) indefinitely. About 10% of patients also received GP IIb–IIIa inhibitors. At 6 months, there was a significant reduction of in-stent LL, intimal hyperplasia, and restenosis for patients receiving the SES compared with the BMS. The significant reduction of in-stent loss also was evident when the proximal and distal edges were evaluated (in-segment loss). During a follow-up period of up to 1 year, the overall rate of major cardiac events was 5.8% in the sirolimus-stent group and 28.8% in the standard-stent group (p < 0.001). The RAVEL study was limited to non-complex lesions. The SIRIUS trial (10), comparing sirolimus DES stents with BMS, recruited patients in the US who had more multivessel disease (40.7%) compared to RAVEL (29%). The study included more patients with diabetes mellitus (26% in SIRIUS vs. 19% in RAVEL), longer lesions (mean 14.4 mm), and 60% of patients received GP IIb–IIIa inhibitors, compared with only 10% of patients in RAVEL. Patients treated with SESs had lower rates of binary (>50% diameter stenosis) angiographic restenosis within the segment (8.9% vs. 36.3% with the BMS; p < 0.001) and within the stent (3.2% vs. 35.4% with the BMS; p < 0.001). SESs were associated with significantly less LLL within the treated segment, within the stent, and within its 5-mm proximal and distal edges (all p < 0.001). The reduction of restenosis with the SES was consistent in patients at risk for restenosis, including those with small vessels, long lesions, and diabetes mellitus (144).

Paclitaxel

Paclitaxel is a compound isolated from the bark of the Pacific yew tree of the northwestern US (*Taxus brevifolia*). Paclitaxel exerts its pharmacologic effect by inhibiting microtubule de-polymerization, resulting in the formation of numerous decentralized and unorganized micro tubules during cell division. This results in inhibition of cellular replication at the G_0/G_1 and G_1/M phase and stops cytokine-mediated induction of cell proliferation and migration.

Paclitaxel (PES) efficacy was demonstrated in the TAXUS II and TAXUS IV trials, which examined patients with low-risk lesions or previously untreated coronary stenosis who randomly received BMS or PES with either a slow or a moderate drug-release rate. All trials resulted in reduction of ISR and TLR (145–148). Furthermore, TAXUS IV demonstrated that these benefits were maintained in subgroups, including patients with vessels <2.5 mm in diameter, those with lesions >20 mm in length, and those with renal insufficiency or diabetes. Pooled and long-term analysis also revealed a reduction in CV events.

Sirolimus versus Paclitaxel-Eluting Stent Trials

The TAXi trial was the first prospective, randomized trial that compared the efficacy of SES (CYPHER) versus PES (TAXUS). Two hundred and two patients with similar demographics were randomized into two groups: the SES (n = 102) group and the PES (n = 100) group. Although the data showed no significant difference in MACE between SES and PES at 6 months, the trial was limited in its sample size to determine any clinical superiority between the two drug-eluting stents (DES) (5).

This was followed by the REALITY trial, a large prospective, randomized trial that compared the polymer-coated Cypher SES to the polymer-coated Taxus PES in terms of safety and efficacy. The study randomized 1,353 patients with similar angiographic and clinical variables into SES (n = 684) and PES (n = 669) groups, with the primary endpoint of the in-lesion restenosis rate at 8 months. At the 8-month angiographic follow-up, significant differences were found in in-stent MLD, percentage diameter stenosis, in-stent LL, and in-stent LL index, all favoring the SES. These observations indicate a significantly greater degree of suppression of NIH achieved by the SES, particularly considering the smaller mean vessel diameter measured immediately after the implantation of the SES. However, the significant differences in several continuous angiographic variables, most importantly in-stent LL, did not translate into significant differences in in-lesion binary restenosis or in TLR (149). Other studies such as SIRTAX suggested superiority of SES to PES, with lower rates of TVR (150). SES also proved superior to PES in suppression of NIH when evaluated by IVUS imaging (151). Long-term follow-up of SIRTAX showed no difference between the two groups, likely attributed to the loss of initial release kinetics of SES compared to PES (152).

Everolimus

Everolimus is the 40-O-(2-hydroxyethyl) derivative of sirolimus and works similarly to sirolimus as an mTOR inhibitor. The purpose of the COMPARE study was to compare the safety and efficacy of the Xience V (Abbott Vascular, Santa Clara, CA) EES with the Taxus Liberté (Boston Scientific, Natick, MA) PES in 1,800 patients (153). This randomized, open-label trial demonstrated a superior clinical outcome of EES over PES at 1 year in all comers. Patients undergoing PCI with limited exclusion criteria were randomly allocated to EES or PES. The 2-year pre-specified endpoints were composites of safety and efficacy and stent thrombosis.

The primary composite of all death, nonfatal MI, and TVR occurred in 9.0% of EES patients and 13.7% of PES patients, with a 37% risk reduction driven by a lower rate of MI (3.9% vs. 7.5%; RR: 0.52; 95% CI: 0.35–0.77) and TLR (3.2% vs. 8.0%; RR: 0.41; 95% CI: 0.27–0.62), in parallel with a lower rate of definite or probable stent thrombosis (0.9% vs. 3.9%; RR: 0.23; 95% CI: 0.11–0.49). The substantial clinical benefit of the EES over the PES with regard to measures of both safety and efficacy is maintained at 2 years in real-life practice with an increasing benefit in terms of safety and efficacy between 1 year and 2. The subgroup analysis showed that significantly more patients had clinically indicated TVR (9.3% vs. 2.0%, RR: 0.20, 95% CI: 0.04–0.70, p = 0.008), and there was a trend toward more TLR in the PES group compared with the EES group (5.8% vs. 2.0%, respectively; p = 0.09).

Differences in stent design, strut thickness, delivery platform, polymer coating, drug, and drug release profile could all play a role in these differences between PES and EES. Other potential explanations may be more rapid reendothelialization with EES, documented in the rabbit iliac model, or the more biocompatible fluorinated copolymer (103).

EES has proven to be non-inferior compared to SES. EXCELLENT was a randomized study comparing both platforms (Xience/Promus) and had the same rate of TVR (3.75% and 3.0% respectively) (154).

Zotarolimus

Zotarolimus, an analogue of sirolimus, was designed to have a shorter in vivo half-life. Zotarolimus was found to be similar to sirolimus in having high-affinity binding to the immunophilin FKBP12 and comparable potency for inhibiting in-vitro proliferation of both human and rat T cells (155). The FDA approved the Endeavor stent platform in 2008 after reviewing the ENDEAVOR clinical program, which included seven studies: three randomized controlled trials and four registries. ENDEAVOR IV was the first trial comparing two different DES platforms and was powered for clinical (target vessel failure) and angiographic (late loss [LL]) endpoints. The study met its primary endpoint: zotarolimus-eluting stent (ZES) was noninferior to PES in target vessel failure at a 9-month clinical follow-up. It did not meet its LL goal, however, because ZES did not achieve noninferiority compared with PES at the 8-month angiographic follow-up. This disparity in outcomes has been suggested to be due to the curvilinear relationship between LL and clinical TLR. Stuart Pocock et al. using data from 11 randomized trials of DES versus BMS showed that the slope appears to be nearly flat between LL values of 0 and 0.7 and then becomes linear at LL values >0.7 (12). In addition, angiographic follow-up has been shown to have a significant impact on revascularization rates. In the ENDEAVOR IV trial, TLR and TVR rates were similar in patients who had clinical follow-up, yet different in those who underwent angiographic follow-up (156).

Serruys et al. sought to investigate the non-inferiority of the Resolute Zotarolimus stent compared to everolimus by randomizing 2,297 patients to either stent. The next-generation Resolute stent, consisted of the same cobalt chromium metallic platform (Driver BMS) and the drug (zotarolimus) as the Endeavor stent, but with a substantially longer polymer drug release kinetics (180 days) compared to 14 days. The primary endpoint was target-lesion failure, defined as a composite of death from cardiac causes, any MI (not clearly attributable to a nontarget vessel), or clinically indicated TLR within 12 months. The secondary angiographic endpoint was the extent of in-stent stenosis at 13 months. The ZES was noninferior to the EES with respect to the primary endpoint, which occurred in 8.2% and 8.3% of patients, respectively (p < 0.001 for noninferiority). There were no significant differences between the groups—group differences in the rate of death from cardiac causes, any MI, or revascularization. The zotarolimus-eluting stent was also noninferior with regard to the degree (±SD) of in-stent stenosis (21.65 ± 14.42% for zotarolimus vs. 19.76 ± 14.64% for everolimus, p = 0.04 for noninferiority). However, the angiographic endpoint of LLL was discovered to be different between the two stents with 0.27 ± 0.43 mm in the zotarolimus-stent group versus 0.19 ± 0.40 mm in the everolimus-stent group, which trended to favor everolimus, but did not achieve statistical significance (157).

The TWENTE trial also compared the Resolute ZES with the Xience V EES in 1,391 patients with complex lesions, of whom 52% presented with acute coronary syndromes. Target vessel failure was similar in both groups around 8% (158). The definitions between studies determine the rates of events; however, they remain low.

Long-term outcomes appear to be key in head-to-head comparisons between stents. The SORT OUT III study provided 5-year follow-up data in 2,332 patients who were randomized to either

ZES or SES. The study showed that the superiority found with SES over ZES at 1-year follow-up was lost after 5 years. In this study, 77% of TLR in the SES group occurred between 1 and 5 years after stent implantation (159).

Coated Balloon Drug Delivery

The PEPCAD-DES Study examined the impact of paclitaxel-coated balloon angioplasty for treatment of drug-eluting stent restenosis compared with uncoated balloon angioplasty. In a prospective, single-blinded, multicenter, randomized trial, 110 patients were randomized to paclitaxel-coated balloon angioplasty or uncoated balloon angioplasty. Dual antiplatelet therapy was prescribed for 6 months. The primary endpoint was 6-month LLL. The secondary endpoint was a composite of cardiac death, MI, or TVR (160). Treatment with a paclitaxel-coated balloon was superior to balloon angioplasty, with LLL approaching 50% reduction. There was an absolute 40% reduction in restenosis rates. These angiographic findings correlated with 30% reduction in events. This is a promising treatment that has been used in Europe and has yet to gain FDA approval.

Therapy for ISR in the DES Era

ISAR-DESIRE was a prospective, randomized, controlled trial that assessed the efficacy of DES in the treatment of ISR in comparison to conventional balloon angioplasty Three hundred patients with similar clinical variables and documented angiographic ISR were randomized to receive either SES (n = 100), PES (n = 100), or balloon angioplasty (n = 100). Angiographic analysis preformed in 275 (92%) patients showed a significant decrease in rates of restenosis in both DES cohorts in comparison to balloon angioplasty at 9 months. A secondary analysis comparing the two DES cohorts showed a significant decrease in LLL (p = 0.004) and in-stent % DS (p = 0.004) in the SES versus the PES group. There were lower rates of in-stent, in-lesion restenosis, and MACE that did not reach significance in the SES group. There was no significant difference in the incidence of death or MI across all three groups (161). This further advanced the notion of using DES for treatment of an existing ISR.

Brachytherapy

Intravascular brachytherapy has shown a reduction in neointimal proliferation and ISR in multiple randomized clinical trials (162–164). The treatment was particularly successful in diabetic patients (165). With the introduction of DES, brachytherapy has become very uncommon. The practical difficulty in scheduling the procedure with radiation oncologists and the catheterization lab, specialized availability at tertiary centers, and increased rates of subacute thrombosis have delayed the wide acceptance of intracoronary radiation into clinical practice (166,167).

Conclusion

Restenosis has been a limiting factor into the clinical success of PCI. The paradigm introduced by Forrester based on the vascular biology of wound healing suggested a three-phase process: an inflammatory phase, a granulation or cellular proliferation phase, and a phase of remodeling involving ECM protein synthesis. The mechanism of inflammation and cell recruitment is a complex cascade with

the aggregation of platelets and the release of chemotactic agents recruiting leucocytes, macrocytes, and monocytes. In turn, these cells stimulate muscular smooth muscle cells from the quiescent phase to active phase. The combination of a local drug delivery strategy combined with antiproliferative agents has been a successful strategy in limiting this particular complication.

Key Points

- Restenosis is part of the vascular biology of wound healing and occurs in three phases in the process: an inflammatory phase, a granulation or cellular proliferation phase, and a phase of remodeling involving ECM protein synthesis.
- The mechanism of inflammation and cell recruitment is a complex cascade, with the aggregation of platelets and the release of chemotactic agents recruiting leukocytes, macrocytes, and monocytes.
- Mechanisms of drugs used to reduce restenosis act to suppress cell division and/or act in a cytotoxic manner.
- Inflammatory cells stimulate muscular SMCs from the quiescent phase to the active phase.
- The combination of a local drug delivery strategy combined with antiproliferative agents has been a successful strategy in limiting restenosis.
- Treatment of DES restenosis is typically with repeat DES placement, followed by brachytherapy for refractory cases.

References

1. Dotter CT, Judkins MP. Transluminal treatment of arteriosclerotic obstruction. description of a new technic and a preliminary report of its application. *Circulation.* 1964;30:654–70.
2. Gruntzig AR, Senning A, Siegenthaler WE. Nonoperative dilatation of coronary-artery stenosis: percutaneous transluminal coronary angioplasty. *N Engl J Med.* 1979;301:61–68.
3. Serruys PW, et al. A comparison of balloon-expandable-stent implantation with balloon angioplasty in patients with coronary artery disease. Benestent Study Group. *N Engl J Med.* 1994;331:489–495.
4. Abbott JD, et al. Unrestricted use of drug-eluting stents compared with bare-metal stents in routine clinical practice: findings from the National Heart, Lung, and Blood Institute Dynamic Registry. *J Am Coll Cardiol.* 2007;50:2029–2036.
5. Goy JJ, et al. A prospective randomized comparison between paclitaxel and sirolimus stents in the real world of interventional cardiology: the TAXi trial. *J Am Coll Cardiol.* 2005;45:308–311.
6. Simonton CA, et al. Comparative clinical outcomes of paclitaxel- and sirolimus-eluting stents: results from a large prospective multicenter registry—STENT Group. *J Am Coll Cardiol.* 2007;50:1214–1222.
7. Cosgrave J, et al. Comparable clinical outcomes with paclitaxel- and sirolimus-eluting stents in unrestricted contemporary practice. *J Am Coll Cardiol.* 2007;49:2320–2328.
8. Roubin GS, King SB III, Douglas JS Jr. Restenosis after percutaneous transluminal coronary angioplasty: the Emory University Hospital experience. *Am J Cardiol.* 1987;60:39B–43B.
9. Mehilli J, et al. Randomized trial of a nonpolymer-based rapamycin-eluting stent versus a polymer-based paclitaxel-eluting stent for the reduction of late lumen loss. *Circulation.* 2006;113:273–279.

10. Morice MC, et al. A randomized comparison of a sirolimus-eluting stent with a standard stent for coronary revascularization. *N Engl J Med.* 2002;346:1773–1780.

11. Dobesh PP, et al. Drug-eluting stents: a mechanical and pharmacologic approach to coronary artery disease. *Pharmacotherapy.* 2004;24:1554–1577.

12. Pocock SJ, et al. Angiographic surrogate end points in drug-eluting stent trials: a systematic evaluation based on individual patient data from 11 randomized, controlled trials. *J Am Coll Cardiol.* 2008;51:23–32.

13. Ruygrok PN, et al. Clinical and angiographic factors associated with asymptomatic restenosis after percutaneous coronary intervention. *Circulation.* 2001;104:2289–2294.

14. Bossi I, et al. In-stent restenosis: long-term outcome and predictors of subsequent target lesion revascularization after repeat balloon angioplasty. *J Am Coll Cardiol.* 2000;35:1569–1576.

15. Chen MS, et al. Bare metal stent restenosis is not a benign clinical entity. *Am Heart J.* 2006;151:1260–1264.

16. Rathore S, et al. A comparison of clinical presentations, angiographic patterns and outcomes of in-stent restenosis between bare metal stents and drug eluting stents. *EuroIntervention.* 2010;5:841–846.

17. Meliga E, et al. Longest available clinical outcomes after drug-eluting stent implantation for unprotected left main coronary artery disease: the DELFT (Drug Eluting stent for LeFT main) Registry. *J Am Coll Cardiol.* 2008;51:2212–2219.

18. Buszman PP, et al. Early and long-term outcomes after surgical and percutaneous myocardial revascularization in patients with non-ST-elevation acute coronary syndromes and unprotected left main disease. *J Invasive Cardiol.* 2009;21:564–569.

19. Serruys PW, et al. Percutaneous coronary intervention versus coronary-artery bypass grafting for severe coronary artery disease. *N Engl J Med.* 2009;360:961–972.

20. Serruys PW, et al. Incidence of restenosis after successful coronary angioplasty: a time-related phenomenon. A quantitative angiographic study in 342 consecutive patients at 1, 2, 3, and 4 months. *Circulation.* 1988;77:361–371.

21. Ellis SG, et al. Risk factors, time course and treatment effect for restenosis after successful percutaneous transluminal coronary angioplasty of chronic total occlusion. *Am J Cardiol.* 1989;63:897–901.

22. Nayak AK, et al. Myocardial infarction as a presentation of clinical in-stent restenosis. *Circ J.* 2006;70:1026–1029.

23. Kastrati A, et al. Predictive factors of restenosis after coronary stent placement. *J Am Coll Cardiol.* 1997;30:1428–1436.

24. Frobert O, et al. Differences in restenosis rate with different drug-eluting stents in patients with and without diabetes mellitus: a report from the SCAAR (Swedish Angiography and Angioplasty Registry). *J Am Coll Cardiol.* 2009;53:1660–1667.

25. Abizaid A, et al. The influence of diabetes mellitus on acute and late clinical outcomes following coronary stent implantation. *J Am Coll Cardiol.* 1998;32:584–589.

26. Aronson D, Bloomgarden Z, Rayfield EJ. Potential mechanisms promoting restenosis in diabetic patients. *J Am Coll Cardiol.* 1996;27:528–535.

27. Ribichini F, et al. Plasma activity and insertion/deletion polymorphism of angiotensin I-converting enzyme: a major risk factor and a marker of risk for coronary stent restenosis. *Circulation.* 1998;97:147–154.

28. Vogiatzi K, et al. Interleukin 8 gene polymorphisms and susceptibility to restenosis after percutaneous coronary intervention. *J Thromb Thrombolysis.* 2010;29:134–140.

29. Richardson A, Kaye SB. Drug resistance in ovarian cancer: the emerging importance of gene transcription and spatio-temporal regulation of resistance. *Drug Resist Updat.* 2005;8:311–321.

30. Huang S, Houghton PJ. Resistance to rapamycin: a novel anticancer drug. *Cancer Metastasis Rev.* 2001;20:69–78.

31. Moreno PR, et al. Macrophage infiltration predicts restenosis after coronary intervention in patients with unstable angina. *Circulation.* 1996;94:3098–3102.

32. Neumann FJ, et al. Neutrophil and platelet activation at balloon-injured coronary artery plaque in patients undergoing angioplasty. *J Am Coll Cardiol.* 1996;27:819–824.

33. Mickelson JK, et al. Leukocyte activation with platelet adhesion after coronary angioplasty: a mechanism for recurrent disease? *J Am Coll Cardiol.* 1996;28:345–353.

34. Cipollone F, et al. Elevated circulating levels of monocyte chemoattractant protein-1 in patients with restenosis after coronary angioplasty. *Arterioscler Thromb Vasc Biol.* 2001;21:327–334.

35. Gibson CM, et al. Comparison of effects of bare metal versus drug-eluting stent implantation on biomarker levels following percutaneous coronary intervention for non-ST-elevation acute coronary syndrome. *Am J Cardiol.* 2006;97:1473–1477.

36. Kim JY, et al. Comparison of effects of drug-eluting stents versus bare metal stents on plasma C-reactive protein levels. *Am J Cardiol.* 2005;96:1384–1388.

37. Segev A, et al. Pre-procedural plasma levels of C-reactive protein and interleukin-6 do not predict late coronary angiographic restenosis after elective stenting. *Eur Heart J.* 2004;25:1029–1035.

38. Yip HK, et al. Serum concentrations of high-sensitivity C-reactive protein predict progressively obstructive lesions rather than late restenosis in patients with unstable angina undergoing coronary artery stenting. *Circ J.* 2005;69:1202–1207.

39. Skowasch D, et al. Progression of native coronary plaques and in-stent restenosis are associated and predicted by increased pre-procedural C reactive protein. *Heart.* 2005;91:535–536.

40. Katsaros KM, et al. High soluble Fas and soluble Fas ligand serum levels before stent implantation are protective against restenosis. *Thromb Haemost.* 2011;105:883–891.

41. Hwang CW, Wu D, Edelman ER. Physiological transport forces govern drug distribution for stent-based delivery. *Circulation.* 2001;104:600–605.

42. Takebayashi H, et al. Nonuniform strut distribution correlates with more neointimal hyperplasia after sirolimus-eluting stent implantation. *Circulation.* 2004;110:3430–3434.

43. Doi H, et al. Classification and potential mechanisms of intravascular ultrasound patterns of stent fracture. *Am J Cardiol.* 2009;103:818–823.

44. Aoki J, et al. Incidence and clinical impact of coronary stent fracture after sirolimus-eluting stent implantation. *Catheter Cardiovasc Interv.* 2007;69:380–386.

45. Lee MS, et al. Stent fracture associated with drug-eluting stents: clinical characteristics and implications. *Catheter Cardiovasc Interv.* 2007;69:387–394.

46. Umeda H, et al. Frequency, predictors and outcome of stent fracture after sirolimus-eluting stent implantation. *Int J Cardiol.* 2009;133:321–326.

47. Dangas GD, et al. In-stent restenosis in the drug-eluting stent era. *J Am Coll Cardiol.* 2010;56:1897–1907.

48. Mehran R, et al. Angiographic patterns of in-stent restenosis: classification and implications for long-term outcome. *Circulation.* 1999;100:1872–1878.

49. Forrester JS, et al. A paradigm for restenosis based on cell biology: clues for the development of new preventive therapies. *J Am Coll Cardiol.* 1991;17:758–769.

50. Park SJ, et al. In-stent neoatherosclerosis: a final common pathway of late stent failure. *J Am Coll Cardiol.* 2012;59:2051–2057.

51. Rensing BJ, et al. Quantitative angiographic assessment of elastic recoil after percutaneous transluminal coronary angioplasty. *Am J Cardiol.* 1990;66:1039–1044.

52. Violaris AG, Serruys PW. New technologies in interventional cardiology. *Curr Opin Cardiol.* 1994;9:493–502.

53. Mintz GS, et al. Intravascular ultrasound assessment of the mechanisms and predictors of restenosis following coronary angioplasty. *J Invasive Cardiol.* 1996;8:1–14.

54. Breeman A, et al. Complications shortly after transluminal angioplasty or following coronary surgery in 183 comparable patients with multi-vessel coronary disease. *Ned Tijdschr Geneeskd.* 1994;138:1074–1080.

55. Fischman DL, et al. A randomized comparison of coronary-stent placement and balloon angioplasty in the treatment of coronary artery disease. Stent Restenosis Study Investigators. *N Engl J Med.* 1994;331:496–501.

56. Hoffmann R, et al. Patterns and mechanisms of in-stent restenosis. A serial intravascular ultrasound study. *Circulation.* 1996;94:1247–1254.

57. Kornowski R, et al. In-stent restenosis: contributions of inflammatory responses and arterial injury to neointimal hyperplasia. *J Am Coll Cardiol.* 1998;31:224–230.

58. Koster R, et al. Nickel and molybdenum contact allergies in patients with coronary in-stent restenosis. *Lancet.* 2000;356:1895–1897.

59. Marcus AJ. Thrombosis and inflammation as multicellular processes: significance of cell–cell interactions. *Semin Hematol.* 1994;31:261–269.

60. Diacovo TG, et al. Neutrophil rolling, arrest, and transmigration across activated, surface-adherent platelets via sequential action of P-selectin and the beta 2-integrin CD11b/CD18. *Blood.* 1996;88:146–157.

61. Yeo EL, Sheppard JA, Feuerstein IA. Role of P-selectin and leukocyte activation in polymorphonuclear cell adhesion to surface adherent activated platelets under physiologic shear conditions (an injury vessel wall model). *Blood.* 1994;83:2498–2507.

62. Ott I, et al. Increased neutrophil-platelet adhesion in patients with unstable angina. *Circulation.* 1996;94:1239–1246.

63. Furman MI, et al. Increased platelet reactivity and circulating monocyte-platelet aggregates in patients with stable coronary artery disease. *J Am Coll Cardiol.* 1998;31:352–358.

64. Farb A, et al. Morphological predictors of restenosis after coronary stenting in humans. *Circulation.* 2002;105:2974–2980.

65. Inoue T, et al. Expression of polymorphonuclear leukocyte adhesion molecules and its clinical significance in patients treated with percutaneous transluminal coronary angioplasty. *J Am Coll Cardiol.* 1996;28:1127–1133.

66. Inoue T, et al. Stent-induced expression and activation of the leukocyte integrin Mac-1 is associated with neointimal thickening and restenosis. *Circulation.* 2003;107:1757–1763.

67. Pietersma A, et al. Late lumen loss after coronary angioplasty is associated with the activation status of circulating phagocytes before treatment. *Circulation.* 1995;91:1320–1325.

68. Gaspardone A, et al. Predictive value of C-reactive protein after successful coronary-artery stenting in patients with stable angina. *Am J Cardiol.* 1998;82:515–518.

69. Cybulsky MI, Gimbrone MA Jr. Endothelial expression of a mononuclear leukocyte adhesion molecule during atherogenesis. *Science.* 1991;251: 788–791.

70. Li H, et al. An atherogenic diet rapidly induces VCAM-1, a cytokine-regulatable mononuclear leukocyte adhesion molecule, in rabbit aortic endothelium. *Arterioscler Thromb.* 1993;13:197–204.

71. Li H, et al. Inducible expression of vascular cell adhesion molecule-1 by vascular smooth muscle cells in vitro and within rabbit atheroma. *Am J Pathol.* 1993;143:1551–1559.

72. Richardson M, et al. Increased expression in vivo of VCAM-1 and E-selectin by the aortic endothelium of normolipemic and hyperlipemic diabetic rabbits. *Arterioscler Thromb.* 1994;14:760–769.

73. Walpola PL, et al. Expression of ICAM-1 and VCAM-1 and monocyte adherence in arteries exposed to altered shear stress. *Arterioscler Thromb Vasc Biol.* 1995;15:2–10.

74. Tanaka H, et al. Sustained activation of vascular cells and leukocytes in the rabbit aorta after balloon injury. *Circulation.* 1993;88:1788–1803.

75. Welt FG, et al. Neutrophil, not macrophage, infiltration precedes neointimal thickening in balloon-injured arteries. *Arterioscler Thromb Vasc Biol.* 2000;20:2553–2558.

76. Rogers C, et al. Monocyte recruitment and neointimal hyperplasia in rabbits. Coupled inhibitory effects of heparin. *Arterioscler Thromb Vasc Biol.* 1996;16:1312–1318.

77. Rogers C, Edelman ER, Simon DI. A mAb to the beta2-leukocyte integrin Mac-1 (CD11b/CD18) reduces intimal thickening after angioplasty or stent implantation in rabbits. *Proc Natl Acad Sci U S A.* 1998;95:10134–10139.

78. Mori E, et al. Essential role of monocyte chemoattractant protein-1 in development of restenotic changes (neointimal hyperplasia and constrictive remodeling) after balloon angioplasty in hypercholesterolemic rabbits. *Circulation.* 2002;105:2905–2910.

79. Libby P, et al. A cascade model for restenosis. A special case of atherosclerosis progression. *Circulation.* 1992;86:III47–III52.

80. Kockx MM, et al. Triphasic sequence of neointimal formation in the cuffed carotid artery of the rabbit. *Arterioscler Thromb.* 1992;12:1447–1457.

81. Jorgensen L, et al. Sequence of cellular responses in rabbit aortas following one and two injuries with a balloon catheter. *Br J Exp Pathol.* 1988;69:473–486.

82. Richardson M, et al. Wound healing in the media of the normolipemic rabbit carotid artery injured by air drying or by balloon catheter de-endothelialization. *Am J Pathol.* 1990;137:1453–1465.

83. Cole CW, et al. A neutrophil derived factor(s) stimulates [3H]thymidine incorporation by vascular smooth muscle cells in vitro. *Clin Invest Med.* 1988;11:62–67.

84. Lloyd AR, Oppenheim JJ. Poly's lament: the neglected role of the polymorphonuclear neutrophil in the afferent limb of the immune response. *Immunol Today.* 1992;13:169–172.

85. Inoue T, et al. Comparison of activation process of platelets and neutrophils after coronary stent implantation versus balloon angioplasty for stable angina pectoris. *Am J Cardiol.* 2000;86:1057–1062.

86. Clowes AW, Clowes MM. Kinetics of cellular proliferation after arterial injury. II. Inhibition of smooth muscle growth by heparin. *Lab Invest.* 1985;52:611–616.

87. Clowes AW, Clowes MM. Kinetics of cellular proliferation after arterial injury. IV. Heparin inhibits rat smooth muscle mitogenesis and migration. *Circ Res.* 1986;58:839–845.

88. Edelman ER, Karnovsky MJ. Contrasting effects of the intermittent and continuous administration of heparin in experimental restenosis. *Circulation.* 1994;89:770–776.

89. Rogers C, Karnovsky MJ, Edelman ER. Inhibition of experimental neointimal hyperplasia and thrombosis depends on the type of vascular injury and the site of drug administration. *Circulation.* 1993;88:1215–1221.

90. Welt FG, et al. Leukocyte recruitment and expression of chemokines following different forms of vascular injury. *Vasc Med.* 2003;8:1–7.

91. Indolfi C, et al. Molecular mechanisms of in-stent restenosis and approach to therapy with eluting stents. *Trends Cardiovasc Med.* 2003;13:142–148.

92. Indolfi C, et al. Activation of cAMP-PKA signaling in vivo inhibits smooth muscle cell proliferation induced by vascular injury. *Nat Med.* 1997;3:775–779.

93. Indolfi C, et al. Inhibition of cellular ras prevents smooth muscle cell proliferation after vascular injury in vivo. *Nat Med.* 1995;1:541–545.

94. Indolfi C, et al. In vivo gene transfer: prevention of neointima formation by inhibition of mitogen-activated protein kinase kinase. *Basic Res Cardiol.* 1997;92:378–384.

95. Schwartz RS, Henry TD. Pathophysiology of coronary artery restenosis. *Rev Cardiovasc Med.* 2002;3(suppl 5):S4–S9.

96. Grewe PH, Deneke T, Machraoui A, et al. Acute and chronic tissue response to coronary stent implantation: pathologic findings in human specimen. *J Am Coll Cardiol.* 2000;35:157–163.

97. Mintz GS, et al. Arterial remodeling after coronary angioplasty: a serial intravascular ultrasound study. *Circulation.* 1996;94:35–43.

98. Lansky AJ, et al. Remodeling after directional coronary atherectomy (with and without adjunct percutaneous transluminal coronary angioplasty): a serial angiographic and intravascular ultrasound analysis from the Optimal Atherectomy Restenosis Study. *J Am Coll Cardiol.* 1998;32:329–337.

99. Kimura T, Nobuyoshi M. Remodelling and restenosis: intravascular ultrasound studies. *Semin Interv Cardiol.* 1997;2:159–166.

100. Scott NA, et al. Identification of a potential role for the adventitia in vascular lesion formation after balloon overstretch injury of porcine coronary arteries. *Circulation.* 1996;93:2178–2187.

101. Wilcox JN, et al. The role of the adventitia in the arterial response to angioplasty: the effect of intravascular radiation. *Int J Radiat Oncol Biol Phys.* 1996;36:789–796.

102. Nakazawa G, et al. The pathology of neoatherosclerosis in human coronary implants bare-metal and drug-eluting stents. *J Am Coll Cardiol.* 2011;57:1314–1322,

103. Joner M, et al. Endothelial cell recovery between comparator polymer-based drug-eluting stents. *J Am Coll Cardiol.* 2008;52:333–342.

104. Nakazawa G, et al. Evaluation of polymer-based comparator drug-eluting stents using a rabbit model of iliac artery atherosclerosis. *Circ Cardiovasc Interv.* 2011;4:38–46.

105. Otsuka F, et al. The importance of the endothelium in atherothrombosis and coronary stenting. *Nat Rev Cardiol.* 2012;9:439–453.

106. Otsuka F, et al. Pathology of second-generation everolimus-eluting stents versus first-generation sirolimus- and paclitaxel-eluting stents in humans. *Circulation.* 2014;129:211–223.

107. Nakazawa G, , et al. Pathophysiology of vascular healing and stent mediated arterial injury. *EuroIntervention.* 2008;4(suppl C):C7–C10.

108. Otsuka F, et al. Contribution of in-stent neoatherosclerosis to late stent failure following bare metal and 1st- and 2nd-generation drug-eluting stent placement: an autopsy study. *J Am Coll Cardiol.* 2014;64:B190–B191.

109. Fitzgerald PJ, et al. Final results of the Can Routine Ultrasound Influence Stent Expansion (CRUISE) study. *Circulation.* 2000;102:523–530.

110. Bittl JA, et al. Meta-analysis of randomized trials of percutaneous transluminal coronary angioplasty versus atherectomy, cutting balloon atherotomy, or laser angioplasty. *J Am Coll Cardiol.* 2004;43:936–942.

111. Martinez-Elbal L, et al. Direct coronary stenting versus stenting with balloon pre-dilation: immediate and follow-up results of a multicentre, prospective, randomized study. The DISCO trial. DIrect Stenting of COronary Arteries. *Eur Heart J.* 2002;23:633–640.

112. Leon MB, et al. A clinical trial comparing three antithrombotic-drug regimens after coronary-artery stenting. Stent Anticoagulation Restenosis Study Investigators. *N Engl J Med.* 1998;339:1665–1671.

113. Schwartz L, et al. Aspirin and dipyridamole in the prevention of restenosis after percutaneous transluminal coronary angioplasty. *N Engl J Med.* 1988;318:1714–1719.

114. Rensing BJ, et al. Luminal narrowing after percutaneous transluminal coronary angioplasty. A study of clinical, procedural, and lesional factors related to long-term angiographic outcome. Coronary Artery Restenosis Prevention on Repeated Thromboxane Antagonism (CARPORT) Study Group. *Circulation.* 1993;88:975–985.

115. Savage MP, et al. Effect of thromboxane A2 blockade on clinical outcome and restenosis after successful coronary angioplasty. Multi-Hospital Eastern Atlantic Restenosis Trial (M-HEART II). *Circulation.* 1995;92:3194–3200.

116. Welt FG, Rogers C. Inflammation and restenosis in the stent era. *Arterioscler Thromb Vasc Biol.* 2002;22:1769–1776.

117. Blindt R, et al. Abciximab inhibits the migration and invasion potential of human coronary artery smooth muscle cells. *J Mol Cell Cardiol.* 2000;32:2195–2206.

118. Liu Y, et al. Cilostazol (pletal): a dual inhibitor of cyclic nucleotide phosphodiesterase type 3 and adenosine uptake. *Cardiovasc Drug Rev.* 2001;19:369–386.

119. Tsutsui M, et al. Effect of cilostazol, a novel anti-platelet drug, on restenosis after percutaneous transluminal coronary angioplasty. *Jpn Circ J.* 1996;60:207–215.

120. Douglas JS Jr, et al. Coronary stent restenosis in patients treated with cilostazol. *Circulation.* 2005;112:2826–2832.

121. Tamhane U, et al. Efficacy of cilostazol in reducing restenosis in patients undergoing contemporary stent based PCI: a meta-analysis of randomised controlled trials. *EuroIntervention.* 2009;5:384–393.

122. Brack MJ, et al. The Subcutaneous Heparin and Angioplasty Restenosis Prevention (SHARP) trial. Results of a multicenter randomized trial investigating the effects of high dose unfractionated heparin on angiographic restenosis and clinical outcome. *J Am Coll Cardiol.* 1995;26:947–954.

123. Grassman ED, et al. A randomized trial of the low-molecular-weight heparin certoparin to prevent restenosis following coronary angioplasty. *J Invasive Cardiol.* 2001;13:723–728.

124. Dangas G, Iakovou I. The end of systemic anticoagulation therapy for restenosis prevention. *J Invasive Cardiol.* 2001;13:729–731.

125. Sarembock IJ, et al. Effectiveness of recombinant desulphatohirudin in reducing restenosis after balloon angioplasty of atherosclerotic femoral arteries in rabbits. *Circulation.* 1991;84:232–243.

126. Serruys PW, et al. A comparison of hirudin with heparin in the prevention of restenosis after coronary angioplasty. Helvetica Investigators. *N Engl J Med.* 1995;333:757–763.

127. Burchenal JE, et al. Effect of direct thrombin inhibition with Bivalirudin (Hirulog) on restenosis after coronary angioplasty. *Am J Cardiol.* 1998;82:511–515.

128. Pepine CJ, et al. A controlled trial of corticosteroids to prevent restenosis after coronary angioplasty. M-HEART Group. *Circulation.* 1990;81:1753–1761.

129. Freed M, et al. Combination of lovastatin, enalapril, and colchicine does not prevent restenosis after percutaneous transluminal coronary angioplasty. *Am J Cardiol.* 1995;76:1185–1188.

130. Schonbeck U, et al. Augmented expression of cyclooxygenase-2 in human atherosclerotic lesions. *Am J Pathol.* 1999;155:1281–1291.

131. Whitworth HB, et al. Effect of nifedipine on recurrent stenosis after percutaneous transluminal coronary angioplasty. *J Am Coll Cardiol.* 1986;8:1271–1276.

132. Hoberg E, Kubler W. Calcium-antagonists in preventing restenosis following coronary angioplasty. *Cardiologia.* 1991;36:225–227.

133. O'Keefe JH Jr, et al. Effects of diltiazem on complications and restenosis after coronary angioplasty. *Am J Cardiol.* 1991;67:373–376.

134. Hillegass WB, et al. A meta-analysis of randomized trials of calcium antagonists to reduce restenosis after coronary angioplasty. *Am J Cardiol.* 1994;73:835–839.

135. Jorgensen E, et al. Predictors of coronary in-stent restenosis: importance of angiotensin-converting enzyme gene polymorphism and treatment with angiotensin-converting enzyme inhibitors. *J Am Coll Cardiol.* 2001;38:1434–1439.

136. Suzuki T, et al. Stent-based delivery of sirolimus reduces neointimal formation in a porcine coronary model. *Circulation.* 2001;104:1188–1193.

137. Farb A, et al. Pathological analysis of local delivery of paclitaxel via a polymer-coated stent. *Circulation.* 2001;104:473–479.

138. Park SJ, et al. A paclitaxel-eluting stent for the prevention of coronary restenosis. *N Engl J Med.* 2003;348:1537–1545.

139. Sousa JE, et al. Lack of neointimal proliferation after implantation of sirolimus-coated stents in human coronary arteries: a quantitative coronary angiography and three-dimensional intravascular ultrasound study. *Circulation.* 2001;103:192–195.

140. Serruys PW, et al. The effect of variable dose and release kinetics on neointimal hyperplasia using a novel paclitaxel-eluting stent platform: the Paclitaxel In-Stent Controlled Elution Study (PISCES). *J Am Coll Cardiol.* 2005;46:253–260.

141. Tanner FC, et al. Expression of cyclin-dependent kinase inhibitors in vascular disease. *Circ Res.* 1998;82:396–403.

142. Poon M, et al. Rapamycin inhibits vascular smooth muscle cell migration. *J Clin Invest.* 1996;98:2277–2283.

143. Moses JW, et al. Sirolimus-eluting stents versus standard stents in patients with stenosis in a native coronary artery. *N Engl J Med.* 2003;349:1315–1323.

144. Popma JJ, et al. Quantitative assessment of angiographic restenosis after sirolimus-eluting stent implantation in native coronary arteries. *Circulation.* 2004;110:3773–3780.

145. Colombo A, et al. Randomized study to assess the effectiveness of slow- and moderate-release polymer-based paclitaxel-eluting stents for coronary artery lesions. *Circulation.* 2003;108:788–794.

146. Halkin A, Stone GW. Polymer-based paclitaxel-eluting stents in percutaneous coronary intervention: a review of the TAXUS trials. *J Interv Cardiol.* 2004;17:271–282.

147. Stone GW, et al. One-year clinical results with the slow-release, polymer-based, paclitaxel-eluting TAXUS stent: the TAXUS-IV trial. *Circulation.* 2004;109:1942–1947.

148. Stone GW, et al. A polymer-based, paclitaxel-eluting stent in patients with coronary artery disease. *N Engl J Med.* 2004;350:221–231.

149. Morice MC, et al. Sirolimus- vs paclitaxel-eluting stents in de novo coronary artery lesions: the REALITY trial: a randomized controlled trial. *JAMA.* 2006;295:895–904.

150. Windecker S, et al. Sirolimus-eluting and paclitaxel-eluting stents for coronary revascularization. *N Engl J Med.* 2005;353:653–662.

151. Ohlmann P, et al. Intravascular ultrasound findings in patients with restenosis of sirolimus- and paclitaxel-eluting stents. *Int J Cardiol.* 2008;125:11–15.

152. Raber L, Serruys PW. Late vascular response following drug-eluting stent implantation. *JACC Cardiovasc Interv.* 2011;4:1075–1078.

153. Smits PC, et al. 2-year follow-up of a randomized controlled trial of everolimus- and paclitaxel-eluting stents for coronary revascularization in daily practice. COMPARE (Comparison of the everolimus eluting XIENCE-V stent with the paclitaxel eluting TAXUS LIBERTE stent in all-comers: a randomized open label trial). *J Am Coll Cardiol.* 2011;58:11–18.

154. Park KW, et al. Everolimus-eluting versus sirolimus-eluting stents in patients undergoing percutaneous coronary intervention: the EXCELLENT (Efficacy of Xience/Promus Versus Cypher to Reduce Late Loss After Stenting) randomized trial. *J Am Coll Cardiol.* 2011;58:1844–1854.

155. Chen YW, et al. Zotarolimus, a novel sirolimus analogue with potent anti-proliferative activity on coronary smooth muscle cells and reduced potential for systemic immunosuppression. *J Cardiovasc Pharmacol.* 2007;49:228–235.

156. Leon MB, et al. A randomized comparison of the Endeavor zotarolimus-eluting stent versus the TAXUS paclitaxel-eluting stent in de novo native coronary lesions 12-month outcomes from the ENDEAVOR IV trial. *J Am Coll Cardiol.* 2010;55:543–554.

157. Serruys PW, et al. Comparison of zotarolimus-eluting and everolimus-eluting coronary stents. *N Engl J Med*. 2010;363:136–146.

158. von Birgelen C, et al. A randomized controlled trial in second-generation zotarolimus-eluting Resolute stents versus everolimus-eluting Xience V stents in real-world patients: the TWENTE trial. *J Am Coll Cardiol*. 2012;59:1350–1361.

159. Maeng M, et al. Differential clinical outcomes after 1 year versus 5 years in a randomised comparison of zotarolimus-eluting and sirolimus-eluting coronary stents (the SORT OUT III study): a multicentre, open-label, randomised superiority trial. *Lancet*. 2014;383:2047–2056.

160. Rittger H, et al. A randomized, multicenter, single-blinded trial comparing paclitaxel-coated balloon angioplasty with plain balloon angioplasty in drug-eluting stent restenosis: the PEPCAD-DES Study. *J Am Coll Cardiol*. 2012;59(15):1377–1382.

161. Kastrati A, et al. Sirolimus-eluting stent or paclitaxel-eluting stent vs balloon angioplasty for prevention of recurrences in patients with coronary in-stent restenosis: a randomized controlled trial. *JAMA*. 2005;293:165–171.

162. Raizner AE, et al. Inhibition of restenosis with beta-emitting radiotherapy: report of the Proliferation Reduction with Vascular Energy Trial (PREVENT). *Circulation*. 2000;102:951–958.

163. Sabate M, et al. Intracoronary brachytherapy after stenting de novo lesions in diabetic patients: results of a randomized intravascular ultrasound study. *J Am Coll Cardiol*. 2004;44:520–527.

164. Coen V, et al. Reno, a European postmarket surveillance registry, confirms effectiveness of coronary brachytherapy in routine clinical practice. *Int J Radiat Oncol Biol Phys*. 2003;55:1019–1026.

165. Baumgart D, et al. Successful reduction of in-stent restenosis in long lesions using beta-radiation—subanalysis from the RENO registry. *Int J Radiat Oncol Biol Phys*. 2004;58:817–827.

166. Amols HI, et al. Dosimetric considerations for catheter-based beta and gamma emitters in the therapy of neointimal hyperplasia in human coronary arteries. *Int J Radiat Oncol Biol Phys*. 1996;36:913–921.

167. Sabate M, et al. Methodological and clinical implications of the relocation of the minimal luminal diameter after intracoronary radiation therapy. Dose Finding Study Group. *J Am Coll Cardiol*. 2000;36:1536–1541.

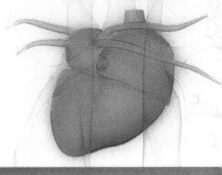

3

Platelet—Inhibitor Agents

José Luis Ferreiro, MD, PhD and Francesco Franchi, MD

The rupture or erosion of an atheromatous plaque and subsequent thrombus formation can lead to an acute coronary syndrome (ACS). The rupture of an atherosclerotic plaque may also be iatrogenic, as occurs in the setting of percutaneous coronary interventions (PCI). The exposure of subendothelial collagen after a plaque rupture or erosion allows platelet adhesion, activation, and aggregation at the site of vessel injury. In addition, exposure of tissue factor triggers the extrinsic pathway of the coagulation cascade (1,2). This is a dynamic process that results in thrombus formation (Fig. 3.1). Advances in the understanding of these complex mechanisms have been pivotal for the development of safer and more efficacious antithrombotic and antiplatelet therapies (1). This chapter is aimed to review currently available antiplatelet therapies in the setting of PCI.

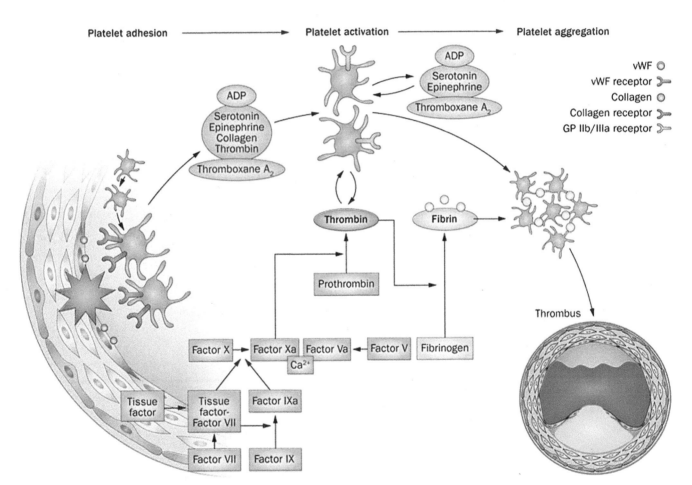

FIGURE 3.1 Platelet-mediated thrombosis. Plaque rupture exposes subendothelial components. Platelet adhesion during the rolling phase is mediated by interactions between vWF and GP Ib/V/IX receptor complexes located on the platelet surface, and between platelet collagen receptors (GP VI and GP Ia) and collagen exposed at the site of vascular injury. Binding of collagen to GP VI induces the release of activating factors (ADP, thromboxane A₂, serotonin, epinephrine, and thrombin), which promote interactions between adherent platelets, as well as further recruitment and activation of circulating platelets. Platelet activation leads to changes in platelet shape, expression of proinflammatory molecules, platelet procoagulant activity, and activation of platelet integrin GP IIb/IIIa. Activated GP IIb/IIIa binds to the extracellular ligands fibrinogen and vWF, leading to platelet aggregation and thrombus formation. Vascular injury also exposes subendothelial tissue factor, which forms a complex with factor VIIa and sets off a chain of events that culminates in formation of the prothrombinase complex. Prothrombin is converted to thrombin, which subsequently converts fibrinogen to fibrin, generating a fibrin-rich clot, and further activates platelets through binding to PAR-1 and PAR-4 receptors. ADP, adenosine diphosphate; GP, glycoprotein; PAR, protease-activated receptor; vWF, von Willebrand factor. (Adapted with permission from: Franchi F, et al. Novel antiplatelet agents in acute coronary syndrome. *Nat Rev Cardiol.* 2015;12:30–47).

Antiplatelet Therapy

Currently, there are three families of antiplatelet agents for the treatment and prevention of recurrent events in patients undergoing PCI (1). These include cyclooxygenase-1 (COX-1) inhibitors, adenosine diphosphate (ADP) P2Y$_{12}$ receptor inhibitors, and glycoprotein (GP) IIb/IIIa inhibitors. Other agents with antiplatelet properties are available, such as vorapaxar, cilostazol, dipyridamole, or pentoxifylline. Vorapaxar is a protease-activated receptor-1 antagonist indicated in secondary prevention for the reduction of thrombotic cardiovascular events as an adjunct to aspirin and/or clopidogrel in patients with a history of myocardial infarction or with peripheral arterial disease. The other mentioned agents do not have a clinical indication for prevention of recurrent ischemic events in coronary artery disease (CAD) patients.

Aspirin

Mechanisms of Action

Aspirin is an irreversible inhibitor of COX activity of prostaglandin H (PGH) synthase 1 and synthase 2, also known as COX-1 and COX-2, respectively (3). These isoenzymes catalyze the conversion of arachidonic acid to PGH$_2$. The latter serves as a substrate for the generation of several prostanoids, including thromboxane A$_2$ (TXA$_2$) and prostacyclin (PGI$_2$). TXA$_2$, an amplifier of platelet activation and a vasoconstrictor, is mainly derived from platelet COX-1 and is highly sensitive to inhibition by aspirin.

Vascular PGI$_2$, a platelet inhibitor and a vasodilator, is derived largely from COX-2 and is less susceptible to inhibition by low doses of aspirin (Fig. 3.2). Only high doses of aspirin can inhibit COX-2, which has anti-inflammatory and analgesic effects, while low doses of aspirin are sufficient to inhibit COX-1 activity, leading to antiplatelet effects (3). Aspirin is rapidly absorbed in the upper gastrointestinal tract and leads to platelet inhibition within 60 minutes. The plasma half-life of aspirin is ~20 minutes; peak plasma levels of aspirin are achieved within 30 to 40 minutes. Enteric-coated aspirin delays absorption and increases plasma levels, which require ~3 to 4 hours. Because aspirin induces an irreversible COX-1 blockade, COX-mediated TXA$_2$ synthesis is prevented for the entire life span of the platelet (~7–10 days) (3).

Indications

Aspirin is the mainstay of antiplatelet therapy for secondary prevention of recurrent ischemic events (3). In high-risk patients, particularly those with ACS and undergoing PCI, aspirin should be given as promptly as possible (4–6). Patients already taking daily aspirin therapy should take 81 to 325 mg prior to PCI, while patients not on aspirin

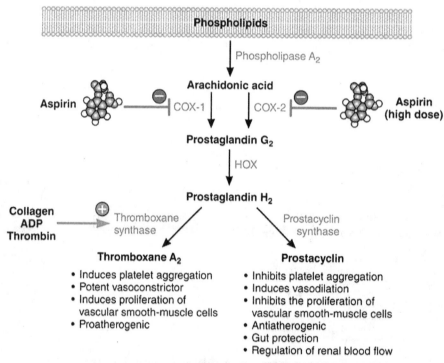

FIGURE 3.2 Mechanism of action of aspirin. Aspirin acts by irreversibly blocking the COX activity of the prostaglandin H synthases 1 and 2, also known as COX-1 and COX-2, respectively. This effect is achieved by acetylating a serine residue (serine 529 in COX-1 and serine 516 in COX-2), which prevents arachidonic acid from reaching the COX catalytic site of the enzyme. This causes the upstream block of prostanoid biosynthesis and, ultimately, inhibition of TXA$_2$ and prostacyclin generation. Mature platelets express only COX-1, whereas vascular endothelial cells express both COX-1 and COX-2 and represent the main site of prostacyclin generation. Low-dose aspirin selectively inhibits COX-1 activity, whereas higher doses inhibit both COX-1 and COX-2. ADP, adenosine diphosphate; COX, cyclooxygenase; HOX, hydroperoxidase; TXA$_2$, thromboxane A$_2$. (Reproduced with permission from: Capodanno D, Angiolillo DJ. Aspirin for primary cardiovascular risk prevention and beyond in diabetes mellitus. *Circulation.* 2016;134:1579–1594.)

therapy should be given 325 mg non-enteric coated aspirin prior to PCI (Class I recommendation, level of evidence: B) (5). Aspirin should be continued indefinitely after PCI (Class I recommendation, level of evidence: B). Nevertheless, the optimal maintenance dose of aspirin for prevention of cardiovascular events has been a subject of controversy. Registry data have shown oral aspirin doses of 75 to 150 mg/day to be as effective as higher doses for long-term prevention of ischemic events (3,7). Importantly, higher doses of aspirin (>150 mg) do not offer greater protection from recurrent ischemic events, whereas bleeding events, in particular gastrointestinal bleeding, are significantly increased (3,7). Such registry data are in line with randomized clinical trial findings (8). Based on these observations, the PCI guidelines state that it is reasonable to consider 81 mg/day in preference to higher maintenance doses as a maintenance regimen (Class IIa recommendation, level of evidence: B) (5).

Side Effects

The side effects of aspirin are primarily gastrointestinal and are dose-related. Using low doses (75–162 mg/day) reduces these side effects (3). Aspirin use can lead to gastric erosions, hemorrhage, and ulcers that can contribute to anemia. Other interactions and side effects related to aspirin include those due to concomitant treatment with some nonsteroidal anti-inflammatory drugs (NSAIDs), such as naproxen and ibuprofen (3). These drugs in fact compete for the COX-1 active site and thus can interfere with the action of aspirin when administered concomitantly, resulting in attenuation of its antiplatelet effects (3).

This may contribute to a reduction in the cardioprotective effects of aspirin. Finally, three types of aspirin sensitivity have been described: respiratory sensitivity (asthma and/or rhinitis), cutaneous sensitivity (urticaria and/or angioedema), and systemic sensitivity (anaphylactoid reaction) (9). Desensitization using escalating doses of oral aspirin can be considered in these patients (9).

P2Y₁₂ Inhibitors

ADP is one of the main platelet-activating factors and is mediated by the $P2Y_1$ and $P2Y_{12}$ receptors (1,10). The $P2Y_1$ and $P2Y_{12}$ are G-coupled receptors and are required for platelet aggregation. ADP-stimulated effects are mediated mainly by $P2Y_{12}$ receptor activation, however, which leads to sustained platelet aggregation and stabilization of the platelet aggregate. Inhibition of the $P2Y_{12}$ signaling pathway is critical, particularly in the setting of PCI, as emerged from seminal studies with ticlopidine, a first-generation thienopyridine. In fact, the combination of aspirin and ticlopidine showed association with better outcomes—in particular, the prevention of thrombotic complications—compared to aspirin monotherapy or aspirin plus warfarin in patients undergoing coronary stenting (11).

Ticlopidine has two major disadvantages: (a) it has a limited safety profile with the nondepreciable rates of agranulocytosis, rash, and gastrointestinal effects; (b) it achieves antiplatelet effects slowly, given that the drug cannot be given under a loading dose because of risk of toxicity. Other oral and intravenous $P2Y_{12}$ receptor inhibitors with more favorable safety and/or efficacy profiles have been developed and are available for clinical use (Table 3.1).

Clopidogrel, a second-generation thienopyridine, has shown to have a more favorable safety profile than that of ticlopidine. Because of this, thienopyridine has become the drug of choice in the setting of PCI in patients with stable CAD (12). Clopidogrel has been evaluated in a large number of clinical investigations over the past decade, supporting its role in the setting of ACS and PCI (13) (Table 3.2). Clopidogrel has limitations, however; the most important of which is its broad range in interindividual antiplatelet drug effects (14). In particular, a considerable number of patients persist with high platelet reactivity despite clopidogrel therapy, exposing them to an increased risk of recurrent ischemic events, including stent thrombosis (ST) (14). This has set the basis for the development of newer generation oral $P2Y_{12}$ receptor inhibitors. These include prasugrel, a third-generation thienopyridine, and ticagrelor, a first-in-class cyclopentyltriazolopyrimidine (CPTP), which has already been approved for clinical use (13). In addition, cangrelor, an adenosine triphosphate (ATP) analog, is the first intravenous $P2Y_{12}$ antagonist available, which has been recently approved by the Food and Drug Administration (FDA) for use in patients with CAD undergoing PCI (15) (Tables 3.1 and 3.3).

A large number of studies associating results of platelet function and genetic phenotype testing with adverse outcomes, particularly in the setting of PCI, initially led guidelines to implement recommendations

TABLE 3.1 Pharmacologic Properties of Currently Approved P2Y₁₂ Receptor Inhibitors

	CLOPIDOGREL	PRASUGREL	TICAGRELOR	CANGRELOR
Group	Thienopyridine	Thienopyridine	CPTP	ATP analog
Receptor blockade	Irreversible	Irreversible	Reversible	Reversible
Adminutesistration	Oral	Oral	Oral	IV
Dosage	Once daily	Once daily	Twice daily	Bolus plus infusion
Prodrug	Yes	Yes	No[a]	No
Onset of action[b]	2–8 hours	30 minutes–4 hours[b]	30 minutes–4 hours[b]	2 minutes
Offset of action	7–10 days	7–10 days	3–5 days	~60 minutes
Approved settings	Stable CAD, ACS, PCI	ACS undergoing PCI	ACS (full spectrum)	P2Y₁₂ receptor inhibitors-naïve patients undergoing PCI

[a]Although ticagrelor is direct-acting, approximately 30% to 40% of its antiplatelet effects are attributed to an active metabolite (AR-C124910XX).
[b]Depending on clinical setting (for oral agents).
ACS, acute coronary syndrome; ATP, adenosine triphosphate; CAD, coronary artery disease; CPTP, cyclopentyltriazolopyrimidine; IV, intravenous; PCI, percutaneous coronary intervention.

TABLE 3.2 Large-Scale Randomized Clinical Trials Evaluating the Efficacy of Dual Antiplatelet Therapy with Aspirin and Clopidogrel in ACS/PCI Patients

TRIAL	PATIENTS (N)	SETTING	TREATMENT ARMS[a]	PRIMARY ENDPOINT	RESULTS[b]
CURE	12,562	UA/NSTE-ACS	Aspirin + clopidogrel vs. aspirin	CV death, non-fatal MI or stroke at 1 year	9.3% vs. 11.4% HR: 0.80 (0.72–0.90)
PCI-CURE	2,658	PCI patients from CURE	Aspirin + clopidogrel vs. aspirin	CV death, MI or revascularization within 30 days	4.5% vs. 6.4% RR: 0.70 (0.50–0.97)
CREDO	2,116	Elective PCI	Aspirin + clopidogrel vs. aspirin	CV death, MI, or stroke at 1 year	8.5% vs. 11.5% RRR: 26.9% (3.9%–44.4%)
COMMIT	45,852	Acute MI (93% STEMI)	Aspirin + clopidogrel vs. aspirin	Death, reinfarction, or stroke at 28 days	9.2% vs. 10.1% OR: 0.91 (0.86–0.97)
CLARITY	3,491	STEMI with fibrinolysis	Aspirin + clopidogrel vs. aspirin	Occluded infarct-related artery, death or recurrent MI before angiography	15.0% vs. 21.7% OR: 0.64 (0.53–0.76)
PCI-CLARITY	1,863	PCI patients from CLARITY	Aspirin + clopidogrel vs. aspirin	CV death, recurrent MI, or stroke at 30 days	3.6% vs. 6.2% OR: 0.54 (0.35–0.85)
CURRENT-OASIS 7	25,087	ACS patients referred invasive strategy	Aspirin + double-dose clopidogrel vs. aspirin + standard-dose clopidogrel	CV death, MI, or stroke at 30 days	4.2% vs. 4.4% HR: 0.94 (0.83–1.06)
CURRENT-OASIS 7 (PCI cohort)	17,263	PCI patients from CURRENT-OASIS 7	Aspirin + double-dose clopidogrel vs. aspirin + standard-dose clopidogrel	CV death, MI, or stroke at 30 days	3.9% vs. 4.5% HR: 0.86 (0.74–0.99)

[a]Clopidogrel was given as a 300-mg loading dose and then 75 mg daily in CURE, PCI-CURE, CREDO, COMMIT, and CLARITY. In CURRENT-OASIS 7, double-dose clopidogrel was defined as a 600-mg loading dose and 150 mg once daily for 7 days, followed by 75 mg once daily; standard-dose clopidogrel was defined as a 300-mg loading dose, followed by 75 mg once daily. Patients were also randomized to receive low-dose (75–100 mg/day) or high-dose (300–325 mg/day) aspirin.
[b]Results are expressed as % of events and association measure (95% confidence interval).
ACS, acute coronary syndrome; CV, cardiovascular; HR, hazard ratio; MI, myocardial infarction; NSTE-ACS, non-ST-segment elevation acute coronary syndrome; OR, odds ratio; PCI, percutaneous coronary intervention; RR, relative risk; RRR, relative risk reduction; STEMI, ST-segment elevation myocardial infarction; UA, unstable angina; CURE, Clopidogrel in Unstable Angina to Prevent Recurrent Events trial; CREDO, Clopidogrel for the Reduction of Events During Observation trial; COMMIT, Clopidogrel and Metoprolol in Myocardial Infarction trial; CLARITY, Clopidogrel as Adjunctive Reperfusion Therapy trial; CURRENT-OASIS-7, Clopidogrel Optimal Loading Dose Usage to Reduce Recurrent Events/Optimal Antiplatelet Strategy for Intervention Trial.

for the use of these tests as a tool to tailor antiplatelet therapy (4,5). Nevertheless, the findings of large-scale clinical trials have, to date, failed to show a benefit in reducing ischemic complications of a strategy of adjusting antiplatelet therapy based on the results of these assays and, therefore, their routine use is not recommended (16).

Mechanisms of Action

Thienopyridines (ticlopidine, clopidogrel, and prasugrel) are oral prodrugs, and thus need to be metabolized by the hepatic cytochrome P450 (CYP) system to give rise to an active metabolite that irreversibly inhibits the $P2Y_{12}$ receptor (**Fig. 3.3**) (13,14). Clopidogrel is a second-generation thienopyridine, which requires a two-step oxidation by the CYP system to generate an active metabolite (13,14). However, ~85% of the prodrug is hydrolyzed by prehepatic esterases to an inactive carboxylic acid derivative, and only ~15% of the prodrug is metabolized by the CYP system into an active metabolite. Multiple CYP enzymes are involved in this process. Among these, CYP2C19 is pivotal because it is involved in both metabolic steps of clopidogrel. This explains why genetic variants associated with reduced metabolic activity of the CYP2C19 enzyme or drugs interfering with its activity, such as certain proton pump inhibitors (PPIs), can reduce the antiplatelet effects of clopidogrel. Prasugrel

is a third-generation thienopyridine, which has a more efficient metabolism than does clopidogrel (17,18). After oral ingestion, the prodrug is exposed to hydrolysis by carboxyesterases, mainly in the intestine, giving rise to an intermediate thiolactone, which then requires only a single-step hepatic metabolism (Fig. 3.3). In turn, the active metabolite is generated more rapidly and effectively (17,18). This more favorable pharmacokinetic profile translates into better pharmacodynamic effects, showing more potent platelet inhibition, lower interindividual variability, and a faster onset of antiplatelet activity than with clopidogrel, even when the latter is used at a high dose ($\geq$600 mg) (17,18). A 60-mg loading dose of prasugrel achieves 50% platelet inhibition by 30 minutes and 80% to 90% inhibition by 1 to 2 hours (17,18). Although clopidogrel and prasugrel active metabolites have a half-life of only ~8 hours, they have an irreversible effect on platelets, which lasts for their life span (7–10 days) (13).

Ticagrelor is the first nonthienopyridine forming part of a new class of $P2Y_{12}$ inhibitors called CPTP approved for clinical use (17,19). Ticagrelor is orally administered and direct-acting, with reversible binding to the $P2Y_{12}$ receptor (Fig. 3.3) (17,19). Although ticagrelor has direct-acting effects (no metabolism required), ~30% to 40% of its effects are attributed to a metabolite generated by the CYP system, in particular by the CYP3A4 isoenzyme. Ticagrelor is

TABLE 3.3 Large-Scale Randomized Clinical Trials Evaluating the Efficacy of Dual Antiplatelet Therapy with Aspirin and New Generation P2Y$_{12}$ Receptor Inhibitors in ACS/PCI Patients

TRIAL	PATIENTS (N)	SETTING	TREATMENT ARMS	PRIMARY ENDPOINT	RESULTS[a]
TRITON-TIMI 38	13,608	ACS patients undergoing PCI	Aspirin + prasugrel vs. aspirin + clopidogrel	CV death, non-fatal MI or non-fatal stroke up to 15 months	9.9% vs. 12.1% HR: 0.81 (0.73–0.90)
ACCOAST	4,033	NSTEMI scheduled for angiography	Pretreatment with prasugrel 30 mg vs. placebo	CV death, MI, stroke, GPI bailout or urgent revascularization at 7 days	10.0% vs. 9.8% HR: 1.02 (0.84–1.25)
PLATO	18,624	ACS	Aspirin + ticagrelor vs. aspirin + clopidogrel	Death from vascular causes, MI or stroke at 12 months	9.8% vs. 11.7% HR: 0.84 (0.77–0.92)
PLATO invasive cohort	13,408	ACS with planned invasive strategy	Aspirin + ticagrelor vs. aspirin + clopidogrel	Death from vascular causes, MI or stroke at 12 months	9.0% vs. 10.7% HR: 0.84 (0.75–0.94)
CHAMPION PHOENIX	11,145	Stable angina or ACS undergoing PCI	Aspirin + cangrelor[c] vs. aspirin + clopidogrel	Death from any cause, MI, IDR, and stent thrombosis at 48 hours	4.7% vs. 5.9% OR: 0.78 (0.66–0.93)
CHAMPION pooled analysis[b]	24,910	Patients undergoing PCI	Aspirin + cangrelor[d] vs. aspirin + clopidogrel	Death from any cause, MI, IDR, and stent thrombosis at 48 hours	3.8% vs. 4.7% OR: 0.81 (0.71–0.91)

[a]Results are expressed as % of events and association measure (95% confidence interval).
[b]Pooled analysis of patient-level data from three CHAMPION trials (CHAMPION-PCI, CHAMPION-PLATFORM, and CHAMPION-PHOENIX) using the PHOENIX definition of MI.
[c]In CHAMPION PHOENIX, patients received 600 mg of clopidogrel at the end of cangrelor infusion; patients in the control arm received 300 or 600 mg of clopidogrel at the time of PCI (before or immediately after PCI, at the discretion of the site investigator).
[d]In CHAMPION PCI, clopidogrel loading dose (600 mg) was administered within 30 minutes before the procedure, whereas in CHAMPION PLATFORM clopidogrel (600 mg) was administered at the end of PCI. In both trials, patients randomized to cangrelor received their loading dose of clopidogrel (600 mg) after stopping cangrelor infusion in order to avoid any possible interaction.
ACS, acute coronary syndrome; CV, cardiovascular; GPI, glycoprotein IIb/IIIa inhibitor; HR, hazard ratio; IDR, ischemia-driven revascularization; MI, myocardial infarction; NSTE, non-ST-elevation; OR, odds ration; PCI, percutaneous coronary intervention. TRITON, Trial to Assess Improvement in Therapeutic Outcomes by Optimizing Platelet Inhibition with Prasugrel; ACCOAST, A Comparison of Prasugrel at PCI or Time of Diagnosis of Non-ST Elevation Myocardial Infarction; PLATO, Platelet Inhibition and Outcomes; CHAMPION, Cangrelor versus standard tHerapy to Achieve optimal Management of Platelet InhibitiON.

rapidly absorbed and exerts its effects on P2Y$_{12}$-mediated signaling, acting as a noncompetitive ADP antagonist and inhibiting platelet inhibition via allosteric modulation of the receptor. Also, ticagrelor has shown faster, more potent, and less variable platelet inhibition than clopidogrel. A 180-mg loading dose of ticagrelor achieves 80% to 90% platelet inhibition in 1 to 2 hours (17,19). Ticagrelor has a half-life of 7 to 12 hours, requiring twice-daily dosing. Although the slope of offset of ticagrelor effects is rapid, ~5 days are needed after ticagrelor withdrawal to return to baseline platelet function because of the profound platelet inhibition during treatment (17,19).

Cangrelor is the first developed intravenous P2Y$_{12}$ antagonist available for clinical use. After being modified from ATP, the final molecule of cangrelor (2-trifluoropropylthio, N-[2-(methylthio) ethyl]-b, g-dichloromethylene ATP) has great affinity for the P2Y$_{12}$ receptor, being directly active after infusion (no metabolic activation into an active metabolite required). In brief, cangrelor has an almost immediate onset of action, reaching steady-state concentrations within a few minutes, and a dose-dependent and very potent effect, achieving a very high degree of platelet inhibition (>90% of the P2Y$_{12}$ signaling pathway). In addition, this compound has a fast offset of action, due to its extremely short half-life (3–5 minutes) caused by a rapid deactivation by plasmatic ectonucleotidases, which allows platelet functions to return to the baseline within 60 to 90 minutes after stopping the infusion (15,20). The recommended dose of cangrelor is a 30 μg/kg bolus, followed by a 4 μg/kg/min infusion for at least 2 hours or the duration of the procedure, whichever is longer (the infusion may be continued for up to 4 hours).

Indications

Adding P2Y$_{12}$ receptor inhibitors to aspirin has shown to be particularly beneficial in the settings of PCI and across the spectrum of ACS manifestations (Tables 3.2 and 3.3) (13). Pivotal issues surrounding the optimal use of P2Y$_{12}$-receptor-inhibiting therapy in patients undergoing PCI include timing of treatment, dosing, and duration of therapy.

Although the optimal timing of the administration of P2Y$_{12}$ antagonists is currently a matter of discussion, a loading dose of a P2Y$_{12}$ receptor inhibitor should be given in patients undergoing PCI with stenting (Class I recommendation; level of evidence: A) (4,6). Of note, treatment with prasugrel is not recommended for "upfront" therapy in patients with non-ST-elevation ACS (6). An important trade-off of starting therapy prior to knowing coronary anatomy is that patients will need to suspend therapy (at least 5–7 days for clopidogrel, 7 days for prasugrel, and 5 days for ticagrelor) if surgical revascularization is needed in order to minimize the risk of bleeding complications (4,6). Guidelines outlining the recommended loading and maintenance dosing regimens of P2Y$_{12}$ inhibitors in patients with and without ACS who are undergoing PCI treated with drug-eluting stents (DESs) or bare-metal stents (BMSs) are summarized in **Table 3.4**. This table also summarizes the optimal duration of dual oral antiplatelet therapy according to the clinical setting (ACS vs. non-ACS) and stent type used (DES vs. BMS). Cangrelor has received FDA approval as an adjunct to PCI for reducing the risk of periprocedural myocardial infarction, repeat coronary revascularization, and ST in patients who have not been treated with a P2Y$_{12}$ platelet inhibitor and are not being given a GP IIb/IIIa.

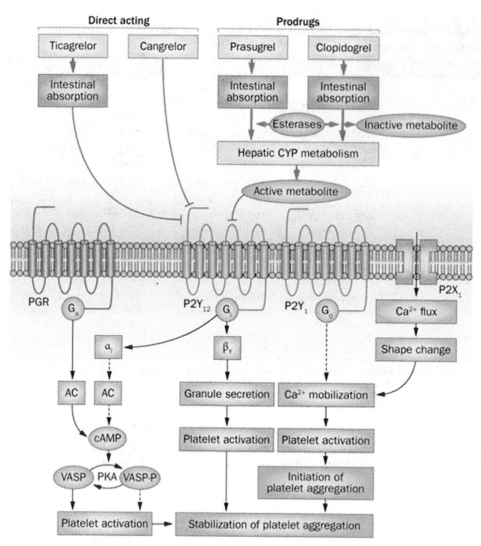

FIGURE 3.3   Mechanisms of action of P2Y$_{12}$ inhibiting agents. Clopidogrel is an oral prodrug and, after intestinal absorption, approximately 85% of clopidogrel is hydrolyzed by carboxylase to an inactive metabolite. The remaining approximately 15% is rapidly metabolized by hepatic cytochrome (CYP) P450 isoenzymes in a two-step oxidation process, with the generation of a highly unstable active metabolite. Prasugrel is also an oral prodrug with a similar intestinal absorption process. Nevertheless, in contrast to clopidogrel, prasugrel is oxidized more efficiently to its active metabolite via a single CYP-dependent step. Direct-acting antiplatelet agents (cangrelor and ticagrelor) have reversible effects and do not require hepatic metabolism for achieving pharmacodynamic activity. Ticagrelor is orally administered and, after intestinal absorption, directly inhibits platelet activation by allosteric modulation of the P2Y$_{12}$ receptor, binding to a site on the receptor distinct from the ADP-binding site. Cangrelor is intravenously administered, and directly inhibits the P2Y$_{12}$ receptor, bypassing intestinal absorption. Platelets express at least two purinergic G-protein-coupled receptors: P2Y$_1$ and P2Y$_{12}$. The activation of P2Y$_{12}$ inhibits AC, causing a decrease in the cAMP level, and the activation of P2Y$_1$ causes an increase in the intracellular Ca^{2+} level, leading to platelet aggregation through the change in the ligand-binding properties of the glycoprotein IIb/IIIa receptor. Clopidogrel, prasugrel, ticagrelor, and cangrelor bind to the P2Y$_{12}$ receptor and ultimately inhibit platelet activation and aggregation processes by modulating intra-platelet levels of cAMP and VASP-P. *Solid black arrows* indicate activation. *Dotted black arrows* indicate inhibition. AC, adenylyl cyclase; ADP, adenosine diphosphate; cAMP, cyclic adenosine monophosphate; CYP, cytochrome P450; PDE, phosphodiesterase; PKA. protein kinases A; VASP, vasodilator-stimulated phosphoprotein; VASP-P, phosphorylation of VASP. (Adapted with permission from: Angiolillo DJ, et al. Optimizing platelet inhibition in clopidogrel poor metabolizers: therapeutic options and practical considerations. *JACC Cardiovasc Interv.* 2011;4:411–414.)

TABLE 3.4 ACC/AHA Guidelines Recommendations for the Use of Oral and Intravenous Antiplatelet Therapy for Patients with Stable Ischemic Heart Disease, NSTE-ACS or STEMI undergoing PCI

RECOMMENDATIONS	CLASS AND LOE
NSTE-ACS	
Oral Therapy	
Non-enteric-coated aspirin (162–325 mg) should be given to all patients promptly after presentation.	I A
Patients not on aspirin therapy should be given non-enteric-coated aspirin 325 mg as soon as possible before PCI.	I B
After PCI, aspirin should be continued indefinitely at a dose of 81–325 mg daily.	I B
A loading dose of a P2Y$_{12}$ receptor inhibitor should be given before the procedure in patients undergoing PCI with stenting. Options include clopidogrel 600 mg (LOE: B), prasugrel 60 mg (LOE: B), ticagrelor 180 mg (LOE: B).	I A
In patients receiving a stent (BMS or DES) during PCI for NSTEACS, P2Y$_{12}$ inhibitor therapy should be given for at least 12 months. Options include clopidogrel 75 mg daily; prasugrel 10 mg daily; ticagrelor 90 mg twice a day.	I B
It is reasonable to choose ticagrelor over clopidogrel for P2Y$_{12}$ inhibition treatment in patients with NSTE-ACS treated with an early invasive strategy and/or coronary stenting.	IIa B
It is reasonable to choose prasugrel over clopidogrel for P2Y$_{12}$ treatment in patients with NSTEACS who undergo PCI who are not at high risk of bleeding complications.	IIa B
After PCI, it is reasonable to use 81 mg/d of aspirin in preference to higher maintenance doses.	IIa B
If the risk of morbidity from bleeding outweighs the anticipated benefit of a recommended duration of P2Y$_{12}$ inhibitor therapy after stent implantation, earlier discontinuation (e.g., <12 months) of P2Y$_{12}$ inhibitor therapy is reasonable.	IIa C
Continuation of DAPT beyond 12 months may be considered in patients undergoing stent implantation.	IIb C
Prasugrel should not be administered to patients with a prior history of stroke or transient ischemic attack.	III B
Intravenous Therapy	
In patients with high-risk features (e.g., elevated troponin) not adequately pretreated with clopidogrel or ticagrelor, it is useful to administer a GP IIb/IIa inhibitor (abciximab, double-bolus eptifibatide, or high-dose bolus tirofiban) at the time of PCI.	I A
In patients with high-risk features (e.g., elevated troponin) treated with UFH and adequately pretreated with clopidogrel, it is reasonable to administer a GP IIb/IIa inhibitor (abciximab, double-bolus eptifibatide, or high-dose bolus tirofiban) at the time of PCI.	IIa B
STEMI	
Oral Therapy	
Aspirin 162–325 mg should be given before primary PCI.	I B
After PCI, aspirin should be continued indefinitely.	I A
A loading dose of a P2Y$_{12}$ receptor inhibitor should be given as early as possible, or at the time of primary PCI, to patients with STEMI. Options include clopidogrel 600 mg, prasugrel 60 mg, and ticagrelor 180 mg.	I B
P2Y$_{12}$ inhibitor therapy should be given for 1 year to patients with STEMI who receive a stent (BMS or DES) during primary PCI, using the following maintenance doses: clopidogrel 75 mg daily, prasugrel 10 mg daily, ticagrelor 90 mg twice a day.	I B
It is reasonable to use 81 mg of aspirin per day in preference to higher maintenance doses after primary PCI.	IIa B
Continuation of a P2Y$_{12}$ inhibitor beyond 1 year may be considered in patients undergoing DES placement.	IIb C
Prasugrel should not be administered to patients with a prior history of stroke or transient ischemic attack.	III B
Intravenous Therapy	
It is reasonable to begin treatment with an intravenous GP IIb/IIIa receptor antagonist such as abciximab (LOE: A), high-bolus-dose tirofiban (LOE: B), or double-bolus eptifibatide (LOE: B) at the time of primary PCI (with or without stenting or clopidogrel pretreatment) in selected patients with STEMI who are receiving UFH.	IIa
It may be reasonable to administer an intravenous GP IIb/IIIa receptor antagonist in the precatheterization laboratory setting (e.g., ambulance, ED) to patients with STEMI for whom primary PCI is intended.	IIb B
It may be reasonable to administer intracoronary abciximab to patients with STEMI undergoing primary PCI.	IIb B

(continued)

TABLE 3.4 ACC/AHA Guidelines Recommendations for the Use of Oral and Intravenous Antiplatelet Therapy for Patients with Stable Ischemic Heart Disease, NSTE-ACS or STEMI undergoing PCI (*continued*)

RECOMMENDATIONS	CLASS AND LOE
Stable Ischemic Heart Disease	
Oral Therapy	
Patients already taking daily aspirin therapy should take 81–325 mg before PCI	I B
Patients not on aspirin therapy should be given non-enteric aspirin 325 mg before PCI.	I B
After PCI, use of aspirin should be continued indefinitely	I A
A loading dose of clopidogrel (600 mg) should be given to patients undergoing PCI with stenting	I B
In patients receiving DES for a non-ACS indication, clopidogrel 75 mg daily should be given for at least 12 months if patients are not at high risk of bleeding.	I B
In patients receiving BMS for a non-ACS indication, clopidogrel should be given for a minimum of 1 month, and ideally up to 12 months (unless the patient is at increased risk of bleeding; then it should be given for a minimum of 2 weeks).	I B
After PCI, it is reasonable to use aspirin 81 mg/d in preference to higher maintenance doses.	IIa B
Continuation of DAPT beyond 12 months may be considered in patients undergoing DES implantation	IIb C
Intravenous Therapy	
In patients undergoing elective PCI treated with UFH and not pretreated with clopidogrel, it is reasonable to administer a GP IIb/IIIa inhibitor (abciximab, double-bolus eptifibatide, or high-bolus dose tirofiban).	IIa B
In patients undergoing elective PCI with stent implantation treated with UFH and adequately pretreated with clopidogrel, it might be reasonable to administer a GP IIb/IIIa inhibitor (abciximab, double-bolus eptifibatide, or high-bolus dose tirofiban).	IIb B

ACC, American College of Cardiology; ACS, acute coronary syndrome; AHA, American Heart Association; BMS, bare-metal stent; DAPT, dual antiplatelet therapy; DES, drug-eluting stent; GP, glycoprotein; LOE, level of evidence; NSTE-ACS, non-ST-segment elevation acute coronary syndrome; PCI, percutaneous coronary intervention; STEMI, ST-elevation myocardial infarction; UFH, unfractionated heparin.

Side Effects

Bleeding complications remain the main concern in patients treated with P2Y$_{12}$ receptor inhibitors (13). Bleeding events are increased with dual antiplatelet therapy, rather than with aspirin alone. In clopidogrel-treated patients, the risk of bleeding is related to the dose of aspirin used, the risk being greater with higher doses of aspirin (21). Other rare complications of thienopyridine use include neutropenia (0.1%) and thrombotic thrombocytopenic purpura, which have been shown mainly with clopidogrel (13).

Spontaneous bleeding is further increased with the more potent P2Y$_{12}$ receptor antagonists prasugrel and ticagrelor (16–19). With prasugrel and ticagrelor, the risk of spontaneous bleeding increases over time, and these drugs are contraindicated in patients at high risk of bleeding. In particular, in prasugrel-treated patients there was no net clinical benefit of prasugrel, because it was offset by the increased bleeding risk, in low-weight (<60 kg) and elderly (≥75 years) patients, which might suggest the need for dose modifications in these settings (e.g., 5 mg) (16,17). The safety of the 5-mg dose has not been prospectively studied, however, and this dose derives from pharmacokinetic findings. It is important to note that in the elderly with diabetes or a prior myocardial infarction (MI), the benefits outweighed the risks, supporting the use of prasugrel at standard dosing in the elderly with these characteristics. Importantly, patients with prior stroke or transient ischemic attack had net clinical harm from prasugrel, which therefore is contraindicated in these patients (16,17). The prasugrel clinical profile has been shown to be unaffected by aspirin doses.

In comparison with clopidogrel, ticagrelor was not associated with a significant increase in overall bleeding events; it was, however, associated with a higher rate of spontaneous non-coronary artery bypass grafting (CABG)-related major bleeding, including more instances of fatal intracranial bleeding (18,19). Ticagrelor is therefore contraindicated in patients at high risk of bleeding and in those with a history of prior intracranial hemorrhage; it is also contraindicated in patients with severe hepatic dysfunction. Also, ticagrelor should be used with low-dose aspirin (<100 mg), as higher doses may limit its efficacy (22). Other nonbleeding adverse events have shown to be higher with ticagrelor than with clopidogrel. These include dyspnea, ventricular pauses, and an increase in serum uric acid and serum creatinine, which have been associated with high rates of treatment discontinuation (18,19). In patients treated with ticagrelor, coadministration of strong CYP3A4 inhibitors (e.g., ketoconazole, itraconazole, voriconazole, clarithromycin, nefazodone, ritonavir, saquinavir, nelfinavir, indinavir, atazanavir, and telithromycin) and strong CYP3A4 inducers (e.g., rifampin, dexamethasone, phenytoin, carbamazepine, and phenobarbital) is not recommended (18,19). Also, simvastatin and lovastatin doses of >40 mg should be avoided in ticagrelor-treated patients, and digoxin levels need to be monitored with initiation of, or any change in, ticagrelor therapy. Ultimately, because ticagrelor is administered twice daily, guidelines recommend cautionary use in patients with a history of poor compliance (5).

Drug-regulating agencies prompted a boxed warning for clopidogrel-treated patients, which was mainly based on post hoc analyses and pharmacodynamic studies showing a drug interaction between PPIs, mainly omeprazole and esomeprazole (because they interfere with CYP2C19 activity), and clopidogrel, as well as the presence of reduced antiplatelet effects among patients carriers of loss-of-function alleles (mainly from CYP2C19) (23,24). Nevertheless, it is unclear whether the pharmacokinetic interaction between PPIs and clopidogrel translates into worse clinical outcomes (25). These drug interactions and genetic modulating effects have not been demonstrated with prasugrel and ticagrelor (17). Guidelines recommend that PPIs should be used in patients with a history of prior gastrointestinal bleeding who require dual antiplatelet therapy, and in these patients with a clear indication for PPI therapy, clinicians may choose to use a PPI that interferes less with CYP2C19 activity, such as pantoprazole (Class I recommendation, level of evidence: C) (5). Guidelines also state that PPI use is reasonable in patients with increased risk of gastrointestinal bleeding (advanced age, concomitant use of warfarin, steroids, NSAIDs, Helicobacter pylori infection, etc.) who require dual antiplatelet therapy (Class IIa recommendation, level of evidence: C). In patients requiring oral anticoagulation and dual antiplatelet therapy, known as triple therapy, the risk of bleeding is increased. In these patients, the use of low-dose aspirin, as well as close monitoring of INR (international normalized ratio), should be reinforced in order to keep this within the lower therapeutic range (2.0–2.5) to minimize bleeding complications (26). The routine use of a PPI is not recommended for patients at low risk of gastrointestinal bleeding, who have much less potential to benefit from prophylactic therapy (Class III recommendation, level of evidence: C) (5). Prasugrel and ticagrelor use in patients treated with drugs associated with increased bleeding potential, including fibrinolytics and oral anticoagulant therapy, may result in an excessive risk of hemorrhages and is therefore discouraged (17).

Cangrelor is administered for a short period of time and has a rapid offset of action, which provides this agent with a good safety profile despite achieving a great platelet inhibition. Nevertheless, the incidence of bleeding is slightly higher with cangrelor compared with clopidogrel (mainly driven by the occurrence of hematomas at the access site), and cangrelor is contraindicated in patients with significant active bleeding (15,20). Nonbleeding adverse reactions include hypersensitivity, renal function impairment, and dyspnea, which has been reported more frequently in patients treated with cangrelor (1.3%) than with control (0.4%) and may lead to discontinuation

of therapy. In addition, caution must be taken when transitioning from cangrelor to thienopyridines in order to minimize the risk of having a gap of insufficient platelet inhibition that could result in thrombotic complications (15). In particular, clopidogrel and prasugrel should be administered at the end of cangrelor infusion. On the other hand, no interaction has been shown with ticagrelor, which can be administered any time before, during, or after cangrelor infusion (15,27).

Glycoprotein IIb/IIIa Inhibitors

Mechanisms of Action

The GP IIb/IIIa receptor is an integrin, a heterodimer consisting of noncovalently associated alpha (αIIb) and beta (β3) subunits (28,29). By competing with fibrinogen and von Willebrand factor (vWF) for GP IIb/IIIa binding, GP IIb/IIIa antagonists interfere with platelet cross-linking and platelet-derived thrombus formation. Because the GP IIb/IIIa receptor represents the final common pathway leading to platelet aggregation, these agents are very potent platelet inhibitors. The lack of benefit, including increased mortality, in patients with ACS or undergoing PCI showed by the oral GP IIb/IIIa inhibitors stopped their investigations, being only parenteral forms available for clinical use (28).

There are three parenteral GP IIb/IIIa antagonists approved for clinical use: abciximab, eptifibatide, and tirofiban (Table 3.5). Abciximab is a large chimeric monoclonal antibody with a high binding affinity that results in a prolonged pharmacologic effect (28). In particular, it is a monoclonal antibody that is a Fab (antigen-binding fragment) of a chimeric human–mouse genetic reconstruction of 7E3. The specific binding site of abciximab is the β3 subunit. Its plasma half-life is biphasic, with an initial half-life of <10 minutes

TABLE 3.5 Pharmacologic Properties and Dosing of Currently Approved Glyprotein IIb/IIIa Antagonists

	ABCIXIMAB	TIROFIBAN	EPTIFIBATIDE
Molecular structure	Fab of a monoclonal antibody	Non-peptide synthetic molecule	Synthetic cyclic heptapeptide
Molecular mass	47.615 Da	495 Da	832 Da
Reversibility	Yes[a]	Yes	Yes
Affinity	Very high	High	Intermediate
Specifity	No[b]	Yes	Yes
Plasmatic half-life	Biphasic: <10 min and ~30 min	~2 hours	~2.5 hours
Duration of antiplatelet effect after discontinuation	Platelet life-span	~4–8 hours	~4 hours
PCI dosing	Bolus: 0.25 mg/kg Infusion: 0.125 μg/kg/min (maximum 10 μg/min)	Bolus: 25 μg/kg Infusion: 0.15 μg/kg/min	Bolus: 180 μg/kg + second 180 μg/kg bolus 10 min after the first one Infusion: 2 μg/kg/min
Renal adjustment	No	In patients with CrCl <30 mL/min, reduce infusion by 50%	In patients with CrCl <50 mL/min, reduce infusion by 50%

[a]Often reported as irreversible due to its great affinity for the receptor.
[b]It also binds to the vitronectin receptor on vascular cells and to the activated MAC-1 receptor on leucocytes.
CrCl, creatinine clearance; Da, Dalton; Fab, antigen-binding fragment; PCI, percutaneous coronary intervention.

and a second-phase half-life of ~30 minutes. Because of its high affinity for the GP IIb/IIIa receptor, it has a biologic half-life of 12 to 24 hours, and because of its slow clearance from the body, it has a functional half-life of up to 7 days; platelet-associated abciximab can be detected for >14 days after treatment discontinuation (28).

Eptifibatide and tirofiban, also called "small-molecule agents," do not induce immune response and have a lower affinity for the GP IIb/IIIa receptor compared with abciximab. Eptifibatide is a reversible and highly selective heptapeptide, which has a rapid onset and a short plasma half-life of 2 to 2.5 hours. After discontinuation of the infusion, the recovery of platelet aggregation occurs within 4 hours (28). Tirofiban is a tyrosine-derived nonpeptide inhibitor that functions as a mimic of the RGD sequence and is highly specific for the GP IIb/IIIa receptor (28). Tirofiban has a rapid onset and short duration of action, with a plasma half-life of ~2 hours. Similar to eptifibatide, tirofiban has significant recovery of platelet aggregation within 4 hours of completion of infusion (28).

Indications

Numerous clinical trials have been conducted over the past decades, and, currently, these agents are indicated only in the setting of PCI (4–6). Nevertheless, clinical trial data showed no benefit in using these agents in the setting of patients with stable CAD undergoing elective PCI, in particular if pretreated with clopidogrel (30). GP IIb/IIIa inhibitors, however, have shown to be of benefit in the setting of ACS patients undergoing PCI (31). Among non-ST-segment elevation ACS patients undergoing PCI, guidelines advise that high-risk patients, especially with positive cardiac biomarkers, should receive a GP IIb/IIIa antagonist (4–6). The small-molecule agents, eptifibatide and tirofiban, may be started 1 to 2 days before and continued during the procedure (upstream) or at the time of PCI (ad hoc), while abciximab is typically recommended for in-lab use. Recent clinical trial data have failed to show any benefit with routine upstream use of these agents over ad hoc GP IIb/IIIa inhibition in ACS patients undergoing PCI (32), and is thus no longer recommended. In patients with ST-segment elevation MI (STEMI) undergoing primary PCI, abciximab has been extensively evaluated. In particular, it has been associated with a significant reduction in the rate of reinfarction, as well as mortality rates at 30 days in the prethienopyridines era (33). Nevertheless, more recent data argue against upstream GP IIb/IIIa inhibitor use in patients pretreated with $P2Y_{12}$ inhibitors undergoing primary PCI, as reflected in practice guidelines (4–6,34). While no renal adjustments are required for abciximab, eptifibatide and tirofiban require dose adjustments in renal dysfunction (Table 3.5) (4–6). Guideline recommendations for the use of GP IIb/IIIa inhibitors are summarized in Table 3.4. The risk of bleeding complications has limited the use of GP IIb/IIIa receptor antagonists. In addition, the reduced utilization of GP IIb/IIIa receptor antagonists in clinical practice is also attributed to the encouraging outcomes associated with bivalirudin, which has shown to significantly reduce bleeding without a trade-off in ischemic events (see Chapter 4).

Side Effects

Bleeding is the primary adverse effect of GP IIb/IIIa receptor antagonists (28), and is increased in elderly patients and in those with chronic kidney disease. This has been frequently attributed to overdosing, underscoring the need for dose adjustments in these settings. In addition, adjusting heparin dosing (50–70 IU/kg) is pivotal to reduce bleeding complications in PCI patients treated with GP IIb/IIIa receptor antagonists.

Thrombocytopenia is also an undesired side effect of GP IIb/IIIa receptor antagonists, which is more common with abciximab than with

eptifibatide and tirofiban. Thrombocytopenia in patients undergoing PCI is associated with more ischemic events, bleeding complications, and transfusions and warrants immediate cessation of therapy (29). Finally, it is important to remember that readministration of abciximab, but not eptifibatide and tirofiban, is associated with a slightly increased risk of thrombocytopenia, considered an immune-related process; thus, its use should be avoided or small-molecule agents should be used in its place.

Conclusions

Platelets play a key role in ischemic complications in patients with ACS and in those undergoing PCI, underscoring the importance of platelet-inhibiting agents. Dual antiplatelet therapy with aspirin and a $P2Y_{12}$ receptor inhibitor is the mainstay of short- and long-term secondary prevention treatment of ACS and PCI patients. Clopidogrel is currently the most utilized $P2Y_{12}$ receptor inhibitor and is indicated in both ACS and non-ACS settings. Prasugrel and ticagrelor are newer and more potent oral $P2Y_{12}$ inhibitors, which are indicated for use only in ACS patients. These agents have shown to reduce ischemic complications, including ST, compared with clopidogrel, although they are associated with an increased risk of bleeding complications, and should therefore be considered the first choice in patients with ACS. In this setting, clopidogrel use should be considered only when both prasugrel and ticagrelor are contraindicated or not available. Cangrelor is a novel and potent intravenous $P2Y_{12}$ antagonist that has recently received indication for use in PCI patients not pretreated with an oral $P2Y_{12}$ blocker and not receiving a GP IIb/IIIa inhibitor for reducing the risk of ischemic adverse events, where it has been proven superior to clopidogrel. GP IIb/IIIa inhibitors (abciximab, eptifibatide, and tirofiban) are available for parenteral administration, and their use is limited for the acute management of high-risk ACS patients. The elevated rates of bleeding complications with GP IIb/IIIa inhibitors, as well as the more favorable safety profiles of other antithrombotic agents, have led to a reduced utilization of these agents in clinical practice.

Key Points

- Platelets play a key role in ischemic complications in patients with ACS and in those undergoing PCI, underscoring the importance of platelet-inhibiting agents.

- Oral antiplatelet therapy is a pivotal component of secondary prevention of acute and long-term events in the settings of ACS and PCI. Dual antiplatelet therapy with aspirin and $P2Y_{12}$ receptor inhibitor is the mainstay of treatment for ACS and PCI patients.

- Clopidogrel is currently the most utilized $P2Y_{12}$ receptor inhibitor and is indicated in both ACS and non-ACS settings. Prasugrel and ticagrelor are newer and more potent $P2Y_{12}$ inhibitors that are only indicated for use in ACS patients.

- Cangrelor is a potent intravenous $P2Y_{12}$ receptor antagonist that has recently received FDA approval as an adjunct to PCI in patients who have not been treated with a $P2Y_{12}$ platelet inhibitor and are not being given a GP IIb/IIIa.

- GP IIb/IIIa inhibitors include abciximab, eptifibatide, and tirofiban. These agents are available for intravenous and intracoronary administration, and their use is limited for the acute management of high-risk ACS settings.

References

1. Angiolillo DJ, Ueno M, Goto S. Basic principles of platelet biology and clinical implications. *Circ J.* 2010;74:597–607.

2. Davì G, Patrono C. Platelet activation and atherothrombosis. *N Engl J Med.* 2007;357:2482–2494.

3. Patrono C, et al. Low-dose aspirin for the prevention of atherothrombosis. *N Engl J Med.* 2005;353:2373–2383.

4. O'Gara PT, et al. 2013 ACCF/AHA guideline for the management of ST-elevation myocardial infarction: a report of the American College of Cardiology Foundation/American Heart Association Task Force on Practice Guidelines. *J Am Coll Cardiol.* 2013;61:e78–e140.

5. Levine GN, et al. 2011 ACCF/AHA/SCAI guideline for percutaneous coronary intervention: executive summary: a report of the American College of Cardiology Foundation/American Heart Association Task Force on Practice Guidelines and the Society for Cardiovascular Angiography and Interventions. *J Am Coll Cardiol.* 2011;58:2550–2583.

6. Amsterdam EA, et al. 2014 AHA/ACC guideline for the management of patients with non-ST-elevation acute coronary syndromes: a report of the American College of Cardiology/American Heart Association Task Force on Practice Guidelines. *J Am Coll Cardiol.* 2014;64:e139–e228.

7. Baigent C, et al; Antithrombotic Trialists' (ATT) Collaboration. Aspirin in the primary and secondary prevention of vascular disease: collaborative meta-analysis of individual participant data from randomised trials. *Lancet.* 2009;373:1849–1860.

8. Mehta SR, et al. Dose comparisons of clopidogrel and aspirin in acute coronary syndromes. CURRENT-OASIS 7 Investigators. *N Engl J Med.* 2010;363:930–942.

9. Rossini R, et al. Aspirin desensitization in patients undergoing percutaneous coronary interventions with stent implantation. *Am J Cardiol.* 2008;101:786–789.

10. Gachet C, Léon C, Hechler B. The platelet P2 receptors in arterial thrombosis. *Blood Cells Mol Dis.* 2006;36:223–227.

11. Leon MB, et al. A clinical trial comparing three antithrombotic-drug regimens after coronary-artery stenting. Stent Anticoagulation Restenosis Study Investigators. *N Engl J Med.* 1998;339:1665–1671.

12. Bertrand ME, et al; CLASSICS Investigators. Double-blind study of the safety of clopidogrel with and without a loading dose in combination with aspirin compared with ticlopidine in combination with aspirin after coronary stenting: the clopidogrel aspirin stent international cooperative study (CLASSICS). *Circulation.* 2000;102:624–629.

13. Vivas D, Angiolillo DJ. Platelet P2Y$_{12}$ receptor inhibition: an update on clinical drug development. *Am J Cardiovasc Drugs.* 2010;10:217–226.

14. Angiolillo DJ, et al. Variability in individual responsiveness to clopidogrel: clinical implications, management, and future perspectives. *J Am Coll Cardiol.* 2007;49:1505–1516.

15. Marcano AL, Ferreiro JL. Role of new antiplatelet drugs on cardiovascular disease: update on cangrelor. *Curr Atheroscler Rep.* 2016;18:66.

16. Franchi F, et al. Platelet function testing in contemporary clinical and interventional practice. *Curr Treat Options Cardiovasc Med.* 2014;16:300.

17. Franchi F, Angiolillo DJ. Novel antiplatelet agents in acute coronary syndrome. *Nat Rev Cardiol.* 2015;12:30–47.

18. Wiviott SD, et al; TRITON-TIMI 38 Investigators. Prasugrel versus clopidogrel in patients with acute coronary syndromes. *N Engl J Med.* 2007;357:2001–2015.

19. Wallentin L, et al; PLATO Investigators. Ticagrelor versus clopidogrel in patients with acute coronary syndromes. *N Engl J Med.* 2009;361:1045–1057.

20. Bhatt DL, et al; CHAMPION PHOENIX Investigators. Effect of platelet inhibition with cangrelor during PCI on ischemic events. *N Engl J Med.* 2013;368:1303–1313.

21. Peters RJ, et al; Clopidogrel in Unstable angina to prevent Recurrent Events (CURE) Trial Investigators. Effects of aspirin dose when used alone or in combination with clopidogrel in patients with acute coronary syndromes: observations from the Clopidogrel in Unstable angina to prevent Recurrent Events (CURE) study. *Circulation.* 2003;108:1682–1687.

22. Mahaffey KW, Wojdyla DM, Carroll K, et al. Ticagrelor compared with clopidogrel by geographic region in the Platelet Inhibition and Patient Outcomes (PLATO) trial. *Circulation.* 2011;124:544–554.

23. Angiolillo DJ, Gibson CM, Cheng S, et al. Differential effects of omeprazole and pantoprazole on the pharmacodynamics and pharmacokinetics of clopidogrel in healthy subjects: randomized, placebo-controlled, crossover comparison studies. *Clin Pharmacol Ther.* 2011;89:65–74.

24. Simon T, et al. Genetic polymorphisms and the impact of a higher clopidogrel dose regimen on active metabolite exposure and antiplatelet response in healthy subjects. *Clin Pharmacol Ther.* 2011;90:287–295.

25. Bhatt DL, et al; COGENT Investigators. Clopidogrel with or without omeprazole in coronary artery disease. *N Engl J Med.* 2010;363:1909–1917.

26. Faxon DP, et al. Antithrombotic therapy in patients with atrial fibrillation undergoing coronary stenting: a North American perspective: executive summary. *Circ Cardiovasc Interv.* 2011;4:522–534.

27. Rollini F, Franchi F, Angiolillo DJ. Switching P2Y$_{12}$-receptor inhibitors in patients with coronary artery disease. *Nat Rev Cardiol.* 2016;13:11–27.

28. Topol EJ, Byzova TV, Plow EF. Platelet GPIIb-IIIa blockers. *Lancet.* 1999;353:227–231.

29. Hantgan RR, Nichols WL, Ruggeri ZM. von Willebrand factor competes with fibrin for occupancy of GPIIb:IIIa on thrombin-stimulated platelets. *Blood.* 1990;75:889–894.

30. Kastrati A, et al. A clinical trial of abciximab in elective percutaneous coronary intervention after pretreatment with clopidogrel. *N Engl J Med.* 2004;350:232–238.

31. Kastrati A, et al. Abciximab in patients with acute coronary syndromes undergoing percutaneous coronary intervention after clopidogrel pretreatment: the ISAR-REACT 2 randomized trial. *JAMA.* 2006;295:1531–1538.

32. Giugliano RP, et al; EARLY ACS Investigators. Early versus delayed, provisional eptifibatide in acute coronary syndromes. *N Engl J Med.* 2009;360:2176–2190.

33. De Luca G, et al. Abciximab as adjunctive therapy to reperfusion in acute ST-segment elevation myocardial infarction: a meta-analysis of randomized trials. *JAMA.* 2005;293:1759–1765.

34. Mehilli J, et al; Bavarian Reperfusion Alternatives Evaluation-3 (BRAVE-3) Study Investigators. Abciximab in patients with acute ST-segment-elevation myocardial infarction undergoing primary percutaneous coronary intervention after clopidogrel loading: a randomized double-blind trial. *Circulation.* 2009;119:1933–1940.

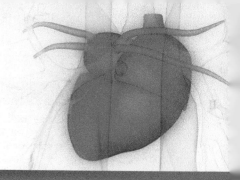

4

Anticoagulant and Fibrinolytic Agents for NSTE-ACS, PCI, and STEMI

Vivian G. Ng, MD and

Ajay J. Kirtane, MD, SM, FSCAI, FACC

Acute coronary syndromes (ACS) are typically characterized by thrombosis superimposed over rupture, erosion, or mechanical disruption of a thin fibrous cap overlying lipid-laden plaque within a culprit coronary artery. Exposure of plaque contents to the bloodstream initiates the activation and upregulation of various mediators of the thrombotic cascade, which further contribute to luminal compromise, resulting in worsening ischemia and reinfarction. Anticoagulant and antiplatelet therapies help minimize and placate the thrombotic process, which is the hallmark of ACS. As such, these agents are the cornerstones of adjunctive pharmacology for ACS. Additionally, anticoagulant and antiplatelet agents can more safely facilitate mechanical therapies such as percutaneous coronary intervention (PCI), which, while aiming to mechanically stabilize the plaque responsible for ACS, are at the same time prothrombotic and constitute an iatrogenic form of plaque rupture similar to natively occurring ACS. This chapter covers the indications and usage of various anticoagulant therapies in the setting of non-ST segment acute coronary syndromes (NSTE-ACS), ST-segment elevation myocardial infarction (STEMI), and during PCI. This chapter also briefly touches upon the interventional aspects of fibrinolytic therapy, when administered to STEMI patients.

process, but is rather a secondary event (e.g., as a result of severe blood loss, trauma, or sepsis, i.e., type 2 infarction).

Several classes of anticoagulants have been shown to be effective in treating patients with ACS: unfractionated heparin (UFH), low-molecular-weight heparins (LMWHs), direct thrombin inhibitors, and Factor Xa inhibitors. The primary function of these agents is to inhibit the coagulation cascade, thereby preventing or minimizing thrombosis in order to alleviate the ischemic effects of ACS. A critical management issue related to the use of anticoagulant agents in ACS is the potential trade-off of more potent anticoagulation (aimed at maximizing anti-ischemic efficacy) for an increase in bleeding complications. The association between ischemic events and late mortality has been recognized historically and well described in studies of ACS; in fact, this is one of the fundamental principles behind the use of anticoagulant therapy in ACS. More recently, a strong linkage between nonfatal bleeding events and subsequent mortality has also emerged in both randomized clinical trials and observational studies on ACS (2–4). Thus, the treating physician must be acutely aware of the joint importance of both ischemic and bleeding complications when selecting the optimal anticoagulant strategy for patients with NSTE-ACS.

Overview of ACC/AHA/SCAI Guideline Recommendations for NSTE-ACS

Anticoagulants in NSTE-ACS

The updated ACC/AHA guidelines (1) summarizing the recommendations for the use of anticoagulant therapy in NSTE-ACS patients first discuss the use of antithrombotic therapies for patients with definite or likely ACS. Once the diagnosis of ACS has been made, patients should be immediately started on anticoagulant therapy, regardless of the management strategy—a Class I recommendation in the ACC/AHA guidelines (Table 4.1). The notable exception to this is for those patients whose ACS is not a consequence of an atherothrombotic

Initial Anticoagulant Use in Patients with Definite NSTE-ACS

In patients with definite NSTE-ACS, parenteral anticoagulation is recommended for all patients regardless of the choice of treatment strategy (early invasive vs. ischemia-guided management). Options include enoxaparin, bivalirudin, fondaparinux or UFH. Dosing is described in Table 4.2.

Anticoagulant Use with an Early Invasive Management Strategy

Patients presenting with NSTE-ACS who are being treated with an early invasive management strategy are usually started on

TABLE 4.1 ACC/AHA Guideline Recommendations for NSTE-ACS

RECOMMENDATION	CLASS OF RECOMMENDATION	LEVEL OF EVIDENCE
SC enoxaparin for duration of hospitalization or until PCI is performed	I	A
Bivalirudin until diagnostic angiography or PCI is performed in patients with early invasive strategy only	I	B
SC fondaparinux for the duration of hospitalization or until PCI is performed	I	B
Administer additional anticoagulant with anti-IIa activity if PCI is performed while patient is on fondaparinux	I	B
IV UFH for 48 hours or until PCI is performed	I	B
IV fibrinolytic treatment not recommended in patients with NSTE-ACS	III	A

IV, intravenous; NSTE-ACS, non-ST segment acute coronary syndrome; PCI, percutaneous coronary intervention; SC, subcutaneous; UFH, unfractionated heparin.

TABLE 4.2 Dosing of Anticoagulant Agents in NSTE-ACS

	UPSTREAM THERAPY FOR NSTE-ACS	DURING PCI (IF UPSTREAM THERAPY GIVEN FOR NSTE-ACS)	DURING PCI (NO UPSTREAM THERAPY GIVEN OR ELECTIVE PCI)
Bivalirudin	0.1 mg/kg IV bolus, 0.25 mg/kg/h IV infusion	0.5 mg/kg IV bolus, increase infusion to 1.75 mg/kg/h If UFH was given, discontinue UFH, wait for 30 minutes, then give 0.75 mg/kg IV bolus, 1.75 mg/kg/h IV infusion	0.75 mg/kg IV bolus, 1.75 mg/kg/h IV infusion
Unfractionated heparin (UFH)	Loading dose of 60 U/kg (max 4,000 U) as IV bolus Maintenance IV infusion of 12 U/kg/h (max 1,000 U/h) to maintain aPTT at 1.5–2.0 times control (approximately 50–70 seconds)	IV GP IIb/IIIa planned: IV bolus doses with target ACT 200–250 seconds No IV GP IIb/IIIa planned: IV bolus doses with target ACT 250–300 seconds for HemoTec; 300–350 seconds for Hemochron	IV GP IIb/IIIa planned: 50–70 U/kg IV bolus with target ACT 200–250 seconds No IV GP IIb/IIIa planned: 70–100 U/kg IV bolus to achieve target ACT of 250–300 seconds for HemoTec; 300–350 seconds for Hemochron
Enoxaparin	Loading dose of 30 mg IV may be given in selected patients Maintenance of 1 mg/kg SC every 12 hours Extend dosing interval to 1 mg/kg SC every 24 hours if estimated CrCl <30 mL/min	Last SC dose within 8 hours: no additional therapy Last SC dose 8–12 h prior or if <2 therapeutic SC doses administered: 0.3 mg/kg IV bolus	0.5–0.75 mg/kg IV bolus
Fondaparinux	2.5 mg SC once daily Avoid for CrCl <30 mL/min	Use another agent with anti-IIa activity considering whether GP IIb/IIIa planned	N/A (use other agent if no prior exposure to fondaparinux)

ACT, activated clotting time; aPTT, activated partial thromboplastin time; CrCl, creatinine clearance; GP, glycoprotein; IV, intravenous; NSTE-ACS, non-ST segment acute coronary syndrome; PCI, percutaneous coronary intervention; SC, subcutaneous.

anticoagulant therapy at the time of diagnosis, and typically taken to the catheterization lab within 48 hours of presentation. Anticoagulant agents that have been shown to be effective in this setting include intravenous bivalirudin, intravenous UFH, subcutaneously administered fondaparinux, or subcutaneously administered enoxaparin. There are limited comparative data among the various Class I agents in this setting, and across-study comparative assessments based upon historical data are often confounded by changes in adjunctive therapies (e.g., antiplatelet agents) over time. Thus, the specific choice of an anticoagulant agent may be a physician- or an institution-dependent decision, modified by patient-specific factors.

NSTE-ACS patients undergoing PCI frequently require uptitration of anticoagulant dosing at the time of PCI in order to minimize the additional thrombogenicity associated with the procedure (Table 4.2). Consistency in anticoagulant choice should be maintained in most circumstances, given that several studies have demonstrated an associated increased risk of bleeding when switching anticoagulant agents, particularly if enoxaparin is used as the initial anticoagulant (5). In rare cases (e.g., in the treatment of intraprocedural thrombotic complications), patients may require the use of more than one anticoagulant agent during PCI. Additionally, because of an increased rate of catheter-related thrombotic complications observed during PCI performed with fondaparinux (2), intraprocedural treatment with an additional anticoagulant should be administered at the time of PCI (1).

Anticoagulant therapy is typically discontinued immediately following PCI because continued administration has demonstrated limited additional anti-ischemic benefits and an increased risk of bleeding.

Anticoagulant Use with an Ischemia-Guided Management Strategy

The goal of anticoagulant therapy in patients with NSTE-ACS is first to placate the activated prothrombotic state. Appropriate patients can then be further risk-stratified with noninvasive testing, which may lead to a more selective use of angiography and/or revascularization. NSTE-ACS patients receiving ischemia-guided management may be treated with various anticoagulants, including UFH, enoxaparin, or fondaparinux. According to the current ACC/AHA guidelines, bivalirudin is not considered part of the armamentarium for an ischemia-guided management strategy because of the limited data with this agent in these patients.

There are limited data regarding the exact duration of anticoagulant therapy in patients receiving ischemia-guided therapy. It is recommended that enoxaparin and fondaparinux should be continued for the duration of the hospitalization, or until PCI is performed. In contrast, UFH is usually continued for only 48 hours or until PCI is performed.

Anticoagulants during PCI

Anticoagulation is generally administered during PCI in order to suppress the thrombotic process that may be precipitated by the introduction of foreign objects into the coronary vasculature (i.e., catheters, wires, balloons, stents). Furthermore, anticoagulants can help suppress activation of the thrombotic cascade following vessel injury during PCI. There are several classes of anticoagulants that have shown to be effective in treating patients undergoing PCI, including UFH; enoxaparin, a LWMH; and direct thrombin inhibitors such as bivalirudin.

Anticoagulants are typically not administered during diagnostic catheterization procedures with the exception of transradially performed diagnostic procedures. If the radial artery is chosen as the access site for angiography, it is recommended that parenteral anticoagulation be started promptly after the arterial sheath is placed, in order to reduce the risk of radial artery occlusion. Spaulding et al. demonstrated a correlation between the dose of UFH therapy used following transradial access and the rate of radial artery occlusion postprocedure in 415 patients; occlusion occurred in 71% of patients with no UFH therapy, 24% in patients treated with 2,000 to 3,000 U of UFH, and 4.3% in those treated with 5,000 U of UFH (6). Whether the use of more modern hydrophilic sheaths, smaller catheter sizes, and shorter procedure times can completely mitigate this effect is unknown.

Once the decision is made to pursue PCI (irrespective of the access site), the ACC/AHA/SCAI guidelines give a Class I recommendation to administer additional parenteral anticoagulation at the time of the procedure (7). Specific recommendations regarding the choice of agent depend upon the clinical scenario. For patients not previously on parenteral anticoagulants, an anticoagulant agent is chosen and typically administered as a parenteral bolus, with an infusion lasting for the duration of the PCI. For patients with NSTE-ACS treated with upstream therapy, the dose of anticoagulation is typically higher during PCI than during maintenance upstream therapy, and several therapies used upstream are not indicated for PCI; thus, specific decisions regarding switching anticoagulants, further bolus dosing, and/or increasing the dose of infusion are required (Table 4.2). Of the anticoagulants used during PCI, UFH is one agent for which intraprocedural monitoring of levels of anticoagulant activity is recommended.

In general, anticoagulant therapy is discontinued immediately following PCI. Decisions regarding management of the vascular access site depend upon several factors: the site of access (e.g., femoral vs. radial), whether use of a vascular closure device is planned, and the particular anticoagulant used. For femoral access, if use of a vascular closure device is planned, it is typically deployed immediately after PCI. For manual compression of a femoral access site, sheaths are usually removed when the activated clotting time (ACT) falls below 150 to 180 seconds in patients treated with UFH; for patients treated with bivalirudin, sheaths are typically removed 2 hours after termination of the infusion. For radial access, sheath removal is typically performed immediately after PCI by applying nonocclusive pressure, typically with a specialized pressure device to achieve patient hemostasis in order to preserve flow in the radial artery.

Specific Anticoagulants

Unfractionated Heparin

UFH is a mixture of polysaccharide chains with molecular weights ranging from 3,000 to 30,000 Da, which exerts its major anticoagulant effect by indirectly inactivating thrombin and the coagulation cascade. UFH facilitates activation of antithrombin III, which then inactivates Factors IIa (thrombin), IXa, and Xa. Bioavailability of UFH varies from patient to patient because of its nonspecific binding to plasma proteins and cells. As a consequence, the anticoagulant response to UFH varies among patients and necessitates the monitoring of the activated partial thromboplastin time (aPTT) or ACT in order to achieve the optimally desired level of anticoagulation.

SUMMARY OF TRIAL DATA

NSTE-ACS

One of the oldest anticoagulants used to treat ACS, UFH has been studied in numerous trials involving NSTE-ACS patients. In a meta-analysis comparing the effect of aspirin plus UFH with that of UFH alone, aspirin plus UFH was shown to reduce early ischemic events, with borderline significance noted in the reduction of early death or myocardial infarction (MI) (**Fig. 4.1**) (8). It should be noted that the effects of UFH regarding the endpoint of death/MI were not significant in any of the individual trials included in this meta-analysis. Furthermore, antiplatelet agents such as adenosine diphosphate (ADP) receptor blockers, which provide an additional anti-ischemic effect, were not included in these trials, so the "true" effect of UFH when used in conjunction with more potent antiplatelet agents compared with no UFH is poorly understood from clinical trials (Fig. 4.1).

Elective PCI

UFH was the sole anticoagulant used in PCI for many years, and because of its widespread and early acceptance, there are limited trial data examining its efficacy and safety compared with a background of no UFH. Clinical experience with the use of UFH suggests that the optimal intensity of anticoagulation is generally greater in patients undergoing PCI than in those who are being medically managed with ACS. Early on in the PCI experience, UFH was given at the beginning of the procedure as a standard dose of 10,000 U intravenously, with further bolus doses administered hourly. Nevertheless, because of variable anticoagulant effects observed with these fixed dosing regimens of UFH, as well as the observation of an increased rate of bleeding complications in patients treated with UFH plus potent antiplatelet agents such as GP IIb/IIIa inhibitors, the measurement of ACT has become integrated as part of the PCI procedure (see below).

UNFRACTIONATED HEPARIN: DOSING STRATEGIES AND THERAPEUTICS

NSTE-ACS

In ACS, UFH is administered as an intravenous bolus followed by a continuous intravenous infusion. Traditionally, UFH is given as a 5,000-U bolus followed by a 1,000 U/hr infusion, with further adjustments made according to the aPTT. Nevertheless, more predictable anticoagulation can be effected through weight-based dosing, which is the current recommendation in the ACC/AHA

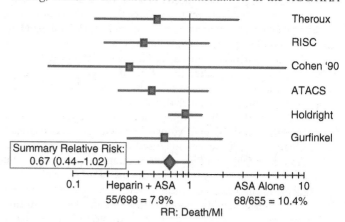

FIGURE 4.1 Meta-analysis of UFH plus aspirin versus aspirin alone in ACS. ACS, Acute coronary syndromes; ASA, aspirin; MI, myocardial infarction; RR, relative risk; UFH, unfractionated heparin. (Adapted from: Oler A, et al. Adding heparin to aspirin reduces the incidence of myocardial infarction and death in patients with unstable angina. A meta-analysis. JAMA. 1996;276:811–815, with permission.)

guidelines. These guidelines recommend an intravenous bolus dose of UFH (60 U/kg not to exceed 4,000 U), followed by an initial 12 U/kg/hr infusion (not to exceed 1,000 U/hr). Further dosing is dictated by monitoring of the aPTT or ACT (the latter for patients undergoing PCI).

Measurement of the aPTT can vary from institution to institution, so it is important to implement an institution-specific nomogram and/or protocol for UFH. Ideally, patients maintained on UFH should have a target aPTT in the range of 1.5 to 2.0 times control. This dosing is thought to optimize the anti-ischemic effects of UFH while minimizing bleeding that can occur at higher achieved levels of anticoagulation (9). For patients undergoing PCI, additional intravenous boluses are typically administered.

The ACC/AHA guidelines recommend the administration of UFH up until the time of angiography for those patients undergoing an early invasive management strategy, but the optimal duration of UFH in ACS patients beyond angiography is unknown. Patients who undergo PCI should have UFH discontinued after PCI; those undergoing coronary artery bypass grafting (CABG) should continue UFH. Patients being treated medically or those not undergoing an invasive management strategy are typically treated with UFH through their hospitalization (at least 48 hours), at which point it can be discontinued.

UFH is a reversible anticoagulant whose effect dissipates over time when the infusion is stopped. In more emergent settings, protamine sulfate can be administered for rapid reversal. A test dose is usually given prior to administering a full dose of protamine to prevent anaphylaxis-type reactions, which have been known to occur in patients with prior exposure to long-acting insulins.

During PCI

For PCI, UFH is administered as an intravenous bolus with therapeutic levels monitored by ACT. Because the intensity of anticoagulation during PCI is greater than during upstream medical therapy, heparin infusions are typically discontinued 30 minutes prior to PCI, and full dosing of UFH is given at the time of PCI. Weight-based dosing should be employed, using doses of 50 to 70 U/kg with a target ACT of 200 to 250 seconds if GP IIb/IIIa inhibitors are used and 70 to 100 U/kg with a target ACT of 300 to 350 seconds if no GP IIb/IIIa inhibitors are used (Table 4.2). In rare cases, such as in retrograde PCI procedures, the current clinical standard is to maintain ACT at the

higher end of this scale so as to mitigate against catheter thrombosis within a large ischemic territory. Patients undergoing PCI with UFH should have the anticoagulant stopped at the end of the procedure.

Chew and colleagues pooled the results from the UFH-only arms of six randomized control trials enrolling 5,216 patients who were primarily treated with balloon angioplasty alone, and then examined the association between ACT and outcomes after PCI (10). In this analysis, patients with ACT values ranging from 350 to 375 seconds had the lowest ischemic event rates (**Fig. 4.2**, left panel); however, major or minor bleeding rates were lowest with ACT values between 300 and 350 seconds (Fig. 4.2, right panel). A pooled analysis of four more recent randomized trials, which included patients treated primarily with stents and GP IIb/IIIa inhibitors, demonstrated no significant correlation between maximal ACT and ischemic complications, with a monotonically increasing risk of bleeding at increasing levels of ACT (11). Based upon these and other studies, current guidelines recommend ACT-based titration of UFH during PCI, with lower levels of ACT for patients treated with concomitant potent antiplatelet therapies.

ADVERSE CONSEQUENCES

As an anticoagulant, UFH is associated with bleeding complications, which must be weighed against the potential anti-ischemic effects of the agent. While bleeding complications can occur despite a therapeutic range aPTT, higher aPTT values are associated with increased bleeding complications. Appropriate dosing and monitoring of UFH should be performed in order to maximize UFH's risk–benefit ratio, as higher doses of both the bolus and infusion have been associated with adverse outcomes (12). In a large observational registry of ACS patients, excess dosing of UFH was found in almost one-third of patients (13).

In addition to bleeding complications, exposure to UFH has also been associated with the development of heparin-induced thrombocytopenia, which can occur with or without thrombosis (1,14). Mild thrombocytopenia may occur in 10% to 20% of patients, whereas significant thrombocytopenia (platelet count < 100,000) occurs in 1% to 5% of patients and typically appears after several days of therapy. Discontinuation of UFH usually resolves the thrombocytopenia. Immune-mediated heparin-induced thrombocytopenia is a more rare complication of UFH treatment (<0.2%), and requires

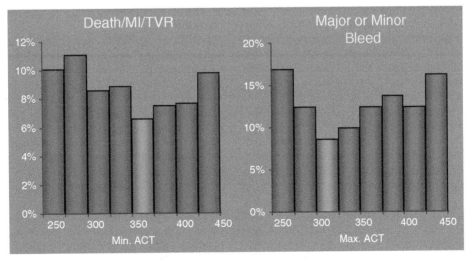

FIGURE 4.2 Optimal levels of anticoagulation with UFH based upon ACT. ACT, activated clotting time; MI, myocardial infarction; TVR, target vessel revascularization; UFH, unfractionated heparin. (Adapted from: Chew DP, et al. Defining the optimal activated clotting time during percutaneous coronary intervention: aggregate results from 6 randomized, controlled trials. *Circulation.* 2001;103:961–966, with permission.)

abrupt withdrawal of UFH and active treatment with a direct thrombin inhibitor to prevent the thrombotic sequelae of the syndrome. Finally, excess thrombin generation (the so-called "rebound effect") has additionally been described following cessation of UFH; the actual adverse clinical sequelae of this effect are largely unknown, particularly in the era of more potent antiplatelet therapies (15).

Low-Molecular-Weight Heparins

LWMHs, ranging from 1,000 to 10,000 Da, are derived from UFH via chemical or enzymatic depolymerization. Similar to UFH, LMWH forms a complex with antithrombin III, converting it from a slow to a rapid inactivator of clotting factors. LMWHs are potent inactivators of Factor Xa and Factor IIa (thrombin). In addition, LMWHs exhibit less binding to plasma proteins and cells, and have a longer half-life. This facilitates more predictable dose responses to LMWH compared with UFH, and allows LMWH to be administered via subcutaneous administration with twice-daily dosing or daily dosing in those with renal impairment (CrCL < 30 mL/min).

SUMMARY OF TRIAL DATA

NSTE-ACS

The FRISC study was the only large randomized trial that compared LMWH with placebos. It randomized 1,506 patients with ACS, and showed that the addition of dalteparin to aspirin reduced the risk of early death or MI (in the first 6 days) from 4.8% to 1.8% (p = 0.001) compared with aspirin alone (16). This study primarily enrolled medically managed patients with ACS, and it should be noted that among patients randomized to dalteparin, therapy was continued for several weeks.

Comparisons of LMWH versus UFH

The majority of data with LMWH in ACS consist of randomized trials comparing the use of LMWH with UFH on a background of aspirin antiplatelet therapy. Although different preparations of LMWH have been studied (including dalteparin and nadroparin), the most positive results have been observed using enoxaparin.

Early data from the TIMI 11B and ESSENCE trials demonstrated reductions in the composite of death, MI, or recurrent ischemia with enoxaparin compared with UFH. These trials supported the use of LMWH in ACS patients managed predominantly with an ischemia-guided strategy rather than with an invasive strategy (17).

These favorable results led to the design of trials comparing the use of LMWH to UFH in invasively managed patients with ACS. In the 10,027-patient SYNERGY trial, the rate of the composite ischemic endpoint of death or MI was 14.0% with enoxaparin versus 14.5% with UFH (nonstatistically different); however, bleeding complications were more frequent with enoxaparin (18). The use of enoxaparin in this trial was in addition to aspirin and, in approximately half of enrolled patients, GP IIb/IIIa inhibitors. In the smaller A-to-Z trial in which patients were randomized to enoxaparin or UFH groups on a background of aspirin and routine GP IIb/IIIa inhibition, treatment with enoxaparin was associated with a nonsignificantly lower rate of death, MI, or recurrent ischemia at 30 days (8.4% vs. 9.4%), with numerically greater rates of bleeding compared with UFH (19). In A-to-Z, however, only half of the patients were managed with an early invasive strategy, and a post hoc subgroup analysis demonstrated that the benefit of enoxaparin was largely confined to patients managed using an ischemia-guided strategy.

A meta-analysis of all enoxaparin versus UFH trials in ACS has been conducted, which demonstrates an approximately 10% reduction in death or MI with enoxaparin over UFH, with no significant differences in major bleeding outcomes (5). It should be noted that this meta-analysis included a number of patients who were managed using an ischemia-guided strategy, and that higher rates of bleeding outcomes were observed with enoxaparin compared with UFH in the SYNERGY trial, the largest trial of invasively managed patients with ACS. A posthoc analysis of the SYNERGY trial showed that the higher rates of bleeding in the enoxaparin arm might have been a consequence of the use of either multiple anticoagulants or the switching of agents in the study. It remains unclear whether maintaining consistency in the use of anticoagulants could have minimized bleeding complications in this trial (20).

Elective PCI

While the use of enoxaparin in PCI is not common in the United States, enoxaparin has a Class IIb indication in the ACC/AHA/SCAI guidelines for elective PCI, largely on the basis of the randomized STEEPLE trial. STEEPLE enrolled over 3,000 patients and compared three intravenously administered anticoagulant regimens in patients undergoing elective PCI: enoxaparin 0.5 mg/kg, enoxaparin 0.75 mg/kg, or UFH 70 to 100 U/kg adjusted for ACT (if GP IIb/IIIa inhibitors were used, then UFH was decreased to 50–70 U/kg) (21). The trial demonstrated a statistically significant reduction in the primary endpoint of non-CABG bleeding with enoxaparin 0.5 mg/kg compared with UFH (5.9% vs. 8.5%, p = 0.01), but no statistically significant difference between enoxaparin 0.75 mg/kg and UFH. The incidence of minor bleeding was significantly reduced in both enoxaparin groups compared with UFH, and there were no statistically significant differences in the rates of death, MI, or urgent target vessel revascularization between study arms.

DIFFERENTIATION BETWEEN LMW HEPARINS

Different formulations of LMWH have varying ratios of anti-factor Xa to anti-factor IIa activity. It is unclear, however, whether these differences have any clinically meaningful effects. Very few trials have directly compared the various LMWHs. Indirect comparisons between agents suggest that enoxaparin is likely the most clinically useful agent, and there is one small randomized trial comparing enoxaparin versus tinzaparin in patients with unstable angina (UA). In the EVET trial, patients treated with enoxaparin had significantly lower rates of ischemic outcomes compared with those treated with tinzaparin, with similar rates of bleeding outcomes (22).

DOSING STRATEGIES

NSTE-ACS

The ACC/AHA guidelines recommend the administration of LMWH up to the time of diagnostic angiography for patients treated according to an invasive management strategy. Patients who undergo PCI should have LWMH discontinued after PCI; those undergoing CABG should discontinue LMWH 12 to 24 hours prior to CABG. Patients being treated medically or those not undergoing an invasive management strategy should be treated with LMWH through hospitalization, at which point the agent can be discontinued.

The anticoagulant effect of LMWH can be measured directly by assessing Factor Xa activity. The aPTT is not a reliable indicator of anticoagulant effect. Because of the predictable effects of LMWH, it is not necessary in clinical practice to monitor the level of anticoagulant effect, making LMWH easier to use compared with intravenously dosed UFH. Caution should be used when administering LMWH in patients with renal dysfunction; a dose reduction to once a day is recommended in patients with creatinine clearance (CrCl) of <30 mL/min. LWMH can also be administered intravenously, which can be useful for PCI, particularly in patients who have not received prior doses of LWMH.

During PCI

Patients who have not received any prior anticoagulant therapy should be loaded with 0.5 to 0.75 mg/kg IV loading dose of enoxaparin. Patients who are being treated initially with subcutaneously administered enoxaparin and undergo PCI within 8 hours of the last dose do not need to have any additional anticoagulant given. Nevertheless, if PCI is undertaken in the 8- to 12-hour period after the last dose of subcutaneous enoxaparin, or if patients have received only one dose of enoxaparin, the guidelines recommend that they be given additional enoxaparin (0.3 mg/kg IV) at the time of PCI (Table 4.2). Those patients undergoing PCI more than 12 hours after the last dose of enoxaparin are typically treated as if they have not received upstream therapy. Once the procedure is completed, further anticoagulation should be stopped.

It is also reasonable to administer intravenous enoxaparin to those patients presenting for elective PCI who have not been given any prior anticoagulation. While direct assessment of factor Xa levels is possible, this test is rarely indicated because of the predictability of enoxaparin's effect. The initial intravenous dose given should be 30 mg. ACT levels are not reliable indicators of anticoagulant effect in patients who were administered enoxaparin.

ADVERSE CONSEQUENCES OF LMWH

LMWH agents, likely UFH, are associated with bleeding complications, which must be weighed against potential anti-ischemic benefits. In a large observational series of patients with ACS, excess dosing of LMWH agents occurred 13.6% of the time, and was associated with increased rates of bleeding (13). Thus, careful attention must be paid to optimal weight-based dosing and dose adjustments based on renal dysfunction for those agents that are primarily renally cleared in order to minimize bleeding complications.

LMWH have been associated with heparin-associated thrombocytopenia, but with a much lower frequency compared with UFH (14). Additionally, LMWH causes less platelet activation and aggregation than UFH. The use of LMWH during PCI has been associated with a low but notable rate of episodes of catheter-related thrombotic complications, despite adequate inhibition of Factor Xa (23). This complication requires treatment with either UFH or a direct thrombin inhibitor. While a "rebound" phenomenon has been observed with cessation of LMWH therapy, LMWH, unlike UFH, can stimulate the release of tissue factor pathway inhibitors, which enhance anti-factor Xa activity and can attenuate the rebound hypercoagulability that has been observed with UFH (24).

Direct Thrombin Inhibitors

Direct thrombin inhibitors offer advantages over UFH and LMWH in that they inhibit thrombin directly, rather than through activation of antithrombin III. Additionally, direct thrombin inhibitors can inhibit both free as well as clot-bound thrombin, provide a very stable level of anticoagulation, and do not cause thrombocytopenia. Hirudin, a naturally occurring anticoagulant derived from the medicinal leech, is made commercially by recombinant DNA technology in a number of formulations (including lepirudin, desirudin), and was used in early studies of ACS. Bivalirudin, another direct thrombin inhibitor, is an analog of hirudin and binds reversibly to thrombin with a short half-life, inhibiting thrombin's activity. Bivalirudin is the most widely studied direct thrombin inhibitor in the contemporary management of ACS and patients undergoing PCI. Argatroban is another monovalent direct thrombin inhibitor that is approved for the treatment of heparin-induced thrombocytopenia, but is not indicated for the treatment of ACS following negative studies with this agent in STEMI.

SUMMARY OF TRIAL DATA

NSTE-ACS

Several early trials evaluated recombinant hirudin versus UFH for patients with ACS. The largest of these trials was GUSTO IIb, enrolling 12,142 patients with both NSTE-ACS and STEMI, including patients treated with fibrinolytic therapy. In this trial, although the 24-hour endpoint of death or MI favored hirudin, the 30-day rate of death or MI was not significantly lower with hirudin compared with UFH, and the rate of moderate bleeding was higher with hirudin (25). Further evaluation of hirudin continued in the 10,141-patient OASIS-2 trial, which again demonstrated improved ischemic outcomes with hirudin (but nonsignificantly so), and higher rates of bleeding (26). Pooling of all the major hirudin trials has demonstrated an overall reduction, ~20%, in ischemic events (death or MI) with hirudin over UFH, but at the cost of an excess of bleeding complications (26,27). Notably, these early trials were conducted on an antiplatelet background of aspirin alone.

Bivalirudin, a synthetic analogue of hirudin, was first studied in the BAT trial, a trial of bivalirudin versus UFH in 4,098 patients undergoing PCI for UA or postinfarction angina. In this trial, bivalirudin did not significantly reduce the incidence of the composite primary ischemic endpoint (a combination of early death, MI, abrupt vessel closure, or clinical deterioration) compared with UFH, but was associated with a reduction in bleeding (28). A subsequent reevaluation of the data from this trial with a more contemporary ischemic endpoint of death, MI, or repeat revascularization demonstrated the benefit of using bivalirudin over UFH (6.2% vs. 7.9%, p = 0.039), with lower rates of bleeding (29). These data and other emerging favorable data for bivalirudin in PCI patients led to a reassessment of the use of bivalirudin for ACS in the ACUITY trial.

ACUITY randomly assigned 13,819 patients with moderate- to high-risk ACS to one of three antithrombotic regimens: UFH (or enoxaparin) plus a GP IIb/IIIa inhibitor, bivalirudin plus a GP IIb/IIIa inhibitor, or bivalirudin monotherapy (30). Patients were managed with an early invasive strategy. In this trial, bivalirudin monotherapy was associated with a similar rate of composite ischemia (7.8% vs. 7.3%, p = 0.32) and significantly reduced major bleeding (3.0% vs. 5.7%, p < 0.001), compared with UFH/enoxaparin plus a GP IIb/IIIa inhibitor (Fig. 4.3). While these results were consistent in most major subgroups of the trial, the 30-day composite ischemic event rate was notably higher with bivalirudin monotherapy than with UFH plus GP IIb/IIIa inhibition among patients not pretreated with an ADP-receptor antagonist (9.1% vs. 7.1%, p = 0.05 for interaction). In ACUITY, treatment with bivalirudin plus routine GP IIb/IIIa inhibition resulted in similar rates of 30-day death, MI, or unplanned revascularization for recurrent ischemia compared with UFH/enoxaparin plus GP IIb/IIIa inhibitors (7.7% vs. 7.3%, p = 0.39) and similar rates of major bleeding (5.3% vs. 5.7%, p = 0.38).

Because both BAT and ACUITY employed invasive management strategies and in the case of ACUITY the time from admission to angiography was short (19.6 hours), current guidelines stress that for patients experiencing more significant delays to catheterization, or patients with recurrent ischemia following the initial treatment strategy, consideration should be given to further escalation of the antithrombotic regimen (e.g., through the addition of a GP IIb/IIIa inhibitor). In fact, some have questioned whether the potential benefits of bivalirudin over UFH alone could be replicated by more aggressive oral antiplatelet therapy (such as ADP-receptor blockade) in conjunction with UFH monotherapy (without a GP IIb/IIIa inhibitor). In the ISAR-REACT 3 study, this strategy was tested among patients undergoing PCI either electively or for UA (31). In this trial on 4,570 patients pretreated with 600 mg of clopidogrel,

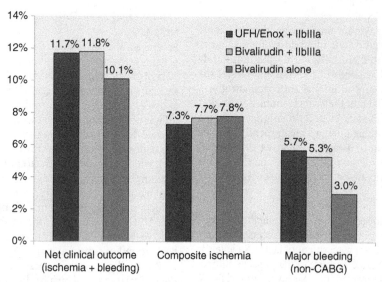

FIGURE 4.3 Thirty-day outcomes from the ACUITY Trial of bivalirudin in acute coronary syndromes (ACS).

the rates of ischemic outcomes were similar for patients treated with bivalirudin or UFH, but bivalirudin-treated patients had a significantly lower rate of bleeding complications (3.1% vs. 4.6%, p = 0.008). Further validation of the ACUITY results, however, has occurred in the ISAR-REACT-4 trial, a trial randomizing 1,721 patients in a double-blind manner to abciximab plus UFH versus bivalirudin. The primary composite endpoint of death, MI, major bleeding, and urgent target-vessel revascularization was similar in both arms, with an increased risk of major bleeding observed with abciximab plus UFH compared with bivalirudin alone (4.6% vs. 2.6%, p = 0.02) (32).

More recently, there have been conflicting data regarding whether the benefits of bivalirudin therapy persist when compared to heparin therapy alone and GP IIb/IIIA inhibitor use is reserved as a bailout therapy. For example, in the MATRIX study, 7,213 patients with ACS were randomized to receive either UFH or bivalirudin. Thirty day major adverse cardiovascular events (MACE) rates (composite of death, MI, or stroke) were similar among patients receiving bivalirudin or heparin (10.3% vs. 10.9%, p = 0.44) (33). Furthermore, in the NSTE-ACS patient subset, there was no significant difference in MACE rates between patients receiving bivalirudin or heparin (15.9% vs. 16.5%, p = 0.74) (34). In contrast, bivalirudin was associated with fewer net adverse clinical events at 30 days compared to heparin (8.8% vs. 13.2%, p = 0.008) in the BRIGHT trial, which included 2,194 AMI patients. Moreover, patients receiving bivalirudin had lower rates of 30-day bleeding compared to those receiving heparin (4.1% vs. 7.5%, p < 0.001) (35). Additional large randomized controlled studies are needed to address this clinical question.

Elective PCI
Early trials such as BAT (see earlier) and REPLACE-1 (36) were conducted to study the use of bivalirudin as an alternative anticoagulant for PCI. REPLACE-1 randomized 1,056 patients undergoing elective or urgent PCI to bivalirudin versus UFH; the majority of patients were pretreated with clopidogrel, and 72% of patients received a GP IIb/IIIa inhibitor. Compared with UFH, bivalirudin was associated with a similar rate of death, MI, or repeat revascularization, with a similar frequency of major bleeding complications. The larger REPLACE-2 trial was designed to further test the use of bivalirudin in 6,000 patients undergoing urgent

or elective PCI; the majority of patients were pretreated with a thienopyridine platelet antagonist (37). Patients were randomized to either bivalirudin and provisional GP IIb/IIIa inhibition (with either eptifibatide or abciximab) or UFH plus routine GP IIb/IIIa inhibition. There were no significant differences in the occurrence of the primary study endpoint of death, MI, urgent revascularization, or in-hospital major bleeding between study arms. Nevertheless, there was a significant reduction of major bleeding events (using a more sensitive bleeding scale) with bivalirudin compared with UFH (2.4% vs. 4.1%; p < 0.001).

DIRECT THROMBIN INHIBITORS
The two direct thrombin inhibitors best studied in ACS are bivalirudin and hirudin. Hirudin and argatroban have limited ischemic efficacy and are presently only approved for those patients who have developed heparin-induced thrombocytopenia. The best-studied agent for use in PCI is bivalirudin. Argatroban can be used during PCI, but given the widespread availability of bivalirudin, its use is limited. Argatroban can be considered in patients with renal insufficiency because of its hepatic clearance. In these cases, the usual dose is an intravenous infusion of 2 μg/kg/min which is adjusted to maintain an aPTT 1.5 to 3 times baseline (but not >100 seconds).

NSTE-ACS
Bivalirudin is given a Class I recommendation from ACC/AHA for the treatment of invasively managed NSTE-ACS patients, but is not currently indicated for NSTE-ACS patients receiving ischemia-guided management. Bivalirudin is administered as an intravenous bolus followed by an infusion (Table 4.2). Due to its excellent bioavailability, there is no need for monitoring of therapeutic effect. Patients undergoing PCI should receive an additional bolus and an increased rate of infusion; dose adjustments should be made for those CrCl < 30 mL/min. The bivalirudin infusion is typically discontinued immediately following cardiac catheterization (and/or PCI), although some have advocated a longer duration of therapy, particularly for patients not adequately treated with thienopyridines. Patients treated with bivalirudin who are medically managed following diagnostic angiography can have the bivalirudin stopped or continued for up to 72 hours at the treating physician's discretion. Patients scheduled to undergo CABG should have the bivalirudin stopped 3 hours prior to CABG and can then be treated with UFH if necessary.

During PCI

For patients undergoing elective PCI (or those with NSTE-ACS not on prior anticoagulation), an intravenous weight-based bolus of 0.75 mg/kg is administered, followed by an intravenous infusion of 1.75 mg/kg/hr (Table 4.2). In patients who have already received UFH, the bolus and intravenous infusion rates should be started after the UFH has been stopped for 30 minutes. In patients who have already been started on a bivalirudin infusion, an additional 0.5 mg/kg loading dose should be given and the intravenous infusion rate should be increased to 1.75 mg/kg/hr during PCI. Switching from another anticoagulant (e.g., enoxaparin or UFH) to bivalirudin during PCI has not been associated with adverse outcomes (38). Due to bivalirudin's excellent bioavailability, there is no need for intraprocedural monitoring. Dose adjustments to the infusion should be made for those patients with a CrCl < 30 mL/min. Once the PCI procedure is complete, the infusion is typically discontinued.

Adverse Events

Bleeding complications are the primary adverse effects that need to be monitored in anticoagulated patients who are being treated with this agent. Unlike UFH, direct thrombin inhibitors cannot be reversed, and bleeding complications that arise need to be managed supportively until the anticoagulant effect has diminished. Despite this, bivalirudin is associated with lower bleeding complications compared with UFH and LMWH, particularly when the latter are coadministered with GP IIb/IIIa inhibitors. This makes bivalirudin an attractive agent to consider in patients who are at higher risk for bleeding complications.

Factor Xa Inhibition with Fondaparinux

Factor Xa inhibitors exert their anticoagulant effect more proximally in the coagulation cascade, and have demonstrated promise in the treatment of ACS. The synthetic pentasaccharide fondaparinux is the best-studied parenteral Factor Xa inhibitor used for patients with ACS. Fondaparinux is structurally similar to the antithrombin-binding portion of UFH (and LMWH), and by reversibly binding to antithrombin III, it indirectly inhibits factor Xa.

SUMMARY OF TRIAL DATA

NSTE-ACS

The largest trial of fondaparinux in NSTE-ACS was the OASIS-5 trial. This trial randomized 20,078 patients with ACS to fondaparinux versus enoxaparin; both agents were administered subcutaneously for a mean of 6 days (2). Patients in this trial were managed more conservatively compared with other contemporary ACS trials: overall, approximately two-thirds of patients underwent diagnostic coronary angiography. Patients undergoing PCI received additional anticoagulant therapy depending on the duration from the last administered study dose (in some cases in the fondaparinux arm, patients received additional intravenously administered fondaparinux). The rate of the primary composite endpoint of death, MI, or refractory ischemia was similar to that of fondaparinux and enoxaparin (5.8% vs. 5.7%), but bleeding events were significantly decreased with the use of fondaparinux (2.2% vs. 4.1%, p < 0.001) (**Fig. 4.4**). These benefits persisted at 30 days; in fact, 30-day mortality was lower with fondaparinux compared with enoxaparin (2.9% vs. 3.5%, p = 0.02).

In the subset of patients undergoing PCI in OASIS-5, fondaparinux was associated with an increased risk of catheter-related thrombus (0.9% vs. 0.3% for enoxaparin), a finding that was also confirmed in the OASIS-6 trial of fondaparinux for STEMI. As a result, operators were permitted to use open-label UFH during PCI for patients already treated with fondaparinux. A subsequent trial, FUTURA/OASIS-8, has examined the effects of UFH dosing during PCI for 2,026 patients treated with fondaparinux for ACS (39). In this trial, there was no difference in outcomes using a low dose of UFH versus a higher dose.

Elective PCI

Fondaparinux has been studied in patients with ACS, but has not been studied in patients undergoing elective PCI.

DOSING STRATEGIES AND ADVERSE EVENTS

Fondaparinux has minimal binding to plasma proteins other than antithrombin (40). Thus, it is readily absorbed, with peak plasma concentrations peaking at around 2 hours. Its long elimination half-life of approximately 17 hours allows for once daily dosing, and there is no need for monitoring. Given that it is renally cleared, fondaparinux is contraindicated in patients with a CrCl < 30 mL/min.

The optimal duration of fondaparinux therapy in ACS patients is unknown, but the ACC/AHA guidelines recommend continuing dosing up to the time of diagnostic angiography for patients undergoing an invasive management strategy. Patients who undergo PCI should have fondaparinux discontinued after PCI. Additional UFH should be given

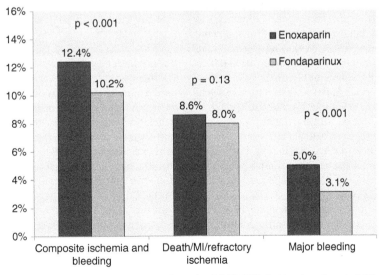

FIGURE 4.4   Thirty-day outcomes from the OASIS-5 Trial of fondaparinux in ACS. ACS, Acute coronary syndromes; MI, myocardial infraction.

particularly during the performance of PCI in fondaparinux-treated patients to avoid the occurrence of catheter-related thrombus formation. Patients undergoing CABG should discontinue fondaparinux 24 hours prior to CABG. Patients being treated medically or those not undergoing an invasive management strategy should be treated with fondaparinux throughout their hospitalization, at which point it can be discontinued.

Other adverse events, such as bleeding complications, have been associated with treatment with fondaparinux, but these were less frequently observed in the OASIS-5 trial compared with enoxaparin, leading to the recommendation in the ACC/AHA guidelines for the use of this agent in patients managed using an ischemia-guided strategy at risk for bleeding.

Owing to the occurrence of catheter-related thrombus during PCI with fondaparinux anticoagulation, the ACC/AHA/SCAI guidelines for PCI give fondaparinux as a sole anticoagulant a Class III (harm) indication for patients undergoing PCI.

Warfarin and Other Oral Anticoagulants for NSTE-ACS

While warfarin and other oral anticoagulants do not provide sufficient levels of anticoagulation for patients to undergo PCI, these agents have been studied as adjunctive add-on therapies for patients with ACS. It is of historical significance to note that early in the stent experience, anticoagulation with warfarin was used as a means of trying to prevent stent thrombosis. The use of warfarin following stent implantation dramatically decreased after several trials demonstrated that dual antiplatelet therapy (DAPT) with aspirin plus the thienopyridine ticlopidine was superior to aspirin plus warfarin following stent implantation (41).

WARFARIN IN NSTE-ACS

Warfarin is an oral anticoagulant whose effect is mediated by inhibiting the formation of vitamin K–dependent coagulation factors (Factors II, VII, IX, X, and proteins C and S). The anticoagulant activity of warfarin is variable, and the agent has a relatively narrow therapeutic window, which requires close monitoring of the prothrombin time/international normalized ratio in order to assure the optimal level of anticoagulation.

Oral anticoagulation with warfarin post-ACS has been examined in several trials, with the rationale that prolonged treatment might extend the benefit of early anticoagulation in NSTE-ACS. The warfarin substudy of the OASIS-2 trial subrandomized 3,712 patients to continued warfarin or standard therapy, including aspirin, following initial presentation and treatment for ACS (42). In this trial, there were no significant differences in the rate of the composite of death, MI, or stroke with either therapy, but major bleeding was increased with warfarin therapy (2.7% vs. 1.3%, p = 0.004). Subanalyses of the OASIS-2 data based upon countries with greater adherence to warfarin therapy (>70% compliance with the therapy at 35 days) demonstrated significant anti-ischemic benefits of warfarin among countries with greater adherence to warfarin therapy, but higher relative risks of bleeding complications. Similar data have been reported from other smaller trials, including patients at potentially higher risk, such as STEMI. In the WARIS-2 trial, which randomized 3,630 post-MI patients to aspirin alone, warfarin alone, or aspirin plus warfarin, treatment with the combination of aspirin and warfarin was associated with the lowest rate of death, MI, or thromboembolic stroke (15.0% with aspirin plus warfarin vs. 16.7% with warfarin alone vs. 20% for aspirin alone, p < 0.001) (43). Nevertheless, the incidence of nonfatal bleeding was increased in both warfarin groups compared with that in aspirin alone.

Notable caveats to these early studies are that they largely excluded patients undergoing early revascularization and were conducted prior to more widespread use of DAPT. Oral antiplatelet agents such as P2Y$_{12}$ receptor antagonists have been demonstrated to reduce ischemic outcomes over therapy with aspirin alone, and are recommended as the standard of care in virtually all patients with NSTE-ACS. Because the combination of warfarin plus aspirin alone has been associated with increased bleeding, and the combination of aspirin, a P2Y$_{12}$ receptor antagonist, and warfarin increases bleeding to an even greater extent, the role of "triple therapy" is generally limited to patients with other indications for warfarin anticoagulation (e.g., mechanical valve, atrial fibrillation, stroke, ventricular thrombus, venous thromboembolism). In these patients, the benefit of preventing thromboembolic events and recurrent ischemic events must be balanced with the risk of bleeding. The WOEST trial investigated the use of antiplatelet medications in patients requiring oral anticoagulant medications who required PCI. This study contained 563 patients (25% with NSTE-ACS) and randomized them to single antiplatelet treatment with clopidogrel or to DAPT with aspirin and clopidogrel. Patients on anticoagulation randomized to clopidogrel alone had significantly fewer bleeding complications than those randomized to Dual anti-platelet therapy (DAPT) (44). Furthermore, there was no significant difference in thrombotic events between the two treatment arms. Thus, when possible, shorter durations of triple therapy are recommended. Although there is no prospective data suggesting decreasing the target INR (international normalized ratio) to between 2.0 and 2.5 improves bleeding complication rates, it is currently a Class IIb recommendation that this may be reasonable in patients requiring triple therapy.

While the data on triple therapy using clopidogrel is limited, even fewer data are available regarding the use of newer P2Y$_{12}$ inhibitors such as prasugrel and ticagrelor in patients requiring oral anticoagulation. These medications are associated with more potent platelet activation and may be associated with increased bleeding (45). In the TRITON-TIMI 38 study, 13,608 patients with ACS undergoing PCI were randomized to either prasugrel or clopidogrel. Patients who received prasugrel had reduced rates of ischemic events, including death from cardiovascular causes, nonfatal myocardial infarction, or nonfatal stroke (9.9% vs. 12.1%; p < 0.001). Nevertheless, they had an increased risk of major bleeding (2.4% vs. 1.8%, p = 0.01), including life-threatening bleeding (1.4% vs. 0.9%, p = 0.01) (45). Thus, it is recommended that these agents be used with caution in patients who require triple therapy.

OTHER ORAL FACTOR Xa INHIBITORS IN NSTE-ACS

There is great current interest in the use of oral Factor Xa inhibitors for the treatment of ACS. It is theorized that many of the post-ACS/PCI cardiovascular events that occur despite aspirin and ADP-receptor antagonist administration may result from increased levels of thrombin generation precipitated by the initial event (46). As stated earlier, anticoagulants targeting Factor Xa have shown great promise in further downmodulating the thrombotic activation in ACS patients. Rivaroxaban, a direct oral factor Xa inhibitor, was studied in the double-blind placebo-controlled ATLAS-TIMI 51 study, which enrolled over 15,000 patients (47). In this trial, stabilized patients with recent ACS in whom the initial management strategy (e.g., revascularization) had already been completed were randomized to rivaroxaban 2.5 mg twice daily, 5 mg twice daily, or a placebo. Treatment with rivaroxaban was associated with a reduction in the primary study endpoint of death from cardiovascular causes, MI, or stroke compared with a placebo for both the 2.5-mg dose (9.1% vs. 10.7% with placebo, p = 0.02) and the 5-mg dose (8.8% vs. 10.7%

with placebo, p = 0.03). Despite these benefits, however, there was an increase in the rates of non-CABG–related major bleeding (2.1% vs. 0.6%, p < 0.001) and intracranial hemorrhage (0.6% vs. 0.2%, p = 0.009) in patients treated with rivaroxaban compared with a placebo, although bleeding complications were less frequent with the 2.5-mg dose of rivaroxaban compared with the 5-mg dose. Notably, the 2.5-mg dose of rivaroxaban was associated with a reduction in all-cause mortality compared with a placebo (2.9% vs. 4.5%, p = 0.002), although the trial was underpowered for this comparison. Furthermore, the PIONEER AF-PCI trial demonstrated that the use of rivaroxaban in patients requiring triple therapy may be safer than the use of warfarin. This study randomized 2,124 patients with atrial fibrillation undergoing PCI to either low-dose rivaroxaban (15 mg once daily), very low-dose rivaroxaban (2.5 mg twice daily), or standard therapy with warfarin. Patients receiving either a low dose or very low dose of rivaroxaban had significantly lower rates of bleeding compared to patients receiving warfarin (16.8% vs. 18.0% vs. 26.7%, p < 0.001). Furthermore, the rates of death from cardiovascular causes, MI, or stroke were similar between all treatment groups (48). This data suggests the safety of using these newer agents with DAPT; however, larger trials are needed. Furthermore, the role of this therapy as a third agent in the treatment of patients with ACS already on more potent dual antiplatelet therapies such as prasugrel or ticagrelor (see Chapter 17) is at present unstudied.

Apixaban, another oral Factor Xa inhibitor, was similarly studied to determine its efficacy in reducing post-ACS cardiovascular events in the APPRAISE-2 trial, a randomized double-blind placebo-controlled trial comparing apixaban 5 mg twice daily with a placebo on a background of aspirin or aspirin plus clopidogrel (49). While the trial managed to enroll over 7,000 patients, the study was stopped early, after review of the data demonstrated an increase in major bleeding events with apixaban compared with the placebo (1.3% vs. 0.5%, p = 0.001), without a counterbalancing reduction in ischemic events.

PCI in Patients on Oral Anticoagulants

It is not unusual to be presented in the catheterization laboratory with a patient fully therapeutic on warfarin or another oral anticoagulant prescribed for another indication (e.g., for stroke prevention in atrial fibrillation). In this scenario, as a general rule, it is recommended that the oral anticoagulant be discontinued (if possible and not contraindicated), and patients can then undergo angiography and/or PCI using standard techniques, including parenterally administered anticoagulation for PCI. For example, for patients undergoing elective PCI who are therapeutic on warfarin, it is recommended to stop warfarin therapy 2 to 3 days prior to the procedure, and once the procedure is complete (using standard parenteral anticoagulation if PCI is needed), patients can resume their home dose of medication. Patients being treated with the oral direct thrombin inhibitor dabigatran should have their medication stopped 1 to 2 days (if CrCl ≥ 50 mL/min) or 3 to 5 days (if CrCl < 50 mL/min) prior to the procedure; patients being treated with rivaroxaban or apixaban should have their medication stopped a day before the procedure. In low-risk patients, oral anticoagulants can typically be resumed after completion of the procedure.

For patients with mechanical valves or other indications requiring "bridging therapy," oral anticoagulation is typically converted to a parenteral agent such as UFH, which is typically maintained through the periprocedural period (and at a higher dose if PCI is required). Once the procedure is complete, the oral agent is typically resumed and the patient maintained on parenteral anticoagulation,

until the oral agent has taken effect. Patients in whom the indication for angiography and/or PCI is more urgent can proceed with these procedures while orally anticoagulated, particularly if a transradial approach is utilized.

Overview of ACC/AHA/SCAI Guideline Recommendations for STEMI

Fibrinolytic Therapy in STEMI

While there is no role for fibrinolytic therapy in UA/NSTEMI patients (1), fibrinolytic therapy plays a critical role in STEMI patients for whom the time delay to achieve successful reperfusion through primary PCI is too great. Fibrinolytic agents activate plasminogen by cleaving it into its active form plasmin, which promotes fibrin degradation. Fibrinolytic therapy is recommended when STEMI patients present to a non-PCI-capable hospital and patients are unable to be transferred to a PCI-capable facility within an anticipated first medical contact to PCI reperfusion time of 120 minutes (50). In addition, current guidelines recommend that fibrinolytic therapy should be administered within 30 minutes of patient presentation. There are specific contraindications to fibrinolytic therapy that should be noted (Table 4.3). Despite the benefits of fibrinolytic therapy in terms of improving reperfusion, fibrinolytic therapy is associated with a constant risk of major bleeding complications, including the most feared complication of intracranial hemorrhage, which occurs in <1% of patients, but with variability based upon patient characteristics (e.g., age).

The use of fibrinolytic therapy in STEMI patients has been well established as a reperfusion strategy (especially for patients with delays to primary PCI). The GISSI-1 trial, containing 11,712 STEMI patients, demonstrated that mortality rates at 21 days were significantly lower in patients treated with streptokinase compared to control patients (10.7% vs. 13%, p = 0.0002) (51). In the ISIS-2 trial, 17,187 patients were randomized to streptokinase alone, aspirin alone, and streptokinase with aspirin or placebo. Patients who received streptokinase with aspirin had lower rates of death (8.0% vs. 13.2%, p < 0.001) and reinfarction (1.8% vs. 2.9%, p < 0.001) compared with patients receiving a placebo (52). Furthermore, in the ASSET trial, which randomized 8,307 AMI patients to either tissue-type plasminogen activator (t-PA) with heparin to heparin alone, patients receiving t-PA had lower rates of 1 month mortality (relative reduction 26%) (53).

In addition, STEMI patients who present within the first 1 to 2 hours of symptom onset may benefit the most from immediate fibrinolytic therapy. In the CAPTIM trial, 840 patients were randomized to either primary PCI or to prehospital fibrinolysis with immediate transfer to PCI-capable facilities. At 30 days, there were no significant differences in outcomes between the two groups. Long-term follow-up

TABLE 4.3 Absolute Contraindications to Fibrinolytic Therapy

   a. Previous hemorrhagic stroke
   b. Ischemic stroke within 3 months (unless within 3 hours)
   c. Closed-head trauma within 3 months
   d. Intracranial neoplasm or AVM
   e. Active internal bleeding (not menses)
   f. Suspected aortic dissection

AVM, arteriovenous malformation.

at 5 years found that all-cause mortality was similar between the two groups; however, patients treated within 2 hours of symptom onset with fibrinolysis had lower rates of all-cause mortality than the primary PCI group (5.8% vs. 11.1%, p = 0.04) (54).

CHOICE OF FIBRINOLYTIC AGENT

The ACC/AHA guidelines recommend that fibrin-specific fibrinolytic agents (tenecteplase, reteplase, alteplase) be used over non-fibrin-specific agents (streptokinase) when available (50). Fibrin-specific agents deplete fibrinogen to a lesser extent than non-fibrin-specific agents, potentially improving the safety profile of these agents. The doses of fibrinolytic agents are detailed in **Table 4.4**. Multiple trials have compared the use of different thrombolytic therapies (55–59). Early studies demonstrated the superiority of t-PA compared to streptokinase. For example, the GUSTO investigators compared the use of t-PA to streptokinase in 41,021 patients with STEMI. Patients receiving t-PA with UFH had lower 30-day mortality rates (6.3% vs. 7.4%, p = 0.001) and death or disabling stroke rates (6.9% vs. 7.8%, p = 0.006) compared to streptokinase with UFH (55). In addition, the rate of infarct-related artery patency at 90 minutes was higher in patients receiving t-PA with intravenous UFH compared to patients receiving streptokinase with UFH (81% vs. 60%, p < 0.001) (57). These findings suggested the superiority of t-PA over streptokinase.

Subsequent trials comparing recombinant plasminogen activator (rPA) and tenecteplase (TNK-tPA) to t-PA failed to show superiority of these agents over t-PA. For example, the GUSTO III trial compared rPA to t-PA in 15,059 STEMI patients. Mortality rates were similar between these two therapies at 30 days (4.5% vs. 7.2%, p = NS) and 1 year (11.2% vs. 11.1%, p = NS) (59). Similarly, the ASSENT-2 trial compared TNK-tPA to t-PA and found no significant difference in mortality between the two randomized groups (6.2% vs. 6.2%, p = NS) (58).

Anticoagulants in STEMI

The ACC/AHA guidelines summarizing the recommendations for the use of anticoagulant therapy in STEMI patients separate anticoagulant management of these patients on the treatment strategy: for primary PCI, as an adjunct to fibrinolytic therapy, or support for PCI after administration of fibrinolytic therapy. Support for PCI after fibrinolytic therapy can occur during a rescue PCI strategy (PCI

after a patient demonstrates signs or symptoms of failed reperfusion after fibrinolytic therapy) or as part of a pharmacoinvasive strategy (after fibrinolytic therapy the patient is transferred to a PCI-capable hospital for early coronary angiography and PCI when appropriate). Treatment strategies for STEMI are discussed in depth in Chapter 18.

Similar to NSTE-ACS, several classes of anticoagulants have been shown to be effective in treating patients with STEMI: UFH, enoxaparin, and direct thrombin inhibitors. Rapid reperfusion in STEMI patients is of utmost importance, and delays to reperfusion are associated with higher mortality rates (60). Thus, the need for rapid reperfusion drives the choice of reperfusion strategy and likely trumps the actual anticoagulant strategy chosen (50). Anticoagulation in STEMI patients is generally administered during PCI in order to suppress the ongoing thrombotic process, or any additional thrombosis that may be precipitated by equipment and vessel injury during PCI. In addition, anticoagulants are used to maintain vessel patency after fibrinolytic therapy.

Anticoagulant Use in Primary PCI

Primary PCI is the recommended reperfusion method when it can be performed within 120 minutes of the patient's presentation to a medical facility (50). In fact, immediate transfer to a PCI-capable hospital for primary PCI is preferred for STEMI patients when a first medical contact to reperfusion time is anticipated to be less than 120 minutes. For STEMI patients undergoing primary PCI, ACC/AHA guidelines recommend supportive anticoagulation with either UFH or bivalirudin (Class I indication). In contrast, fondaparinux should not be used as a sole anticoagulant in these patients (Class III indication) for reasons of possible increased catheter thrombosis as described earlier.

CHOICE OF ANTICOAGULANT

UFH during primary PCI for STEMI has been routinely used and has been widely accepted. As a result, there are limited trial data examining its efficacy and safety compared with a background of no UFH. The HORIZONS-AMI trial demonstrated the effectiveness of bivalirudin use in STEMI patients (61) by randomizing 3,602 STEMI patients undergoing primary PCI to either heparin with GP IIb/IIIa therapy or to bivalirudin alone. Patients treated with bivalirudin had similar rates of major adverse cardiovascular events (5.4% vs. 5.5%, p = 0.95) compared to patients receiving heparin; however, patients treated with bivalirudin had significantly lower rates of major bleeding (4.9% vs. 8.3%, p < 0.001). Thus, bivalirudin is a possible alternative for anticoagulation during primary PCI, especially in patients who are at higher risk of bleeding.

While bivalirudin has been established as an anticoagulant choice in STEMI patients, the optimal anticoagulant therapy has not been established. Prior studies compared the use of bivalirudin to heparin with routine GP IIb/IIIa inhibition. Recent studies have provided conflicting data regarding whether patients receiving bivalirudin have better outcomes compared with heparin when both patient populations receive GP IIb/IIIa only as a bailout therapy and GP IIb/IIIa is not a mandated therapy. The first study to investigate this question was the single center HEAT-PPCI trial which randomized 1,829 STEMI patients in a single center to either bivalirudin or heparin therapy. At 28 days, patients receiving bivalirudin had higher rates of the composite primary endpoint (all-cause mortality, cerebrovascular accidents, reinfarction, or unplanned target lesion revascularization) compared to patients receiving heparin (8.7% vs. 5.7%, p = 0.01) (62). Stent thrombosis was also increased with the bivalirudin-only regimen. Since HEAT-PPCI, additional multicenter trials such as MATRIX and BRIGHT have investigated this clinical question and

TABLE 4.4	Dosing of Fibrinolytic Agents in STEMI
FIBRINOLYTIC AGENT	**DOSE**
Tenecteplase	Single weight-based bolus <60 kg: 30 mg 60–69 kg: 35 mg 70–79 kg: 40 mg 80–89 kg: 45 mg ≥90 kg: 50 mg
Reteplase	10 U plus 10 U IV boluses given 30 minutes apart
Alteplase	90 min weight-based infusion Bolus 15 mg, infusion 0.75 mg/kg for 30 min (max 50 mg) then 0.5 mg/kg (max 35 mg) over next 60 minutes; total dose not to exceed 100 mg
Streptokinase	1.5 million units IV given over 30–60 minutes

IV, intravenous.

have provided conflicting results as described in the NSTE-ACS section. Postulated reasons for these differences in outcomes have included the following: differences between the practice patterns captured within single center versus multicenter studies; differences in included patient populations across studies; type of access (femoral vs. radial) used; doses of anticoagulant; and the duration of anticoagulation (with longer durations of the bivalirudin infusion seeming to mitigate the acute stent thrombosis seen with bivalirudin monotherapy). The VALIDATE-SWEDEHEART trial is an ongoing multicenter, prospective, randomized, registry-based, controlled clinical trial of AMI patients investigating whether bivalirudin use in patients receiving contemporary dual anti-platelet therapy (ticagrelor, prasugrel, or cangrelor) have improved outcomes compared to patients receiving heparin (63). This large trial, enrolling 6,000 patients, will provide important data to help answer this question.

There is limited data on the role of enoxaparin use in STEMI patients receiving primary PCI. In the ATOLL study, in which 910 patients were randomized to receive either enoxaparin or UFH, treatment with enoxaparin had similar rates of the composite primary endpoint, including death, complication of MI, procedure failure, or major bleeding (28% vs. 34%, p = 0.06) (64). Furthermore, there were no differences in the rates of the individual component events. As a result, enoxaparin is not a recommended anticoagulant for STEMI patients undergoing primary PCI.

DOSING STRATEGY

Dosing of UFH during primary PCI is dependent on whether GP IIb/IIIa use is planned (Table 4.5). When GP IIb/IIIa use is not anticipated, a bolus of 70 to 100 U/kg heparin bolus is given to achieve a recommended ACT target of 250 to 300 seconds (HemoTec device) or 300 to 350 seconds (Hemochron device). With GP IIb/IIIa use, a lower initial bolus of UFH is given (50–70 U/kg IV bolus) with a goal ACT between 200 and 250 seconds.

For primary PCI, bivalirudin is given as 0.75 mg/kg IV bolus followed by a 1.75 mg/kg/hr infusion regardless of prior treatment with UFH. An additional bolus of 0.3 mg/kg may be given if needed. Because this medication is renally cleared, the bivalirudin infusion should be reduced to 1 mg/kg/hr if the patient has a CrCl <30 mL/min.

Anticoagulant Use with Fibrinolytic Therapy

Regardless of the choice of fibrinolytic agent, patients who have received fibrinolytic therapy should receive additional anticoagulation for the duration of the hospitalization (up to 8 days or until revascularization is performed) and for a minimum of 48 hours. In these cases, anticoagulation is used to maintain coronary vessel patency after clot lysis with fibrinolytic therapy. After fibrinolytic therapy, recurrent clot formation may occur as a result of increased thrombin activity, which can lead to recurrent coronary thrombosis (65). This may be suppressed by either UFH, enoxaparin, or fondaparinux.

Choice of Anticoagulant

Early studies demonstrated that concurrent treatment with heparin in patients receiving fibrinolytic therapy resulted in improved coronary patency rates. In a study containing 84 patients, patients

TABLE 4.5 Dosing of Anticoagulant Agents in STEMI

	DURING PRIMARY PCI	AFTER FIBRINOLYTIC THERAPY	DELAYED PCI AFTER FIBRINOLYTIC THERAPY
Bivalirudin	0.75 mg/kg IV bolus then 1.75 mg/kg/h infusion with or without prior UFH treatment. Additional 0.3 mg/kg bolus if needed. Reduce infusion to 1 mg/kg/h if CrCl <30 mL/min.	NA	NA
Unfractionated heparin (UFH)	IV GP IIb/IIIa planned: 50–70 U/kg IV bolus to achieve target ACT 200–250. No IV GP IIb/IIIa planned: 70–100 U/kg bolus to achieve target ACT 250–300	Weight-adjusted IV bolus and infusion to obtain activated partial thromboplastin time 1.5–2.0 times the control. 60 U/kg (max 4,000 U) IV bolus followed by 12 U/kg/h infusion (max 1,000 U).	Continue through PCI with additional doses to achieve therapeutic ACT
Enoxaparin	NA	If age <75 y, 30 mg IV bolus followed in 15 minutes by 1 mg/kg SC injection every 12 hours (max 100 mg for the first two doses). If age ≥75 years, 0.75 mg/kg SC every 12 hours (max 75 mg for the first two doses). Regardless of age, if CrCl <30 mL/min, use 1 mg/kg SC every 12 hours.	Last dose within 8 hours: no additional dose required. Last dose 8–12 hours earlier: 0.3 mg/kg IV bolus.
Fondaparinux	Should not be used as sole agent	Initial 2.5 mg IV dose followed by 2.5 mg SC injections in 24 if CrCl >30 mL/min	Should not be used as sole agent

ACT, activated clotting time; CrCl, creatinine clearance; GP, glycoprotein; IV, intravenous; PCI, percutaneous coronary intervention; SC, subcutaneous.

were randomized to receiving tissue plasminogen activator with and without heparin anticoagulation. All patients underwent coronary angiography 3 days after fibrinolytic therapy to document vessel patency. Patients who received concurrent heparin had higher rates of vessel patency after fibrinolytic therapy (71% vs. 43%, p = 0.015) (66). Furthermore, in the HART trial, 205 patients were randomized to either aspirin or heparin after fibrinolysis with t-PA. Patients underwent angiography 7 to 24 hours after fibrinolysis. Patients receiving heparin had higher rates of infarct-related artery patency compared to patients only receiving aspirin (82% vs. 52%, p < 0.0001) (67).

The use of enoxaparin after fibrinolytic therapy has been studied against heparin therapy. In the ASSENT-3 trial, containing 6,095 STEMI patients receiving fibrinolytic therapy, patients receiving enoxaparin had lower rates of the composite 30-day endpoint of mortality, in-hospital reinfarction, or in-hospital refractory ischemia compared to patients receiving heparin (11.4% vs. 15.4%, p = 0.0002) (68). In addition, patients receiving enoxaparin had lower rates of in-hospital intracranial hemorrhage or major bleeding complications (13.7% vs. 17.0%, p = 0.0037). As a result of these findings, enoxaparin is recommended after fibrinolytic therapy and is the preferred anticoagulation therapy over heparin after 48 hours.

A subgroup analysis of the OASIS-6 trial demonstrated the benefit of using fondaparinux in STEMI patients undergoing fibrinolytic therapy (69). Of the 5,436 patients included in this analysis, 2,692 patients received fondaparinux. Treatment with fondaparinux was associated with lower rates of death and MI at 30 days (HR 0.79 [95% CI: 0.68–0.92]) compared to patients receiving UFH. Furthermore, the risk of severe bleeding was reduced among patients receiving fondaparinux (HR 0.62 [95% CI: 0.40–0.94]).

DOSING STRATEGY

For patients receiving fibrinolytic therapy, UFH should be administered as a weight-adjusted intravenous bolus and infusion to obtain an activated partial thromboplastin time of 1.5 to 2.0 times the control for 48 hours or until revascularization (Table 4.5). An IV bolus of 60 U/kg (maximum 4,000 U) followed by an infusion of 12 U/kg/hr (maximum 1,000 U). Enoxaparin should be given as an IV bolus, followed in 15 minutes by a SC injection. If the patient's age is <75, a 30-mg IV bolus is administered, followed in 15 minutes by 1 mg/kg subcutaneously every 12 hours (maximum 100 mg for the first two doses). If the patient's age is ≥75, a bolus is not given and only a 0.75 mg/kg SC injection every 12 hours (maximum 75 mg for the first two doses) is administered. If the patient has impaired renal function (CrCl < 30 mL/min), only a 1 mg/kg SC injection every 24 hours of enoxaparin should be administered, regardless of the patient's age. Fondaparinux should be administered with an initial intravenous dose, followed by daily SC injections if the patient's CrCl is greater than 30 mL/min. An initial dose of fondaparinux 2.5 mg IV, and then 2.5 mg SC daily starting the following day, may be used for the duration of the hospitalization up to 8 days or until revascularization.

Anticoagulant Use with Delayed PCI after Fibrinolytic Therapy

Despite appropriate doses of fibrinolytic therapy, a proportion of patients will still require PCI because of evidence of failed reperfusion or reocclusion of the target vessel. In these situations, anticoagulation should be continued uninterrupted from the time after fibrinolytic therapy to the time of the PCI procedure. Patients may be switched from UFH to bivalirudin for PCI. In addition, if the last dose of enoxaparin was >12 hours prior to PCI, the patient may be switched to either UFH or bivalirudin.

There are limited data comparing anticoagulation strategies in STEMI patients undergoing PCI after receiving fibrinolytic therapy. The EXTRACT-TIMI 25 trial compared the using of enoxaparin to UFH in 20,479 STEMI patients undergoing PCI after fibrinolytic therapy. Patients who received enoxaparin had lower rates of death or recurrent MI through 30 days compared to patients receiving UFH (10.7% vs. 13.8%, p < 0.001) and there were no differences in major bleeding. Thus, enoxaparin use is an effective anticoagulant strategy in these patients.

DOSING STRATEGY

ACT monitoring should be performed on patients receiving UFH undergoing PCI after fibrinolytic therapy. Additional boluses of heparin should be administered in order to achieve appropriate ACT targets, depending on whether concomitant GP IIb/IIIa receptor antagonists are administered (Table 4.5). Patients receiving enoxaparin prior to PCI do not need additional anticoagulation dosing if the PCI is performed within 8 hours of the last enoxaparin administration. If PCI is performed 8 to 12 hours after the last dose of enoxaparin, an additional enoxaparin 0.3 mg/kg IV bolus should be administered.

Future Directions

Because of their antithrombotic effects, anticoagulants remain a cornerstone of therapy for patients with NSTE-ACS and STEMI. Despite an abundance of trial data on the use of anticoagulants for ACS and PCI, further trials are ongoing in an attempt to bring to market newer anticoagulants that will help improve the management and treatment of high-risk patients with atherothrombotic disease. Several of these agents are within the classes of agents discussed earlier, and other agents belong to novel classes of agents, with different mechanisms of action. Clearly affecting the development of novel anticoagulants is the increasing recognition of the complementary importance of both ischemic and bleeding events. The development of novel anticoagulant agents has therefore focused upon attempts to either provide incremental gains in anti-ischemic benefits without further increases in bleeding risk or preserve the anti-ischemic benefits of current agents while incrementally lowering bleeding risks. In light of the decreasing event rates in clinical trials of antithrombotic therapy because of the advances already made in this space, the margins through which these potential incremental clinical benefits can be measured are slim, and the clinical trial sizes required to demonstrate these gains with statistical confidence often can be daunting. Nonetheless, further study of novel anticoagulant agents remains an area of active interest and investigation.

Key Points

■ All NSTE-ACS and STEMI patients (without contraindications) should be started on an anticoagulant as soon as possible after presentation (Class I). Similarly, all PCI patients should be started on a parenteral anticoagulant at the time of PCI (Class I).

■ The duration of anticoagulation for patients undergoing PCI is up until (but not after) the PCI is performed.

■ Four different agents are recommended as Class I upstream options for UA/NSTEMI patients being managed with an invasive strategy: UFH, enoxaparin, bivalirudin, or fondaparinux.

■ At the time of PCI, agents with Class I recommendations include bivalirudin and UFH in NSTE-ACS and STEMI patients.

■ Use of fondaparinux alone as an anticoagulant during PCI is contraindicated. Patients treated with upstream fondaparinux who require PCI should be treated with UFH at the time of the PCI to avoid catheter-related thrombus.

■ The benefits and risks of triple antithrombotic therapy with aspirin, clopidogrel, and warfarin in NSTE-ACS have not been clearly established. Such therapy should be selected for clear indications for extended duration of oral anticoagulation, and given for the shortest duration of time, at the minimally effective doses necessary to achieve protection.

■ Time to reperfusion in STEMI patients is of upmost importance and may be more important than reperfusion strategy (primary PCI vs. fibrinolytic therapy).

■ Fibrin-specific agents (tenecteplase, reteplase, alteplase) are preferred agents over non-fibrin-specific fibrinolytics (streptokinase) in STEMI patients undergoing fibrinolysis.

■ Three different anticoagulant agents are recommended as Class I options for STEMI patients receiving fibrinolytic therapy: UFH, enoxaparin, or fondaparinux.

References

1. Amsterdam EA, et al. 2014 AHA/ACC guideline for the management of patients with non-ST-elevation acute coronary syndromes: a report of the American College of Cardiology/American Heart Association Task Force on Practice Guidelines. *J Am Coll Cardiol.* 2014;64:e139–228.
2. Yusuf S, et al. Comparison of fondaparinux and enoxaparin in acute coronary syndromes. *N Engl J Med.* 2006;354:1464–1476.
3. Rao SV, et al. Bleeding and blood transfusion issues in patients with non-ST-segment elevation acute coronary syndromes. *Eur Heart J.* 2007;28:1193–1204.
4. Mehran R, et al. Associations of major bleeding and myocardial infarction with the incidence and timing of mortality in patients presenting with non-ST-elevation acute coronary syndromes: a risk model from the ACUITY trial. *Eur Heart J.* 2009;30:1457–1466.
5. Petersen JL, et al. Efficacy and bleeding complications among patients randomized to enoxaparin or unfractionated heparin for antithrombin therapy in non-ST-Segment elevation acute coronary syndromes: a systematic overview. *JAMA.* 2004;292:89–96.
6. Spaulding C, et al. Left radial approach for coronary angiography: results of a prospective study. *Cathet Cardiovasc Diagn.* 1996;39:365–370.
7. Levine GN, et al. 2011 ACCF/AHA/SCAI guideline for percutaneous coronary intervention: executive summary: a report of the American College of Cardiology Foundation/American Heart Association Task Force on practice guidelines and the society for cardiovascular angiography and interventions. *Catheter Cardiovasc Interv.* 2012;79:453–495.
8. Oler A, et al. Adding heparin to aspirin reduces the incidence of myocardial infarction and death in patients with unstable angina. A meta-analysis. *JAMA.* 1996;276:811–815.
9. Anand SS, et al. Relationship of activated partial thromboplastin time to coronary events and bleeding in patients with acute coronary syndromes who receive heparin. *Circulation.* 2003;107:2884–2888.
10. Chew DP, et al. Defining the optimal activated clotting time during percutaneous coronary intervention: aggregate results from 6 randomized, controlled trials. *Circulation.* 2001;103:961–966.
11. Brener SJ, et al. Relationship between activated clotting time and ischemic or hemorrhagic complications: analysis of 4 recent randomized clinical trials of percutaneous coronary intervention. *Circulation.* 2004;110:994–998.
12. Melloni C, et al. Unfractionated heparin dosing and risk of major bleeding in non-ST-segment elevation acute coronary syndromes. *Am Heart J.* 2008;156:209–215.
13. Alexander KP, et al. Excess dosing of antiplatelet and antithrombin agents in the treatment of non-ST-segment elevation acute coronary syndromes. *JAMA.* 2005;294:3108–3116.
14. Arepally GM, Ortel TL. Clinical practice. Heparin-induced thrombocytopenia. *N Engl J Med.* 2006;355:809–817.
15. Granger CB, et al. Rebound increase in thrombin generation and activity after cessation of intravenous heparin in patients with acute coronary syndromes. *Circulation.* 1995;91:1929–1935.
16. Low-molecular-weight heparin during instability in coronary artery disease, Fragmin during Instability in Coronary Artery Disease (FRISC) study group. *Lancet.* 1996;347:561–568.
17. Antman EM, et al. Assessment of the treatment effect of enoxaparin for unstable angina/non-Q-wave myocardial infarction. TIMI 11B-ESSENCE meta-analysis. *Circulation.* 1999;100:1602–1608.
18. Ferguson JJ, et al. Enoxaparin vs unfractionated heparin in high-risk patients with non-ST-segment elevation acute coronary syndromes managed with an intended early invasive strategy: primary results of the SYNERGY randomized trial. *JAMA.* 2004;292:45–54.
19. Blazing MA, et al. Safety and efficacy of enoxaparin vs unfractionated heparin in patients with non-ST-segment elevation acute coronary syndromes who receive tirofiban and aspirin: a randomized controlled trial. *JAMA.* 2004;292:55–64.
20. Drouet L, Bal dit Sollier C, Martin J. Adding intravenous unfractionated heparin to standard enoxaparin causes excessive anticoagulation not detected by activated clotting time: results of the STACK-on to ENOXaparin (STACKENOX) study. *Am Heart J.* 2009;158:177–184.
21. Montalescot G, et al. Enoxaparin versus unfractionated heparin in elective percutaneous coronary intervention 1-year results from the STEEPLE (SafeTy and efficacy of enoxaparin in percutaneous coronary intervention patients, an international randomized evaluation) trial. *JACC Cardiovasc Interv.* 2009;2:1083–1091.
22. Michalis LK, et al. Enoxaparin versus tinzaparin in non-ST-segment elevation acute coronary syndromes: the EVET trial. *Am Heart J.* 2003;146:304–310.
23. Dana A, et al. Macroscopic thrombus formation on angioplasty equipment following antithrombin therapy with enoxaparin. *Catheter Cardiovasc Interv.* 2007;70:847–853.
24. Gori AM, et al. Tissue factor and tissue factor pathway inhibitor levels in unstable angina patients during short-term low-molecular-weight heparin administration. *Br J Haematol.* 2002;117:693–698.
25. Global Use of Strategies to Open Occluded Coronary Arteries (GUSTO) IIb investigators. A comparison of recombinant hirudin with heparin for the treatment of acute coronary syndromes. *N Engl J Med.* 1996;335:775–782.
26. Effects of recombinant hirudin (lepirudin) compared with heparin on death, myocardial infarction, refractory angina, and revascularisation procedures in patients with acute myocardial ischaemia without ST elevation: a randomised trial. Organisation to Assess Strategies for Ischemic Syndromes (OASIS-2) Investigators. *Lancet.* 1999;353:429–438.
27. Direct Thrombin Inhibitor Trialists' Collaborative Group. Direct thrombin inhibitors in acute coronary syndromes: principal results of a meta-analysis based on individual patients' data. *Lancet.* 2002;359:294–302.
28. Bittl JA, et al. Treatment with bivalirudin (Hirulog) as compared with heparin during coronary angioplasty for unstable or postinfarction angina. Hirulog Angioplasty Study Investigators. *N Engl J Med.* 1995;333:764–769.
29. Bittl JA, et al. Bivalirudin versus heparin during coronary angioplasty for unstable or postinfarction angina: final report reanalysis of the Bivalirudin Angioplasty Study. *Am Heart J.* 2001;142:952–959.
30. Stone GW, et al. Bivalirudin for patients with acute coronary syndromes. *N Engl J Med.* 2006;355:2203–2216.

31. Kastrati A, et al. Bivalirudin versus unfractionated heparin during percutaneous coronary intervention. *N Engl J Med*. 2008;359:688–696.

32. Kastrati A, et al. Abciximab and heparin versus bivalirudin for non-ST-elevation myocardial infarction. *N Engl J Med*. 2011;365:1980–1989.

33. Valgimigli M, et al. Bivalirudin or unfractionated heparin in acute coronary syndromes. *N Engl J Med*. 2015;373:997–1009.

34. Leonardi S, et al. Bivalirudin or unfractionated heparin in patients with acute coronary syndromes managed invasively with and without ST elevation (MATRIX): randomised controlled trial. *BMJ*. 2016;354:i4935.

35. Han Y, et al. Bivalirudin vs heparin with or without tirofiban during primary percutaneous coronary intervention in acute myocardial infarction: the BRIGHT randomized clinical trial. *JAMA*. 2015;313:1336–1346.

36. Lincoff AM, et al. Comparison of bivalirudin versus heparin during percutaneous coronary intervention (the Randomized Evaluation of PCI Linking Angiomax to Reduced Clinical Events [REPLACE]-1 trial). *Am J Cardiol*. 2004;93:1092–1096.

37. Lincoff AM, et al. Bivalirudin and provisional glycoprotein IIb/IIIa blockade compared with heparin and planned glycoprotein IIb/IIIa blockade during percutaneous coronary intervention: REPLACE-2 randomized trial. *JAMA*. 2003;289:853–863.

38. Gibson CM, et al. Association of prerandomization anticoagulant switching with bleeding in the setting of percutaneous coronary intervention (A REPLACE-2 analysis). *Am J Cardiol*. 2007;99:1687–1690.

39. Steg PG, et al. Low-dose vs standard-dose unfractionated heparin for percutaneous coronary intervention in acute coronary syndromes treated with fondaparinux: the FUTURA/OASIS-8 randomized trial. *JAMA*. 2010;304:1339–1349.

40. Paolucci F, et al. Fondaparinux sodium mechanism of action: identification of specific binding to purified and human plasma-derived proteins. *Clin Pharmacokinet*. 2002;41(suppl 2):11–18.

41. Leon MB, et al. A clinical trial comparing three antithrombotic-drug regimens after coronary-artery stenting. Stent Anticoagulation Restenosis Study Investigators. *N Engl J Med*. 1998;339:1665–1671.

42. Effects of long-term, moderate-intensity oral anticoagulation in addition to aspirin in unstable angina. The Organization to Assess Strategies for Ischemic Syndromes (OASIS) Investigators. *J Am Coll Cardiol*. 2001;37:475–484.

43. Hurlen M, et al. Warfarin, aspirin, or both after myocardial infarction. *N Engl J Med*. 2002;347:969–974.

44. Dewilde WJ, et al. Use of clopidogrel with or without aspirin in patients taking oral anticoagulant therapy and undergoing percutaneous coronary intervention: an open-label, randomised, controlled trial. *Lancet*. 2013;381:1107–1115.

45. Wiviott SD, et al. Prasugrel versus clopidogrel in patients with acute coronary syndromes. *N Engl J Med*. 2007;357:2001–2015.

46. Merlini PA, et al. Persistent activation of coagulation mechanism in unstable angina and myocardial infarction. *Circulation*. 1994;90:61–68.

47. Mega JL, et al. Rivaroxaban in patients with a recent acute coronary syndrome. *N Engl J Med*. 2012;366:9–19.

48. Gibson CM, et al. Prevention of bleeding in patients with atrial fibrillation undergoing PCI. *N Engl J Med*. 2016;375:2423–2434.

49. Alexander JH, et al. Apixaban with antiplatelet therapy after acute coronary syndrome. *N Engl J Med*. 2011;365:699–708.

50. O'Gara PT, et al. 2013 ACCF/AHA guideline for the management of ST-elevation myocardial infarction: executive summary: a report of the American College of Cardiology Foundation/American Heart Association Task Force on Practice Guidelines: developed in collaboration with the American College of Emergency Physicians and Society for Cardiovascular Angiography and Interventions. *Catheter Cardiovasc Interv*. 2013;82:E1–E27.

51. Effectiveness of intravenous thrombolytic treatment in acute myocardial infarction. Gruppo Italiano per lo Studio della Streptochinasi nell'Infarto Miocardico (GISSI). *Lancet*. 1986;1:397–402.

52. Randomised trial of intravenous streptokinase, oral aspirin, both, or neither among 17,187 cases of suspected acute myocardial infarction: ISIS-2. ISIS-2 (Second International Study of Infarct Survival) Collaborative Group. *Lancet*. 1988;2:349–360.

53. Wilcox RG, et al. Trial of tissue plasminogen activator for mortality reduction in acute myocardial infarction. Anglo-Scandinavian Study of Early Thrombolysis (ASSET). *Lancet*. 1988;2:525–530.

54. Bonnefoy E, et al. Comparison of primary angioplasty and pre-hospital fibrinolysis in acute myocardial infarction (CAPTIM) trial: a 5-year follow-up. *Eur Heart J*. 2009;30:1598–1606.

55. The GUSTO investigators. An international randomized trial comparing four thrombolytic strategies for acute myocardial infarction. *N Engl J Med*. 1993;329:673–682.

56. Bode C, et al. Randomized comparison of coronary thrombolysis achieved with double-bolus reteplase (recombinant plasminogen activator) and front-loaded, accelerated alteplase (recombinant tissue plasminogen activator) in patients with acute myocardial infarction. The RAPID II Investigators. *Circulation*. 1996;94:891–898.

57. The GUSTO Angiographic Investigators. The effects of tissue plasminogen activator, streptokinase, or both on coronary-artery patency, ventricular function, and survival after acute myocardial infarction. *N Engl J Med*. 1993;329:1615–1622.

58. Van De Werf F, et al. Single-bolus tenecteplase compared with front-loaded alteplase in acute myocardial infarction: the ASSENT-2 double-blind randomised trial. *Lancet*. 1999;354:716–722.

59. Topol EJ, et al. Survival outcomes 1 year after reperfusion therapy with either alteplase or reteplase for acute myocardial infarction: results from the Global Utilization of Streptokinase and t-PA for Occluded Coronary Arteries (GUSTO) III Trial. *Circulation*. 2000;102:1761–1765.

60. Rathore SS, et al. Association of door-to-balloon time and mortality in patients admitted to hospital with ST elevation myocardial infarction: national cohort study. *BMJ*. 2009;338:b1807.

61. Stone GW, et al. Bivalirudin during primary PCI in acute myocardial infarction. *N Engl J Med*. 2008;358:2218–2230.

62. Shahzad A, et al. Unfractionated heparin versus bivalirudin in primary percutaneous coronary intervention (HEAT-PPCI): an open-label, single centre, randomised controlled trial. *Lancet*. 2014;384:1849–1858.

63. Erlinge D, et al. Bivalirudin versus heparin in non-ST and ST-segment elevation myocardial infarction-a registry-based randomized clinical trial in the SWEDEHEART registry (the VALIDATE-SWEDEHEART trial). *Am Heart J*. 2016;175:36–46.

64. Montalescot G, et al. Intravenous enoxaparin or unfractionated heparin in primary percutaneous coronary intervention for ST-elevation myocardial infarction: the international randomised open-label ATOLL trial. *Lancet*. 2011;378:693–703.

65. Eisenberg PR. Role of heparin in coronary thrombolysis. *Chest*. 1992;101:131S–139S.

66. Bleich SD, et al. Effect of heparin on coronary arterial patency after thrombolysis with tissue plasminogen activator in acute myocardial infarction. *Am J Cardiol*. 1990;66:1412–1417.

67. Hsia J, et al. A comparison between heparin and low-dose aspirin as adjunctive therapy with tissue plasminogen activator for acute myocardial infarction. Heparin-Aspirin Reperfusion Trial (HART) Investigators. *N Engl J Med*. 1990;323:1433–1437.

68. Assessment of the Safety and Efficacy of a New Thrombolytic Regimen (ASSENT)-3 Investigators. Efficacy and safety of tenecteplase in combination with enoxaparin, abciximab, or unfractionated heparin: the ASSENT-3 randomised trial in acute myocardial infarction. *Lancet*. 2001;358:605–613.

69. Peters RJ, et al. The role of fondaparinux as an adjunct to thrombolytic therapy in acute myocardial infarction: a subgroup analysis of the OASIS-6 trial. *Eur Heart J*. 2008;29:324–331.

5

Vasoactive and Antiarrhythmic Drugs in the Catheterization Laboratory

Gilbert Zoghbi, MD, FSCAI, FACC

Vasoactive Drugs

Vasodilators

Coronary vasodilators are generally classified into endothelium-dependent or endothelium-independent based on their mode of action (**Table 5.1**). The endothelium-dependent drugs act via a healthy endothelium to convert L-arginine into nitric oxide, which in turn relaxes the vascular smooth muscle cells (VSMCs), causing vasodilation. The endothelium-independent drugs bypass the endothelium and act directly on the VSMCs to convert guanosine-5′-triphosphate (GTP) into cyclic guanosine monophosphate (GMP), leading to vascular smooth muscle relaxation and subsequent vasodilation (1).

NITROGLYCERIN

Nitroglycerin is metabolized in the VSMCs into nitric oxide, which is in turn converted to S-nitrosothiol that activates guanylate cyclase and generates cyclic GMP, resulting in smooth muscle relaxation and vasodilatation of the various venous and coronary or noncoronary vessels. Nitroglycerin has a more pronounced effect on the venous compared to the arterial circulation. In patients with angina, nitroglycerin's anti-ischemic effect is more related to venodilatation and preload reduction, which reduces myocardial wall stress, which in turn decreases myocardial oxygen demand and indirectly improves sub-endocardial myocardial flow and collateral flow when present. Nitroglycerin dilates both normal and diseased coronary arteries; however, this action is of uncertain clinical importance except in patients who have vasospastic angina.

Nitroglycerin has a rapid onset of action and a short duration. It can be administered via the sublingual, intra-arterial (IA), intravenous (IV), intra-coronary (IC), or intra-ventricular route. Nitroglycerin is generally used in the catheterization laboratory to prevent or treat arterial spasm, and is used during coronary angiography or percutaneous coronary interventions (PCIs) to improve coronary flow, prevent or alleviate coronary spasm, provoke myocardial bridging, relieve angina, or reduce preload in patients with elevated filling pressures (1).

Prophylactic administration of IC nitroglycerin is commonly used before intravascular ultrasound (IVUS) or rotablation device activation. Nitroglycerin is also used in the pharmacologic cocktail given via the radial artery to prevent or treat radial artery spasm during transradial procedures. Sublingual nitroglycerin is administered as a 0.4-mg tablet or spray. IV, IA, or IC nitroglycerin is commonly administered in 50- to 400-μg boluses. Higher doses can result in hypotension and reflex tachycardia without further augmentation in coronary blood. Nitroglycerin should not be administered to patients with a systolic blood pressure of <90 mm Hg, or to patients who have taken phosphodiesterase-5 inhibitors within 24 (sildenafil [Viagra or Revatio], avanafil [Stendra or Spedra] and vardenafil [Levitra]) to 48 hours (tadalafil [Cialis or Adcirca]) (2). It should be administered very cautiously to patients with severe aortic stenosis, hypertrophic cardiomyopathy, severe left main disease, right ventricular infarctions, volume depletion, or volume-dependent pathology (such as restrictive cardiomyopathy) due to increased risk of an exaggerated and deleterious hypotensive response (1,3,4). Hypotension caused by the administration of nitroglycerin can be treated with administration of IV fluids or α agonists.

NITROPRUSSIDE

Nitroprusside is a direct nitric oxide donor that activates guanylate cyclase and generates cyclic GMP, resulting in smooth muscle relaxation and subsequent vasodilatation of the various venous and arterial beds. Unlike nitroglycerine, nitroprusside has a more potent effect on the arterial beds compared to the venous beds. Nitroprusside can be

TABLE 5.1 Properties and Hemodynamic Effects of the Adrenergic Agonists (1,29,31)							
	RECEPTOR				EFFECT		
	D	β1	β1	β2	BP	CI	HR
Dopamine							
Low (<3 μg/kg/min)	++	0	+	0	0	0–↑	0–↑
Medium (3–7 μg/kg/min)	++	++	++	+	↑	↑	↑
High (>7 μg/kg/min)	++	++++	++++	+	↑↑	↑↑	↑↑
Dobutamine	0	0/+	++++	+++	0–↓	↑↑↑	↑
Epinephrine	0	++++	++++	++	↑↑↑	↑↑	↑↑↑
Norepinephrine	0	++++	++++	+	↑↑↑	↑↑	↑↑
Phenylephrine	0	++++	0	0	↑↑	0	0
Isoproterenol	0	0	++++	++++	0–↓	↑↑↑	↑↑↑

BP, blood pressure; CI, cardiac index, HR: heart rate.

used to treat hypertensive crisis and acute heart failure, particularly due to acute mitral regurgitation. The IV nitroprusside dose starts at 0.25 to 0.3 μg/kg/min and can be titrated by 0.5 μg/kg/min every few minutes to achieve the desired hemodynamic effects (maximum dose of 10 μg/kg/min). Nitroprusside has been used to treat slow flow or no-reflow during PCIs and is given in 25- to 200-μg IC boluses with a quick saline flush of up to 1,000 μg (1,5).

Calcium Channel Blockers

Calcium channel blockers inhibit the L-type calcium channel on VSMCs and the slow-responding myocardial cells. Calcium channel blockers are classified as either dihydropyridines or nondihydropyridines. Dihydropyridines (such as amlodipine, felodipine, isradipine, nicardipine, and nifedipine) have a predominant vasodilator effect with very little or no effect on cardiac contractility or conduction. In contrast, nondihydropyridines (such as verapamil and diltiazem) have a lesser vasodilator effect and a more pronounced effect on reducing cardiac contractility and conduction. Nicardipine is the only dihydropyridine that can be given IV or IA. In general, calcium channel blockers decrease peripheral vascular resistance (PVR), decrease blood pressure, alleviate coronary spasm, and increase coronary blood flow. Calcium channel blockers can be used in the catheterization laboratory to treat supraventricular and atrial arrhythmias (nondihydropyridines), hypertensive crisis (nicardipine), radial or coronary spasm, and slow flow or no-reflow (nondihydropyridines and nicardipine). Common side effects include hypotension, reflex tachycardia (dihydropyridines), negative inotropy (more pronounced with the nondihydropyridines), and conduction disturbances such as A-V nodal blocks or sinus arrest (nondihydropyridines). The nondihydropyridines are generally contraindicated in left or right ventricular dysfunction due to their myocardial depression effects (more pronounced with verapamil compared to diltiazem) (1,5–8).

1. Diltiazem: IV bolus of 0.25 mg/kg (15–20 mg) over 2 minutes, followed by a maintenance rate of 5 to 20 mg/hr for supraventricular tachycardia (SVT)/atrial tachycardias; 2.5- to 5-mg IA for prophylactic treatment or treatment of radial artery spasm; 0.5- to 2-mg IC boluses for treatment of slow flow or no-reflow.
2. Verapamil: IV bolus of 2.5 to 5 mg over 2 minutes; second dose of 5 to 10 mg (~0.15 mg/kg) may be given 15 to 30 minutes later (for SVT/atrial tachycardias); 2.5- to 5-mg IA for prophylactic treatment or treatment of radial artery spasm; 50- to 200-μg slow IC boluses, for 2 to 4 boluses, if needed for treatment of slow flow or no-reflow (60%–100% success).
3. Nicardipine: IV infusion of 5 mg/hr (maximum dose of 15–20 mg/hr) for treating hypertension; 200-μg IC boluses, for 2 to 4 boluses, for the treatment of slow flow or no-reflow (99% success in one study; some benefit in prophylactic administration to prevent no-reflow in saphenous vein graft (SVG) PCIs and rotational atherectomy); 2.5- to 5-mg IA for prophylactic treatment or treatment of radial artery spasm during trans-radial procedures.

Adenosine Agonists

Adenosine is a nonselective adenosine receptor agonist. Adenosine binding to the A2A receptors on arteriolar smooth muscle cells (SMCs) increases the production of cyclic adenosine monophosphate (AMP), which leads to SMC relaxation and arteriolar vasodilation (9). Adenosine produces coronary hyperemia, and has been used in conjunction with nuclear myocardial perfusion imaging and for

assessing coronary flow reserve (CFR) and fractional flow reserve (FFR) in the catheterization laboratory (9). Adenosine can be administered as an IC bolus (50–100 μg for the right coronary artery [RCA] and 100–200 μg for the left coronary artery [LCA]) or IV infusion (140 μg/kg/min) over 2 to 3 minutes for FFR or CFR evaluation. Higher doses of IC adenosine boluses (doses of 120, 180, 360, and 720 μg) were well-tolerated and progressively increased the frequency of patients with an FFR < 0.75 from 30% with a dose of 60 μg, to 51% with a dose of 720 μg (10).

A more recent dose-response study of adenosine showed that an IC adenosine bolus injection of 100 μg in the RCA and 200 μg in the LCA induced maximal hyperemia with minimal side effects (11). The peak hyperemic effect of IC adenosine is achieved within a few seconds of its bolus administration, with a sustained plateau of hyperemia of around 5 seconds. The peak hyperemic effect of IV adenosine is reached within 2 minutes of its administration and lasts for <30 seconds from its termination. IV adenosine permits measuring a pullback FFR and has been shown in one study to cause more hyperemia than IC adenosine (12). Adenosine has also been used in the catheterization laboratory in vasodilator challenge testing in patients with pulmonary hypertension, where IV adenosine is initially infused at 50 μg/kg/min and is increased by 50 μg/kg/min every 2 minutes to a maximum dose of 250 μg/kg/min (13).

Regadenoson is a selective adenosine A2A receptor agonist that is administered as a single 0.4-mg IV bolus and is used as a stress agent in conjunction with nuclear myocardial perfusion imaging. Peak hyperemia is reached within seconds of its administration and lasts for around 2 minutes from its administration. Regadenoson single IV bolus of 0.4 mg was compared to an IV adenosine infusion at 140 μg/kg/min for evaluation of coronary stenoses using FFR (14,15). Regadenoson was as effective as adenosine in measuring FFR, with a strong linear correlation with adenosine and similar frequency in detecting FFR ≤ 0.8, a similar hemodynamic response, more rapid hyperemia, more ease of use, and an excellent side-effect profile (14,15). Regadenoson is a promising agent for use in the catheterization laboratory due to its ease of administration, obviating the use of an infusion pump. IC adenosine boluses of 24 to 60 μg with a quick saline flush have been used to treat slow flow or no-reflow during coronary and SVG PCIs, with a 90% success rate.

Common side effects of adenosine include bronchospasm, chest pain, dyspnea, flushing, Atrioventricular (AV) block, modest hypotension, and modest increases in heart rate. The side effects are short lived and can be reversed with 50 to 100 mg of IV aminophylline if they become severe and prolonged. Adenosine is contraindicated in patients with heart transplantation or in patients with second- or third-degree heart block in the absence of a functional pacemaker. Adenosine should be used cautiously in patients with bronchospastic lung disorders due to the risk of adenosine-induced bronchoconstriction.(1,9–11,14,16–19).

Papaverine

Papaverine is a potent arterial vasodilator, whose mechanism of action is thought to be due to inhibition of a phosphodiesterase enzyme that results in increasing cyclic AMP in smooth muscle cells, with resultant smooth muscle relaxation and arterial vasodilatation. IC papaverine is used to induce coronary hyperemia for assessment of CFR or FFR. Its onset of action is within 10 to 30 seconds and its duration is for 45 to 60 seconds from time of administration. Commonly used IC bolus doses are 12 to 16 mg for the RCA and 16 to 20 mg for the LCA. Papaverine (30-mg intra-renal bolus) was also used to "stress" the kidney and measure hyperemic renal artery FFR and hyperemic renal artery systolic gradients (HSGs). An HSG of 21 mm Hg and a renal FFR of 0.90 have been considered to represent a hemodynamically significant renal artery stenosis. Papaverine can prolong the QT segment and cause torsades de pointes. Papaverine can cause crystallization when combined with some of the ionic contrast agents, and can also increase coronary venous lactate production, which may cause myocardial ischemia (1,12,17,20–22).

Coronary Vasoconstrictors

ACETYLCHOLINE

Acetylcholine is an endogenous neurotransmitter that stimulates muscarinic receptors on endothelial cells and causes endothelial-dependent vasodilatation via release of nitric oxide and other vasoactive substances in the presence of a normal endothelium and causes vasoconstriction via direct activation of receptors on smooth muscle cells in the presence of an abnormal endothelium (1). IC acetylcholine administration constricts diseased coronary arteries (endothelial dysfunction or atherosclerosis) and vasodilates normal coronary arteries (normal endothelial function). The net effect is a balance between vasodilation and vasoconstriction. Acetylcholine has been used to diagnose variant (Prinzmetal) angina, particularly in patients who have normally apparent coronary arteries on coronary angiography.

Acetylcholine has also been used to assess epicardial and microvascular vasomotor responses, which can lead to ischemia in patients with stable angina who have normal or minimal coronary artery disease without features of variant angina (1). In one study of patients with stable angina and normal or minimal coronary artery disease, two-thirds of the patients had an abnormal test where 45% of the patients had epicardial spasm (≥75% coronary narrowing with symptom production) and 55% of the patients had microvascular spasm (symptom reproduction with ischemic ECG changes and no epicardial spasm) (23). IC incremental doses of acetylcholine of 20, 50, and 80 μg are usually injected into the RCA, and 20, 50, and 100 μg are injected into the LCA. Spasm is defined as total or subtotal occlusion after acetylcholine administration. Spasm caused by low doses of acetylcholine is usually more proximal and focal and is more associated with more stent thrombosis (ST) elevation and the clinical findings of variant angina. Spasm caused by higher acetylcholine doses is associated with more distal and diffuse spasm and is associated with less ST elevation and less characteristics of variant angina.

Acetylcholine is very short-acting and rapidly inactivated. Continuous infusions of 0.02 to 2.2 μg (10^{-8}, 10^{-7}, 10^{-6} M) have been used to identify normal endothelial coronary artery function manifesting as vasodilatation. Marked bradycardia, heart block, and vasospasm are common with acetylcholine, and thus temporary pacing is recommended during its administration. Serious side effects such as sustained ventricular tachycardia (VT), shock, and cardiac tamponade occurred in 4 of 715 patients (0.56%) in one study, although no death or irreversible complications occurred (1,24–26).

ERGONOVINE

Ergonovine is an ergot derivative that causes smooth muscle cell contraction and is commonly used to induce uterine contractions to treat or prevent postpartum hemorrhage. It can also be used in the coronary tree to provoke coronary spasm and evaluate patients with angina pectoris who have normal coronaries or minimal coronary artery disease on coronary angiography (1). Ergonovine can be administered IC as an infusion of 10 μg/min over 4 minutes for a maximal dose of 40 μg in the RCA, and as 16 μg/min over

4 minutes for a total dose of 64 μg in the LCA (27). Alternatively, ergonovine can be administered by slow IC injections over 1 minute each of sequential doses of 1, 5, 10, and 30 μg at 3- to 5-minute intervals with a maximum cumulative dose of 50 μg (28). An electrocardiography (ECG) is obtained at the end of each interval or if the patient develops angina symptoms.

Angiography of the right and left coronary arteries should be promptly performed when angina symptoms occur. Diffuse coronary narrowing is a physiologic response to ergonovine, whereas a severe (> 75% narrowing in some studies and subtotal to total occlusion in other studies) focal coronary narrowing is considered a response indicative of coronary spasm when associated with ischemic ECG changes or typical symptoms (27). Ergonovine-induced spasm can be reversed with the administration of IC nitroglycerine. In one study, IC acetylcholine-induced spasm (873 patients) was compared to IC ergonovine-induced spasm (635 patients). In patients without ischemic heart disease, acetylcholine-induced spasm were significantly more common than ergonovine-induced spasm (11% vs. 6%). Additionally, acetylcholine significantly provoked more spasms in patients without fixed stenosis than ergonovine (36.2% vs. 25.5%). Major complications occurred in 1.4% of patients with the acetylcholine test, and in 0.2% of patients with the ergonovine test, with no occurrence of any MI or death with either test (1,27).

Vasopressors and Inotropes

Vasopressor drugs generally cause peripheral vasoconstriction, leading to an increase in systemic vascular resistance (SVR) and mean arterial pressure (MAP). Inotropic drugs, on the other hand, increase cardiac contractility and chronotropy. Some of the vasopressor drugs have both vasopressor and inotropic effects, depending on the receptors they stimulate (1). Stimulation of peripheral $\alpha 1$ receptors causes vasoconstriction, and stimulation of cardiac $\alpha 1$ receptors augments inotropy. Stimulation of $\beta 1$ receptors (located mainly on myocytes) augments inotropy and chronotropy. Stimulation of the $\beta 2$ receptors (located mainly in the vasculature) augments vasodilatation. Stimulation of the dopaminergic receptors DA1 causes vasodilatation in the renal, splanchnic cerebral, and coronary beds (1,29–31). These drugs can be used in the catheterization laboratory depending on the situation encountered and the desired effect (Table 5.1) (1,29,31).

PHENYLEPHRINE (NEOSYNEPHRINE)

Phenylephrine is a pure α receptor agonist. Its main effect is peripheral vasoconstriction, with minimal cardiac inotropy and minimal effect on cardiac output. Phenylephrine is used in hypotension with low SVR, such as sepsis, neurologic disorders, and anesthesia- or medication-induced hypotension. It is commonly used in the catheterization laboratory to correct medication-related hypotension (nitrates, nitroprusside, calcium, or channel blockers) or transient hypotension related to ischemia or during carotid stenting. It is also used in patients with severe aortic valve stenosis or hypertrophic obstructive cardiomyopathy who develop hypotension. It can be given as 100- to 200-μg rapid boluses to correct sudden onset hypotension or as an IV drip (Table 5.2). Phenylephrine can cause marked increase in blood pressure (especially in patients on nonselective β blockers), reflex-mediated bradycardia, and severe peripheral and visceral vasoconstriction. (1,29,31).

NOREPINEPHRINE (LEVOPHED)

Norepinephrine predominantly stimulates the $\alpha 1$ and $\beta 1$ receptors with less effect on the $\beta 2$ receptors. It thus has a significant vasoconstrictor effect and minimal inotropic and chronic effects, and as such is used

TABLE 5.2 Indications and Doses of the Various Vasopressors and Inotropes (1,31,35,36)

DRUG	INDICATION AND DOSE
Epinephrine	ACLS/cardiac arrest: 1 mg (1:10,000) IV/IO q 3–5 minutes; 2–2.5 mg (1:1,000) ET tube q 3–5 minutes
	Symptomatic bradycardia or heart block unresponsive to atropine or pacing/shock (cardiogenic/vasodilatory): 2–10 μg/min IV maintenance
	Anaphylaxis/bronchospasm: 0.1–0.5 mg (1:1,000) SC/IM q 5–15 minutes or 0.1–0.25 mg (1:10,000) IV q 5–15 minutes
Norepinephrine	Shock (vasodilatory/cardiogenic): Start 0.5–1 μg/min IV, maintenance 2–12 μg/min up to 30 –g/min
Phenylephrine	Shock (vagally mediated/medication-induced), hypotension in aortic valve stenosis and HOCM): 100–500 μg IV bolus q 10–15 minutes, maintenance 40–60 μg/min IV infusion up to 200 μg/min
Isoproterenol	Brady-arrhythmias (especially in torsade des pointes and Brugada syndrome): 20–60 μg IV bolus, 2–10 μg/min IV maintenance
Dopamine	Heart failure: 1–3 μg/kg/min
	Symptomatic bradycardia unresponsive to atropine or pacing: 2–10 μg/kg/min
	Shock (cardiogenic/vasodilatory): 2–20 μg/kg/min (up to 50 μg/kg/min for refractory shock)
Dobutamine	Low cardiac output (decompensated heart failure, cardiogenic shock, sepsis-induced myocardial dysfunction)/ symptomatic bradycardia unresponsive to atropine or pacing: 2–10 μg/kg/min (up to 20 μg/kg/min)
Milrinone	Low cardiac output (decompensated heart failure/post-cardiotomy): 50 μg/kg IV bolus followed by 0.375–0.75 μg/kg/min (decrease dose based on Cr clearance)
Vasopressin	ACLS/cardiac arrest: 40 units IV × 1; 80–100 units ET tube
	Shock (vasodilatory/cardiogenic): 0.01–0.10 units/min IV maintenance

ACLS, advanced cardiac life support; ET, endotracheal; HOCM, hypertrophic obstructive cardiomyopathy; IO, intraosseous; IV, intravenous.

to treat severe cardiogenic shock, septic shock, or shock refractory to other pressors, particularly in low SVR states. Norepinephrine can cause peripheral ischemia, arrhythmias, and increase SVR and blood pressure (especially in patients with non selective β blockers) (Table 5.2) (1,29,31).

EPINEPHRINE

Epinephrine has equipotent effects on the α1 and β1 receptors and modest effects on the β2 receptors. At lower doses, epinephrine increases cardiac output with a minimal decrease in SVR and variable effect on MAP (due to equal stimulation of α1 and β2 receptors). At higher doses, stimulation of the α1 receptors predominates over β2 receptor stimulation, resulting in more peripheral vasoconstriction than vasodilatation and increases in SVR. Epinephrine is the first-line drug used in cardiac arrest (asystole, pulseless electrical activity, and ventricular fibrillation [VF]) and anaphylactic shock and is a second-line drug for treating septic shock or severe cardiogenic shock. It is commonly used to treat hypotension following cardiac surgery (Table 5.2). Epinephrine can cause tachycardia, ventricular arrhythmias, increased oxygen demand, cardiac ischemia, increased SVR, and severe hypertension that can cause cerebrovascular hemorrhage (1,29,31).

DOPAMINE

Dopamine stimulates various receptors and produces its effects in a dose-dependent manner. At a low dose of 1 to 2 μg/kg/min, it activates the dopamine receptors (renal DA1 and peripheral DA2 receptors) with resultant vasodilatation in the renal, splanchnic, coronary, and cerebral circulations. Low-dose dopamine augments renal blood flow and natriuresis. Medium-dose dopamine (2–7 μg/kg/min) stimulates the β1 receptors and has variable effects on SVR and blood pressure, depending on the balance of peripheral vasodilatation and the increased cardiac output. High-dose dopamine (>7–10 μg/kg/min) predominantly stimulates the α1 receptors, resulting in vasoconstriction and increases in SVR and MAP. Dopamine is commonly used to treat

hypotension due to nonprofound septic or cardiogenic shocks, poor tissue perfusion states (oliguria, anuria, altered level of consciousness), or symptomatic bradycardia. Dopamine, particularly at high doses, can cause tachycardia, arrhythmias, renal vasoconstriction, and tissue ischemia at high doses (Table 5.2) (1,29,31).

DOBUTAMINE

Dobutamine is a predominant β1 receptor agonist with less effect on the β2 receptor, and as such it is an inotrope rather than a pressor drug. Dobutamine is mainly used to treat low cardiac output congestive heart failure (CHF) by augmenting cardiac output and decreasing SVR and cardiac filling pressures. It has no effect or a minimal decrease in MAP. It can cause tachycardia, increase ventricular response in atrial arrhythmias, ventricular arrhythmias, cardiac ischemia, and occasionally hypotension (Table 5.2) (1,29,31).

ISOPROTERENOL (ISUPREL)

Isoproterenol is a pure β1 and β2 agonist with predominant chronotropic effect and a lesser effect on inotropy and peripheral vasodilatation. It is mainly used in the electrophysiology laboratory to induce tachycardia, and to stimulate the sinus node in some situations of resistant bradycardia unresponsive to atropine and dopamine, as well as in hypotension related to bradycardia or postcardiac transplantation. Continuous IV isoproterenol infusion can cause a significant increase in heart rate and inotropy, a decrease in diastolic blood pressure and SVR, and increased myocardial work. It can also cause ventricular arrhythmias, cardiac ischemia, and hypertension or hypotension (Table 5.2) (1,29,31).

PHOSPHODIESTERASE INHIBITORS

Phosphodiesterase inhibitors such as milrinone are inotropes that inhibit phosphodiesterase III and increase intracellular cyclic AMP, independent of the β-adrenergic receptors. Milrinone has equipotent inotropic effects, and both a more potent central and peripheral vasodilator effect and a lesser chronotropic effect compared to dobutamine. It is used to treat low cardiac output heart failure. It can cause ventricular arrhythmias, hypotension, cardiac ischemia, and torsades des pointes (Table 5.2) (1,29,31).

VASOPRESSIN

Vasopressin is an antidiuretic hormone that has vasopressor effects. It stimulates V1 receptors on VSMCs and V2 receptors in the renal collecting duct system. It can be used as a second-line drug for catecholamine-refractory septic or anaphylactic shock, or as a first-line drug during cardiac arrest instead of epinephrine. It can cause arrhythmias, hypertension, cardiac ischemia, decreased cardiac output (at high doses), and severe peripheral ischemia leading to splanchnic, and skin vasoconstriction (Table 5.2) (1,29,31,32).

SIDE EFFECTS

The vasopressors and inotropes have potential serious complications. Stimulation of the α receptors can cause significant peripheral vasoconstriction and decreased perfusion with resultant limb ischemia, renal hypoperfusion and renal ischemia, mesenteric ischemia, gastritis, and shock liver. Stimulation of the $\beta1$ receptor augments chronotropy that can result in sinus tachycardia, and atrial or ventricular arrhythmias. Chronotropic and inotropic augmentation can also lead to myocardial ischemia, particularly in patients with underlying coronary artery disease. Extravasation of vasopressors into surrounding skin and connective tissue can cause local vasoconstriction with subsequent skin and tissue necrosis (1,31).

Antiarrhythmic Drugs

Antiarrhythmic drugs are classified based on their predominant mechanism of action, such as with the modified Vaughn-Williams classification (33,34). **Table 5.3** summarizes the different antiarrhythmic drugs, with their properties, indications, and side effects. The antiarrhythmic drugs commonly used in the cardiac catheterization are those needed to treat or control acute ventricular or supraventricular arrhythmias (1).

Procainamide

Procainamide is a Class IA antiarrhythmic drug with eletrophysiologic properties similar to quinidine, but without the vagolytic and α receptor effects. Procainamide has a ganglionic blocker effect that accounts for some of the hypotension noted with its IV administration. N-acetyl procainamide (NAPA) is a major procainamide metabolite that also blocks the K channel, similar to the parent drug. Procainamide is hepatically metabolized to NAPA, and both the parent compound and its metabolite are renally excreted. The significant side-effect profile of procainamide precludes its long-term use. Procainamide is indicated for hemodynamically stable monomorphic VT or pre-excited atrial fibrillation. The loading dose is infused at 20 to 50 mg/min or 100 mg every 5 minutes until the arrhythmia is controlled, hypotension occurs, the QRS widens by 50% of its original width, or a total of 17 mg/kg is given. The maintenance infusion is 1 to 4 mg/min. Procainamide should not be administered if the QT is prolonged or if the patient has CHF (1,33–36).

TABLE 5.3 Classification and Properties of Antiarrhythmic Drugs (1,33,34)

	ACTION	USE	SIDE EFFECTS
Class IA	Na channel blocker; slows conduction velocity, prolongs action potential duration		
Quinidine	K channel blocker, α blocker, vagolytic activity	Conversion of Afib, Aflutter and maintenance of sinus rhythm, life-threatening ventricular arrhythmias	Proarrhythmias, QT prolongation, torsades de pointes, GI intolerance, tinnitus, headache, thrombocytopenia, SLE, worsening myasthenia gravis, hypotension and sinus tachycardia with IV use or high oral dose
Procainamide	K channel blocker, ganglionic blocker	Ventricular arrhythmias, reentrant SVT, Afib or Aflutter associated with WPW	QT prolongation, drug-induced lupus, rash, arthlargia, fever, pericardial and pleural effusions, bone marrow aplasia, agranulocytosis, hypotension with IV dose or high serum levels
Disopyramide	K channel blocker, vagolytic activity of primary metabolite	Ventricular arrhythmias, SVT, HCM (reduce LVOT gradient)	Anticholinergic effects, constipation, urinary retention, dry mouth, GERD, glaucoma exacerbation, worsening CHF (negative inotropic effect)
Class IB	Na channel blocker, no effect on conduction velocity		
Lidocaine	Shortens action potential, minimal effect on QT	Ischemia-induced ventricular arrhythmias or recurrent ventricular arrhythmias	CNS symptoms such as tremor, paresthesias, hearing abnormalities, slurred speech, depressed mentation, seizure, coma, and nausea
Mexilitine	Derivative of Lidocaine with similar properties	Refractory ventricular arrhythmias	CNS symptoms such as tremor, dizziness, dysphoria, and GI intolerance

(continued)

TABLE 5.3 Classification and Properties of Antiarrhythmic Drugs (1,33,34) (continued)

	ACTION	USE	SIDE EFFECTS
Class IC	Slows conduction velocity, minimal prolongation of action potential duration		
Flecainide	Late opening Na channels, delayed rectifier K channel and calcium channel blocker; prolong action potential at fast rates, no effect on QT	Prevention of PAF and SVT in patients without structural heart disease, prevention of life-threatening ventricular arrhythmias	Blurred vision and dry eyes, CHF exacerbation with abnormal LV function
Propafenone	Fast Na channel blocker, decrease membrane excitability and spontaneous automaticity, β blocker activity	SVT, Afib in patients without structural heart disease, ventricular arrhythmias	Metallic taste, GI intolerance, dizziness, blurred vision, fatigue, hepatotoxicity, lupus, blood dyscrasias, bronchospasm, proarrhythmia in patients with depressed LV function or history of ventricular arrhythmias
Class II	β Blockers, β1 receptor blocker, sinus rate and AV nodal slowing, decreased contractility	SVT, rate control of Afib and Aflutter, ventricular arrhythmias	
Class III	Delayed K rectifier channel blocker; prolong action potential duration, no effect on conduction velocity		QT prolongation, torsades de pointes
Amiodarone	Class I, II, and IV action	Suppressing and preventing ventricular and supraventricular arrhythmias, tolerated in patients with depressed LV function	GI intolerance, hypotension and phlebitis (IV administration), pulmonary and hepato toxicities, hyper or hypothyroidism, peripheral neuropathy, skin discoloration, and corneal deposits
Dronedarone	Similar to amiodarone	Preventing Afib (PAF)	Similar to amiodarone, contraindicated in patients with permanent Afib, or history or current heart failure or LV dysfunction
Sotalol	β Blockade	Ventricular arrhythmias, conversion and maintenance of Afib	Proarrhythmias, QT prolongation, torsades de pointes, close monitoring during initiation
Ibutilide	Analogue of sotalol, IV administration only	Conversion of Afib or Aflutter	Proarrhythmias, QT prolongation, torsades de pointes
Dofetilide	Prolong repolarization	Conversion and maintenance of Afib	Proarrhythmias, QT prolongation, torsades de pointes, close monitoring during initiation and in patients with renal dysfunction
Class IV			
Verapamil/ Cardizem	Non-dihydropyridine calcium channel blockers; slow Ca channel blockers in sinus and AV nodes; negative inotropic effects	Acute and chronic treatment of SVT, rate control of Afib and Aflutter	Caution in patients with LV dysfunction and patients with WPW

Afib, atrial fibrillation; Aflutter, atrial flutter; AV, atrio-ventricular; IV, intravenous; CHF, congestive heart failure; CNS, central nervous system; HCM, hypertrophic cardiomyopathy; GERD, gastroesophageal reflux disorder; GI, gastrointestinal; LV, left ventricular; LVOT, left ventricular outflow tract; PAF, paroxysmal atrial fibrillation; SLE, systemic lupus erythematosis; SVT, supraventricular tachycardia; WPW, Wolf Parkinson White.

Lidocaine

Lidocaine is a Class IB antiarrhythmic drug that has minimal effect on the QT compared to other Class I drugs. Lidocaine's suppressive effects are mainly on the depolarized myocardium, and it is used to treat ventricular arrhythmias induced by ischemia. Lidocaine is metabolized in the liver into two metabolites that have less antiarrhythmic effects than the parent drug. Lidocaine levels should be monitored closely to prevent toxicities, particularly in patients with CHF or liver dysfunction. In the catheterization laboratory, lidocaine can be given as an IV bolus of 50 to 100 mg before ventriculography to suppress ventricular ectopy or to treat ischemia-induced ventricular arrhythmias during cardiac catheterization or PCI. Lidocaine is indicated for VF or pulseless VT if amiodarone is not available, and for hemodynamically stable VT. Lidocaine is administered as a 1- to 1.5-mg/kg IV bolus, with a repeat bolus of 0.5 to 0.75 mg/kg every

5 to 10 minutes (the maximum cumulative dose is 3 mg/kg) for refractory VF or pulseless VT, followed by a maintenance infusion of 1 to 4 mg/min. An intra-tracheal loading dose of 2 to 3.75 can be used (1,33–36).

Amiodarone

Amiodarone is a Class III antiarrhythmic drug that also has Class I, II, and IV effects. Desethylamioda-rone (DEA), the main metabolite of amiodarone, is a potent Na channel blocker. Amiodarone requires a solvent (polysorbate-80) for its IV administration. The solvent, as well as the β and calcium channel blocker effects of amiodarone, can decrease the heart rate and reduce the blood pressure, particularly during IV bolus administration. Amiodarone is metabolized in the liver, with minimal renal elimination and a very long elimination half-life (mean of 54 days). Amiodarone can decrease the hepatic or renal clearance of other antiarrhythmic drugs such as flecainide, procainamide, and quinidine. Concomitant use of amiodarone with other antiarrhythmic drugs (mexiletine, propafenone, quinidine, disopyramide, procainamide), tricyclic antidepressants, and some of the antipsychotic drugs can prolong the QT interval and induce torsades de pointes. Warfarin and digoxin doses should be reduced by half when used long term with amiodarone. Amiodarone should be used with caution in conjunction with antihypertensives, β blockers, or calcium channel blockers. Amiodarone is indicated for VF or pulseless VT and is given as a 300-mg IV bolus, with a supplemental 150-mg IV bolus dose if VF or pulseless VT continues after defibrillation, or if it recurs. Amiodarone is infused at 1 mg/min for 6 hours, followed by 0.5 mg/min for 18 hours after the return of spontaneous circulation. Amiodarone is also indicated for stable VT or for pharmacologic conversion or rate control of supraventricular or atrial arrhythmias. A 150-mg IV bolus is infused over 10 minutes, followed by a maintenance dose infused at 1 mg/min for 6 hours followed by 0.5 mg/min for 18 hours (1,33–36).

β Blockers

β blockers belong to the Class II antiarrhythmic drugs. β blockers can be used in the catheterization laboratory for rate control of fast supraventricular or atrial arrhythmias, as well as for suppression of ventricular arrhythmias, particularly with long-term use. Metoprolol or lopressor can be administered as 2.5- to 5-mg IV boluses every 2 to 5 minutes for a maximum of 15 mg. Esmolol is the β blocker of choice for a maintenance IV infusion. Esmolol is given as a 500-μg/kg bolus over 1 minute, followed by a maintenance infusion at 50 μg/kg/min that can be titrated upward in 50 μg/kg/min increments every 4 minutes, to a maximum of 200 μg/kg/min (1).

Calcium Channel Blockers

The nondihydropyridine calcium channel blockers belong to the Class IV antiarrhythmic agents. Similar to the β blockers, they can be used in the catheterization laboratory for rate control of fast supraventricular or atrial arrhythmias (discussed in the "Vasodilators" section earlier).

Adenosine

Adenosine (Adenocard) is indicated for pharmacologic conversion of AV nodal reentrant SVT. Adenosine has a very short half-life of a few seconds. Adenosine is administered as a rapid IV bolus of 6 mg that can be repeated in 1 to 2 minutes as a 12-mg rapid IV bolus if the first dose was ineffective (1).

Key Points

- Nitroglycerin causes more venous than arterial vasodilatation. It improves coronary flow, prevents or alleviates coronary spasm, provokes myocardial bridging, relieves angina, reduces preload in patients with elevated filling pressures, and prevents or treats radial artery spasm.

- Nitroprusside, a direct nitric oxide donor, can be used to treat hypertensive emergencies, acute heart failure particularly due to acute mitral regurgitation, and no-reflow during PCIs.

- Dihydropyridines calcium channel blockers (such as amlodipine, felodipine, isradipine, nicardipine, and nifedipine) have a predominant vasodilator effect, with very little or no effect on cardiac contractility or conduction.

- Nondihydropyridines calcium channel blockers (such as verapamil and diltiazem) have a lesser vasodilator effect and a more pronounced effect on reducing cardiac contractility and conduction.

- Calcium channel blockers decrease PVR, decrease blood pressure, alleviate coronary spasm, and increase coronary blood flow.

- Calcium channel blockers can be used to treat supraventricular and atrial arrhythmias (nondihydropyridines). They are also used in prophylactic treatment or treatment of radial or coronary spasm and no-reflow (nondihydropyridines and nicardipine).

- Adenosine, a nonselective adenosine receptor agonist, produces coronary hyperemia for assessing CFR and FFR. It can also be used for vasodilator testing in patients with pulmonary hypertension.

- Regadenoson, a selective adenosine A2A receptor agonist, is administered as a single 0.4-mg IV bolus for assessing CFR and FFR.

- Papaverine, a potent arterial vasodilator, is used to induce coronary hyperemia for assessment of CFR or FFR, or to induce renal artery hyperemia for assessment of hyperemic renal artery FFR and HSG.

- Papaverine's onset of action is within 10 to 30 seconds, and its duration is for 45 to 60 seconds from time of administration.

- Acetylcholine, an endogenous neurotransmitter, causes endothelial-dependent vasodilatation via the release of nitric oxide and other vasoactive substances in the presence of a normal endothelium, and causes vasoconstriction via direct activation of receptors on smooth muscle cells in the presence of an abnormal endothelium.

- IC acetylcholine administration constricts diseased coronary arteries (endothelial dysfunction or atherosclerosis) and vasodilates normal coronary arteries (normal endothelial function). It is used to assess epicardial and microvascular vasomotor responses and to diagnose Prinzmetal angina.

- Ergonovine, an ergot derivative, causes smooth muscle cell contraction and is used in the coronary tree to provoke coronary spasm and evaluate patients with angina pectoris who have normal coronaries or minimal coronary artery disease on coronary angiography.

- Diffuse coronary narrowing is a physiologic response to ergonovine, whereas a severe (>75% narrowing in some studies and subtotal to total occlusion in other studies) focal coronary narrowing is considered a response indicative of coronary spasm when associated with ischemic ECG changes or typical symptoms.

- Phenylephrine, a pure α receptor agonist, produces peripheral vasoconstriction with minimal cardiac inotropy and minimal effect on cardiac output. Phenylephrine is used to treat hypotension with low SVR, medication-related hypotension, or transient hypotension related to ischemia or carotid stenting.

- Norepinephrine predominantly stimulates the $\alpha1$ and $\beta1$ receptors, with less effect on the $\beta2$ receptors, and is used to treat septic shock or severe cardiogenic shock. Epinephrine has equipotent effects on the $\alpha1$ and $\beta1$ receptors, and modest effects on the $\beta2$ receptors. It is used as a first-line drug in cardiac arrest and anaphylactic shock, and as a second-line drug for treating septic shock or severe cardiogenic shock, or when treating hypotension following cardiac surgery.

- Dopamine's effects depend on its infusion dose. Medium to high dopamine doses further stimulate the $\alpha1$ receptors, in addition to the $\beta1$ receptors, and are used to treat nonprofound septic or cardiogenic shocks, or symptomatic bradycardia.

- Dobutamine is a predominant $\beta1$ receptor agonist with less effect on the $\beta2$ receptor. It is used as an inotrope to treat low cardiac output CHF.

- Isoproterenol is a pure $\beta1$ and $\beta2$ agonist with a predominant chronotropic effect and a lesser effect on inotropy and peripheral vasodilatation. It is mainly used to induce tachycardia during electrophysiology studies, to treat hypotension related to bradycardia, or to stimulate the sinus node postcardiac transplantation.

- Phosphodiesterase inhibitors, such as milrinone, are inotropes that inhibit phosphodiesterase III and increase intracellular cyclic AMP, independent of the β adrenergic receptors.

- Vasopressin, an antidiuretic hormone, is used as a second-line drug for catecholamine-refractory septic or anaphylactic shock, or as a first-line drug instead of epinephrine during cardiac arrest.

References

1. Zoghbi G. Vasoactive and antiarrhythmic drugs in the catheterization laboratory. In: Kern M, ed. *SCAI Interventional Board Review*. 2nd ed. Philadelphia, PA: Lippincott Williams & Wilkins; 2014:49–56.
2. Kloner RA. Cardiovascular effects of the 3 phosphodiesterase-5 inhibitors approved for the treatment of erectile dysfunction. *Circulation*. 2004;110:3149–3155.
3. Abrams J. Hemodynamic effects of nitroglycerin and long-acting nitrates. *Am Heart J*. 1985;110:216–224.
4. Chen Z, Zhang J, Stamler JS. Identification of the enzymatic mechanism of nitroglycerin bioactivation. *Proc Natl Acad Sci U S A*. 2002;99:8306–8311.
5. Wong DT, et al. Myocardial 'no-reflow': diagnosis, pathophysiology and treatment. *Int J Cardiol*. 2013;167:1798–1806.
6. Fischell TA, et al. Nicardipine and adenosine "flush cocktail" to prevent no-reflow during rotational atherectomy. *Cardiovasc Revasc Med*. 2008;9:224–228.
7. Huang RI, et al. Efficacy of intracoronary nicardipine in the treatment of no-reflow during percutaneous coronary intervention. *Catheter Cardiovasc Interv*. 2006;68:671–676.
8. Caputo RP, et al. Transradial arterial access for coronary and peripheral procedures: executive summary by the Transradial Committee of the SCAI. *Catheter Cardiovasc Interv*. 2011;78:823–839.
9. Zoghbi GJ, Iskandrian AE. Coronary artery disease detection: pharmacologic stress SPECT. In: Zaret BL, Beller GA, eds. *Clinical Nuclear Cardiology: State of the Art and Future Directions*. Philadelphia, PA: Mosby Elsevier; 2010:225–266.
10. De Luca G, et al. Effects of increasing doses of intracoronary adenosine on the assessment of fractional flow reserve. *JACC Cardiovasc Interv*. 2011;4:1079–1084.
11. Adjedj J, Toth GG, Johnson NP, et al. Intracoronary adenosine: dose-response relationship with hyperemia. *JACC Cardiovasc Interv*. 2015;8:1422–1430.
12. De Bruyne B, et al. Intracoronary and intravenous adenosine 5'-triphosphate, adenosine, papaverine, and contrast medium to assess fractional flow reserve in humans. *Circulation*. 2003;107:1877–1883.
13. McLaughlin VV, et al. ACCF/AHA 2009 expert consensus document on pulmonary hypertension: a report of the American College of Cardiology Foundation Task Force on Expert Consensus Documents and the American Heart Association developed in collaboration with the American College of Chest Physicians; American Thoracic Society, Inc.; and the Pulmonary Hypertension Association. *J Am Coll Cardiol*. 2009;53:1573–1619.
14. Nair PK, et al. Clinical utility of regadenoson for assessing fractional flow reserve. *JACC Cardiovasc Interv*. 2011;4:1085–1092.
15. Prasad A, et al. Use of regadenoson for measurement of fractional flow reserve. *Catheter Cardiovasc Interv*. 2014;83:369–374.
16. Casella G, et al. Are high doses of intracoronary adenosine an alternative to standard intravenous adenosine for the assessment of fractional flow reserve? *Am Heart J*. 2004;148:590–595.
17. McGeoch RJ, Oldroyd KG. Pharmacological options for inducing maximal hyperaemia during studies of coronary physiology. *Catheter Cardiovasc Interv*. 2008;71:198–204.
18. Assali AR, et al. Intracoronary adenosine administered during percutaneous intervention in acute myocardial infarction and reduction in the incidence of "no reflow" phenomenon. *Catheter Cardiovasc Interv*. 2000;51:27–31.
19. Fischell TA, et al. Reversal of "no reflow" during vein graft stenting using high velocity boluses of intracoronary adenosine. *Cathet Cardiovasc Diagn*. 1998;45:360–365.
20. Kapoor N, et al. Physiological assessment of renal artery stenosis: comparisons of resting with hyperemic renal pressure measurements. *Catheter Cardiovasc Interv*. 2010;76:726–732.
21. Subramanian R, et al. Renal fractional flow reserve: a hemodynamic evaluation of moderate renal artery stenoses. *Catheter Cardiovasc Interv*. 2005;64:480–486.
22. van der Voort PH. Comparison of intravenous adenosine to intracoronary papaverine for calculation of pressure-derived fractional flow reserve. *Cathet Cardiovasc Diagn*. 1996;39:120–125.
23. Ong P, et al. High prevalence of a pathological response to acetylcholine testing in patients with stable angina pectoris and unobstructed coronary arteries: the ACOVA Study (Abnormal COronary VAsomotion in patients with stable angina and unobstructed coronary arteries). *J Am Coll Cardiol*. 2012;59:655–662.
24. Sueda S, et al. Clinical and angiographical characteristics of acetylcholine-induced spasm: relationship to dose of intracoronary injection of acetylcholine. *Coron Artery Dis*. 2002;13:231–236.
25. Sueda S, et al. Frequency of provoked coronary vasospasm in patients undergoing coronary arteriography with spasm provocation test of acetylcholine. *Am J Cardiol*. 1999;83:1186–1190.
26. Sueda S, et al. Major complications during spasm provocation tests with an intracoronary injection of acetylcholine. *Am J Cardiol*. 2000;85:391–394.
27. Sueda S, et al. Clinical impact of selective spasm provocation tests: comparisons between acetylcholine and ergonovine in 1508 examinations. *Coron Artery Dis*. 2004;15:491–497.

28. Coma-Canella I, et al. Ergonovine test in angina with normal coronary arteries. Is it worth doing it? *Int J Cardiol.* 2006;107:200–206.

29. Holmes CL. Vasoactive drugs in the intensive care unit. *Curr Opin Crit Care.* 2005;11:413–417.

30. Diamond LM. Cardiopulmonary resuscitation and acute cardiovascular life support—a protocol review of the updated guidelines. *Crit Care Clin.* 2007;23:873–880.

31. Overgaard CB, Dzavik V. Inotropes and vasopressors: review of physiology and clinical use in cardiovascular disease. *Circulation.* 2008;118:1047–1056.

32. Leone M, Martin C. Vasopressor use in septic shock: an update. *Curr Opin Anaesthesiol.* 2008;21:141–147.

33. Kowey PR. Pharmacological effects of antiarrhythmic drugs. Review and update. *Arch Intern Med.* 1998;158:325–332.

34. Kowey PR, et al. Classification and pharmacology of antiarrhythmic drugs. *Am Heart J.* 2000;140:12–20.

35. Field JM, et al. Part 1: executive summary: 2010 American Heart Association Guidelines for Cardiopulmonary Resuscitation and Emergency Cardiovascular Care. *Circulation.* 122:S640–S656.

36. Hazinski MF, et al. Part 1: executive summary: 2010 International Consensus on Cardiopulmonary Resuscitation and Emergency Cardiovascular Care Science With Treatment Recommendations. *Circulation.* 2010;122:S250–S275.

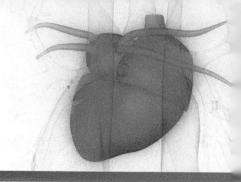

Fundamentals of X-ray Imaging, Radiation Safety, and Contrast Media

Jeremy D. Rier, DO and Charles E. Chambers, MD, MSCAI

The interventional cardiologist is required to master many skills. Most of these provide immediate positive or negative feedback. Procedural best practices in radiation safety and contrast usage, while essential, provide less immediate feedback. The operator may not "see" when imaging in steep angles impacts dose, nor appreciate the importance of contrast management until either skin or renal injury is identified in post-case follow-up. Therefore, the interventionist must have the knowledge base to manage radiation and contrast dose with an appreciation of the need to do this from the outset of the procedure, not when a high dose of either "agent" is reached. To that end, this chapter is written as a concise, schematic look at these intertwined issues of radiation and contrast management for the purposes of interventional cardiology board review with the additional hope to impact best practice.

Image Formation, Equipment Use, and Cine Storage

The Physics of Imaging

Imaging systems have seen significant evolution over the years, all while the basic principles of image formation remain in play. The general concept of what happens between the generator and the x-ray tube when forming x-rays is shown in **Figure 6.1** (1). The x-ray tube is a vacuum tube with a cathode coil (or coils) facing a spinning anode. Electrons are sent to the cathode from the generator, and the cathode becomes white hot (about 3,000°F). At this temperature, the electrons virtually boil off (thermionic emission). The generator also sets up a voltage potential across the x-ray tube. The electrons

from the cathode cross from the cathode to the anode as a result of this voltage potential. The maximal (peak) voltage across the x-ray tube is referred to as the kVp, representing the energy of the photons. The number of photons that cross from the cathode to the anode is mA (milliamperes). Radiation dose is determined by variations in mA and kVp and ultimately impacts image quality.

Most of the electrons that cross from the cathode to the anode produce heat, with only a small percentage actually striking the anode to produce x-rays. Early generation x-ray tubes were limited due to the challenges of heat production. Current systems control the heat generated, with the anode rotating rapidly (3,500–10,000 rpm) in conjunction with oil circulating around the x-ray tube to help cool it. Photons that strike the tungsten anode produce x-rays that emerge from a point source called the x-ray beam focal spot. Because low-frequency x-rays are not clinically useful and only contribute to noise, many of them are absorbed by copper and aluminum filters added at the output of the x-ray tube. Collimation helps shape the x-ray beam as it emerges, as well as reduce scatter and decrease exposure. *Scatter radiation from Compton interactions* within the patient is directly related to dose, degrades image quality, and serves as the primary source of radiation exposure to the operator and staff (2).

Creation of an image has similarly seen significant advances in recent years with the evolution from the image intensifier to flat-panel microprocessor technology. "Flat-panel" detectors have replaced the image intensifier and television camera in traditional analog imaging chains for improved efficiency of the image formation process (Fig. 6.2). In a *flat-panel* system, the clumps of photons are converted to electrons by a layer of photodiodes. This technology incorporates detectors with a charge-coupled visible-light device that is in direct contact with the input phosphor. This signal is then digitized and sent directly from the panel to the monitor for display. This direct digital video signal is generated from the original visible-light fluorescence without an intervening stage. *The fewer steps in image transfer, the less the image is degraded. This results in enhanced image uniformity, uniform brightness, and dynamic range when compared to the multiple image transfer required in the image intensifier.* The avoidance of another conversion of energy to light, and then to electricity, improves the overall performance of the flat-panel system. Improved image quality through reduced image transfer allows for dose reduction. Although "analog" and "digital" systems share similar x-ray tube technologies, it is the "detector" that has fundamentally changed the way images are formed and processed (3).

X-rays diverge as they leave the x-ray tube and travel through the table and patient toward the image detector (Fig. 6.2). Most of the x-rays never make it to the image detector, because they are absorbed, attenuated, or scattered by the patient and the table. While continuous emission of the x-rays has traditionally been used during fluoroscopy and pulsing of the x-ray beam used during cineangiographic acquisition, newer systems now pulse the fluoroscopic beam as well. Pulsing the fluoroscopic beam reduces total x-ray exposure, with many studies in adults now utilizing fluoroscopic rates of 7.5 frames/s. To assure adequate image quality, the image detector is

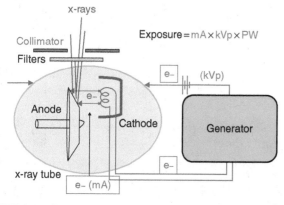

FIGURE 6.1 The x-ray tube is depicted. A potential is set up across the x-ray tube that encourages electrons from the cathode inside the vacuum tube to jump to the anode. The peak voltage across the x-ray tube is referred to as the kVp of the system, and the number of electrons that jump is referred to as the mA. The exposure equation is defined as the mA × kVp × pulse width. Collimators and filters help shape and filter out unusable x-rays.

Exposure = mA × kVp × PW

programmed to provide feedback to the x-ray tube based on the output voltage (automatic dose-rate exposure control). *This internally modulated x-ray production is designed to utilize the least possible dose so as to produce an acceptable image quality.*

Flat-panel technology has significantly improved the prior challenges with dynamic range that resulted in blooming over denser bones, where more exposure was required, than the lungs. Patient characteristics, such as an obese patient, and procedure requirements, such as steep angulated views, require an increased dose to satisfy the exposure equation. Magnification increases dose, although to a lesser degree in the current era of flat-panel technology. These parameters are initially set by the manufacturer, with modification required based upon individual laboratory needs. Resolution is dependent upon field size. With small field-of-view imaging, the resolution may increase. However, with a larger field of view, image processing bundles pixels to achieve magnification. Because the image may actually lose resolution, an increase in x-ray dose is required to keep the signal-to-noise ratio satisfactory (4).

Basic Operation of an X-ray Cine/Fluoroscopic Unit

With a basic understanding of image formation, it is important to understand how this process is modulated so as to maximize image quality while minimizing dose, *recognizing that image quality can almost always be improved by increasing dose.* **Figure 6.3** shows a block diagram of the key elements of an interventional fluoroscope,

emphasizing the role of the physician in maximizing image quality and minimizing dose. An essential component in this process, not seen in the diagram, is the presence of high-resolution, in-room, table-side monitors. Careful attention must be paid to the calibration, resolution (contrast and spatial), and dynamic range of these monitors. Complete system operation is determined by the combination of operator-selectable parameters and feedback elements that stabilize system performance and imaging. The operator is the center for many of these control loops.

Multiple imaging parameters influence exposure associated with a cine/fluoroscopic examination (2,4). These include the following:

1. *X-ray image detector dose per pulse:* This is the dose for each x-ray pulse (typically measured in nanogray) that reaches the detector. It is important to note that the detector dose is considerably smaller than the subject dose, given that generally 5% or less of the incident radiation penetrates the subject and reaches the detector.
2. *X-ray unit framing (pulsing) rate:* This is the number of pulses the x-ray system generates per unit of time. It is an operator-selectable parameter that ranges between 4 and 30 pulses/s and is a determinant of image *temporal* resolution.
3. *Imaging field size:* This is the area of the x-ray beam that impinges on the subject. It is discussed in greater depth later under "kerma area product (KAP)" in the "Assessment of Dose in Fluoroscopic Procedures" section.

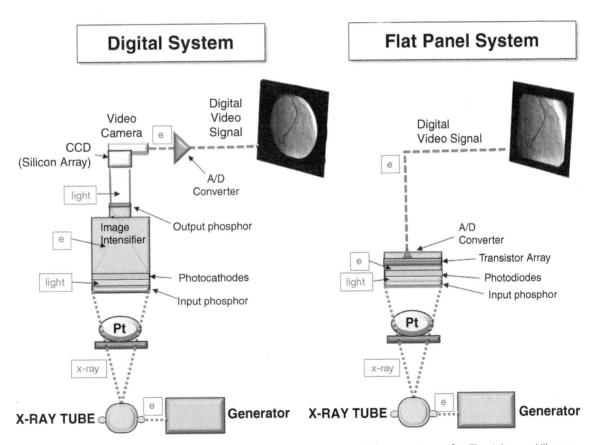

FIGURE 6.2 The left panel represents the older digital imaging system with the image intensifier. The right panel illustrates the current flat-panel system. Electrons generated are converted to x-rays, pass through the patient, and are sensed on the input phosphor and converted to light in both systems. The limitation with the *image intensifier* is the multiple steps involved. Light photons are converted back to electrons, accelerated, and strike the output phosphor. The image is then picked up by the CCD chips, converted to a video signal, digitized in the A/D converter and sent to the monitor. In the *flat-panel system,* the light is converted to electrons, sensed by a transistor array, digitized, and sent directly to the monitor.

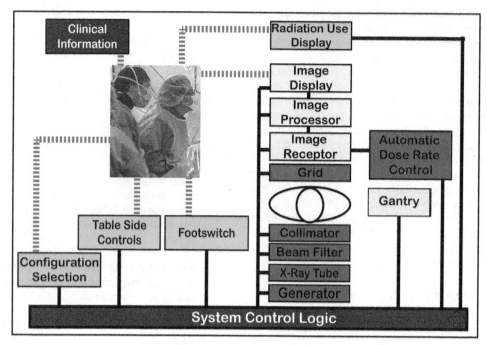

FIGURE 6.3 This is a diagrammatic representation of an x-ray fluoroscopy system illustrating the pathway from x-ray production through image formation. This emphasizes the role of a knowledgeable physician recognizing the appropriate feedback loops in controlling radiation dose and image quality.

4. *X-ray beam filtration:* An x-ray tube produces a spectrum of x-ray photon energies. The lower-energy photons (photon energies <30 keV) have insufficient penetrating power to reach the detector, and thus expose the subject without contributing to image formation. These "undesirable" photons are typically "filtered" out of the x-ray beam by interposing layers of aluminum and copper in the x-ray tube exit port.

Image Storage

While high-quality, real-time fluoroscopic imaging is required for procedure performance, cineangiographic acquisition for post-procedure review, as well as long-term access, is similarly necessary. Digital imaging allows for high-resolution image data to be made immediately available. However, this increase in information content that occurs with digital imaging requires a significant increase in system "bandwidth" to facilitate "on-line" and post-acquisition review and archiving of studies. Newer systems all have the system bandwidth for storage and transfer of large amounts of data. Once in a digital format, the data are then written to the disk using the DICOM (Digital Communication in Medicine) standard, established in the 1990s. This format provides for "seamless" image access of this digital data for viewing across internal and external network connections. Additionally, this provides a medium for short- and long-term image storage on a variety of archival media devices, including disaster recovery technology to prevent data loss. Initially limited by large expensive storage capabilities, the duration of digital image storage, previously defined in the film era as 7 years, was continued. However, as the cost of digital storage has dropped, with ready availability of terabytes for large media storage, the long-term availability of these cine images for case review has become less of a concern and has often been extended (2).

Radiation Dose

Terminology

Confusion often exists regarding the various terms used to describe radiation, radiation absorption, and radiation exposure. The traditional use of the *ALARA (As Low As Reasonably Achievable)* principle is still required, as no dose of ionizing radiation is without harm. The basic unit of radiation ionization is the roentgen (R). It is the amount of ionization that a defined mass of air undergoes when bombarded by x-rays or γ-rays. The amount of energy actually absorbed by material is the *radiation absorbed dose (rad)* and varies according to the type of radiation and atomic number of the material. Radiation protection units are simply rads times some quality factor that is dependent on the type of radiation, and these units are called *rems* (Roentgen equivalent man, rem dose = rad dose $\times$ QF $\times$ other modifying factors). In cardiology, the quality factor is 1.0 for both x-rays and γ-rays, so rems and rads are equal.

The following is a list of commonly used terms:

Exposure: Exposure is rarely used as a quantity, with *air kerma* now preferred for measuring the amount of radiation present at a location. The Système Internationale (SI) units of the measurement of exposure are coulombs of charge produced per kilogram of air (C/kg). However an older obsolete unit, the roentgen (abbreviated R, and equal to 2.58×10^{-4} C/kg), is sometimes reported.
Kerma: This is Kinetic Energy Released in Material, used to measure units of energy per mass in mGy.
Air kerma: This is the above-defined kerma delivered to air.
Dose: Radiologic *dose* is the local concentration of energy, extracted from a radiation field, when it interacts with matter. It refers to the absorption of energy in matter following interactions with ionizing radiation.
Absorbed dose: This is energy absorbed per mass of material measured in mGy. It is directly related to the severity of reactions (skin effects).

Effective dose: This is the hypothetical equivalent of *whole-body dose* that produces the same magnitude of cancer risk as dose from an actual absorbed/equivalent dose delivered to a limited portion of the body. The effective dose represents a sum of equivalent doses from different tissues adjusted for the radiation absorption capacity of each tissue. *Equivalent dose:* This is a term needed for dosimetry of neutrons. In cardiology, while equivalent dose for a specific organ exposed may be used interchangeably with absorbed dose, it often creates confusion due to different units/quantities of measure. *Therefore, caution is recommended in using this term in fluoroscopic imaging.*

Example, 10 mGy (absorbed dose) = 10 mSv (equivalent dose), with 1 mSv = 100 mrem. Air kerma, 1 rad (1 cGy) represents radiation in air. Absorbed dose, 1 rad (1 cGy), represents the energy deposited in tissue. Effective dose, 1 rem (10 mSv), represents whole-body risk. Equivalent dose, 1 rem (10 mSv), represents dose quantity for biologic damage.

Assessment of Dose in Fluoroscopic Procedures

Because all fluoroscopic equipment sold in the US since 2006 is required to measure and display dose parameters, current guidelines recommend recording all relevant patient procedure radiation dose data (4–6). These measures include the following:

Total air kerma at the interventional reference point (IRP) ($K_{a,r}$, Gy) is the procedural cumulative air kerma (x-ray energy delivered to air) at the IRP. This point is 15 cm on the x-ray tube side of isocenter, which is the primary x-ray beam intersection with the rotational axis of the "C" arm gantry. $K_{a,r}$ is used to monitor patient dose burden because it is associated with threshold-dependent deterministic skin effects. This is also referred to as cumulative air kerma (CAK).

Air KAP (P_{KA}, Gycm^2) is the product of instantaneous air kerma and x-ray field area. Unlike $K_{a,r}$, P_{KA} is impacted by collimation because it includes the field exposed. P_{KA} is used to monitor the linear, non-threshold patient dose burden associated with potential stochastic/cancer effects. This is also referred to as dose area product (DAP) and KAP.

Peak skin dose (PSD, Gy) is the maximum dose received by any area of a patient's skin. While some systems provide these estimates, the most accurate assessments of PSD are obtained by a qualified physicist if air kerma and x-ray geometry details are known.

Fluoroscopic time (FT, min), once a time-honored parameter to follow, is now recognized as not being a measure of procedural radiation, as are these other true dose parameters. This is time-, not dose-dependent, and does not include cine imaging, nor reflect dose changes with angulation or frame rate. Steeper angulations, larger patients, and patient extremities in the field of view will significantly increase dose without affecting FT. The operator who utilizes store fluoroscopy, minimizes angles, and reduces frame rate will decrease dose. However, when compared based on FT to other operators and labs, these improvements will not be seen (7).

Procedural Radiation Awareness

In interventional cardiology, the importance of a radiation-conscious environment is essential, where protection of the patient, in turn, protects the staff, and vice versa (6). Methods for measuring patient dose, monitoring staff dose, implementing appropriate training, and managing radiation dose from the outset of the procedure are all important components of a cardiac catheterization laboratory's radiation safety program (6,8,9). High-level factors that should be considered include:

- *Equipment:* Fluoroscopes are general-purpose instruments. Appropriate configuration to accommodate the current clinical task is essential to the procedure. Unacceptable patient irradiation and/or image quality will occur if the equipment is inappropriately configured.
- *Operator:* The total dose delivered to a patient is influenced by an operator's ability to manage radiation appropriately. Therefore, operators must be mindful of radiation use to justify continuing with the procedure based on their assessment of benefit and risk.
- *Patient:* Complex patients are the norm in current interventional practice. Assessing risk based upon the patient's prior procedures, body habitus, co-morbidities, and lesion characteristics allows the operator in managing radiation dose from procedure onset.

Biologic Effects from X-ray Exposure

Radiation-induced changes have a common mechanism: molecular damage caused by particles or photons of sufficient energy to induce atomic ionization (10). This is the basis of the term "ionizing radiation." X-rays are classified as a form of ionizing radiation because each x-ray photon contains enough energy to ionize atoms and disrupt molecular bonds. *Direct ionization* means the radiation disrupts the atomic structure of the material it strikes, producing chemical and biologic changes. X-rays (and γ-rays) are *indirectly ionizing*. When absorbed, they produce fast-moving particles that can ionize other atoms, breaking vital chemical bonds. The biologic effects due to the production of free radicals result from either a single-stranded break or a double-strand DNA break. Single-strand breaks are readily healed, with no cell death, but if they are incorrectly repaired, a mutation may occur. Double-strand breaks are less common, but more serious. If enough cell damage occurs to prevent normal function, necrosis occurs, appearing within days to months following the exposure. However, if DNA damage occurs without necrosis, carcinogenesis may occur, becoming evident many years following the exposure. Although significant radiation-induced injury from isolated episodes is typically limited, all radiation exposure confers risk, classified as *Deterministic and Stochastic* (2,4).

Deterministic effects are dose-dependent direct health effects of radiation, for which a threshold exists, *linear with threshold*. These tissue reactions can cause cell necrosis, preventing normal function, including repair. If extensive enough damage occurs, clear tissue injury will occur (11). Skin injury is the most common tissue reaction observed in cardiovascular imaging, and may lead to significant tissue necrosis, typically presenting weeks after exposure (Fig. 6.4). Patient factors associated with skin injury include light-colored skin, smoking, poor nutrition, obesity, hyperthyroidism, diabetes, connective tissue disorders, chemotherapy, and recent radiation exposure or previous high-dose radiation tissue injury.

Air kerma at the IRP, $K_{a,r}$, is used to approximate the patient's entrance skin dose relating to skin injury listed (Table 6.1). Dose-dependent skin injury occurs with a time delay that can impede correct early recognition (Table 6.2). Therefore, all patients who receive a $K_{a,r}$ greater than 5 Gy should be told of potential skin injury and provided follow-up. X-ray-induced skin injuries are often best managed with good dermatologic care, without biopsy if possible, to prevent further tissue damage that may not heal (4).

Stochastic effects of radiation occur by chance in a population of exposed persons, for which no clear threshold exists. Probability is proportional to radiation dose, and the severity is independent of dose, *linear, non-threshold*. A stochastic injury occurs when there is non-fatal injury to the DNA backbone that does not properly

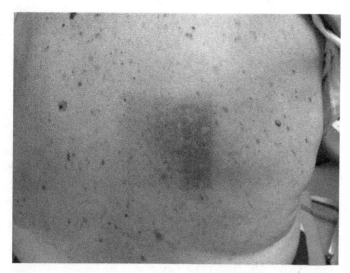

FIGURE 6.4   Tissue injury is seen 1 month following a complex PCI. Notice the characteristic square configuration, as well as the variation in coloration. FT was 104 minutes with no dose recorded. This color variation represents variations in skin exposure produced by alterations in angles and or collimation. This produced representative skin dose injury that is likely 5 Gy at the least intense coloration and exceeding 10 Gy at the most intense color changes. FT, fluoroscopic time; PCI, percutaneous coronary intervention.

heal itself, resulting in mutation, which leads to either cancer or a genetic abnormality. The risk is related to the dose delivered and the volume of tissue exposed and requires time for one transformed cell to multiply into a malignancy with a latent period in years (average 20 years). Therefore, the stochastic risk from a given radiation exposure is greater in the young and, at a given age, greater in females than males. Knowing the individual's age and sex, as well as the organs at greatest risk, assists the operator in assessing individual patient risk. This may be inconsequential if the patient's expected survival is less than the latent period for the adverse effect to occur.

Each of the body's organs has a variable susceptibility to radiation injury; the more biologically active organs are more susceptible to radiation. Models have been created to calculate coefficients that estimate the excess relative/absolute risk per sievert of exposure. The BEIR VII model for incidence and mortality for all solid cancers (excluding thyroid and non-melanoma skin) lists the associated risk with a dose of one sievert (12). The risk estimates for ages greater than 60 is limited by small sample sizes in the studied population. The data clearly demonstrate the direct age-relationship for sensitivity to radiation-induced cancer. These are gender averaged and thus do not reflect differences between males and females.

TABLE 6.1   Chronology and Severity Thresholds of Tissue Reactions from Single-Delivery Radiation Dose

SINGLE SITE (Gy) ACUTE SKIN DOSE	PROMPT <2 WKS	EARLY 2–8 WKS	MID TERM 6–52 WKS	LONG TERM >52 WKS
0–2	No observable effects expected.			
2–5	Transient erythema	Epilation	Recovery from hair loss	None expected
5–10	Transient erythema	Erythema, epilation	Recovery; high doses cause Prolonged erythema and Permanent partial epilation	Recovery; higher Dose cause dermal Atrophy/induration
10–15	Transient erythema	Erythema, epilation Dry/moist desquamation	Prolonged erythema Permanent epilation	Telangietasia; dermal Atrophy/induration
>15	Transient erythema; Very high-dose causes Edema/ulceration	Erythema, epilation Moist desquamation	Dermal atrophy with Secondary ulceration; Late surgical repair likely	Telangiectasia; dermal Atrophy/induration; Skin breakdown Surgical repair likely

Modified from Balter S, Schuler BA, Miller DL, et al. NCRP radiation dose management for fluoroscopically guided interventional medical procedures. National Council on Radiation Protection and Measures, NCRP Report No.168, NCRP, 2011. http://www.ncrppublications.org/Reports/168.

TABLE 6.2   Suggested Values for First and Subsequent Notifications and the Substantial Radiation Dose Level (SRDL)

DOSE METRIC	FIRST NOTIFICATION	SUBSEQUENT NOTIFICATIONS (INCREMENTS)	SRDL
$D_{skin,max}$[a]	2 Gy	0.5 Gy	3 Gy
$K_{a,r}$[b]	3 Gy	1 Gy	5 Gy[b]
P_{KA}[c]	300 Gy cm^2 [d]	100 Gy cm^2 [d]	500 Gy cm^2 [d]
Fluoroscopy time	30 min	15 min	60 min

[a]$D_{skin,max}$ is peak skin dose, requiring calculations by physicist.
[b]$K_{a,r}$ is total air kerma at the reference point.
[c]P_{KA} is air kerma area product.
[d]Assuming a 100 cm^2 field at the patient's skin. For other field sizes, the P_{KA} values should be adjusted proportionally to the actual procedural field size (e.g., for a field size of 50 cm^2, the SRDL value for P_{KA} would be 250 Gy cm^2).
Modified from Balter S, Schuler BA, Miller DL, et al. NCRP radiation dose management for fluoroscopically guided interventional medical procedures. National Council on Radiation Protection and Measures, NCRP Report No.168. NCRP, 2011. http://www.ncrppublications.org/Reports/168.

Radiation Exposure in Interventional Cardiology

The majority of radiation an individual receives annually comes from background radiation. However, the advances in medical diagnosis and treatment have occurred in the setting of increasing radiation exposure (10). Although interventional cardiology contributes a relatively small component to this increase, efforts have focused on establishing a radiation safety program for all cardiac catheterization laboratories, where dose reduction for the patient similarly benefits the operator and staff.

Patient Exposure and Risk

The annual patient radiation dose from medical imaging has increased threefold since 1982, with cardiovascular dose alone increasing approximately 20%. This risk includes a threefold increase in patient medical radiation exposure over the past 25 years. Nineteen percent of the entire patient annual radiation exposure is attributed to cardiovascular imaging (6.2 mSv total, 3.0 mSv all medical imaging, 1.2 mSv cardiac) (10). This dramatic increase in radiation from medical imaging has appropriately heightened concerns for radiation safety. Table 6.3 outlines the typical effective doses for invasive and non-invasive cardiac procedures (13).

Patients receive approximately 20 mSv/min from continuous fluoroscopy alone, correlating to 100 to 200 chest x-rays/min of fluoroscopy (14). Unlike chest x-rays, where >90% of a patient's exposure is within the body, a patient's actual radiation exposure from fluoroscopy occurs inside the imaging field (15). This illustrates the challenges of comparing these two forms of x-ray exposure regarding stochastic risk. While vascular injury from high-dose radiation for cancer therapy can lead to premature cardiovascular disease, particularly in young adults, these events suggest an endothelial component to radiation-induced vascular injury, *which has not been identified from cine-fluoroscopic exposure.*

Exposure and Risk to Operator and Staff

Compared to a patient, an operator's single procedure exposure is significantly less. However, high lifetime exposure from repeated procedures is not uncommon. Operator exposure is expressed as *equivalent dose* for organ-specific exposure and as *effective dose* for whole-body exposure. The effective dose represents a sum of equivalent doses from different tissues adjusted for the radiation absorption capacity of each tissue. Note that the total recommended maximal dose for an invasive cardiologist is 50 mSv (rem)/y, and the total accumulative dose is age × 10 mSv (age × total rems) (16). Table 6.4 lists the National Council on Radiation Protection (NCRP) recommendations for occupational radiation dose limits. The International Council for Radiation protection (ICRP) has lowered their limits to 20 mSv not only for total body annual but also for the eye (17). This is based upon concerns that eye injury occurs at doses lower than previously reported. NCRP has not altered their recommendations as of February 2017.

An interventional cardiologist, utilizing best practices for radiation protection, receives about 1 to 10 mSv/y (18), dependent upon volume and case section. This is significantly below the U.S. occupational dose limit of 50 mSv/y. However, a busy interventionalist doing complex cases may receive in excess of 50 mSv/y; this emphasizes the importance of personnel dosimeters and best practices for radiation safety. Nurses and technologists, dependent upon their role and location during the procedure, receive approximately 2 mSv/y.

TABLE 6.3 Typical Effective Doses for Cardiac Procedures (13)

MODALITY	PROTOCOL	EFFECTIVE DOSE (mSv)
MDCT	CT angio.: prospective triggering	0.5–7
MDCT	CT angio.: high-pitch helical	<0.5–3
MDCT	CT angio., pre-TAVR (multi-phase)	5–50
MDCT	Calcium scoring	1–5
SPECT	10/30 mi Ci 99m Tc sestamibi St/Rst	11
SPECT	10/30 mi Ci 99m Tc tetrofosmin St/Rst	9
SPECT	Dual isotope (3.5 mi Ci Tl/30 mi Ci Tc)	22–23
PET	50 mCi 82 Rb rest/50 mCi 82 Rb stress	4
Inv. Dx	Dx cath: coronaries and ventriculography	2–20
Inv. Inter.	PCI Intervention, with or without Dx cath	5–57
TAVR	Early data (?):, trans apical and trans femoral	12–>50?
EP	Diagnostic	0.1–3.2
EP	Ablation	1–25
EP	Device insertion	0.2–8

TABLE 6.4 Recommended Dose Limits from the NCRP

BACKGROUND RADIATION	3.6 mSv (0.36 rem)
Chest x-ray	0.02–0.04 mSv
Annual Dose Limits	
Stochastic effects	
Cumulative	10 mSv × age (rem × age)
Annual	50 mSv (5 rems)
Deterministic effects (Annual)	
Eye	150 mSv/y (15 rem)
Skin	500 mSv/y (50 rem)
Embryo or fetus	0.5 mSv/mo (0.05 rem)

Adapted from Hall EJ. Radiation protection. In: Hall EJ, ed. *Radiobiology for the Radiologist.* Philadelphia, PA: Lippincott Williams & Wilkins; 2000:234–248; International Commission on Radiation Units and Measurements. Recommendations. Report 60. New York, NY: Pergamon Press; 1991; National Council on Radiation Protection and Measurement. Recommendations for limits on exposure to ionizing radiation. Report 116. Bethesda, MD: National Council on Radiation Protection and Measurement, 1993.

The cumulative additional risk for cancer in those exposed to occupational radiation is about 0.004% × mSv (or 0.04% × rem). If a busy interventionist receives 25 mSv/y and practices for 20 years, his total dose would be about 500 mSv (50 rem), with an added risk of 500 × 0.004% or 2%. This additional radiation exposure would increase the cancer risk 20% to 22% from baseline (18).

Maternal and fetal risks are reviewed in several multi-societal papers (19,20). Radiation exposure to the fetus is particularly an issue during the first trimester. However, radiation exposure within 2 weeks of uterine implantation of the fertilized egg may be less critical, because all of the cells at that point are pluripotent. The United Nations Scientific Committee on the Effects of Atomic Radiation (UNSCEAR) suggests that the risk of a fetal congenital malformation or a malignancy is about 0.0002% per mSv (0.002% per rem) exposure. A dose of 100 mSv (10 rem) during the most sensitive period (10 days to 26 weeks) is often regarded as the cutoff point for considering a therapeutic abortion.

While invasive/interventional cardiology is appropriately focused on patient outcomes, the risks to the profession have received far less attention and differ significantly from other medical disciplines. In addition to the potential radiation concerns, which include cataract formation (21), brain tumors (22), skin injury, and inheritable defects, orthopedic injuries from protective attire are frequent. These are often categorized as anecdotal and are thus underestimated (23). Individuals entering into interventional cardiology often have limited understanding of these issues. Recognizing that techniques utilized to reduce patient dose will reduce operator dose, the interventional cardiologist should assess this benefit; that is, the risk analysis for the patient comes in understanding that operator and staff benefits must be considered in the context of maximal patient safety. As interventional cardiologists, we need to continue to strive for the safest environment for our patients, staff, and ourselves.

Personnel Dosimetry and Patient Lifetime Exposure

Radiation exposure to the operator is usually measured with either a TLD (thermoluminescent dosimeter) badge or an OSL (optically simulated luminescent) badge. The TLD badge has a LiF crystal that absorbs x-rays. When heated, it releases light photons in proportion to the amount of x-ray absorbed. The OSL badge is similar, but the substrate is aluminum oxide doped with carbon, and it releases light in proportion to the amount of x-ray absorbed when struck with a laser. The badges have different filters to mimic attenuation for different parts of the body. The results are usually reported for shallow, lens, or deep dose exposure. It is an individual's responsibility to wear a dosimeter for personal benefit, although state regulations are in place to enforce this practice.

While a single dosimeter worn outside the collar can be used and is acceptable, two dosimeters, when properly worn (one under the garment and one at the collar outside the protective garment), is a better reflection of effective dose (6,8). Real-time operator dose monitoring has been studied and shown to be effective in procedural dose reduction (24). The pregnant worker should wear a dosimeter under the lead collar, as well as on the thyroid collar, with no more than 0.5 mSv (0.05 rem)/mo, not to exceed 5 mSv (0.5 rem) total exposures, once the pregnancy is declared. Legal precedent supports a pregnant worker remaining in the laboratory if she chooses, but counseling from the radiation safety officer is recommended (16,19,20).

No system is currently in place to monitor an *individual patients'* *cumulative lifetime radiation exposure*. The availability and ACCF/AHA/SCAI-recommended reporting of all relevant patient procedure radiation dose data—including FT (minute), total air kerma at the IRP (Gy), and air KAP (Gy cm²)—make such a monitoring system possible (25). However, the dispersion of patient radiation exposures across multiple care sites with separate medical records will require a comprehensive program to document an individual patient's cumulative radiation exposure.

Radiation Dose Management in the Catheterization Laboratory

In 2010, the FDA called for radiation reduction in medical imaging (26). Equipment manufacturers responded with system modifications and best practice protocols in fluoroscopic imaging, which will be discussed later. Organization and societies have published their recommendations on radiation dose management in the cardiac catheterization laboratory (4,6).

Training

The interventional cardiology board certification examination includes physics and radiation safety. Although only certain states mandate fluoroscopy training, everyone should receive radiation safety training commensurate to their responsibilities. This catheterization laboratory radiation safety education program should be coordinated in conjunction with the hospital radiation safety officer and include the following NCRP components (4):

1. Initial didactic training that should include the following topics: physics of x-ray production; equipment technology with modes of operation; image quality in fluoroscopy; dosimetry, quantities and units; biological effects of radiation; principles of radiation safety; applicable federal, state, and local regulations; requirements and techniques to minimize patient and staff dose
2. Periodic, annual, updates on radiation safety
3. Hands on training for newly hired operators and current operators on new equipment

Minimizing Radiation Exposure: Radiation Dose Management

A successful cardiac catheterization laboratory must have a radiation safety program committed to reducing patient and staff radiation exposure to a level that reflects the ALARA principle (27). Procedure *justification and dose optimization* are key concepts. The first step is avoiding unnecessary use of ionizing radiation by requiring justification for exposure. Recognizing the role for Appropriate Use Criteria and preventing repetitive procedures is essential for all imaging modalities. Once justified, dose optimization is essential. The interventional imaging team, physicians, technologists, physicists, and other medical personnel should be responsible for developing protocols, implementing regular equipment quality control tests, and monitoring patients' radiation doses. This requires a *quality assurance program* emphasizing and monitoring best practices in radiation management (5).

A procedure-based review of radiation dose management is essential, including pre-procedure, procedure, and post-procedure best practice recommendations, outlined in **Table 6.5** (4,6). *Pre-procedure* planning includes identifying the high-risk patient (obese, complex disease, or fluoroscopic procedures needed within 30–60 days) and obtaining informed consent. *During the case*, the physician should manage dosage from the outset, monitoring key components of this optimal procedure. Dose management is reviewed below. Staff must

TABLE 6.5 Components of Radiation Dose Management in PCI

Pre-Procedure

Obtain patient's radiation history; check patient's skin if positive Hx

Extend radiation aspects of informed consent when appropriate especially for high-risk cases (CTO)

Plan alternative beam orientations for forthcoming case when necessary

Time Out

Verify that fluoroscopic system settings are correct for the planned procedure

All staff should be wearing their personal radiation monitors (staff safety item)

All staff wearing their radiation and non-radiation PPE (staff safety item)

Ancillary radiation shielding devices present in lab (staff safety item)

During Procedure

Minimizing radiation exposure to the patient (Table 6.6)

Time, distance, and shielding for occupational dose reduction (see Text)

Remember: Best practices to reduce patient dose benefit operator and staff.

Regular radiation dose notification by staff with brief pause to assess benefit-risk

Post-Procedure

Complete patient dosimetry recorded in medical record and case report

Substantial dose of radiation justified in medical record when appropriate

Patient notified if substantial dose of radiation was used; and given their initial follow-up processes.

Patents receiving substantial doses followed as appropriate.

Radiation safety issues must be a part of the Cardiac Catheterization Laboratory Quality Program.

TABLE 6.6 Minimizing Radiation Exposure to the Patient

Proper collimation
Minimize the beam "on-time"
Use filters at the output of the x-ray tube
Keep the kVp as high as possible to maintain good image contrast
Minimize mA
Use the minimal number of views
Keep the image intensifier as close to the patient as possible
Keep the source-to-image distance as narrow as possible
Use the lowest framing rate possible
Use pulsed fluoroscopy
Limit "high-dose" fluoroscopy
Keep the number of magnified views to a minimum
Use direct shielding of gonadal organs
Vary views to distribute radiation over a wider area

important to use fluoroscopy only when looking at the monitor and limit cine imaging. Steep angles (28), frame rate, collimation, protective shielding, and table and image receptor height are all important variables during the procedure. Operator and staff must maximize their distance from the x-ray tube (using the inverse square law). All appendages of the operator and patient should be out of the imaging field.

The acronym "DRAPED" provides a practical approach to reducing radiation exposure:

D	Distance	Inverse square law; i.e., utilize tubing extensions as needed
R	Receptor	Keep image receptor close to patient and collimate
A	Angles	Avoid steep angles
P	Pedal	Keep foot off pedal except when looking at the monitor
E	Extremities	Keep patient and operator extremities out of the beam
D	Dose	Limit cine, adjust frame rate, wear personal dosimeter

Three basic tenets for minimizing *occupational exposure* are *time, distance, and shielding.* Keep the studies as short as possible. Although a minute of fluoroscopy may only result in one tenth the dose of 1 minute of cineangiography, most of the radiation exposure in the laboratory is due to fluoroscopy. In fact, the operator typically receives about six times the dose from fluoroscopy than from cine. Remember the inverse square law and stay as far from the x-ray source as possible. Extension tubing should be attached to catheters to allow operators to be farther from the x-ray source. Distance may impact radial cases with increased operator dose but usually only for the less experienced operators (29).

Operators and staff should routinely utilize all available personal protective apparel and in-room shielding. Protective garments and aprons with thyroid shielding stop approximately 95% of scatter radiation. Ceiling- and table-mounted shields are available and are effective in operator dose reduction. With posterior sub-capsular cataract formation a proven risk for those exposed to significant eye radiation, protective glasses are effective in reducing this risk but must fit properly, have 0.25-mm lead-equivalent protection, and additional side shielding (30). Radiation caps, both disposable and reusable, are available as lead and lead-equivalent options, and have been shown to reduce cranial radiation, but long-term benefits are

provide periodic dose updates to assist the operator with radiation awareness. *Post-procedure*, all cardiac catheterization reports should include available radiation parameters: FT (min), $K_{a,r}$, (Gy), and P_{KA}, (Gy cm^2). Patient notification, chart documentation, and communication with the primary care provider should be routine for high-dose procedures. ($K_{a,r}$ >5 Gy, P_{KA} >500 Gy cm^2). Patients should be educated regarding potential skin changes with a 2 to 4 week phone call follow-up or office visit as required. For $K_{a,r}$ >10 Gy (P_{KA} >1,000 Gy cm^2), a qualified physicist should promptly calculate PSD. The Joint Commission identifies PSD >15 Gy as a sentinel event; hospital risk management and regulatory agencies should be contacted within 24 hours.

Keys to Optimal Procedural Dose Management

Operator dose is directly proportional to patient dose, thus reducing the dose to the patient will benefit the operator and staff. Developing good techniques is essential to minimize radiation dose through meticulous application of established best practices. Minimizing patient exposure benefits operator and staff (**Table 6.6**). It is less well-established (31). Sterile protective disposable drapes will decrease operator scatter but may increase patient dose.

Additional cath lab options have been developed to reduce operator dose. More extensive protective shielding is available, both ceiling suspended as well as table-mounted, to surround the operator with a weightless environmental radiation shield. Robotic systems offer a radiation-free environment for the operator in a remote/non-in-procedure room laboratory location. Embracing these, as well as improving and developing further options, will offer potentially improved safety in the work place.

Advancement in X-ray Systems

In 2010, as previously noted, the Food and Drug Administration published recommendations for enhanced imaging safety, challenging industry to improve equipment and imaging protocols (26). Current imaging equipment for invasive fluoroscopic imaging is designed to both monitor and minimize dose to produce the appropriate image for the specific procedure. In total, these changes in the imaging chain are significant:

a. *X-ray generator*: electronic control/high-frequency/high-output; automatic dose control (ADC); pulse and continuous—modes of operation with a large selection of "stations" for different procedure types, as well as multiple dose/exposure settings for each procedure.
b. *X-ray tube*: high-heat-capacity tubes with efficient anode cooling mechanism; more effective collimation (automatic) and spectral filtration ("beam hardening"); use of wedge filters.
c. *Image processing*: recursive filtering, edge enhancement, and "smoothing" algorithms.
d. *Image display*: liquid crystal display (LCD) flat-panel monitors; improved dynamic range.
e. *Dose monitoring*: DAP monitoring/display, IRP cumulative dose monitoring/display/reporting (FDA-mandated since 2006).
f. *Dose management*: virtual collimation permitting collimator settings without fluoroscopy; fluoroscopic last-image-hold; retrospective storage of fluoroscopy data.

These improved performance characteristics impact x-ray dose. Operators need to be aware of these dose-monitoring capabilities and should consult with a qualified medical physicist and the equipment manufacturer to optimize the settings for efficient x-ray use. The operator must remember that image quality is inversely related to "image noise." This point-to-point variation in image brightness can be decreased by increasing dose, thereby improving image quality. However, this increased dose is at the expense of increased radiation to the patient, staff, and operator. *As image quality and radiation dose are interwoven, the operator must know the patient/procedure, own and properly operate the equipment to its highest potential, and learn the necessary skills for radiation dose management in order to obtain the appropriate image quality at the lowest required radiation dose.*

Contrast Media

Background

The introduction of radiodinated contrast has been indispensable in the evaluation of cardiac structure and function in the cardiac catheterization laboratory. Although necessary, the use of contrast agents can result in complications that can be broadly categorized as hypersensitivity and chemotoxic reactions. Advances in the understanding of the structure and properties of contrast media has

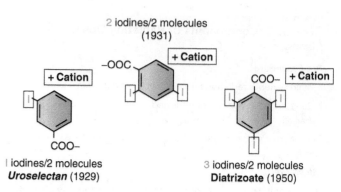

FIGURE 6.5 Ionic, high-osmolar contrast agents. Each ring has a progressive increase in the number of iodines attached. The more iodines present per molecule, the fewer the number of molecules in solution and the lower the osmolality.

led to improvement in prevention and management of complications that result from contrast agents (32).

Structure and Properties of the Contrast Media Agents

Contrast media was first introduced for urinary tract visualization in 1923. All contrast media agents have a basic structure consisting of a benzene ring (one benzene ring-monomeric; two rings dimeric), which has iodine (located at positions 2, 4, 6) and side chains (located at positions 1, 3, and 5) that differentiate the various contrast media agents (**Figs. 6.5–6.7**). The two major classifications of contrast agents for cardiovascular imaging are based on their ability to either dissociate into ionic particles in solution (ionic) or not dissociate (non-ionic). The ionic agents were the first group developed, with sodium diatrizoate and iothalamate anions as the iodine carriers, such as Renografin, Hypaque, and Angiovist. Non-ionic contrast agents began to impact clinical practice in the 1980s and now are the contrast agent of choice. While most are non-ionic monomers, there are two dimeric compounds: one ionic dimer and one non-ionic dimer. These are listed in **Table 6.7**.

In addition to iconicity, contrast agents are characterized by two additional properties: osmolality and viscosity. Osmolality refers to the concentration of a solution expressed as the number

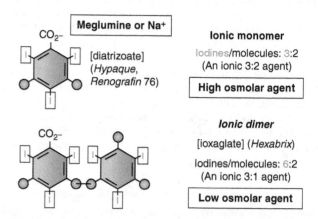

FIGURE 6.6 Ionic contrast agents. The top represents the 3:2 agent, the high-osmolar diatrizoate. The bottom combines these two into a larger molecule that still ionizes, but now has six iodines per molecule (a 6:2 or 3:1 agent) ioxaglate. Because the combination results in fewer molecules in solution, it is referred to as a low-osmolar agent.

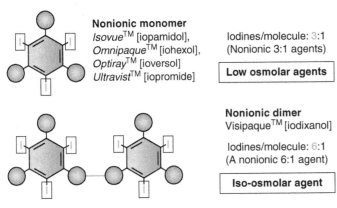

Nonionic monomer
Isovue™ [iopamidol],
Omnipaque™ [iohexol],
Optiray™ [ioversol]
Ultravist™ [iopromide]

Iodines/molecule: 3:1
(Nonionic 3:1 agents)

| Low osmolar agents |

Nonionic dimer
Visipaque™ [iodixanol]

Iodines/molecule: 6:1
(A nonionic 6:1 agent)

| Iso-osmolar agent |

FIGURE 6.7   The non-ionic contrast agents. The top panel represents the non-ionic agents, each with three iodines attached. Because there are fewer molecules in solution, these are considered low-osmolar agents. The bottom panel attaches two of these together and results in a 6:1 agent. Although a large molecule (increased viscosity), the number of molecules in solution is much lower and not too dissimilar to serum. It is referred to as an iso-osmolar agent.

of osmotically active molecules per fluid mass. Contrast media are characterized most commonly by their osmolality in reference to the normal blood osmolality (280 mOsm/kg H_2O) and include high-osmolar, low-osmolar, and iso-osmolar contrast agents (IOCM). Ionic contrast media has anionic (usually a carboxyl group) and cationic (usually sodium) components that dissociate in solution resulting in a higher osmolality. Because non-ionic contrast media do not ionize in solution, they have a lower osmolality (**Table 6.7**). A non-ionic agent may further increase their iodine carrying capacity/molecule and thereby further decrease there osmolality by becoming a dimer. Viscosity refers to the resistance of the contrast media to flow. Viscosity is directly related to particle size and is inversely related to osmolality and temperature.

High-osmolar contrast media (HOCM) are rarely used in the catheterization laboratory today (32,33). HOCM consist of ionic monomers (single benzene ring) and has an osmolality of >1,400 mOsm/kg H_2O. The HOCM agents have a ratio of three iodine atoms for every ion in solution (3:2) (Fig. 6.5). Many of the side effects, which include arrhythmic and hemodynamic side effects, are thought to result from the hypertonicity and ability to chelate calcium (34).

Low-osmolar contrast media (LOCM) have an osmolality of 500 to 1,000 mOsm/kg H_2O, which is lower than the prior generation of contrast media but is hypertonic relative to normal blood plasma. The earliest developed LOCM agent, ioxaglate, is an ionic dimer. Ioxaglate has six iodines for every two molecules (6:2 or 3:1) (Fig. 6.6). Subsequent LOCM contrast agents (iopamidol, iohexol, ioxilan, ioversol, iopromide) were developed and are non-ionic monomers that have a 3:1 ratio of iodine per ion. The newest generation of contrast media agents is the IOCM. Iodixanol (visipaque) is a non-ionic dimer that has a 6:1 ratio of iodine per ion (Fig. 6.7). While its osmolality is similar to that of plasma, its larger molecular size results in a higher viscosity than that of the older-generation contrast agents. Warming the agent can reduce the viscosity of this agent.

Physiologic Effects of Contrast Media
DIRECT CARDIOVASCULAR EFFECTS

Contrast media can directly affect the cardiovascular system, which can manifest as impaired contractility/myocardial depression, peripheral vasodilation with hypotension, fluid overload, vasovagal response, and arrhythmias (bradycardia, atrioventricular [AV] conduction delay with heart block, QRS prolongation, and ventricular arrhythmias) (34). The increased osmolality and calcium binding capacity of higher osmolality agents are thought to be responsible for these cardiovascular effects. These effects are transient and much less common with LOCM agents.

COAGULATION ISSUES

Both ionic and non-ionic agents have anticoagulant and antiplatelet effects, these being pronounced with ionic agents. With the introduction of non-ionic contrast media, there was a concern for potential thrombus formation in angiographic catheters. Initial in vitro and randomized clinical trials presented conflicting evidence regarding the pro-coagulant and antithrombotic effects of non-ionic compared to ionic contrast media. However, further studies have identified no difference between ionic and non-ionic agents regarding thrombotic complications of either type of agent (35). Although minute thrombi may form when blood and non-ionic contrast remain in a syringe, clinical sequelae have not been noted. In light of current anticoagulation regimens, possible differences in thrombogenic potential are likely negligible.

TABLE 6.7   Contrast Agents (Non-ionic Both Monomeric and Dimeric)

PRODUCT	TYPE OF CONTRAST AGENT	CONCENTRATION mg/mL	OSMOLALITY mOsm/kg WATER
Monomers			
iohexol (Omnipaque)	non-ionic LOCM	350	844
iopamidol (Isovue)	non-ionic LOCM	370	796
ioxilan (Oxilan)	non-ionic LOCM	350	695
iopromide (Ultravist)	non-ionic LOCM	370	774
ioversol (Optiray)	non-ionic LOCM	350	792
Dimers			
iodixanol (Visipaque)	non-ionic IOCM	320	290
ioxaglate (Hexabrix)	ionic LOCM	320	600

Ultravist is a registered trademark of Berlex Laboratories; Isovue is a registered trademark of Bracco Diagnostics; Omnipaque and Visipaque are registered trademarks of Nycomed Inc; Optiray is a registered trademark of Mallinckrodt Medical, Inc; Hexabrix is a registered trademark of Guerbet, S.A.
LOCM, low-osmolality contrast media; IOCM, isosmolar contrast media.

HYPERTHYROIDISM

Although the true incidence is unknown and likely very rare, the use of iodinated contrast media has been associated with both hyperthyroidism and hypothyroidism. The iodine load from contrast media is involved in the development of this pathologic state. The patients who are at the highest risk of developing thyrotoxicosis after contrast medium are patients with Graves' disease, multinodular goiter, and patients living in areas of iodine deficiency (36). The highest risk patients may benefit from an endocrinology evaluation.

Complications from the Use of Contrast Agents

Contrast media adverse reactions are infrequent and range from 5% to 12% for HOCM and from 1% to 3% for LOCM (34). When only serious adverse events are considered, the incidence for HOCM agents is estimated at about 1.0% compared with about 0.05% for LOCM agents. **Table 6.8** outlines the common complications associated with contrast agents in the cardiac catheterization laboratory. They include cardiovascular complications (both electrophysiologic and hemodynamic), hypersensitivity reactions (both acute and delayed), coagulation issues, hyperthyroidism, contrast-induced nephrotoxicity, and metformin-related lactic acidosis.

Anaphylactoid Reactions

IMMEDIATE

Allergic reactions to iodinated CM occur in ≤1% of all procedures. Contrast reactions are not truly anaphylactic because they are not IgE mediated (34,37,38). The best characterization is that they are anaphylactoid, in that they involve degranulation of mast cells and circulating basophils through direct complement activation. Therefore, CM reactions can occur even without previous exposure to contrast agents. These reactions are idiosyncratic, generally occur within 20 minutes of contrast administration, and are independent of contrast volume. This negates the potential benefits of "test dosing" to determine potential reactivity. Hypersensitivity reactions occur at a higher incidence with HOCM compared to LOCM agents. Anaphylactoid reactions are more frequent in patients with a history of atopy (asthma, allergic rhinitis, atopic dermatitis or food allergies) (three to five times), patients with previous reactions (four to six times), patients with cardiovascular and renal disease, and individuals on β-blockers (37,38). It is a common misconception that shellfish

allergies are associated with an allergy to iodinated contrast media. Although it was thought to be an "iodine" allergy, shellfish-specific tropomyosin is thought to be responsible for shellfish allergies (39). Therefore, prophylaxis is not recommended in these patients (25).

Although infrequent, serious contrast mediated anaphylactoid reactions occur, so the symptoms and treatment are important to review (**Table 6.9**). The clinical presentation of anaphylactoid reactions may be mild (skin rash, itching, nasal discharge, nausea, and vomiting), moderate (persistence of mild symptoms, facial or laryngeal edema, bronchospasm, dyspnea, tachycardia, or bradycardia), or severe (life-threatening arrhythmias, hypotension, overt bronchospasm, laryngeal edema, pulmonary edema, seizure, syncope, and death). Severe reactions must be recognized and treated immediately with aggressive fluid resuscitation, antihistamines, and, if required, epinephrine (repeat boluses or infusion if necessary). Intubation may be necessary if there is evidence of airway compromise. Patients who are on β-blockers may not respond to epinephrine and should be treated with glucagon (boluses as needed every 5 minutes, followed by an infusion if necessary) if symptoms are refractory.

Pre-treatment for prevention of acute/immediate reactions is recommended for patients with a known prior allergy to contrast and potentially considered for the patient with a strong atopic history (37–38). The recurrence rate of anaphylactoid reactions was initially estimated at 35%, a figure that originates from a single study in which a high-osmolar agent, Urografin, was used in aortic root injection. Several different treatment protocols exist, which may include glucocorticoids, H1 blocker, and H2 blockers (**Table 6.10**). Current regimens include oral prednisone 50 mg (13, 7, and 1 hour prior to the procedure) for non-urgent cases, often with the addition of H1 blockers (diphenhydramine, 50 mg). The benefit of H2 blocker therapy (cimetidine/ranitidine) is less well-substantiated. With prophylaxis, recurrent reactions may occur but are unlikely.

TABLE 6.8 Complications from Radiographic Contrast Media

Hypersensitivity reactions
  Anaphylactoid
  Delayed
Direct cardiovascular effects
  Hemodynamic and myocardial
  Electrophysiologic
Potential coagulopathy
Contrast nephropathy
Others
  Hyperthyroidism
  Encephalopathy
  Compartment syndrome (extravasation)

TABLE 6.9 Presentation and Treatment of Hypersensitivity Reactions (33)

SEVERITY	SYMPTOMS	MANAGEMENT
Mild	Urticarial rash Pruritus	Stop infusion Diphenhydramine 50 mg IV Observe for progression to severe
Severe	Hives Angioedema Laryngospasm causing stridor Bronchospasm with wheezing Respiratory distress Circulatory collapse (hypotension and tachycardia)	Stop CM infusion IM epinephrine 0.3–0.5 mg Intubation if clinically indicated Supplemental oxygen (at least 8–10 L) Normal saline boluses for hypotension Methyl prednisone 125 mg IV Diphenhydramine 50 mg IV Ranitidine 50 mg IV
Refractory symptoms	Patients with inadequate response to IM epinephrine and IV saline	Epinephrine continuous infusion, 2–10 µg/min Additional pressor if needed If patient on β-blockers and not responding to epinephrine: glucagon 1–5 mg IV over 5 min

TABLE 6.10 Prevention of Hypersensitivity Reactions from CM (33)

PATIENT STATUS	RECOMMENDED PROTOCOL
No previous history of CM reaction	Premedication not recommended
Previous history of adverse reaction (elective procedure)	Prednisone 50 mg orally 13 h, 7 h, and 1 h prior to procedure Diphenhydramine 50 mg PO 1 h prior to procedure
Previous history of adverse reaction (emergent procedure)	Hydrocortisone 200 mg IV once Diphenhydramine 50 mg IV

Limited data are available for emergent procedures in patients with known contrast-induced anaphylactoid reaction. Rapidly administering high-dose intravenous steroid or IV glucocorticoid (hydrocortisone or methylprednisolone) immediately upon recognizing the indication for the procedure, combined with the H1 blocker diphenhydramine, is an approach utilized when delaying the procedure is not an option (33).

DELAYED

The delayed reactions commonly occur within 2 days but can occur up to 5 days following contrast injection. Symptoms most commonly include rash, fever, fatigue, congestion, abdominal pain, diarrhea, constipation, and polyarthropathy (34,37,38). These reactions are common (5–8%) but frequently not identified due to the heterogeneous nature of their symptoms. Atopy has been well documented as an associated risk factor for the occurrence of both delayed and immediate reactions. Reactions such as the Koebner response, iodine sialadenitis, toxic epidermal necrolysis, and fatal acute vasculitis have all been reported as delayed reactions to contrast media. It is important to recognize this condition to prevent the unnecessary discontinuation of important medications, such as P2Y12 inhibitors, on the assumption the symptoms may be because of a new medication. Because these reactions are IgE and IgA mediated, they are generally self-limiting but often respond well to antihistamines. Steroids are rarely necessary. It is important to elicit any history of delayed contrast reaction, because these patients are at risk for immediate hypersensitivity on repeat exposure to contrast agents.

Acute Kidney Injury: Contrast-Induced Nephropathy/Contrast-Induced Acute Kidney Injury

EPIDEMIOLOGY

Acute kidney injury (AKI), is a major complication that may affect as many as 16% of patients undergoing cardiac catheterization (40,41). While it is unclear if it is a marker of a patient's overall underlying disease severity, AKI after catheterization has been associated with worse outcomes, which include: prolonged hospital stays, greater inpatient costs, short-term and long-term adverse outcomes (42). There are many potential etiologies of AKI after catheterization, including dehydration, hemodynamic instability, drug toxicity, athero-embolic disease/cholesterol embolization syndrome, and contrast-induced nephropathy (CIN), also referred to as contrast-induced acute kidney injury (CI-AKI).

The cause of CI-AKI has not been well-defined. Direct cytotoxic effects to the renal tubules and ischemic injury to the renal medulla may develop secondary to the viscosity of contrast, vasoconstriction, or decreased vasodilation (43). The loss of nitric oxide production secondary to oxidative stress may cause CI-AKI; this has been targeted

in prevention (44). The true incidence of CI-AKI after catheterization is unknown due to variations in definitions and populations studied. It is estimated to be around 3% (45). CI-AKI has been defined as a rise in serum creatinine of at least 0.5 mg/dL or a 25% increase from baseline within 48 to 72 hours after contrast administration (46). The Kidney Disease Improving Global Outcomes (KDIGO) working group has defined CI-AKI as any of the following: increase in serum creatinine by $\geq$0.3 mg/dL ($\geq$26.5 μmol/L) within 48 hours; increase in serum creatinine to $\geq$1.5 times baseline, which is known or presumed to have occurred within the prior 7 days; or urine volume <0.5 mL/kg/h for 6 hours (47). The clinical course of CI-AKI is usually benign, with creatinine levels peaking approximately at 48 to 72 hours and returning to baseline within 1 to 2 weeks (48). Occasionally, CI-AKI may progress, requiring hemodialysis in approximately 1% of patients who develop CI-AKI; this is higher in a patient with risk factors (49,50).

Chronic kidney disease (CKD) is the most powerful predictor of subsequent CI-AKI. The risk of CI-AKI increases with the decrease in estimated glomerular filtration rate (eGFR), with increased risk defined as an eGFR <60 mL/min/1.73 m². Other important risk factors include presentation (acute coronary syndrome, heart failure, and cardiogenic shock), age, and history of diabetes mellitus, anemia, and volume of contrast used during the procedure. Risk models (by Mehran et al., Gurm et al., and Tsai et al.) have been developed to predict the risk of CI-AKI (51–53). The amount of contrast used can also predict the risk of developing CI-AKI. A volume of contrast to creatinine clearance ratio (V/CrCl) of >3.7 is an independent

TABLE 6.11 Preventive Strategies for CIN

PREVENTIVE STRATEGY	RECOMMENDATION
Hydration with normal saline	Strongly recommended for all patients
Hydration with sodium bicarbonate	No additional benefit over normal saline
Minimize amount of CM	Strongly recommended for all patients
Use of non-ionic LOCM or IOCM	Recommended for all patients, especially if renal impairment is present
Hemodialysis	Not recommended
Continuous veno-venous hemofiltration	Likely beneficial but not cost-effective
Systemic fenoldopam	Not recommended
Intrarenal fenoldopam	Further studies are required to establish effectiveness
Theophylline	Controversial—currently not recommended
N-acetylcysteine	No proven benefit Considering that it is safe and inexpensive, we do not recommend against its use
Ascorbic acid	Not recommended
Statins	Likely beneficial—further studies are required
RenalGuard System	Investigational device—not available for commercial use

Adapted from Christodoulidis et al. (33)

predictor of increase in creatinine (54). A maximal radiographic contrast dose (MCRD), has been defined as MRCD = 5 mL × body weight (kg)/serum creatinine (mg/dL). This formula, developed by Freeman et al., represents the volume of contrast that predicts the risk of nephropathy requiring hemodialysis (49).

PREVENTION

With limited treatment options for CI-AKI, it is most important to reduce the risk with the goal to ultimately prevent its occurrence. However, despite significant advances in identification of risk, as well as therapeutic approaches for reduction of risk, CI-ARI is not preventable in the high-risk patient requiring contrast administration.

Therefore, protocols must be in place to assure best practice for risk reduction and assessment of occurrence if prevention is not possible in the extremely high-risk patient.

Identification of the high-risk patient with assurance of adequate hydration is essential. Several prevention strategies that have been employed with negative or mixed results include increased diuresis (mannitol, furosemide), renal vasodilators (dopamine, theophylline, fenoldopam, calcium channel blockers, endothelin receptor antagonist, atrial natriuretic peptide, prostacyclins), antioxidants (acetylcysteine, vitamin C, trimetazidine), hypothermia, and iso-osmolar contrast (**Table 6.11**). Because of the risk for nephrogenic systemic fibrosis, gadolinium is not an alternative.

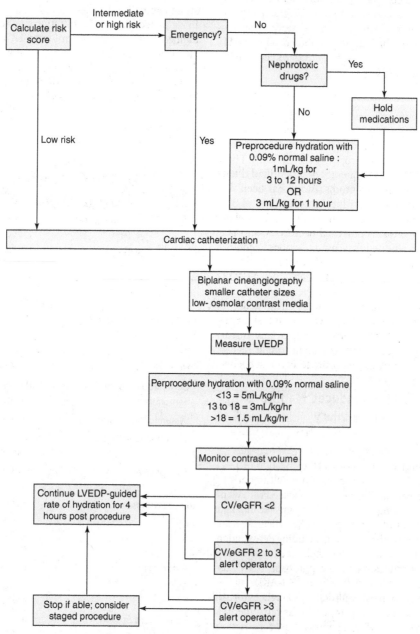

FIGURE 6.8 Algorithm for preventing/decreasing risk of CIN/ARI from contrast media. CIN, contrast-induced nephropathy.

The primary strategy that has yielded consistent results has been peri-procedural hydration. Although several treatment regimens have been proposed, the CI-AKI Consensus Working Panel recommends intravenous volume expansion with isotonic crystalloid (1.0–1.5 mL/kg/h) for 3 to 12 hours pre-procedurally, and continuing for 6 to 24 hours post-procedurally (55). Close observation is required in the patient with reduced ventricular function prone to heart failure. While there has been interest in encouraging oral hydration pre-procedurally, results of trials have shown a potential increased risk of CI-AKI with only oral hydration (56). However, appropriate reassessment of prolonged NPO periods pre-procedure often need to be reassessed. In situations where there is evidence of inadequate peri-procedural hydration, algorithms have been proposed for LVEDP-guided peri-procedural hydration rates (57). Isotonic sodium bicarbonate results in alkalization, which may protect from free radical injury. While results of clinical trials evaluating sodium bicarbonate have shown some promise, meta-analysis suggests a limited additional benefit over intravenous saline (58).

N-acetylcysteine (NAC) has been used as an antioxidant in the prevention of CI-AKI with conflicting results. Meta-analysis has not shown a significant benefit in reduction in CI-AKI with the use of NAC. Although this agent has not obviously shown a benefit, some advocate continued use for patients at the highest risk of developing nephropathy due to limited risk of therapy. Despite the fact that contrast is eliminated primarily via the kidneys, hemodialysis has not been shown to be effective in prevention of CI-AKI. Continuous veno-venous hemofiltration (CVVH) has been shown to be protective against nephropathy but is invasive and arguably not cost-effective. High-dose statins have shown promise in prevention of CI-AKI (59), although meta-analyses have questioned the benefit of statins in patients with baseline CKD (60), with further studies needed to determine their role in therapy.

There are several strategies that can be employed to prevent CI-AKI. Figure 6.8 outlines the current approaches to reduce the incidence of contrast nephropathy (25,61). Use of LOCM or IOCM agents has clearly resulted in decreased rates of CI-AKI. While theoretically more advantageous, the use of IOCM has not consistently reduced the rates of CI-AKI, although controversy still exists (62). Limiting contrast volume is essential. Both before and during the procedure, the maximal contrast dose should be discussed with contrast dose management key. If available, biplane coronary angiography should be considered to reduce the contrast administered. Additionally, the contrast volume can be minimized by avoiding "test" injections, use of smaller French size catheters, careful selection of diagnostic imaging, and elimination of ventriculography/angiography. Performing ad hoc percutaneous coronary intervention (PCI) might not be best in the patient at risk for developing CI-AKI. If clinically appropriate, the patient should return for a "staged" procedure if there is concern about the volume of contrast administered. Staged procedures should allow for the 48- to 72-hour identification of possible CI-AKI and then deferred if needed until renal function recovers. The catheterization laboratory quality improvement program should oversee local protocols for prevention and processes for patient follow-up (25).

METFORMIN-ASSOCIATED LACTIC ACIDOSIS

Metformin-associated lactic acidosis is a rare condition associated with renal failure in patients who take metformin. Although its onset occurs after the development of renal failure, *metformin is not related to CI-AKI.* It may have a mortality rate as high as 50%. Given that diabetics are at increased risk of developing CI-AKI, diabetic patients should not take their metformin on the day of the procedure, and should resume it at 48 hours or when the creatinine has returned to a normal level (63).

Conclusions

As a text for board review, the authors were tasked to provide a basic understanding of radiation and contrast with facts and concepts more as a learning resource than as a practice tool. The physics of imaging and the biochemistry of contrast constitute a basic knowledge base required for the interventionist to intelligently manage the dose of these entities in the context of a multi-faceted interventional procedure. The hope for this chapter is that it also provides the reader with the opportunity to incorporate this basic understanding of radiation and contrast, necessary for board review preparation, to best practice in the catheterization laboratory.

Acknowledgments

This chapter could not have been completed without full access to the excellent prior chapter written by Dr. Thomas Bashore. He permitted access to the prior text, tables, and figures, which allowed for appropriate updates to an excellent earlier manuscript. Additional thanks are extended to Dr. Stephen Balter for his shared expertise in the field of radiation physics.

Key Points

X-ray Formation

- Knowledge of the physics of imaging allows one to utilize the x-ray system to achieve the best image quality at the lowest dose through a balance of mA, kVp, and pulse width.

- Flat-panel image receptor technology provides for direct contact with the input phosphor, resulting in less image transfer creating the potential for improved image quality.

- Magnification in the flat-panel system differs from prior technology. Although now pixel-based, it still requires increase dose to minimize noise and improve imaged quality.

- Understanding that image quality is directly related to dose allows the operator to accept the image quality required for the procedure to appropriately minimize radiation exposure.

- The current era of image acquisition and storage requires rapid Ethernet-transmission speeds for the acquiring images at mega-pixel resolution that are then "processed," "filtered," and presented for review, utilizing high-resolution monitors and cost-effective long-term terabyte capacity archival DICOM-based digital image storage with disaster recovery.

Radiation Safety

- Basic terminology requires an understanding of different kinds of assessments, appreciating that *absorbed* and *equivalent dose* is interchangeable in cardiac imaging and applies to the targeted organ, while *effective* dose extrapolates this to the potential total body doses.

- Fluoroscopy time is not an accurate assessment of dose because it does not account for cine, frame rate, patient size, image angulations, etc. Therefore, total air kerma at the IRP (CAK) and air KAP (DAP) should be measured and reported for all invasive interventional cardiac procedures.

- All ionizing radiation has the potential to produce breaks in the DNA backbone, single or double stranded, and either directly or indirectly result in two risk classifications.

- Deterministic events require a well-defined, linear, dose-dependent threshold effect resulting in tissue injury (i.e., skin). Stochastic events (cancers, mutations) are probability based, linear to dose (the higher the radiation dose, the higher the probability of an event), but not threshold dependent (no specific dose for an individual to produce a defined event).

- Air KAP is a measure of the total radiation delivered to a body area and correlates more with stochastic injury. Total air kerma at the IRP is a point dose in space, approximating skin dose, and correlating with deterministic injury.

- Pre, during, and post-case dose management is required with initial patient assessment, in lab radiation dose management, and appropriate post-case follow-up when a high dose is utilized.

- Best practices in the lab require dose management from the outset of the case. Patient dose exposure can be minimized by using collimation, limiting magnified views, using the fewest number of frames, avoiding steep angles, keeping the image receptor close to the patient, spending the least amount of "on pedal time," and limiting unnecessary cine acquisition.

- Operator/staff exposure requires an understanding of time, distance, and shielding with best practices for the patient safety correlating to operator and staff safety.

- Personnel Dosimeters should be worn by all for individual assessment of risk. While two badges, outside at collar and inside at waist, are often recommended, one badge at collar worn correctly is an adequate assessment and is better than two badges worn incorrectly.

- Pregnant women may continue to work in the catheterization laboratory as long as they see a radiation safety officer and wear an additional badge under their lead.

- The maximal dose of occupational radiation exposure is 50 mSv/y or your age × 10 mSv for a lifetime to reduce stochastic effects. The annual cutoff is 150 mSv/y for deterministic effects (eye); however, eye injury may be evident at lower exposure.

Contrast Media

- Osmolality relates to the number of molecules in solution, with the terms ionic and non-ionic referring to whether they dissociate or do not dissociate in solution, respectively. By not ionizing, the three iodine benzene ring is a low-osmolar 3:1 agent (i.e., iopamidol, iohexol). Creating a non-ionic dimer produces a 6:1 agent (iodixanol) that is iso-osmolar to serum.

- The most clinically impactful complications from contrast media include immediate and delayed hypersensitivity, and CI-AKI. These complications have decreased significantly since the introduction of LOCM.

- Treatment of anaphylactoid reactions includes generous fluid administration, epinephrine (severe reactions), and other supportive measures. Glucagon can be given if the patient is on β-blockers. These reactions are idiosyncratic and more common in atopic individuals. Shellfish allergy invokes a separate allergen; therefore, pre-treatment is not required.

- Pre-treatment with steroids is effective in reducing the incidence of an anaphylactoid reaction but necessitates initiation of therapy at least 12 to 13 hours prior to contrast. H1 blockers are often combined with steroids. However, H2 blockers are often used but with little data.

- CIN, also known as CI-AKI after administration of contrast agents is most commonly seen in high-risk patients with baseline impaired renal function and diabetes. Protocols must be in place to assure these patients are identified pre-procedure, with methods to reduce the risk employed.

- If AKI/CIN is not prevented, it is associated with worse outcomes, including increased morbidity and mortality, and/or prolonged hospital stays with associated costs.

- Methods to reduce and ideally prevent AKI/CIN are primarily focused on ensuring adequate hydration pre- and post-procedure, as well as limiting procedural contrast load. Because renal impairment is seldom evident until 48 to 72 hours post-contrast, a follow-up program should be in place to identify these high-risk patients.

References

1. Bashore TM. Fundamentals of X-ray imaging, radiation safety, and contrast media. In: Kern MJ, ed. *SCAI 2012 Interventional Cardiology Review Book*. 2nd ed. 57–68.
2. Hirshfeld JW Jr, et al. ACCF/AHA/HRS/SCAI clinical competence statement on physician knowledge to optimize patient safety and image quality in fluoroscopically guided invasive cardiovascular procedures: A report of the American College of Cardiology Foundation/American Heart Association/American College of Physicians Task Force on clinical competence and training. *Circulation*. 2005;111:511–532.
3. Chida K, et al. Radiation dose of Interventional radiology system using a flat-panel detector. *AJR Am J Roentgenol*. 2009;193:1680–1685.
4. Balter S, et al. NCRP radiation dose management for fluoroscopically guided interventional medical procedures. National council on radiation protection and measures, NCRP Report No.168, NCRP, 2011. http://www.ncrppublications.org/Reports/168.
5. Balter S, et al. Administrative policies for managing substantial dose procedures and tissue reactions associated with fluoroscopically guided interventions (FGI), SC 4-6, NCRP, 2014.
6. Chambers CE, et al. Radiation safety program for the cardiac catheterization laboratory. *Catheter Cardiovasc Interv*. 2011;77:546–556.
7. Chambers CE. Radiation dose monitoring in the cath lab: Is fluoroscopy time enough? *Catheter Cardiovasc Interv*. 2013;82:1106–1107.
8. Duran A, et al. Recommendations for occupational radiation protection in interventional cardiology. *Catheter Cardiovasc Interv*. 2013;82:29–42.
9. Christopoulus G, et al. Optimizing radiation safety in the cardiac catheterization laboratory: a practical approach. *Catheter Cardiovasc Interv*. 2016;87(2):291–301.
10. National Council on Radiation Protection and Measurement. Ionizing radiation exposure of the population of the United States, NCRP Report No 160. Bethesda, MD: National Council on Radiation Protection and Measurements, 2009.
11. Balter S, Miller DL. Patient skin reactions from interventional fluoroscopy procedures. *AJR Am J Roentgenol*. 2014;202(4):W335–W342.

12. The National Academics of Sciences Engineering Medicine. Health risks from exposure to low levels of ionizing radiation: BEIR VII Phase 2. Consensus Study Report. http://www.nap.edu/catalog.php?record_id=11340#toc.

13. Einstein AJ, et al. Patient-centered imaging: shared decision making for cardiac imaging procedures exposure to ionizing radiation. *J Am Coll Cardiol.* 2014;63:1480–1489.

14. Lobotessi H, et al. Effective dose to a patient undergoing coronary angiography. *Radiat Prot Dosimetry.* 2001;94:173–176.

15. Kato M, et al. Evaluating the maximum patient radiation dose in cardiac interventional procedures. *Radiat Prot Dosimetry.* 2011;143:69–73.

16. National Council on Radiation Protection and Measurement. Recommendations for limits on exposure to ionizing radiation, NCRP Report No. 116. Bethesda, MA: National Council on Radiation Protection and Measurement, 1993. http://www.ncrponline.org/Publications/Press_Releases/116press.html.

17. International Commission on Radiation Units and Measurement. Recommendations 60. Updated 2013. http://www.iaea.org/ns/tutorials/regcontrol/intro/resources.htm.

18. Kim KP, et al. Occupational radiation doses to operators performing cardiac catheterization procedures. *Health Phys.* 2008;94:211–227.

19. Best PJ, et al. SCAI consensus document on occupational radiation exposure to the pregnant cardiologist and technical personnel. *EuroIntervention.* 2011;77:232–241.

20. Dauer LT, et al. Occupational radiation protection of pregnant or potentially pregnant workers in interventional radiology. A joint guideline of the Society of Interventional radiology and the Cardiovascular and Interventional Radiological Society of Europe. *J Vasc Interv Radiol.* 2015;26(2):171–181. doi: 10.1016/j.jvir.2014.11.026.

21. Ciraj-Bjelac O, et al. Radiation-induced eye lens changes and risk for cataract in interventional cardiology. *Cardiology.* 2012;123:168–171.

22. Reeves RR, et al. Invasive cardiologists are exposed to greater left sided cranial radiation: the BRAIN study (brain radiation exposure and attenuation during invasive cardiology procedures). *JACC Cardiovasc Interv.* 2015;8:1197–1206.

23. Klein LW, et al. Occupational health hazards in interventional cardiologists in the current decade. *Catheter Cardiovasc Interv.* 2015;86(5):913–924. doi: 10.1002/ccd.25927.

24. Christopoulos G, et al. Effect of a real-time radiation monitoring device on operator radiation exposure during cardiac catheterization: the radiation reduction during cardiac catheterization using real-time monitoring (RadiCure) study. *Circ Cardiovasc Interv.* 2014;7:744–750.

25. Levine GL, et al. 2011 ACCF/AHA/SCAI guidelines for percutaneous coronary intervention. *J Am Coll Cardiol.* 2011;58:44–122. doi: 10.1016/j.jacc.2011.08.007.

26. FDA Center for Devices and Radiologic Health. Initiative to reduce radiation exposure from medical imaging. FDA Library Publication, February 2010.

27. Fetterly KA, et al. Radiation dose reduction in the invasive cardiovascular laboratory. Implementing a culture and philosophy of radiation safety. *JACC Cardiovasc Interv.* 2012;5(8):866–873.

28. Agarwal S, et al. Relationship of beam angulation and radiation exposure in the cardiac catheterization laboratory. *JACC Cardiovasc Interv.* 2014;7:558–566.

29. Abdelaal E, et al. Effectiveness of low rate fluoroscopy at reducing operator and patient radiation dose during transradial coronary angiography and interventions. *JACC Cardiovasc Interv.* 2014;7:567–574.

30. Maeder M, et al. Impact of a lead glass screen on scatter radiation to eyes and hands in interventional cardiologists. *Catheter Cardiovasc Interv.* 2006;67:18–23.

31. Karadag B, et al. Effectiveness of a lead cap in radiation protection of the head in the cardiac catheterisation laboratory. *EuroIntervention.* 2013;9:754–756

32. Georgios C, Baber U, Mehran R. Contrast selection. In: Bhatt DL. *Cardiovascular Intervention: A Companion to Braunwald's Heart Disease.* Philadelphia, PA: Saunders; 2015:105–112.

33. Klein LW, et al. The use of radiographic contrast media during PCI: a focused review: a position statement of the Society of Cardiovascular Angiography and Interventions. *Catheter Cardiovasc Interv.* 2009;74:728–746.

34. Bottinor W, Polkampally P, Jovin I. Adverse reactions to iodonated contrast media. *Int J Angiol.* 2013;22(3);149–154.

35. Reiner JS. Contrast media and clotting: what is the evidence? *Catheter Cardiovasc Interv.* 2010;75(suppl 1):S35–S38.

36. Lee SY, et al. A review: radiographic iodinated contrast media-induced thyroid dysfunction. *J Clin Endocrinol Metab.* 2015;100:376–383.

37. Idee JM, et al. Allergy-like reactions to iodinated contrast agents. A critical analysis. *Fundam Clin Pharmacol.* 2005;19:263–281.

38. Brockow K, Ring J. Anaphylaxis to radiographic contrast media. *Curr Opin Allergy Clin Immunol.* 2011;11:326–331.

39. Huang SW. Seafood and iodine: an analysis of a medical myth. *Allergy Asthma Proc.* 2005;26:468–469.

40. Fox CS, et al. Short-term outcomes of acute myocardial infarction in patients with acute kidney injury: a report from the national cardiovascular data registry. *Circulation.* 2012;125:497–504.

41. Tsai TT, et al. Contemporary incidence, predictors, and outcomes of acute kidney injury in patients undergoing percutaneous coronary interventions: insights from the NCDR Cath-PCI registry. *JACC Cardiovasc Interv.* 2014;7:1–9.

42. Allen SF, Nallamothu BK, Patel UD. Contrast-induced acute kidney injury and the role of chronic kidney disease in percutaneous coronary intervention. In: Topol EJ, Teirstein PS, eds. *Textbook of Interventional Cardiology.* 7th ed. Philadelphia, PA: Elsevier - Health Sciences Division; 2015:108–117.

43. Persson PB, Tepel M. Contrast medium-induced nephropathy: the pathophysiology. *Kidney Int Suppl.* 2006:S8–S10. doi: 10.1038/sj.ki.5000367.

44. Katholi RE, et al. Oxygen free radicals and contrast nephropathy. *Am J Kidney Dis.* 1998;32:64–71.

45. Rihal CS, et al. Incidence and prognostic importance of acute renal failure after percutaneous coronary intervention. *Circulation.* 2002;105:2259–2264.

46. McCullough PA, et al. Epidemiology and prognostic implications of contrast-induced nephropathy. *Am J Cardiol.* 2006;98:5K–13K.

47. Kidney Disease: Improving Global Outcomes (KDIGO) Acute Kidney Injury Work Group. KDIGO clinical practice guideline for acute kidney injury. *Kidney Inter.* 2012;(suppl):1–138.

48. Thomsen HS, Morcos SK. Contrast media and the kidney: European Society of Urogenital Radiology (ESUR) guidelines. *Br J Radiol.* 2003;76:513–518.

49. Freeman RV, et al. Nephropathy requiring dialysis after percutaneous coronary intervention and the critical role of an adjusted contrast dose. *Am J Cardiol.* 2002;90:1068–1073.

50. Nikolsky E, et al. Impact of chronic kidney disease on prognosis of patients with diabetes mellitus treated with percutaneous coronary intervention. *Am J Cardiol.* 2004;94:300–305.

51. Mehran R, et al. A simple risk score for prediction of contrast-induced nephropathy after percutaneous coronary intervention: development and initial validation. *J Am Coll Cardiol.* 2004;44:1393–1399.

52. Gurm HS, et al. A novel tool for reliable and accurate prediction of renal complications in patients undergoing percutaneous coronary intervention. *J Am Coll Cardiol.* 2013;61:2242–2248.

53. Tsai TT, et al. Validated contemporary risk model of acute kidney injury in patients undergoing percutaneous coronary interventions: insights from the National Cardiovascular Data Registry Cath-PCI Registry. *J Am Heart Assoc.* 2014;3(6):e001380.

54. Laskey WK, et al. Volume-to-creatinine clearance ratio: a pharmacokinetically based risk factor for prediction of early creatinine increase after percutaneous coronary intervention. *J Am Coll Cardiol.* 2007;50:584–590.

55. Caixeta A, Mehran R. Evidence-based management of patients undergoing PCI: contrast-induced acute kidney injury. *Catheter Cardiovasc Interv.* 2010;75(suppl 1):S15–S20.

56. Trivedi HS, et al. A randomized prospective trial to assess the role of saline hydration on the development of contrast nephrotoxicity. *Nephron Clin Pract.* 2003;93:C29–C34.

57. Howe M, Gurm HS. A practical approach to preventing renal complications in the catheterization laboratory. *Interv Cardiol Clin.* 2014;3:429–439.

58. Subramaniam RM, et al. Effectiveness of prevention strategies for contrast-induced nephropathy: a systematic review and meta-analysis. *Ann Intern Med.* 2016;164:406–416.

59. Leoncini M, et al. Early high-dose rosuvastatin for contrast-induced nephropathy prevention in acute coronary syndrome: results from the PRATO-ACS Study (Protective effect of Rosuvastatin and antiplatelet therapy on contrast-induced

acute kidney injury and myocardial damage in patients with Acute Coronary Syndrome). *J Am Coll Cardiol*. 2014;63:71–79.

60. Zhang BC, Li WM, Xu YW. High-dose statin pretreatment for the prevention of contrast-induced nephropathy: a meta-analysis. *Can J Cardiol*. 2011;27:851–858.

61. Amsterdam EA, et al. 2014 AHA/ACC guideline for the management of patients with non–st-elevation acute coronary syndromes: a report of the American College of Cardiology/American Heart Association Task Force on Practice Guidelines. *J Am Coll Cardiol*. 2014;64:e139–e228.

62. Biondi-Zoccai G, et al. Nephropathy after administration of iso-osmolar and low-osmolar contrast media: evidence from a network meta-analysis. *Int J Cardiol*. 2014;172(2):375–380.

63. DeFronzo R, et al. Metformin-associated lactic acidosis: current perspectives on causes and risk. *Metabolism*. 2016;65:20–29.

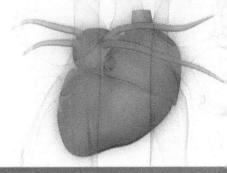

7

Coronary Hemodynamics: Pressure and Flow

Morton J. Kern, MD, MSCAI, FAHA, FACC,

Amir S. Lofti, MD, and Arnold H. Seto, MD, MPA,

FSCAI, FACC

Coronary physiologic lesion assessment in the cath lab is required to overcome the inability of anatomy (either angiographic or intravascular ultrasound imaging) to accurately predict the ischemic potential of a coronary luminal narrowing. Measurements of coronary pressure and flow in the cath lab are now used in daily clinical practice and associated with improved clinical outcomes over angiographic decision making alone.

Coronary Blood Flow and Resistance

Coronary arterial resistance (R, pressure/flow) is the summed resistances of the epicardial coronary conductance (R1), precapillary arteriolar (R2), and intramyocardial capillary (R3) resistance circuits (Fig. 7.1). Normal epicardial coronary arteries in humans typically taper gradually from the base of the heart to the apex. The epicardial vessels (R1) do not offer significant resistance to blood flow in their normal non-diseased state. Coronary epicardial resistance would be manifest as a pressure drop along the length of human epicardial arteries (1). Epicardial vessel resistance (R1) is trivial until atherosclerotic obstructions develop.

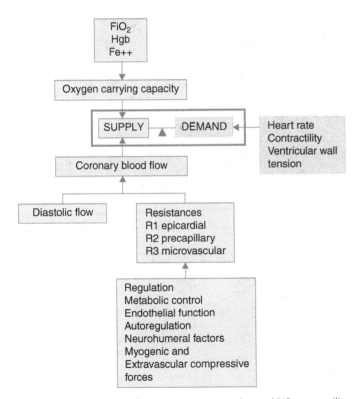

FIGURE 7.1 Myocardial flow increases to meet demand (HR, contractility and LV wall stress. Sources of perfusion: R1 = epicardial; R2 = precapillary arterioles; R3 = myocardial (microcirculation). HR, heart rate; LV, left-ventricular.

Precapillary arterioles (R2) are small (100–500 μm in size) resistive vessels connecting epicardial arteries to myocardial capillaries and are the main controllers of coronary blood flow (1). Precapillary arterioles autoregulate the perfusion pressure at their origin within a finite pressure range.

The microcirculatory resistance (R3) consists of a dense network of capillaries perfusing each myocyte adjacent to a capillary. Several conditions, such as left-ventricular (LV) hypertrophy, myocardial ischemia, or diabetes, can impair the microcirculatory resistance (R3) and blunt the normal increases in coronary flow in response to demand or pharmacologic agents. Increased R3 resistance may increase resting blood flow, resulting in reduced coronary flow reserve (CFR) (i.e., the hyperemic/basal flow ratio).

Coronary vasodilator flow reserve (CFR), the ratio of maximal hyperemic to resting coronary flow or flow velocity, is the ability of the coronary vascular bed to increase flow from a basal level to a maximal (or near maximal) hyperemic level in response to a mechanical or pharmacologic stimuli. Normal CFR ranges from 2× to 5× resting flow in man (2).

Gould et al. (3) showed that increasing coronary stenosis severity was associated with a predictable decline in CFR. CFR begins to decline at about a 60% artery diameter narrowing. Hence, it was thought that such stenoses carried physiologic importance; a truth in the animal, but not the human, experiment models. At diameter stenoses >80% to 90%, all available coronary reserve has been exhausted, and resting flow begins to decline (Fig. 7.2). Factors responsible for reduced CFR in absence of epicardial stenosis are shown in Table 7.1.

Pressure Loss across a Stenosis

As blood traverses a diseased arterial segment, turbulence, friction, and separation of laminar flow cause energy loss, resulting in a pressure gradient (ΔP) across the stenosis. Morphologic features of the stenosis are also responsible for resistance to flow changing exponentially with lumen cross-sectional area (the most commonly used measure of severity) and linearly with lesion length (4) (Fig. 7.3). Additional factors contributing to stenosis resistance include the shape of the entrance and exit orifices. Using a simplified Bernoulli formula for fluid dynamics, pressure loss across a stenosis can be estimated from blood flow as follows:

$$\Delta P = fQ + sQ^2$$

where ΔP is the pressure drop across a stenosis (mm Hg) and Q is the flow across the stenosis (ml/sec). The components of these two terms are shown next:

The first term (f) accounts for energy losses owing to viscous friction of laminar flow, while the second term (s) reflects energy loss when normal arterial flow is accelerated to high-velocity flow in the stenosis and then back to slower turbulent non-laminar distal flow on exiting the stenosis. A_s = stenotic segment cross-sectional area, p = blood density, μ = blood viscosity, L = stenosis length, A_n = normal artery cross-sectional area.

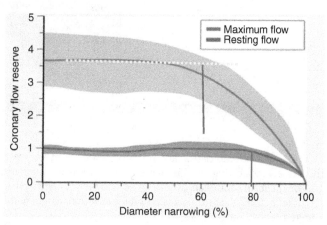

FIGURE 7.2 Relationship of coronary flow reserve to percent diameter narrowing from experimental dog model. CFR is preserved until percent narrowing exceeds 60%, and resting flow is not affected until narrowing exceeds 80%. In patients, this relationship is not strong because the percent diameter stenosis is not accurate from the angiogram, and because patients have microvascular disease and thus can have an impaired CFR despite a normal coronary artery. The shaded area represents the limits of variability of data about the mean. CFR, coronary flow reserve. (From: Gould KL, Lipscomb K, Hamilton GW. Physiologic basis for assessing critical coronary stenosis: instantaneous flow response and regional distribution during coronary hyperemia as measures of coronary flow reserve. *Am J Cardiol*. 1974;33:87–94.)

TABLE 7.1 Factors Responsible for Microvascular Disease and Reduction of Coronary Flow Reserve

Abnormal vascular reactivity
Abnormal myocardial metabolism
Abnormal sensitivity toward vasoactive substances
Coronary vasospasm
Myocardial infarction
Hypertrophy
Vasculitis syndromes
Hypertension
Diabetes
Recurrent ischemia

Adapted from Baumgart D, et al. Current concepts of coronary flow reserve for clinical decision making during cardiac catheterization. *Am Heart J*. 1998;136:136–149.

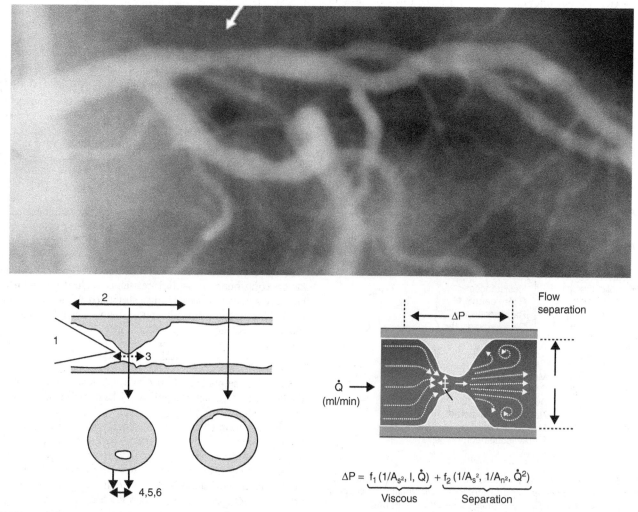

$$\Delta P = \underbrace{f_1\left(1/A_{s}^2, \, l, \, \dot{Q}\right)}_{\text{Viscous}} + \underbrace{f_2\left(1/A_{s}^2, \, 1/A_{n}^2, \, \dot{Q}^2\right)}_{\text{Separation}}$$

FIGURE 7.3 Factors contributing to pressure loss across a stenosis involve total morphology of the narrowing, not just the most narrowed diameter. White arrow identifies intermediate lesion. lower left, 1, entrance angle, 2 lesion length, 3 stenosis length, 4,5,6 lesion shape, 7 area of normal reference vessel.

Because of the second term, the increases in coronary blood flow increase the associated pressure gradient in a quadratic manner. As an additional consequence, for a given stenosis with potentially variable area and size of reference normal vessel, there may be a family of pressure–flow relationships reflecting altered stenosis diameter and variable distending pressure.

Fractional Flow Reserve

Pijls et al. (5) derived an estimate of the percentage of normal coronary blood flow expected to go through a stenotic artery from the distal/aortic pressure ratio at maximal hyperemia, called the fractional flow reserve (FFR) (Fig. 7.4). FFR can be subdivided into three components describing the flow contributions by the coronary artery (FFR_{cor}), the myocardium (FFR_{myo}), and the collateral supply. FFR of the coronary artery is thus: $FFR_{cor} = FFR_{myo} - FFR_{cor}$. The following equations are used to calculate the FFR of a coronary artery and its dependent myocardium:

$$(FFR_{myo}) = 1 - \Delta P/P_a - P_v = (P_d - P_v)/(P_a - P_v)$$

$$(FFR_{cor}) = 1 - \Delta P/(P_a - P_w) = (P_d - P_w)/(P_a - P_w)$$

$$(FFR_{coll}) = FFR_{myo} - FFR_{cor}$$

where P_a is mean aortic pressure; P_d is mean distal coronary pressure; ΔP is mean translesional pressure gradient; P_v is mean right atrial pressure; and P_w is mean coronary wedge pressure or distal coronary pressure during balloon inflation (6). Because FFR_{cor} uses P_w, it can be calculated only during balloon coronary angioplasty. For daily clinical practice, FFR can be easily calculated by a simplified ratio of pressures and expressed as:

$$FFR \approx P_d/P_a$$

The FFR is simplified to P_d/P_a, assuming P_v is negligible relative to P_a.

The normal value for FFR is unequivocally one for each patient, coronary artery, myocardial distribution, and microcirculatory status. An FFR value of <0.75 in patients with stable angina is strongly related to provocable myocardial ischemia using multiple stress testing methods. Because it is independent of hemodynamic and loading conditions (Fig. 7.5), the FFR is a more epicardial lesion-specific measurement compared with CFR or resting trans-stenotic pressure gradients. FFR reflects both antegrade and collateral perfusion. Because it is calculated only at peak hyperemia, it excludes the microcirculatory resistance from the computation. FFR is largely independent of basal flow, driving pressure, heart rate, systemic blood pressure, or status of the microcirculation (7).

FFR is strongly related to provocable myocardial ischemia using different clinical stress testing modalities in patients with stable angina as the comparative standard. The nonischemic threshold value for FFR used in most recent clinical outcome studies is >0.80 for deferral of percutaneous coronary intervention (PCI). Even in patients with an abnormal microcirculation, a normal FFR indicates the epicardial conduit resistance (i.e., a stenosis) is not a major contributing factor to perfusion impairment, and that focal conduit enlargement (e.g., stenting) would not restore normal perfusion. Errors and pitfalls of measuring FFR have been described in detail elsewhere (5).

Technique of Angioplasty Sensor-Guidewire Use

After diagnostic angiography, the sensor pressure guidewire is set to atmospheric pressure on the cath table. It is then passed through the guide catheter to the central aortic position, and the two pressure signals are matched. Heparin (60 U/kg) is given before inserting the guidewire. Intracoronary (IC) nitroglycerin (100–200 μg) is given to vasodilate and block vasoconstriction of the artery. Nitroglycerin has no effect on hemodynamic measurements unless the stenosis is vasoconstricted (5).

After the sensor wire is passed beyond the lesion, baseline aortic and guidewire pressures are recorded, followed immediately by induction of coronary hyperemia, continuously recording both guide catheter and sensor-wire pressures. FFR is computed as the ratio distal coronary to aortic pressure at maximal hyperemia, occurring at the lowest distal coronary pressure.

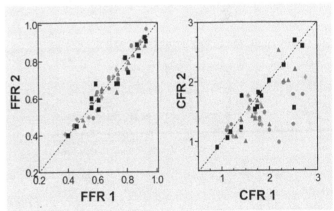

FIGURE 7.5 Reproducibility of fractional flow reserve (FFR) compared with (B) coronary flow reserve (CFR) in the same patients. Blue boxes represent baseline conditions. Violet diamonds represent changes in blood pressure induced by infusion of nitroprusside. Blue triangles represent changes in heart rate induced by pacing. Pink circles represent changes in contractility induced by infusion of dobutamine. Despite variations in heart rate of 40%, blood pressure of 35%, and contractility of 50%, FFR but not CFR was unaffected by these changes. Reproduced with permission from De Bruyne B, et al. Simultaneous coronary pressure and flow velocity measurements in humans. Feasibility, reproducibility, and hemodynamic dependence of coronary flow velocity reserve, hyperemic flow versus pressure slope index, and fractional flow reserve. *Circulation* 1996;94:1842–9.

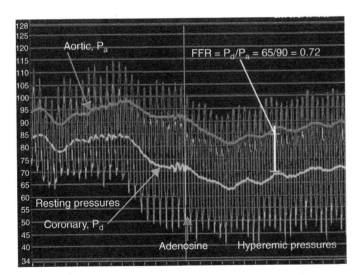

FIGURE 7.4 Aortic (*red*) and coronary (*green*) pressure tracings used to calculate FFR. Adenosine intracoronary bolus is given at the red arrow, and FFR is computed at the nadir of the distal pressure in steady state. In this example, FFR is P_d/P_a = 65/90 = 0.72. FFR, fractional flow reserve.

	Adenosine	Adenosine	Papaverine	NTP
Route	IV	IC	IC	IC
Dosage	140 mcg/kg/min	100–200 mcg LCA 50–100 mcg RCA	15 mg LCA 10 mg RCA	50–100 mcg
T 1/2	1–2 min	30–60 sec	2 min	1–2 min
Time to max	≤1–2 min	5–10 sec	30–60 sec	10–20 sec
Advantage	Gold Standard	Short action	Short action	Short action
Disadvantage	↓BP by 10–15%, Chest burning	AV delay, ↓BP	Torsades, severe ↓BP	↓BP by 10–15%

FIGURE 7.6 Pharmacologic agents for inducing hyperemia in the measurement of FFR and CFR. AV, atrioventricular; CFR, coronary flow reserve; FFR, fractional flow reserve.

Coronary Hyperemia for Stenosis Assessment

The most accurate stenosis severity assessment is made during maximal hyperemia. At maximal hyperemia, autoregulation is abolished and microvascular resistance fixed and minimal. Under these conditions, coronary blood flow is directly related to coronary pressure and forms the basis for the derivation of pressure-derived FFR.

The most widely used coronary hyperemic drug for FFR is adenosine, a potent short-acting hyperemic stimulus. Adenosine is benign in the appropriate dosages (50–100 μg in the right coronary artery and 100–200 μg in the left coronary artery or infused intravenously at 140 μg/kg/min). Because of a sustained hyperemia, weight-based dosing, and lack of operator interaction, IV is preferable to IC adenosine. IV and IC adenosine produce equivalent hyperemia. **Figure 7.6** lists the characteristics of pharmacologic hyperemia-inducing agents that can be used in coronary flow studies. IC nitroprusside (50-, 100-μg bolus) produces nearly identical results to IV and IC adenosine (8).

Resting Translesional Index of Stenosis Severity— Coronary Pulse-Wave Analysis

Davies et al. (9) reported that coronary resistance is low and constant during part of the diastolic period in which coronary forward and backward traveling waves are absent; i.e., a wave-free period. Instantaneous wave-free ratio (iFR) was derived from wave-intensity analysis and involves estimation of the trans-stenotic pressure gradient at rest during a time interval starting 25% into diastole and ending 5 ms before the onset of systole using a trademarked algorithm (**Fig. 7.7**). As described in the 2011 ADVISE study, an iFR cut-off value of 0.83 was equivalent to an FFR value of 0.80 (10,11) (**Fig. 7.8**). A hybrid iFR-FFR strategy has also been proposed, which could potentially increase the adoption of physiologically guided PCI by reducing the need for vasodilator administration. The randomized controlled trials, which compare the clinical outcomes between iFR- and FFR-guided strategy, DEFINE-FLAIR *NCT02053038* (12) and

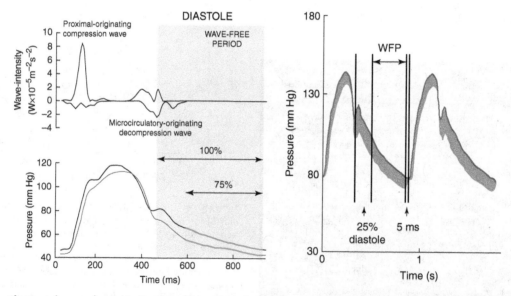

FIGURE 7.7 Identification of a wave-free period in the cardiac cycle. *Left, top:* Wave-intensity analysis demonstrates the proximal and microcirculatory (distal) originating waves generated during the cardiac cycle. A wave-free period can be seen in diastole when no new waves are generated (*shaded*). This corresponds to a time period in which there is minimal microcirculatory (distal)–originating pressure, minimal and constant resistance, and a nearly constant rate of change in flow velocity. *Right:* Pressure tracings showing the portion of the cardiac cycle, with the wave-free period (WFP) used to calculate the instantaneous wave-free ratio. (Modified from: Sen S, et al. Diagnostic classification of the instantaneous wave-free ratio is equivalent to fractional flow reserve and is not improved with adenosine administration. *J Am Coll Cardiol.* 2013;61(13):1409–1420. doi:10.1016/j.jacc.2013.01.034.)

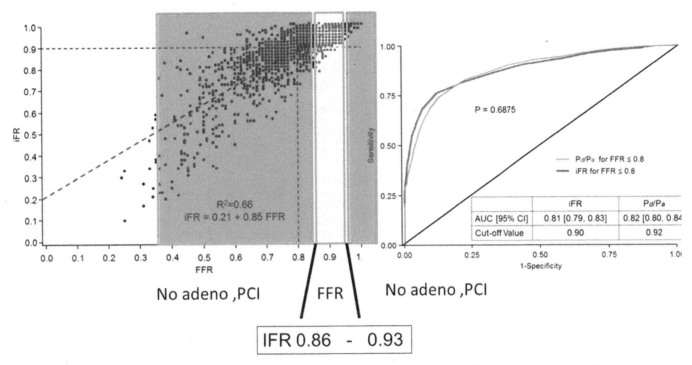

FIGURE 7.8 The ADVISE study. Several studies investigated the iFR to see if it was comparable to FFR. In the Advise II study, FFR was appointed as a reference standard. A hybrid approach seems reasonable based on iFR <0.86 and >0.93 designated as adenosine-free areas. Recent DEFINE-FLAIR and SWEDEHEART studies support a single dichotomous threshold of >0.89 as not needing treatment. FFR, fractional flow reserve; iFR, Instantaneous wave-free ratio. (From: Sen S, et al. Development and validation of a new adenosine-independent index of stenosis severity from coronary wave-intensity analysis: results of the ADVISE [ADenosine Vasodilator Independent Stenosis Evaluation] study. *J Am Coll Cardiol.* 2012;59:1392–1402.)

SWEDEHEART *NCT02166736* (13), presented in 2017, provide a dichotomous iFR of 0.89 as the threshold for non-inferior 1-year outcomes relative to FFR in low-risk coronary artery disease (CAD) populations (**Fig. 7.9**).

CORONARY FLOW RESERVE

Coronary flow reserve (CFR), also known as coronary vasodilatory reserve (CVR) or coronary flow velocity reserve (CFVR), was

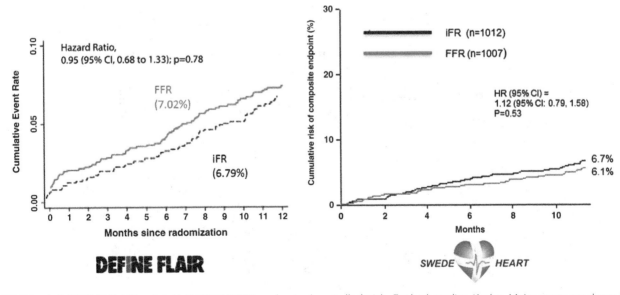

FIGURE 7.9 *Left*, DEFINE-FLAIR and *right*, SWEDEHEART randomized controlled trials. For both studies, Kaplan–Meier curves are shown for the cumulative risk of the composite of death from any cause, nonfatal myocardial infarction, or unplanned revascularization within 12 months after the index procedure. Both studies used a single cut-off of 0.89 for the threshold of treatment. (From: Davies JE, et al. Use of the instantaneous wave-free ratio or fractional flow reserve in PCI. *N Engl J Med.* 2017;376(19):1824–1834; Götberg M, et al. Instantaneous wave-free ratio versus fractional flow reserve to guide PCI. *N Engl J Med.* 2017;376(19):1813–1823.)

described previously and is defined as the ratio of maximal to basal coronary flow. CFR is a measure of both the epicardial artery and the microvascular resistances. Hence, a normal CFR requires both components to be normal. CFR may be abnormal if one or both are abnormal, and for this reason, an abnormal CFR cannot be determined to be solely due to a coronary stenosis.

There are two methods available for measuring coronary blood flow reserve in the catheterization laboratory: IC Doppler flow velocity and coronary artery thermodilution.

Coronary Doppler Flow Velocity

Unlike the pressure wire, measuring flow velocity with the Doppler sensor wire requires no zeroing or central signal matching. Once sensor connections and the velocity settings on the screen display are set, the Doppler wire is passed beyond the stenosis, with the Doppler guidewire tip (Fig. 7.10) positioned at least 5 to 10 artery-diameter lengths (>2 cm) beyond the target stenosis. Resting flow velocity is recorded, and then coronary hyperemia is induced by IC or IV adenosine (or other suitable agents) with continuous recording of the flow velocity signals. CFR is computed as the ratio of maximal hyperemic to basal average peak velocity. Because of the highly position-dependent signal, poor signal acquisition may occur in 10% to 15% of patients even within normal arteries. As with transthoracic echo Doppler studies, the operator must adjust the guidewire position (sample volume) to optimize the velocity signal.

Guidewire Thermodilution Blood Flow Technique

The coronary thermodilution technique uses thermistors on a pressure-sensor angioplasty guidewire and measures the arrival time of room temperature saline bolus indicator injections through the guiding catheter into the coronary artery (14,15). The shaft of the angioplasty pressure-monitoring guide wire (St. Jude Medical Systems) has a temperature-dependent electrical resistance and acts as a proximal thermistor, which allows for the detection of the start of the indicator (saline) injection (Fig. 7.11). Thermodilution CFR (CFR_{thermo}) is defined as the ratio of hyperemic flow divided by resting coronary flow (F).

$$CFR = \frac{Fat\ hyperemia}{Fat\ rest}$$

Simultaneous measurements of CFR and FFR are currently obtained for research studies on coronary and myocardial resistance. When combined with pressure measurements, CFR measurements can provide a complete description of the pressure–flow relationship and the response of the microcirculation.

Normal Coronary Flow and Flow Velocity Reserve

The range of normal absolute coronary flow velocities, both at baseline and during hyperemia, is large. Nonetheless, normal CFR in young patients with normal arteries commonly exceeds 3.0. In adult patients with chest pain undergoing cardiac catheterization with angiographically normal vessels, the CFR averages 2.7 ± 0.64 (16). CFR values <2.0 have been associated with inducible myocardial ischemia on stress testing. Changes in heart rate, blood pressure, and contractility alter CFR by changing resting basal flow or maximal hyperemic flow or both (17).

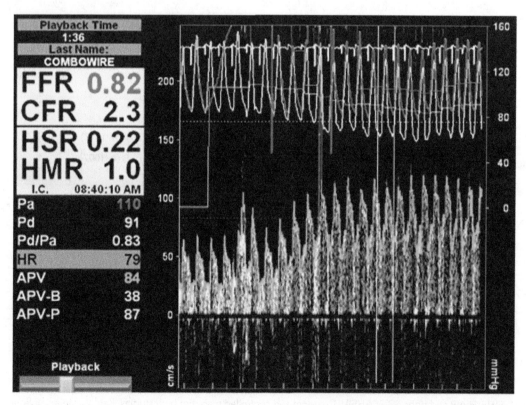

FIGURE 7.10 Pressure and Doppler flow measurements during adenosine-induced hyperemia. Top of figure displays aortic (*red*) and coronary (*yellow*) pressure tracings. Doppler tracings below are outlined in *blue* as the maker of instantaneous average peak velocity. The peak response is at the right side of the figure. CFR, coronary vasodilator flow reserve; FFR, fractional flow reserve; HMR, hyperemic myocardial resistance; HSR, hyperemic stenosis resistance.

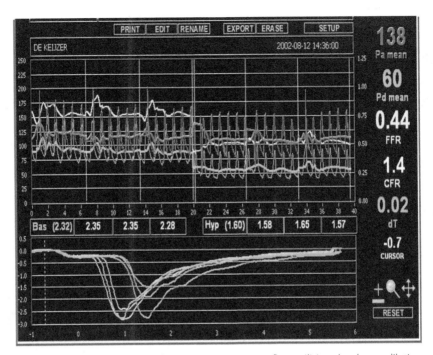

FIGURE 7.11 An example of determining coronary flow utilizing the thermodilution technique from the St. Jude Medical pressure-wire system. As can be seen on the top of the figure, the *red* signals reflect the guide catheter pressure (P_a), the *green* signals reflect the coronary pressure (P_d), and the *yellow line* represents the calculated FFR for the corresponding pressures. The particulars of the measurement of coronary flow can be seen on the bottom of the figure. The curves at the bottom represent the thermodilution temperature changes during rest and subsequently at maximal hyperemia. The numbers just above the curves depict the calculated transit time corresponding to the color-coded thermodilution curve. The average of the baseline and hyperemic transit times are then used to calculate the coronary flow reserve, as shown on the right side of the figure. FFR, fractional flow reserve.

CLINICAL APPLICATIONS OF CORONARY BLOOD FLOW MEASUREMENTS

The physiologic criteria for a hemodynamically significant coronary lesion include post-stenotic absolute CVR <2.0 when using flow velocity, and the FFR threshold is <0.80 when using pressure-sensor guidewires.

Validation and Threshold of Ischemia

FFR values <0.75 are associated with ischemic stress testing in numerous comparative studies with high sensitivity (88%), specificity (100%), positive predicted value (100%), and overall accuracy (93%). FFR values >0.80 are associated with negative ischemic results with a predictive accuracy of 95%. Single stress-testing comparisons with variations in testing methods and patient cohorts have produced a zone of FFR with overlapping positive and negative results (0.75–0.80). The use of FFR in this zone requires clinical judgment. A meta-analysis of 31 studies (18) found that QCA had a random effects sensitivity of 78% and a specificity of 51% against FFR (<0.75 cut-off), compared with non-invasive imaging (21 studies, 1,249 lesions), FFR versus perfusion scintigraphy (976 lesions, sensitivity 75%, specificity 77%), and dobutamine stress echocardiography (273 lesions, sensitivity 82%, specificity 74%). From the ischemia validation studies over the last 15 years, FFR can be used as a vessel-specific index of ischemia.

Although no longer commonly used for stenosis assessment, an abnormal CFR (<2.0) corresponded to reversible myocardial perfusion imaging defects with high sensitivity (86%–92%), specificity (89%–100%), predictive accuracy (89%–96%), and positive and negative predictive values (84%–100% and 77%–95%, respectively) (15).

Simultaneous Pressure–Flow Velocity Measurements

Combined pressure and flow data have produced a novel set of invasive physiologic tools for epicardial lesion assessment, such as hyperemic stenosis resistance (HSR), and for microvascular assessment, such as index of microcirculatory resistance (IMR) and hyperemic myocardial resistance (HMR) (Fig. 7.11). Defined as the hyperemic change in pressure across a stenosis divided by the hyperemic distal velocity, HSR may have better predictive value than FFR for detecting noninvasive ischemia (19). Minimum hyperemic microvascular resistance (HMR, the ratio of mean distal pressure to average peak blood flow velocity during hyperemia) was significantly higher in patients with FFR >0.75 and CFR <2.0. A HSR index (defined as the ratio of hyperemic stenosis pressure gradient [mean aortic minus mean distal pressure] to hyperemic average peak flow velocity) had better agreement with single-photon emission computed tomography (SPECT) scanning in lesions with discordant FFR and CVR (20,21). Table 7.2 summarizes the characteristics of physiologic measurements used in the cath lab. A summary of coronary physiologic measurements and derivations is provided in Table 7.3.

TABLE 7.2 Comparison of Physiologic Measurements

	HEMODYNAMIC INDEPENDENCE	INDEPENDENT OF MICROCIRCULATION ABNORMALITIES	UNEQUIVOCAL NORMAL VALUES	USE IN MULTIVESSEL CAD	USE FOR COLLATERAL MEASUREMENTS
CFR	−	−	Range > 2.0	+	+
IMR	+	+	Range (> 0.8)	−	−
FFR	+	+	1.0	+	+
iFR	−	−	Range (> 0.89)	+	−

+, useful; −, not useful. CFR, coronary flow reserve; FFR, fractional flow reserve; iFR, instantaneous wave-free ratio; IMR, index of microvascular resistance.
Adapted from: Kern MJ. Coronary physiology revisited: practical insights from the cardiac catheterization laboratory. *Circulation.* 2000;101:1344–1351. Used with permission.

TABLE 7.3 Indices of Coronary Pressure and Flow Measurements

BSR	$(P_{aorta} - P_{distal})$/APV (basal condition)
HSR	$(P_{aorta} - P_{distal})$/APV (during hyperemia)
Resting P_d/P_a	mean P_{distal}/mean P_{aorta} (basal condition)
FFR	mean P_{distal}/mean P_{aorta} (during hyperemia)
iFR	mean P_{distal}/mean P_{aorta} (wave-free period basal condition)
CFR	$APV_{hyperemia}/APV_{basal}$
HMR	$P_d/APV_{hyperemia}$
IMR	$P_d \times T_{mn\ hyperemia}$

APV, average peak flow velocity; BSR, basal stenosis resistance index; CFR, coronary flow reserve; FFR, fractional flow reserve; HSR, hyperemic stenosis resistance index; HMR, hyperemic myocardial resistance; iFR, instantaneous wave-free ratio; IMR, index of microcirculatory resistance; P_{aorta}, aortic pressure; P_{distal}, distal coronary pressure; T_{mn}, mean transit time.

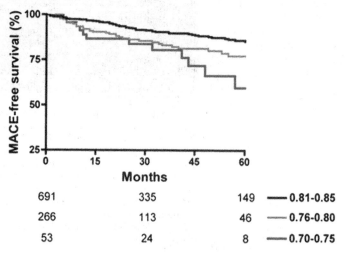

691	335	149	0.81-0.85
266	113	46	0.76-0.80
53	24	8	0.70-0.75

FIGURE 7.12 Results of the DEFER study at 5 years. Survival and adverse events. *Top:* Kaplan–Meier survival curves for freedom from adverse cardiac events during 5 years follow-up for the three groups. *Middle:* Cardiac death and acute myocardial infarction rate in the three groups after a follow-up of 5 years. *Bottom:* Percentage of patients free from chest pain in the three groups at baseline and during follow-up. *p = 0.028; **p = <0.001; ***p = 0.021. (From: Adjedj J, et al. Significance of Intermediate Values of Fractional Flow Reserve in Patients With Coronary Artery Disease. *Circulation.* 2016;133:502–8. DOI: 10.1161/CIRCULATIONAHA.115.018747.)

Clinical Outcomes and FFR

FFR can be used to determine the appropriateness of angioplasty. For example, the DEFER study randomized 325 patients scheduled for PCI into three groups and reported the 5-year outcomes (22). If FFR was ≥0.75, patients were randomly assigned to the deferral group (n = 91, medical therapy for CAD) or the PCI performance group (n = 90, PCI with stents). If FFR was <0.75, PCI was performed as planned and patients were entered into the reference group (n = 144). The event-free survival was not different between the deferred and performed group (80% and 73%, respectively, p = 0.52), and both were significantly better than in the reference PCI group (63%, p = 0.03). The composite rate of cardiac death and acute myocardial infarction (MI) in the deferred, performed, and reference groups was 3.3%, 7.9%, and 15.7%, respectively (p = 0.21 for deferred vs. performed and p = 0.003 for reference vs. both of the deferred and performed groups) (**Fig. 7.12**).

Multivessel CAD

In a larger prospective randomized, multicenter trial, Tonino et al. (23) for the FAME (FFR vs. Angiography for Multivessel Evaluation study) investigators tested outcomes for two PCI strategies: a physiologically guided PCI approach (FFR-PCI) compared to a conventional angiographically guided PCI (Angio-PCI) in patients with multivessel CAD. After identifying which of the multiple lesions

required treatment, 1,005 patients undergoing PCI with drug-eluting stents were randomly assigned to one of the two strategies. For the FFR-PCI group, all lesions had FFR measurements and were only stented if the FFR was <0.80. The primary endpoints of death, MI, and repeat revascularization (coronary artery bypass grafting [CABG] or PCI) were obtained at 1 year. Of the 1,005 patients, 496 were assigned to the Angio-PCI, while 509 were assigned to the FFR-PCI group. Clinical characteristics and angiographic findings were similar in both groups. The SYNTAX (Synergy between PCI with Taxus and Cardiac Surgery) scores for gauging risk in multivessel disease involvement were identical (14.5), indicating low- to intermediate-risk patients.

Compared to the Angio-PCI group, the FFR-PCI group used fewer stents per patient (1.9 ± 1.3 vs. 2.7 ± 1.2; p < 0.001) and less contrast, and had lower procedure costs and shorter hospital stays. More importantly, at the 2-year follow-up, the FFR-PCI group had fewer MACE (13.2% vs. 18.4%; p = 0.02), fewer combined deaths, or MI

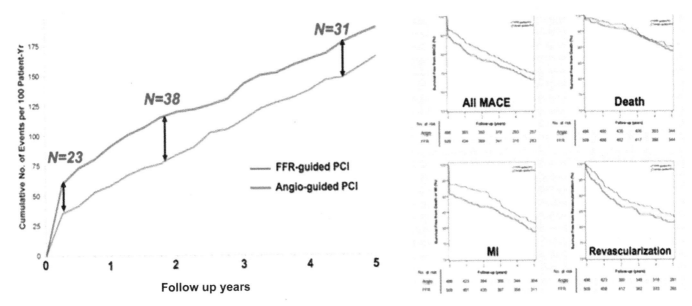

FIGURE 7.13   The FAME study 2-year survival free of MACE. The patients randomized to the angiographically guided treatment strategy had a significantly higher rate of death or MI (12.7% vs. 8.4%; p = 0.03) and a higher rate of needing CABG or repeat PCI (9.5% vs. 6.1%; p = 0.03). CABG, coronary artery bypass grafting; MI, myocardial infarction; PCI, percutaneous coronary intervention.

(7.3% vs. 11%; p = 0.04), and a lower total number of MACE (76 vs. 113; p = 0.02), compared with the Angio-PCI group (Fig. 7.13).

The FAME study also demonstrated that not all angiographic three-vessel CAD is physiologic three-vessel CAD. A functional SYNTAX score (SYNTAX grading excluding any vessel that has FFR >0.80) adds the prognostic value of FFR to angiographic grading in patients with multivessel CAD. The economic impact of the FFR-guided strategy produces superior results at a lower cost.

FAME II (FFR vs. Angiography for Multivessel Evaluation 2) was a randomized trial of 888 stable angina patients, testing whether optimal medical therapy (OMT) alone, compared to OMT and coronary revascularization with stenting, was better in patients with demonstrated ischemia in at least one vessel (i.e., FFR <0.80). Patients with angiographically assessed one-, two-, or three-vessel coronary artery disease that was amenable to PCI had FFRs measured and were randomized to OMT or OMT + PCI if FFR was <0.80, or if FFR >0.80 was assigned to a registry and was followed. Enrollment in the study was terminated after 19 months due to a highly significant difference in MACE between the groups. At this time, 12.7% of the patients with OMT, compared to only 4.3% of the FFR-guided PCI group, reached the primary endpoint (24). This result was primarily driven by a 7-fold increase in the need for urgent revascularization, which included unstable angina (52%), but also MI or unstable angina with electrocardiographic changes in 48%. A registry group of participants with documented coronary disease, but no functionally significant stenosis by FFR, did not receive PCI and shared the low event rates seen in the PCI group (Fig. 7.14). FFR-guided PCI dramatically reduced the need for urgent revascularization in ischemic patients treated with only medical therapy.

Left Main Stenosis

The assessment of left main (LM) CAD lesions based on angiography alone should be strongly questioned because the consequences of an incorrect decision carry a large penalty of either unnecessary surgery or perhaps premature death if a significant LM is untreated. The most accurate decision requires the support of adjunctive lesion assessment modalities.

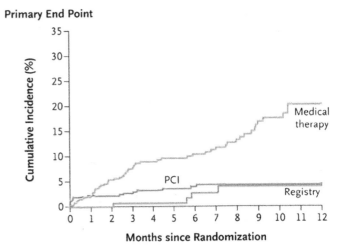

FIGURE 7.14   The FAME II study. Is optimal medical therapy better than PCI + OMT for patients with abnormal FFR (i.e., ischemia)? FFR, fractional flow reserve; OMT, optimal medical therapy; PCI, percutaneous coronary intervention. (From: De Bruyne B, et al. Fractional flow reserve–guided PCI versus medical therapy in stable coronary disease. N Engl J Med. 2012;367:991–1001.)

Non-ischemic FFR values (>0.80) in LM lesions are associated with excellent long-term outcomes. The largest and longest follow-up trial published to date by Hamilos et al. (25) found a low incidence of MACE, including cardiac death or MI between groups with FFR >0.80 (treated medically), compared to those undergoing CABG when FFR <0.80. Reporting their 5 year outcomes with the use of FFR for LM stenoses treated with medical or surgical therapy based on FFR <0.80 (Fig. 7.15), Hamilos et al. (25) found similar low MACE rates, using FFR to assign suitable surgical revascularization or continued medical therapy.

For assessment of the LM with downstream CAD, such as an additional significant left anterior descending (LAD) stenosis, it is necessary to understand the relationship of the myocardial bed size and the FFR. The LM FFR reflects flow to the entire left heart

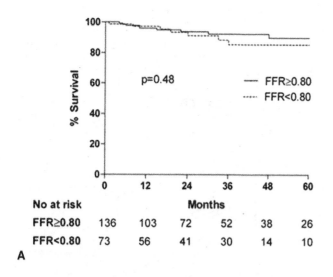

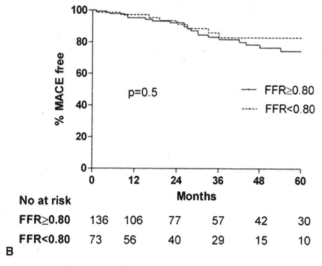

FIGURE 7.15 Figure depicting the survival (**A**) and MACE (**B**) of patients with intermediate left main disease assessed by FFR. Those patients whose FFR of the left main was found to be >0.80 were treated medically, while those patients who had FFR values <0.80 received revascularization. The two patient groups had nearly identical outcomes over a 60-month period. FFR, fractional flow reserve. (From: Hamilos M, et al. Long-term clinical outcome after fractional flow reserve-guided treatment in patients with angiographically equivocal left main coronary artery stenosis. *Circulation.* 2009;120:1505–1512.)

myocardial bed through both the LAD and the circumflex coronary artery (CFX). To compute LM FFR, maximal flow in the bed supplied by the target vessel is required. Thus, the myocardial bed for the LM is the summed territories of both the LAD and the CFX (Fig. 7.16). The LM bed can be even larger if the RCA is occluded and if collateral is supplied from the left coronary system. In this case, the flow through the LM would involve supply to the inferior LV, as well as the anterior LV. An LM narrowing without other disease (i.e., no LAD, CFX, or RCA stenoses; top left, Fig. 7.16) reflects the physiologic significance of just the LM narrowing. An LM narrowing plus LAD stenosis (top right, Fig. 7.16) could produce a higher LM FFR, however, because the LM bed is decreased due to the LAD stenosis. The same considerations would apply in the setting of a CFX narrowing. The LM FFR alone cannot be accurately measured just when there are serial lesions. The impact of downstream disease

on FFR measurement of LM, was demonstrated by Fearon and colleagues (26) in 25 patients by creating intermediate LMCA stenosis, and LAD or CFX stenosis with deflated balloon catheters after PCI of the LAD/CFX, or both. Because downstream disease usually overestimates FFR, a numerical value of <0.75 will accurately identify LMCA stenosis that requires revascularization. If the LAD and CFX are hemodynamically insignificant, the LM FFR will be accurate.

Finally, in the setting of LM narrowing plus totally occluded RCA with collaterals from LCA and no LAD or CFX disease (bottom left, Fig. 7.16), the LM FFR would reflect the flow through the entire left and right ventricular myocardium. After recanalization of the RCA with resolution of collateral flow, the LM FFR would increase because LM myocardial bed size is reduced (bottom right, Fig. 7.16), as illustrated by Sachdeva et al. (27) and Iqbal et al. (28) The overestimation of the LM FFR in the presence of a second lesion downstream depends on the severity of the additional lesion and on the mass of myocardium distal to this second lesion.

Serial Epicardial Lesions

An accurate FFR requires maximum translesional flow across the stenosis. This condition cannot be met in serial lesions wherein the blood flow through one stenosis will be submaximal because of the second stenosis. The FFR can assess the summed effect across any series of stenosis, but individual lesion FFR in the series will be more difficult to appreciate without special calculations (29).

The most practical technique to assess serial lesions involves passing the pressure wire distal to the last lesion and measuring the summed FFR across all lesions. If the FFR = 0.84, then no lesion would need treatment. If the summed FFR is <0.80, then a wire pullback during IV adenosine hyperemia can identify the largest change in gradient (ΔP) between lesions. Stenting should then start with the lesion with the most significant gradient (largest ΔP). After treating this lesion, the remaining lesion(s) can be measured using the standard FFR technique (**Fig. 7.17**).

FFR and Acute Coronary Syndrome (ACS)

ACS is a dynamic condition, with evolving lesion and myocardial bed characteristics making treatment decisions independent of physiology in the acute setting. FFR has value in lesion assessment in the recovery phase of MI and in the assessment of lesions in the remote non-infarct-related vessels.

De Bruyne et al. (30) compared SPECT myocardial perfusion imaging and FFR obtained before and after PCI in 57 MI patients >6 days (mean, 20 days) prior to evaluation. Patients with positive SPECT before PCI had a significantly lower FFR than patients with negative SPECT (0.52 ± 0.18 vs. 0.67 ± 0.16; p = 0.0079), but a significantly higher left ventricular ejection fraction ($63\% \pm 10\%$ vs. $52\% \pm 10\%$; p = 0.0009), despite a similar percent diameter stenosis ($67\% \pm 13\%$ vs. $68\% \pm 16\%$; p = NS). The sensitivity and specificity for FFR of <0.75 to detect a defect on SPECT were 82% and 87%, respectively. In a similar study, Samady et al. (31) compared FFR to SPECT and myocardial contrast echo (MCE) in 48 patients 3.7 ± 1.3 days after infarction. To identify true reversibility, follow-up SPECT was performed 11 weeks after PCI. The sensitivity, specificity, and concordance of FFR <0.75 for detecting true reversibility on SPECT were 88%, 93%, and 91% (chi-square p < 0.001), and for detecting reversibility on MCE were 90%, 100%, and 93% (chi-square p < 0.001), respectively. The optimal FFR value for discriminating inducible ischemia on non-invasive imaging was also 0.78, similar to De Bruyne et al. (30)

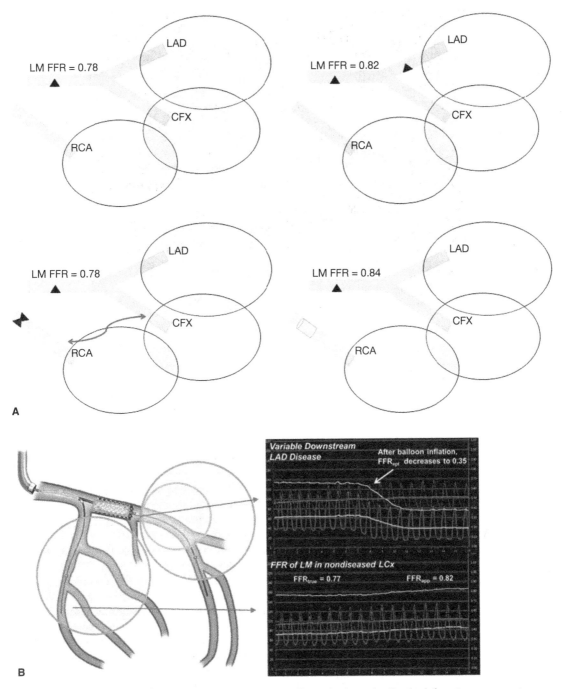

FIGURE 7.16 **A:** A schematic demonstration of how the perfusion bed supplied by the left main coronary artery may play a large role in determining the physiologic significance of a similar left main coronary lesion. **B:** Cartoon of experimental layout demonstrating deflated ("winged") balloon in the left main coronary artery, variably inflated balloon within the newly placed left anterior descending coronary artery (LAD) stent, and pressure wires down the LAD and the left circumflex coronary artery. (From: Fearon W, et al. *J Am Coll Cardiol* Intv. 2015;8(3):398–403.)

FFR in STEMI

In a study by Ntalianis et al. (32), even at 35 days after acute MI, FFR measured in the non-culprit vessel during the acute phase did not change. Hence, in STEMI patients with multivessel disease, FFR measured in the non-culprit vessel in an acute setting may be useful to guide revascularization. DANAMI–3–PRIMULTI (33) is an open-label, randomized trial involving 627 patients with STEMI and multivessel disease. After PCI of the culprit vessel, patients were randomized into two groups: FFR-guided complete revascularization 2 days later prior to discharge, or no further invasive treatment. At 1 year, the rate of primary events (composite of all-cause mortality, non-fatal re-infarction, and ischemia-driven revascularization) was significantly lower in FFR-guided complete revascularization patients (13% vs. 22%; p = 0.004). This difference was predominantly driven by repeat revascularization rates, and there was no significant difference in all-cause mortality or non-fatal MI between the two groups.

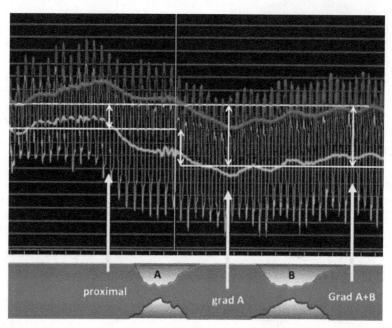

FIGURE 7.17   Measurement of lesions in tandem. Aortic pressure (*red*) and distal pressure wire tracing (*green*) shows gradients between A_o and P_d (*white arrows*) across each lesion A and B. Below is a schematic depiction of the artery with two serial stenosis: "A" and "B." The typical FFR formula cannot be used to calculate individual stenosis on FFR because the first lesion interferes with hyperemia recorded across the second, and vice versa. To assess the lesions, use the largest gradient, and then treat and remeasure the final single vessel FFR. FFR, fractional flow reserve.

ACS-Non-ST Segment Myocardial Infarction

In a subgroup analysis of 328 patients enrolled in FAME with unstable angina or NSTEMI by Sels et al. (34), the absolute risk reduction in major cardiovascular events using an FFR-guided revascularization strategy was similar in patients with NSTEMI and stable angina (5.1% vs. 3.7%; p = 0.92). The only multicenter, randomized trial conducted specifically among NSTEMI patients to evaluate the outcomes of FFR-guided revascularization is FAMOUS NSTEMI (35). In this study, 350 NSTEMI patients with more than 30% stenosis in at least one vessel were randomized to FFR-guided revascularization strategy or angiography-guided standard care. In the FFR-guided group, the operator was disclosed the FFR results, while in the other group, although FFR was measured, it was not disclosed to the operator. Based on the FFR results, the treatment plan was changed in 21.6% of patients. The number of patients who underwent revascularization at index hospitalization was significantly lower in the FFR-guided group (77.3% vs. 86.8%; p = 0.02), with no difference between the two groups in major cardiovascular events.

The PRAMI (36) and CvLPRIT (37) studies found improved outcomes, with complete revascularization performed at the same time or within the index hospitalization. The non-infarct-related arteries (IRA, also called the culprit vessel) were treated based on the angiographic appearance of the lesions, an approach that has the potential to over- or under-treat the non-IRA because of the well-known limitations of equating angiographic visual severity to hemodynamic lesion significance.

In the PRIMULTI study (38), following the PCI of the culprit STEMI vessel, FFR was used to measure the hemodynamic lesion severity in any non-infarct arteries considered angiographically significant, and treated the artery based on an FFR <0.80. A total of 627 patients were enrolled in the study; 313 patients were in the culprit-only group and had no further invasive treatment after primary PCI of the IRA, while 314 patients were assigned to complete revascularization, and only those non-IRA vessels with positive FFR <0.80. At a follow-up of 27 months (range, 12–44 months), the primary endpoint (composite of death, MI, urgent revascularization) was present in 68 patients (22%) of the culprit-only group compared to 40 patients (13%) in the FFR-guided STEMI revascularization group (hazard ratio 0.56, 95% CI 0.38–0.83; p = 0.004). The follow-up events related to the untreated non-IRA vessels are pending.

Despite the fact that the ischemia (FFR)-guided group in the PRI-MULTI study had a lower MACE rate, there is a question whether FFR will be reliable in the ACS setting. The FFR—i.e., the translesional distal to aortic pressure ratio (P_d/P_a) at maximal hyperemia—measures the percent of maximal flow across an epicardial lesion compared to flow through the same vessel in the theoretical absence of the lesion. FFR is directly related to flow; flow is directly related to the myocardial territory or mass supplied by the stenotic vessel. For a given stenosis, the higher the flow, the lower the FFR, and vice versa. Thus, for the same stenosis at two points in time, the FFR could decrease if the flow were measured at a later time and had increased due to myocardial bed changes, as might be expected with infarct healing (Fig. 7.18). Moreover, even in stable anginal patients, the amount of flow to a specific territory across a stenosis explains a common problem related to accepting the FFR. This problem—the "visual functional mismatch between the angiographic stenosis and the FFR"—is commonly seen with severe angiographic lesions in small branches supplying a small mass that has a high FFR, or in mild lesions in large branches supplying a large myocardial mass that has a low FFR.

Because of a changing myocardial bed during the recuperation phase after an acute infarction, FFR is not used in the STEMI culprit artery until 4 to 6 days after the event, when myocardial function is believed to stabilize (30,31). For the non-IRA in STEMI/NSTEMI

The Visual-Functional Mismatch
Myocardial Mass and FFR

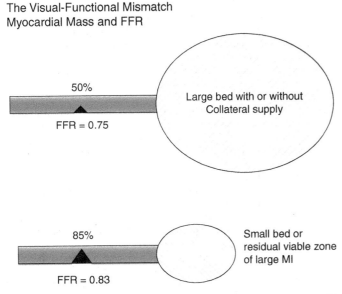

FIGURE 7.18 Influence of myocardial bed size on FFR. *Top:* A mild lesion of 50% supplying a large territory of myocardium can have a low FFR of 0.75. *Bottom:* In contrast, a severe angiographic narrowing of 85% supplying a small myocardial territory can have a high FFR of 0.83. In a STEMI patient, the lower panel might represent the acute phase, and the upper panel the recuperation phase, with changing FFR values influencing the decision making at the time of STEMI. Similar conditions may exist for the non-infarct-related artery assessments. FFR, fractional flow reserve STEMI, ST elevation myocardial infarction.

patients, the zone of myocardial injury of the culprit vessel is unknown, but may extend close to the region supplied by the non-IRA. Thus, a normal FFR at the time of STEMI might be lower several days later if the myocardial flow improves to the remote non-IRA zone, changing the initial treatment decision based on a high FFR. To address the stability of FFR in the non-infarct artery in STEMI/NSTEMI patients, we can look at the ACS patient subset of the FAME study (32). A total of 101 patients undergoing PCI for both STEMI and NSTEMI had 112 non-culprit lesions assessed by FFR at the index procedure and was again repeated 35 ± 4 days later. The FFR of these non-culprit stenoses was 0.77 ± 0.13 during the index procedure and was identical 0.77 ± 0.13 at the time of follow-up. In those with unstable angina or NSTEMI, there was no evidence for a changing FFR over 3 months of follow-up. In the FAME study, FFR-guided interventions for both the stable angina and the NSTEMI patients produced similar relative risk reductions of MACE and death (34). One of the confounding features of decisions to treat the non-IRA, in addition to variable myocardial dysfunction, is the heightened biologic activity of lesions with a stimulated inflammatory and prothrombotic state, and active myocardial compensatory contractile responses in the non-infarct territories. How much these factors play a role in whether a non-infarct vessel should be treated even if FFR is negative remains unknown.

The preliminary data from the COMPARE-ACUTE multicenter trial (39) reported on results in 408 patients with multi-vessel disease and STEMI undergoing primary PCI. A total of 613 FFR measurements were made in non-culprit lesions. FFR measured in a non-culprit lesion was negative in 57% (>0.80) and positive in (43%), highlighting the fact that non-culprit lesions identified during STEMI may be innocent bystanders and may not need to be treated.

References

1. Chilian WM. Coronary microcirculation in health and disease. Summary of an NHLBI workshop. *Circulation.* 1997;95:522–528.
2. Kern MJ, Samady H. Current concepts of integrated coronary physiology in the cath lab. *J Am Coll Cardiol.* 2010;55:173–85.
3. Gould KL, Kirkeeide RL, Buchi M. Coronary flow reserve as a physiologic measure of stenosis severity. *J Am Coll Cardiol.* 1990;15:459–474.
4. Siebes M, Campbell CS, D'Argenio DZ. Fluid dynamics of a partially collapsible stenosis in a flow model of the coronary circulation. *J Biomech Eng.* 1996;118:489–497.
5. Pijls NH, et al. Practice and potential pitfalls of coronary pressure measurement. *Catheter Cardiovasc Interv.* 2000;49:1–16.
6. Pijls NH, et al. Fractional flow reserve: a useful index to evaluate the influence of an epicardial coronary stenosis on myocardial blood flow. *Circulation.* 1995;92:3183–3193.
7. De Bruyne B, et al. Simultaneous coronary pressure and flow velocity measurements in humans: feasibility, reproducibility, and hemodynamic dependence of coronary flow velocity reserve, hyperemic flow versus pressure slope index, and fractional flow reserve. *Circulation.* 1996;94:1842–1849.
8. Parham WA, et al. Coronary hyperemic dose responses to intracoronary sodium nitroprusside. *Circulation.* 2004;109:1236–1243.
9. Davies JE, Sen S, Dehbi HM, et al. Use of the instantaneous wave-free ratio or fractional flow reserve in PCI. *N Engl J Med.* 2017;376:1824–34. doi: 10.1056/NEJMoa1700445.
10. Sen S, et al. Development and validation of a new adenosine-independent index of stenosis severity from coronary wave-intensity analysis: results

of the ADVISE (ADenosine Vasodilator Independent Stenosis Evaluation) study. *J Am Coll Cardiol.* 2012;59:1392–1402.

11. Jeremias A, et al. Multicenter core laboratory comparison of the instantaneous wave-free ratio and resting Pd/Pa with fractional flow reserve: the RESOLVE study. *J Am Coll Cardiol.* 2014;63(13):1253–1261.

12. Davies JE, et al. Use of the instantaneous wave-free ratio or fractional flow reserve in PCI. *N Engl J Med.* 2017;376(19):1824–1834.

13. Götberg M, et al. Instantaneous wave-free ratio versus fractional flow reserve to guide PCI. *N Engl J Med.* 2017;376(19):1813–1823.

14. Kern MJ, et al. Variations in normal coronary vasodilatory reserve stratified by artery, gender, heart transplantation and coronary artery disease. *J Am Coll Cardiol.* 1996;28:1154–1160.

15. Kern MJ. Coronary physiology revisited: practical insights from the cardiac catheterization laboratory. *Circulation.* 2000;101:1344–1351.

16. Davies JE, et al. Evidence of a dominant backward-propagating "suction" wave responsible for diastolic coronary filling in humans, attenuated in left ventricular hypertrophy. *Circulation.* 2006;113:1768–1778.

17. Sen S, et al. Diagnostic classification of the instantaneous wave-free ratio is equivalent to fractional flow reserve and is not improved with adenosine administration. *J Am Coll Cardiol.* 2013;61(13):1409–1420. doi:10.1016/j.jacc.2013.01.034.

18. Christou MA, et al. Meta-analysis of fractional flow reserve versus quantitative coronary angiography and noninvasive imaging for evaluation of myocardial ischemia. *Am J Cardiol.* 2007;99(4):450–456.

19. Meuwissen M, et al. The prognostic value of combined intracoronary pressure and blood flow velocity measurements after deferral of percutaneous coronary intervention. *Catheter Cardiovasc Interv.* 2008;71:291–297.

20. Escaned J, et al. Assessment of microcirculatory remodeling with intracoronary flow velocity and pressure measurements: validation with endomyocardial sampling in cardiac allografts. *Circulation.* 2009;120(16):1561–1568.

21. Takagi A, et al. Clinical potential of intravascular ultrasound for physiological assessment of coronary stenosis: relationship between quantitative ultrasound tomography and pressure-derived fractional flow reserve. *Circulation.* 1999;100(3):250–255.

22. Pijls NH, et al. Percutaneous coronary intervention of functionally non-significant stenoses: 5-year follow-up of the DEFER study. *J Am Coll Cardiol.* 2007;49:2105–2111.

23. Tonino PAL, et al. Fractional flow reserve versus angiography for guiding percutaneous coronary intervention. *N Engl J Med.* 2009;360(3):213–224.

24. De Bruyne B, et al. Fractional flow reserve–guided PCI versus medical therapy in stable coronary disease. *N Engl J Med.* 2012;367:991–1001.

25. Hamilos M, et al. Long-term clinical outcome after fractional flow reserve-guided treatment in patients with angiographically equivocal left main coronary artery stenosis. *Circulation.* 2009;120:1505–1512.

26. Fearon WF, et al. The impact of downstream coronary stenosis on fractional flow reserve assessment of intermediate left main coronary artery disease: human validation. *JACC Cardiovasc Interv.* 2015;8(3):398–403.

27. Sachdeva R, Uretsky BF. The effect of CTO recanalization on FFR of the donor artery. *Catheter Cardiovasc Interv.* 2011;77(3):367–369.

28. Iqbal MB, et al. Reduction in myocardial perfusion territory and its effect on the physiological severity of a coronary stenosis. *Circ Cardiovasc Interv.* 2010;3(1):89–90.

29. Pijls NH, et al. Coronary pressure measurement to assess the hemodynamic significance of serial stenoses within one coronary artery validation in humans. *Circulation.* 2000;102:2371–2377.

30. De Bruyne B, et al. Fractional flow reserve in patients with prior myocardial infarction. *Circulation.* 2001;104(2):157–162.

31. Samady H, et al. Fractional flow reserve of infarct-related arteries identifies reversible defects on noninvasive myocardial perfusion imaging early after myocardial infarction. *J Am Coll Cardiol.* 2006;47(11):2187–2193.

32. Ntalianis A, et al. Fractional flow reserve for the assessment of nonculprit coronary artery stenoses in patients with acute myocardial infarction. *JACC Cardiovasc Interv.* 2010;3(12):1274–1281.

33. Engstrøm T, et al. Complete revascularisation versus treatment of the culprit lesion only in patients with ST-segment elevation myocardial infarction and multivessel disease (DANAMI-3—PRIMULTI): an open-label, randomised controlled trial. *Lancet.* 2015;386(9994):665–671.

34. Sels JW, et al. Fractional flow reserve in unstable angina and non-ST-segment elevation myocardial infarction experience from the FAME (Fractional flow reserve versus Angiography for Multivessel Evaluation) study. *JACC Cardiovasc Interv.* 2011;4(11):1183–1189.

35. Layland J, et al. Fractional flow reserve vs. angiography in guiding management to optimize outcomes in non-ST-segment elevation myocardial infarction: the British Heart Foundation FAMOUS-NSTEMI randomized trial. *Eur Heart J.* 2015;36(2):100–111.

36. Wald DS, et al. Randomized trial of preventive angioplasty in myocardial infarction. *N Engl J Med.* 2013;369(12):1115–1123.

37. Gershlick AH, et al. Randomized trial of complete versus lesion-only revascularization in patients undergoing primary percutaneous coronary intervention for STEMI and multivessel disease: the CvLPRIT trial. *J Am Coll Cardiol.* 2015;65:963–972.

38. Engstrøm T. The Third DANish study of optimal acute treatment of patients with ST-segment elevation myocardial infarction: PRImary PCI in MULTI-vessel Disease. Presented at: American College of Cardiology/i2 Scientific Session; March 16, 2015; San Diego, CA.

39. Smits PC, et al. Fractional flow reserve-guided multivessel angioplasty in myocardial infarction. *N Engl J Med.* 2017;376(13):1234–1244. doi:10.1056/NEJMoa1701067.

8

Intravascular Ultrasound, Optical Coherence Tomography, and Near-Infrared Spectroscopy

Sonia R. Samtani, MD and Arnold H. Seto, MD, MPA, FSCAI, FACC

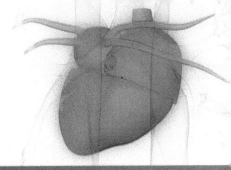

INTRAVASCULAR ULTRASOUND

- Intravascular Ultrasound should be in heading A style
- Optical Coherence Tomography should also be in heading A style
- Near Infared Spectroscopy should also be in heading A style
- The rest can be in B headings.

Intravascular ultrasound (IVUS) allows direct visualization of coronary and vascular anatomy during diagnostic and interventional cardiac catheterization. Unlike angiography, which merely depicts a silhouette of the coronary lumen, IVUS provides a tomographic, cross-sectional perspective. This facilitates direct measurements of the lumen dimensions, including the minimum and maximum diameter and cross-sectional area (1). By employing an automated timed pullback, length measures can also be obtained. Ultrasound-derived measurements are more accurate than quantitative angiographic dimensions (2). IVUS is unique in being able to image the characteristics of full thickness of the arterial wall, enabling characterization of atheroma size, plaque distribution, and lesion composition (3). IVUS can detect the presence or absence of structural abnormalities of the vessel wall after mechanical interventions, including dissections, tissue flaps, intramural hematomas, perforations, and irregular surface features. Since intracoronary ultrasound was first performed in 1988, it has been instrumental to our understanding of coronary anatomy and pathophysiology and has allowed detailed evaluation of interventional procedures (4).

INTRAVASCULAR ULTRASOUND DEVICES

IVUS offers a tomographic view of the arterial wall similar to that of a pathologic section. To achieve this detail, it utilizes higher ultrasound frequencies (40–60 MHz) than that of standard echocardiography, providing axial resolution that ranges from 40 to 150 μm. IVUS requires two components: a catheter incorporating a miniaturized transducer and a console containing the necessary electronics to reconstruct the ultrasound image. Catheters typically range in size from 2.9F to 3.5F, (0.96–1.17 mm), and are thus compatible with 6F guide catheters. Two technical approaches to transducer design have emerged: mechanically rotated imaging devices and a multi-element electronic phased-array device. Most systems use a monorail design to facilitate rapid catheter exchange. In clinical practice, both devices provide sufficiently accurate information for guiding patient care, although rotational IVUS images are typically of higher quality.

ARTIFACTS AND LIMITATIONS

Mechanical transducers may exhibit variations in rotational speed arising from mechanical drag on the catheter driveshaft, creating non-uniform rotational distortion (NURD) and producing visible distortion. NURD is most evident when the driveshaft is bent into a small radius of curvature by a tortuous vessel and is recognized as circumferential "stretching" of a portion of the image with "compression" of the contralateral vessel wall. An additional artifact, transducer ring-down, appears in virtually all medical ultrasound devices. This artifact arises from acoustic oscillations in the piezoelectric transducer material, resulting in high-amplitude signals that obscure near-field imaging. In mechanical systems, this artifact may be merged with the imaging sheath artifact. In electronic array catheters, this artifact may be largely removed by mask subtraction. All intravascular imaging systems are vulnerable to geometric distortion produced by oblique imaging. Thus, when the ultrasound beam interrogates a plane not orthogonal to the vessel walls, an artery with a circular lumen appears elliptical in shape. Most transducer designs position the guide wire external to the transducer, thereby introducing an obligatory "wire artifact." In general, higher-frequency transducers have a lower penetration depth. In practice, this is not usually an issue for coronary imaging, but may become evident if peripheral arterial imaging is attempted. Alternative catheters with a lower ultrasound frequency are used for large-vessel peripheral imaging and for intracardiac examination.

SAFETY OF CORONARY ULTRASOUND

Although IVUS requires intracoronary instrumentation, the technique has been shown to be safe, and no acceleration of atherosclerosis due to catheter-induced endothelial damage has been demonstrated (5). The imaging transducer can transiently occlude the coronary when advanced into a tight stenosis or a small distal vessel, but patients generally do not experience chest pain if the catheter is promptly withdrawn. Pre-instrumentation nitroglycerine is advised to prevent spasm and induce maximal vasodilation. Adequate anticoagulation is required prior to catheter insertion; an activated clotting time of greater than 250 seconds is recommended. Despite the relative safety of coronary ultrasound, any intracoronary instrumentation carries the potential risk of intimal injury or acute vessel dissection.

QUANTITATIVE LUMINAL MEASUREMENTS

Diagnostic and interventional practitioners routinely use luminal measurements to evaluate the severity of stenoses, determine the size of the "normal" reference segment, and assess the gain in lumen size achieved by revascularization (**Fig. 8.1**). Comparisons of vessel dimensions by angiography and IVUS generally reveal a limited correlation, particularly for vessels with an eccentric luminal shape, presumably owing to the inability of angiography to accurately portray the complex, irregular cross-sectional profiles of atherosclerotic vessels. In general, angiography overestimates lumen dimensions compared to IVUS, even after symmetric stent implantation and quantitative angiographic analysis. By performing a timed or calibrated pullback through the vessel, the length of artery involved can also be measured, allowing the calculation of the lumen, vessel, and plaque volume, as

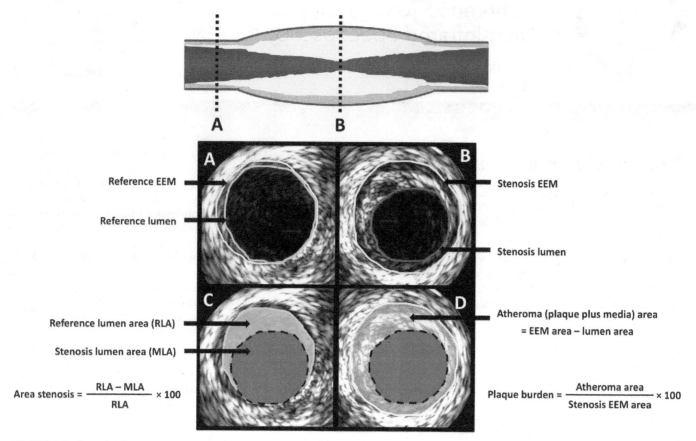

FIGURE 8.1 Basic IVUS measurements. **A** is from the proximal reference, and **B** is from the most severe stenosis representing the minimal lumen area. **C** illustrates the calculation of area stenosis, which compares the stenosis lumen to the reference lumen. This is in contrast to plaque burden **(D)**, which compares the stenosis lumen to the stenosis external elastic membrane (EEM). Due to arterial remodeling, the plaque burden is not the same as area stenosis, and therefore should not be used to assess stenosis severity. MLA, minimal lumen area; RLA, reference lumen area. (Adapted from McDaniel MC, et al. *JACC Cardiovasc Interv.* 2011;4:1155–1167, with permission.)

well as plaque composition. The maximum and minimum luminal diameters are most widely used in clinical practice.

ANGIOGRAPHICALLY UNRECOGNIZED DISEASE

IVUS commonly detects atherosclerotic abnormalities at angiographically normal coronary sites. The long-term implications of these findings remain uncertain. In the Prospective Natural-History Study of Coronary Atherosclerosis Trial (PROSPECT), Stone et al. demonstrated that, after an acute coronary syndrome, most major adverse cardiovascular events involving non-culprit lesions at follow-up were caused by angiographically mild lesions (32.3% ± 20.6% stenosis at baseline), of which 30.2% were angiographically inconspicuous (less than 30% stenosis) (3). Accordingly, the presence of angiographically occult coronary disease may have important prognostic significance. Studies are currently underway to determine the predictive value of IVUS in determining the prognosis in patients with coronary disease. In PROSPECT, a plaque burden of 70% or greater, a minimal lumen area (MLA) of 4.0 mm^2 or less (in the proximal epicardial vessels), and thin-cap fibroatheromas by radiofrequency IVUS were more likely to be associated with recurrent events, but the positive predictive value was too weak to justify preventative stenting.

Using volumetric intracoronary ultrasound, minor changes in plaque and lumen volume can be reliably detected. By comparing baseline and repeat studies, the effects of drug therapy (statins, PCSK09 inhibitors) on atheroma volume can be assessed. Due to the precise measures, such methodology allows pharmaceutical studies to be completed using far fewer patients than necessary if only clinical endpoints are collected (4).

CALCIFICATION

Calcium is frequent in target lesions (75%), but poorly detected by fluoroscopy and angiography (sensitivity only 40%) (5). Calcification markedly increases both the periprocedural risks (dissection, acute closure) and post-procedural outcomes (restenosis, stent thrombosis) after coronary stenting. Calcium is best identified by IVUS, which can accurately determine whether the calcium is circumferential or superficial and if it is likely to require atherectomy prior to stent implantation.

LESIONS OF UNCERTAIN SEVERITY

Despite thorough radiographic examinations with multiple projections, angiographers commonly encounter lesions that elude accurate characterization. Coronary atherosclerosis can be associated with vessel expansion (positive remodeling), thus the angiographic appearance of the vessel may be normal despite significant accumulation of plaque. Lesions of uncertain severity often include ostial lesions and moderate stenoses (40%–70% diameter stenosis). Bifurcation lesions are particularly difficult to assess by angiography because overlapping side branches often obscure the lesion. For these ambiguous lesions, IVUS provides tomographic measurements, enabling quantification of the stenosis independent of the radiographic projection.

Based on earlier studies, a MLA ≥ 4.0 mm^2 can be safely used as a cutoff for identifying non-ischemic lesions for which percutaneous coronary intervention (PCI) can be deferred (6). Nevertheless, using a cutoff MLA to predict which lesions will result in stress-induced ischemia (or a low fractional flow reserve [FFR]) should be avoided, because other lesion characteristics, such as length, area stenosis, plaque burden, reference vessel size, and location are important contributors to the hemodynamic significance of a lesion (7). The Fractional Flow Reserve and Intravascular Ultrasound Relationship (FIRST) study aimed to determine the optimal MLA by IVUS that correlates with FFR. In this study, anatomic measurements in 350 patients obtained by IVUS showed only a moderate correlation with FFR measurements. The correlation between MLA cutoff and FFR values was dependent on vessel size, with the correlation higher in larger vessels. Plaque composition assessed by IVUS did not correlate with FFR (8). In most situations, physiologic measures, such as FFR, are better suited for determination of ischemia and should be considered the gold standard for assessing the significance of intermediate lesions, or decisions regarding revascularization.

LEFT MAIN LESIONS

Unlike in other coronary arteries where IVUS MLA has modest correlation with physiology, the left main has a reasonably high correlation between IVUS and FFR. The lower limit of normal, non-diseased left main luminal area is 7.5 mm^2 (9). The best cut points for predicting an FFR <0.75 is an IVUS left main minimal diameter of <2.8 mm or MLA <5.9 mm^2 (10). Further, in the large, non-randomized, 354-patient LITRO study, a left main MLA cutoff of 6 mm^2 was prospectively validated to be safe for determining which patients require revascularization. In this study, the 179 patients with a left main MLA above 6 mm^2 for whom left main revascularization was deferred had similar outcomes to the revascularized group. Only eight patients required subsequent left main revascularization after 2 years of follow-up (11). The 2011 ACC/AHA/SCAI guidelines for PCI assign a Class IIa recommendation for performing IVUS to assess angiographically indeterminate left main lesions (12). FFR is also appropriate for assessment of intermediate left main lesions, but can be challenging to interpret when distal disease is present.

IVUS guidance during the intervention may affect long-term outcomes after left main stenting. In an analysis of the MAIN-COMPARE registry using propensity-score matching, IVUS guidance was associated with reduced 3-year mortality (in the subset of patients receiving diethylstilbestrol [DES]) compared to angiographic guidance (4.7% vs. 16%, p = 0.048) (13). Prospective randomized data regarding IVUS guidance for left main stenting are currently lacking, although the current consensus is that IVUS should be used during all unprotected left main interventions.

CORONARY STENT DEPLOYMENT

In everyday practice, the most important measurements to be obtained from IVUS include the reference lumen diameter, the post-stent lumen area, and the lesion length. The reference lumen diameter is

TABLE 8.1 Target Lumen Areas Based on Vessel Diameter or Chosen Balloon (Stent) Size

LUMEN DIAMETER (BALLOON SIZE) (mm)	EXPECTED LUMEN CSA (mm^2)
2.00	3.14
2.25	3.98
2.50	4.90
2.75	5.94
3.00	7.07
3.25	8.30
3.50	9.62
3.75	11.00
4.00	12.57

used to determine the appropriate stent diameter, the lesion length (measured from a timed pullback), the stent length, and the stent lumen area the adequacy of expansion and apposition. Operators should be familiar with the relationship between the diameter and areas of commonly used devices within coronary intervention. (Table 8.1). Use of the package inserts listing expected balloon (or stent) diameters at given pressures should be discouraged, because the extent of expansion at any given pressure is dependent on the compliance of the vessel. Direct measurement by IVUS will detect the actual degree of expansion following balloon dilatation.

The criteria for optimal IVUS-guided stent deployment have been extensively explored (14). To minimize restenosis, most authorities recommend that operators attempt to achieve a minimum stent lumen cross-sectional area of over 8 mm^2 when vessel size will allow (15). High-pressure (>16 atm) and upsized balloons (by 0.25–0.5 mm) are frequently necessary to achieve these results.

It is generally accepted that angiographic appearance after intervention can be deceiving, and IVUS can be very useful in determining suboptimal stent expansion and quantifying the additional gain achieved by higher-pressure or larger-diameter repeat balloon dilation. The use of IVUS-guidance has been the subject of multiple randomized and observational trials. A recent meta-analysis of 26,503 patients from three randomized trials and 14 observational studies suggested that IVUS guidance after drug-eluting stent implantation was associated with larger and longer stents and larger post-procedural minimal luminal diameter. These interventions resulted in significantly lower rates of MACE (OR 0.74, p < 0.001), death (OR 0.61, p < 0.001), myocardial infarction (MI) (OR 0.57, p < 0.001), stent thrombosis (OR 0.59, p < 0.001), and target lesion revascularization (OR 0.81, p = 0.046) (16) (Fig. 8.2).

Additional studies have documented benefits for ultrasound guidance in small vessels (17) and long lesions (18), as well as high-risk bifurcation and left main lesions (13,19). The finding that many "small" vessels are actually not small but severely diseased has justified oversized stenting in these positively remodeled vessels. Definitive evidence to support routine IVUS guidance of *all* stent procedures is lacking, although positive studies in varied subgroups suggest that IVUS can be of benefit in many stent procedures.

Data from core laboratories with careful clinical follow-up have allowed investigation of particular IVUS findings. Minor stent malposition (20) or small edge tears (21) have not adversely affected patient outcome after stenting, and may be left untreated.

Major Adverse Cardiovascular Events

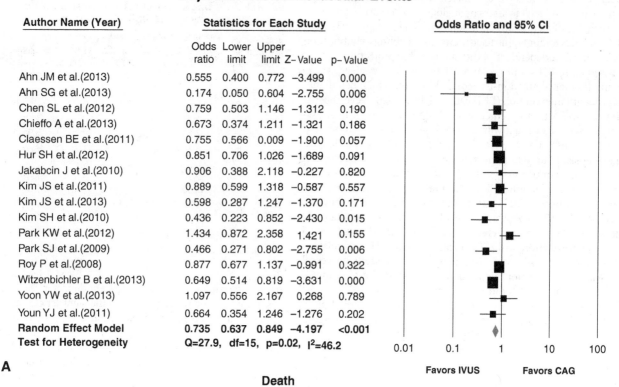

Author Name (Year)	Odds ratio	Lower limit	Upper limit	Z–Value	p–Value
Ahn JM et al.(2013)	0.555	0.400	0.772	−3.499	0.000
Ahn SG et al.(2013)	0.174	0.050	0.604	−2.755	0.006
Chen SL et al.(2012)	0.759	0.503	1.146	−1.312	0.190
Chieffo A et al.(2013)	0.673	0.374	1.211	−1.321	0.186
Claessen BE et al.(2011)	0.755	0.566	0.009	−1.900	0.057
Hur SH et al.(2012)	0.851	0.706	1.026	−1.689	0.091
Jakabcin J et al.(2010)	0.906	0.388	2.118	−0.227	0.820
Kim JS et al.(2011)	0.889	0.599	1.318	−0.587	0.557
Kim JS et al.(2013)	0.598	0.287	1.247	−1.370	0.171
Kim SH et al.(2010)	0.436	0.223	0.852	−2.430	0.015
Park KW et al.(2012)	1.434	0.872	2.358	1.421	0.155
Park SJ et al.(2009)	0.466	0.271	0.802	−2.755	0.006
Roy P et al.(2008)	0.877	0.677	1.137	−0.991	0.322
Witzenbichler B et al.(2013)	0.649	0.514	0.819	−3.631	0.000
Yoon YW et al.(2013)	1.097	0.556	2.167	0.268	0.789
Youn YJ et al.(2011)	0.664	0.354	1.246	−1.276	0.202
Random Effect Model	**0.735**	**0.637**	**0.849**	**−4.197**	**<0.001**
Test for Heterogeneity	Q=27.9,	df=15,	p=0.02,	I^2=46.2	

A

Death

Author Name (Year)	Odds ratio	Lower limit	Upper limit	Z–Value	p–Value
Ahn SG et al.(2013)	1.095	0.174	6.898	0.097	0.923
Ahn JM et al.(2013)	0.477	0.301	0.756	−3.152	0.002
Chen SL et al.(2012)	0.554	0.216	1.422	−1.227	0.220
Chieffo A et al.(2013)	0.198	0.009	4.170	−1.041	0.298
Claessen BE et al.(2011)	0.656	0.376	1.147	−1.478	0.139
Hur SH et al.(2012)	0.486	0.358	0.661	−4.604	0.000
Jakabcin J et al.(2010)	1.515	0.259	8.874	0.461	0.645
Kim SH et al.(2010)	0.172	0.050	0.590	−2.802	0.005
Kim JS et al.(2011)	0.857	0.425	1.725	−0.433	0.665
Kim JS et al.(2013)	1.578	0.254	9.784	0.490	0.624
Park SJ et al.(2009)	0.259	0.107	0.629	−2.982	0.003
Park KW et al.(2012)	1.673	0.506	5.533	0.844	0.399
Roy P et al.(2008)	0.791	0.539	1.160	−1.200	0.230
Witzenbichler B et al.(2013)	0.875	0.636	1.204	−0.818	0.413
Yoon YW et al.(2013)	0.248	0.039	1.587	−1.472	0.141
Youn YJ et al.(2011)	0.210	0.026	1.698	−1.463	0.143
Random Effect Model	**0.613**	**0.478**	**0.786**	**−3.861**	**<0.001**
Test for Heterogeneity	Q=25.9,	df=15,	p=0.039,	I^2=42.2	

B

FIGURE 8.2 Forest plot of OR for MACEs **(A)**, death **(B)**, MI **(C)**, TVR **(D)**, TLR **(E)**, and ST **(F)** in IVUS- versus angiography-guided PCI. Squares are the effect size of the individual studies; diamonds, the summarized effect size; horizontal lines, the upper and lower border of the 95% confidence interval. CAG, coronary angiography; df, degrees of freedom. IVUS, intravascular ultrasound; MI, myocardial infarction; PCI, percutaneous coronary intervention. (From Ahn JM, et al. Meta-analysis of outcomes after intravascular ultrasound-guided versus angiography-guided drug-eluting stent implantation in 26,503 patients enrolled in three randomized trials and 14 observational studies. *Am J Cardiol.* 2014;113(8):1338–1347, with permission.)

Myocardial Infarction

Author Name (year)	Statistics for Each Study					Odds Ratio and 95% CI
	odds ratio	Lower limit	Upper limit	Z-Value	p-Value	
Ahn JM et al.(2013)	0.373	0.131	1.061	−1.849	0.064	
Ahn SG et al.(2013)	0.126	0.014	1.154	−1.833	0.067	
Chen SL et al.(2012)	0.494	0.257	0.948	−2.120	0.034	
Chieffo A et al.(2013)	0.810	0.338	1.941	−0.472	0.637	
Claessen BE et al.(2011)	0.399	0.214	0.744	−2.893	0.004	
Hur SH et al.(2012)	0.497	0.247	1.004	−1.949	0.051	
Jakabcin J et al.(2010)	0.242	0.028	2.094	−1.288	0.198	
Kim SH et al.(2010)	0.139	0.017	1.150	−1.830	0.067	
Kim JS et al.(2011)	0.189	0.054	0.665	−2.596	0.009	
Kim JS et al.(2013)	0.209	0.010	4.414	−1.006	0.315	
Park SJ et al.(2009)	0.757	0.369	1.550	−0.762	0.446	
Park KW et al.(2012)	3.043	1.125	8.234	2.191	0.028	
Roy P et al.(2008)	0.670	0.369	1.218	−1.313	0.189	
Witzenbichler B et al.(2013)	0.660	0.508	0.858	−3.110	0.002	
Yoon YW et al.(2013)	0.666	0.083	5.317	−0.383	0.701	
Youn YJ et al.(2011)	0.640	0.167	2.458	−0.650	0.516	
Random Effect Model	**0.571**	**0.435**	**0.751**	**−4.011**	**<0.001**	
Test for Heterogeneity	Q=22.9, df=15, p=0.086, I^2=34.5%					

0.01   0.1   1   10   100

Favors IVUS   Favors CAG

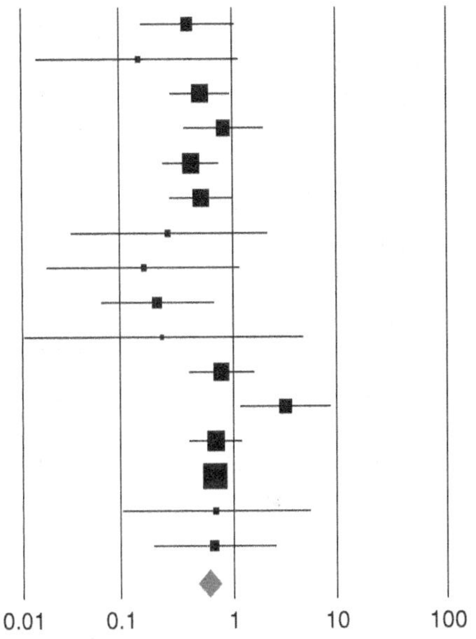

C

Target Vessel Revascularization

Author Name (year)	Statistics for Each Study					Odds Ratio and 95% CI
	odds ratio	Lower limit	Upper limit	Z-Value	p-Value	
Ahn JM et al.(2013)	0.703	0.455	1.086	−1.588	0.112	
Chen SL et al.(2012)	0.728	0.447	1.185	−1.277	0.201	
Chieffo A et al.(2013)	0.592	0.289	1.212	−1.434	0.152	
Claessen BE et al.(2011)	0.851	0.619	1.169	−0.997	0.319	
Hur SH et al.(2012)	1.135	0.895	1.438	1.046	0.296	
Kim JS et al.(2013)	0.667	0.316	1.409	−1.062	0.288	
Park SJ et al.(2009)	0.720	0.310	1.668	−0.767	0.443	
Park KW et al.(2012)	0.929	0.491	1.758	−0.226	0.821	
Roy P et al.(2008)	0.928	0.668	1.290	−0.445	0.656	
Witzenbichler B et al.(2013)	0.590	0.455	0.766	−3.961	0.000	
Yoon YW et al.(2013)	1.409	0.663	2.992	0.891	0.373	
Youn YJ et al.(2011)	0.881	0.453	1.716	−0.372	0.710	
Random Effect Model	**0.824**	**0.698**	**0.972**	**−2.297**	**0.022**	
Test for Heterogeneity	Q=17.9, df=11, p=0.08, I^2=38.5					

0.01   0.1   1   10   100

Favors IVUS   Favors CAG

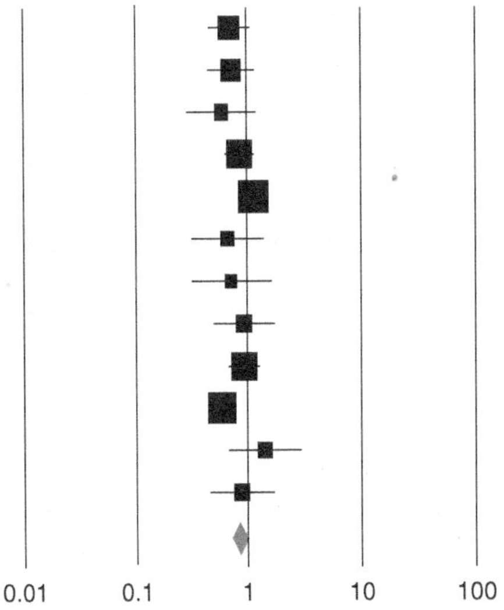

D

FIGURE 8.2 *(continued)*

Target Lesion Revascularization

Author Name (Year)	Statistics for Each Study					Odds Ratio and 95% CI
	Odds ratio	Lower limit	Upper limit	Z-Value	p-Value	
Ahn SG et al. (2013)	0.025	0.001	0.452	−2.501	0.012	
Ahn JM et al. (2013)	0.708	0.449	1.118	−1.481	0.139	
Chen SL et al. (2012)	0.603	0.362	1.003	−1.949	0.051	
Chieffo A et al. (2013)	0.750	0.350	1.608	−0.739	0.460	
Hur SH et al. (2012)	1.133	0.881	1.458	0.974	0.330	
Jakabcin J et al. (2010)	1.000	0.320	3.124	0.000	1.000	
Kim SH et al. (2010)	0.875	0.364	2.105	−0.298	0.765	
Kim JS et al. (2011)	1.113	0.681	1.819	0.427	0.670	
Park KW et al. (2012)	0.954	0.462	1.967	−0.129	0.898	
Roy P et al. (2008)	0.693	0.467	1.027	−1.829	0.067	
Witzenbichler B et al. (2013)	0.636	0.457	0.884	−2.696	0.007	
Youn YJ et al. (2011)	1.014	0.449	2.287	0.033	0.974	
Random Effect Model	**0.811**	**0.660**	**0.996**	**−1.998**	**0.046**	
Test for Heterogeneity	Q=18.7, df=11, p=0.067, I²=41.2					

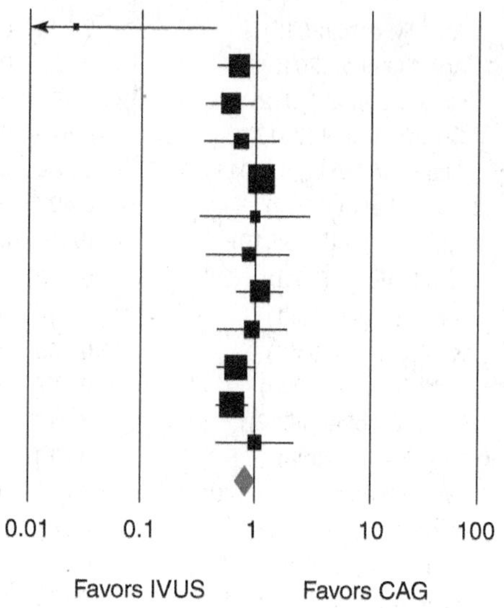

E

Favors IVUS   Favors CAG

Definite or Probable Stent Thrombosis

Author Name (Year)	Statistics for Each Study					Odds Ratio and 95% CI
	Odds ratio	Lower limit	Upper limit	Z-Value	p-Value	
Ahn SG et al. (2013)	0.163	0.017	1.557	−1.575	0.115	
Ahn JM et al. (2013)	0.199	0.037	1.079	−1.872	0.061	
Chen SL et al. (2012)	0.164	0.055	0.489	−3.240	0.001	
Chieffo A et al. (2013)	3.009	0.121	74.609	0.672	0.501	
Claessen BE et al. (2011)	0.553	0.149	2.051	−0.885	0.376	
Hur SH et al. (2012)	0.855	0.558	1.308	−0.723	0.470	
Jakabcin J et al. (2010)	0.653	0.184	2.314	−0.661	0.509	
Kim SH et al. (2010)	0.263	0.059	1.179	−1.745	0.081	
Kim JS et al. (2011)	0.332	0.033	3.300	−0.941	0.347	
Kim JS et al. (2013)	1.000	0.070	14.371	0.000	1.000	
Park SJ et al. (2009)	1.000	0.406	2.465	0.000	1.000	
Park KW et al. (2012)	0.498	0.091	2.719	−0.804	0.421	
Roy P et al. (2008)	0.583	0.392	0.867	−2.666	0.008	
Witzenbichler B et al. (2013)	0.497	0.289	0.855	−2.529	0.011	
Yoon YW et al. (2013)	1.000	0.106	9.393	0.000	1.000	
Youn YJ et al. (2011)	0.854	0.210	3.468	−0.221	0.825	
Random Effect Model	**0.592**	**0.468**	**0.750**	**−4.358**	**<0.001**	
Test for Heterogeneity	Q=15.7, df=15, p=0.40, I²=4.63%					

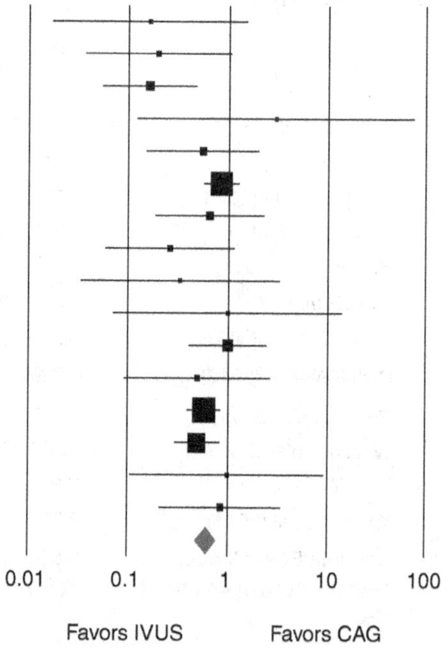

F

Favors IVUS   Favors CAG

FIGURE 8.2 *(continued)*

IVUS INSIGHTS FOR IN-STENT RESTENOSIS

Several multicenter clinical trials have shown that certain findings on ultrasound, such as MLA, plaque composition, and plaque burden, can predict restenosis after intervention (22). Although stent placement abolishes negative remodeling and recoil after angioplasty, it stimulates intimal hyperplasia, which is the primary mechanism of in-stent restenosis (ISR).

The major predictor of ISR has repeatedly been shown to be the final minimal stent area (MSA). In a combined analysis of IVUS sub-studies of six trials involving 1,580 patients treated with both DES (1,098 patients) and BMS (482 patients), post-intervention IVUS MSA was the only independent predictor of ISR at 9 months in the DES-treated patients after multivariate analysis. In BMS-treated patients, post-intervention IVUS-defined MSA and the number of stents implanted were the only two predictors of ISR after multivariate analysis (24). In BMS, areas over 8 to 10 mm^2 are generally associated with target lesion revascularization rates of 10% or less (15). Due to the near-complete suppression of neointimal hyperplasia, the MSA required to prevent target lesion revascularization is less for DES than for BMS (23), allowing sustained success in smaller vessels. In a study of 550 patients receiving DES (sirolimus), the only two IVUS predictors of angiographic restenosis were a MSA <5.5 mm^2 and stent length >40 mm (24). Restenosis following DES placement, although infrequent, is generally due to continued intimal hyperplasia. The site of restenosis is also most often associated with the stented portion having the smallest post-deployment MSA (25).

In addition to frequent inadequate expansion, nearly 5% of all stent implant cases are found to have significant mechanical implantation abnormalities, such as severe stent under-expansion or misplacement (26) (**Figs. 8.3** to **8.6**). Lesion calcification (as noted

earlier) impairs expansion and may lead to significant underexpansion, despite high-pressure post-dilation (**Fig. 8.7**).

Treatment of ISR with various balloon and other devices can be effectively monitored by IVUS (27). Maximizing the MSA is of paramount importance regardless of the technique used. Many experts recommend that all cases of ISR be interrogated by intravascular ultrasound to define the mechanism and guide therapy. The 2011 ACC/AHA/SCAI guidelines for PCI assign a Class IIa recommendation for performing IVUS for ISR (12).

CARDIAC ALLOGRAFT DISEASE

Identification of atherosclerotic lesions in cardiac allograft recipients represents a particularly challenging task. These patients may have diffuse vessel involvement that conceals the disease from angiography. Many large transplant centers now routinely perform IVUS as part of an annual catheterization in cardiac transplant recipients. Studies have revealed two pathways to transplant-associated atherosclerosis, with some patients receiving atherosclerotic plaques from the donor heart, whereas others develop immune-mediated vasculopathy. Rapidly progressive vasculopathy detected by IVUS was found to be a powerful predictor of death and MI in cardiac transplant recipients (28). The 2011 ACC/AHA/SCAI guidelines for PCI assign a Class IIa recommendation for performing IVUS 4 to 6 weeks and 1 year after cardiac transplantation to exclude donor CAD, detect rapidly progressive cardiac allograft vasculopathy, and provide prognostic information (12).

Chronic Total Occlusion Lesions (CTOs)

IVUS can be useful in CTO interventions, for which a short-tipped IVUS catheter is helpful. During intervention, if a side branch is

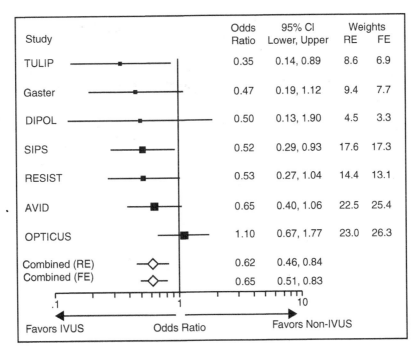

Study	Odds Ratio	95% CI Lower, Upper	Weights RE	Weights FE
TULIP	0.35	0.14, 0.89	8.6	6.9
Gaster	0.47	0.19, 1.12	9.4	7.7
DIPOL	0.50	0.13, 1.90	4.5	3.3
SIPS	0.52	0.29, 0.93	17.6	17.3
RESIST	0.53	0.27, 1.04	14.4	13.1
AVID	0.65	0.40, 1.06	22.5	25.4
OPTICUS	1.10	0.67, 1.77	23.0	26.3
Combined (RE)	0.62	0.46, 0.84		
Combined (FE)	0.65	0.51, 0.83		

Favors IVUS — Odds Ratio — Favors Non-IVUS

FIGURE 8.3 Stent malapposition. Representative IVUS images of stent malapposition at the time of a subacute ST (*left panel*). Stent malapposition (*red arrows*) is clearly evident in the region of angiographic thrombus. Following appropriate-sized balloon re-inflation (*right panel*), the stent is fully apposed. IVUS, intravascular ultrasound.

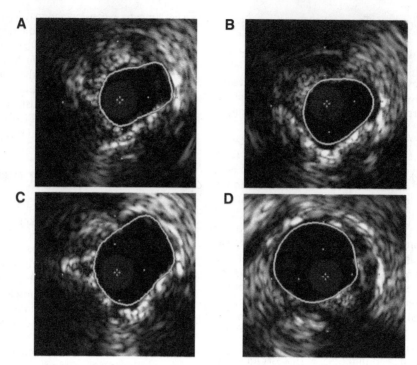

FIGURE 8.4   Stent underexpansion. An example of underexpansion in a 3.0-mm stent at an area of calcified plaque **(A)**. After successive high-pressure inflations with 0.25 mm **(B)** and 0.5-mm larger balloons **(C)**, the minimal stent area improved from 3.7 to 6.2 mm^2. Despite this, the minimal stent area is still less than the well-expanded stent area of 7.0 mm^2 **(D)**.

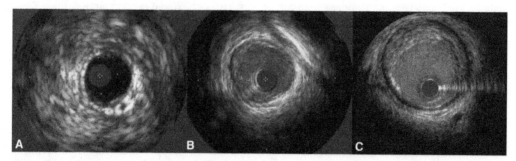

FIGURE 8.5   IVUS device types. Images from **(A)** phased array IVUS (Philips Volcano Eagle Eye), **(B)** rotational IVUS (Philips Volcano Revo), and **(C)** high-definition IVUS (Acist HDi). Phased array IVUS has the lowest-quality images, but tends to be the fastest to set up. IVUS, intravascular ultrasound.

noted near the entrance of the CTO, then IVUS can be placed in this side branch to help determine targets for wire penetration. In addition, the IVUS catheter can be inserted into the subintimal space to determine the direction of the true lumen because it can discern the true lumen with all three layers of the vessel (29). A risk of IVUS for the CTO procedure would be that of enlarging the subintimal space, but IVUS would offer information regarding the extent of intramural hematoma.

Optical Coherence Tomography (OCT)

OCT generates tomographic images from backscattered reflections of infrared light. OCT uses similar principles of pulse-echo ultrasonography imaging, but instead of sound, it uses light (30). As a result of the short wavelength of light, OCT has superior resolution compared with IVUS.

Intravascular OCT catheters consist of a fiberoptic core encapsulated in an optically transparent imaging sheath. Near-infrared light is directed onto the vessel wall, which is reflected off the internal microstructure of the tissue. The intensity of returning waves is used to construct an image of the vessel wall. OCT has an axial resolution of 10 to 15 mm, with a lateral resolution of 20 to 40 mm, and a maximal scan diameter of 7 mm. Quantitative assessment of diameter and area measurements by OCT can be done in a similar fashion to IVUS after adequate calibration for refractive index and z-offset.

A significant limitation of OCT is the need to clear blood from the arterial lumen because OCT cannot image through a blood-filled field (30). Iodinated contrast can be used to displace blood, as can dextran solutions. Due to the difficulty clearing blood from the ostia of coronary arteries, ostial lesions of the left main or right coronary arteries are poorly imaged with OCT. Contrast injections must be injected at high and constant flow and pressure to clear the blood

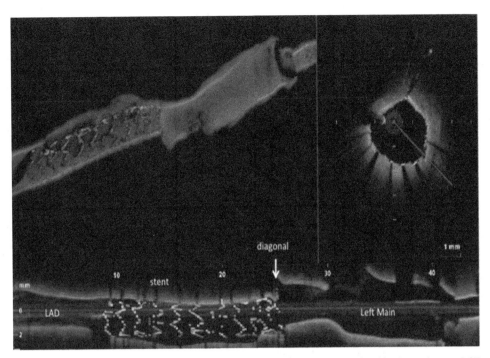

FIGURE 8.6 OCT imaging. Three-dimensional reconstruction (*upper left*) of high-resolution OCT tomographic image (*upper right*) allows for detailed understanding of the relationship between stented segment and coronary branches. Further image analysis (*bottom*) highlights the areas of stent malapposition in *red*. OCT, optical coherence tomography.

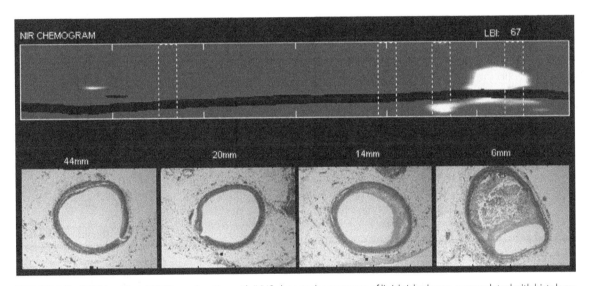

FIGURE 8.7 NIRS imaging. NIRS in conjunction with IVUS detects the presence of lipid-rich plaque, as correlated with histology. NIRS, near-infrared spectroscopy. (From: Gardner CM, et al. Detection of lipid core coronary plaques in autopsy specimens with a novel catheter-based near-infrared spectroscopy system. *JACC Cardiovasc Imaging.* 2008;1:638–648. Used with permission.)

pool sufficiently. Timing OCT imaging with occasions when contrast angiography is desired can help minimize the amount of additional contrast used.

In comparison to IVUS, OCT provides improved resolution by an order of magnitude, but at the expense of a decrease in the depth of imaging (from 10 mm with IVUS to 1–2.5 mm with OCT). Despite this limitation, OCT can be helpful in plaque characterization. Fibrous plaques exhibit homogenous signal-rich images. Calcified plaques have signal-poor regions with sharply delineated upper and lower boards. Lipid-rich plaques are known to have poorly defined diffuse borders with signal-poor regions. The thickness of the fibrous cap can be measured primarily by OCT, and much less so with IVUS due to the limited resolution. As a result, OCT has a potential role in vulnerable plaque imaging, as well as revealing the site of plaque rupture during acute coronary syndromes.

OCT has important uses in acute coronary syndromes. It has a 100% sensitivity in detecting intraluminal thrombus when compared with coronary angioscopy. This is in comparison to the 33% sensitivity seen in IVUS imaging (31). OCT can be used to help differentiate thrombus from calcium and other causes of radiolucency.

OCT has also been used to determine the etiology of acute coronary syndrome, demonstrating in one study that plaque fibrous cap erosion was a relatively frequent cause (31%) of MI, comparable with the conventional frank plaque rupture (43%) (32).

OCT can be used for procedure planning in PCI. Lesion preparation is vital for adequate stent expansion and becomes even more important with the use of bioresorbable scaffolds (33). Bioresorbable scaffolds have thicker struts and mass when compared with current drug-eluting stents. Thus, bioresorbable scaffolds necessitate lesion preparation with calcium debulking or creation of dissection planes in the plaque to allow for ideal expansion and embedding of struts within the vessel wall.

Studies have shown potential benefit with OCT for PCI optimization. The ILUMIEN III: OPTIMIZE PCI trial was a three-arm study that randomized 450 patients to OCT-guided PCI, IVUS-guided PCI, or angiography-guided PCI. The primary endpoint was the post-PCI median MSA, measured by OCT in all patients and blinded to the operators. For this endpoint, OCT guidance was found to be statistically non-inferior to IVUS or angiography. The secondary endpoints involving stent expansion (minimal stent expansion, mean stent expansion, and proportion with acceptable stent expansion) were improved with OCT and IVUS compared with angiography. Thus, it was concluded that OCT matches IVUS in terms of PCI optimization, at the cost of more contrast than IVUS, as well as more time and balloons, compared with angiography alone (34). Compared with IVUS, OCT was also associated with fewer major dissections or areas of major stent malapposition, which may lead to fewer clinical events long term. A clinical outcomes trial (ILUMIEN IV) is planned.

Near-Infrared Spectroscopy (NIRS)

NIRS uses light from the near-infrared region of the electromagnetic spectrum, which can be projected toward the wall of the coronary artery, reflected to a collector, and analyzed according to known spectrographic references (30). Currently, NIRS is commercially available as a combined system with IVUS. NIRS is used to characterize the lipid burden of atherosclerotic plaques. The NIRS spectra is processed by an algorithm and used to create a longitudinal image of the arterial segment, called a chemogram or map of the probability of the lipid being present. NIRS can generate a lipid core burden index (LCBI), which quantifies the amount of lipid core plaques in a scanned arterial segment on a 1 to 1,000 scale. This has been validated histologically, leading to FDA approval of the device and technology prior to any clinically apparent benefit.

Clinically, it had been noted that PCI involving areas with a high burden of lipid core plaques carry an increased rate of post-PCI MI, in part because of distal embolization and stent thrombosis. NIRS could potentially predict those interventions that are more vulnerable to such a complication and allow for further planning of the procedure to help prevent such an event. The data for such practice remains in question, however. Data from the COLOR registry showed that in 1,168 patients, pre-intervention NIRS was performed and the clinical outcomes tracked. Culprit lesion-related major adverse cardiac events were 6.3% for patients with a low LCBI, as compared with 5.4% for patients with a high LCBI. It was noted that the LCBI was not independently associated with major adverse cardiac events (35). As a result, the COLOR registry results did not define any particular benefit of NIRS imaging in predicting post-PCI complications, however additional studies are needed to determine the clinical significance of NIRS-defined lipid-rich plaques. PROSPECT II is expected to use NIRS to image potential vulnerable plaques and define their natural history.

SUMMARY

IVUS adds significantly to day-to-day decision making in the catheterization laboratory. Optimal techniques for stent placement have been developed using IVUS. IVUS is particularly useful in small vessels, complicated anatomy, and long lesions. OCT has better axial and longitudinal resolution, but poorer depth penetration. NIRS generates a chemogram of the probability of lipid core plaque burden, but its routine clinical utility is questionable. Therefore, interventionalists should have a good working knowledge of IVUS and OCT to determine how they can be best used to optimize PCI.

Key Points

- There are two types of IVUS transducer designs: mechanical and electronic array (also known as phased-array or solid state).
- IVUS imaging is safe, with no long-term untoward effects.
- There is a limited correlation with regard to vessel dimension between angiography and IVUS.
- Angiography frequently overestimates vessel dimensions before and after stent implantation.
- Important calculations, such as reference lumen area (RLA), MLA, area stenosis, plaque burden, and lesion length can be obtained from IVUS, which help in planning and guiding interventions.
- IVUS can detect atherosclerotic plaque in angiographically normal coronary arteries.
- In the PROSPECT study, a plaque burden of 70% or greater, a MLA of ≤ 4.0 mm^2, and thin-cap fibroatheromas were more likely to be associated with recurrent events.
- For non-left main lesions, a MLA ≥ 4.0 mm^2 generally identifies non-ischemia producing lesions for which PCI can be safely deferred.
- For lesions with a MLA <4.0 mm^2, physiologic measures such as FFR or stress testing should be used to assess if the lesion is ischemia-producing.
- The 2011 ACC/AHA/SCAI guidelines for PCI assign a Class IIa recommendation for performing IVUS to assess angiographically indeterminate left main disease.
- In the non-randomized LITRO study, patients with a left main MLA ≥ 6 mm^2 for whom left main revascularization was deferred, had similar outcomes to the revascularized group at 2 years.
- In the propensity-score matched MAIN-COMPARE registry, IVUS guidance for left main stenting was associated with reduced 3-year mortality (in the subset of patients receiving DES) compared to angiographic guidance.
- To minimize the risk of restenosis, IVUS guidance, high-pressure balloon inflations, upsized balloons, and rotational atherectomy (in severely calcified lesions) may be required.
- IVUS is useful in specific lesion subsets, such as small vessels, long lesions, high-risk bifurcation, and left main lesions.

- Large propensity-score matched registry data and several randomized trials suggest that IVUS guidance is associated with reduced rates of MI, death, ST, and overall MACE.

- The only consistent IVUS predictor of ISR in both BMS and DES is the post-intervention MSA.

- It is a Class IIa recommendation for performing IVUS for investigation of ISR.

- Rapidly progressive vasculopathy detected by IVUS was found to be a powerful predictor of death and MI in cardiac transplant recipients.

- The 2011 ACC/AHA/SCAI guidelines for PCI assign a Class IIa recommendation for performing IVUS 4 to 6 weeks and 1 year after cardiac transplantation.

- OCT has better axial and lateral resolution, but poorer depth of imaging when compared to IVUS imaging.

- OCT requires the arterial lumen to be clear of blood for imaging.

- OCT matches IVUS in terms of PCI optimization but at the cost of more contrast usage.

- OCT and IVUS are important in pre-treatment of a lesion, which becomes essential with implementation of bioresorbable scaffold systems.

- NIRS uses near-infrared light to generate a chemogram of the probability of lipid core plaque burden within an arterial segment.

- Routine use of NIRS did not show a significant difference in clinical outcomes when the COLOR registry data was analyzed.

ACKNOWLEDGMENTS

The authors and editors acknowledge the authors of the prior version of this chapter, Dr. Vitalie Crudu and Dr. John McB. Hodgson, whose writing served as the basis for this updated chapter.

References

1. Mintz GS, et al. ACC clinical expert consensus document on standards for the acquisition, measurement and reporting of intravascular ultrasound studies: a report of the American College of Cardiology Task Force on Clinical Expert Consensus Documents. *J Am Coll Cardiol*. 2001;37:1478–1492.

2. Jensen LO, et al. Comparison of intravascular ultrasound and angiographic assessment of coronary reference segment size in patients with type 2 diabetes mellitus. *Am J Cardiol*. 2010;101:590–595.

3. Stone GW, et al. A prospective natural history of coronary atherosclerosis. *N Engl J Med*. 2011;364:226–235.

4. Schoenhagen P, Nissen SE. Coronary atherosclerotic disease burden: an emerging endpoint in progression/regression studies using intravascular ultrasound. *Curr Drug Targets Cardiovasc Haematol Disord*. 2003;3:218–226.

5. Mintz GS, et al. Determinants and correlates of target lesion calcium in coronary artery disease: a clinical, angiographic and intravascular ultrasound study. *J Am Coll Cardiol*. 1997;29:268–274.

6. Abizaid AS, et al. Long-term follow-up after percutaneous transluminal coronary angioplasty was not performed based on intravascular ultrasound findings: importance of lumen dimensions. *Circulation*. 1999;100(3):256–261.

7. Park SJ, Ahn JM, Kang SJ. Paradigm shift to functional angioplasty: new insights for fractional flow reserve and intravascular ultrasound-guided percutaneous coronary intervention. *Circulation*. 2011;124(8):951–957.

8. Waksman R, et al. FIRST: Fractional Flow Reserve and Intravascular Ultrasound Relationship Study. *J Am Coll Cardiol*. 2013;61(9):917–923.

9. Fassa A, et al. Intravascular ultrasound-guided treatment for angiographically indeterminate left main coronary artery disease. *J Am Coll Cardiol*. 2005;45:204–211.

10. Jasti V, et al. Correlations between fractional flow reserve and intravascular ultrasound in patients with an ambiguous left main coronary artery stenosis. *Circulation*. 2004;110:2831–2836.

11. de la Torre Hernandez JM, et al. Prospective application of pre-defined intravascular ultrasound criteria for assessment of intermediate left main coronary artery lesions: results from the multicenter LITRO study. *J Am Coll Cardiol*. 2011;58(4):351–358.

12. Levine GN, et al. 2011 ACCF/AHA/SCAI guideline for percutaneous coronary intervention: a report of the American College of Cardiology Foundation/American Heart Association Task Force on Practice Guidelines and the Society for Cardiovascular Angiography and Interventions. *J Am Coll Cardiol*. 2011;58(24):e44–e122.

13. Park SJ, et al. Impact of intravascular ultrasound guidance on long-term mortality in stenting for unprotected left main coronary artery stenosis. *Circ Cardiovasc Interv*. 2009;2:167–177.

14. Stone GW, et al. Analysis of the relation between stent implantation pressure and expansion. Optimal stent implantation (OSTI) investigators. *Am J Cardiol*. 1999;83:1397–1400.

15. Morino Y, et al. An optimal diagnostic threshold for minimal stent area to predict target lesion revascularization following stent implantation in native coronary lesions. *Am J Cardiol*. 2001;88:301–303.

16. Ahn JM, et al. Meta-analysis of outcomes after intravascular ultrasound-guided versus angiography-guided drug-eluting stent implantation in 26,503 patients enrolled in three randomized trials and 14 observational studies. *Am J Cardiol*. 2014;113(8):1338–1347.

17. Park SW, et al. Randomized comparison of coronary stenting with optimal balloon angioplasty for treatment of lesions in small coronary arteries. *Eur Heart J*. 2000;21:1785–1789.

18. Hong SJ, et al. Effect of intravascular ultrasound-guided vs angiography-guided everolimus-eluting stent implantation: the IVUS-XPL randomized clinical trial. *JAMA*. 2015;314(20):2155–2163.

19. Kim JS, et al. Impact of intravascular ultrasound guidance on long-term clinical outcomes in patients treated with drug-eluting stent for bifurcation lesions: data from a Korean multicenter bifurcation registry. *Am Heart J*. 2011;161(1):180–187.

20. Mintz GS, Shah VM, Weissman NJ. Regional remodeling as the cause of late stent malapposition. *Circulation*. 2003;107:2660–2663.

21. Sheris SJ, Canos MR, Weissman NJ. Natural history of intravascular ultrasound-detected edge dissections from coronary stent placement. *Am Heart J*. 2000;139:59–63.

22. Doi H, et al. Impact of post-intervention minimal stent area on 9-month follow-up patency of paclitaxel-eluting stents. An integrated intravascular ultrasound analysis from the TAXUS IV, V, and VI and TAXUS ATLAS workhorse, long lesion, and direct stent trials. *JACC Cardiovasc Interv*. 2009;2(12):1269–1275.

23. Sonoda S, et al. Impact of final stent dimensions on long-term results following sirolimus-eluting stent implantation: serial intravascular ultrasound analysis from the SIRIUS trial. *J Am Coll Cardiol*. 2004;43:1959–1963.

24. Hong MK, et al. Intravascular ultrasound predictors of angiographic restenosis after sirolimus-eluting stent implantation. *Eur Heart J*. 2006;27(11):1305–1310.

25. Fujii K, et al. Contribution of stent underexpansion to recurrence after sirolimus-eluting stent implantation for in-stent restenosis. *Circulation*. 2004;109:1085–1088.

26. Castagna MT, et al. The contribution of "mechanical" problems to in-stent restenosis: an intravascular ultrasonographic analysis of 1090 consecutive in-stent restenosis lesions. *Am Heart J*. 2001;142:970–974.

27. Wu Z, et al. Impact of the acute results on the long-term outcome after the treatment of in-stent restenosis: a serial intravascular ultrasound study. *Catheter Cardiovasc Interv*. 2003;60:483–488.

28. Tuzcu EM, et al. Intravascular ultrasound evidence of angiographically silent progression in coronary atherosclerosis predicts long-term morbidity tomd mortality after cardiac transplantation. *J Am Coll Cardiol*. 2005;45(9):1538–1542.

29. Moscucci M. *Grossman & Baim's Cardiac Catheterization, Angiography, and Intervention.* 8th ed. Philadelphia, PA: Wolters Kluwer, 2015.

30. Groves EM, Seto AH, Kern MJ. Invasive testing for coronary artery disease: FFR, IVUS, OCT, NIRS. *Heart Fail Clin.* 2016;12(1):83–95.

31. Kubo T, et al. Assessment of culprit lesion morphology in acute myocardial infarction: ability of optical coherence tomography compared with intravascular ultrasound and coronary angioscopy. *J Am Coll Cardiol.* 2007;50:933–939.

32. Higuma T, et al. A Combined optical coherence tomography and intravascular ultrasound study on plaque rupture, plaque erosion, and calcified nodule in patients with ST-segment elevation myocardial infarction: incidence, morphologic characteristics, and outcomes after percutaneous coronary intervention. *JACC Cardiovasc Interv.* 2015;8(9):1166–1176.

33. Serruys PW, et al. A bioabsorbable everolimus-eluting coronary stent system (ABSORB): 2-year outcomes and results from multiple imaging methods. *Lancet.* 2009;373:897–910.

34. Ali ZA, et al. Optical coherence tomography compared with intravascular ultrasound and with angiography to guide coronary stent implantation (ILUMIEN III: OPTIMIZE PCI): a randomised controlled trial. *Lancet.* 2016;388(10060):2618–2628.

35. Weisz G, et al. COLOR: a prospective, multicenter registry evaluating the relationship between lipid-rich plaque and two-year outcomes after stent implantation in patients with coronary artery disease. Presented at: TCT 2016; November 1, 2016; Washington, DC.

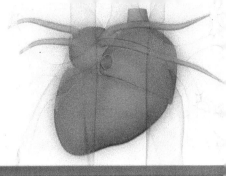

9

Vulnerable Plaque Imaging

Eric A. Osborn, MD, PhD, FSCAI, FACC and
Farouc A. Jaffer, MD, PhD, FSCAI, FACC

omplications related to atherosclerotic vascular disease remain a leading cause of cardiovascular morbidity and mortality in the United States and around the globe (1). While atherosclerosis is recognized as a systemic disease that warrants aggressive medical therapy and lifestyle changes (2,3), individual atheromas harbor a spectrum of risk phenotypes that range from stable, quiescent plaques to unstable, "vulnerable" plaques at high risk of future complication due to thrombosis overlying plaque rupture of thin-capped fibroatheroma (TCFA), plaque erosion, and calcific nodules (4–6). Because high-risk atheroma predates the majority of acute coronary syndrome (ACS) events, there has been substantial interest and resources applied across the cardiovascular field to image-vulnerable plaque phenotypes (Fig. 9.1). The potential to prevent devastating cardiovascular events arising from vulnerable plaques provides a strong rationale to pursue pre-complication plaque imaging in human coronary arteries. As conveyed by an expert consensus document on high-risk atherosclerotic plaque imaging (7), vulnerable plaque imaging holds significant potential to improve risk stratification of patients and plaques that may be at heightened risk for adverse cardiac outcomes, by delineating key characteristics of plaques prone to rupture and thrombosis.

Over the past decade, non-invasive and intravascular, coronary artery–targeted imaging technologies have furnished new insights into the pathophysiology of vulnerable plaque complications. To date, the largest focus of vulnerable plaque imaging revolves around assessing structural features, specifically the detection of thin fibrous caps, lipid pools, and neovascularization (8–10). Structural imaging alone appears insufficient to precisely identify vulnerable plaques, however, motivating the development of a number of new imaging approaches, such as near-infrared spectroscopy (NIRS), photoacoustics, and fluorescence lifetime imaging. More recently, molecular imaging, a field devoted to imaging specific molecules or cells through specialized imaging agents, is emerging clinically to provide new pathobiologic insights that may improve risk stratification and tailored atherosclerosis pharmacotherapy (11,12). This chapter showcases key concepts in vulnerable plaque imaging, focusing on clinically available and emerging intravascular imaging approaches.

The Vulnerable Plaque Foundation

The predominant cause of atherosclerosis-based heart attack, stroke, and sudden cardiac death is vulnerable plaque (13). As opposed to the severely obstructive coronary lesions identified by coronary angiography that are the common targets for percutaneous or surgical revascularization in symptomatic patients, vulnerable plaques are subclinical and typically non-obstructive, mild-to-moderately stenotic lesions in asymptomatic patients (14–16).

Although x-ray angiography, stress testing, and even invasive measures such as fractional flow reserve (FFR) are often normal in patients harboring vulnerable plaques, a subset of these plaques can rapidly progress and cause cardiovascular events within an accelerated time frame (17–22). Local biologic mediators and mechanical stressors can destabilize such vulnerable plaques, leading to frank ACS, or progressive luminal stenosis. At the time of clinical ACS presentation, disrupted or eroded vulnerable plaques identified by coronary angiography may present as complex atherothrombotic lesions exhibiting plaque ulcerations, lumen irregularities and haziness, contrast dye staining, and filling defects within the lumen indicating thrombus (23), findings that correlate with plaque disruption by intravascular imaging (24).

In contrast, angiography is highly insensitive for identifying subclinical (nondisrupted) coronary vulnerable plaques. This limitation of angiography is due to its inability to image the arterial wall (9,25,26). Positively remodeled plaques may contain a substantial plaque burden, yet maintain relatively normal lumen dimensions, and thus be invisible to angiography alone. The limitations of coronary angiography have motivated a new era of vulnerable plaque imaging approaches to interrogate high-risk plaque features resident within the vessel wall, rather than focus solely on the severity of lumen stenosis.

Histopathology of Vulnerable Plaques

Detailed autopsy studies of patients suffering sudden death have elucidated the histopathologic underpinnings of vulnerable atheroma (4,17,18), and thus the sphere of vulnerable plaque imaging targets (25,27). The prototypical vulnerable plaque is denoted as the TCFA, a structure comprised of a large, thrombogenic lipid-rich core with necrotic elements constrained by a thin fibrous cap measuring less than 65 μm in thickness (17,28). TCFAs are the etiologic precursor in approximately two-thirds of ACS cases. In combination with local biomechanical forces, fibrous cap inflammation (characterized by infiltrating macrophages that liberate destabilizing tissue proteases) can promote plaque rupture, followed by extrusion of the lipid contents, and consequent atherothrombosis and ACS events (Fig. 9.2). Geographically, TCFAs are most often located in the proximal one-third of the major epicardial coronary arteries (29,30), and thus they often subtend a large area of at-risk myocardium.

As outlined in Table 9.1, vulnerable plaque pathology includes inflammatory cellular elements, leaky neovessels, intraplaque hemorrhage, microcalcifications, and possibly penetrating cholesterol crystals. Intimal neovessels recruited to the plaque interior that lack normal vascular supporting structures result in extravasation of blood contents, which has been linked to plaque progression and the development of advanced atheroma (31). Calcified nodules near the luminal surface increase biomechanical stress of the plaque ultrastructure, and may promote plaque disruption by hemodynamic forces exerted on the vessel wall (17,18). Finally, inflammation is a driver of collagenolysis and subsequent plaque disruption (32,33), as evidenced by a greater number of ACS events in patients with underlying chronic inflammatory disorders (34). Many of these vulnerable features can occur in combination within an individual

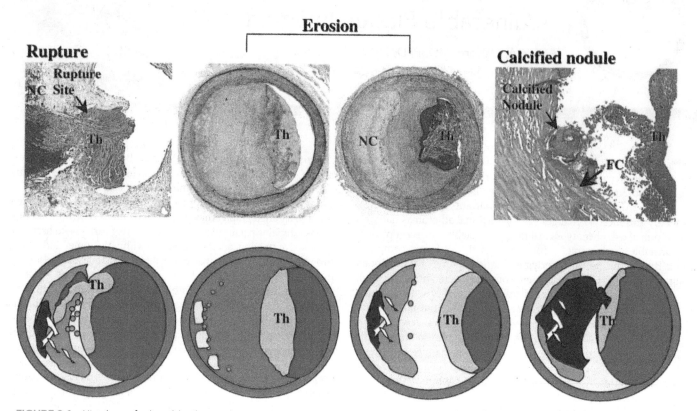

FIGURE 9.1 Histology of vulnerable plaque phenotypes associated with acute coronary ischemia. Prototypical ruptured plaques (*left panels*) exhibit a thin fibrous cap <65 μm overlying a large necrotic core (NC). In plaque erosion (*middle panels*), lesions tend to be fibrotic and proteoglycan-rich, and associate with luminal endothelial compromise and overlying thrombus (Th). Necrotic cores or lipid pools may occasionally be present in plaque erosion, but are located deep to the lumen surface. Calcified nodules (*right panels*), the least common phenotype, may penetrate the surface fibrous cap (FC), leading to plaque mechanical instability and thrombus formation. (Reproduced with permission from: Virmani R, et al. Lessons from sudden coronary death: a comprehensive morphological classification scheme for atherosclerotic lesions. *Arterioscler Thromb Vasc Biol.* 2000;20:1262–1275.)

plaque (4), and can evolve over time (35). The emerging field of intravascular molecular imaging aims to image specific molecules and cells within human coronary artery disease, to complement intravascular ultrasound (IVUS) and optical coherence tomography (OCT) structural imaging and enhance the precision of vulnerable plaque detection (36–42).

TABLE 9.1　Histopathologic Features Associated with Plaque Vulnerability

Large necrotic/lipid core

Fibrous cap covering the necrotic core
　Thin cap (<65 μm)
　High macrophage density
　Few smooth muscle cells

Expansive remodeling preserving the lumen

Large plaque burden

Neovascularization from vasa vasorum

Intraplaque hemorrhage

Adventitial/perivascular inflammation

Spotty calcification

Penetrating cholesterol crystals

Adapted with permission from: Bentzon JF, et al. Mechanisms of plaque formation and rupture. *Circ Res.* 2014;114:1852–1866.

Intravascular Structural Imaging of Vulnerable Plaque

As a result of its long-standing clinical familiarity, and its ability to image the entire coronary arterial wall through blood, IVUS, and its newer derivative virtual histology IVUS (VH-IVUS), have been the most widely applied structural plaque imaging technologies to assess vulnerable plaque features in humans. More recent intravascular optical imaging approaches such as high-resolution OCT and NIRS have provided additional structural and chemical assessments of high-risk plaques, including fibrous cap thickness, neovasculature, subclinical thrombus, and lipid-rich atheroma. A summary of existing clinical intravascular plaque imaging technologies is presented in **Table 9.2**.

Intravascular Ultrasound/Virtual Histology

Conventional grayscale IVUS (Boston Scientific, Natick, MA; Volcano Corporation, Rancho Cordova, CA) can delineate plaque structure, lumen dimensions, and stent complications in human coronary arteries. IVUS has several attributes underlying its long-term clinical utility, including through-blood imaging without flushing, sensitive calcium detection, and outstanding tissue depth penetration, allowing determination of positive and negative plaque remodeling (43,44). Additionally, IVUS can derive plaque burden (100% * [total vessel volume-lumen volume]/total vessel volume), a key plaque predictor of ACS (19–21). Prototypical vulnerable plaques identified by

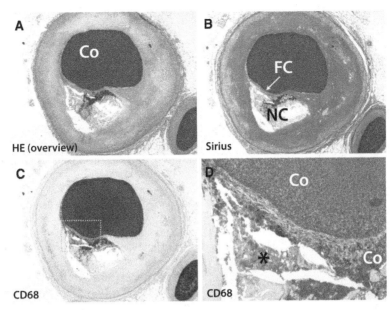

FIGURE 9.2   Inflamed thin-cap fibroatheroma (TCFA). **A** and **B**: A representative histologic TCFA exhibiting a very thin fibrous cap (FC) overlying a necrotic core (NC). **(C)** Low- and **(D)** high-magnification views of the FC after CD68 macrophage immunostaining demonstrates inflammatory macrophage cell infiltration (*red/pink* areas) localized to the thin FC region, associated with zones of dead macrophages(*). Post-mortem injection of iodinated contrast (Co) into the lumen reveals extravasation of Co material from the lumen into the superficial NC, indicating the presence of fibrous cap compromise. HE, hematoxylin-eosin. (Reproduced with permission from: Bentzon JF, et al. Mechanisms of plaque formation and rupture. *Circ Res.* 2014;114:1852–1866.)

IVUS are therefore often large, high (>65%) plaque burden lesions with evidence of positive (expansive) remodeling. In ACS patients, unstable culprit plaques may demonstrate rupture with an empty cavity remnant indicating an extruded lipid core, an intimal flap, and/or luminal thrombus (**Fig. 9.3**).

Nevertheless, the 100- to 200-μm moderate axial resolution of IVUS often limits the discrimination of finer plaque ultrastructural features, such as the fibrous cap thickness, especially in cases where the cap thickness is <65 μm, a classic criterion of histologic TCFA

(17). High-definition IVUS imaging systems utilizing higher frequency 60 MHz (as opposed to conventional 40 MHz) transducers are under development, and may eventually allow more precise structural assessment approaching the level of intravascular OCT imaging. Furthermore, while grayscale IVUS can delineate calcific versus non-calcific lesions, it is unable to accurately discern different soft plaque tissue subtypes, such as lipid-rich versus fibrotic lesions, nor distinguish specific molecular or cellular inflammatory components that drive TCFA complications.

TABLE 9.2 Comparison of Intracoronary Imaging Modalities

	GRAYSCALE IVUS	VH-IVUS	OCT	NIRS	ANGIOSCOPY	NIRF
Resolution, axial (μm)	100–200	150–250	10–20	–	10–50	–
Depth penetration	++	++	+	+	±	+
Fibrous cap	+	+	++	–	+	–
Necrotic/lipid core	±	+	+	++	++	–
TCFA	±	+	++	–	++	–
Expansive remodeling	++	++	±	–	–	–
Calcium	++	++	+	–	–	–
Thrombus	±	±	+	–	++	++
Inflammation	–	–	±	–	–	++

++, excellent; +, good; ±, possible; –, not currently possible.
IVUS, intravascular ultrasound; NIRF, near-infrared fluorescence; NIRS, near-infrared spectroscopy; OCT, optical coherence tomography; TCFA, thin-capped fibroatheroma; VH-IVUS, virtual histology IVUS.
Adapted with permission from: Suh WM, et al. Intravascular detection of the vulnerable plaque. *Circ Cardiovasc Imaging.* 2011;4:169–178.

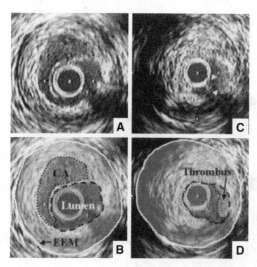

FIGURE 9.3 Plaque rupture and thrombosis identified by IVUS imaging. **A:** Grayscale IVUS reveals an empty plaque rupture cavity above and to the left of the imaging catheter. The zone of signal loss observed at the bottom right of the image is secondary to the wire shadow artifact. **B:** Manual segmentation of the axial IVUS image highlights the borders of the external elastic membrane (EEM) and ruptured plaque cavity (CA), compared to the lumen boundaries. **C** and **D:** At the location of minimum lumen, focal thrombus (*arrow*) was observed. IVUS, intravascular ultrasound. (Reproduced with permission from: Fujii K, et al. Intravascular ultrasound assessment of ulcerated ruptured plaques: a comparison of culprit and nonculprit lesions of patients with acute coronary syndromes and lesions in patients without acute coronary syndromes. *Circulation.* 2003;108:2473–2478.)

Because certain plaque compositional features appear integral in driving vulnerable plaque complications, imaging advancements beyond standalone grayscale IVUS have been developed to better discriminate plaque composition. VH-IVUS (Philips Volcano Corporation) is a newer IVUS technology that employs radiofrequency signal backscatter spectral analysis to further atheroma tissue characterization (45–47). Via post-processing algorithms of the reflected ultrasound signal, VH-IVUS categorizes plaque constituents into four categories: fibrous, fibrofatty, necrotic core (NC), and dense calcium (**Fig. 9.4**). Each plaque tissue type is then color-coded for display purposes, allowing rapid ease of image interpretation.

Validation studies of VH-IVUS compared to human coronary autopsy histology revealed good representation of plaque substructures. Nevertheless, VH-IVUS plaque characterization is limited in heavily calcified lesions where the high signal reflectivity does not permit ultrasound penetration, and VH-IVUS cannot discriminate between immature lipid pools and the NC elements that form the hallmark of advanced risk histologic fibroatheroma. In addition, technical trade-offs inherent to the 20-MHz VH-IVUS phased-array ultrasound transducer design result in a lower axial resolution of 150 to 250 μm, compared to 100 to 200 μm for 40-MHz IVUS. Despite VH-IVUS resolution constraints being below that for histologic TCFA detection, the concept of a VH-TCFA surrogate as a precursor vulnerable plaque phenotype has been postulated and defined as a lesion on three consecutive IVUS slices harboring >40% plaque burden associated with a confluent NC ≥10% that covers a >30° arc directly abutting the lumen surface (47).

CLINICAL OUTCOME STUDIES

IVUS structural and VH-TCFA features were evaluated as predictors of future cardiovascular events in the landmark PROSPECT trial

(Providing Regional Observations to Study Predictors of Events in the Coronary Tree), a natural history atherosclerosis clinical study of 697 ACS patients presenting to the cardiac catheterization laboratory (21). The PROSPECT investigators performed three-vessel VH-IVUS in patients undergoing percutaneous coronary intervention (PCI) of culprit lesions, as well as guideline-directed medical therapy for non-culprit lesions. Subjects were then followed for recurrence of cardiovascular events as a means to prospectively identify baseline VH-IVUS structural plaque characteristics linked to future events. A strength of the PROSPECT study is that most follow-up events were adjudicated by x-ray angiography, which was critical to assign plaque-specific outcomes. Over the 3.4-year median follow-up period, 20% of the enrolled subjects experienced 177 repeat adverse events, despite aggressive medical therapy. Approximately one-half of the events occurred due to nonculprit plaque progression, leading to unstable angina and urgent revascularization (without death or cardiac arrest). The other half of events mostly related to culprit stent complications of restenosis (85%) or thrombosis (15%). By multivariate analysis, a nonculprit VH-TCFA significantly predicted an increased likelihood of subsequent events (hazard ratio [HR] 3.35), although events occurred in only 26 of 595 (4.4%) of identified non-culprit VH-TCFA. In addition, IVUS morphologic measurements revealed that bulky (large plaque burden >70%; HR 5.03) and stenotic (minimum lumen area <4.0 mm²; HR 3.21) lesions also significantly predicted a recurrent, nonculprit plaque-specific event. In combination, lesions exhibiting all three predictors (plaque burden >70%, lumen area <4.0 mm², and VH-TCFA morphology) portended the greatest future risk (HR 11.05). Nevertheless, in practice, few lesions exhibited all three VH-IVUS imaging high-risk features (4.2% prevalence), and yet such patients still only had an 18% recurrent event rate over 3.4 years (48), demonstrating that new imaging approaches beyond IVUS-VH are needed for accurate detection of high-risk vulnerable plaques.

While subsequent prospective VH-IVUS studies (VIVA: VH-IVUS in Vulnerable Atherosclerosis; ATHEROREMO: European Collaborative Project on Inflammation and Vascular Wall Remodeling in Atherosclerosis) confirmed the prognostic capacity of VH-TCFA for future cardiovascular events (19,20), the overall low positive predictive value of VH-IVUS has limited its clinical translation for vulnerable plaque detection (48). Some have therefore suggested that invasive imaging of vulnerable plaques should therefore be abandoned (49,50). Nevertheless, newer methods incorporating multimodal microstructural, molecular, and flow-based methods are positioned to substantially improve the positive predictive value of intravascular imaging readouts (51,52), and therefore the final chapter on invasive imaging remains to be written.

Currently, IVUS still serves a role in clinical research of high-risk plaques. In particular, new investigations are examining the natural history of non-culprit, non-obstructive, lipid-rich atheroma by combination NIRS-IVUS (PROSPECT II trial), and the impact of performing preventative PCI on these lesions with bioabsorbable vascular scaffolds (PROSPECT Absorb). While there are no outcomes studies evaluating the potential benefit of preventative PCI of non-culprit vulnerable lesions, a small pilot study using a self-expanding bare-metal stent to treat VH-TCFA demonstrated good procedural success and short-term clinical safety, with a 4-fold increase in OCT fibrous cap thickness 6 months after stent implantation (53). The PROSPECT Absorb trial will inform on this concept further using bioabsorbable scaffolds that may diminish the inherent long-term risks of permanent metal stents, including neoatherosclerosis, as well as late-stent restenosis and thrombosis.

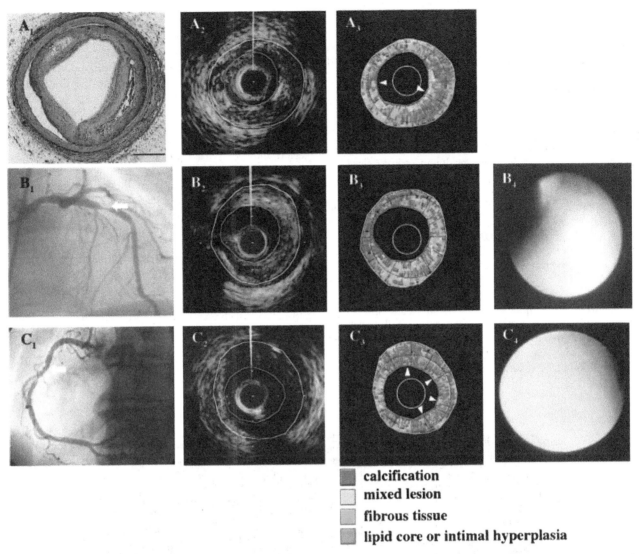

calcification
mixed lesion
fibrous tissue
lipid core or intimal hyperplasia

FIGURE 9.4   Multi-modality intracoronary vulnerable plaque imaging with IVUS, VH-IVUS, and angioscopy. (**A₁–A₃**) Comparison of grayscale IVUS and VH-IVUS with a cadaveric coronary histology section (Masson's trichrome stain, scale bar = 1 mm), demonstrating correspondence of lipid pools between histology (*yellow* * in **A₁**) and VH-IVUS (*blue* pseudocolor, *). VH-IVUS imaging confirms the presence of a thick fibrous cap (*arrowheads* in **A₃**) composed of fibrous (*green* pseudocolor) and mixed (*yellow* pseudocolor) plaque. Of note, the plaque composition visualized by VH-IVUS is unable to be appreciated by conventional grayscale IVUS imaging. (**B₁**) Left coronary angiography with 60% mid LAD stenosis (*arrow*). Co-registered axial grayscale IVUS (**B₂**), VH-IVUS (**B₃**), and angioscopy (**B₄**) images of the plaque shown in **A₁** revealing a predominately fibrotic plaque by VH-IVUS (*green* pseudocolor, F) and angioscopy (*white* appearance). (**C₁–C₃**) Similar intravascular imaging evaluation of an angiographic 40% RCA lesion (*arrow* in **C₁**) reveals a large lipid core (*blue* pseudocolor, * in **C₃**) by VH-IVUS corroborated by an angioscopic appearance of a lipid-rich plaque with thin overlying fibrous cap (*yellow* appearance in **C₄**). IVUS, intravascular ultrasound; LAD, left anterior descending; VH-IVUS, virtual histology IVUS. (Reproduced with permission from: Kawasaki M. In vivo quantitative tissue characterization of human coronary arterial plaques by use of integrated backscatter intravascular ultrasound and comparison with angioscopic findings. *Circulation*. 2002;105:2487–2492.)

Optical Coherence Tomography

OCT (St. Jude Medical, Saint Paul, MN) is a high-resolution optical intravascular imaging technique that has revolutionized visualization of intracoronary plaque and stent structures (8,25,26,54). Utilizing reflected near-infrared (NIR) light at ~1,300 nm emanating from tissues of different optical density, OCT achieves 10- to 20-μm axial resolution, an approximate 10-fold increase compared to conventional grayscale IVUS imaging systems operating at 40 MHz. In addition, OCT image datasets are rapidly collected in a few seconds during catheter pullback speeds of 20 to 40 mm/s, compared to the standard 0.5 to 1.0 mm/s pullback speed for IVUS catheters. As the NIR light required in OCT does not penetrate through blood, a drawback of OCT is the need to displace luminal blood from the imaging field in order to visualize the arterial wall. Blood displacement is typically achieved by manual or automated injection of iodinated contrast (or possibly saline or dextrose) through a properly engaged coronary artery guiding catheter.

Overall, high-resolution OCT imaging provides superb intracoronary images of the luminal plaque surface in vivo (10,54), showing very good overall agreement (κ statistic 0.84) with histologic fibrous, fibrocalcific, and lipid-rich coronary plaques at autopsy (55). In particular, OCT can visualize the thin fibrous caps of TCFA and provide quantitative measurements on par with that observed at histology (**Fig. 9.5**). OCT is the current gold standard for detecting coronary plaque rupture, erosion, and spotty calcification that are otherwise unrecognized on x-ray angiography or IVUS imaging (56–58). In addition, OCT can detect red (red blood cell-rich) and white (platelet-rich) thrombus, neovessels, and potentially identify macrophage accumulations resident in plaques (54,59). Mechanisms of ACS have been further elucidated by clinical intravascular OCT registries, revealing that plaque erosion, rather than rupture, may represent a significantly more frequent ACS etiology in non-ST elevation myocardial infarction (NSTEMI) (56), whereas the traditional plaque rupture paradigm remains dominant in ST elevation myocardial infarction (STEMI) (60).

Due to OCT light's inability to penetrate the arterial wall more than 1 to 2 mm, OCT is limited in assessing important vulnerable plaque attributes such as plaque burden and positive (expansive) plaque remodeling, which are significant VH-IVUS predictors of subsequent cardiovascular events (19–21). Combination IVUS-OCT catheters may overcome these limitations and are an exciting development in the field of intravascular imaging (61). Building upon registry data suggesting ACS patients have more OCT vulnerable plaque features at non-culprit coronary atheroma than subjects with stable angina (62), natural history studies assessing OCT-vulnerable plaque features to predict subsequent events will be needed in order to determine the utility of intracoronary OCT plaque imaging as a predictor of future plaque complications.

Near-Infrared Spectroscopy

Intravascular NIRS imaging (Infraredx, Burlington, MA) is a sensitive method to detect lipid-core coronary plaques (25,26,63). From a technical perspective, NIRS imaging employs an optical fiber integrated with a conventional rotational IVUS catheter that detects the specific chemical signature associated with plaque lipid NIR light absorption by cholesterol moieties, as well as IVUS plaque structure. The spectroscopic NIRS signal is then decoded by the imaging software into a relative probability of LPR being present at a particular coronary region, and displayed as a pseudocolor lookup table ranging from red (low probability of lipid) to yellow (high-probability of lipid), termed a "chemogram" (**Fig. 9.6**). Beyond the local angular lipid content display on axial images, a block chemogram is also presented on the longview pullback image that sums the probability of a coronary lipid plaque being present for each 2-mm distance throughout the length of the catheter pullback. Because NIRS contains no inherent information on plaque architecture, NIRS has been successfully integrated with grayscale IVUS to provide simultaneous structural information that complements NIRS lipid data (64,65).

Early studies validated NIRS interrogation of lipid-containing plaques against coronary autopsy specimens (66), with a subsequent in vivo trial in ACS patients supporting NIRS lipid plaque detection benchmarked to cadaveric coronary plaque NIRS spectra by multivariate analysis (67). Since the initial validation, NIRS has been

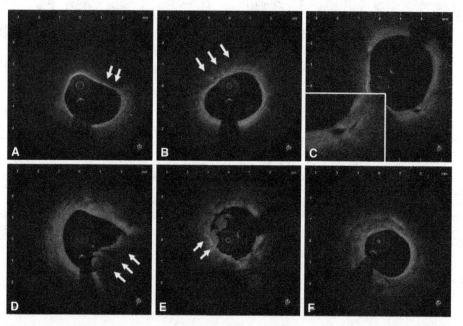

FIGURE 9.5 *Vulnerable plaque features detected by intravascular OCT imaging.* **A:** Example of an OCT-identified thin-cap fibroatheroma (TCFA), where the lipid-rich core is delineated by the low-signal region with diffuse borders. The fibrous cap thickness was measured to be 60 μm (*arrows*). **B:** Regions of plaque macrophage accumulations can be observed as bright reflectors (*arrows*). **C:** Neovessels may be seen as dark voids embedded in the plaque architecture (highlighted by inset). The presence of **(D)** *red* (red-blood-cell-rich, *arrows*) and **(E)** *white* (platelet-rich, *arrows*) thrombus exhibit characteristic high- and low-attenuation OCT appearances, respectively. **F:** Calcified plaque regions demonstrate low OCT signal but with sharp borders at the interface of surrounding fibrous tissue, in contrast to that observed for lipid-rich plaque regions where the borders are more diffuse. OCT, optical coherence tomography. (Reproduced with permission from: Kato K, et al. Nonculprit plaques in patients with acute coronary syndromes have more vulnerable features compared with those with non-acute coronary syndromes: a 3-vessel optical coherence tomography study. *Circ Cardiovasc Imaging.* 2012;5:433–440.)

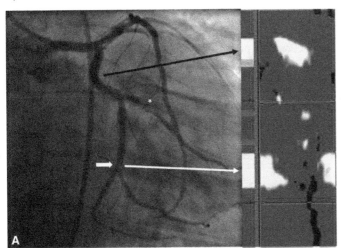

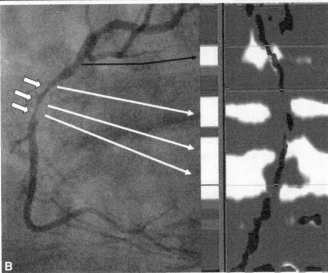

FIGURE 9.6 Intracoronary NIRS imaging of lipid-core plaque. **A:** NIRS imaging of a culprit (*short white arrow*) LCx lesion in a patient with unstable angina reveals high probability of lipid-core plaque (*yellow color*) on the NIRS chemogram. A remote, mildly stenotic proximal LCx stenosis (*black arrow*) by angiography also exhibits a high NIRS lipid signal. **B:** A second unstable angina patient with a culprit RCA stenosis (*short white arrows*) associated with a high degree of lipid by NIRS throughout most of the plaque, separated by a short intervening lipid-free segment (*red color*). A NIRS-positive lipid-core non-culprit mild stenosis (*black arrow*) is also detected. NIRS, near-infrared spectroscopy; RCA, right coronary artery. (Reproduced with permission from: Madder RD, et al. Composition of target lesions by near-infrared spectroscopy in patients with acute coronary syndrome versus stable angina. *Circ Cardiovasc Interv.* 2012;5:55–61.)

investigated in several clinical trials aiming to uncover relationships between potentially vulnerable lipid-core plaques residing within the coronary vasculature and cardiovascular outcomes. Lipid-core coronary plaques detected by NIRS imaging before PCI have been associated with an increased risk of peri-procedural myocardial infarction (68), indicating that NIRS-positive lipid atheroma may indicate higher-risk atheroma populations. Compared to patients with stable angina undergoing PCI, ACS patients were more likely to have LPRs at the culprit PCI location (84.4% vs. 52.8%), as well as a significantly greater frequency of remote, non-target NIRS lipid-positive plaques (69), implying that NIRS reports on the systemic vulnerability of coronary disease in general. NIRS has also demonstrated that intensive lipid-lowering pharmacotherapy with

rosuvastatin reduces intracoronary NIRS LPR content in patients after only 7 weeks (70), supporting clinical trial data that statins can have a rapid stabilizing effect on vulnerable atheroma and reduce coronary events. In a prospective analysis of non-culprit plaques from a mix of approximately 200 stable angina and ACS patients imaged with standalone NIRS in the ATHEROREMO trial, coronary atheroma with greater than the median positive NIRS signal (reported as the lipid core burden index) were associated with a significantly increased 1 year risk of adverse cardiovascular events (HR 4.04), driven predominately by urgent revascularization (71). The ongoing NIRS-IVUS LPR and PROSPECT II trials are evaluating the natural history of lipid-rich atheroma and subsequent cardiac events, and will shed important light on the ability of intracoronary NIRS imaging to detect vulnerable plaques.

Angioscopy

Intracoronary angioscopy utilizes a catheter equipped with color fiber optic video imaging capability to directly interrogate the coronary artery wall. Angioscopy is mainly performed in Japan, and similar to OCT, it requires displacement of blood from the imaging field (typically via saline injection). Angioscopy has provided important insights into coronary atherosclerosis pathophysiology (9,10,26), where it can detect the presence of luminal thrombus (red-blood-cell-enriched red thrombus or platelet-predominant white thrombus) and plaque ulcerations, or frank disruptions, as well as color variations in the surface of intact atheroma that indicate plaque lipid composition and fibrous cap thickness. White-colored plaques by angioscopy reflect plaques with high fibrous tissue content, whereas those with progressively more yellow hues signify LPRs with thinner overlying fibrous caps, a finding validated by intracoronary OCT, where in one study plaques with the highest yellow coloration had a measured fibrous cap thickness of 40 ± 14 μm (72). Angioscopic glistening yellow plaques are therefore considered equivalent to histologic TCFA (Fig. 9.4), and accordingly have been associated with an increased likelihood of ACS presentation at 1 year in a small prospective clinical study of patients with baseline stable angina (22). In comparison, subjects with white or non-glistening yellow angioscopic lesions had a lower frequency of ACS in this study. In patients suffering recent ACS, clinical angioscopy not only revealed frequent thrombus formation in the culprit vessel, but also evidence of diffuse yellow plaques (3–4 per artery, on average) equally distributed between the infarct-related and non-infarct-related arteries, suggesting that angioscopy can also detect vulnerable plaques and patient populations (73). The addition of color fluorescence plaque imaging with selective visible light wavelength filters may increase the detection capability of angioscopy for vulnerable plaque features, including collagen content and oxidized low-density lipoprotein (LDL) (74). Angioscopy thus holds promise for prospective vulnerable plaque identification, and while it has not achieved the widespread adoption that would allow validation in larger patient populations, it has advanced the field of intravascular vulnerable plaque imaging.

Intravascular Near-Infrared Fluorescence Molecular Imaging

Currently available clinical intravascular imaging modalities—IVUS, OCT, and NIRS—are able to interrogate vulnerable plaque structural features, but they lack the ability to report on important plaque biologic factors inherent in plaque instability. For example, plaque inflammation, characterized by inflammatory cytokines and proteases produced by infiltrating tissue macrophages, is a credible mechanism underlying plaque complications. The "inflammatory hypothesis of atherosclerosis" is being tested in several ongoing large clinical trials of FDA-approved and novel anti-inflammatory pharmacotherapies such as methotrexate or canakinumab (32,33). Molecular imaging technology is now transforming to enable imaging of plaque inflammation and other key molecular and cellular biologic processes using highly selective imaging agents that are injected intravenously. After circulating, these molecular imaging agents bind or interact with their target, and then stably localize, allowing detection by non-invasive approaches (e.g., MRI, CT, ultrasound) and invasive (e.g., near-infrared fluorescence, NIRF) imaging systems (11).

Nevertheless, noninvasive molecular imaging approaches (e.g., PET, MRI) have insufficient resolution or sensitivity for coronary artery molecular imaging. To address this unmet need, intravascular NIRF molecular imaging has been developed as a translatable coronary imaging approach for quantitative, high-resolution plaque and stent biologic imaging (8,75). NIRF imaging has several beneficial attributes for intracoronary applications, including through-blood imaging without the need for flushing, no ionizing radiation exposure, good tissue penetration of NIR light wavelengths, low background tissue autofluorescence, and a high-sensitivity for NIR fluorophore-labeled probes that leads to excellent signal-to-noise characteristics. In addition, because intracoronary optical imaging (i.e., OCT, NIRS) is routinely employed in many catheterization laboratories, intravascular NIRF molecular imaging is attractive clinically.

Multi-modality imaging catheters combining co-registered NIRF and OCT (42), and NIRF and IVUS (36), have been developed. NIRF approaches to detect plaque inflammatory protease activity and macrophages have been explored in preclinical atheroma models (**Fig. 9.7**) (37–39,76), and NIRF imaging has been successful in imaging intravascular fibrin in thrombi and that associated with coronary stents (77,78). More recently, first-in-human studies in carotid atheroma with targeted NIRF imaging agents (41), and an intracoronary demonstration of the safety of NIR autofluorescence (NIRAF) detection in patients undergoing PCI has been performed (40), enhancing the prospects of larger clinical trials testing intracoronary NIRF plaque imaging.

Guidelines for Intravascular Plaque Imaging

Given the lack of currently available evidence supporting the clinical utility of vulnerable plaque imaging, routine use of intravascular imaging to identify vulnerable plaque features should not be performed. Society consensus guidelines have been developed to address the use of IVUS imaging in patients (79). While guidelines have not yet commented on the appropriate role of OCT imaging in decision-making, recently an expert consensus statement was provided to guide clinical intravascular OCT imaging use (80). No present guidelines exist regarding use of NIRS or the other intravascular imaging modalities. **Table 9.3** provides a summary of available society guidelines and expert consensus statement recommendations. Because intracoronary imaging is a rapidly evolving field, society guidelines are very likely to include new clinical trial data and new intravascular imaging technologies in future recommendations.

Conclusions

Vulnerable plaque imaging continues to generate significant interest from a clinical and research perspective in the cardiovascular and interventional community. The hypothesis driving vulnerable plaque imaging is predicated on the concept that early identification of specific structural and/or biologic high-risk plaque features will allow prediction and prevention of future major adverse cardiovascular events. Through continued research and development of vulnerable plaque imaging approaches, including the key benefits of merging imaging technologies with different strengths into multi-modality intravascular catheter imaging systems (51), prospective vulnerable plaque detection offers hope for the development of new therapeutic strategies to treat plaque complications before they occur.

Key Points

- Autopsy studies of individuals suffering cardiac death demonstrate vulnerable plaque features, including thin fibrous caps, lipid-rich NCs, neovessels, intraplaque hemorrhage, inflammation, and calcific nodules.

- Correlation between intracoronary imaging findings and gold-standard histopathology has in general been good, but the sensitivity and specificity of individual vulnerable plaque feature detection is variable.

- Each intracoronary vulnerable plaque imaging modality has strengths and weaknesses, and no single imaging modality is currently able to detect all vulnerable plaque features.

- Intracoronary imaging with IVUS, VH-IVUS, OCT, and NIRS are clinically available intravascular imaging technologies that can characterize important structural features of vulnerable plaques.

- The PROSPECT trial, which is the largest prospective natural history atherosclerosis intracoronary imaging study performed to-date, revealed that non-culprit VH-IVUS TCFA, as well as plaque burden $\geq 70\%$ and minimum lumen area $\leq 4\ mm^2$, were independent predictors of subsequent adverse cardiovascular events. Nevertheless, the low positive predictive value of these variables has precluded clinical application of routine VH-IVUS vulnerable plaque imaging.

- Emerging intracoronary NIRF biologic imaging offers a new approach to investigate in vivo plaque biology such as inflammation.

- Current society guideline recommendations do not recommend routine intravascular imaging to detect vulnerable plaque.

- At present, there have been no studies demonstrating that preventative PCI of vulnerable plaque improves cardiovascular outcomes.

Acknowledgments

This work was supported by National Institutes of Health R01 HL122388 (FAJ) and K08 HL130465 (EAO), and the MGH Hassenfeld Research Scholar Fund (FAJ).

Disclosures

Dr. Jaffer received research funding from Siemens and Canon, and has consulting agreements with Boston Scientific and Abbott Vascular. Massachusetts General Hospital has a patent licensing arrangement with Canon Corporation. Dr. Jaffer has the right to receive royalties through this licensing arrangement. Dr. Osborn has consulting agreements with DynaMed and St. Jude Medical.

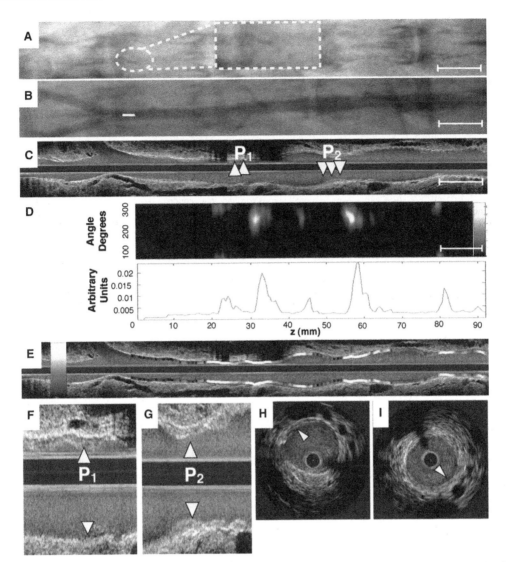

FIGURE 9.7 Intravascular NIRF molecular imaging of atherosclerosis inflammation. Experimental atherosclerosis induced within the rabbit aorta imaged with **(A)** x-ray fluoroscopy, **(B)** contrast angiography, and **(C)** grayscale IVUS reveals scattered mild plaque formation (examples *yellow arrowheads* P_1 and P_2 on the longview IVUS image in **C**). **(D)** Intravascular NIRF imaging performed 24 hours following IV administration of Prosense VM110, a cathepsin protease targeted NIRF molecular imaging agent, identifies locations of aortic plaque protease inflammatory activity (*yellow/white* = high inflammation; *black* = low inflammation). A quantitative one-dimensional plot of the average NIRF signal per axial slice is shown directly below. The NIRF inflammation map in **(D)** is anatomically co-registered with images **(A–C)**, where the starting catheter pullback position in the aorta immediately proximal to the iliac bifurcation is highlighted by the *dashed yellow line* and inset in **(A)** and *yellow solid line* in **(B)**. **(E)** A fusion image of co-registered NIRF protease inflammation and IVUS plaque morphology. **(F** and **G)** High magnification and **(H** and **I)** axial IVUS images at plaque regions P_1 and P_2 from panel **(B)**. IVUS, intravascular ultrasound; NIRF, near-infrared fluorescence. (Reproduced with permission from: Jaffer FA, et al. Two-dimensional intravascular near-infrared fluorescence molecular imaging of inflammation in atherosclerosis and stent-induced vascular injury. *J Am Coll Cardiol.* 2011;57:2516–2526.)

TABLE 9.3 Guideline Recommendations on Intracoronary Imaging

ACC/AHA/SCAI IVUS Consensus Guidelines[a]

Class IIa

- IVUS is reasonable for the assessment of angiographically indeterminate left main coronary artery disease (CAD). (Level of evidence: B)
- IVUS and coronary angiography are reasonable 4–6 weeks and 1 year after cardiac transplantation to exclude donor CAD, detect rapidly progressive cardiac allograft vasculopathy, and provide prognostic information. (Level of evidence: B)

IVUS is reasonable to determine the mechanism of stent restenosis. (Level of evidence: C)

Class IIb

- IVUS may be reasonable for the assessment of non–left main coronary arteries with angiographically intermediate coronary stenoses (50%–70% diameter stenosis). (Level of evidence: B)
- IVUS may be considered for guidance of coronary stent implantation, particularly in cases of left main coronary artery stenting. (Level of evidence: B)

(continued)

TABLE 9.3 **Guideline Recommendations on Intracoronary Imaging** (*continued*)

IVUS may be reasonable to determine the mechanism of stent thrombosis. (Level of evidence: C)

Class III: NO BENEFIT
- IVUS for routine lesion assessment is not recommended when revascularization with PCI or CABG is not being contemplated. (Level of evidence: C)

SCAI OCT Expert Consensus Statement[b]
- *Probably Beneficial:* Determination of optimal stent deployment (sizing, apposition, and lack of edge dissection), with improved resolution compared with IVUS.
- *Possibly Beneficial:* OCT can be useful for the assessment of plaque morphology.
- *No Proven Value / Should Be Discouraged:* OCT should not be performed to determine stenosis functional significance.

[a]Reference, Levine GN, et al. 2011 ACCF/AHA/SCAI guideline for percutaneous coronary intervention: a report of the American College of Cardiology Foundation/ American Heart Association Task Force on Practice Guidelines and the Society for Cardiovascular Angiography and Interventions. *Circulation.* 2011;124:e574–e651.
[b]Reference, Lotfi A, et al. Expert consensus statement on the use of fractional flow reserve, intravascular ultrasound, and optical coherence tomography: a consensus statement of the Society of Cardiovascular Angiography and Interventions. *Catheter Cardiovasc Interv.* 2014;83:509–518.
ACC/AHA, American College of Cardiology / American Heart Association; CABG, coronary artery bypass grafting; IVUS, intravascular ultrasound; OCT, optical coherence tomography; PCI, percutaneous coronary intervention; SCAI, Society for Cardiovascular Angiography and Interventions.

References

1. Mozaffarian D, et al. Heart disease and stroke statistics-2015 update: a report from the american heart association. *Circulation.* 2015;131:e29–e322.
2. Naghavi M, et al. From vulnerable plaque to vulnerable patient: a call for new definitions and risk assessment strategies: Part I. *Circulation.* 2003;108:1664–1672.
3. Naghavi M, et al. From vulnerable plaque to vulnerable patient: a call for new definitions and risk assessment strategies: Part II. *Circulation.* 2003;108:1772–1778.
4. Falk E, et al. Update on acute coronary syndromes: the pathologists' view. *Eur Heart J.* 2013;34:719–728.
5. Libby P. Mechanisms of acute coronary syndromes and their implications for therapy. *N Engl J Med.* 2013;368:2004–2013.
6. Bentzon JF, et al. Mechanisms of plaque formation and rupture. *Circ Res.* 2014;114:1852–1866.
7. Fleg JL, et al. Detection of high-risk atherosclerotic plaque: report of the NHLBI Working Group on current status and future directions. *JACC Cardiovasc Imaging.* 2012;5:941–955.
8. Osborn EA, Jaffer FA. Imaging atherosclerosis and risk of plaque rupture. *Curr Atheroscler Rep.* 2013;15:359–368.
9. Suh WM, et al. Intravascular detection of the vulnerable plaque. *Circ Cardiovasc Imaging.* 2011;4:169–178.
10. Vancraeynest D, et al. Imaging the vulnerable plaque. *J Am Coll Cardiol.* 2011;57:1961–1979.
11. Osborn EA, Jaffer FA. The advancing clinical impact of molecular imaging in CVD. *JACC Cardiovasc Imaging.* 2013;6:1327–1341.
12. Jaffer FA, Weissleder R. Molecular imaging in the clinical arena. *JAMA.* 2005;293:855–862.
13. Arbab-Zadeh A, et al. Acute coronary events. *Circulation.* 2012;125:1147–1156.
14. Muller JE, Tofler GH, Stone PH. Circadian variation and triggers of onset of acute cardiovascular disease. *Circulation.* 1989;79:733–743.
15. Ambrose JA, et al. Angiographic progression of coronary artery disease and the development of myocardial infarction. *J Am Coll Cardiol.* 1988;12:56–62.
16. Maddox TM, et al. Nonobstructive coronary artery disease and risk of myocardial infarction. *JAMA.* 2014;312:1754–1763.
17. Virmani R, et al. Pathology of the vulnerable plaque. *J Am Coll Cardiol.* 2006;47:C13–C18.
18. Virmani R, et al. Lessons from sudden coronary death: a comprehensive morphological classification scheme for atherosclerotic lesions. *Arterioscler Thromb Vasc Biol.* 2000;20:1262–1275.
19. Calvert PA, et al. Association between IVUS findings and adverse outcomes in patients with coronary artery disease: the VIVA (VH-IVUS in Vulnerable Atherosclerosis) Study. *JACC Cardiovasc Imaging.* 2011;4:894–901.
20. Cheng JM, et al. In vivo detection of high-risk coronary plaques by radio-frequency intravascular ultrasound and cardiovascular outcome: results of the ATHEROREMO-IVUS study. *Eur Heart J.* 2014;35:639–647.
21. Stone GW, et al. A prospective natural-history study of coronary atherosclerosis. *N Engl J Med.* 2011;364:226–235.
22. Uchida Y, et al. Prediction of acute coronary syndromes by percutaneous coronary angioscopy in patients with stable angina. *Am Heart J.* 1995;130:195–203.
23. Goldstein JA, et al. Multiple complex coronary plaques in patients with acute myocardial infarction. *N Engl J Med.* 2000;343:915–922.
24. Fujii K, et al. Intravascular ultrasound assessment of ulcerated ruptured plaques: a comparison of culprit and nonculprit lesions of patients with acute coronary syndromes and lesions in patients without acute coronary syndromes. *Circulation.* 2003;108:2473–2478.
25. Muller JE, Weissman NJ, Tuzcu EM. The year in intracoronary imaging. *JACC Cardiovasc Imaging.* 2010;3:881–891.
26. Suter MJ, et al. Intravascular optical imaging technology for investigating the coronary artery. *JACC Cardiovasc Imaging.* 2011;4:1022–1039.
27. Narula J, et al. Histopathologic characteristics of atherosclerotic coronary disease and implications of the findings for the invasive and noninvasive detection of vulnerable plaques. *J Am Coll Cardiol.* 2013;61:1041–1051.
28. Kolodgie FD, et al. The thin-cap fibroatheroma: a type of vulnerable plaque: the major precursor lesion to acute coronary syndromes. *Curr Opin Cardiol.* 2001;16:285–292.
29. Cheruvu PK, et al. Frequency and distribution of thin-cap fibroatheroma and ruptured plaques in human coronary arteries: a pathologic study. *J Am Coll Cardiol.* 2007;50:940–949.
30. Wang JC, et al. Coronary artery spatial distribution of acute myocardial infarction occlusions. *Circulation.* 2004;110:278–284.
31. Kolodgie FD, et al. Intraplaque hemorrhage and progression of coronary atheroma. *N Engl J Med.* 2003;349:2316–2325.
32. Libby P. Inflammation in atherosclerosis. *Arterioscler Thromb Vasc Biol.* 2012;32:2045–2051.
33. Libby P, et al. Inflammation and its resolution as determinants of acute coronary syndromes. *Circ Res.* 2014;114:1867–1879.
34. Mason JC, Libby P. Cardiovascular disease in patients with chronic inflammation: mechanisms underlying premature cardiovascular events in rheumatologic conditions. *Eur Heart J.* 2015;36:482–9c.
35. Kubo T, et al. The dynamic nature of coronary artery lesion morphology assessed by serial virtual histology intravascular ultrasound tissue characterization. *J Am Coll Cardiol.* 2010;55:1590–1597.
36. Bozhko D, et al. Quantitative intravascular biological fluorescence-ultrasound imaging of coronary and peripheral arteries in vivo. *Eur Heart J Cardiovasc Imaging.* 2016. doi:10.1093/ehjci/jew222.
37. Jaffer F, et al. Optical visualization of cathepsin K activity in atherosclerosis with a novel, protease-activatable fluorescence sensor. *Circulation.* 2007;115:2292–2298.
38. Jaffer FA, et al. Two-dimensional intravascular near-infrared fluorescence molecular imaging of inflammation in atherosclerosis and stent-induced vascular injury. *J Am Coll Cardiol.* 2011;57:2516–2526.
39. Jaffer FA, et al. Real-time catheter molecular sensing of inflammation in proteolytically active atherosclerosis. *Circulation.* 2008;118:1802–1809.

40. Ughi GJ, et al. Clinical characterization of coronary atherosclerosis with dual-modality OCT and near-infrared autofluorescence imaging. *JACC Cardiovasc Imaging.* 2016;9:1304–1314.

41. Verjans JW, et al. Targeted near-infrared fluorescence imaging of atherosclerosis: clinical and intracoronary evaluation of indocyanine green. *JACC Cardiovasc Imaging.* 2016;9:1087–1095.

42. Yoo H, et al. Intra-arterial catheter for simultaneous microstructural and molecular imaging in vivo. *Nat Med.* 2011;17:1680–1684.

43. Mintz GS, et al. American College of Cardiology Clinical Expert Consensus Document on Standards for Acquisition, Measurement and Reporting of Intravascular Ultrasound Studies (IVUS). A report of the American College of Cardiology Task Force on Clinical Expert Consensus Documents. *J Am Coll Cardiol.* 2001;37:1478–1492.

44. Mintz GS, et al. Clinical expert consensus document on standards for acquisition, measurement and reporting of intravascular ultrasound regression/progression studies. *EuroIntervention.* 2011;6:1123–1130.

45. Garcia-Garcia HM, et al. Tissue characterisation using intravascular radiofrequency data analysis: recommendations for acquisition, analysis, interpretation and reporting. *EuroIntervention.* 2009;5:177–189.

46. Kawasaki M, et al. Noninvasive quantitative tissue characterization and two-dimensional color-coded map of human atherosclerotic lesions using ultrasound integrated backscatter: comparison between histology and integrated backscatter images. *J Am Coll Cardiol.* 2001;38:486–492.

47. Maehara A, et al. Definitions and methodology for the grayscale and radiofrequency intravascular ultrasound and coronary angiographic analyses. *JACC Cardiovasc Imaging.* 2012;5:S1–S9.

48. Kaul S, Diamond GA. Improved prospects for IVUS in identifying vulnerable plaques? *JACC Cardiovasc Imaging.* 2012;5:S106–S110.

49. Ahmadi A, et al. Prognostic determinants of coronary atherosclerosis in stable ischemic heart disease: anatomy, physiology, or morphology? *Circ Res.* 2016;119:317–329.

50. Arbab-Zadeh A, Fuster V. The myth of the "vulnerable plaque": transitioning from a focus on individual lesions to atherosclerotic disease burden for coronary artery disease risk assessment. *J Am Coll Cardiol.* 2015;65:846–855.

51. Bourantas CV, et al. Hybrid intravascular imaging: recent advances, technical considerations, and current applications in the study of plaque pathophysiology. *Eur Heart J.* 2017;38(6):400–412.

52. Koskinas KC, et al. Intracoronary imaging of coronary atherosclerosis: validation for diagnosis, prognosis and treatment. *Eur Heart J.* 2016;37:524–535a–c.

53. Wykrzykowska JJ, et al. Plaque sealing and passivation with a mechanical self-expanding low outward force nitinol vShield device for the treatment of IVUS and OCT-derived thin cap fibroatheromas (TCFAs) in native coronary arteries: report of the pilot study vShield Evaluated at Cardiac hospital in Rotterdam for Investigation and Treatment of TCFA (SECRITT). *EuroIntervention.* 2012;8:945–954.

54. Tearney GJ, et al. Consensus standards for acquisition, measurement, and reporting of intravascular optical coherence tomography studies: a report from the international working group for intravascular optical coherence tomography standardization and validation. *J Am Coll Cardiol.* 2012;59:1058–1072.

55. Yabushita H, et al. Characterization of human atherosclerosis by optical coherence tomography. *Circulation.* 2002;106:1640–1645.

56. Jia H, et al. In vivo diagnosis of plaque erosion and calcified nodule in patients with acute coronary syndrome by intravascular optical coherence tomography. *J Am Coll Cardiol.* 2013;62:1748–1758.

57. Prati F, et al. OCT-based diagnosis and management of STEMI associated with intact fibrous cap. *JACC Cardiovascular Imaging.* 2013;6:283–287.

58. Kubo T, et al. Assessment of culprit lesion morphology in acute myocardial infarction: ability of optical coherence tomography compared with intravascular ultrasound and coronary angioscopy. *J Am Coll Cardiol.* 2007;50:933–939.

59. Tearney GJ, et al. Quantification of macrophage content in atherosclerotic plaques by optical coherence tomography. *Circulation.* 2003;107:113–119.

60. Higuma T, et al. A combined optical coherence tomography and intravascular ultrasound study on plaque rupture, plaque erosion, and calcified nodule in patients with ST-segment elevation myocardial infarction: incidence, morphologic characteristics, and outcomes after percutaneous coronary intervention. *JACC Cardiovasc Interv.* 2015;8:1166–1176.

61. Li J, et al. Integrated IVUS-OCT for real-time imaging of coronary atherosclerosis. *JACC Cardiovasc Imaging.* 2014;7:101–103.

62. Kato K, et al. Nonculprit plaques in patients with acute coronary syndromes have more vulnerable features compared with those with non-acute coronary syndromes: a 3-vessel optical coherence tomography study. *Circ Cardiovasc Imaging.* 2012;5:433–440.

63. Caplan JD, et al. Near-infrared spectroscopy for the detection of vulnerable coronary artery plaques. *J Am Coll Cardiol.* 2006;47:C92–C96.

64. Schultz CJ, et al. First-in-man clinical use of combined near-infrared spectroscopy and intravascular ultrasound: a potential key to predict distal embolization and no-reflow? *J Am Coll Cardiol.* 2010;56:314.

65. Pu J, et al. In vivo characterization of coronary plaques: novel findings from comparing greyscale and virtual histology intravascular ultrasound and near-infrared spectroscopy. *Eur Heart J.* 2012;33:372–383.

66. Gardner CM, et al. Detection of lipid core coronary plaques in autopsy specimens with a novel catheter-based near-infrared spectroscopy system. *JACC Cardiovasc Imaging.* 2008;1:638–648.

67. Waxman S, et al. In vivo validation of a catheter-based near-infrared spectroscopy system for detection of lipid core coronary plaques: initial results of the SPECTACL study. *JACC Cardiovasc Imaging.* 2009;2:858–868.

68. Goldstein JA, et al. Detection of lipid-core plaques by intracoronary near-infrared spectroscopy identifies high risk of periprocedural myocardial infarction. *Circ Cardiovasc Interv.* 2011;4:429–437.

69. Madder RD, et al. Composition of target lesions by near-infrared spectroscopy in patients with acute coronary syndrome versus stable angina. *Circ Cardiovasc Interv.* 2012;5:55–61.

70. Kini AS, et al. Changes in plaque lipid content after short-term intensive versus standard statin therapy: the YELLOW trial (reduction in yellow plaque by aggressive lipid-lowering therapy). *J Am Coll Cardiol.* 2013;62:21–29.

71. Oemrawsingh RM, et al. Near-infrared spectroscopy predicts cardiovascular outcome in patients with coronary artery disease. *J Am Coll Cardiol.* 2014;64:2510–2518.

72. Takano M, et al. In vivo comparison of optical coherence tomography and angioscopy for the evaluation of coronary plaque characteristics. *Am J Cardiol.* 2008;101:471–476.

73. Asakura M, et al. Extensive development of vulnerable plaques as a pan-coronary process in patients with myocardial infarction: an angioscopic study. *J Am Coll Cardiol.* 2001;37:1284–1288.

74. Uchida Y, et al. Detection of vulnerable coronary plaques by color fluorescent angioscopy. *JACC Cardiovasc Imaging.* 2010;3:398–408.

75. Osborn EA, Jaffer FA. Imaging inflammation and neovascularization in atherosclerosis: clinical and translational molecular and structural imaging targets. *Curr Opin Cardiol.* 2015;30:671–680.

76. Vinegoni C, et al. Indocyanine green enables near-infrared fluorescence imaging of lipid-rich, inflamed atherosclerotic plaques. *Sci Transl Med.* 2011;3:84ra45.

77. Hara T, et al. Molecular imaging of fibrin deposition in deep vein thrombosis using fibrin-targeted near-infrared fluorescence. *JACC Cardiovasc Imaging.* 2012;5:607–615.

78. Hara T, et al. Intravascular fibrin molecular imaging improves the detection of unhealed stents assessed by optical coherence tomography in vivo. *Eur Heart J.* 2015. pii: ehv677.

79. Levine GN, et al. 2011 ACCF/AHA/SCAI guideline for percutaneous coronary intervention: a report of the American College of Cardiology Foundation/American Heart Association Task Force on Practice Guidelines and the Society for Cardiovascular Angiography and Interventions. *Circulation.* 2011;124:e574–e651.

80. Lotfi A, et al. Expert consensus statement on the use of fractional flow reserve, intravascular ultrasound, and optical coherence tomography: a consensus statement of the Society of Cardiovascular Angiography and Interventions. *Catheter Cardiovasc Interv.* 2014;83:509–518.

10 Hemodynamics for Interventional Cardiologists

Morton J. Kern, MD, MSCAI, FAHA, FACC and

Arnold H. Seto, MD, MPA, FSCAI, FACC

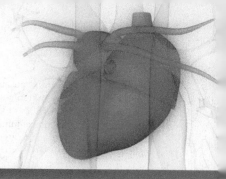

Hemodynamics can confirm or establish the etiology of many surgically correctable cardiac diseases, but diagnoses can be inaccurate if the data are poorly collected or inaccurately obtained. Hemodynamic data play a critical role in teaching cardiovascular pathophysiology, and should be a continued point of excellence for invasive cardiologists.

This chapter will review the essential hemodynamics applicable to coronary and structural interventions in the cardiac catheterization laboratory. Complete reviews of hemodynamics, both in general and those specifically applicable to complex conditions, can be found elsewhere (1–4). An excellent summary of hemodynamics in the cath lab is presented by Nishimura and Carabello (5).

The Cardiac Cycle

All pressure waves of the cardiac cycle can be understood by reviewing the electrical and mechanical activity of the heart, as shown in Dr. Wiggers' diagram (Fig. 10.1). The timing of mechanical events, such as contraction and relaxation and the generation of transvalvular and ventricular pressure gradients can be obtained from the ECG matched to the corresponding pressure waveform. Each electrical event (e.g., P wave, QRS, T wave) is followed normally by a mechanical function (either contraction or relaxation), resulting in a specific pressure wave.

While the ECG "P" wave correlates with the beginning of atrial contraction, the QRS with ventricular activation, and the "T" wave with ventricular relaxation, the normal sequence of contraction and relaxation of the heart muscle is disturbed by arrhythmias and conduction defects. Normal cardiac function may become inefficient or ineffective, as can be demonstrated with associated hemodynamic alterations.

Normal Pressure Wave Forms

Beginning the cardiac cycle, the P wave signals and initiates atrial contraction. Atrial systole and diastole are denoted as the "a" wave (Fig. 10.1, point a), followed by the "x" descent, respectively. The P wave, and the "A/x" pressures, are followed by the QRS, signaling depolarization of the ventricles (point b). The left ventricular (LV) pressure after the "a" wave is the end diastolic pressure, also known as LVEDP, and corresponds to the R wave (vertical line) intersection with the LV pressure (point b). About 15 to 30 ms after the QRS, the ventricles contract, the LV (and right ventricular [RV]) pressure increases rapidly during the isovolumetric contraction period (interval b–c). When LV pressure rises above aortic pressure, the aortic valve (AV) opens (point c). Systolic ejection continues until repolarization, signaled by the "T" wave (point d). After the "T" wave, the LV relaxation produces a fall in the LV and aortic pressure. When the LV pressure falls below the aortic pressure, the AV closes (point e). The ventricular

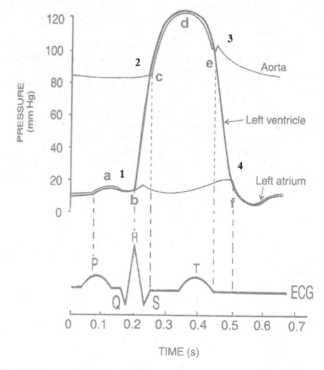

FIGURE 10.1 The Wiggers diagram. Pressure curves of the left atrium and left ventricle are superimposed with the corresponding portions of the electrocardiogram at bottom. Points 1, 2, 3, 4 represent the closure of the AV valves, 2 the opening of the semi-lunar valves (aortic in this case), 3 the closure of the aortic valve, 4 the opening of the AV (mitral valve). AV, aortic valve.

pressure continues to fall, and when it falls below the left atrial (LA) pressure, the mitral valve (MV) opens and the LA empties into the LV (point f).

Returning to the atrial pressure wave across the cycle, after the a wave, atrial pressure slowly rises, with atrial filling during systole, continuing to increase until the end of systole when the pressure and volume of the LA are nearly maximal, producing a ventricular filling wave: the "v" wave. The "v" wave peak (point 4) is followed by a rapid fall, labeled "Y" descent, when the MV opens. The peaks and troughs of the atrial pressure waves are changed by pathologic conditions such as acute valvular regurgitation, heart failure, and infarction.

Right Hemodynamics

The normal right atrial (RA) and pulmonary capillary wedge (PCW) pressure wave forms are shown in Figure 10.2. RA pressure normally decreases with intrathoracic pressure during spontaneous inspiration

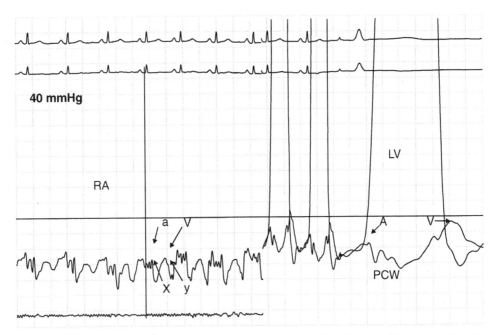

FIGURE 10.2   Normal RA (*left*) and PCW with LV pressure waveforms (*right*) demonstrate the "a" wave of LV pressure (a) and the "a" wave delayed of pulmonary capillary wedge (PCW) pressure ("a") and "v" wave of the PCW pressure (v) noted by large arrows. Normal RA pressures show typical "a" and "v" waves with corresponding "x" and "y" descents. LV = left ventricle, 0 to 40 mm Hg scale.

(Fig. 10.3, top). Nevertheless, in patients with congestive heart failure or other conditions impairing venous return to the right heart (e.g., pericardial constriction), RA pressure during inspiration may fail to decrease, or might even increase during inspiration (Fig. 10.3, Kussmaul's sign), reflecting impaired filling of the RV and elevated pressures. **Figure 10.4** shows rapid "Y" descents during inspiration, with no change in mean RA pressure.

Pressure waves in the atria are a function of the pressure/flow relationship or compliance of the chamber. A poorly compliant chamber (i.e., stiff) may demonstrate a large v wave despite normal flow, while a very compliant chamber may not register marked pressure wave changes despite torrential flow. A low compliance LA can be seen by the pressure waves in a patient with mitral stenosis. **Figure 10.5** shows LA and RA pressures together. The high LA pressure is due to both

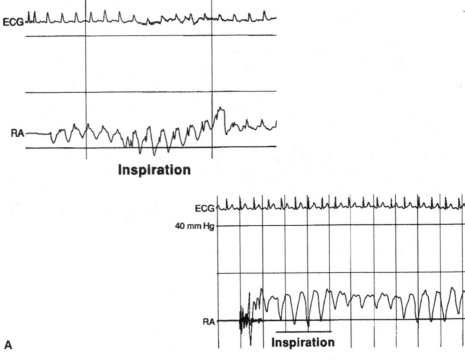

FIGURE 10.3   Top: Right atrial (RA) pressure during inspiration. Note the fall in pressure as the negative intrathoracic pressure is transmitted to RA. **Bottom:** RA pressure in patient with congestive heart failure showing failure to decrease with inspiration (Kussmal's sign).

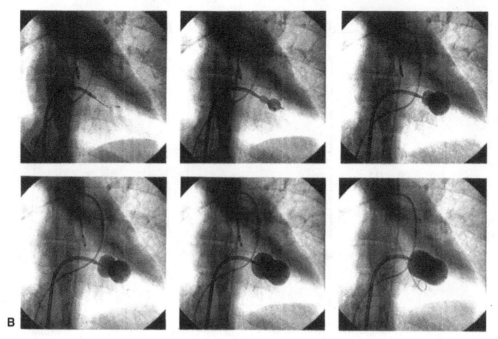

B

FIGURE 10.3   (continued)

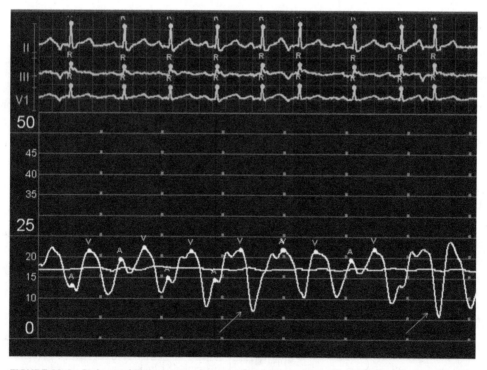

FIGURE 10.4   Right atrial (RA) pressure during inspiration in patient with CHF. The failure to decrease RA pressure during inspiration is Kussmal's sign. Note exaggeration of "v" waves during inspiration. CHF, congestive heart failure.

mitral stenosis and a stiff left atrium after rheumatic inflammation. The LA pressure waveform also has a marked v wave, which is due not to regurgitation but to the poor compliance of the atrium. In this example, atrial fibrillation is present, showing a lack of "a" waves and the presence of a "c" notch preceding the large "v" wave, demonstrating how arrhythmias may distort atrial and ventricular waveforms.

Normal RA waveforms have smaller "a" and "v" waves than the left atrium, but these become distorted in the setting of significant valve dysfunction. In patients with tricuspid regurgitation, the RA wave loses its characteristic "a" and "v" waves, which are replaced by a large and broad "s" (systolic) wave of blood reflux from the RV back into the LV. Figure 10.6 shows the RA waveform of a 67-year-old woman with dyspnea at rest, with systolic murmur, which varies with respiration. In Figure 10.7A, note the corresponding pattern of RV and RA in a patient with severe tricuspid regurgitation (TR). The RV angiogram of this patient is shown in Figure 10.7B.

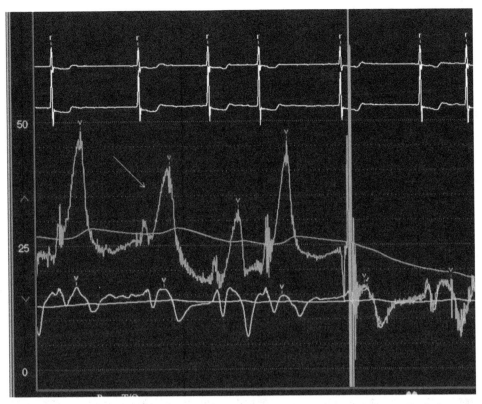

FIGURE 10.5 Left atrial (*orange*) and right atrial (*blue*) pressure tracings during pullback from the LA to the RA in a patient with mitral stenosis. Note the significantly higher LA pressure and large v waves (*arrow*). In the absence of mitral regurgitation, large v waves are a measure of LV compliance. After pulling back across the intra-atrial septum (vertical line artifact), the pressure wave from the LA matches the RA. Note the effect of the cardiac rhythm distorting the atrial waveforms. LA, left atrial; LV, left ventricular; RA, right atrial.

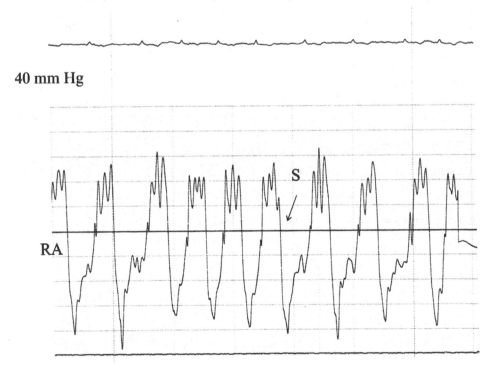

FIGURE 10.6 Right atrial (RA) waveform of a 67-year-old woman with dyspnea at rest and systolic murmur that varies with respiration. S, regurgitant wave.

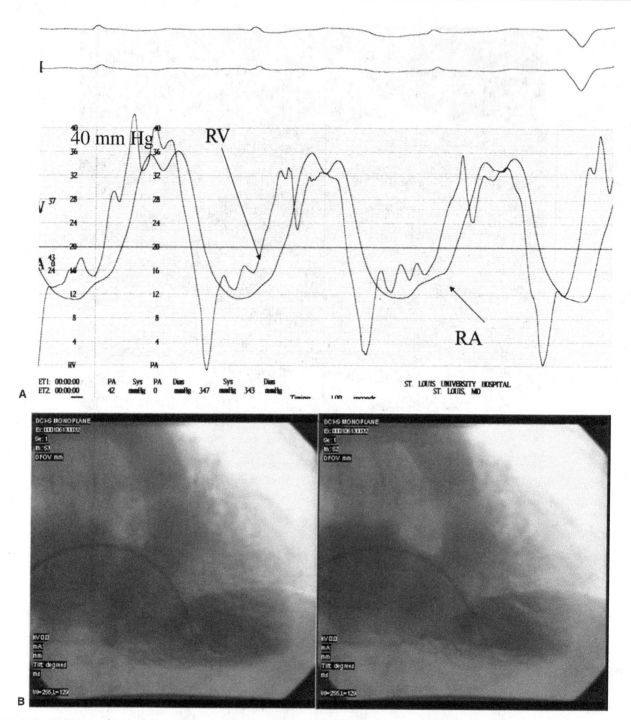

FIGURE 10.7 **A:** Pattern of RV and RA pressures in a patient with severe TR. The regurgitant RA waves are called the "s" waves of TR. Pressure scale 0 to 40 mm Hg. **B:** Cineangiographic frames from right ventriculography showing severe tricuspid regurgitation with reflux of contrast media into the right atrium. RA, right atrial; RV, right ventricular; TR, tricuspid regurgitation.

Fundamental Observations of Pressure-Volume Loops

Pressure Volume Relationships

Cardiac ventricular hemodynamics can be represented by a pressure-volume (PV) loop, which plots the changes of these variables over a cardiac cycle (6–8). The shape of the PV loop is specific for the ventricle/arterial circuit coupling. The PV loop (**Fig. 10.8**) for the left ventricle/aorta is different than the PV loop for the right ventricle/pulmonary artery, but each represents one cardiac cycle. Beginning at end-diastole (point a), LV volume has received the atrial contribution and is maximal. Isovolemic contraction ("a"–"b") increases LV pressure, with no change in volume. At the end of isovolemic contraction, LV pressure exceeds aortic pressure, the AV opens, and blood is ejected from the LV into the aorta (point b). Over the systolic ejection phase, LV volume decreases, and as ventricular repolarization occurs, LV ejection ceases and relaxation

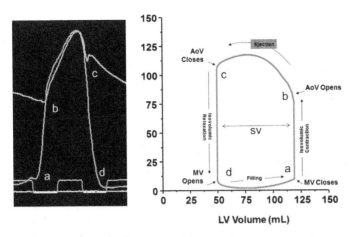

FIGURE 10.8 The pressure volume (PV) loop characterizes the changes in pressure flow over the course of one cardiac cycle. *Left panel*, the left ventricular and aortic pressure as measured during cardiac catheterization. *Right panel*, the pressure volume loop derived from the hemodynamics of LV pressure and volume. Point A, left ventricular end-diastolic pressure is followed by isovolumetric contraction ending at point B, the aortic valve opening. Ejection continues until the repolarization of the LV produces a fall in LV ejection. LV pressure falls past point C, aortic valve closure, and continues to fall along the line of isovolumetric relaxation to point D, mitral valve opening. Changes in the shape of the pressure volume loop demonstrate changes in contractility, cardiac output. LV, left ventricular; SV, stroke volume.

begins. When LV pressure falls below aortic pressure, the AV closes, a point also known as the end-systolic pressure-volume point (ESPV) (point c). Isovolemic relaxation occurs until LV pressure decreases below the atrial pressure, opening the MV (point d).

The stroke volume (SV) is represented by the width of the PV loop, the difference between end-systolic and end-diastolic volumes. The area within the loop represents stroke work. Load-independent LV contractility, also known as E_{max}, is defined as the maximal slope of the ESPV points under various loading conditions, the line of these points is the ESPV relationship (ESPVR). Effective arterial elastance (E_a), a measure of LV afterload, is defined as the ratio of end-systolic pressure to SV. Under steady state conditions, optimal LV contractile efficiency occurs when the ratio of E_a:E_{max} approaches 1.

The PV loop describes contractile function, relaxation properties, SV, cardiac work, and myocardial oxygen consumption. Hemodynamic alterations and interventions change the PV relationship in predictable ways, and comparisons of various hemodynamic interventions can be made more precisely by examining the PV loop (Figs. 10.9 and 10.10).

Acute changes in cardiac function, such as might occur with acute myocardial infarction, are also easily demonstrated (Fig. 10.11). In acute myocardial infarction (AMI), LV contractility (E_{max}) is reduced; LV pressure, and SV and LV stroke work may be unchanged or reduced; and LVEDP is increased. In cardiogenic shock, Emax is severely reduced; LV afterload (E_a) may be increased; LV end-diastolic volume (LVEDV) and LVEDP are increased; and SV is reduced, findings easily seen to display reduced LV contractile function, acute diastolic dysfunction, elevated LVEDV and LVEDP, and increased LV work (oxygen demand). In more severe cases of myocardial infarction that evolve into cardiogenic shock, LV contractile function is more

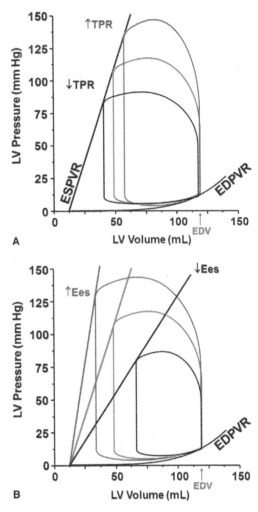

FIGURE 10.10 A: The effects of increasing afterload or total peripheral vascular resistance (TPR) decreases stroke volume (SV), increases aortic pressure and minimally modifies LVEDP. EDPVR, end-diastolic pressure volume relationship; EDV, end-diastolic volume; ESPVR, end-systolic pressure–volume relationship; LVEDP, left ventricular end-diastolic pressure. (Courtesy of Dr. Dan Burkhoff, Columbia University, New York, NY.) **B:** The effect of increasing contractility. The increasing slope of the line of Ees, increases SV, aortic pressure, with minimal effect on LVEDP. Ees, end-systolic elastance; EDPVR, end-diastolic pressure volume relationship; LV, left ventricular. (Courtesy of Dr. Dan Burkhoff, Columbia University, New York, NY.)

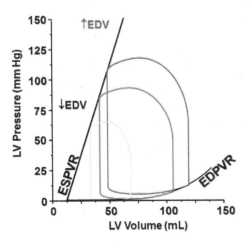

FIGURE 10.9 Effect of changes in left ventricular preload. Increasing the left ventricular end-diastolic pressure along the line of the end-diastolic pressure volume relationship (EDPVR). As volume is increased, left ventricular end-diastole (LVED), stroke volume, and aortic pressure increase. EDV, end-diastolic volume; ESPVR, end-systolic pressure–volume relationship. (Courtesy of Dr. Dan Burkhoff, Columbia University, New York, NY.)

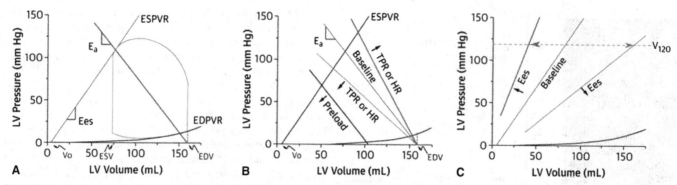

FIGURE 10.11   Overview of pressure–volume loops (PVLs) and relations. **A:** Normal PVL, is bounded by the end-systolic pressure–volume relationship (ESPVR) and end-diastolic pressure–volume relationship (EDPVR). ESPVR is approximately linear with slope end-systolic elastance (Ees) and volume–axis intercept (Vo). Effective arterial elastance (E_a) is the slope of the line extending from the end-diastolic volume (EDV) point on the volume axis through the end-systolic pressure–volume point of the loop. **B:** Slope of the E_a line depends on total peripheral resistance (TPR) and heart rate (HR), and its position depends on EDV. **C:** The ESPVR shifts with changes in ventricular contractility, which can be a combination of changes in Ees and Vo. Changes in contractility can be indexed by V120, the volume at which the ESPVR intersects 120 mm Hg. ESV, end-systolic volume; LV, left ventricular. Load-independent LV contractility also known as E_{max}, is defined as the maximal slope of the end-systolic pressure volume (ESPV) point under various loading conditions, known as the ESPV relationship (ESPVR). Effective arterial elastance (E_a) is a measure of LV afterload and is defined as the ratio of end-systolic pressure and stroke volume. (From: Burkhoff D et al. Hemodynamics of mechanical circulatory support. *J Am Coll Cardiol.* 2015;66(23):2663.)

severely reduced with associated significant increases in end-diastolic P and V. The LV impairment results in a markedly reduced SV, with an increased myocardial oxygen demand.

The most common applications of pressure-volume loops characterize only left ventricular hemodynamics. For research into right ventricular function or extra-cardiac problems, the standard PV loops become complex and affected by the unique factors altering the right-sided PV loop configuration. Interpretation of this is beyond the scope of this review.

Intracardiac Shunts

Blood moves across atrial, ventricular, and other anatomic communications due to differences in pressure over the cardiac cycle. For the most common shunt, the atrial septal defects (ASD), the pressure changes across the atrial septum determine the flow across the shunt.

The LA pressure is typically lower than RA pressure until after birth when the lungs expand with air and the right ventricular flow raises the LA pressure and closes the patent foramen ovale. Immediately after birth, the right atrium and right ventricle see the lower resistance of the pulmonary circuit, compared to the left atrium and ventricle which receive more blood but also must pump across the higher resistance of the systemic circulation. This relationship is evident in a patient with aortic stenosis in whom transseptal LA to RA pressure pullback can be recorded showing large LA "v" waves compared to the lower RA pressure with much reduced "a" and "v" waves (Fig. 10.7). Nevertheless, in certain situations, especially during the Valsalva maneuver, the RA pressure can transiently increase above the LA pressure, which in the presence of a patent foramen ovale (PFO) produces right-to-left shunting and possible transit of emboli-producing clinical sequelae.

Intracardiac Shunts: Atrial Septal Defects

Percutaneous closure of ASD and PFO are performed routinely in many labs by experienced operators. PFOs may be closed out of concern for paradoxical embolism, while ASDs are generally closed due to excessive volume loading of the right heart. Measurement of

atrial hemoglobin oxygen saturations enable precise quantification of the severity of interatrial shunting and is the gold standard for defining which ASDs require closure. Oxygen saturations from multiple locations are obtained during a diagnostic "saturation run" in a rapid but systematic manner. A standard balloon-tipped Swan-Ganz–type catheter is satisfactory, but a large-bore end-hole or side-hole catheter (multipurpose) catheter performs better rapid sampling, particularly from left-sided structures. A left-to-right shunt is suggested when an oxygen step-up, or increase in oxygen content, in a chamber or vessel exceeds that of a proximal compartment. A step-up in oxygen saturation at the pulmonary artery (PA) by more than 7% above the RA saturation is indicative of a significant left-to-right shunt at the atrial level. Similarly, the desaturation of arterial blood samples from the left heart chambers and aorta suggests a right-to-left shunt. In determining the site of the right-to-left shunt, sequential samples from the pulmonary veins, LA, LV, and aorta can be easily obtained when an interatrial septal defect is present

Mixed venous oxygen saturation can be assumed to be fully mixed PA blood in the absence of a shunt. If there is a left-to-right shunt, mixed venous blood is measured one chamber proximal to the step-up. In the case of an atrial septal defect, the mixed venous oxygen content is computed from the weighted average of vena caval blood (i.e., as the sum of three times the superior vena cava (SVC) plus one inferior vena cava (IVC). Oxygen content, divided by four). When pulmonary venous blood is not collected, PVO_2 (pulmonary vein) percentage saturation is assumed to be 95%.

Shunt Calculation

The Fick or left-sided indicator dilution methods of CO determination are employed to measure systemic flow. Using the Fick method, the following formulas apply:

1. Systemic flow

$$Q_s \ (L/min) = \frac{O_2 \ consumption(mL/min)}{(arterial - mixed \ venous) \ O_2 \ content}$$

2. Pulmonary flow

$$Q_p \ (L/min) = \frac{O_2 \ consumption(mL/min)}{(pulmonary \ venous - pulmonary \ arterial)}$$
$$O_2 \ content$$

3. The effective pulmonary blood flow (EPB)

$$Q_{EPB} = \frac{O_2 \ consumption(mL/min)}{(pulmonary \ venous - mixed \ venous) \ O_2 \ content}$$

Normally, the effective pulmonary blood flow is equal to the systemic blood flow. In a left-to-right shunt, the effective pulmonary blood flow is increased (by the amount of the shunt) as follows:

$$Q_{EPB} = systemic \ flow + shunt \ flow, \ (left-to-right) \quad (1)$$

In a right-to-left shunt, the effective pulmonary blood flow is decreased (by the amount of the shunt):

$$Q_{EPB} = systemic \ flow - shunt \ flow, \ (right-to-left) \quad (2)$$

The shunt volume is determined by use of Equations (1) and (2). Intracardiac shunt calculations are summarized on Figures 10.12 to 10.14. The ratio of pulmonary to systemic flow

Left-to-Right Shunt Detection and Quantification
Suspicion and Detection: Search for oxygen saturation "step-ups".
Intrinsic mixing requires significant change in oxygen saturations to be of concern:

SVC/IVC to RA	min 7%	ASD/PAPVR
RA to RV	min 5%	VSD
RV to PA	min 5%	PDA
Any (SVC to PA)	min 7%	Anywhere

FIGURE 10.12 Intracardiac shunt calculations. ASD, atrial septal defect; IVC, inferior vena cava; PA, pulmonary artery; PDA, posterior descending artery; RA, right atrial; RV, right ventricular; SVC, superior vena cava; VSD, ventricular septal defect.

Bidirectional Shuts

- Effective Blood flow:
- $Q_{eff} = O_2$ consumption/(PVO$_2$-MV O$_2$)
- Left to right shunt: Q_p- Q_{eff}
- Right to left shunt: Q_s- Q_{eff}

FIGURE 10.14 Bidirectional shunt calculations.

(called Q_p/Q_s) for a left-to-right shunt is called the shunt fraction. A $Q_p/Q_s > 1.5$ is considered the threshold shunt fraction that makes closure indicated.

Aortic Stenosis

Before reviewing hemodynamics of aortic stenosis, review the normal LV and Aortic Pressure obtained with a micromanometer dual transducer catheter shows nearly ideal waveforms of aortic and left ventricular pressure (Fig. 10.15). As an aside, also note the normal LV filling pattern over the diastolic period. The normal LV pressure has an anachronism shoulder and a normal small impulse outflow tract gradient (red arrow). The pressure tracings most commonly used in clinical practice are acquired with electronic transducers and fluid-filled catheters such as the 5F pigtail catheter and 6F femoral artery (FA) sheath side arm (right side, Fig. 10.15). Note the resonant artifact (whip, fling, or ringing) compared to the high-fidelity tracings. It should be recalled that the FA pressure is not only higher due to resonant signal amplification but also delayed in time as the wave travels from the aortic location to the FA location. This is a normal finding of all peripheral pressures compared to central aortic pressures.

The hemodynamic assessment of aortic stenosis and the subsequent success of valve therapies begin with accurate transvalvular gradient and cardiac output measurements. Many clinical cath lab measurements use the FA to represent aortic pressure. Due to resonance and peripheral pressure amplification, the FA systolic

---

Quick Method to Calculate Severity of Left-to-Right Shunt (Qp/Qs) Using Only Oxygen Saturation Values

$$\frac{PBF}{SBF} = \frac{\dfrac{O_2 \ Consumption}{PV(\%)-PA(\%)}}{\dfrac{O_2 \ Consumption}{AO(\%)-MV(\%)}} = \frac{AO-MV}{PV-PA}$$

Example:

$$\left.\begin{array}{l} MV=60\% \\ PA=80\% \\ PV=95\% \\ AO=95\% \end{array}\right\} \quad \frac{95-60}{95-80} = \frac{35}{15} = 2.33$$

FIGURE 10.13 Left-to-right shunt calculations. MV, mitral valve; PA, pulmonary artery; PBF, pulmonary blood flow; PV, pressure volume; SBF, systemic blood flow.

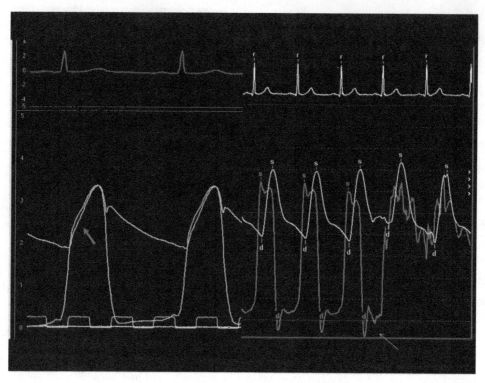

FIGURE 10.15   Normal left ventricular (LV) and aortic pressures. (*Left*) micromanometer dual transducer pressure catheter with near ideal wave forms of aortic and left ventricular pressure. *Red arrow* denotes anachrotic shoulder and small normal impulse LV outflow tract gradient. (*Right*) side shows pressures measured with fluid-filled transducer systems using 5F pigtail catheter through a 6F femoral artery sheath side arm. Note the resonant artifact (fling or ringing, *white arrow*).

pressure is higher and delayed relative to central aortic pressure, which artefactually decreases the mean gradient relative to the LV. When using femoral pressure, precise pressure gradients cannot be obtained in patients with peripheral vascular disease at the level of the aortic bifurcation or lower. For improved accuracy in measuring the LV-Ao gradient, a double lumen catheter or two arterial catheters are required.

There is considerable new information on the mechanisms of aortic stenosis and its hemodynamic manifestations. Pibarot P and Dumesnil (9) reviewed critical characteristics of blood flow and pressure across the AV (Fig. 10.16). The ejection of blood from the LV is forced through the fixed reduced aortic orifice area (i.e., the anatomic orifice area [AOA]). Energy is lost due to resistance (i.e., a portion of the potential energy of the blood pressure), resulting in a pressure drop and acceleration of flow. After crossing the AV (i.e., the effective orifice area [EOA]), part of the kinetic energy is reconverted back to potential energy, and the pressure increases (also called the "pressure recovery"). Doppler echocardiography measures the peak instantaneous gradient across the entire outflow tract and aorta and is thus able to capture this phenomenon of pressure recovery. Catheter-based measurements of aortic pressure are typically several cm distal in the aorta after pressure recovery has already occurred. There are several specialized measures of the relationship between hemodynamic load and arterial resistance or impedance to flow. The global hemodynamic load imposed on the left ventricle results from the summation of the valvular load and the arterial load. These subjects are addressed in detail elsewhere (ref).

In simple terms, aortic stenosis is characterized by a delayed upslope of aortic pressure and a large LV-Aortic pressure gradient (Fig. 10.17). The mean pressure gradient is the area between the aortic (Ao) and LV pressure tracings during systolic ejection. To quickly assess the significance of the LV-Ao pressure gradient, operators frequently use the peak-to-peak LV and aortic pressure difference (8). The peak-to-peak gradient is not equivalent to the mean gradient for mild and moderate stenosis but is often close to mean gradient for severe stenosis. The peak-to-peak gradient should not be confused with the peak instantaneous gradient. Because of pressure recovery, catheter-based measurements of the peak instantaneous gradient are often lower than echocardiographic measurements.

When using the FA pressure, more accurate valve areas are obtained with unshifted LV-Ao pressure tracings (Fig. 10.17, right side), as the delay in FA pressure partially corrects for the effects of peripheral amplification. If the FA pressure is shifted back to match the upstroke of the LV, femoral pressure overshoot (amplification) reduces the true gradient. For the highest accuracy, pressures should be measured immediately above and below the AV with a dual lumen catheter or two catheters, especially for patients with low cardiac output and a low transvalvular gradient.

Valve Area Calculations

Stenotic valve areas are calculated from pressure tracings and cardiac output (12). Cardiac outputs are measured by thermodilution or from the Fick calculation. The Fick calculation uses either assumed

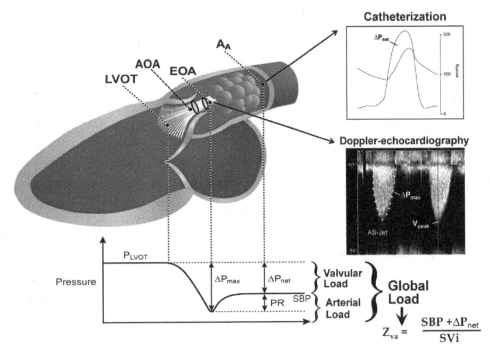

FIGURE 10.16 Pathophysiology of aortic stenosis (AS). Blood flow and pressure across LVOT, aortic valve, and ascending aorta during systole. When the blood flow contracts to pass through a stenotic orifice (i.e., the anatomic orifice area [AOA]), a portion of the potential energy of the blood, namely, pressure, is converted into kinetic energy, namely, velocity, thus resulting in a pressure drop and acceleration of flow. Downstream of the vena contracta (i.e., the effective orifice area [EOA]), a large part of the kinetic energy is irreversibly dissipated as heat because of flow turbulences. The remaining portion of the kinetic energy that is reconverted back to potential energy is called the "pressure recovery" (PR). The global hemodynamic load imposed on the left ventricle results from the summation of the valvular load and the arterial load. This global load can be estimated by calculating the valvuloarterial imped-ance. In patients with medium- or large-sized ascending aorta, the impedance can be calculated with the standard Doppler mean gradient in place of the net mean gradient. A_A, cross-sectional area of the aorta at the level of the sinotubular junction; ΔP_{max}, maximum transvalvular pressure gradient recorded at the level of vena contracta (i.e., mean gradient measured by Doppler); ΔP_{net}, net transvalvular pressure gradient recorded after pressure recovery (i.e., mean gradient measured by catheterization); LVOT, left ventricular outflow tract; P_{LVOT}, pressure in the LVOT; SBP, systolic blood pressure; SVi, stroke volume index; V_{peak}, peak aortic jet velocity; Z_{va}, valvuloarterial impedance. (From: Philippe Pibarot P, Dumesnil JG. Improving assessment of aortic stenosis. *J Am Coll Cardiol.* 2012;60(3):169–180.)

oxygen consumption (3 mL/kg O_2 or 125 mL/min/m^2) or, for best accuracy, direct oxygen consumption with a metabolic oximeter.

The Gorlin formula (10) can be applied to both aortic and MVs:

$$\text{Valve area (cm}^2) = \frac{\text{value flow(mL/s)}}{K \times C \times \sqrt{MVG}},$$

where MVG is mean valvular gradient (mm Hg); K (44.3) is a derived constant by Gorlin and Gorlin; C is an empirical constant that is 1 for semi-lunar valves and tricuspid valves, and 0.85 for MVs; and valve flow is measured in milliliters per second during the diastolic or systolic flow period. For MV flow, the diastolic filling period is used,

$$\frac{CO\,(mL/min)}{(diastolic\ filling\ period)(HR)}$$

For AV flow, the systolic ejection period (SEP) is used:

$$\frac{CO\,(mL/min)}{(systolic\ ejection\ period)(HR)}$$

where SEP (s/min) = systolic period (s/beat) × HR. Computerized hemodynamic systems are generally used to perform these measure-ments and calculations.

A simplified formula (also known as the Hakke formula [11]) can provide a quick in-laboratory determination of AV area, estimated as:

Quick valve area = CO/$\sqrt{LV}$-aortic peak-to-peak pressure difference.

For example, peak-to-peak gradient = 65 mm Hg, CO = 5 L/min

$$\text{Quick valve area} = \frac{5\ L/min}{\sqrt{65}} = \frac{5\ L/min}{8} = 0.63\,cm^2$$

The quick formula differs from the Gorlin formula by 18% ± 13% in patients with bradycardia (<65 beats/min) or tachycardia

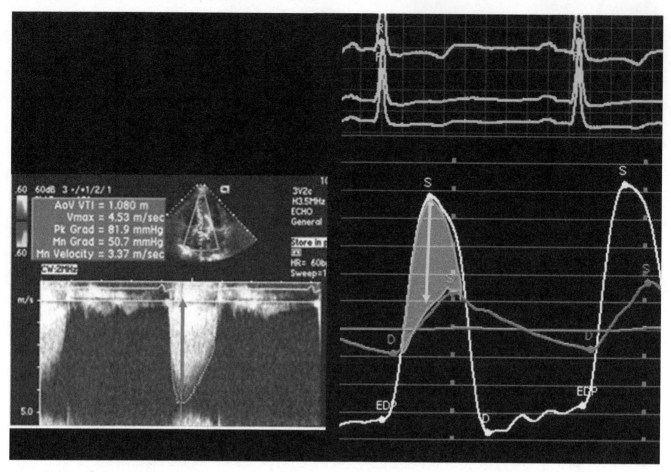

FIGURE 10.17 **Left:** Doppler velocity of the left ventricular outflow tract (LVOT) in patient with AS and corresponding hemodynamic LV-Ao pressure tracings. The peak instantaneous velocity (*red arrow*) is used to compute the transvalvular pressure gradient ($4V^2$) which should correspond to the hemodynamic pressure gradient (*shaded area*) in moderate and severe stenosis. This relationship is weaker in some mild to minimal stenoses. EDP, end-diastolic pressure.

(>100 beats/min). The Gorlin equation overestimates the severity of valve stenosis in low-flow states.

Hemodynamics of Transcatheter Aortic Valve Replacement (TAVR)

Hemodynamic measurements before and after TAVR may demonstrate the effectiveness of the implant and also identify valvular regurgitation or LV dysfunction (see the section titled "Aortic Insufficiency" later in this chapter). An example of a patient's hemodynamics before and after TAVR is shown in **Figure 10.18**. Features denoting successful implantation are the reduction of the LV-Ao gradient (80–0 mm Hg), an increase in aortic systolic pressure (105–122 mm Hg), and the absence of newly widened pulse pressure, which would suggest aortic insufficiency. In addition, after TAVR, there is restoration of a dicrotic notch (Fig. 10.18, point d) and anachrotic shoulder (Fig. 10.18, point a). The rapidly rising LV diastolic pressure may represent unmasked diastolic dysfunction (Fig. 10.18, point dd). The aortic pulse pressure suggests minimal or no aortic insufficiency.

Aortic Regurgitation

Aortic regurgitation occurs when there is inadequate closure or malcoaptation of the AV leaflets, allowing blood to enter the left ventricular cavity from the aorta during diastole (**Fig. 10.19**). The typical hemodynamics findings of aortic insufficiency include an elevated LV end-diastolic pressure (EDP) (Fig. 10.19, arrow), widened aortic pulse pressure (Fig. 10.19, arrowheads), and near equalization of LV and aortic EDP (12). Depending on the extent of the valve leaflet and/or aortic root disruption, some patients may require urgent valve replacement. **Figure 10.20** shows a patient with mixed aortic stenosis and regurgitation. Note the LV-Ao gradient, wide pulse pressure, and rapid LV diastolic filling slope up to the LVEDP and near equilibration of aortic diastolic pressure with LVEDP. **Figure 10.21** illustrates the hemodynamics of a paravalvular leak following a TAVR procedure with an increase in LVEDP and the slope of diastolic pressure rise.

Evaluation of Aortic Stenosis in Patients with Low Gradient and Low Ejection Fraction (EF)

A continuing dilemma exists in patients with low cardiac output and small aortic-left ventricular gradients (e.g., the patient with dyspnea, poor left ventricular function, and a 20-mm-Hg aortic-left ventricular gradient with cardiac output of 3 L/min; AV area = 0.7 cm²). Should this valve be replaced with a prosthetic valve that has an intrinsic gradient of 10 to 20 mm Hg? Because the Gorlin formula

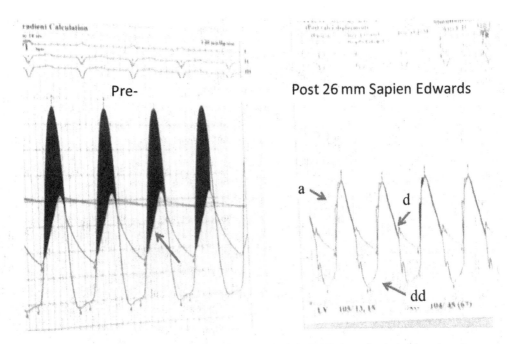

FIGURE 10.18   **Left panel:** LV-Ao pressure tracings before TAVR show classical delayed aortic pressure upstroke (*arrow*) and large pressure gradient (*black shaded area*), scale is 0 to 200 mm Hg. Aortic valve area was 0.6 cm². **Right panel:** Hemodynamics immediately after TAVR. Note the elimination of the pressure gradients, restoration of a dicrotic notch (d) and anachrotic shoulder (a). The rapidly rising LV diastolic pressure may represent unmasked diastolic dysfunction (dd) or mild aortic insufficiency. The aortic pulse pressure suggests minimal or no aortic insufficiency. LV-Ao, left ventricular and aortic; TAVR, transcatheter aortic valve replacement.

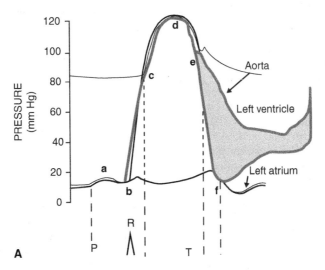

FIGURE 10.19   **A:** Hemodynamics of aortic insufficiency. Important findings include (1) the largest diastolic gradient occurs early; (2) LV retrograde filling increases LV volume and pressure with rapid increase in LV pressure over diastole, left ventricular end-diastolic pressure (LVEDP) will have rapid upstroke until LV size compensates for increased volume; (3) there is wide aortic pulse pressure. **B:** Hemodynamic tracing showing elevated left ventricular (LV) end-diastolic pressure (*arrow*), widened aortic pulse pressure (*arrowheads*), and near equalization of LV and aortic end-diastolic pressures. (From: Ren X, Banki NM. Classic hemodynamic findings of severe aortic regurgitation. *Circulation.* 2012;126:e28–e29.)

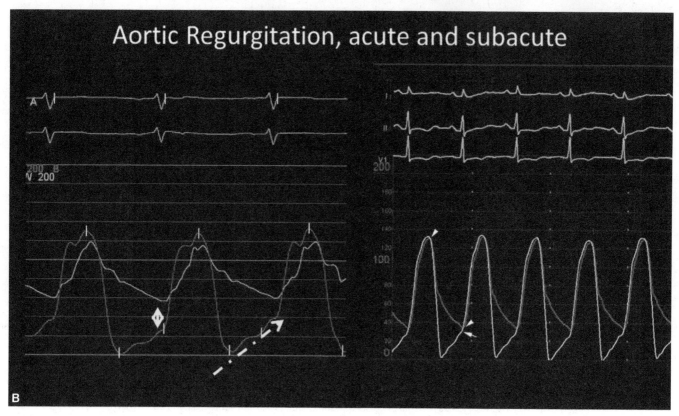

FIGURE 10.19 *(continued)*

for AV area calculations uses an empiric constant (K) the true valve area may be variable under low-flow conditions (13).

To assess whether low-gradient/low-flow aortic stenosis (AS) is due to cardiomyopathy or true fixed valve stenosis, a dobutamine challenge is necessary to increase cardiac output and reassess gradients and valve area. **Figures 10.22** and **10.23** illustrate hemodynamic changes observed under low- and high-flow states. In this example, a 62-year-old man undergoes cardiac catheterization for AS. On examination of the hemodynamic tracings (Fig. 10.22), there is a left ventricular-aortic gradient of 30 mm Hg with a cardiac output of 3.2 L/min and a calculated AV area of 0.7 mm^2. Dobutamine was then infused (Fig. 10.22) at 10 μg/min (with pacing), and then 20 μg/min, with an increased pacing rate of 95 beats/min. The LV-Ao gradient increased to 50 mm Hg, cardiac output of 4.2 L/min, and aortic valve area (AVA) remained fixed at 0.6 cm^2. Figure 10.23 shows a plot of the relationship between the mean gradient (y-axis) and the transvalvular flow (x-axis, bottom), according to the Gorlin formula for three different values of AVA (0.7, 1.0, and 1.5 cm^2). Cardiac output (x-axis, top) is also shown, assuming a heart rate of 75 beats/min and a SEP of 300 ms. At low transvalvular flows, the mean gradient is low at all three valve areas. Two different responses to the dobutamine challenge are illustrated for a hypothetical patient with a baseline flow of 150 mL/s, mean gradient of 23 mm Hg, and calculated AVA 0.7 cm^2. In one scenario (dob 1), flow increases to 225 mL/s, mean gradient increases to 52 mm Hg, and AVA remains 0.7 cm^2, consistent with fixed AS. In a second scenario, flow increases to 275 mL/s, mean gradient increases to 38 mm Hg, and AVA increases to 1.0 cm^2. This patient has changed to a different curve, consistent with relative or pseudo-AS. HR indicates heart rate; SEP, systolic ejection period.

Based on the response to Dobutamine, aortic valve replacement (AVR) is therefore appropriate for this patient, despite a low resting gradient and low EF.

Hypertrophic Obstructive Cardiomyopathy (HOCM)

The hemodynamic evaluation of hypertrophic obstructive cardiomyopathy centers on the degree of left ventricular outflow tract (LVOT) obstruction. LVOT obstruction in hypertrophic cardiomyopathy (HCM) is dynamic and exquisitely sensitive to ventricular loading conditions and contractility, often producing disparate findings between echocardiographic and invasive measurements, and at different times and under different conditions. The LVOT gradient at rest should be compared to dynamic and provocable gradients (e.g., variation with respiration, post-premature ventricular contraction [PVC] accentuation) before committing to alcohol septal ablation.

The assessment of the LVOT gradient is identical to that used for the assessment of AV stenosis. While acceptable in most circumstances, a pigtail catheter with shaft side holes should be replaced by an end hole or HALO (out of plane pigtail) catheter, because pigtail catheters have shaft side holes that may be positioned above the intracavitary obstruction, producing an erroneously low LVOT gradient. A HALO catheter with no shaft side holes is preferred. The most accurate hemodynamic assessment of LVOT obstruction uses a transseptal approach with a balloon-tipped catheter placed at the left ventricular inflow region and a pigtail catheter in the ascending aorta for simultaneous measurement of the LVOT gradient. The transseptal approach helps to avoid catheter entrapment, which can be confused for left ventricular pressure of LVOT obstruction. Use of an 8F Mullins sheath for transseptal access also enables the recording of left atrial pressure via the sidearm for assessment for concomitant diastolic dysfunction.

A typical HOCM pressure wave form at rest is shown in **Figure 10.24**. The demonstration of LVOT obstruction, compared to intrinsic AV obstruction, is made by pullback of the LV catheter from apex to

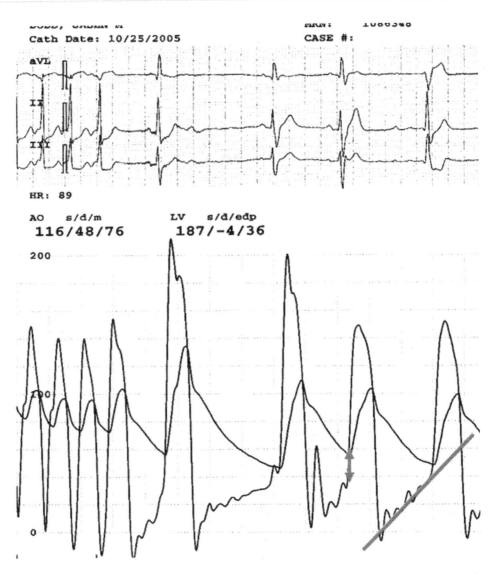

FIGURE 10.20 Hemodynamics of combined mixed AS and AI with LV-Ao systolic gradient and rapidly increasing diastolic LV filling pressure (*diagonal line*), wide pulse pressure, and close approximation of aortic diastolic pressure with LVEDP (*double arrow head*). AS, aortic stenosis; Top, A(i) hemodynamics before and A(ii) after TAVR. LV-Ao, left ventricular and aortic; LVEDP, left ventricular end-diastolic pressure.

base. The large LV aortic gradient disappears when the catheter is positioned just above the mid-cavity obstruction (Fig. 10.24).

Because of the dynamic nature of HOCM obstruction and its sensitivity to loading conditions, the hemodynamic recordings during a premature ventricular contraction (PVC) can unmask the pathophysiology. The post-PVC hemodynamic tracings in a patient with HOCM (Fig. 10.25) is associated with three distinct features: (1) the rapid upstroke of aortic pressure, (2) a narrow aortic pulse pressure, and (3) a spike and dome configuration of early vigorous LV ejection, followed by delay in ejection of the remaining LV volume, with the resulting outflow gradient. Another method to demonstrate the severity of LVOT obstruction in hypertrophic obstructive cardiomyopathy (HOCM) patients is to perform a Valsalva maneuver. At the beginning of the Valsalva strain phase, there is an increase in LVEDP and reduced arterial pulse pressure. The LVOT gradient begins to appear. It is most pronounced during the plateau phase and may be dramatic during a PVC in this setting.

Both aortic stenosis and HOCM are associated with systolic outflow obstruction with systolic murmurs. AS can be easily differentiated from HOCM by examining the response to a PVC. A comparison of the post-PVC hemodynamic responses between HOCM and AS is shown in Figure 10.26. In aortic stenosis, the post-PVC hemodynamic tracings show a larger pulse pressure, a consistently slow aortic upstroke of fixed valve obstruction, and no change in the aortic waveform, all in contrast to the HOCM hemodynamics, which show a reduced pulse pressure, brisk aortic pressure upstroke (parallel to LV pressure), and deformation of the aortic waveform with a spike and dome of rapid early ejection with secondary outflow obstruction.

MV Stenosis

Rheumatic mitral stenosis restricts LA outflow, increases LA pressure, and limits cardiac output. Characteristic changes include thickening of the cusps and retraction of the subvalvular apparatus (Fig. 10.27).

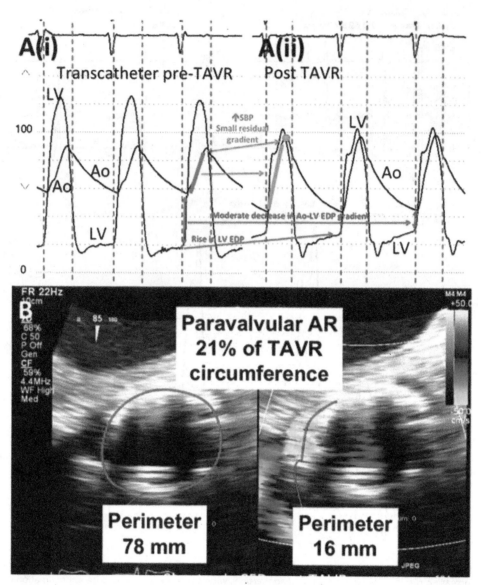

FIGURE 10.21   An illustration of the hemodynamics of a paravalvular leak following a TAVR procedure with an increase in LVEDP and the slope of a diastolic pressure rise. *Lower panel* shows echocardiographic images of Doppler paravalvular leakage. LVEDP, left ventricular end-diastolic pressure; TAVR, transcatheter aortic valve replacement. (Courtesy of Dr. Raj Makkar.)

Figure 10.28 is a schematic representation of LV, aortic, and LA pressures, showing normal relationships and alterations with mild and severe mitral stenosis (MS). Corresponding classic auscultatory signs of MS are shown at the bottom. Compared with mild MS, with severe MS the higher left atrial "v" wave causes earlier pressure crossover and earlier MV opening, leading to a shorter time interval between AV closure and the opening snap (OS). The higher left atrial EDP with severe MS also results in later closure of the MV. With severe MS, the diastolic rumble becomes longer and there is accentuation of the pulmonic component (P_2) of the second heart sound (S_2) in relation to the aortic component (A_2).

The hemodynamic assessment of the stenotic MV is performed initially with combined left and right heart hemodynamics, most often using a PCW pressure, compared to a simultaneous LV pressure at rest. In patients with borderline hemodynamic results, measurements should be made during exercise (e.g., arm lifting with weights). The PCW pressure often overestimates LA pressure in patients with

mitral stenosis or prosthetic MVs due to delayed and poor pressure transmission, making correct alignment of pressure tracings difficult.

For patients with elevated PCW pressure and suspected MV abnormalities, use of direct LA pressure by transseptal puncture is the most accurate method and should be used prior to MV surgery or valvuloplasty. **Figure 10.29** shows a PCW pressure (red) and LA pressure (orange) demonstrating different timing of v waves and a higher mean for PCW, which would falsely increase MV gradient measurement. Nevertheless, if the PCW/LV pressure tracings show no significant gradients, transseptal catheterization is often unnecessary.

If the medical treatment for mitral stenosis is ineffective, then percutaneous balloon mitral valvuloplasty (PBMV) is indicated. **Figure 10.30** illustrates a case of mitral stenosis treated with PBMV. Successful procedures produce an average decrease in MV gradient of approximately 50% to 75% of the baseline gradient, and a doubling of the MV area: on average, about 2 cm^2.

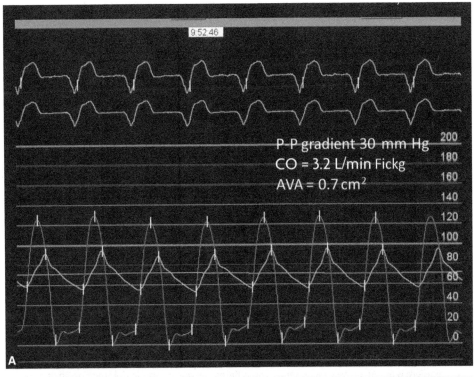

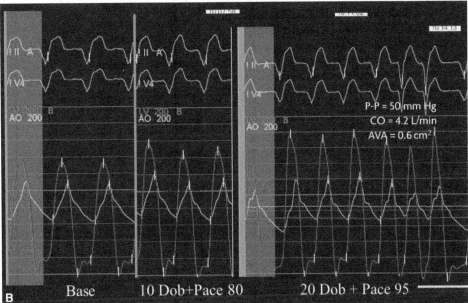

FIGURE 10.22 **A:** Patient with low pressure gradient AS and reduced LVEF (25%). There is no CAD. The peak-to-peak (P-P) gradient is 30 mm Hg with a cardiac output (CO) of 3.2 L/min Fick, resulting in aortic valve area (AVA) of 0.7 cm². Is this fixed AS or cardiomyopathy? **B:** Dobutamine challenge in patient with low-gradient/low-flow AS. After infusion of dobutamine 10 μg/min and 20 μg/min with ventricular pacing, the P-P gradient is now 50 mm Hg, CO is 4.2 L/min, and AVA is 0.6 cm² AS is fixed despite increased CO. Valve replacement is appropriate. AS, aortic stenosis; LVEF, left ventricular ejection fraction.

Mitral Regurgitation

Mitral regurgitation is the result of the inability to maintain leaflet coaptation during systole. The mitral apparatus consists of the annulus, the anterior and posterior leaflets, and their tethers of the thin chordae tendinae attached to the papillary muscles. Failure of any of these structures can result in malcoaptation of the mitral leaflets and valvular regurgitation.

Acute mitral regurgitation (MR) produced by stretching or tearing of leaflets is characterized by a new and large "v" wave (Fig. 10.31). A new large "v" wave after PBMV is MR until proven otherwise. Nevertheless, the quality of "v" waves depends upon the compliance of the chamber, and large "v" waves can be seen in absence of MR (Fig. 10.32). The PCW "v" wave is thus of limited value in the accurate identification of true mitral regurgitation. Figure 10.33 shows LA hemodynamics, with a large "v" wave due to a paravalvular mitral prosthetic valve leak.

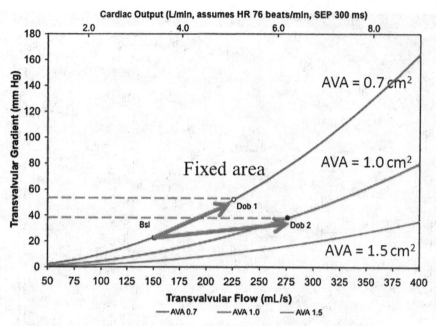

FIGURE 10.23 Shows the plot of the relationship between mean gradient (y-axis) and transvalvular flow (x-axis, *bottom*) according to the Gorlin formula for three different values of AVA (0.7, 1.0, and 1.5 cm²). Cardiac output (x-axis, *top*) is also shown, assuming a heart rate of 75 beats/min and a systolic ejection period of 300 ms. At low transvalvular flows, the mean gradient is low at all three valve areas. Two different responses to the dobutamine challenge are illustrated for a hypothetical patient (Bsl) with a baseline flow of 150 mL/s, mean gradient of 23 mm Hg, and calculated AVA 0.7 cm². In one scenario (dob 1), flow increases to 225 mL/s, mean gradient increases to 52 mm Hg, and AVA remains 0.7 cm², consistent with fixed AS. In a second scenario, flow increases to 275 mL/s, mean gradient increases to 38 mm Hg, and AVA increases to 1.0 cm². This patient has changed to a different curve, consistent with relative or pseudo-AS. AS, aortic stenosis; AVA, aortic valve area; HR indicates heart rate; SEP, systolic ejection period. (From: Grayburn PA. Assessment of low-gradient aortic stenosis with dobutamine. *Circulation.* 2006;113:604–606.)

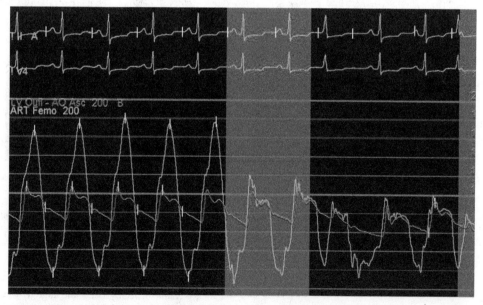

FIGURE 10.24 Hemodynamic left ventricular (*blue*) and aortic (*red*) pressure tracings in patient with hypertrophic cardiomyopathy. The LV catheter is pullback from distal LV (*left side*) to subaortic position (*right side*). Note the reduction in LV-Ao pressure gradient while still recording LV pressure. In addition, one can appreciate the configuration of the aortic pressure with a typical "spike and dome" appearance. LV, left ventricular.

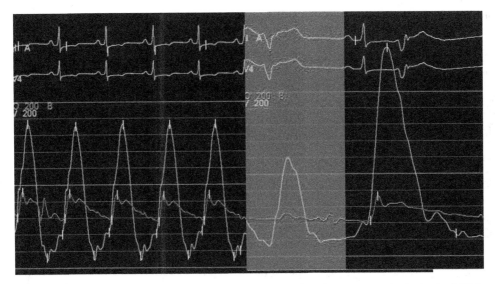

FIGURE 10.25 Hemodynamics in a patient with hypertrophic obstructive cardiomyopathy (HCM). LV (*blue*) and aortic (*red*) pressure tracings demonstrate the vertical upstroke of aortic pressure with a rapid early ejection and mid systolic delay (*spike and dome pattern*). Following a PVC (*shaded bar*), the post-PVC reduction of the aortic pulse pressure is evident (called the Brockenbrough Braunwald Morrow sign) with a marked increase in the LVOT pressure gradient. LVOT, left ventricular outflow tract; PVC, premature ventricular contraction.

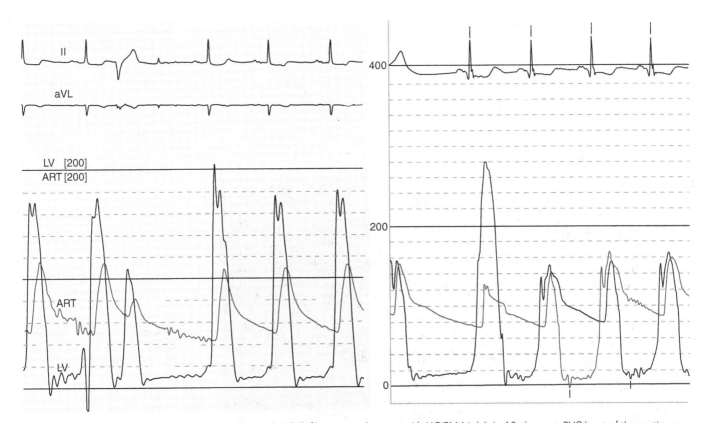

FIGURE 10.26 Hemodynamic tracings in a patient with AS (*left*) compared to one with HOCM (*right*). In AS, the post-PVC beat of the aortic pressure wave has a slow upstroke, wide pulse pressure, and the same waveform as normal beats. In HOCM, the post-PVC aortic pressure has a vertical upstroke, a narrow pulse pressure, and the typical alteration of the aortic pressure of obstruction with the spike and dome contour. AS, aortic stenosis; HOCM, hypertrophic obstructive cardiomyopathy; PVC, premature ventricular contraction.

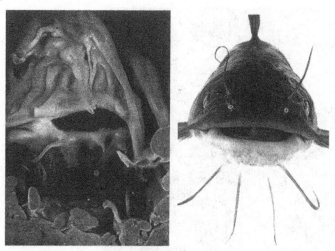

FIGURE 10.27 Rheumatic mitral stenosis with thickening of the cusps and retraction of the subvalvular apparatus. The right side is a fish-mouth shape similar to that of the mitral stenotic valve.

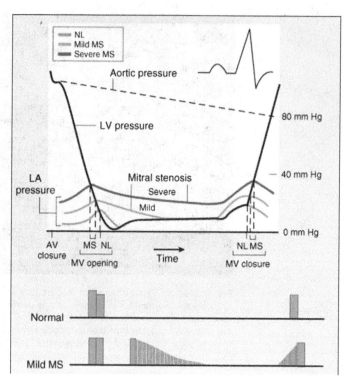

FIGURE 10.28 Schematic representation of the left ventricular (LV), aortic, and left atrial (LA) pressures, showing normal relationships and alterations with mild and severe mitral stenosis (MS). Corresponding classic auscultatory signs of MS are shown at the bottom. Compared to mild MS, severe MS has a higher left atrial "v" wave, causing earlier pressure crossover and an earlier mitral valve (MV) opening, leading to a shorter time interval between aortic valve (AV) closure and the opening snap (OS). The higher left atrial end-diastolic pressure with severe MS also results in later closure of the mitral valve. With severe MS, the diastolic rumble becomes longer and there is accentuation of the pulmonic component (P₂) of the second heart sound (S₂) in relation to the aortic component (A₂).

Constrictive and Restrictive Cardiac Hemodynamics

Dyspnea, elevated neck veins, ascites, and pedal edema suggest right-sided heart failure with a potential differential diagnosis that includes both restrictive and constrictive pathophysiologic diseases. The traditional hemodynamic criteria for the diagnosis of constrictive pericardial disease have been based largely on diastolic equalization of ventricular pressures, with a characteristic abrupt cessation of ventricular filling early in diastole and restriction of further filling demonstrated by a plateau of diastolic left and right ventricular pressure (Fig. 10.34). Dynamic respiratory changes in right and left ventricular pressures in patients with constrictive

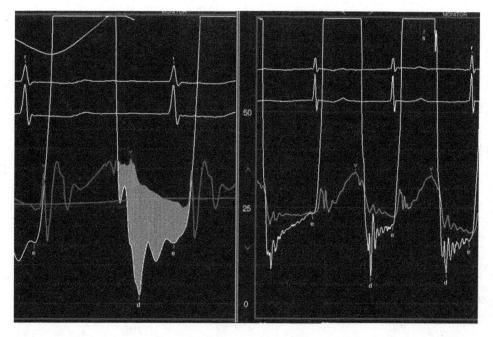

FIGURE 10.29 Hemodynamic tracings in a patient with mitral stenosis. The LV and PCW (left side) tracings show a large mitral valve gradient of approximately 20 mm Hg (pressure scale is 0–50 mm Hg). On the right panel, LV and directly measured LA pressures (via transseptal approach) show higher fidelity pressure wave forms and marked reduction in the mitral pressure gradient (6 mm Hg). Note the "c" notch and "v" wave are distinct compared to the wave forms on the PCW. PCW does not always equal LA. LA, left atrial; LV, left ventricular; PCW, pulmonary capillary wedge.

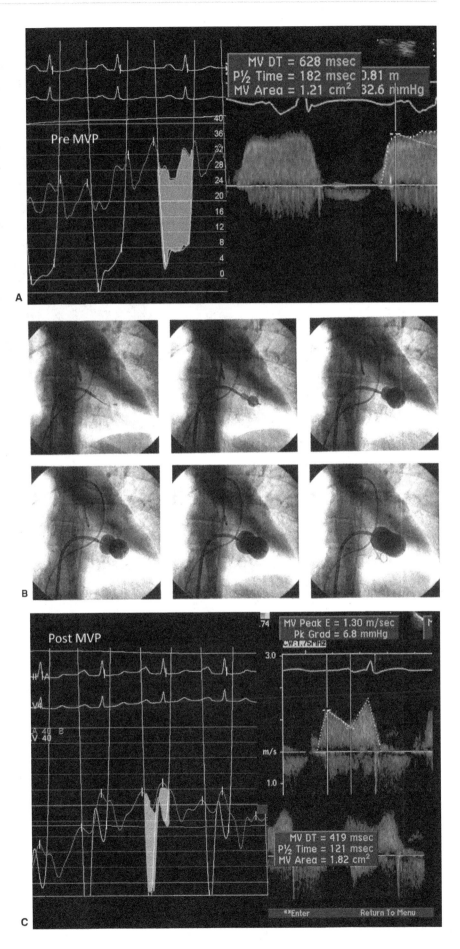

FIGURE 10.30 A: Hemodynamics and Doppler echo findings before mitral valve balloon valvuloplasty (PMBV). **Left:** LV (*blue tracing*) and LA (*red tracing*) demonstrate a large diastolic mitral valve gradient (*yellow*). **Right:** The Doppler velocity across the mitral valve shows a mitral valve area of 1.21 cm² with a 32-mm-Hg gradient. After evaluation by 2D echo and TEE, the results were a low Wilken's score (<8) and no LA thrombus; mitral balloon valvuloplasty was performed. **B:** Cine frames of Inoue balloon expansion during Inoue mitral balloon valvuloplasty. Hemodynamics after PBMV are shown in **C. C:** Hemodynamic and Doppler echo findings after PMBV. **Left:** LV and LA pressures show marked reduction of diastolic mitral gradient. Doppler flow after the procedure likewise shows reduced peak transvalvular velocities, an improved pressure half time, and an increased mitral valve area of 1.82 cm². LA, left atrial; LV, left ventricular; PBMV, percutaneous balloon mitral valvuloplasty; TEE, transesophageal echocardiograms.

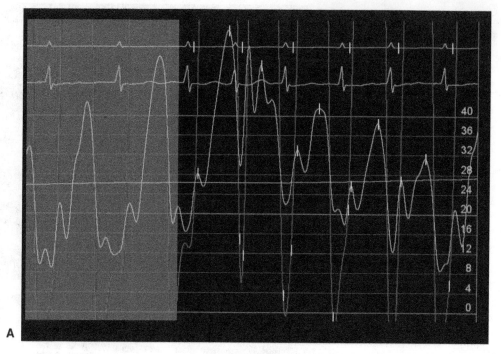

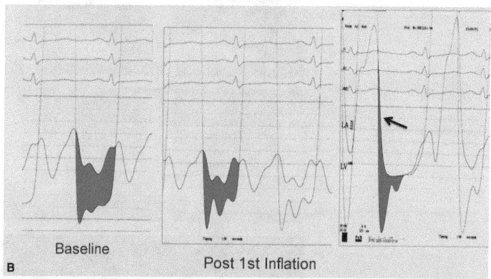

Baseline

Post 1st Inflation

B

FIGURE 10.31 Transesophageal echocardiogram showed 1 small anterolateral and a larger posteromedial leak **(A,)**. Under 3-dimensional echocardiographic guidance **(B)**, 3 Amplatzer vascular plugs (Plymouth, MN, USA) were deployed to close the posteromedial leak, and 1 additional device was placed in the antero-lateral leak (C). The procedure was uncomplicated, with marked reduction in paravalvular prosthetic mitral regurgitation (D). There was significant hemodynamic (E and F) and clinical improvement post-procedure. Percutaneous device closure is an effective procedure for the treatment of clinically significant paravalvular prosthetic regurgitation (1). AO, aorta; LA, left atrium; LAA, left atrial appendage; LV, left ventricle. (Courtesy of Vuyisile T. Nkomo, Sorin V. Pislaru, Paul Sorajja and Allison K. Cabalka, citation is unchange.)

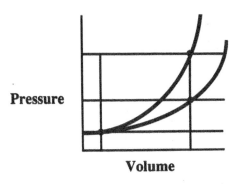

FIGURE 10.32 Pressure volume relationship can produce different compliance curves. This graph illustrates the effect of high and lower compliance on a "v" wave. A highly compliant system (*lower curve*) produces little pressure change as volume increases, whereas a low compliant or "stiff" (*top curve*) system produces large pressure increases during similar volume infusion.

pericarditis, as proposed by Hurrell et al. (14), have the highest sensitivity and specificity for true constrictive pericardial disease. (Table 10.1).

With constrictive physiology, upon inspiration there is a decrease in the early transmitral gradient, demonstrating a dissociation of the intrathoracic and intracardiac pressures. The right and left ventricular systolic pressures move *discordantly* due to ventricular interdependence (i.e., when the RV fills, the LV volume decreases, and vice versa). With inspiration, the left ventricular systolic pressure decreases and the right ventricular systolic pressure increases. Figure 10.35 shows an example of normal RV/LV dynamic pressure responses in a normal patient (left) and the discordant systolic pressure during respiration in a patient with constrictive pericardial disease (right).

In restrictive cardiomyopathy, the RV/LV systolic pressures move together during respiration because ventricular volumes can expand together (Fig. 10.36).

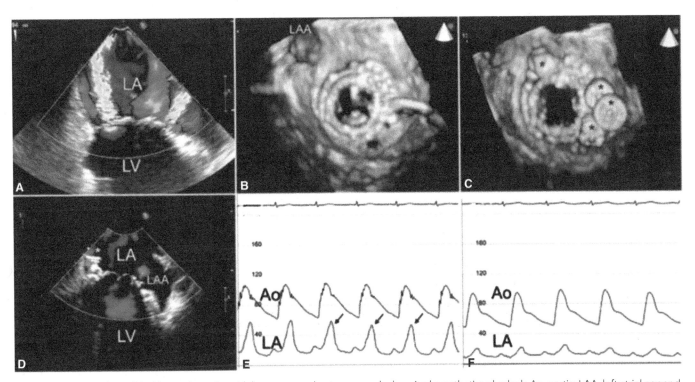

FIGURE 10.33 Left atrial (LA) hemodynamics with large v wave due to a paravalvular mitral prosthetic valve leak. Ao, aortic; LAA, left atrial appendage; LV, left ventricular. (From: Sorajja P, et al. Plugged! *J Am Coll Cardiol*. 2013;61(3):356. doi:10.1016/j.jacc.2012.05.071.)

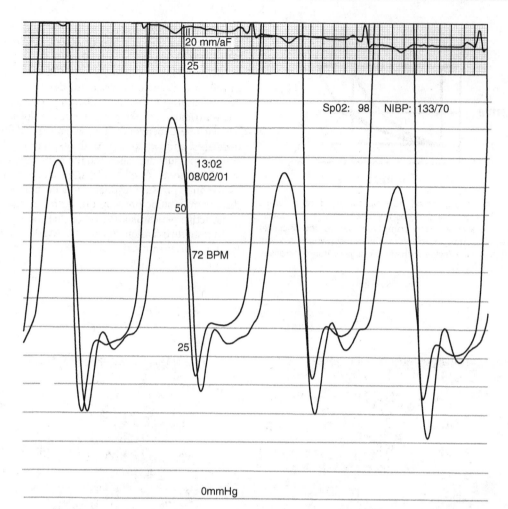

FIGURE 10.34 Hemodynamics of constrictive/restrictive physiology. LV and RV tracings (0–40 mm Hg scale) show an abrupt cessation of diastolic filling, with a dip and plateau configuration. This pattern is common but not diagnostic for constrictive pericarditis. LV, left ventricular; RV, right ventricular.

TABLE 10.1 Comparison of Traditional and Dynamic Respiratory Criteria for Diagnostic Constrictive Pericarditis

	CRITERIA	SENSITIVITY (%)	SPECIFIC (%)	PPV	NPV
Traditional	LVEDP vs. RVEDP <5	60	38	4	57
	RVEDP vs. RVSP >1/3	93	38	52	89
	PASP <55	93	24	47	25
	Right ventricular free wall >7 mm	93	57	61	92
	Respiratory: Change of right atrial pressure <3 mm Hg	93	48	58	92
Dynamic respiratory factors	Pulmonary capillary wedge versus LV >5 mm Hg	93	81	78	94
	LV/RV interdependence	100	95	94	100

LVEDP – RVEDP, left and right ventricular end-diastolic pressure; RVSP, right ventricular systolic pressure; PASP, pulmonary artery systolic pressure; PPV, positive predictive value; NPV, negative predictive value; RFW, rapid filling wave; RAP, right atrial pressure; PCWP, pulmonary capillary wedge pressure; RV, right ventricular. (From Hurrell et al. Value of dynamic respiratory changes in left and right ventricular pressures for the diagnosis of constrictive pericarditis. *Circulation.* 1996;93:2007–2013.)

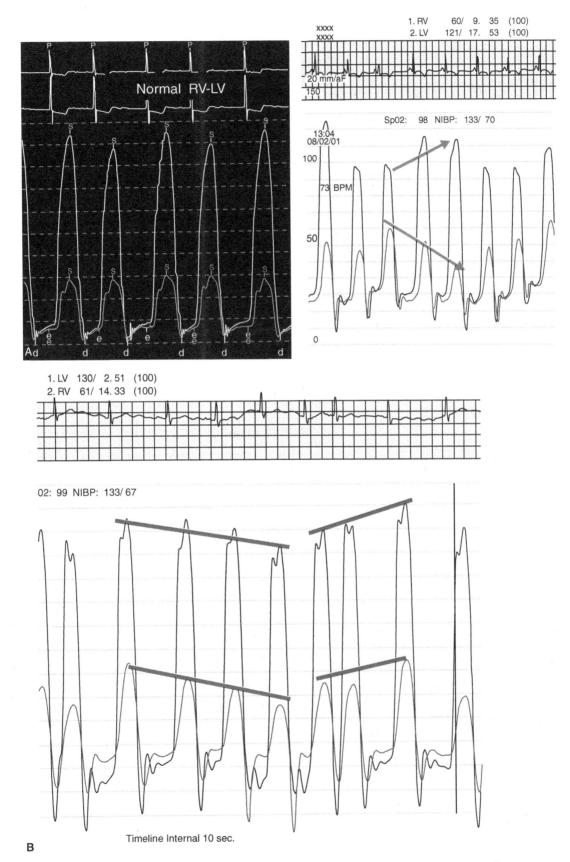

FIGURE 10.35   A: *Left,* normal LV/RV relationship over the respiratory cycle. *Right,* Dynamic respiratory variation of systolic RV and LV pressures demonstrates discordant respiratory motion. The discordant respiratory variation of pressures shown here is diagnostic for constrictive pericardial physiology. **B:** Dynamic respiratory variation of systolic RV and LV pressures demonstrates concordant respiratory motion. The concordant respiratory variation of pressures shown here is diagnostic for restrictive cardiomyopathy. LV, left ventricular; RV, right ventricular.

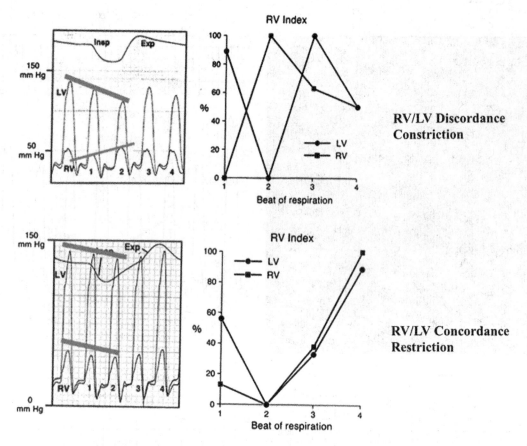

FIGURE 10.36 Dynamic respiratory variation of LV and RV systolic pressures differentiate constrictive from restrictive physiology. **Top:** RV/LV Discordance = Constriction. **Bottom:** RV/LV Concordance = Restriction. LV, left ventricular; RV, right ventricular. (From: Hurrell DG, et al. Value of dynamic respiratory changes in left and right ventricular pressures for the diagnosis of constrictive pericarditis. *Circulation.* 1996;93:2007–2013.)

Cardiac Tamponade

Cardiac tamponade is the most severe form of diastolic dysfunction and is associated with compression of the heart and an inability to fill due to pericardial pressure exceeding intracardiac pressure. Tamponade may occur during or after structural, coronary, or electrophysiologic interventions. A high index of suspicion is critical to rapidly detect and treat this life-threatening condition with pericardiocentesis. Fluid accumulating in the pericardial space produces an elevation of pericardial pressure. The magnitude of pericardial pressure increase depends on the rate of fluid accumulation and the compliance of the pericardium. Compression of the heart, as well as prevention of adequate ventricular filling, reduces SV, cardiac output, arterial pressure, and may rapidly progress to cardiogenic shock and death without intervention. Both tamponade and constriction may be associated with a paradoxical pulse (>10 mm Hg reduction in arterial pressure during inspiration) (Fig. 10.37), low cardiac output, tachycardia, and hypotension. Cardiac tamponade and constrictive pericarditis have important pathophysiologic differences. In constriction, early diastolic filling is very rapid, as the ventricle rapidly recoils after ejection. This results in the characteristic brisk "Y" descent that is almost universally observed. In contrast, elevated pericardial pressure in cardiac tamponade limits filling throughout all of diastole, and the "Y" descent is characteristically blunted. Figure 10.38 illustrates the hemodynamics of cardiac tamponade and its relief after pericardiocentesis.

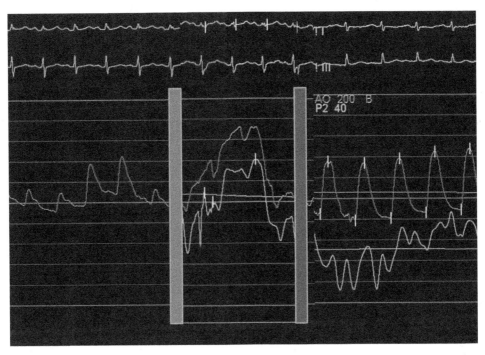

FIGURE 10.37 Hemodynamic findings in cardiac tamponade. **Left:** Aortic pressure (0–200 mm Hg scale) before pericardiocentesis in patient with clinical and echocardiographic findings of tamponade. **Middle:** RA and pericardial pressures (0–40 mm Hg scale) before pericardiocentesis. **Right:** Aortic pressure (0–200 mm Hg scale) and pericardial pressure (0–40 mm Hg scale) after pericardiocentesis. Note restoration of arterial pulse with loss of marked respiratory variance (Pulsus paradoxus) and reduction of pericardial pressure from 22 to 12 mm Hg. RA, right atrial.

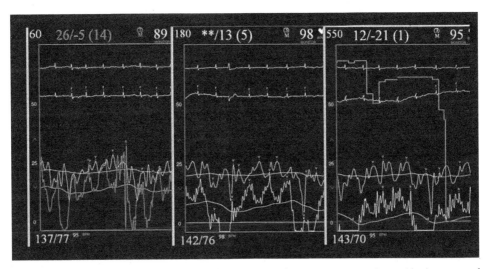

FIGURE 10.38 Hemodynamic tracings during pericardiocentesis in a patient with shortness of breath and pericardial effusion. The presumed cause of dyspnea was tamponade. *Left panel*, baseline hemodynamics. RA pressure is yellow tracing. *Middle panel*, RA and pericardial pressure after 180 mL removed. *Right panel*, pressures after 550 mL fluid removed from pericardium. Nevertheless, the relief of pericardial pressure by pericardiocentesis demonstrated no change in RA pressure. No cardiac tamponade is present. The diagnosis is effusive constrictive pericardial disease with LV dysfunction. LV, left ventricular; RA, right atrial.

Key Points

- The cardiac cycle and pressure—volume loops can be used to assess the effects of interventions on cardiac output (SV) and filling pressures.

- Right hemodynamics and shunt calculations are important to placement of closure devices.

- Left heart hemodynamics are used to identify ventricular function, relaxation, and outflow obstruction due to valvular, subvalvular, or supravalvular lesions.

- Hypertrophic obstructive cardiomyopathy may be confused with aortic stenosis in some patients.

- MV hemodynamics are critical to understand applications of balloon valvuloplasty and mitral clip for regurgitation.

- Pericardial hemodynamics must differentiate among constrictive, restrictive, and tamponade physiology.

- Basic hemodynamics and pressure wave interpretation can be appreciated from review of Wiggers' diagram.

- Valvular heart disease: Pressure waveforms demonstrate transvalvular gradients and identify mechanisms of valve function. HOCM versus AS has unique post-PVC hemodynamic configuration.

- Diastolic dysfunctional hemodynamics: constriction versus restriction.

- Diastolic "dip and plateau" configuration is present in several types of diastolic dysfunction whether due to pericardium or myocardium. The most specific differentiating features of the two disease states involve the dynamic respiratory interaction of left and right ventricular systolic pressure. Concordant respiratory systolic pressure changes are associated with restrictive cardiomyopathy, whereas discordant respiratory pressure changes are associated with constrictive pericardial disease.

References

1. Kern MJ, Lim MJ, Goldstein JA, eds. *Hemodynamic Rounds: Interpretation of Cardiac Pathophysiology from Pressure Waveform Analysis.* 4th ed. Hoboken, NJ: Wiley-Blackwell; 2017.
2. Kern MJ, ed. *The Cardiac Catheterization Handbook.* 6th ed. Philadelphia, PA: Elsevier; 2015.
3. Kern MJ, ed. *Interventional Cardiac Catheterization Handbook.* 4th ed. St Louis, MO: Elsevier; 2017.
4. Moscucci M. *Grossman and Baim's Cardiac Catheterization, Angiography, and Intervention.* 8th ed. Philadelphia, PA: Wolters Kluwer/Lippincott Williams & Wilkins; 2013:223–272.
5. Nishimura RA, Carabello BA. Hemodynamics in the cardiac catheterization laboratory of the 21st century. *Circulation.* 2012;125:2138–2150.
6. Borlaug BA, Kass DA. Invasive hemodynamic assessment in heart failure. *Heart Fail Clin.* 2009;5(2):217–228.
7. Burkhoff D, Mirsky I, Suga H. Assessment of systolic and diastolic ventricular properties via pressure-volume analysis: a guide for clinical, translational, and basic researchers. *Am J Physiol Heart Circ Physiol.* 2005;289(2):H501–H512.
8. Remmelink M, et al. Acute left ventricular dynamic effects of primary percutaneous coronary intervention from occlusion to reperfusion. *J Am Coll Cardiol.* 2009;53(17):1498–1502.
9. Pibarot P, Dumesnil JG, Improving assessment of aortic stenosis. *J Am Coll Cardiol.* 2012;60(3):169–180.
10. Gorlin R, Gorlin SG. Hydraulic formula for calculation of stenotic mitral valve, other cardiac valves, and central circulatory shunts. *Am Heart J.* 1951;41;1–29.
11. Hakki AH, et al. A simplified valve formula for the calculation of stenotic cardiac valve areas. *Circulation.* 1981;63:1050.
12. Ren X. Classic hemodynamic findings of severe aortic regurgitation. *Circulation.* 2012;126:e28–e29.
13. Grayburn PA. Assessment of low-gradient aortic stenosis with dobutamine. *Circulation.* 2006; 113:604–606.
14. Hurrell DG, et al. Value of dynamic respiratory changes in left and right ventricular pressures for the diagnosis of constrictive pericarditis. *Circulation.* 1996;93:2007–2013.

11 Coronary Angiography for PCI

Morton J. Kern, MD, MSCAI, FAHA, FACC and
Arnold H. Seto, MD, MPA, FSCAI, FACC

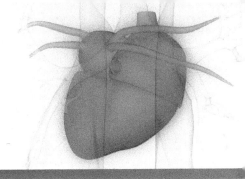

Coronary angiography for percutaneous coronary intervention (PCI) should establish the precise lesion length, morphology, and degree of calcification (or thrombus), as well as the relationship to side branches and their associated ostial involvement with atherosclerosis. Knowledge of optimal angiographic projections will assist in guide catheter selection, visualizing the target vessel course and angle for optimal treatment, the distribution of collateral supply, and estimating the true (maximally vasodilated) dimensions of the PCI artery.

Optimal definition of the ostial and proximal coronary segment is critical to guide PCI catheter selection. Assessment of calcium from angiography is less reliable than from intravascular ultrasound imaging (IVUS), but still serves a useful purpose in determining the need for rotational atherectomy. Coronary angiography defines the risks associated with the procedure and demonstrates a successful intervention; thus, it is of subtantial prognostic value.

For chronic total vessel occlusion (CTO) PCI feasiblity, the distal vessel should be visualized as clearly as possible. For the procedure, this may require the simultaneous injection of collateral supply arteries with cineangiography of sufficient duration to visualize late collateral vessel filling and the length of the occluded segment. A complete understanding of basic angiographic techniques, angulations, and access are necessary to appreciate the approach to PCI that can be found elsewhere (1–4).

Radiation exposure is higher in PCI than diagnostic procedures (5–7). Continued awareness of the inverse square law of radiation propagation will reduce the exposure to patients, operators, and cath lab teams. Obtaining quality images should not necessitate increasing the ordinary procedural radiation exposure to either the patient or catheterization personnel.

Common Angiographic Views for PCI

The nomenclature for angiographic views will be reviewed briefly here, emphasizing the interventionalist's thinking for visualizing anatomy for appropriate revascularization. Classic terminology for angiographic projections with regard to left and right anterior oblique, cranial and caudal angulation, and lateral projections remains as defined in previous discussions of diagnostic coronary angiography.

Anteroposterior Imaging

The image intensifier is directly over the patient, with the beam perpendicular to the patient lying flat on the x-ray table (Figs. 11.1 and 11.2). The anteroposterior (AP) view or shallow right anterior oblique (RAO) displays *the left main coronary artery* in its entire perpendicular length. In this view, the branches of the left anterior descending (LAD) and left circumflex coronary artery branches overlap. In patients with acute coronary syndromes, starting with this view to exclude left main stenosis will facilitate PCI. The AP cranial view is also excellent for visualizing the entire LAD, with

septals moving to the left (on screen) and diagonals to the right, helping wire placement.

Right Anterior Oblique Imaging

The RAO caudal view shows the left main coronary artery bifurcation, with the origin and course of the circumflex/obtuse marginals, ramus intermediate branch, and proximal LAD segment being well seen. The LAD beyond the proximal segment is often obscured by overlapped diagonals. The RAO cranial or AP cranial views are used to open the diagonals along the mid and distal LAD. The diagonal branches are projected upward.

For the right coronary artery (RCA), the RAO view shows the mid RCA and the length of the posterior descending artery and posterolateral branches. patent ductus arteriosus (PDA) septals may show an occluded LAD via collaterals. The posterolateral branches overlap and may be best displayed with cranial angulation.

Left Anterior Oblique (LAO) Imaging

The LAO cranial view shows a foreshortened left main coronary artery and the full course of the LAD. Septal and diagonal branches are separated clearly. The circumflex and marginals are foreshortened and overlapped. Cranial angulation tilts the left main coronary artery down and permits visualization of the LAD/circumflex bifurcation.

For the RCA, the LAO cranial view shows the origin of the artery, its entire length, and the posterior descending artery bifurcation (crux). Cranial angulation tilts the posterior descending artery down to reduce foreshortening.

The LAO caudal view ("spider" view) shows a foreshortened left main coronary artery but excellent visualization of the bifurcation of the circumflex and LAD. Proximal and midportions of the circumflex and the origins of obtuse marginal branches are well seen. The LAD is markedly foreshortened in this view (Fig. 11.3).

A left lateral view shows the mid and distal LAD best. This view is best to see coronary artery bypass graft (CABG) conduit anastomosis to the LAD. The LAD and circumflex are well-separated. Diagonals usually overlap. The course of the (ramus) intermediate branch is also well visualized.

For the RCA, the lateral view also shows the origin (especially in those with more anteriorly oriented orifices) and the mid RCA well. The posterior descending artery and posterolateral branches are foreshortened.

Angulations for Saphenous Bypass Grafts

Coronary artery saphenous vein grafts are visualized in at least two views (LAO and RAO). It is important to show the aortic anastomosis, the body of the graft, and the distal anastomosis. The distal runoff and continued flow or collateral channels are also critical. The graft vessel anastomosis is best seen in the view that depicts the native vessel best (Table 11.1). The graft views can be summarized as follows:

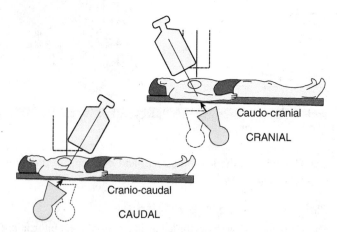

FIGURE 11.1 Nomenclature for angiographic views. (Modified from: Paulin S. Terminology for radiographic projections in cardiac angiography. *Cathet Cardiovasc Diagn.* 1981;7:341.)

1. RCA graft: LAO cranial/RAO, and lateral
2. LAD graft (or internal mammary artery): lateral, RAO cranial, LAO cranial, and AP (the lateral view is especially useful to visualize the anastomosis to the LAD)
3. Circumflex (and obtuse marginals) grafts: LAO and RAO caudal

Angiographic TIMI Classification of Blood Flow

The Thrombolysis in Myocardial Infarction (TIMI) group's system of flow grading has been used to assess, in a qualitative fashion, the degree of perfusion before and after thrombolysis or angioplasty in patients with acute myocardial infarction. **Table 11.2** provides descriptions used to assign TIMI flow grades.

Classification of Distal Angiographic Contrast Runoff

The distal runoff is classified into four stages (also known as TIMI grade):

- Normal distal runoff (TIMI 3)
- Good distal runoff (TIMI 2)
- Poor distal runoff (TIMI 1)
- Absence of distal runoff (TIMI 0).

TIMI flow grades 0 to 3 have become a standard description of coronary blood flow in clinical trials. TIMI grade 3 flows have been associated with improved clinical outcomes.

TIMI Frame Count

Contrast runoff can be performed quantitatively by using cine frame counts. The method uses cineangiography with 6F catheters and filming at 30 frames/s. The number of cine frames from the introduction of dye in the coronary artery to a predetermined distal landmark is counted. The TIMI frame count (TFC) for each major vessel is thus standardized according to specific distal landmarks (8).

Typically, a normal contrast frame count reflecting normal flow is 24 ± 10 frames. The TFC can further be corrected for the length of the LAD. The TFC in the LAD requires normalization or correction for comparison to the two other major arteries. This is called corrected TIMI frame count (CTFC). High TFC (i.e., slow blood flow) may be associated with microvascular dysfunction despite an open epicardial artery. A CTFC of <20

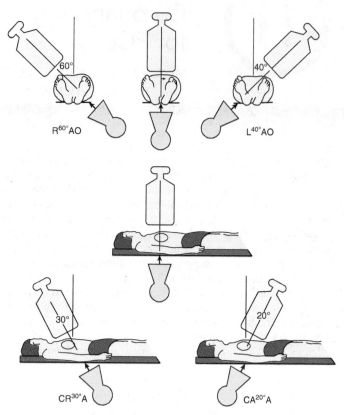

FIGURE 11.2 Diagrammatic view of image intensifier for common angiographic projections.

frames has been associated with a low risk for adverse events in patients following myocardial infarction. The TFC method provides valuable information relative to clinical response after coronary intervention.

TIMI Myocardial Blush Grades (MBGs)

Washout of contrast from the microvasculature in the acute infarction patient is coupled to prognosis. Improved blush scores indicate a larger amount of myocardial salvage, while failure to improve the MBG suggests microvascular dysfunction or occlusion. The MBG scoring system is showing in Table 11.2.

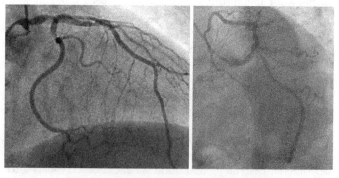

FIGURE 11.3 Frame from cineangiogram showing LM narrowing in RAO (*left*) and LAO caudal (*right*). Ostial CFX was not well seen until LAO caudal was reviewed. CFX, circumflex artery; LAO, left anterior oblique; LM, left main; RAO, right anterior oblique.

TABLE 11.1 Recommended "Key" Angiographic View for Specific Coronary Artery Segments

CORONARY SEGMENT	ORIGIN/BIFURCATION	COURSE/BODY
Left main	AP	AP
	LAO cranial	LAO cranial
	LAO caudal[a]	
Proximal LAD	LAO cranial	LAO cranial
	RAO caudal	RAO caudal
Mid LAD	LAD cranial	
	RAO cranial	
	Lateral	
Distal LAD	AP	
	RAO cranial	
	Lateral	
Diagonal	LAO cranial	RAO cranial, caudal, or straight
	RAO cranial	
Proximal circumflex	RAO caudal	LAO caudal
	LAO caudal	
Intermediate	RAO caudal	RAO caudal
	LAO caudal	Lateral
Obtuse marginal	RAO caudal	RAO caudal
	LAO caudal	
	RAO cranial (distal marginals)	
Proximal RCA	LAO	
	Lateral	
Mid RCA	LAO	LAO
	Lateral	Lateral
	RAO	RAO
Distal RCA	LAO cranial	LAO cranial
	Lateral	Lateral
PDA	LAO cranial	RAO
Posterolateral	LAO cranial	RAO cranial
	RAO cranial	RAO cranial

AP, anteroposterior; LAD, left anterior descending artery; LAO, left anterior oblique; PDA, posterior descending artery (from RCA); RAO, right anterior oblique; RCA, right coronary artery.
[a]Horizontal hearts.
Adapted from: Kern MJ, ed. *The Cardiac Catheterization Handbook*. St Louis, MO: Mosby, 1995:286.

Angiographic Classification of Collateral Flow

Collateral flow can be seen and classified angiographically. The late opacification of a totally or subtotally (99%) occluded vessel through antegrade or retrograde channels will assist in correct guidewire placement, lesion localization, and a successful procedure. The collateral circulation is graded angiographically, as established by Rentrop:

- Grade 0: No collateral branches seen.
- Grade 1: Very weak (ghostlike) opacification.
- Grade 2: Opacified segment is less dense than the source vessel and filling slowly.
- Grade 3: Opacified segment is as dense as the source vessel and filling rapidly.

Collateral visualization may help establish the size of the recipient vessel for the purposes of selecting an appropriately sized balloon, but may underestimate the true size of the vessel because it is underpressurized. Determining whether the collateral circulation is ipsilateral (e.g., proximal RCA to distal RCA collateral supply) or contralateral (e.g., circumflex to distal RCA collateral supply) and exactly which region will be affected should collateral supply be disrupted is important to be able to gauge procedural risk. Grade 0 and 1 collaterals provide minimal protection from ischemia, whereas Grade 2 and 3 collaterals may be sufficient to prevent angina.

Assessment of Coronary Stenoses

The degree of an angiographic narrowing (stenosis) is reported as the estimated percentage lumen reduction of the most severely narrowed segment compared to the adjacent angiographically normal vessel segment, as seen in the x-ray projection that creates the most severely narrowed appearance. Because the operator uses visual estimations, an exact evaluation is impossible. There is a ±20% variation between readings of two or more experienced angiographers. Stenosis severity alone should not always be assumed to be associated with abnormal physiology (flow) and ischemia.

Moreover, coronary artery disease is a diffuse process and thus minimal luminal irregularities on angiography may represent significant, albeit non-obstructive, coronary artery disease (CAD) at the time of angiography. The stenotic segment lumen is compared with a nearby lumen that does not appear to be obstructed but that may have diffuse atherosclerotic disease. This explains why postmortem examinations, as well as IVUS, describe much more plaque than is seen on angiography (Fig. 11.4). Because coronary arteries normally taper as they travel to the apex, proximal segments are always larger than distal segments, often explaining the large disparity between several observers' estimates of stenosis severity. *Area stenosis* is always greater than *diameter stenosis* and assumes the lumen is circular, whereas the lumen is usually eccentric. Assessment of the physiologic impact of a coronary stenosis to produce ischemia requires objective evidence acquired either from stress testing or fractional flow reserve (FFR) measurement.

Quantitative Coronary Angiography

The degree of coronary stenosis reported from the cineangiogram in clinical practice is a visual estimation of the percentage of diameter narrowing. While widely applicable in clinical practice, visual assessment is inadequate for PCI research studies. Quantitative methodologies use digital calipers or automated or manual edge detection systems. Densitometric analysis with digital angiography also provides quantitative lesion measurements.

Coronary Lesion Descriptions for PCI

There are at least three different major classifications of lesion characteristics (Table 11.3), which were derived from large studies in which the characteristics of the lesions were associated with different clinical outcomes and used to assess the risk for adverse cardiac events in the performance of PCI.

General characteristics of the lesion and of the artery proximal to the lesion are as follows:

TABLE 11.2 Thrombolysis in Myocardial Infarction (TIMI) Flow: Grade and Blush Scores

TIMI FLOW GRADE	DESCRIPTION
Grade 3 (complete reperfusion)	Anterograde flow into the terminal coronary artery segment through a stenosis is as prompt as anterograde flow into a comparable segment proximal to the stenosis. Contrast material clears as rapidly from the distal segment as from an uninvolved, more proximal segment.
Grade 2 (partial reperfusion)	Contrast material flows through the stenosis to opacify the terminal artery segment. Nevertheless, contrast enters the terminal segment perceptibly more slowly than more proximal segments. Alternatively, contrast material clears from a segment distal to a stenosis noticeably more slowly than from a comparable segment not preceded by a significant stenosis.
Grade 1 (penetration with minimal perfusion)	A small amount of contrast flows through the stenosis, but fails to fully opacify the artery beyond.
Grade 0 (no perfusion)	There is no contrast flow through the stenosis.

Myocardial Blush Grade

0 No myocardial blush or contrast density. Myocardial blush persisted ("staining").
1 Minimal myocardial blush or contrast density.
2 Moderate myocardial blush or contrast density but less than that obtained during angiography of a contralateral or ipsilateral noninfarct-related coronary artery.
3 Normal myocardial blush or contrast density, comparable with that obtained during angiography of a contralateral or ipsilateral noninfarct-related coronary artery.

Modified from: Sheehan F, et al. The effect of intravenous thrombolytic therapy on left ventricular function: a report on tissue-type plasminogen activator and streptokinase from the Thrombolysis in Myocardial Infarction (TIMI) Phase I Trial. *Circulation.* 1987;72:817–829.

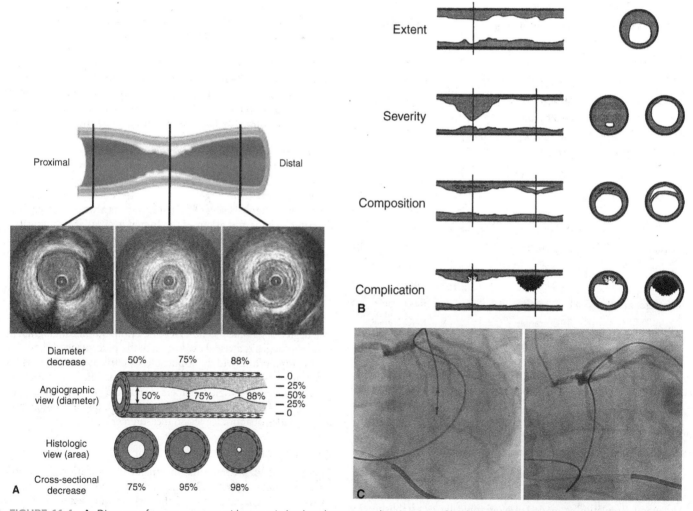

FIGURE 11.4   A: Diagram of coronary artery with stenosis (*top*) and corresponding intravascular ultrasound (IVUS) images demonstrating diffuse nature of coronary artery disease. The percent narrowing is compared only to the "normal" appearing angiographic lumen, which may not be normal at all. **B:** Characteristics of different angiographic lesions. **C:** Frame from cineangiogram showing clot in left main segment as lucent filling defect. View best seen was RAO caudal. RAO, right anterior oblique.

TABLE 11.3 Major Classifications of Lesion Characteristics (see attached table)

ACC/AHA LESION-SPECIFIC CHARACTERISTICS		
TYPE A **LOW RISK**	**TYPE B** **MEDIUM RISK**	**TYPE C** **HIGH RISK**
Discrete (<10 mm length) Concentric Readily accessible Non-angulated segment <45 degrees Smooth contour Little or no calcification Less than totally occlusive Not ostial in location No major branch involvement Absence of thrombus	Tubular (10–20 mm length) Eccentric Moderate tortuosity of proximal segment Moderately angulated segment, 45–90 degrees Irregular contour Moderate to heavy calcification Ostial in location Bifurcation lesions requiring double guidewires Some thrombus present Total occlusion <3 months old	Diffuse (length >2 cm) Excessive tortuosity of proximal segment Extremely angulated segments >90 degrees Total occlusions >3 months old ± bridging collaterals Inability to protect major side branches Degenerated vein grafts with friable lesions
Procedure success rate 92% Complication rate 2%	Procedure success rate 76% Complication rate 10%	Procedure success rate 61% Complication rate 21%

Note: If more than two medium-risk factors are present, lesion is classified as type B2 and is considered complex.
Adapted from: National Cardiovascular Disease Registry Cath PCI Registry v4.3.1 Coder's Data Dictionary, 2008.

SCAI LESION-SPECIFIC CHARACTERISTICS			
TYPE I	**TYPE II**	**TYPE III**	**TYPE IV**
Patent and does not meet criteria for ACC/AHA type C lesion	Patent and meets any criteria for type C lesion	Occluded and does not meet any criteria for type C lesion	Occluded and meets any criteria for type C lesion
Procedure success rate 98% Complication rate 2.4%	Procedure success rate 94% Complication rate 5.1%	Procedure success rate 91% Complication rate 9.8%	Procedure success rate 80% Complication rate 10.1%

Note: Major complications were the composite of in-hospital death, acute myocardial infarction, emergency angioplasty, or emergency coronary artery bypass surgery. Lesion success was defined as a >20% decrease in stenosis, with a residual stenosis of <50%.
Adapted from: Krone RJ, Shaw RE, Klein LW, et al. Evaluation of the American College of Cardiology/American Heart Association and the Society for Coronary Angiography and Interventions lesion classification system in the current stent era of coronary interventions (from the ACC-National Cardiovascular Data Registry). *Am J Cardiol.* 2003;92:389–394.

ELLIS LESION-SPECIFIC CLASSIFICATION			
CLASS I **LOW RISK**	**CLASS II** **MODERATE RISK**	**CLASS III** **HIGH RISK**	**CLASS IV** **HIGHEST RISK**
No risk factors	1–2 moderate correlates and the absence of strong correlates	≥3 moderate correlates and the absence of strong correlates	Either of the strongest correlates
Complication rate 2.1%	Complication rate 3.4%	Complication rate 8.2%	Complication rate 12.7%

Moderately strong correlates:
Length ≥10 mm
Lumen irregularity
Large filling defect
Calcium + angle ≥45 degrees
Eccentric
Severe calcification
SVG age ≥10 years

Strongest correlates:
Non-chronic total occlusion
Degenerated SVG

Note: Complication defined as death, myocardial infarction, or emergent coronary artery bypass grafting.
SVG, Saphenous vein graft.
Adapted from: Ellis SG, et al. Relation between lesion characteristics and risk with percutaneous intervention in the stent and glycoprotein IIb/IIIa era—an analysis of results from 10,907 lesions and proposal for new classification scheme. *Circulation.* 1999;100:1971–1976.

1. Tortuosity:

None/mild = straight proximal segment or only one bend of ≥60 degrees.
Moderate = two bends of 60 degrees or more proximal to the lesion.
Severe = three or more bends of 60 degrees or more proximal to the lesion.

2. Arterial calcification:

Light = proximal artery wall calcification (not necessarily the lesion) seen as thin line(s).
Heavy = easily seen calcification.

3. Arrangement of the lesion(s):

Tandem = two lesions separated by one balloon length (i.e., both lesions can be covered during a single balloon inflation).
Sequential = two lesions located at a distance longer than the balloon

4. Length:

Discrete = <10 mm in length.
Tubular = 10 to 20 mm in length.
Diffuse = >20 mm in length.

5. Eccentricity:

Concentric = lumen axis is located along the long axis of the artery or on either side of it, but by no more than 25% of the normal arterial diameter.

6. Contour: Smooth, irregular, or ulcerated
7. Thrombus:

Definite = intraluminal, round filling defect, visible in two views, largely separated from the vessel wall and/or documentation of embolization of this material.
Possible = other filling defects not associated with calcification, lesion haziness, irregularity with ill-defined borders, intraluminal staining at the total occlusion site.

The SYNTAX Score

Angiographic lesion quantification for PCI risk relative to CABG risk was reported in 2009 by the SYNTAX trial, which compared multivessel PCI (including patients with left main narrowings) to CABG surgery (9–11). The SYNTAX score is an angiographic grading tool used in the trial to stratify the complexity of coronary artery disease encountered. The results of this randomized study demonstrated that patients who had high SYNTAX scores (>34) did better with CABG compared to PCI than those with lower SYNTAX scores, in whom PCI had similar major adverse cardiac events with lower stroke rates.

The SYNTAX score is the sum of the points assigned to each individual coronary lesion with >50% diameter narrowing in vessels >1.5 mm diameter. The coronary tree is divided into 16 segments according to the American Heart Association (AHA) classification (Fig. 11.5A and Table 11.4). Each segment is given a score of 1 or 2 based on the presence of disease, and this score is then weighted based on the amount of myocardium at risk, with values ranging from 3.5 for the proximal LAD artery to 5.0 for the left main, and 0.5 for smaller branches. Branches <1.5 mm in diameter, despite having severe lesions, are not included in the SYNTAX score. The percent diameter stenosis is not a consideration in the SYNTAX score, only the presence of a stenosis from 50%–99% diameter, <50% diameter narrowing or the total occlusion. A multiplication factor of 2 is used for non-occlusive lesions, while 5 is used for occlusive lesions, reflecting the difficulty of PCI.

Table 11.4 summarizes the SYNTAX grade categories. A computerized algorithm is then queried and a summed value is produced. The SYNTAX score is a useful differentiator for the outcome of patients undergoing multivessel PCI. The SYNTAX scores can be divided into three tertiles. High scores have the worst prognosis for revascularization with PCI compared to CABG surgery. Equivalent or superior outcomes for percutaneous intervention were noted in comparison to CABG surgery for patients in the lowest two tertiles (Figs. 11.5 and 11.6). The best discriminating feature of the SYNTAX score was between the lowest and highest tertiles of grading.

Radiographic Contrast Media for PCI

The contrast material is selected from several commercially available solutions with varying features of osmolarity, viscosity, and sodium content found to be appropriate for the specific procedure to be conducted. The most common contrast media for PCI is non-ionic, low-osmolar contrast agents because of safety, patient tolerance, and cost. Selection of a specific non-ionic, low-osmolar contrast agent for the particular interventional procedure is, to a large extent, a matter of personal preference. Iso-osmolar agents (iodixanol) may be better tolerated in peripheral vascular procedures and in patients with prior contrast reactions, but carry an equal risk of contrast nephropathy.

Peripheral Vascular Angiography

Renal Arteriography

Non-selective renal arteriography (e.g., aortic flush) is used to evaluate the renal artery origins and vasculature (12). The origins of the arteries usually arise at the L1 vertebra (just below the T12 ribs). Selective renal arterial injections provide the most detail. The LAO projection often provides the best view of the renal artery ostia in a majority of patients. Acutely angled origins of the renal artery may require specially shaped catheters or an upper extremity arterial approach. Atherosclerotic disease of the renal artery usually involves the proximal one-third of the renal artery and is seldom present without abdominal atherosclerotic plaques.

TABLE 11.4 The SYNTAX Score Algorithm

1. Dominance
2. Number of lesions
3. Segments involved per lesion, with lesion characteristics
4. Total occlusions with subtotal occlusions:
   a. Number of segments
   b. Age of total occlusions
   c. Blunt stumps
   d. Bridging collaterals
   e. First segment beyond occlusion visible by antegrade or retrograde filling
   f. Side branch involvement
5. Trifurcation, number of segments diseased
6. Bifurcation type and angulation
7. Aorto-ostial lesion
8. Severe tortuosity
9. Lesion length
10. Heavy calcification
11. Thrombus
12. Diffuse disease, with number of segments

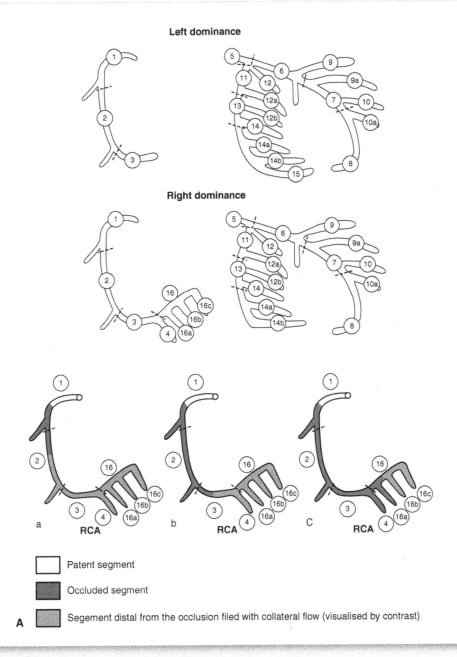

Definition of the coronary tree segments

1. RCA proximal: From the ostium to one half the distance to the acute margin of the heart.
2. RCA mid: From the end of the first segment to the acute margin of the heart.
3. RCA distal: From the acute margin of the heart to the origin of the posterior descending artery.
4. Posterior descending artery: Running in the posterior interventricular groove.
5. Left main: From the ostium of the LCA through bifurcation into the left anterior descending and left circumflex branches.
6. LAD proximal: Proximal to and including first major septal branch.
7. LAD mid: LAD immediately distal to origin of first septal branch and extending to the point where LAD forms an angle (RAO view). If this angle is not identifiable, this segment ends at one half the distance from the first septal to the apex of the heart.
8. LAD apical: Terminal portion of LAD, beginning at the end of the previous segment and extending to or beyond the apex.
9. First diagonal: The first diagonal originating from segment 6 or 7.
9a. First diagonal a: Additional first diagonal originating from segment 6 or 7, before segment 8.
10. Second diagonal: Originating from segment 8 or the transition between segment 7 and 8.
10a. Second diagonal a: Additional second diagonal originating from segment 8.
11. Proximal circumflex artery: Main stem of the circumflex, from its origin of the left main, and including the origin of its first obtuse marginal branch.

FIGURE 11.5 A: SYNTAX diagram. **B:** An example of the SYNTAX score and the specific angiographic anatomy. LAD, left anterior descending; LM, left main; RCA, right coronary artery.

12. Intermediate/anterolateral artery: Branch from the trifurcating left main other than the proximal LAD or LCX. It belongs to the circumflex territory.
12a. Obtuse marginal a: First side branch of the circumflex, running in general to the area of the obtuse margin of the heart.
12b. Obtuse marginal b: Second additional branch of the circumflex, running in the same direction as 12.
13. Distal circumflex artery: The stem of the circumflex distal to the origin of the most distal obtuse marginal branch, and running along the posterior left atrioventricular groove. The caliber may be small or the artery absent.
14. Left posterolateral: Running to the posterolateral surface of the left ventricle. May be absent or a division of obtuse marginal branch.
14a. Left posterolateral a: Distal from 14 and running in the same direction.
14b. Left posterolateral b: Distal from 14 and 14a and running in the same direction.
15. Posterior descending: Most distal part of the dominant left circumflex when present. It gives origin to septal branches. When this artery is present, segment 4 is usually absent. (From: Sianos G, Morel MA, Kappetein AP, et al. The SYNTAX score: an angiographic tool grading the complexity of coronary artery disease. *EuroInterv.* 2005;1:219–227.)
16. Posterolateral branch from RCA: The posterolateral branch originating from the distal coronary artery distal to the crux.
16a. Posterolateral branch from RCA: The first posterolateral branch from segment 16.
16b. Posterolateral branch from RCA: The second posterolateral branch from segment 16.
16c. Posterolateral branch from RCA: The third posterolateral branch from segment 16.

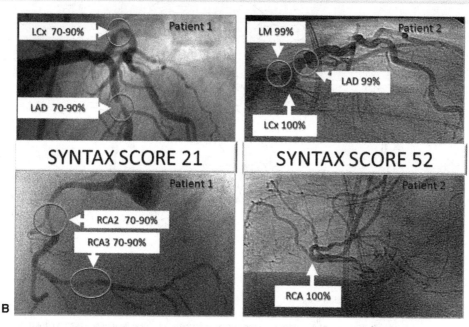

FIGURE 11.5 *(continued)*

Aortography of the thoracic and abdominal aorta is used to assess disease, dissections, and the course of the vessel in order to perform and plan interventions. In high-risk PCI, abdominal aortography with visualization of common iliac arteries is useful prior to insertion of intra-aortic balloon pump (IABP) or left ventricular (LV) support devices, and as part of evaluation for percutaneous aortic valvuloplasty or replacement.

Lower Extremity Angiography

Angiography of the lower extremities is typically performed with small-diameter (5F–6F) catheters and reduced contrast volumes (10–20 mL over 1–2 seconds) which are injected, panning down and following the artery course to the most distal locations. Angulated views may be necessary to open bifurcations and overlying vessels that obscure the vessel origin. Even with the imaging equipment to the side of the patient, the ability to pan down to the ankle should be tested before injection. Digital subtraction techniques are commonly available in modern laboratories, but preclude the use of panning.

Non-ionic, iso-osmolar contrast agents are less painful than other types for peripheral angiography.

The area most frequently involved in peripheral atherosclerotic disease is the distal superficial femoral artery at the abductor canal (**Fig. 11.7**). The calf (tibial) and knee (popliteal) arteries are the next most commonly involved vessels after the superficial femoral artery. Disease in the deep femoral artery (femoral profunda) is rare. Pathways of collateralization are often rich and varied in patients with chronic distal femoral artery disease, especially in total occlusion of the superficial femoral artery that reconstitutes at or below the knee, close to the branching trifurcation of the tibial and deep peroneal arteries. Magnified images focusing on the area of interest are frequently needed.

Angiography of Common Coronary Anomalies

Misdiagnosis of an unsuspected anomalous origin of the coronary arteries is a potential problem for the angiographer. It is an error to assume that a vessel is occluded when it has not been visualized because of

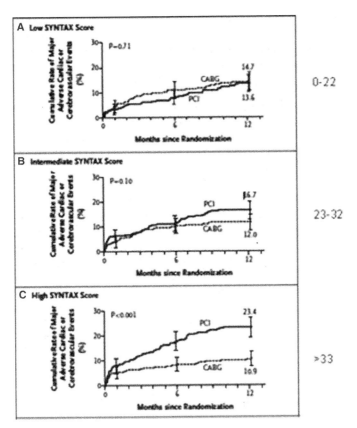

FIGURE 11.6 Outcomes of PCI versus CABG by SYNTAX scores. CABG, coronary artery bypass graft; PCI, percutaneous coronary intervention. (From: Serruys PW, et al. Percutaneous coronary intervention versus coronary artery bypass grafting for severe coronary artery disease [the SYNTAX trial]. *N Engl J Med.* 2009;360:961–972.)

an anomalous origin. Even experienced angiographers have difficulty delineating the true course of the anomalous vessel. While computed tomography angiography is a superior technique to angiography, the diagnosis often is still required in the cath lab. **Figure 11.8** diagrams five pathways of anomalous coronary arteries (13).

Anomalous Origin of the Left Main Coronary Artery from the Right Sinus of Valsalva

For the most common critical coronary anomaly, the left main anomalous origin from the right cusp, a simple "dot and eye" method for determining the proximal course of the anomalous artery from RAO ventriculogram, RAO aortogram, or selective RAO injection is proposed. When the LMCA arises from the right sinus of Valsalva or the proximal RCA, it may follow one of four pathways: (**Fig. 11.9** and **Table 11.5**)

1. Septal course (benign variant). The LMCA runs an intramuscular course through the septum along the floor of the right ventricular (RV) outflow tract.
2. Anterior free wall course (benign variant). The LMCA crosses the anterior free wall of the right ventricle, and then divides at the mid-septum into the LAD and circumflex arteries.
3. Retroaortic course (benign course). The LMCA passes posteriorly around the aortic root to its normal position on the anterior surface of the heart. (It is also seen with anomalous origin of circumflex from the right sinus.)

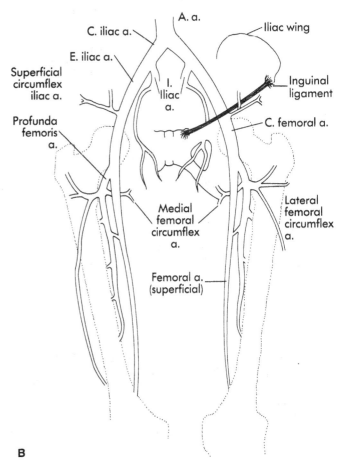

FIGURE 11.7 **A** and **B:** Pelvic and proximal femoral arterial branches. (From: Johnsrude IS, et al. *A Practical Approach to Angiography.* 2nd ed. Boston, MA: Little, Brown & Co., 1987.)

4. Interarterial course (malignant). The LMCA courses between the aorta and PA to its normal position on the anterior surface of the heart. During RAO ventriculography, aortography, or coronary angiography, the LMCA is seen "on end," anterior to the aorta, and appears as a radio-opaque dot to the left of the aortic root.

The interarterial course of the LMCA originating from the right sinus of Valsalva has been associated with exertional angina, syncope,

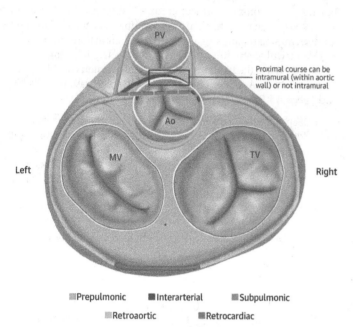

FIGURE 11.8 Pathways of the anomalous coronary arteries. (From: Cheezum MK, et al. Anomalous aortic origin of a coronary artery from the inappropriate sinus of Valsalva. *J Am Coll Cardiol.* 2017;69:1592–1608.)

and sudden death at a young age. The mechanism causing myocardial ischemia appears to be the slit-like opening in the aortic wall that narrows further during activity with dynamic compression of the obliquely arising LMCA ostium as it courses between the aortic root and the root of the pulmonary trunk. When this anomaly is identified, coronary revascularization (especially with surgical "unroofing" or bypass) is indicated in patients with myocardial ischemia. The need for revascularization in older patients with this anomaly is less clear. A decision for revascularization should be based on the severity of concomitant obstructive coronary disease and inducible myocardial ischemia. **Figure 11.10** summarizes the methods and techniques used to assess the anomalous LMCA.

Anomalous Origin of the Circumflex Coronary Artery

The most common coronary anomaly is the circumflex artery arising from the proximal RCA (**Fig. 11.11**). This feature is often suggested during left coronary angiography when the operator sees a long LMCA segment with a small or trivial circumflex branch. When the circumflex coronary artery arises from the right coronary cusp or the proximal RCA, it invariably follows a retroaortic course and passes posteriorly around the aortic root to its normal position. During RAO ventriculography, aortography, or coronary angiography, the circumflex artery is seen "on end," appearing as a radio-opaque dot posterior to the aorta.

Anomalous Origin of the RCA from the Left Sinus of Valsalva

When the RCA arises from the left coronary cusp or the proximal LMCA, it generally follows only one path, although other courses are theoretically possible. The RCA courses between the aorta and PA to its normal position. During RAO ventriculography, aortography, or coronary angiography, the RCA is seen "on end," anterior to the aorta,

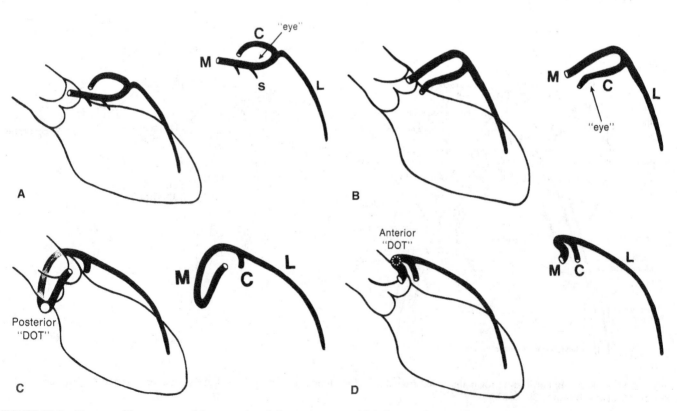

FIGURE 11.9 Diagram of four courses of the anomalous left coronary artery. M, Left main; C, circumflex; L, left anterior descending artery.

TABLE 11.5 Radiographic Appearance of Anomalous Origin of the Left Main Coronary Artery from the Right Sinus of Valsalva

COURSE OF ANOMALOUS	RAO AORTOGRAPHY OR VENTRICULOGRAPHY			
Left Main Coronary	Dot	Eye	LAD length	Septal branches arising from LMCA
Septal (lower LMCA)	–	+ (upper CFX)	Short	Yes
Anterior (lower CFX)	–	+ (upper LMCA)	Short	No
Retroaortic	+ (posterior)	–	Normal	No
Interarterial	+ (anterior)	–	Normal	No

+, Present; –, absent. Posterior and anterior are in reference to the aorta root.
CFX, circumflex coronary artery; LAD, left anterior descending coronary artery; LMCA, left main coronary artery.

and appears as a radio-opaque dot. This coronary anomaly has been associated with symptoms of myocardial ischemia, particularly when the RCA is dominant. Coronary revascularization should be considered when this anomaly is associated with symptoms of myocardial ischemia.

Anomalous RCA above the Sinus of Valsalva or from the Anterior Aortic Wall

The RCA may arise from an anterior location or high above the sinus of Valsalva. Aortic root flush injection helps locate the ostium

for proper, subselective catheter selection (e.g., Amplatz left 2 or multipurpose). This variant is benign.

LAD and Circumflex Coronary Arteries from Separate Ostia in the Left Aortic Sinus

When the LAD and circumflex coronary arteries arise from separate ostia in the left coronary cusp, the normal proximal course is followed. Also, a conus branch has a separate ostium arising from the right coronary cusp.

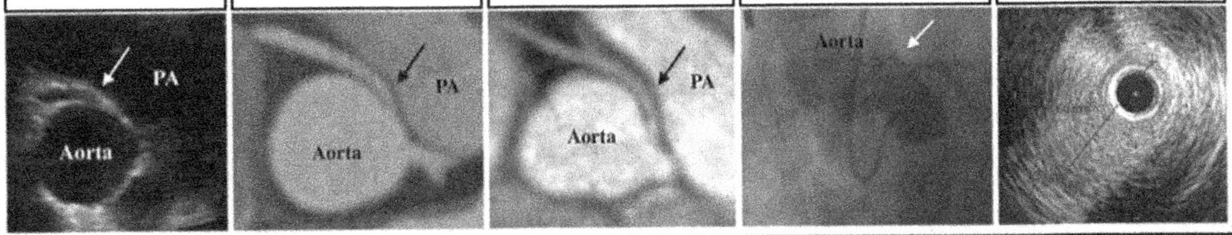

	Echo	CTA	MRA	ICA	IVUS
Indication for AAOCA Imaging	-	Class I	Class I	Class IIa	Class IIa
Spatial Resolution	0.8 × 1.5 mm (4-MHz transducer)	0.5 mm (isotropic)	1.0 mm (volumetric)	0.3 mm	0.15 × 0.25 mm
Temporal Resolution	30 msec	75-175 msec	60–120 msec	7-20 msec	Variable
Visualize surround structures	Limited	✔✔	✔	X	X
Dynamic imaging	Limited	Limited	Limited	✔ (Limited at ostium)	✔✔
Strengths	✓ Noninvasive, rapid ✓ Widely available ✓ Low cost	✓ Noninvasive, rapid ✓ Visualize takeoff + course + surrounding structures ✓ Evaluate CAD ✓ Examine multiple AAOCA features *	✓ Noninvasive ✓ Visualize takeoff + course + surrounding structures ✓ Evaluate cardiac function, perfusion and prior MI ✓ Avoid radiation & iodinated contrast	✓ Availability ✓ Improved spatial and temporal resolution ✓ Ancillary techniques (IVUS, OCT, FFR)	✓ Dynamic imaging ✓ Evaluation of proximal narrowing
Limitations	✕ Limited accuracy for detection of AAOCA ✕ Dependent on body habitus and operator technique	✕ Limited availability ✕ Iodinated contrast ✕ Radiation (low dose, e.g. 2-8 mSv now routine)	✕ Limited availability ✕ Cost and scan-time increased vs. CTA ✕ Spatial resolution decreased vs. CTA	✕ Invasive; Cost ✕ Contrast and radiation ✕ Limited visualization of ostium, proximal course, surrounding structures	✕ Invasive ✕ Cost ✕ Difficulty engaging anomalous vessel

FIGURE 11.10 Methods and techniques to assess the anomalous coronary artery AAOCA, Anomalous aortic origin of the coronary artery; CAD, coronary artery disease; FFR, fractional flow reserve; IVUS, intravascular ultrasound imaging; OCT, optical coherence tomography. (From: Cheezum MK, et al. Anomalous aortic origin of a coronary artery from the inappropriate sinus of Valsalva. *J Am Coll Cardiol.* 2017;69:1592–1608.)

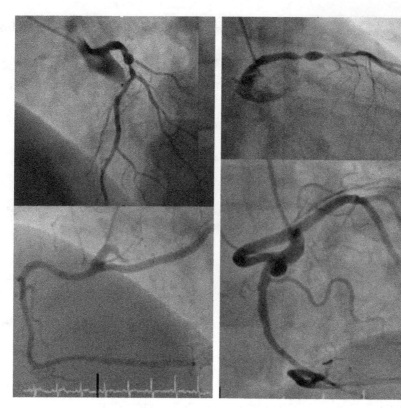

FIGURE 11.11 Frames from cineangiogram showing (*top, left and right*) the elongated LAD in the LAO cranial and RAO caudal views and (*bottom, left and right*) the right coronary artery with the circumflex originating in the RCA ostium in the LAO and RAO views. The retroaortic course is evident in the RAO view as a "dot" of density because the circumflex is in the viewer's plane as it runs behind the aorta. LAO, left anterior oblique; RAO, right anterior oblique; RCA, right coronary artery.

Key Points

- All lesions should be visualized in at least two angiographic views to establish severity.

- The working view should be selected to optimally visualize the lesion, guide catheter, and distal vessel, while minimizing vessel foreshortening.

- The TIMI flow grade, CTFC, and MBGs are useful measures of coronary and microvascular flow that have prognostic implications.

- The presence and quality of collaterals may affect the risk and potential benefits of PCI.

- Visual estimation of stenosis severity has a high interobserver variability, and should not be considered a diagnostic of ischemia.

- The characteristics of the lesion and proximal vessel can help determine the risk of PCI.

- The SYNTAX score takes into account lesion characteristics and the myocardium at risk, and is useful in choosing between multivessel PCI and CABG.

- Peripheral angiography requires specific techniques and equipment.

- Knowledge of typical coronary artery anomalies is important in order to determine between benign and malignant conditions.

References

1. Kern MJ, Lim MJ, Sorraja P, eds. *The Interventional Cardiac Catheterization Handbook*. 3rd ed. Philadelphia, PA: Elsevier, 2012:450–454.
2. Kern MJ, ed. *The Cardiac Catheterization Handbook*. 6th ed. Philadelphia, PA: Elsevier-Saunders, 2014:145–218:chap 3.
3. Shroff A, et al. *Transradial Angiography and Intervention Handbook: Principles and Applications*. Malvern, PA: HMP Communications, 2011:185.
4. Green NE, et al. Angiographic views used for percutaneous coronary interventions: a three-dimensional analysis of physician-determined vs. computer-generated views. *Catheter Cardiovasc Interv*. 2005;64:451–459.
5. Balter S, Moses J. Managing patient dose in interventional cardiology. *Catheter Cardiovasc Interv*. 2007;70:244–249.
6. Kaul P, et al. Ionizing radiation exposure to patients admitted with acute myocardial infarction in the United States. *Circulation*. 2010;122:2160–2169.
7. Hirshfeld JW Jr, et al. ACCF/AHA/HRS/SCAI clinical competence statement on physician knowledge to optimize patient safety and image quality in fluoroscopically guided invasive cardiovascular procedures. A report of the American College of Cardiology Foundation/American Heart Association/American College of Physicians Task Force on Clinical Competence and Training. *J Am Coll Cardiol*. 2004;44:2259–2282.
8. Gibson CM, et al. TIMI frame count: a quantitative method of assessing coronary artery flow. *Circulation*. 1996;93:879–888.
9. Valgimigli M, et al. Cyphering the complexity of coronary artery disease using the SYNTAX score to predict clinical outcome in patients with three-vessel lumen obstruction undergoing percutaneous coronary intervention. *Am J Cardiol*. 2007;99(8):1072–1081.

10. Serruys PW, et al. Percutaneous coronary intervention versus coronary artery bypass grafting for severe coronary artery disease (the SYNTAX trial). *N Engl J Med.* 2009;360:961–972.

11. Sianos G, et al. The SYNTAX score: an angiographic tool grading the complexity of coronary artery disease. *EuroInterv.* 2005;1:219–227.

12. White CJ, et al. Indications for renal angiography at the time of coronary angiography: a science advisory from the American Heart Association Committee on Diagnostic and Interventional Cardiac Catheterization, Council on Clinical Cardiology, and the Councils on Cardiovascular Radiology and Intervention and on Kidney in Cardiovascular Disease. *Circulation.* 2006;114:1892–1895.

13. Cheezum MK, et al. Anomalous aortic origin of a coronary artery from the inappropriate sinus of Valsalva. *J Am Coll Cardiol.* 2017;69(12):1592–1608.

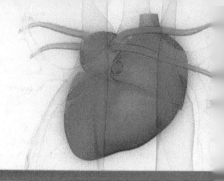

Introduction to Statistics in Clinical Research for Interventional Cardiology

Robert A. Harrington, MD, FSCAI, FACC and
Karen S. Pieper, MS

Clinical cardiologists, including interventional specialists, need to understand the quantitative issues in clinical research so they are capable of choosing therapies and technologies that have proven benefit for their patients, while avoiding therapies and technologies that are either harmful or unlikely to provide benefit to these patients. In this chapter, we discuss the basic concepts of evidence-based medicine, address basic issues of designing clinical studies, and discuss common analytical techniques. All of these topics should be familiar to clinicians, whether or not they are engaged in clinical investigation. Interventional cardiology is a continuous learning process; an ability to read and interpret the medical literature with facility is an important part of one's professional life.

Clinical research provides the evidence upon which the practice of medicine is best and most reliably based. The results of clinical studies are typically subjected to peer review before being published in leading medical journals. Nevertheless, the individual clinician needs to have a level of comfort with, and an understanding of, basic quantitative methods to evaluate the at-times conflicting sources of evidence in order to make the best medical decision for his or her patients.

Evidence-Based Medicine

Evidence-based medicine has been defined as combining quantitative evidence about medical practice with expert judgment in an effort to ensure that medical care is provided with reproducibly high quality (1). In addition to understanding the concept of evidence-based medicine, those preparing for the Interventional Cardiology Board examinations must be familiar with the various American College of Cardiology/American Heart Association (ACC/AHA) guidelines for clinical practice.

The ACC/AHA Guidelines Committees have issued a series of evidence-based practice recommendations that cover a variety of diseases and cardiac procedures, including percutaneous coronary intervention (PCI) and coronary bypass surgery (2,3). These guidelines are constructed using a defined, objective methodology that begins with the accumulation and weighing of evidence. All recommendations are accompanied by an assigned evidence grade (A, B, or C) (Table 12.1). Grade A means that the data have been derived from many trials, or at least a single large, randomized clinical trial. Grade B indicates that the data have been derived from smaller randomized trials or nonrandomized observational studies. The lowest weight of evidence is a grade C, which denotes expert consensus.

After weighing the evidence, guideline writers, including clinical experts, statisticians, and policy makers, assign classes of recommendations (I, II, or III) (Table 12.1). Class II recommendations are further subdivided into IIa and IIb. For the purposes of Board preparation, the candidate must be particularly familiar with Class I and III recommendations. Class I recommendations are those in which the intervention is felt to be useful and effective; Class III denotes interventions that are not deemed useful or effective, and may in fact be harmful. The Class II recommendations indicate situations where the evidence has been more controversial. A Class IIa recommendation is given when

TABLE 12.1 Levels of Evidence for Clinical Practice Recommendations

MEASURE	DESCRIPTION
Class of Recommendation	
I	Intervention is useful and effective
IIa	Evidence conflicts/opinions differ but lean toward efficacy
IIb	Evidence conflicts/opinions differ but lean against efficacy
III	Intervention is not useful/effective and may be harmful
Level of Evidence	
A	Data from many randomized clinical trials
B	Data from single randomized trial or nonrandomized studies
C	Expert consensus

Adapted from: Gibbons RJ, et al. American College of Cardiology/American Heart Association clinical practice guidelines: part I: where do they come from? *Circulation.* 2003;107:2979–2986, with permission.

the evidence conflicts or opinions differ, but, overall, the evidence leans toward benefit; a Class IIb recommendation indicates that the evidence conflicts or opinions differ, but the weight of the evidence leans against benefit. Despite a wealth of information from clinical trials supporting many of the major decisions in cardiovascular medicine, including interventional cardiology, the majority of recommendations in the ACC/AHA guidelines are Class II recommendations, suggesting that a limited amount of evidence exists even for interventions considered routine in clinical practice.

Types of Study Designs

There are two main types of study design: *observational studies and experimental studies* (4). In observational studies, patients or groups of patients are observed over a period of time, and their characteristics are recorded. In an experimental design, an intervention such as a drug, procedure, or technology is introduced into the population, and the effect on the study subjects is observed.

Types of observational studies vary. We will consider a few with which the reader should be familiar. These include case–control studies and cohort studies. Regarding experimental studies, we will mainly consider randomized controlled trials.

Case–Control Studies

A case–control study is typically performed on previously collected, retrospective data. In these studies, there are five steps to consider. First, one begins with either the presence or absence of an outcome of

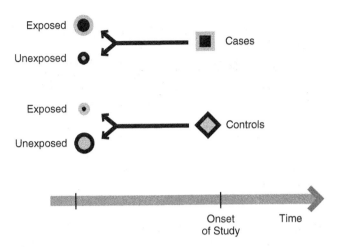

FIGURE 12.1   Example of a case–control study design.

interest. Second, one defines a group of cases that have this measure of interest—typically, this is a disease or an outcome event. Third, a control group is identified that does not have the disease or the measure of interest, but may be matched on common characteristics such as age or gender. Fourth, the investigator looks at the history of cases to detect possible causes or risk factors that were not controlled for in the matching process. Step five is an attempt to answer the question of what happened or what is the difference between the cases and the controls that might explain the outcome of interest. A case–control study might be useful, for example, to consider whether the use of a medication is related to the development of a disease. When considering a treatment, the cases and controls should be carefully matched on important risk factors in order to be as certain as possible that only the treatment effect varies between the two groups. **Figure 12.1** and **Table 12.2** show examples.

Case–control studies have certain advantages and disadvantages. This may be the best design for studying diseases or conditions that develop over a long time or are extremely rare. They may be very useful for investigating a preliminary hypothesis, because they are typically a very rapid way of performing a study, provided the data on the population have already been collected. The major disadvantage is that the case–control study depends on existing records, which may have been collected for other reasons. This particular study design is subject to a fair degree of bias or error, because the data are typically collected in advance of the question being asked, so one is limited by the existing data. For example, factors associated with

the outcome may not be equally distributed between the two treatments. If these factors are not available to be examined, one cannot test whether the differences in the factors, rather than the treatment being studied, are responsible for any statistically significant treatment results. In addition, patient care may have changed since the data were collected, making the results no longer applicable. Choosing an appropriate control group (including one that is matched for certain characteristics) is critical, but may prove to be quite difficult.

Cohort Studies

In a cohort study, information is collected on a group of subjects who have something in common and who remain part of that group for an extended period of observation or follow-up. Typically, in this type of design, one begins with the identification of an exposure to some event that is felt to be relevant to the development of some outcome in the future. One then identifies two groups of subjects: the exposed group and the non-exposed group. One then looks forward in time from the exposure to determine the effect of the defining characteristics or exposure on the outcome of interest. This design attempts to answer the prospective question: What will happen?

An example of a cohort study design is seen in **Figure 12.2** and **Table 12.3**. A cohort study is a good design when one is interested in studying the particular causes of a condition, the course of a particular disease, or the impact of risk factors over time. The Framingham Heart Study, which has provided much critical information on the understanding

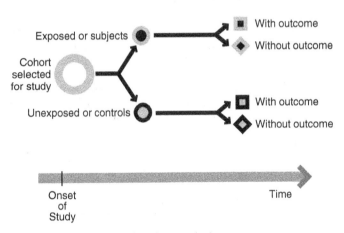

FIGURE 12.2   Example of a cohort study design.

TABLE 12.2 Example of a Case–Control Study: Is There an Association between the Use of Aspirin and the Development of Reye's Syndrome?

We have 30 patients with Reye's syndrome, of whom 28 used aspirin. There were 60 patients drawn from a large population of patients with minor viral illnesses, but not Reye's syndrome. Of these, 35 used aspirin.

Odds of exposure in cases: 28/2 = 14

Odds of exposure in controls: 35/25 = 1.4

Odds ratio: 14/1.4 = 10

Interpretation: Odds of being on aspirin is 10 times greater with Reye's syndrome than without.

TABLE 12.3 Example of a Cohort Study Design

The association of smoking with coronary heart disease (CHD) is investigated by selecting a group of 3,000 smokers (exposed) and a group of 5,000 nonsmokers (unexposed) who, in both groups, are free of heart disease at the beginning of the study. Both groups are followed for the development of CHD, and the incidence in the groups is compared. Suppose CHD develops in 84 smokers and 87 nonsmokers.

Risk of CHD in smokers: 84/3,000 = 2.8%

Risk of CHD in nonsmokers: 87/5,000 = 1.74%

Risk Ratio: 2.8/1.74 = 1.61

Interpretation: The risk of CHD is 61% times greater in patients who smoke than those who do not.

of the association between cardiac risk factors and cardiac outcome, is an example of a cohort study (5). One of the major disadvantages of a cohort design is that studies such as the Framingham study may take a long time to conduct. Because of this, they tend to be resource-intensive. It is also a difficult methodology when one is interested in causation: one may define association, but because there is no intervention being introduced into the population, it is difficult to prove causation. It may also be a difficult design when a disease is rare in the population, because the requisite large sample size may be prohibitive.

Experimental Studies

There are two types of experimental studies: the controlled and the uncontrolled study. In a controlled study, an experimental drug, procedure, or technology is typically compared with at least one other drug, procedure, or technology. This might include a comparison with placebo. In an uncontrolled study, an investigator will describe the experience with the experimental drug or procedure, but not compare it directly with another treatment. This type of experiment has less validity and is less likely to allow one to conclude that there are differences between the treatments.

Controlled clinical trials may be further grouped into two types: *randomized* and *nonrandomized experiments*. In each of these, the trial is conducted with concurrent controls. There are typically two groups: the experimental group, who receive the experimental drug or procedure, and the control group, who receive placebo or a standard drug or procedure. Randomized clinical trials provide the strongest evidence for reaching a conclusion of causation, whereas in the nonrandomized trial, when the assignment to a treatment group is not random, there may be biases introduced that render conclusions questionable.

The randomized clinical trial is distinguished from other types of research by the process of randomization and the introduction of an intervention. The question being asked is, does the intervention make a difference? Because the treatments are randomly allocated, risk factors should occur fairly equally in the two groups. Thus, only the intervention is left to be different. **Figure 12.3** shows an example of a randomized clinical trial, while **Table 12.4** shows some of the

TABLE 12.4 Randomized Clinical Trials versus Observational Studies	
EFFICACY (RCTS)	**EFFECTIVENESS (OBSERVATIONAL)**
Experimental setting (reduced bias → causality)	Clinical practice setting
"Ideal" Circumstances	
Limited population	Broad range of patients/ providers
Optimal care	Community standard of care

differences between randomized trials and observational studies. Both types of research have complementary value, and the methodology employed will largely depend upon the question of interest.

In the next section, we will discuss a variety of issues relevant to randomized clinical trials, including study endpoints; the calculation of sample size; superiority, equivalence, and non-inferiority trials; and the concept of "intention to treat" (ITT).

Study Endpoints

In any clinical study, the investigator is typically interested in the outcome events, or endpoints. In very broad terms, endpoints may be thought of as consisting of two types: hard or soft endpoints. Soft endpoints are those that may be affected by individual views or interpretations, and thus may be difficult to define or measure. Examples of this include quality of life, symptom scales, and clinical impression. Conversely, hard endpoints are those that are well-defined, measurable, and objective, including death, myocardial infarction (MI), stroke, revascularization, or rehospitalization. Hard clinical endpoints are typically required to make more definitive statements about the value of a therapy or technology in the clinical setting.

Composite Endpoints

Because some outcome events may occur infrequently, investigators commonly combine the endpoints into a composite that will increase the number of anticipated outcome events and therefore decrease the potential sample size. Examples of this include the composites of death or MI; death, MI, or revascularization; and death or heart failure hospitalization. Typically, in a composite endpoint, one measures the occurrence of any one of the events versus that of none of the events. In such an analysis, one must be vigilant and careful that endpoints of differing severity do not cancel each other out and potentially obscure any potential treatment effect. One should also be sure that information is recorded for all of the endpoints; in the presence of a missing component, the composite status cannot be determined. For example, a patient was known to be alive at 30 days, but information about MI was not obtained. For this patient, one would have to either make an assumption about MI status or list the composite as missing. A secondary analysis that reports the individual rates of the component events by treatment groups should always be planned.

A different way to view the composite endpoint is to have a ranked composite endpoint. In such an analysis, each component is assigned a severity score. For example, death would be assigned a higher score, and a nonfatal event like rehospitalization, a lower score. Although such an approach has intuitive appeal, the ranking scale must be properly defined. The best case for ranking would be

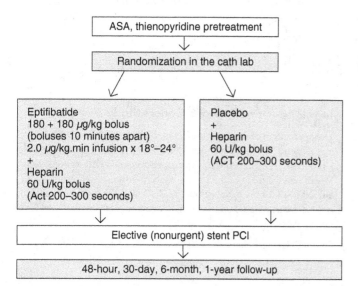

FIGURE 12.3 Example of a randomized clinical trial; in this case, the ESPRIT study. ESPRIT was a randomized, double-blind, placebo-controlled, parallel group study on 2,064 patients scheduled to undergo percutaneous coronary intervention with stent implantation. ESPRIT, European/Australasian Stroke Prevention in Reversible Ischaemia Trial.

with a general survey of the group of interest: cardiologists, family physicians, patients, and/or the general public. Nevertheless, these surveys are difficult, expensive, and rarely given to a diverse sample of the potential users of the scale.

Sample Size

A proper calculation of sample size is a critical part of clinical research. Understanding this process is essential for understanding the validity of clinical research findings. The calculation of sample size depends on multiple factors, including the Type I error rate, Type II error rate, endpoint to be analyzed, estimated value for the endpoint occurring in the control arm, estimated improvement in the treatment arm, amount of variation in the endpoint measured, and statistical method to be used in analyzing the endpoint. In particular, clinicians should feel comfortable in understanding both Type I and Type II errors (**Table 12.5**). The Type I error (α) occurs when one observes an effect, when in truth no effect exists. The Type II error (β) occurs when one observes no treatment effect, when in fact a treatment effect does exist. One minus the Type II error ($1-\beta$) is also the trial's power. By understanding the risk of a Type II error or, conversely, the importance of power in examining clinical trials results, one can appreciate whether or not a trial actually has adequate power to answer the desired question. Yusuf et al. first pointed this out in the cardiovascular clinical literature nearly 20 years ago (6). **Table 12.6** summarizes his thesis and the importance of sample size in allowing clinicians to determine whether the population was adequate to answer the question the study sought to answer.

Sample size is also dependent upon what type of trial is planned. We will briefly discuss three types of trials: superiority, non-inferiority, and equivalence (7). In a superiority trial, the experiment is designed to test for a statistically significant and clinically meaningful improvement (or harm) from the use of the experimental treatment over that of the standard of care. In an equivalence trial, the experiment is designed to evaluate whether the difference in outcome for the experimental treatment compared with standard care falls within the boundary of a clinically defined minimally important difference (MID). The MID is the largest difference that one would accept between the outcome of the two groups while still considering them clinically similar or comparable. In a non-inferiority trial, the results are evaluated assuming that the experimental treatment is not worse than the standard of care by a clinically meaningful amount. Although one still uses the MID to determine the boundary of non-inferiority, unlike equivalence studies, a non-inferiority study does not look for small improvements over the standard therapy. Essentially, one might view this as a one-sided test, as opposed to the two-sided evaluation that is the hallmark of equivalence. One can see graphically in **Figure 12.4** the results of a variety of studies and the potential results in superiority, equivalence, and non-inferiority studies.

Several recent examples from cardiology literature demonstrate the concept of non-inferiority. Both the Superior Yield of the New strategy of Enoxaparin, Revascularization and GlYcoprotein IIb/IIIa inhibitors (SYNERGY) (8) and the Rivaroxaban Once Daily Oral Direct Factor Xa Inhibition Compared with Vitamin K Antagonism for Prevention of Stroke and Embolism (ROCKET) (9) trials were designed to demonstrate the superiority of an experimental therapy over the standard of care. Nevertheless, in both cases, it was prespecified that if superiority was not met, then the treatments would be compared for non-inferiority. In ROCKET, the hypothesis was that a once-daily dose of oral rivaroxaban was superior to dose-adjusted warfarin for the prevention of stroke and systemic embolism in moderate-to-high-risk patients with nonvalvular atrial fibrillation. While the trial did not show the superiority of rivaroxaban in the ITT population, it did demonstrate non-inferiority, with the upper boundary of the 95% CI being less than the prespecified non-inferiority boundary of 1.46. Similarly, SYNERGY did not demonstrate that enoxaparin was superior to unfractionated heparin among patients presenting with non–ST elevation acute coronary syndromes. Nevertheless, the protocol defined inferiority criteria that were met when the upper boundary of the CI did not exceed the prespecified ratio of 1.1.

In an era when multiple active therapies are available for patients with acute cardiovascular disease, equivalence and non-inferiority trials are becoming increasingly important in the evaluation of new therapies. Non-inferiority and equivalence trials have most of their value when the experimental therapy is felt to be unlikely to be better than the established therapy, but could offer incremental benefit with regard to, for example, improved safety, greater ease of administration, or reduced cost. The challenge for non-inferiority and equivalence studies is the establishment of the MID boundary.

Although a number of recent large-scale trials have used the equivalence or non-inferiority methodology, there is no firmly accepted definition of the MID. Consequently, in interpreting the medical literature, one

TABLE 12.5 Sample Size Estimation: Type I and II Errors

		TEST RESULTS	
		NO TREATMENT EFFECT	TREATMENT HAS AN EFFECT
Truth	No treatment effect	—	Type 1 error (α)
	Treatment has an effect	Type II error (β)	Power ($1-\beta$)

TABLE 12.6 Sample Size Calculations

DEATHS	PTS. RANDOMIZED RISK = 10%)	CHANCE OF TYPE II ERROR[a]	COMMENTS ON SAMPLE SIZE
0–50	<500	>0.9	Utterly inadequate
50–150	1,000	0.7–0.9	Probably inadequate
150–350	3,000	0.3–0.7	Possibly inadequate
350–650	6,000	0.1–0.3	Probably adequate
>650	10,000	<0.1	Adequate

[a]Probability of failing to achieve p <0.01 if risk reduction = 25%.
Reprinted from: Yusuf S, et al. Beta blockade during and after myocardial infarction: an overview of the randomized trials. *Prog Cardiovasc Dis.* 1985;27:335–371, with permission.

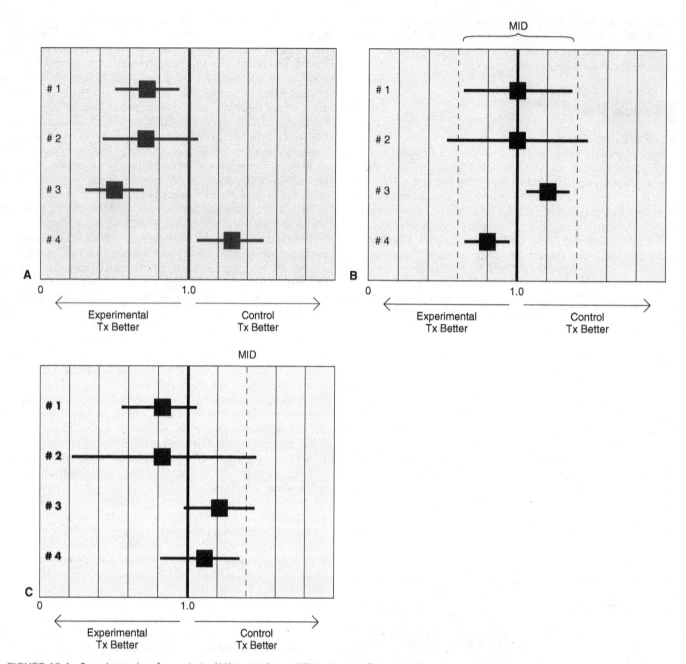

FIGURE 12.4 Sample results of superiority (4A), equivalence (4B), and non-inferiority (4C) studies. In **(A)**, studies #1 and #3 show that the experimental therapy is statistically significantly *superior* to the control therapy, while in study #4, the control therapy is statistically better. Study #2 does not show statistical significance at all because the confidence interval crosses the line of no difference. In **(B)**, study #1 shows that the experimental therapy is clinically and statistically *equivalent* to the control therapy, because the confidence interval crosses the line of no difference and falls within the minimally important difference (MID). In study #2, the experimental therapy cannot be considered either statistically equivalent or different because the confidence interval crosses both the line of no difference and the MID. Studies #3 and #4 show statistical equivalence as well; had these results come from a superiority trial, the experimental therapy would be considered clinically equivalent but statistically inferior (#3) or superior (#4). In **(C)**, studies #1 and #4 show that the experimental treatment is *noninferior* to the control therapy, because the confidence interval does not cross the MID. The confidence interval of study #2 is too wide to draw a conclusion. Study #3 crosses the MID, indicating that the experimental treatment is inferior to the control. MID, minimally important difference

must pay particular attention to how that boundary was constructed. If the MID is quite large, the validity of a non-inferiority or equivalence claim can be questioned. On the other hand, if the boundary is overly narrow, very little is gained by choosing a non-inferiority or equivalence design over a more traditional superiority design. The boundary of the MID can be a clinically determined one, owing to

a fair bit of subjectivity as to what constitutes an acceptable clinical deviation. It can also be derived mathematically by determining the expected treatment effect for the standard treatment over placebo. The MID boundary is derived such that it will not be crossed if at least 50% of this treatment effect over placebo would be maintained by using the experimental rather than the control treatment.

ITT Analysis

An important concept in the evaluation of clinical studies is the notion of performing an analysis on the basis of the ITT principle. Broadly, ITT is the notion that patients are randomly assigned to a treatment group and then analyzed as if they received that treatment, regardless of whether they actually did. The purest form of ITT means that any patient who signs an informed consent and who is assigned a randomized treatment remains in that treatment arm for the purposes of analysis, even if they drop out before any treatment was received or if they received a treatment different from the allocated one.

A commonly performed analysis, preferably in blinded studies, is the ITT-treated analysis, sometimes called modified ITT. In this adaptation of the ITT principle, the patients remain in the group that they were randomized into for the purposes of analysis, but only those patients who actually received the treatment are considered in the primary analysis. In order for this analytical method to be as valid as possible, the investigator must be blinded to the treatment that the patient had been randomized to receive when the decision is made not to give them the treatment. This helps to assure that factors other than the allocation assignment itself are responsible for the patient not receiving the assigned therapy. An example of this in PCI trials is a patient who has been randomized prior to the final decision to perform percutaneous intervention. Another example was the Cangrelor versus Standard Therapy to Achieve Optimal Management of Platelet Inhibition (CHAMPION) PCI (10). To test the use of Cangrelor versus clopidogrel in the setting of PCI, the CHAMPION PCI study excluded a fairly small group of randomized patients (8.7%) because they had an ST-segment elevation MI (STEMI), did not receive any study medication, or were not suitable for PCI; the majority of them were excluded because they were STEMI patients. The potential therapeutic effect of Cangrelor might best be considered when one evaluates the patients who actually received any amount of study drug. The results remained nonsignificant, regardless of the type of ITT population observed (10).

The decision to use an ITT analysis versus using a modified ITT analysis has particular importance in the interpretation of non-inferiority trials. In a non-inferiority trial, the most essential and appropriately robust analysis considers only those patients who have actually received therapy. This is because, paradoxically, non-compliance actually improves the chances of declaring a noninferior result. An extreme example would be if in a randomized trial, none of the patients received the assigned therapy, then the two groups would likely not appear different from one another, thus fulfilling the criteria of non-inferiority.

Considerations in Analysis Method

In order to understand what analysis method one might choose when considering clinical data, one should be familiar with the scales used to measure data. Data can be described as nominal, ordinal, or continuous. Nominal data are made up of discrete categories that have no particular order (e.g., gender). Ordinal data are categorical, but with an inherent order—for example, the number of diseased vessels in patients with coronary artery disease (one, two, or three vessels). Finally, continuous data are those in which the differences between numbers have actual meaning. Examples of continuous data include age and weight. When dealing with continuous measures, in addition to considering the scales of measurement, one should also consider the shape of the distribution. For example, are the data points normally distributed, like a bell-shaped or symmetric

curve? Are they skewed? Or do they have a bimodal distribution? The latter two may also be referred to as a non-normal distribution of continuous data.

In describing continuous data, one might refer to measures of the center of the distribution. For example, one refers to the mean, which is the average of the measures, or to the median, which is the middle value of the distribution. Also important are measures of the variability around the center. This can be described as the range of the data (maximum value–minimum value), the standard deviation or variance, or the percentile (e.g., the 25th–75th range).

There are a number of ways to perform statistical tests that compare two groups. When the data are nominally distributed, these include the chi-square test, Fisher's exact test, or logistic regression. The results are often presented as rates, odds ratios, or risk ratios. Odds ratios and risk ratios are frequently confused for one another. Although these are among the most common ways to compare two groups, it is worth understanding how they are calculated. **Table 12.7** provides examples for calculating an odds ratio and a risk ratio. Finally, a clinically important number to understand that is frequently reported in the medical literature is the so-called "number needed to treat" (NNT). The NNT refers to the number of patients who need to be treated with a therapy to prevent one adverse outcome. This is calculated by dividing 1 by the absolute risk reduction. For example, if the absolute difference between two therapies is 1.5%, the NNT is 1 divided by 0.015, which equals 67 patients.

p-Values

A p-value is the probability of obtaining the results you have observed (or even more extreme results) if the effect is really because of random chance alone (11). For example, a p-value of ≤ 0.05 indicates that a difference of at least the amount observed in the experiment would occur in fewer than 50 out of 1,000 similar experiments if the treatment studies had absolutely no effect on the measured outcome. In designing a clinical study, particularly a randomized clinical trial, the investigators must state the hypothesis that is being tested, the statistical test that will be used on this hypothesis (to reject the null hypothesis, meaning the rejection of the statement that there is no

TABLE 12.7 Examples of Calculating Odds Ratios and Risk Ratios in the ASCEND-HF Trial

One of the two primary endpoints—death from any cause or hospitalization for heart failure to 30 days—was compared in patients receiving intravenous nesiritide vs. placebo. In the nesiritide group, 321 out of 3,496 patients experienced an event. In the placebo group, 345 out of 3,511 experienced an event.

Odds Ratios

Odds in the nesiritide group: 321/3,175 = 0.101

Odds in the placebo group: 345/3,166 = 0.109

Odds ratio: 0.101/0.109 = 0.929

Risk Ratios

Risk in the nesiritide group: 321/3,496 = 9.2%

Risk in the placebo group: 345/3,511 = 9.8%

Risk ratio: 9.2/9.8 = 0.934

Adapted from: O'Connor CM, et al. Effect of nesiritide in patients with acute decompensated heart failure. *N Engl J Med.* 2011;365:32–43, with permission.

difference between the treatment groups), and the critical (or nominal) value for declaring significance (the Type I error rate).

In most clinical research, the critical value to declare significance is set at 0.05. As this is mostly by convention, it is appropriate for certain types of studies to set a different level of nominal significance—for example, at 0.025 or 0.001. When one states a nominal level of significance, then the prestated declaration must be followed. For example, if the nominal level of significance has been set at 0.05, then for a final study p-value of 0.053, one cannot declare statistical significance, whereas if the results provide a p-value of 0.048 under the same conditions, then one could declare a statistically significant difference between the treatment groups. Understanding clinical trial results requires careful reading of the clinical study methods and understanding of the Type I error that has been prospectively set for a clinical experiment. Violation of this conservation approach through activities such as data mining until one obtains a desired p-value is particularly troublesome and has been termed "random research" (12).

Confidence Intervals

As with p-values, a reader of the clinical research literature must be facile in an understanding of confidence intervals. The p-value and CI provide complementary information. For example, consider the 95% CI. This suggests that if one were to perform the same study an infinite number of times, then 95% of the estimates of the effect would fall within the bounds of the interval. A ratio of two rates that are the same gives a value of 1. Thus, a CI that overlaps 1 implies that the treatment difference is not statistically significant. An interval that does not include 1 implies statistical significance. When the p-value and the CI are calculated using

the same test statistic, they will give the same interpretation for statistical significance. Data are frequently presented in ratio plots displaying the point estimate and the associated 95% CI. **Figure 12.5** demonstrates study results using ratio plots that include superiority and uncertainty results.

Further Interpretation

When interpreting clinical study results, it is insufficient to consider only the conclusion that the results are statistically significant. The reader should ask a series of questions to better understand the meaning of that claim. Is the effect size clinically meaningful and important? Is the study sample very homogeneous? Can these results be generalized to broader populations? How statistically robust are the results? For example, how close is the actual p-value to the nominal level of significance? When the results are displayed as a ratio plot, do the CIs include the estimate of no difference (1 for an odds ratio, 0 for absolute differences, or % change)? How wide are the CIs? Other questions to ask in interpreting the results of a clinical trial are delineated in **Table 12.8**.

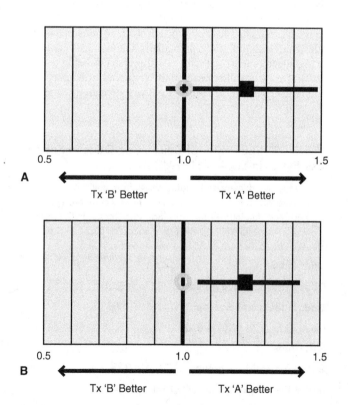

FIGURE 12.5   Interpreting the ratio plots. If the confidence interval crosses the value of no difference (1.0 for a ratio), as in **(A)**, then the p-value is >0.05. If it does not, as in **(B)**, the p-value is <0.05 and the comparison is statistically significant, which, in this case, shows that Treatment A is better.

TABLE 12.8 Questions to Ask When Reading and Interpreting the Results of a Clinical Trial

ARE THE RESULTS OF THE STUDY VALID?

Primary Guides

Was the assignment of patients to treatment randomized?

Were all patients who entered the study properly accounted for at its conclusion?

Was follow-up complete?

Were patients analyzed in the groups to which they were randomized?

Secondary Guides

Were patients, their clinicians, and study personnel blinded to treatment?

Were the groups similar at the start of the trial?

Aside from the experimental intervention, were the groups treated equally?

What Were the Results?

How large was the treatment effect?

How precise was the treatment effect (confidence intervals)?

Will the Results Help Me in Caring for My Patients?

Does my patient fulfill the enrollment criteria for the trial? If not, how close is the patient to the enrollment criteria?

Does my patient fit the features of a subgroup in the trial report? If so, are the results of the subgroup analysis in the trial valid?

Were all the clinically important outcomes considered?

Are the likely treatment benefits worth the potential harm and costs?

Reprinted from: Califf RM, Topol EJ. Considerations in the design and conduct of clinical studies and the interpretation of quantitative evidence. In: Topol EJ, ed. *Textbook of Cardiovascular Medicine.* 2nd ed. Philadelphia, PA: Lippincott Williams & Wilkins; 2002, with permission. Adapted from: Gibbons RJ, et al. American College of Cardiology/American Heart Association clinical practice guidelines: part I: where do they come from? *Circulation.* 2003;107:2979–2986, with permission.

Conclusion

Clinicians need familiarity with common quantitative issues in order to fairly and appropriately interpret the medical literature. The essence of evidence-based medicine is thoughtful clinical care guided by the best available data on the topic. Interventional cardiologists preparing for their Board exams should understand basic statistical topics, as well as how the commonly used ACC/AHA Practice Guidelines are constructed and employed.

Key Points

- Critical to understanding statistics is identifying the types of study designs:
  - A case–control study is typically performed on previously collected, retrospective data.
  - A cohort study consists of information collected on a group of subjects who have something in common and who remain part of that group for an extended period.
  - Experimental studies may be either a controlled or uncontrolled study.

- Study endpoints determine the importance of the study.
  - Consider soft and hard endpoint.
  - Composite endpoints are used to increase the number of anticipated outcome events, and therefore decrease the potential sample size.

- Sample size calculations depends on multiple factors, including the Type I error rate, Type II error rate, estimated incidence of events/endpoints in the control arm, estimated improvement in the treatment arm, amount of variation in the endpoint measured, and statistical method for data analysis.

- An ITT analysis versus using a modified ITT analysis has particular importance in the interpretation of non-inferiority trials.

References

1. Sackett DL, et al. Evidence-based medicine: what it is and what it is not. *BMJ*. 1996;312:71–72.
2. Gibbons RJ, et al. American College of Cardiology/American Heart Association clinical practice guidelines: part I: where do they come from? *Circulation*. 2003;107:2979–2986.
3. Gibbons RJ, Smith SC Jr, Antman E. American College of Cardiology/American Heart Association clinical practice guidelines: part II: evolutionary changes in a continuous quality improvement project. *Circulation*. 2003;107:3101–3107.
4. Bailer JC, Mosteller F. *Medical Uses of Statistics*. 2nd ed. Boston, MA: New England Journal of Medicine Books; 1992:149–151.
5. Fox CS, et al. Temporal trends in coronary heart disease mortality and sudden cardiac death from 1950 to 1999: the Framingham heart study. *Circulation*. 2004;110:522–527.
6. Yusuf S, et al. Beta blockade during and after myocardial infarction: an overview of the randomized trials. *Prog Cardiovasc Dis*. 1985;27:335–371.
7. Friedman LM, Furberg CD, DeMets DL. *Fundamentals of Clinical Trials*. 3rd ed. St. Louis, MO: Mosby-Year Book Inc; 1996:55–56.
8. Mahaffey KW, Ferguson JJ. Exploring the role of enoxaparin in the management of high-risk patients with non–ST-elevation acute coronary syndromes: the SYNERGY trial. *Am Heart J*. 2005;149:S81–S90.
9. Patel MR, et al. Rivaroxaban versus warfarin in nonvalvular atrial fibrillation. *N Engl J Med*. 2011;365:883–891.
10. Harrington RA, et al. Platelet inhibition with cangrelor in patients undergoing PCI. *N Engl J Med*. 2009;361:2318–2329.
11. Moyé LA. P-value interpretation, and alpha allocation in clinical trials. *Ann Epidemiol*. 1998;8:351–357.
12. Moyé LA. Random research. *Circulation*. 2001;103:3150–3153.

13

Equipment Selection for Coronary Interventions

Keshav Nayak, MD, FSCAI, FACC, Arnold H. Seto, MD, MPA, FSCAI, FACC, Jeffrey Cavendish, MD, FSCAI, and Morton J. Kern, MD, MSCAI, FAHA, FACC

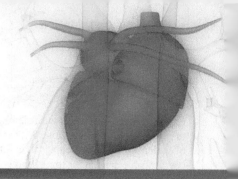

The initial decisions regarding the selection of guide catheters and guide wires, and the need for other ancillary equipment, are critical. Often, the difference between an apparently effortless coronary intervention and one that appears laborious or challenging revolves around obtaining adequate guide support and guide-wire mobility.

Percutaneous coronary intervention (PCI) equipment consists of three basic elements: the guiding catheter, the balloon–stent catheter, and the coronary guide wire. Typically, the choice of equipment remains the same regardless of whether the procedure is performed from the femoral or radial approach, although adequate support may be more difficult to obtain from the radial approach. This chapter will highlight equipment essential to any PCI procedure: coronary guide catheters, balloon catheters, and coronary guide wires. Details of coronary stent design and use are discussed in Chapter 14 (Stents). Specialized equipment for vascular access and closure, rotational atherectomy, laser atherectomy, cutting balloons, and structural heart disease are also addressed separately. This chapter also includes specialized equipment for PCI from the radial approach, due to the resurgence in the radial artery approach as a result of improved patient comfort, reduced major bleeding, and all-cause mortality benefit in ACS patients (1,2). A recent report of the NCDR CathPCI registry demonstrated an increasing proportion of procedures performed using the radial access site (3).

Guiding Catheters

Guide catheters are dedicated large-bore catheters used to deliver coronary guide wires and balloon catheters to the target vessel. Sizes of catheters are shown in **Figure 13.1A**. The traditional guide catheter was constructed with three layers: an outer nylon layer, a middle braided wire mesh layer, and an inner hydrophilic coated layer (**Fig. 13.1B**). Compared with simple diagnostic catheters, the braided guide catheter has thinner walls and a larger internal diameter (ID) through which balloon and stent delivery catheters can be inserted. Guide catheters are stiffer than diagnostic catheters, which enables them to provide support for balloon or stent catheters to traverse coronary stenoses. Manipulation of guide catheters differs from that of diagnostic catheters. The tip of the guide catheter is larger and not tapered, making it more likely to obstruct the coronary ostium,

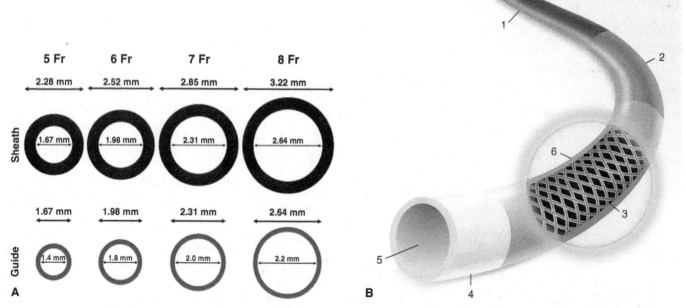

FIGURE 13.1 A: Sheath sizes and guide catheter inner and outer diameters. (From: From AM, et al. Sheathless transradial intervention using standard guide catheters. *Catheter Cardiovasc Interv.* 2010;76(7):911–916, with permission.) **B:** Layers of guide catheter. Illustration of a guiding catheter shows stiffer body (1); variable softer primary curve (2); wire braiding (3); atraumatic tip (4); large lumen (optional radiopaque marker) (5); lubrious coating (6) (Boston Scientific, Inc.).

TABLE 13.1 Factors to Consider in Choosing Guide Catheters

French size (6, 7 or 8)	Complex procedure, CTO, calcified and tortuous vessel, requires extra support—choose 7 or 8 Fr
Shape of the guide (need for back wall support)	Aorta is dilated or enlarged, tortuous—choose longer length between primary and secondary curve for left guides
Length	PCI through long bypass grafts or the LIMA into the native arteries—choose 90-cm guide
Side holes	Small ostia, pressure will damp or ventricularize, need to deeply intubate guide—choose a guide with side holes

AORTIC CONFIGURATION	RCA GUIDES
Normal	JR 3.5,4 AL 0.75, 1 Hockey Stick AR 1
Dilated	JR 4.5, 4 AL 1.5,2, AR 2
Narrow	JR 3, LIMA

AORTIC CONFIGURATION	LEFT CORONARY GUIDES
Normal	EBU/XB 3.5-4, JL4, AL 1.5-2
Dilated	EBU/XB 4 or >, JL 4.5 or >, Voda
Narrow	EBU/XB 3-3.5, JL 3-3.5

OTHER CIRCUMSTANCES THAT WILL DICTATE GUIDE SELECTION	
Coronary Anatomy and Orientation	
Ostial disease	Use side holes, use guide that will be easy to disengage
Short left main / dual left coronary ostial	Need to subselect LAD or LCX
Shepherd's Crook right	Need extra support, consider AL guide
Bypass Grafts Orientation	
To right coronaries	Horizontal or inferior
To left coronaries	Horizontal or superior

CTO, chronic total occlusion; LAD, left anterior descending; LIMA, left internal mammary artery; PCI, percutaneous coronary intervention; RCA, right coronary artery.

causing pressure dampening upon engagement (4–6). Therefore, careful manipulation of guiding catheters is important to avoid guide catheter–related ostial dissection or disruption.

Guide catheter choice depends upon many factors (Table 13.1), such as the patient's body habitus; age; anatomy of the ascending aorta and aortic root; coronary artery anatomic variants; diseased native coronary arteries or bypass grafts; ostial, proximal, or distal location of the target lesions; bifurcation disease; degree of tortuosity; and calcification in the coronary artery. The French size, the shape, the need for side holes, and the length of the catheter are also important factors. Many manufacturers supply a wide variety of preshaped guide catheters with various sizes and features (Table 13.2).

Guide catheters can be used as either active or passive guides. Most guide catheters are designed to provide passive support, meaning they are placed at the ostium of the vessel. They provide adequate support to facilitate the intervention through their stiffness, back support against the aortic wall, and shape. An active guide is one that is smaller (≤6 Fr) and more flexible and that can be deeply seated or advanced past the ostium down into the vessel to provide additional support. This technique is less commonly used because there is a risk of damage to the vessel and ischemia to the territory supplied. Nevertheless, in difficult cases, active support may be required to pass equipment. Mother-daughter extension catheters, such as the Guideliner or Guidezilla devices, provide a form of enhanced active support (7).

Guide Catheter Sizes

Today, 6-Fr guiding catheters are the most commonly used catheters. Larger guiding catheters (7 Fr or 8 Fr) may be needed for kissing balloons/stents, rotablator burrs larger than 2 mm, and some cutting balloons (Table 13.3). Because the limitation of the device is its external diameter, it is important to know the ID of the guides you select. Many of the newer 6-Fr guide catheters have the braided wire mesh embedded into the nylon outer layer, increasing the ID

TABLE 13.2 Guide Catheter Styles and Lengths

Standard Shapes (cm)

Right Judkins/Femoral—JR or FR (3.0, 3.5, 4.0, 4.5, 5.0, 6.0)

Left Judkins/Femoral—JL or FL (3.0, 3.5, 4.0, 4.5, 5.0, 6.0)

Right Amplatz—AR1, 2

Left Amplatz—AL 0.75, 1, 1.5, 2, 3

Multipurpose

Specialty Curves

Right bypass

Left bypass

Internal mammary

"Q" curve

Voda curve

"C" curve (3.0, 3.5, 4.0, 4.5, 5.0)

Hockey stick

Extra backup support—EBU or XB (3.0, 3.5, 3.75, 4.0)

TABLE 13.3 Guide Catheter Diameter Requirements

DEVICE	GUIDE CATHETER
Rotational Atherectomy	
Burr size	
1.25 mm (0.049″)	6 Fr
1.50 mm (0.059″)	6 Fr
1.75 mm (0.069″)	7 Fr
2.00 mm (0.079″)	8 Fr
2.15 mm (0.085″)	8 Fr
2.25 mm (0.089″)	8 Fr
2.50 mm (0.098″)	9 Fr
AngioJet	
XMI catheter	6 Fr
XVG catheter	7 Fr
Frontrunner chronic occlusion device	8 Fr
Kissing balloons	6–8 Fr
Kissing stents	7–8 Fr
Covered stents	7–8 Fr
Stent or balloon needing extra support	7–8 Fr

or lesions requiring two simultaneous over-the-wire (OTW) systems. In some labs, 7-Fr guides are used as a compromise. A variety of periprocedural complications (bleeding, dissection) are associated with the use of 7- or 8-Fr guides than with 6-Fr guides. Although patients receiving larger guides almost certainly have more complex lesions and comorbidities, mortality rates appear higher with larger guides (Fig. 13.2). Hence, the general adage is "bigger is not better" (7,8).

Procedural complexity should strongly influence the decision to choose the larger 7- or 8-Fr guides. Chronic total occlusions (CTO), left main disease, bifurcation stenting, rotational atherectomy, and any need for extra backup support in tortuous and/or calcified vessels are situations that should make the interventional cardiologist strongly consider 7- or 8-Fr guides (Table 13.3). While larger guides may have a higher risk of complications, the importance of facilitating a successful percutaneous intervention cannot be understated. Larger lumen guides, particularly 8-Fr guides, give the interventional cardiologist much more support to deliver balloons and stents, as well as the option to perform rotational atherectomy, bifurcation stenting, or even covered stent placement, especially in the rare event of a perforation.

Guide Catheter Shapes

After considering the size, the shape of the tip of the guide is selected in order to provide the optimal combination of support, coaxial alignment, and reach. The anatomy of the ascending aorta and tortuosity of the aorta and iliac arteries can lead to challenges in coaxial guide catheter engagement in the coronary artery. In the majority of patients with normal anatomy, the left coronary ostia can be engaged with standard Judkins left guide catheters (JLs), guide catheters that have a "U" shape (CLS, Q, Voda) or a back wall supportive curve (XB, EBU, Amplatz). Judkins right guides are commonly used for the right coronary artery (RCA), but often provide little support. In circumstances where back wall support is needed, a variety of other shapes are available (HS, AR, AL) (Figs. 13.3 and 13.4, Table 13.2).

significantly (up to 0.071 inch) (Fig. 13.1). As a result, the vast majority of interventions can now be performed with a 6-Fr guide.

From both the femoral and the radial approach, sheath and guide catheter diameter impacts the procedural outcomes and complications. The 6-Fr guide is preferred for routine procedures that do not require large devices. The 8-Fr guides are reserved for larger devices

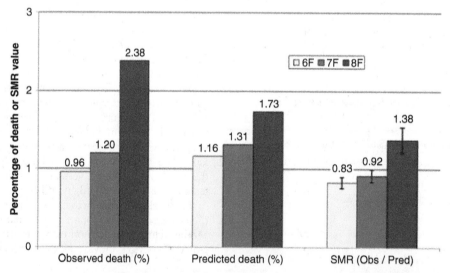

FIGURE 13.2 **Standardized mortality rate in patients undergoing PCI based upon the guide catheter size.** The observed and predicted mortality of 8-Fr guide catheter PCI patients was higher than the observed mortality of the 6- and 7-Fr guide catheter PCI patients (p <0.05 for both). The observed mortality in patients treated with 8-Fr guide catheters was higher than the predicted mortality (p <0.05), and the observed mortality of those who underwent PCI with a 6-Fr guide was lower than the predicted mortality (p <0.05). The SMR (a ratio of observed mortality to predicted mortality) of patients treated with an 8-Fr guide was significantly higher than that of patients who underwent PCI with a 6- or 7-Fr catheter (p <0.05). PCI, percutaneous coronary intervention; SMR, standardized mortality rate. (From: Grossman, et al. Percutaneous coronary intervention complications and guide catheter size. *JACC Cardiovasc Interv.* 2009;2(7):636–644, with permission.)

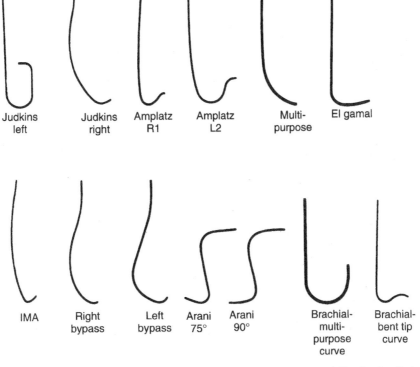

FIGURE 13.3 Basic guide catheter shapes and support. (From: Kern, ed. *The Cardiac Catheterization Handbook*. 5th ed. Philadelphia, PA: Saunders Elsevier; 2011, with permission.)

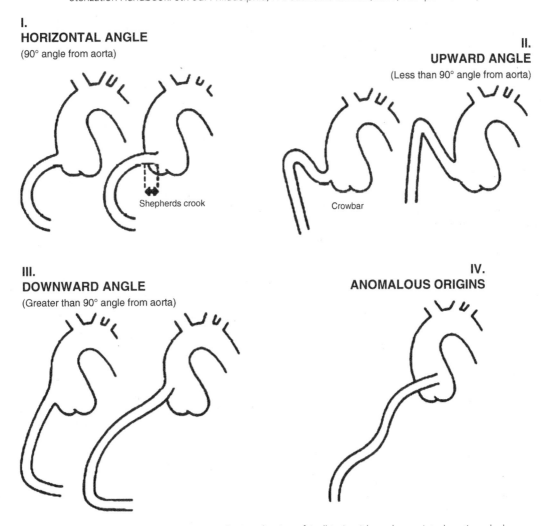

I. HORIZONTAL ANGLE
(90° angle from aorta)

Shepherds crook

II. UPWARD ANGLE
(Less than 90° angle from aorta)

Crowbar

III. DOWNWARD ANGLE
(Greater than 90° angle from aorta)

IV. ANOMALOUS ORIGINS

FIGURE 13.4 Anatomic variations to consider in selection of Judkins' guide and associated aortic arch shape.

For the left coronary artery, the length of the secondary curve depends on the patient's body habitus, age, and aorta. In general, smaller patients with narrow ascending aortas will need a shorter curve, whereas larger patients and those with dilated or tortuous aortas will require longer ones. As a rule of thumb, guide catheters should be sized a quarter to half times smaller than their equivalent diagnostic catheters. For example, if a JL 4 diagnostic catheter fits well in the left main, a JL 3.5 or EBU 3.5 would also likely fit well. Finally, oversizing the secondary curve of a left coronary guide catheter may tend to direct the catheter toward the left circumflex artery.

Side Holes for Guide Catheters

Use of side holes in guide catheters can be helpful in cases where ostial stenoses are being treated or where the guide catheter will be deeply seated for extra backup support. In guide catheters of size close to that of the coronary ostium, pressure wave damping may occur along with flow obstruction. Side holes will allow some limited perfusion into the coronary artery and permit accurate central aortic pressure monitoring. Nevertheless, side holes will tend to increase the amount of iodinated contrast used, and may give a false impression of adequate coronary perfusion. Side hole guides can create pressure artifacts when measuring fractional flow reserve.

Guide Catheter Length

The standard length of guide catheters is 100 cm; shorter guides are used if the stenosis being treated is located very distally, usually through a long saphenous vein graft into the native coronary artery or through the left internal mammary artery (IMA) into the left anterior descending coronary artery. The shorter guide, usually 90 cm, allows the angioplasty balloon catheters and stents to reach the lesion without exceeding the shaft length with 100-cm guides. Shorter guides are also commonly used now for chronic total occlusion (CTO) recanalization, especially for the donor artery in dedicated retrograde approach procedures.

Guide Catheters for the Left Internal Mammary Artery and Saphenous Vein Bypass Grafts (SVG)

Consider Judkins right, IMA, or left coronary bypass guide shapes for left IMA–left anterior descending (LIMA-LAD) interventions. Left radial access is preferable for such interventions due to proximity to the LIMA conduit as well as previously mentioned benefits with respect to bleeding and mortality. Additionally, side holes are beneficial if the LIMA is small or prone to spasm. The 90-cm guide is often chosen when the lesion is beyond the LIMA-LAD anastomosis.

Bypass grafts to the RCA often take off the aorta in an inferior or downward angle. Multipurpose guides, right coronary bypass guides, or Judkins right (JR) guides are commonly used. Bypass grafts to the left coronary arteries come off the aorta at a horizontal or upward angle. As the anatomy can be quite variable, JR, Amplatz, Hockey Stick, left coronary bypass, LIMA, and extra backup guides may be used.

Guide Catheters for Radial Access

In general, guide catheters that work well from the leg—EBU, XB, Judkins, and Amplatz shapes—also work well from the radial approach. This is particularly the case in the left radial access, which has similar approach geometry as the femoral approach. From the right radial approach, the extent of back support is limited, and catheter shapes that provide extra backup support (XB/EBU, AL, XBR, AR) are preferred.

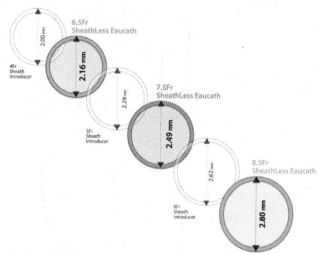

FIGURE 13.5 Comparison of inner and outer diameters of introducer sheaths and sheathless guide catheters.

Specialized shapes specifically designed to provide extra support from the radial approach include the Ikari left and right catheter. The Ikari left guide is particularly appealing during primary PCI for utility as a "single catheter" guide that can selectively cannulate either the left or right coronary main stem. The Ikari left guide also enables active support in the power position. The Amplatz left guide can be used for right coronary artery PCI due to deeper engagement, although it increases the risk for ostial and proximal coronary dissection if care is not taken in achieving a stable coaxial position.

Availability of commercially produced sheathless guide catheters now allows complex interventions to be accomplished via the transradial route. Because the outer diameter of a sheathless guide is equivalent to the outer diameter of a standard sheath approximately 2 Fr sizes smaller, most radial arteries can accommodate 7.5-Fr sheathless guides to perform complex left main or bifurcation lesion interventions (**Fig. 13.5**).

Balloon Catheters

Three types of angioplasty balloon systems are useful to dilate the target lesions before delivering a stent (**Fig. 13.6**): OTW, monorail, and fixed-wire systems. The OTW and monorail systems are also fitted with stents of various types (see Chapter 14). The OTW and monorail systems are the most commonly used systems in daily practice, whereas the fixed-wire system is reserved for the rare case of the extremely severe, difficult-to-cross stenosis. Rotational atherectomy has obviated the use of the fixed-wire balloon in nearly all cases.

A standard OTW balloon catheter has a central lumen throughout the length of the catheter for the guide wire and a separate lumen for the balloon inflation. These catheters are approximately 145 to 155 cm long and can be used with long or short guide wires, usually 0.014 inch. In contrast to monorail catheters, OTW catheters allow for the exchange of workhorse wires to stronger, stiffer, or hydrophilic guide wires. This is particularly helpful for tortuous lesions or CTO. The wire lumen can also be used to inject contrast to confirm intraluminal positioning of the catheter, or to inject intracoronary medications.

A limitation of the OTW balloon catheters is the need to extend the guide wire to keep distal wire position during balloon catheter exchanges. A 300-cm exchange wire is therefore commonly used for most OTW applications.

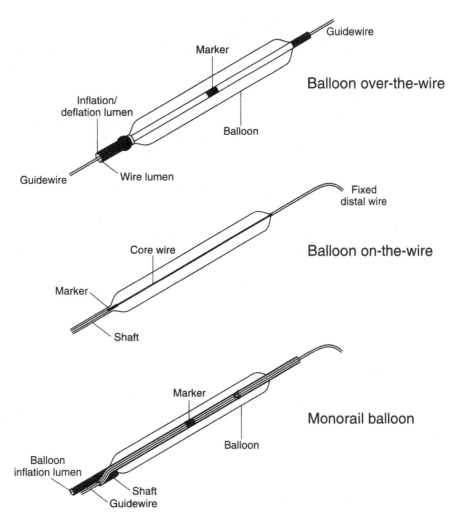

FIGURE 13.6   Three common types of coronary balloon angioplasty catheter design. **Top:** Over-the-wire balloon catheter construction. **Middle:** fixed tip wire balloon catheter. **Bottom:** Monorail balloon catheter construction. (Modified from: Freed, et al., eds. *Manual of Interventional Cardiology.* Birmingham, MI: Physicians' Press; 1992:29, with permission.)

Monorail catheters, also called rapid-exchange (RX) or single-operator balloon catheters, are the most popular catheters used today. Monorail catheters allow a single operator to exchange the PCI catheters unassisted. The monorail catheter differs from OTW catheters in that only a specific length of the shaft has two lumens. One lumen is for balloon inflation and the other, which extends through only a portion of the catheter shaft, houses the guide wire. Because only a limited portion of the balloon requires dual lumens, the catheter shafts can be made smaller than OTW systems. This allows for better deliverability and the ability to perform bifurcation balloon angioplasty using a 6-Fr guide catheter. Monorail balloon catheters obviate the need for 300-cm exchange wires, but do not allow for the exchange of guide wires. Monorail catheters also have limitations, requiring additional stronger guiding catheter support and greater diligence in the manipulation of the guide wire, balloon catheter, and guiding catheter.

diameter when inflated at high pressure. These "soft" balloons are generally used for predilatation of coronary lesions because they are inflated at lower pressures and are more flexible in crossing stenoses. They are only partially effective against vessels that are fibrotic or calcified, or in dilating a stent to full size, because they will preferentially dilate more-compliant or less-resistant areas of the vessel.

Noncompliant or "stiff" balloons are designed to expand to the target diameter; they expand only minimally with high-pressure inflation. This ensures that the pressure in the balloon is distributed equally in all directions within the vessel. These balloon catheters are useful in dilating stents to their full capacity, or for resistant lesions. Postdilatation of stents with a high-pressure balloon inflation ensures optimal stent expansion and apposition from media to media of the treated vessel.

Compliant versus Noncompliant Balloons

Balloons are generally divided into compliant and noncompliant categories. Compliance is the change in unit volume for every change in unit pressure. Compliant balloons therefore expand more in

Coronary Guide Wires

Coronary angioplasty guide wires (**Fig. 13.7**) are small-caliber (0.010–0.018 inch, typically 0.014 inch) steerable wires, advanced into the coronary artery beyond the target lesion. Extra-long guide

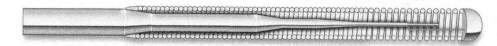

FIGURE 13.7   Schematic of coronary guide wire construction.

wires (300 cm) are used to exchange OTW balloon catheters. The tip flexibility and torque-control characteristics of these coronary guide wires vary. The softer wires are largely safer and easier to advance into tortuous branches, whereas the stiffer wires are especially useful for crossing severe or total occlusions.

Guide wires can be divided into three basic categories on the basis of their usage: "workhorse" (routine use) wires, support wires, and specialty wires (primarily for CTO). Several key factors are important for guide-wire selection: support, tip stiffness, steerability, trackability, lubricity, and torquability. With experience, every interventional cardiologist becomes accustomed to a particular guide wire he or she prefers to use in a majority of cases, thereby making it an all-purpose wire or workhorse guide wire. The majority of operators choose a guide wire that has a flexible tip and medium support as their workhorse.

Most 0.014-inch coronary wires are available from the manufacturers with a straight tip with a shaping ribbon. This allows the tip to be manually shaped into a curve by the operator. Some wires with hydrophilic coatings come preshaped from the factory. Guide wires can be safely advanced through the coronary vessel using a "torque device" for 1:1 steerability and torquability. Care should be taken when advancing the guide wire through a stenotic lesion so as to prevent dissection into the lesion, entering a subintimal space, or raising a flap, which may cause acute closure of the artery. Difficulty in crossing a lesion with a workhorse wire can be overcome by using a soft-tipped hydrophilic wire. A second wire or "buddy" wire can be used to provide extra support when difficulty is encountered in passing interventional equipment such as balloons or stents.

Polymers distinguish each coronary guide wire by its hydrophilicity. Coatings allow for increased lubricity, thereby reducing friction of the wire because it is in direct contact with the vessel wall, or in allowing delivery of interventional equipment. Hydrophilic coated wires are useful

to cross severely stenosed or subtotaled lesions, access side branches, traverse tortuous vessels, or access a side branch "jailed" by a stent.

Workhorse Wires

Standard or workhorse coronary wires are selected on the basis of their basic components, which include the central core, guide wire tip, and coating. Steerability is often enhanced in a guide wire with a central core composed of stainless steel, whereas flexibility can be expected in guide wires with nitinol central cores. Newer guide wires combine the benefits of steerability and flexibility by using a central core composed of stainless steel and nitinol. The central core is critically important for support when delivering devices such as balloons, microcatheters, or stents. The shaft or core stiffness can be increased to provide a better "rail" over which equipment can be delivered. Nevertheless, the increase in shaft stiffness can decrease steerability and cause pseudostenosis or straightening artifacts of the coronary artery. The core is ground down, and tapers toward the tip of the wire juxtaposed with a platinum spring coil, which yields flexibility and contributes to the floppiness of the wire tip. The degree of the grind to the tip will determine the flexibility, steerability, or stiffness of the tip, and therefore various guide-wire-tip designs will alter the degree of tip stiffness.

Recent advances in wire manufacturing, such as Inner Coil technology (Boston Scientific), have resulted in composite core construction, with an added inner coil, which increases wire durability, wire shape retention, rail support, and torque response. See **Figure 13.8**.

Support Wires

Extra stiff shafts are features of some wires, and these are needed to assist in delivering equipment down the coronary artery. Various support wires are available either as a primary wire or as a second or "buddy" wire placed alongside the initial wire across the stenosis.

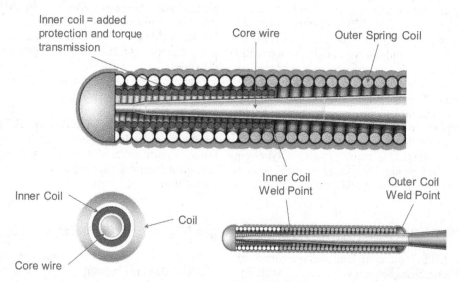

FIGURE 13.8   Schematic of Inner Coil technology of coronary guide wire construction.

The wiggle wire is a particularly helpful wire that provides great support and allows stents to be delivered across tortuous and stiff vessels (9).

Specialty Wire

Guide wires with extra tip stiffness allow the operator to traverse severely stenosed vessels, access side branches through stent struts, and cross CTO. The variety of wires to approach CTOs continues to increase. The distal wire-tip tapering and stiffness have increased, and these characteristics and the addition of hydrophilic coatings to some CTO wires have greatly enhanced the possibility of crossing the CTO. By equal measure or more, the risk of perforations and complications increases as well.

Specific Guide Wire–Related Complications

Operators should be familiar with specific coronary guide wire–related complications and their management. Rarely, coronary guide wires can get entrapped in the distal coronary circulation as a result of calcification, stenting over the wire, or jailing the wire. An OTW balloon can be helpful in dislodging the entrapped wire and allows safe removal. Attempts to retrieve any sheared components of the guide wire can be carried out using snares.

Stiff guide wires can cause a straightening artifact in tortuous vessels, producing an accordion effect or "pseudostenosis." The sudden appearance of a new lesion not present during diagnostic angiography in a tortuous vessel likely represents a straightening artifact or pseudolesion. Withdrawal of the wire (at least to the flexible tip) or changing to softer wire can relieve these pseudo-obstructions, thereby avoiding unnecessary treatment (10,11).

Coated coronary guide wires are more frequently associated with coronary artery perforation, which occurs with an incidence of 0.2% to 0.8%. Coronary perforation can lead to cardiac tamponade, emergency surgery, or death. The highest risk is seen when hydrophilic wires with stiffer tips are used in challenging cases (tortuous severe lesions and CTO), especially in conjunction with glycoprotein 2B3A inhibitors.

Wire perforations can occur when the wire tip is inadvertently advanced distally in the terminal portion of the artery or one of its side branches. Diagnosis is made angiographically when extravascular contrast stain or blush is noted outside the coronary vascular tree. The mainstay of successful treatment includes balloon occlusion of the vessel, immediate reversal of anticoagulation, and pericardiocentesis, if necessary. Surveillance echocardiography is

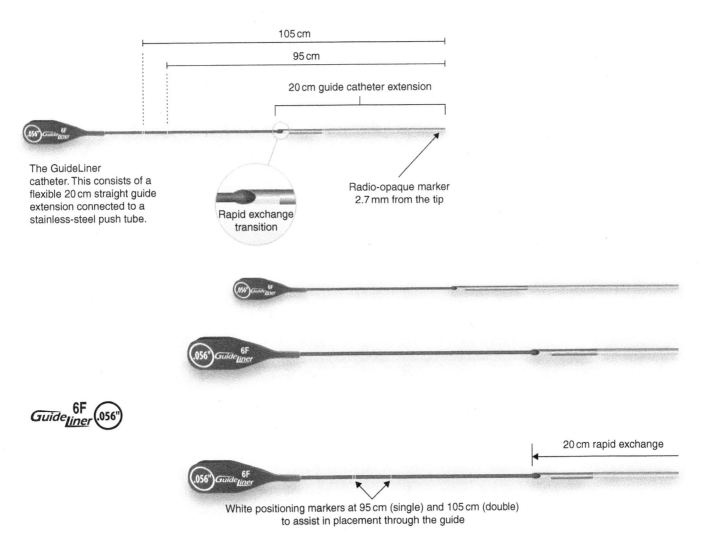

FIGURE 13.9 **Guideliner design.** This catheter extension consists of a flexible 20-cm straight extension tube connected to a stainless-steel push tube. (Vascular Solutions, Inc.)

warranted for both early and late management. Coil embolization, thrombin injection, or gel foam can be effective in sealing a distal wire perforation (12).

Adjunctive Equipment

Guide Catheter Extension—The Guideliner

The Guideliner (**Fig. 13.9**) is a monorail "guide extension" that is inserted into a guide over a 0.014-inch guide wire that is already down the coronary artery across the stenosis. The Guideliner can be advanced down the coronary artery, intubating the vessel and providing active support. This provides the added support that can then facilitate stent delivery across calcified and/or tortuous vessels. The Guideliner has been modified into a two-in-one device to include a trapping balloon, aptly named the TrapLiner, which when inflated

can maintain guidewire position. The Guideliner and TrapLiner are available in various sizes (see **Fig. 13.10**).

Microvascular Catheters for CTO

A variety of microvascular catheters are now available that can assist coronary interventions. Many catheters, such as the Transit catheter, are just single-lumen catheters used to either exchange out a wire or inject through. Other catheters available are discussed in the context of treating CTO: The Quick cross, FineCross, Turnpike, Caravel, Corsair, and Tornus catheters all have special features that can facilitate revascularizing CTOs (**Fig. 13.11**). The Corsair Pro builds on the original Corsair with hub design changes that allow improved catheter durability during crossing of septal channels or CTO segments (see **Fig. 13.12A** and **B**).

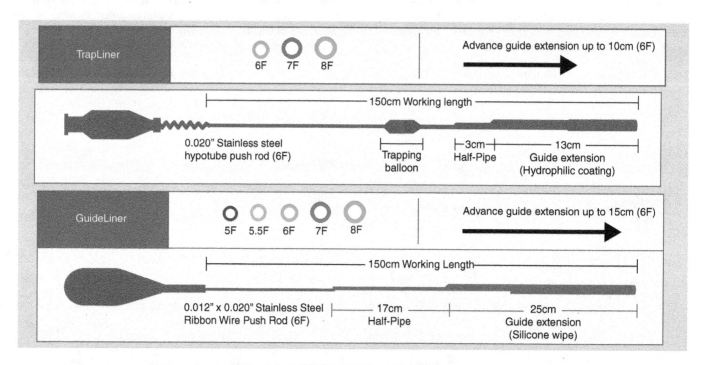

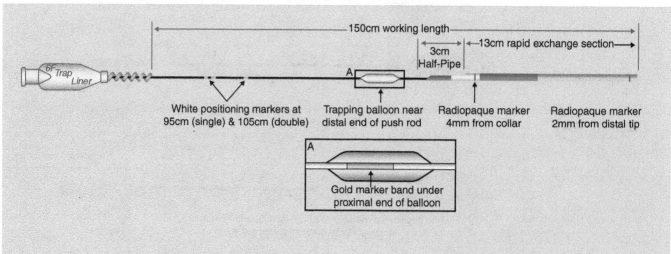

FIGURE 13.10 Comparison of TrapLiner and GuideLiner catheters.

| Micro Catheter | Outer diameter | | | Length |
	Entry	Distal shaft	Proximal shaft	
Fine cross	1.8 Fr	1.8 Fr	2.6 Fr	135/150
	.60mm	.60mm	.87mm	
Micro 14	1.6 Fr	1.9 Fr	2.5 Fr	155
	.53mm	.64mm	.83mm	
Caravel	1.4 Fr	1.9 Fr	2.6 Fr	135/150
	.53mm	.64mm	.83mm	
Turnpike LP	1.6 Fr	2.2 Fr	2.9 Fr	135/150
	.53mm	.74mm	.97mm	
Corsair	1.3 Fr	2.6 Fr	2.8 Fr	135/150
	.42mm	.87mm	.93mm	
Turnpike	1.6 Fr	2.6 Fr	3.1 Fr	135/150
	.53mm	.86mm	1.02mm	

FIGURE 13.11 Whisker plot of odds ratio of cumulative revascularization and MACE rates at 360 days from randomized clinical trials comparing cutting balloon angioplasty (ablation) to percutaneous coronary angioplasty (PTCA). (Adapted from: Bittl JA, et al. Meta-analysis of randomized trials of percutaneous transluminal coronary angioplasty versus atherectomy, cutting balloon atherectomy, or angioplasty. *J Am Coll Cardiol*. 2004;43(6):936–942, with permission.)

SuperCross Microcatheters

The SuperCross family of microcatheters are 0.014-inch guide-wire support catheters composed of a full-length stainless-steel braid with a polytetrafluoroethylene (PTFE) inner layer. The former allows for excellent flexibility and pushability, while the latter allows for optimal guide-wire movement and exchange. The distal 40 cm of the catheter has a hydrophilic coating, which improves deliverability. Unique to this family of microcatheters is the seamless, conical, tapered distal tip, which greatly enhances tip flexibility. The distal tip also has an embedded gold marker band allowing for adequate radiopacity, similar to the FineCross catheter. The SuperCross catheters are available in 130-cm and 150-cm working lengths. These microcatheters come in angled-tip versions of 45°, 90°, and 120°, markedly improving the ease of guide-wire insertion in tortuous vessels, especially at bifurcation points, or easing direct wire placement through stent struts. The distal angled-tip portion of the catheter is composed of a platinum/tungsten coil, which improves curve retention and radiopacity. The combination of improved flexibility, pushability, and radiopacity with an angled-tip version makes these catheters

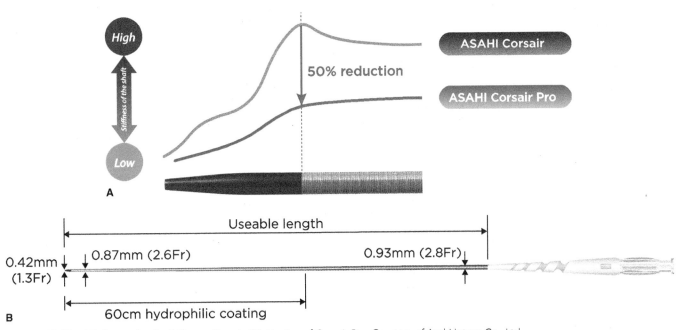

FIGURE 13.12 **(A)** Corsair Pro flexibility vs. Corsair; **(B)**, Design of Corsair Pro. Courtesy of Asahi Intecc Co., Ltd.

an ideal option to successfully traverse tortuous coronary anatomy when attempting to treat a distal lesion.

Venture Catheter for Tortuous Vessels

The Venture catheter (Fig. 13.8) is an OTW or RX accessory catheter that is used in cases where there is great difficulty steering the guide wire down the coronary and across the target lesion. Angulation of the catheter can be obtained by torquing and deflecting the tip, allowing passage of a guide wire across tortuous vessels. The Venture catheter is helpful in passing wires down the retrograde limb of a SVG, obtaining access to a tortuous acute-angled side branch, as well as passing a wire down a left circumflex that comes off the left main at a very sharp angle.

■ The majority of operators choose a guide wire that has a flexible tip and medium support as their workhorse.

■ Ideal workhorse coronary guide wire includes the following:
- Soft, flexible, and atraumatic tip
- Excellent torque transfer, 1:1
- Exquisite tactile feel
- Retains shape
- Steerability and pushability
- Supportive, but tracks well in tortuous vessels
- Facilitates balloon and stent delivery

■ The increase in shaft stiffness can help facilitate equipment delivery. Nevertheless, it will decrease steerability and cause pseudostenosis or straightening artifacts of the coronary artery.

Key Points

■ The choice of radial or femoral approach depends on operator experience and the need for extra guide support.

■ The transradial route is preferable for PCI during acute coronary syndrome.

■ Sheathless guides permit performance of complex transradial interventions.

■ The majority of PCIs can be performed through a 6-Fr guide.

■ The 8-Fr guides are associated with higher morbidity and mortality than 6-Fr guides.

■ For complex procedures, an 8-Fr guide will give the operator added support and more options and room for ancillary equipment.

■ The anatomy of the ascending aorta plays a pivotal role in guide selection.

■ Guides with side holes may be helpful for hemodynamic monitoring and can provide additional coronary perfusion.

■ Balloon catheters typically come in OTW and monorail formats.

■ OTW balloons are useful for total occlusions and tortuous lesions.

■ Compliant balloons expand with inflation and are used for predilatation of lesions prior to stenting.

■ Noncompliant balloons expand less with high-pressure inflation, and are useful for resistant lesions and for optimal postdilatation of stents.

References

1. Vranckx P, et al. Radial versus femoral access in patients with acute coronary syndromes with or without ST-segment elevation. *Eur Heart J.* 2017;38(14):1069–1080.
2. Valgimigli M, et al. Radial versus femoral access in patients with acute coronary syndromes undergoing invasive management: a randomized multicenter trial. *Lancet.* 2015;385(9986):2465–2476.
3. Masoudi F, et al. Trends in U.S. Cardiovascular Care 2016 Report from 4 ACC National Cardiovascular Data Registries. *J Am Coll Cardiol.* 2017;69(11):1427–1450.
4. Rakhit RD, et al. Five French versus six French PCI: a case control study of efficacy, safety and outcome. *J Invasive Cardiol.* 2002;14(11):670–674.
5. Takeshita S, Tanaka S, Saito S. Coronary intervention with 4 French catheters. *Catheter Cardiovasc Interv.* 2010;75(5):735–739.
6. Mizuno S, et al. Percutaneous coronary intervention using a virtual 3 French guiding catheter. *Catheter Cardiovasc Interv.* 2010;75(7):983–988.
7. Grossman PM, et al. Percutaneous coronary intervention complications and guide catheter size. *JACC Cardiovasc Interv.* 2009;2:636–644.
8. Applegate RJ, et al. Trends in vascular complications after diagnostic cardiac catheterization and percutaneous coronary interventions via the femoral artery 1998–2007. *JACC Cardiovasc Interv.* 2008;1:317–326.
9. Burzotta F, et al. Use of a second buddy wire during percutaneous coronary interventions: a simple solution for some challenging situation. *J Invasive Cardiol.* 2005;17:171–174.
10. Alfonso F, et al. Pressure wire kinking, entanglement, and entrapment during intravascular ultrasound studies: a potentially dangerous complication. *Catheter Cardiovasc Interv.* 2000;50:221–225.
11. Gouveia D, et al. De-novo reversible stenoses in tortuous arteries during coronary angioplasty due to the accordion effect. A clinical case and review of the literature [in Portuguese]. *Rev Port Cardiol.* 1997;16:1037–1042, 957.
12. Gunning MG, et al. Coronary artery perforation during percutaneous intervention: incidence and outcome. *Heart.* 2002;88:495–498.

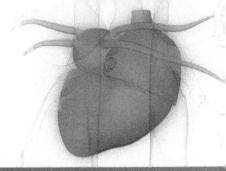

14

Niche Devices: Atherectomy, Cutting and Scoring Balloons, and Laser

P. Matthew Belford, MD, FACC, FSCAI, and

Robert J. Applegate, MD, FACC, FAHA, MSCAI

Rotational Atherectomy

DEVICE

The rotablator (Boston Scientific; Marlboro, MA) is an over-the-wire (OTW) system that consists of a nickel-plated, diamond-coated brass burr attached to a drive shaft that can achieve speeds up to 200,000 rpm driven by compressed gas (Fig. 14.1). The 20- to 30-μm-sized diamond chips are located only on the front half of the olive-shaped burr. Much like a high-speed sander, the rotablator burr ablates and creates microparticulate debris when the burr comes into contact with relatively inelastic tissue. The turbine unit is cooled using a saline flush solution that also helps irrigate the vessel during activation of the burr, helping disperse the microparticulate debris through the vasculature. The reusable console can be adjusted to achieve burr speeds up to 200,000 rpm in the fully activated mode, and speeds of 80,000 rpm when used in the Dynaglide mode (used almost solely for the purpose of removing the burr from the guide catheter). Each burr and drive shaft come as a separate unit and are attached to a disposable advancer using a locking mechanism. The advancer has a control knob that allows the operator to advance or retract the spinning burr, and has a range of 10 cm before the burr position needs to be moved if additional atherectomy is desired. The burr and drive shaft accommodate a 0.09 inch guide wire with a floppy tip of 30 cm that has a 0.21 olive at the joint between the flexible tip and the shaft of the guide wire to prevent the burr from advancing to the flexible tip of the guide wire. A special wire clip is attached at the end of the guide wire as it exits the advancer, and helps prevent the wire from spinning during the high-speed rotation. The advancer also has an internal brake that prevents the wire from spinning or advancing, which can be manually overridden by a "brake defeat" button at the back end of the device.

Principles of Atherectomy

The atheroablative effect of the rotablator system is based on the concept of differential cutting that is selective ablation of relatively inelastic materials such as calcified or heavily fibrotic atheromatous plaque versus sparing of elastic non-diseased vessel segments. The analogy of rotablation is shaving with the razor preferentially cutting hair (inelastic tissue) and not skin (elastic tissue). The microparticulate debris generated during atherectomy range from 5 to 12 μm depending on the atherectomy speed and composition of the plaque. The debris passes through the coronary microcirculation and is ultimately taken up by the reticulo endothelial system of the spleen and liver. The rate and volume of microparticulate debris in relation to coronary flow will ultimately determine whether or not microvascular obstruction occurs, overwhelming the capacity of the capillary system. The rotablator device also takes advantage of

Console and foot pedal

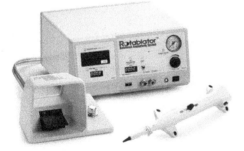

Advancer and catheter

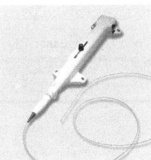

Cartoon of burr in vessel

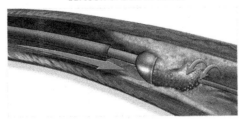

FIGURE 14.1 Composite images of the components (console and foot pedal; and advancer and catheter) of the rotablator system. The 0.009-inch guide wire used to deliver the burr to the lesion site is not shown. A cartoon of the burr within a lesion is shown on the bottom.

orthogonal displacement of friction as a result of the high rotational speeds, which essentially eliminates the longitudinal friction component of resistance. This characteristic distinguishes it from simple balloon and stent catheter passive movement within the coronary arterial system and guide catheter.

The optimal speed during an atherectomy procedure has undergone extensive evaluation (1). Extremely low speeds potentially generate larger microparticulate debris and are inefficient in ablation, while very high speeds are associated with significant local rises in temperature and potentially thermal-mediated vascular changes, including a propensity for flow reduction. Rates of 140,000 to 160,000 appear to provide an optimal compromise between the efficiency and extent of atherectomy in relation to local thermal effects and are the currently recommended range of speed for most atherectomy procedures.

Procedure

BURR SELECTION

Burr selection has undergone a substantial evolution since the introduction of rotational atherectomy (RA). Initially, the device was used to debulk arteries, followed by balloon angioplasty. With the advent and success of intracoronary stents, and lack of data demonstrating that RA reduced restenosis rates, RA has been used almost exclusively for lesion preparation, prior to stenting, when a lesion is undilatable or extensive calcification is present. In contemporary use, burr sizes of 1.25 to 1.75 mm generally provide appropriate lesion preparation prior to stenting and it would only be under unusual circumstances that burr sizes beyond this would be chosen. In general, the greater the vessel angulation and/or extent of calcification, the smaller the burr sizes that would be chosen. The operator's comfort level will also help dictate whether the procedure will start with a 1.25- or 1.5-mm burr. One technical note bears mentioning: the 1.25 burr has a more tubular shape than the larger, more-olive shaped burrs, with many experts believing that the smallest burr is more prone to "jump forward" and potentially get lodged in the vessel.

GUIDE CATHETER SELECTION

Guide catheter selection for RA requires coaxial alignment, appropriate sizing to allow advancement and retraction of the burrs, and some measure of coronary flow during the procedure to help move microparticulate debris through the coronary microvasculature. The internal diameter of the guide catheter should be 0.04 inches larger than the burr to minimize difficulty during advancement and retraction of the burr. In addition, guide shapes require gentle transition from the shaft of the burr to the tip because acute angles, such as may be seen with a typical Judkins catheter, can impede the advancement and/or retraction of the burrs at the primary and secondary curves of the catheter. Finally, side holes may be useful so that continued flow occurs around the drive shaft of the rotablator device even during activation and advancement.

Procedural Technique

Atherectomy is begun approximately 1 cm proximal to the target lesion with constant flush through the drive shaft, controlled by a foot pedal connected to the console in an on-and-off fashion (**Table 14.1**). Expert consensus opinion is that optimal RA involves slow advancement of the burr with contact with the stenotic plaque for approximately 10 to 15 seconds, and then withdrawal of the burr from the lesion allowing coronary flow to occur, followed by resumption of 10 seconds of atherectomy. Total atherectomy runs are recommended to last no more than 30 to 45 seconds to minimize the potential of overwhelming the microvasculature with the microparticulate debris. Atherectomy is continued with multiple runs until the lesion has been successfully crossed, the full extent of the 10-cm range of the advancer has been exhausted, or it appears that continued efforts would be futile with the burr chosen.

Adjunctive Techniques

The composition of the fluid used to cool the turbine of the advancer is often augmented to include nitroglycerin as a vasodilator, as well as Roto-glide (Boston Scientific; Marlboro, MA) as a coronary lubricant.

TABLE 14.1 Contemporary Rotational Atherectomy

	TRADITIONAL	CONTEMPORARY
Arterial access	Femoral 8 Fr	Radial (6–7.5 Fr) or femoral (6–8 Fr), depending upon burr size requirement and operator experience.
Guiding catheter	Judkins catheters	Single curve with strong support. Operator preference but stable catheter position required.
Guide wire	Floppy rotawire or extra support rotawire for aorto-ostial lesions	Rotawire placement not always straightforward. Use of regular wire placement, with exchange using microcatheter placement is often required.
Burr size	Debulking up to 0.7 vessel ratio	Plaque modification with small burrs (1.25–1.5 mm) as initial strategy is default position. A step-up approach is encouraged to limit debris size and complications.
Ablation speed	180,000–200,000 rpm	Plaque modification usually achieved at low speeds (135,000–180,000 rpm) to reduce risk of complications.
Temporary pacemaker	Always for dominant RCA and left main PCI	Smaller burrs at lower speeds have led to lower incidence of transient heart block. Many operators use atropine to treat, avoiding any complications of temporary pacemaker placement.
Rotablation flush	Rotablation cocktail with verapamil, nitrates, and heparin in saline recommended.	Rotablation cocktail with verapamil, nitrates, and heparin in saline recommended.

RCA, right coronary artery; PCI, percutaneous coronary intervention.

TABLE 14.2 Indications and Contraindications for Rotational Atherectomy

INDICATIONS	CONTRAINDICATIONS
Single-vessel atherosclerotic CAD[a]	Lesion cannot be crossed with guide wire[a]
Multi-vessel atherosclerotic CAD[a]	Last remaining vessel with compromised LV function[a]
Restenotic lesions[a]	Saphenous vein grafts[a]
Native vessel CAD with lesion length <25 mm[a]	Angiographic evidence of thrombus[a]
Heavily calcified lesions	Angiographic evidence of dissection at lesion site[a]
Undilatable lesions	

[a] Per instructions for use.
CAD, coronary artery disease; LV, left ventricular.

The latter consists of a sterile egg white and olive oil emulsion, which in animal testing appeared to minimize heat generation, permitting a higher rate of rotation of the burr if needed. General expert consensus also recommends liberal use of vasopressors to maintain an adequate perfusion pressure during RA. Practically, this is most easily performed with 100-μg bolus injections of Neo-Synephrine. Additionally, liberal use of nitroglycerin throughout the procedure is recommended to enhance coronary flow and minimize microparticulate obstruction of the microvasculature. Prophylactic pacemakers have been used

by some to counteract the bradycardia, which can be severe at times, that may accompany rotablation. Nevertheless, some operators use aminophylline and/or atropine to minimize atherectomy-associated bradycardia without use of temporary pacemakers.

Indications and Contraindications for Use

The manufacturers' and generally accepted clinical indications and contraindications for use of RA are shown in **Table 14.2**. Operator experience will dictate comfort levels with these parameters. Accepted indications are heavily calcified lesions able to be crossed with the rotablator guide wire, as well as undilatable lesions. In contemporary practice, RA has shown a resurgence in use due to a more elderly population enriched with more calcific disease, as well as use in more complex percutaneous coronary intervention (PCI) and chronic total occlusions. Accepted contraindications include severe lesion entry or exit angulation, and angiographically visible thrombus or dissection.

Outcomes

The studies evaluating the clinical efficacy and safety of RA were performed in the late 1990s (2–4). As a result of these studies, RA was shown to be at most non-inferior to percutaneous transluminal coronary angioplasty (PTCA) with respect to restenosis, and associated with higher rates of adverse cardiac events. More recently, Arora and colleagues (5) published the results of PCI with and without RA from a nationwide patient sample from 107,131 cases in 2012, and showed higher overall complication rates with RA (12.7%) compared to without RA (9.1%), p < 0.01 (**Table 14.3**). With the advent of the stent era, continued interest in debulking prior to

TABLE 14.3 Incidence of Periprocedural Complications of Percutaneous Coronary Intervention

	ATHERECTOMY		OVERALL	p-VALUE
	NO	YES		
Overall (unweighted)	103,759 (96.85)	3,372 (3.15)	107,131	
Overall (weighted)	518,795 (96.85)	16,860 (3.15)	535,655	
Any complication[a]	9.05%	12.66%	9.16%	<0.001
Any complication or death	9.73%	13.5%	9.85%	<0.001
Any vascular complication	1.06%	1.57%	1.08%	<0.001
Postoperative hemorrhage requiring transfusion	0.4%	0.3%	0.4%	<0.001
Vascular injury	0.7%	1.28%	0.71%	<0.001
Cardiac complications	2.07%	4.06%	2.14%	<0.001
Iatrogenic cardiac complications	1.83%	3.56%	1.88%	<0.001
Pericardial complications	0.13%	0.3%	0.13%	<0.001
Open heart surgery	0.16%	0.24%	0.16%	0.01
Respiratory complications (postoperative respiratory failure)	5.46%	7.12%	5.51%	<0.001
Postoperative stroke/TIA	0.14%	0.12%	0.14%	0.507
Acute renal failure requiring dialysis	0.18%	0.24%	0.18%	0.107
Postoperative DVT/PE	0.52%	0.71%	0.53%	0.001
Postoperative infectious complications	1.44%	1.66%	1.45%	0.019

[a] Any peri-procedural complication listed in supplemental table 1.
DVT, deep venous thrombosis; PE, pulmonary embolism; TIA, transient ischemic attack.
Adapted from: Arora S, et al. Coronary atherectomy in the United States (from a nationwide inpatient sample). *Am J Cardiol.* 2016;117:555–562.

TABLE 14.4 2011 ACCF/AHA/SCAI PCI Guidelines

Coronary Atherectomy: Recommendations

- Class IIa
  - Rotational atherectomy is reasonable for fibrotic or heavily calcified lesions that might not be crossed by a balloon catheter or adequately dilated before stent implantation (*Level of Evidence: C*).
- Class III: NO BENEFIT
  - Rotational atherectomy should not be performed routinely for de-novo lesions or in-stent restenosis (*Level of Evidence: A*).

TABLE 14.5 Complication Management—Avoid with Good Technique

	TECHNIQUE TO AVOID	STRATEGY FOR RESOLUTION
Slow-flow	Small burrs and lower speeds	Optimize BP if low
	Be patient between ablation runs	Use of intracoronary nitrates/verapamil/adenosine/nitroprusside all described
		Use of flush cocktail
Dissection	Careful case selection to avoid excessive tortuosity	Avoid further rotablation if dissection identified
		Dissection management as for any PCI
Burr entrapment	Rare complication usually avoided with careful case selection and good technique	Controlled push and pull of rotablation shaft
		Position second wire to allow balloon placement
		Cautious deep intubation with mother-in-child catheter for more support
		Cardiothoracic surgical resolution occasionally required
Perforation	Commonly related to poor technique (oversizing of burr, too angulated, inappropriate speed)	Standard techniques to resolve any perforation, including emergency pericardiocentesis and use of covered stents

BP, blood pressure; PCI, percutaneous coronary intervention.

stent placement led to the evaluation of atherectomy as an adjunct to stenting. In the SPORT trial, patients with moderate to heavily calcified lesions were randomized to either RA, followed by stenting, or PTCA followed by stenting (6). The trial was stopped early, but available data were presented that showed the primary endpoint of restenosis at 9 months was similar between the two groups, while major adverse cardiac events were higher with RA. More recently, outcomes after Taxus stent placement, with or without RA, were evaluated in 240 patients in the ROTAXUS trial (7). They also did not observe a decrease in late lumen loss after RA, compared to balloon angioplasty.

As a result of these clinical trials, in the 2011 update of PCI guidelines (**Table 14.4**), coronary atherectomy was given a Class IIa recommendation for preparation of fibrotic or heavily calcified lesions that might not be crossed by a balloon catheter or adequately dilated prior to stent implantation (level of evidence: C). Coronary atherectomy was given a Class III indication (harm) in the routine treatment of de novo or in-stent restenosis (level of evidence: A) (8).

Complications

The operator should be aware of several procedural complications that are relatively common with the use of coronary atherectomy (**Table 14.5**). Bradycardia can accompany RA and can be severe. It most commonly is associated with treatment of the right coronary artery but can be seen with treatment of both the left anterior descending (LAD) and circumflex coronary arteries as well. Although some operators favor pre-procedural placement of a temporary pacemaker, this is often not required with the use of aminophylline and atropine, as mentioned earlier, and can result in cardiac tamponade as a result of ventricular perforation. Coronary slow flow or no flow is a well-recognized complication of coronary atherectomy. Multiple preventive strategies have been outlined. Factors that have been implicated in slow flow include excessive burr speeds, prolonged atherectomy, as well as burr "deceleration" during atherectomy. The latter is defined as a decrease in more than 5,000 rpm below the average working atherectomy speed and is signaled in the change in the frequency generated by the device during atherectomy. Although very uncommon, burr entrapment can occur as the burr deeply engages the vessel and plaque, causing stalling or complete cessation of rotation of the device. Once this occurs, coronary ischemia will develop due to flow obstruction. Because the device performs atherectomy in a clockwise fashion, it has been suggested that detachment of the burr from the advancer, and counterclockwise manual rotation of the burr, can help facilitate removal of the device. In extreme circumstances, it may be necessary to perform emergency surgery to remove the device.

Finally, coronary perforation remains one of the feared complications of coronary RA. In the largest cohort study to date of perforations associated with RA use, the incidence of coronary perforations was 1.3% (103/8,047), and in multivariate analysis had an odds ratio of 2.37 (95%; CI 1.80–3.11; p < 0.001) for predicting a perforation (9). In spite of differential cutting, the position of the guide wire across an angulated segment of the vessel may still result in ablation and ultimately perforation. The propensity for the guide wire to lay within the coronary vessel in the straightest path has been termed "wire bias" and may bring the burr into contact with non-diseased elements of the vessel wall (1). Type I and Type II perforations can often be managed with adjunct balloon angioplasty. Free-flowing Type III perforations are much more difficult to treat and may often necessitate pericardiocentesis and/or emergency surgery. Although a covered stent would be attractive in these situations, these perforations often occur at severe angulations of vessels, in heavily calcified vessels and in more distal locations of the coronary circulation, making placement of the bulky covered stents difficult at best. It should be noted that direct thrombin inhibitors were not used at the time of the initial experience with RA. In today's practice, direct thrombin inhibitors are frequently used and are potentially problematic with use of RA because their effect cannot be reversed in the setting of a perforation, and unfractionated heparin is the consensus recommendation of experts regarding use of this device.

Orbital Atherectomy

Device

The orbital atherectomy system (OAS) (Cardiovascular Systems, Inc., St. Paul, Minnesota) is an OTW system that has similarities to rotational atherectomy (RA), but with notable differences in the mechanism of atherectomy and technique (Fig. 14.2). The single, eccentrically mounted diamond-coated crown orbits on the wire rather than spins, utilizing the mechanism of centrifugal force, which presses the crown against the lesion, resulting in differential sanding. An advantage of the system is it is able to exert sanding motions with both forward and backward advancement of the burr. The subsequent microparticulate debris is smaller than with RA (<2 vs. 5–10 μm). The entire system consists of four components: the device (OAD, orbital atherectomy device), which is an OTW sheath-covered drive shaft and crown; a guide wire; a reusable external pump system; and a lubricant solution. The OAD has a single crown size that can be used for all cases. It is 6-Fr guide-compatible, but can be used with a 7-Fr guide for more robust support. The radius of atherectomy is altered using the speed of orbit: 80,000 and 120,000 rpm. An advancer unit allows the operator to advance or retract the burr at a target travel rate of between 1 and 10 mm per second. Similar to the rotablator, the pump infuses a mixture to cool and lubricate the mechanism, reducing friction between the drive shaft and the glide wire. The glide wire is a stainless steel 0.012-inch wire with a silicon coating and spring tip, which measures 0.014 inch,

in contrast to the body of the 0.009-inch rotablator wire. This tip must angiographically be at least 10 cm distal to the target lesion.

Principles of Orbital Atherectomy

The underlying mechanism of differential sanding is similar to that of RA (see earlier) in that there is selective ablation of inelastic materials, including heavily calcified or fibrotic plaque versus normal vessel. The notable differences involve the single crown size and orbit compared to the potentially larger burr sizes with RA.

Procedure

BURR SELECTION

In contrast to RA where burr size is a complex choice and has been well-studied, in orbital atherectomy (OA) this is a far more straightforward choice. Most cases are accomplished with one crown size (fixed "classic crown" of 1.25 mm), but the orbital path and speed allow for varied depth of orbital cutting.

GUIDE CATHETER SELECTION

Guide catheter selection requires significant coaxial guide support and appropriate sizing. Extra backup guides for the left coronary system, and a MAC 3.0 (Medtronic) or the Amplatz Left curve guides, work well for the right coronary system. This can be accomplished through a 6- or 7-Fr system.

Procedural Technique

OA is begun by positioning the crown over the wire 1 cm proximal to the target lesion, visualizing that the tip is not within the lesion

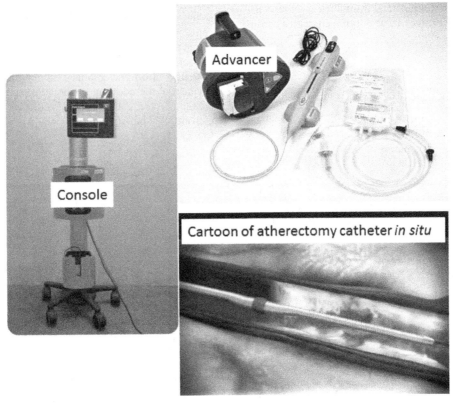

FIGURE 14.2 Composite images of the components (console; and advancer and catheter) of the orbital atherectomy system. The guide wire used to deliver the burr to the lesion site is not shown. A cartoon of the crown within a lesion is shown on the bottom.

when the crown and drive shaft begin to spin. The advancement begins after ensuring that 5 mm exists between the proximal end of the guide wire spring tip and the OAD drive shaft at the distal end of the lesion. The break lever is engaged and the control knob and button is used to turn on the device and control the forward advancement of the burr. A slow rate of travel through the lesion, between 1 and 10 mm per second, is desired in a slow forward-and-backward motion for a total of no more than 30 seconds—with a maximal treatment time of 5 minutes. An equal period of rest between runs is recommended, and the system provides an audible alarm at 25 seconds. Unlike RA, additional runs or passes with the device will provide further gain in luminal area due to the different mechanism of action and the contribution of increasing centrifugal force on the lesion. Longer lesions will require additional passes, not just longer-duration passes.

Adjunctive Techniques

The system includes ViperSlide (Cardiovascular Systems, Inc.; St. Paul, MN), which is an emulsion comprised of soybean oil, egg yolk phospholipids, glycerin, sodium hydroxide, and water. This decreases heat and friction between the OAD and the guide wire. Similar to RA, prophylactic pacemaker placement should be considered in right coronary artery (RCA) lesions, or in left dominant circumflex lesions.

Indications and Contraindications for Use

The manufacturer's generally accepted clinical indication is to facilitate stent delivery in patients with coronary artery disease who are acceptable candidates for PTCA or stenting due to, de novo, severely calcified coronary artery lesions (**Table 14.6**). The accepted contraindications include an inability to pass the wire, a target in a bypass graft, a stent or last remaining conduit, and an angiographically visible dissection or thrombus. A strong relative contraindication would be that of severe tortuosity, with a particular focus on lesion entry or exit angles.

Outcomes

The data evaluating the clinical safety and efficacy of OA are derived from the ORBIT I and ORBIT II studies. There is no randomized controlled trial directly comparing RA with OA. The ORBIT I trial was a two-center, prospective, non-randomized feasibility study in 50 patients (10). Device success was 98%, and procedural success

was 94%. Major adverse events occurred in 4% in-hospital; in 6% at 30 days; and in 8% at 6 months. The ORBIT II trial (Chambers) was a prospective multicenter non-blinded single-arm trial in 443 patients with severely calcified lesions. Successful stent delivery after OA occurred in 97.7% of patients. The rates of slow flow and no-reflow were very low, occurring in less than 1% of patients. In-hospital MI occurred in 0.7% of patients, target vessel revascularization in 0.7%, and cardiac death in 0.2%. Guidelines for use of OA were not included in the 2011 PCI AHA/ACC/SCAI guidelines.

Complications

The overall mix of complications with OA is similar to that of RA, including bradycardia, particularly in patients with culprit RCA or left-dominant large circumflex lesions; dissection; slow flow or no reflow; and, most alarmingly, coronary perforation. In the ORBIT II trial, the rate of any of these complications was low: 0.9% post-OA and 1.8% overall (8/443).

Cutting Balloon Angioplasty

Device

The Flextome Cutting Balloon Device (Boston Scientific, Minneapolis, MN) is a novel device that features three or four longitudinally aligned atherotomes (microsurgical blades) fixed to a balloon (**Fig. 14.3**). The atherotomes measure 10 to 15 mm in length by 0.011 to 0.013 inches in height, with a width of 0.04 to 0.06 inches—depending on balloon diameter and length. Balloon sizes from 2.0 to 3.25 mm have three atherotomes, while those balloon sizes 3.5 to 4.0 have four atherotomes. These atherotomes are folded within the balloon material along its long axis in the deflated position and are slowly deployed over approximately 1 minute. This process creates controlled longitudinal incisions as a result of the deployment process. When the balloon is deflated, the atherotomes are folded within the balloon material to minimize the risk of trauma as the balloon is withdrawn from the coronary circulation. It should be noted that, because of the addition of the atherotomes, the balloons have a crossing profile that is larger than either compliant or noncompliant conventional balloons.

Procedure

The general preparation for the cutting balloon procedure is similar to that for a simple balloon angioplasty (11). The one caveat may be that guides with additional backup support might be necessary to cross some lesions because of the bulkier nature of the cutting balloon compared to a conventional balloon. Similar to simple balloon angioplasty, the lesion is initially crossed with a coronary guide wire and the cutting balloon is advanced to the lesion site. As can be recognized by the short working lengths, the device is designed to treat short lesions. Once the lesion is crossed, the balloon is inflated at 2-atm increments, over 10 to 20 seconds, until a final deployment pressure of 4 to 8 atm is achieved. Deflation is performed similar to balloon angioplasty and the device withdrawn into the guide catheter. In some circumstances when the result is suboptimal, upsizing an additional half size may be necessary to achieve optimal enlargement of the vessel at the lesions site.

Indications for Use

The manufacturer's and generally accepted clinical indications and contraindications for use of cutting balloon angioplasty are shown

---

TABLE 14.6 Indications and Contraindications for Orbital Atherectomy

INDICATIONS	CONTRAINDICATIONS
To facilitate stent delivery in patients with coronary artery disease who are acceptable candidates for PTCA or stenting due to de-novo, severely calcified coronary artery lesions[a]	Inability to pass wire[a]
	Target in a bypass graft, stent, or last remaining conduit[a]
	Angiographically visible thrombus[a]

[a]Per instructions for use.
PTCA, percutaneous transluminal coronary angioplasty.

Cutting balloon OTW and monorail catheters

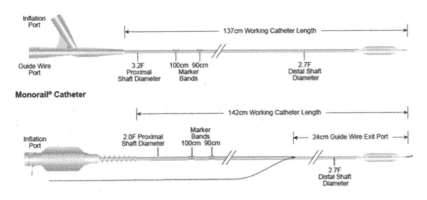

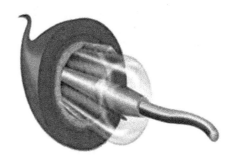

Cartoon of inflated cutting balloon *in situ*

Magnified view of inflated cutting balloon

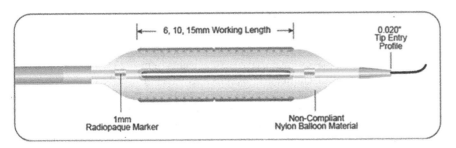

FIGURE 14.3 Schematics of an over-the wire (*top*) and monorail cutting balloon are shown. A magnified image of an inflated cutting balloon showing the exposed atherotomes fixed to the long axis of the balloon is shown on the bottom. A cartoon of an inflated cutting balloon in a vessel is shown on the right.

in Table 14.7. Generally accepted indications are for focal-resistant lesions, in-stent restenosis, and ostial and bifurcation lesions. Contraindications are angiographically visible thrombus and concentric severe calcification. The manufacturer warns about using the cutting balloon distal to a stent, or through a stent strut, because the device may become entangled in the stent and be difficult to remove and/or disrupt the stent architecture.

TABLE 14.7 Indications and Contraindications for Cutting Balloon Angioplasty

INDICATIONS	CONTRAINDICATIONS
High-pressure, balloon-resistant lesion[a]	Angiographic evidence of thrombus[a]
Discrete (<15 mm) or tubular (<10–20 mm) lesions[a]	Angiographic evidence of calcification[a]
References vessel diameter 2–4 mm[a]	Vessel angulation > 45 degrees[a]
In-stent restenosis	Use through stent struts or a lesion distal to a recently implanted stent[a]
Bifurcation lesions	Presence of coronary spasm[a]
Ostial lesions	

[a] Per instructions for use.

Outcomes

The cutting balloon was introduced in the mid-1990s and underwent evaluation in comparison to simple balloon angioplasty for de novo coronary artery lesions (12). In the CAPAS (13) trial, angiographic restenosis was lower than with balloon angioplasty, but in the much larger global restenosis trial (GST) (14) and REDUCE I (15) trial, angiographic restenosis at 9 months was similar for both devices. Overall cumulative rates of major adverse clinical events were similar for both devices, although there was a trend in favor of the cutting balloon.

In the RESCUT trial, the cutting balloon was compared to balloon angioplasty for treatment of in-stent restenosis, with binary restenosis as a primary endpoint again (16). In this trial, 9-month angiographic restenosis rates were similar for the two devices, as was cumulative major adverse cardiac events at 1 year.

Based on the results of these three randomized clinical trials, cutting balloon angioplasty was not felt to be superior to simple balloon angioplasty, and should be reserved for difficult-to-treat in-stent restenosis or ostial lesions of side branches. In a 2011 update of the PCI guidelines, cutting balloon angioplasty received a Class IIb indication to avoid slippage-induced coronary artery trauma during PCI for in-stent restenosis or ostial lesions in the side branches (level of evidence: C) (Table 14.8). It received a Class III (no benefit) recommendation for routine PCI (level of evidence: A) (8).

Complications

The complications associated with cutting balloon angioplasty are in general similar to those of simple balloon angioplasty. Although

TABLE 14.8 2011 ACCF/AHA/SCAI PCI Guidelines

Cutting Balloon Angioplasty: Recommendations

Class IIb
- Cutting balloon angioplasty might be considered to avoid slippage-induced coronary artery trauma during PCI for in-stent restenosis or ostial lesions in side branches (*Level of Evidence: C*).
- Class III: NO BENEFIT
- Cutting balloon angioplasty should not be performed routinely during PCI (*Level of Evidence: A*).

PCI, percutaneous coronary intervention.

the device is intended to create controlled dissections, extensive dissections nonetheless have been observed. Additionally, perforations and other ischemic complications have been observed similar to simple balloon angioplasty.

Scoring Balloon Angioplasty

Device

The AngioSculpt scoring balloon (Spectranetics; Colorado Springs, CO) is a novel balloon catheter consisting of a semi-compliant balloon catheter, around which three rectangular nitinol scoring wires are wrapped in a helical fashion. The balloon catheter can be expanded to 20 atm of pressure, allowing greater force to be applied focally compared to standard balloon angioplasty. The device is a 0.014-inch guide wire and is 6-Fr guide catheter–compatible. It is available in diameters of 2.0, 2.5, 3.0, and 3.5 mm, and lengths of 6, 10, and 15 mm.

Procedure

The general preparation for the scoring balloon procedure is similar to that for a simple balloon angioplasty (11). The tip of the original scoring balloon has been reengineered to have a better tip transition to facilitate lesion crossing. Similar to simple balloon angioplasty, the lesion is initially crossed with a coronary guide wire, and the scoring balloon is advanced to the lesion site. Once the lesion is crossed, the balloon is inflated at 2-atm increments, over 10 to 20 seconds, until a final deployment pressure of 4 to 8 atm is achieved. The scoring balloon has the potential advantage over conventional balloons in restenotic lesions where slippage with conventional balloons occurs frequently. With its helical cage design and square, rather than round, wire shape, the scoring balloon provides circumferential scoring and helps minimize slippage, locking the device within the lesion (**Fig. 14.4**). Deflation is performed similar to balloon angioplasty, and the device is withdrawn into the guide catheter. In some circumstances when the result is suboptimal, upsizing an additional half size may be necessary to achieve optimal enlargement of the vessel at the lesion's site.

Indications for Use

The AngioSculpt scoring balloon catheter is indicated for use in the treatment of hemodynamically significant coronary artery stenosis, including in-stent restenosis and complex type C lesions, for the purposes of improving myocardial perfusion (**Table 14.9**).

Outcomes

The results of a US multicenter trial evaluating the safety and efficacy of the AngioSculpt scoring balloon indicated a high success

Magnified view of nitinol helical scoring wires

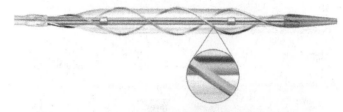

Cartoon of scoring balloon *in situ*

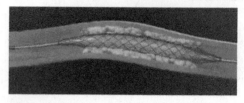

FIGURE 14.4 Magnified view of the nitinol helical scoring wires, with a blowup of the wire itself. On the bottom an illustration of the scoring balloon within a lesion is shown.

rate and low incidence of coronary dissections (13.7%) (17). In an observational trial of 299 patients, ultrasound was used to assess drug-eluting stent placement (Cypher or Taxus) after direct stenting, pre-dilatation with a conventional balloon, and after scoring balloon pre-treatment. Use of the scoring balloon resulted in greater luminal gain and a higher percentage of lesions achieving a final stent diameter >5.0 mm^2, compared to either direct stenting or pre-dilation with a conventional balloon (18). Outcomes after use of a drug-coated balloon, with or without pre-treatment with a scoring balloon, are being evaluated in the ISAR-DESIRE 4 trial (NCT01632371), with results potentially available late in 2017 (http://ichgcp.net/clinical-trials-registry/NCT01632371). Finally, the scoring balloon was used to treat the side branch of bifurcation lesions treated with a drug-eluting stent in 93 patients in the AGILITY trial (19). The post-scoring balloon dissection rate was 6.0% (2.1% after stenting); and the 9-month major adverse cardiac events (MACE) rate was 5.4%. Guidelines for use of the scoring balloon were not included in the 2011 PCI ACC/AHA/SCAI guidelines.

TABLE 14.9 Indication and Contraindications for Scoring Balloon Angioplasty

INDICATIONS	CONTRAINDICATIONS
Use in the treatment of hemodynamically significant coronary artery stenosis, including in-stent restenosis, and complex type C lesions for the purpose of improving myocardial perfusion[a]	Use through stent struts or a lesion distal to a recently implanted stent[a]
Bifurcation lesions	Presence of coronary spasm[a]
Ostial lesions	Excessive vessel angulation
Lesion preparation in conjunction with bioresorbable stents	Angiographic evidence of thrombus

[a] Per instructions for use.

Complications

The complications associated with scoring balloon angioplasty are in general similar to those of simple balloon angioplasty and cutting balloon angioplasty. Although the device is intended to create controlled dissections, extensive dissections nonetheless have been observed. Additionally, perforations and other ischemic complications have been observed similar to simple balloon angioplasty.

Lasers

Device

The excimer laser coronary atherectomy (ELCA) system (Spectranetics, Colorado Springs, CO) consists of a multi-fiber catheter and a CVX-300 console, which emits light at ultraviolet wavelengths of 308 nm (Fig. 14.5). It is 0.014-inch guide wire–compatible and is available in either Rx or OTW configurations. Catheters are available in sizes ranging from 0.9 to 2.0 mm for the Rx configuration, and 0.9 mm in the OTW configuration. Fluence of 30 to 60 mJ/mm^2 are available for all catheters, while the 0.9-mm X-80 has the unique quality of delivering fluence up to 80 mJ/mm^2. The catheters are 6- to 8-Fr compatible, depending on the catheter size.

Principles of Laser Angioplasty

Laser-mediated coronary angioplasty was developed and offered for clinical application in order to approach lesions that were challenging for routine balloon angioplasty, such as non-dilatable lesions, as well as chronic total occlusions. Most interventionalists are familiar with the general concept of laser performance because it is used in multiple medical applications, including lead extraction for pacemaker lead removal. Lasers produce intense electromagnetic energy delivered through coaxial optical fibers bundled inside a coronary delivery catheter. The optimal lasing technique involves delivery of the tip of the laser catheter to the area of interest. Activation of the device produces a cone of laser energy that extends no more than 50 µm beyond the tip of the catheter and leads to vaporization of plaque. The vaporization of organic material such as plaque is achieved by photochemical, photomechanical, and photothermal effects (the reader is referred to this chapter's references section for details of laser–tissue interactions). The laser beam does not interact with inorganic material, such as calcium or steel, thus it can be used safely near a guide wire or stent. Not surprisingly, the tremendous energy generated by the laser beam can also lead to gas bubbles and acoustic effects, which have the untoward effect of possible dissection and perforation, but which can be minimized by good technique and saline clearance of the vessel.

Laser Technique

Optimal lasing requires guide wire positioning across a lesion, as well as coaxial movement within the coronary circulation. Lasing also generates a tremendous amount of heat, which is dissipated a number of ways: via control of the energy intensity used to deliver the energy, limiting the length of each of the lasing sequences, and the liberal use of a heparin flush throughout the procedure. The lasing technique currently used is similar to that reported in the LEONARDO trial, a prospective registry evaluating the safety and efficacy of fluence rates up to 80 mJ/mm^2 in patients with complex coronary lesions using the X-80 laser catheter (20). Initial lasing was initiated at 60 mJ/mm^2 (40 Hz) and increased to 80 mJ/mm^2 (80 Hz) for resistant lesions.

The laser pulse length is 185 nanoseconds, with cycles of 5 seconds on, and 10 seconds off (except for the X-80 catheter which uses a 10 seconds on and 5 seconds off cycle). Successful coronary laser angioplasty is followed by stenting.

Indications for Use

The manufacturer's and generally accepted clinical indications and contraindications for use of laser angioplasty are shown in Table 14.10. Current indications are for occluded saphenous vein bypass grafts; ostial lesions; long lesions; moderately calcified

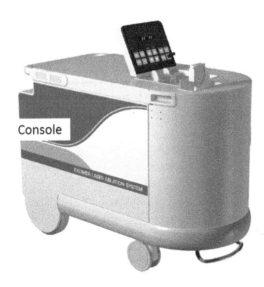

Console

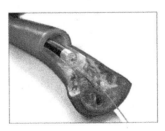

Cartoon of laser *in situ*

FIGURE 14.5 The excimer laser ablation system console is shown on the left. An illustration of the laser within a lesion is shown on the right.

TABLE 14.10 Indications and Contraindications for Coronary Laser Angioplasty

INDICATIONS	CONTRAINDICATIONS
Occluded SVGs[a]	Lesion in unprotected LM[a]
Ostial lesions[a]	Lesion is beyond acute bends or is in a location where the catheter cannot traverse[a]
Long lesions >20 mm[a]	Lesion cannot be reached by catheter[a]
Moderately calcified stenoses[a]	Bifurcation lesion[a]
CTOs crossable by guide wire[a]	Patient is not a CABG candidate[a]
Lesion that previously failed PTCA[a]	
Restenosis in 316L stainless-steel stents, prior to the administration of intravascular brachytherapy[a]	

[a] Per instructions for use.
CABG, coronary artery bypass grafting; CTO, chronic total occlusion; LM, left main; PTCA, percutaneous transluminal coronary angioplasty; SVG, saphenous vein graft.

lesions; CTOs; lesions that previously failed balloon angioplasty; and restenosis in 316L stainless-steel stents. Contraindications include inability to cross the lesion with a guide wire; lesion located within a bifurcation; excessive lesion entry and exit angulation of the lesion and vessel; and lesion is located in an unprotected left main artery.

Outcomes

DE NOVO CORONARY ARTERY LESIONS

In the AMRO (6) and LAVA (21) trials, laser and balloon angioplasty were evaluated with a primary endpoint of 6-month clinical outcomes. Rates of revascularization were higher with laser versus balloon angioplasty and were also associated with a significant increase in rates of coronary complication compared to simple balloon angioplasty alone. Based on these studies, routine use of laser angioplasty is not recommended for de novo coronary lesions.

IN-STENT RESTENOSIS, CHRONIC TOTAL OCCLUSIONS, THROMBUS RICH LESIONS, AND UNDILATABLE STENTS

Prior to the advent of drug-eluting stents, restenosis after simple balloon angioplasty and after bare-metal stenting remained a clinical challenge. Because of the physical characteristics of the restenotic material, use of simple balloon angioplasty was challenging because of the propensity of the balloon to slip (watermelon seed) within the stenotic region. A number of devices, such as the rotablator and cutting balloon, were developed specifically to address this limitation of balloon angioplasty. Laser angioplasty, similarly, was also added to the devices attempting to treat this specific lesion subset. Successful treatment of in-stent restenosis has been reported in single-center registries, but no trial has been conducted to determine its efficacy and safety compared to other modalities. Optimal use of the laser angioplasty is performed in an OTW fashion. Nevertheless, some lesions are not amenable to wire crossing, such as chronic total occlusion, and so present a unique clinical challenge. A laser-tipped wire was developed to facilitate passage through an occluded vessel. In the TOTAL randomized trial, laser-assisted angiography and

TABLE 14.11 2011 ACCF/AHA/SCAL PCI Guidelines

Laser Angioplasty: Recommendations
- Class IIb
  - Laser angioplasty might be considered for fibrotic moderately calcified lesions that cannot be crossed or dilated with conventional balloon angioplasty (*Level of Evidence: C*).
- Class III: NO BENEFIT
  - Laser angioplasty should not be used routinely during PCI (*Level of Evidence: A*).

stenting was successful in 91% of cases (22). Six-month angiographic restenosis rates were similar and high for both groups, including a 20% reocclusion rate. MACE was similar for both groups.

Recent experience in patients with stents inadequately expanded using high-pressure noncompliant balloons indicates that ELCA can be useful to facilitate full stent expansion, presumably by ablating organic elements within the vessel wall, thus constraining calcium within the vessel wall (23). Additionally, interest in use of ELCA for thrombotic lesions, especially in degenerated vein grafts and in acute myocardial infarction patients, has grown as the safety and feasibility of ELCA in these settings has been described (24,25).

Based on the data obtained, although limited, the ACCF/AHA has issued the following recommendations: There is a Class IIb recommendation for laser angioplasty, which might be considered fibrotic or moderately calcified lesions that cannot be crossed or dilated with conventional balloon angioplasty (level of evidence: C) (**Table 14.11**). A Class III recommendation (no benefit) has been issued for routine use during PCI (level of evidence: A) (8).

Complications

Similar to most other coronary interventional devices, the use of laser angioplasty is associated with potential dissection, perforation, and acute closure. The use of saline flushes in conjunction with compulsive attention to technique and a methodical approach to laser angioplasty has minimized the potential for these complications, but given the intense energy at the tip of the catheter, the potential for serious coronary complications persists. The treatment of these complications is similar to that for complications arising from other interventional devices. Similar to the potential concern for coronary perforation during coronary RA, general expert consensus is that anticoagulation accompanying the use of laser angioplasty should be unfractionated heparin because it can be readily reversed with protamine.

Key Points

■ RA
- Rotational atherectomy (PTCRA) achieves atheroablation with an OTW diamond-tipped burr spinning at >140,000 rpm based on the concept of differential cutting; i.e., selective ablation of relatively inelastic materials such as calcified or heavily fibrotic atheromatous plaque versus sparing of elastic non-diseased vessel segments.
- PTCRA was not superior to PTCA or laser atherectomy in reducing restenosis in multiple clinical trials in de novo or restenotic lesions.

- As a result of these clinical trials and the 2011 update of PCI guidelines, coronary atherectomy is given a Class IIa recommendation for preparation of fibrotic or heavily calcified lesions that might not be crossed by a balloon catheter or adequately dilated prior to stent implantation (level of evidence: C). Coronary atherectomy was given a Class III indication (harm) in the routine treatment of de novo or in-stent restenosis (level of evidence: A).
- Contemporary practice uses PTCRA for lesion preparation prior to stenting, particularly in calcified vessels.

■ OA
- The mechanism of differential sanding occurring during OA is similar to that of RA with selective ablation of inelastic materials, including heavily calcified or fibrotic plaque, and sparing of elastic tissue.
- The safety and efficacy of OA was evaluated in ORBIT I and ORBIT II trials, both prospective registries of patients undergoing PCI of heavily calcified vessels. Procedural success was high, and complication rates were similar to, or lower than, historical studies of RA.
- Similar to PTCRA, OA is used for lesion preparation prior to stenting, particularly in moderate to severely calcified lesions.

■ Scoring balloon angioplasty
- The scoring balloon (AngioSculpt) is composed of three rectangular nitinol wires wrapped in a helical fashion about a semi-compliant balloon. On inflation, there is circumferential scoring of the vessel while minimizing slippage, which is ideal for treating restenotic lesions.
- The AngioSculpt balloon is indicated for treatment of in-stent restenosis and complex type C lesions.

■ Cutting balloon angioplasty
- Cutting balloon atherectomy achieves vessel dilation with three or four atherotomes attached to the surface of a conventional angioplasty balloon by controlled longitudinal incision of the vessel wall.
- In three randomized clinical trials, cutting balloon angioplasty was not felt to be superior to simple balloon angioplasty for reducing restenosis in de novo or in-stent restenotic lesions.
- In the 2011 update of the PCI guidelines, cutting balloon angioplasty received a Class IIb indication to avoid slippage-induced coronary artery trauma during PCI for in-stent restenosis or ostial lesions in the side branches (level of evidence: C). It received a Class III (no benefit) recommendation for routine PCI (level of evidence: A).
- The cutting balloon is used in contemporary practice for lesion preparation in restenotic or ostial main or branch vessel disease.

■ Laser atherectomy
- Lasers produce intense electromagnetic energy at ultraviolet wavelengths of 308 nm delivered through coaxial optical fibers bundled inside a coronary delivery catheter. Vaporization of plaque is achieved by photochemical, photomechanical, and photothermal effects.
- Based on limited clinical data, the 2011 update of the PCI guidelines has issued the following recommendations: There is a Class IIb recommendation for laser angioplasty that might be considered for fibrotic or moderately calcified lesions that cannot be crossed or dilated with conventional balloon angioplasty (level of evidence: C). A Class III recommendation (no benefit) has been issued for routine use during PCI (level of evidence: A).
- Contemporary practice with a laser is useful for lesion preparation in lesions that have failed PTCA, or that have restenosis of 316L stainless-steel stents. Lasers can also be useful in mild to moderately calcified lesions, or long lesions, and in CTOs, including occluded vein grafts.

References

1. Reisman M, et al. Analysis of heat generation during high-speed rotational ablation: technical implications. *J Am Coll Cardiol.* 1996;27:292A.
2. Whitlow PL, et al. Results of the study to determine rotablator and transluminal angioplasty strategy (STRATAS). *Am J Cardiol.* 2001;87:699–705.
3. Dill T, et al. A randomized comparison of balloon angioplasty versus rotational atherectomy in complex coronary lesions (COBRA study). *Eur Heart J.* 2000;21:1759–1766.
4. Reifart N, et al. Randomized comparison of angioplasty of complex coronary lesions at a single center: excimer laser, rotational atherectomy, and balloon angioplasty comparison (ERBAC) study. *Circulation.* 1997;96:91–98.
5. Arora S, et al. Coronary atherectomy in the United States (from a nationwide inpatient sample). *Am J Cardiol.* 2016;117:555–562.
6. Buchbinder M, et al. Debulking prior to stenting improves acute outcomes: early results from the SPORT trial. *J Am Coll Cardiol.* 2000;35:8A.
7. Abdel-Wahab M, et al. High-speed rotational atherectomy before paclitaxel-eluting stent implantation in complex calcified coronary lesions: the randomized ROTAXUS (Rotational Atherectomy Prior to Taxus Stent Treatment for Complex Native Coronary Artery Disease) trial. *JACC Cardiovasc Interv.* 2013;6:10–19.
8. Levine GN, et al. 2011 ACCF/AHA/SCAI guideline for percutaneous coronary intervention: a report of the American College of Cardiology Foundation/American Heart Association Task Force on Practice Guidelines and the Society for Cardiovascular Angiography and Interventions. *J Am Coll Cardiol.* 2011;58:e44–e122.
9. Kinnaird T, et al. Incidence, determinants, and outcomes of coronary perforation during percutaneous coronary intervention in the United Kingdom between 2006 and 2013: an analysis of 527,121 cases from the British Cardiovascular Intervention Society database. *Circ Cardiovasc Interv.* 2016;9. pii: e003449. doi:10.1161/CIRCINTERVENTIONS.115.003449.
10. Parikh K, et al. Safety and feasibility of orbital atherectomy for the treatment of calcified coronary lesions: the ORBIT I trial. *Catheter Cardiovasc Interv.* 2013;81:1134–1139.
11. Lee MS, et al. Cutting balloon angioplasty. *J Invasive Cardiol.* 2002;14:552–556.
12. Barath P, et al. Cutting balloon: a novel approach to percutaneous angioplasty. *Am J Cardiol.* 1991;68:1249–1252.
13. Izumi M, et al. Final results of the CAPAS trial. *Am Heart J.* 2001;142:782–789.
14. Mauri L, et al. Cutting balloon angioplasty for the prevention of restenosis: results of the cutting balloon global randomized trial. *Am J Cardiol.* 2002;90:1079–1083.
15. Bittl JA, et al. Meta-analysis of randomized trials of percutaneous transluminal coronary angioplasty versus atherectomy, cutting balloon atherotomy, or laser angioplasty. *J Am Coll Cardiol.* 2004;43:936–942.
16. Albiero R, et al. Cutting balloon versus conventional balloon angioplasty for the treatment of in-stent restenosis: results of the restenosis cutting balloon evaluation trial (RESCUT). *J Am Coll Cardiol.* 2004;43:943–949.
17. Mooney MR, et al. Final results from the U.S. multi-center trial of the AngioSculpt scoring balloon catheter for the treatment of complex coronary artery lesions. *Am J Cardiol.* 2006;98:121M.
18. Costa JD Jr, et al. Nonrandomized comparison of coronary stenting under intravascular ultrasound guidance of direct stenting without predilation versus conventional predilation with a semi-compliant balloon versus predilation with a new scoring balloon. *Am J Cardiol.* 2007;100:812–817.

19. Weisz G, et al. A provisional strategy for treating true bifurcation lesions employing a scoring balloon for the side branch: final results of the AGILITY trial. *Catheter Cardiovasc Interv.* 2013;82:352–359.

20. Ambrosini V, et al. Early outcome of high energy Laser (Excimer) facilitated coronary angioplasty ON hARD and complex calcified and balloOn-resistant coronary lesions: LEONARDO study. *Cardiovasc Revasc Med.* 2015;16:141–146.

21. Stone GW, et al. Prospective, randomized, multicenter comparison of laser-facilitated balloon angioplasty versus stand-alone balloon angioplasty in patients with obstructive coronary artery disease. The Laser Angioplasty Versus Angioplasty (LAVA) trial investigators. *J Am Coll Cardiol.* 1997;30:1714–1721.

22. Serruys PW, et al. Total occlusion trial with angioplasty by using laser guidewire. The TOTAL trial. *Eur Heart J.* 2000;21:1797–1805.

23. Badr S, et al. The state of the excimer laser for coronary intervention in the drug-eluting stent era. *Cardiovasc Revasc Med.* 2013;14:93–98.

24. Nishino M, et al. Indication and outcomes of excimer laser coronary atherectomy: efficacy and safety for thrombotic lesions—the ULTRAMAN registry. *J Cardiol.* 2017;69:314–319.

25. Giugliano GR, et al. A prospective multicenter registry of laser therapy for degenerated saphenous vein graft stenosis: the COronary graft Results following Atherectomy with Laser (CORAL) trial. *Cardiovasc Revasc Med.* 2012;13:84–89.

15 Coronary Stents

F. David Russo, MD and Sunil V. Rao, MD, FSCAI, FACC

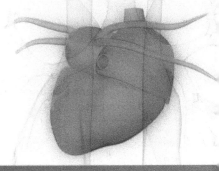

With the first successful balloon angioplasty performed by Andreas Gruentzig in 1977 in Zurich, Switzerland, the era of percutaneous coronary intervention officially began. Numerous technologic and procedural advances have occurred throughout the following decades, enabling millions of subsequent coronary interventions to occur since that time. This chapter will discuss the role of coronary stents, ranging from their initial development to their modern usage in various clinical populations.

Measures of Device and Procedural Success

It is important to provide an overview regarding various clinical trial terminology in order to better understand our current understanding of differences in stent technology. Various studies investigating stent effectiveness have assessed both angiographic and clinical outcomes (1,2). An understanding of a few terms will aid in the understanding of some of these differences as outlined by prior clinical trials.

Angiographic outcomes (see **Fig. 15.1**):

Acute gain = post minus pre minimal lesion diameter, often measured in millimeters

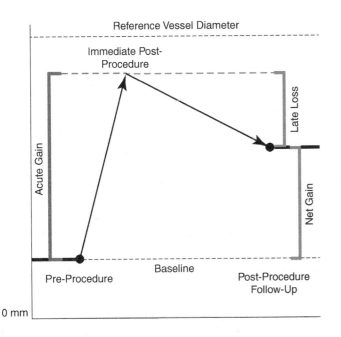

FIGURE 15.1 Acute gain, late loss, and net gain. Prior to coronary intervention, a stenotic segment has a minimal lumen diameter. The intervention results in an *acute gain*, illustrated by the upward arrow showing improvement in minimal lumen diameter. In subsequent angiographic follow-up, the minimal lumen diameter decreases, a phenomenon referred to as *late loss*. The resultant overall improvement in minimal lumen diameter is referred to as *net gain*.

Late loss = post minus late minimal lesion diameter (usually measured 6–9 months after initial procedure)
Late loss index = late loss divided by acute gain
Net gain = late minus pre minimal lesion diameter
Angiographic (binary) restenosis is typically defined as a late lesion diameter stenosis ≥50%.

Clinical outcomes:

Target lesion revascularization (TLR): Any repeat revascularization of the original lesion, which includes the stented segment and 5 mm proximal and distal to the stent, usually measured 6 to 12 months after the procedure
Target vessel revascularization (TVR): Any repeat revascularization involving the previously treated vessel
Major adverse cardiac events (MACE): Although the definition varies slightly with different clinical trials, it is classically defined as death, Q-wave myocardial infarction (MI), or target vessel or lesion revascularization.
Target vessel failure (TVF): Composite of TVR or MACE

Overview of Stent Design

Coronary stents may be classified based on mode of implantation, material composition, scaffold configuration, and stent coatings.

Mode of implantation—self-expanding or balloon-expandable stents. While the initial coronary stent was self-expanding, the vast majority of coronary stents today are balloon-expandable, utilizing various processes to tightly crimp the stent on the balloon until it is deployed.

Material composition—the specific stent material used to construct the scaffold. Until recently, the most widely used material was 316L stainless steel. Nevertheless, cobalt chromium, nickel chromium, and platinum chromium alloys have been employed in more recent balloon-expandable designs. Other compositions include nitinol, a nickel/titanium alloy, often used in self-expanding stents, and biodegradable polymers, often used in bioabsorbable stents. A multitude of additional materials have been utilized. Furthermore, the material composition can be further characterized by strut thickness, which may impact deliverability, visibility, as well as short- and long-term stent outcomes.

Scaffold configuration—refers to the shape and construction of the stent design. Traditionally, stents can be assigned to one of three subgroups: wire coils, modular, or slotted tube/multicellular (most commonly used). Several iterations of configurations have been designed to enhance radial strength, wall coverage, flexibility/deliverability, and to prevent deformation. Furthermore, multicellular stents can be subclassified as open cell or closed cell. Open cell designs often have varying cell sizes and shapes, allowing for increased flexibility, deliverability, and side-branch access. Closed cell designs typically provide more uniform wall coverage with less tendency for plaque prolapse.

TABLE 15.1 Stent Coatings Designed to Reduce Stent Thrombosis

Carbon
Ionic oxygen
Gold
Nitric oxide scavengers
Heparin
IIb/IIIa inhibitors
Activated protein C
Hirudin and bivalirudin
Prostacyclin
CD34 antibody
Phosphorylcholine
Fluorinated copolymer
Biolinx polymer
Trifluoroethanol (Polyzene-F)
Protein coating
PET fiber mesh

Stent coatings—Stents may be uncoated (bare metal), contain passive coatings such as polytetrafluoroethylene (PTFE), or contain polymers to reduce thrombogenicity and/or allow for controlled delivery of antiproliferative drug therapy. A multitude of stent coatings have been designed and studied in an attempt to prevent vascular complications, as outlined in **Table 15.1**. These polymers may be further classified as durable, bioresorbable, and may have varying degrees of biocompatibility and vascular responses.

When these factors are considered, one can theoretically envision an "ideal" stent. This stent would be easily deliverable, conform to vessel size with adequate lesion coverage, maintain sufficient radial strength while conforming to vessel bends, allow for side-branch access, and resist deformation. These stents would need to be visible enough to facilitate precise placement without obscuring angiographic vessel detail. Furthermore, the ideal stent would demonstrate enhanced biocompatibility in a manner that would maximize short- and long-term efficacy while minimizing stent-related complications such as thrombosis. Finally, the ideal stent would be able to overcome commonly associated factors associated with restenosis, which are summarized in Table 15.2.

TABLE 15.2 Factors Associated with In-Stent Restenosis or Target Lesion Revascularization after Drug-Eluting Stent Implantation

PATIENT	Age
	Female
	Diabetes mellitus
	Multivessel coronary artery disease
LESION	In-stent restenosis
	Bypass graft
	Chronic total occlusion
	Small vessels
	Calcified lesion
	Ostial lesion
	Left anterior descending lesion
PROCEDURE	Treatment of multiple lesions
	Type of drug-eluting stents
	Final diameter stenosis

The complexity of coronary stents underscores the number of variables that affect device efficacy, applicability, and safety. Changes or additions to one aspect of a stent can affect its other properties. A thick-strut, drug-eluting stent may be difficult to deliver and have inferior clinical outcomes to a thin-strut, drug-eluting stent. On the other hand, both will likely be superior to a bare-metal stent. These various properties should be kept in mind when considering the clinical application of various coronary stents.

Bare-Metal Stent Overview

Prior to the development of coronary stents, balloon angioplasty was utilized to improve coronary stenosis. Mechanistically, this entailed plaque fracture involving the media, expansion of the external elastic media, and axial plaque redistribution. While the majority of vessels treated with balloon angioplasty demonstrated good success rates, the results of balloon angioplasty were often unpredictable (3). Specifically, two major limitations were identified: acute vessel closure (which often occurred immediately or within the first several days after angioplasty) and restenosis (which often occurred within months of the procedure due to a combination of vessel recoil and vascular remodeling). As a result, the concept of the coronary stent was developed as a scaffold that would improve on the early and late results of balloon angioplasty.

In 1986, Ulrich Sigwart and colleagues implanted the first stents in coronary arteries (4). The Wallstent (Medinvent, Lausanne, Switzerland) was a sheathed, self-expanding metallic scaffold that was placed in the coronary and peripheral arteries of eight patients. Although further experience with these stents demonstrated high rates of thrombotic occlusion and late mortality, angiographic restenosis rates appeared modestly improved from those observed with balloon angioplasty (5).

The first United States Food and Drug Administration (FDA)–approved balloon-expandable stent was developed in 1988 by Cesare Gianturco and Gary Roubin, gaining FDA approval in 1993 for reversal of postangioplasty acute or threatened vessel closure. These 316L stainless-steel, wire-coil stents with a strut thickness of 127 μm generally lacked axial and radial strength (6), and often resulted in less sufficient coverage compared with other stent designs (7). Subsequently, the development of the stainless-steel Palmaz-Schatz stent (Johnson and Johnson, Interventional Systems, Warrant NJ), which consisted of a balloon-expandable, slotted, stainless-steel tube with a central connecting bridge, soon became the dominant stent design for coronary use after the results of two simultaneous randomized multicenter studies (STRESS and BENESTENT) comparing balloon angioplasty alone with elective Palmaz-Schatz stenting (8,9).

The STRESS study assigned 401 patients to Palmaz-Schatz stent or balloon angioplasty with a primary endpoint of angiographic restenosis at 6 months. Those patients receiving the Palmaz-Schatz stent experienced improved procedural success and larger acute gain upon implantation. At 6 months, those receiving stenting experienced a higher rate of late loss compared with angioplasty, but had a lower overall rate of restenosis and larger net gain. There was a trend toward less TVR (10.2% vs. 15.4%, p = 0.06) in the stented patients (8).

BENESTENT was a multicenter randomized controlled trial performed in Europe, where 520 patients with stable angina were randomized to a Palmaz-Schatz stent versus balloon angioplasty, with a primary clinical endpoint of TVF (defined as death, cerebrovascular accident, MI, and TVR). Similar to the STRESS study, patients receiving the Palmaz-Schatz stent demonstrated larger acute gain, increased late loss, and decreased restenosis. There was a trend toward larger net gain (p = 0.09). Clinically, those patients receiving stents demonstrated decreased TVF, driven by decreased rates of TVR (13.5% vs. 23.3%) (9).

These results led to FDA approval of the Palmaz-Schatz stent in 1994. Long-term follow-up of these stents have demonstrated few late clinical or angiographic recurrences from years 1 to 5 after implantation, with progressive decrements in luminal diameter beyond 10 years (10). While initial rates of stent thrombosis occurred in approximately 3% of patients, the utilization of dual-antiplatelet therapy and refinements in stent deployment technique (including more frequent intravascular ultrasound guidance and routine high-pressure dilation) resulted in low overall stent thrombosis rates of 1.5% at 15 years (10).

In summary, while coronary stents increase acute luminal diameters more than balloon angioplasty, an exaggerated post-stent implantation response of neointimal hyperplasia results in greater decreases in luminal diameter compared with balloon angioplasty alone. Despite the late loss observed with stenting, net gain remains favorable compared with angioplasty (resulting in less overall restenosis), leading to the consistently observed association between improved acute results following stent placement and lower rates of subsequent restenosis.

These early coronary stents were a significant improvement over balloon angioplasty with respect to abrupt closure, the need for emergency coronary artery bypass graft (CABG), and long-term restenosis. Nevertheless, TLR and stent thrombosis were still issues (11). Specific physical properties of these devices were likely responsible (12,13). Namely, many early stent designs contained thick struts (>120 μm) (14), with the exception of the Palmaz-Schatz stent, which had thinner struts. The ISAR-STEREO trial compared the thick strut acute coronary syndrome (ACS) Multi-Link Duet stent (strut thickness 140 μm) with the think strut ACS Rx Multi-Link (strut thickness 50 μm) in 651 patients undergoing PCI of native coronary vessels >2.8 mm in diameter. Use of the thin strut stent resulted in a 42% reduction in 6-month angiographic binary restenosis and a 38% reduction in 6-month clinical restenosis (15). The two stents compared in this trial had similar overall designs (interconnected rings), and the ISAR-STEREO 2 trial compared the ACS Rx Multi-Link stent with the thick strut BX Velocity stent. The BX Velocity had a strut thickness of 140 μm and utilized a closed

cell design. The thin strut stent was again superior with respect to clinical and angiographic restenosis, underscoring the importance of strut thickness on outcomes (16).

One drawback of the thin-strut 316L stainless-steel bare-metal stents (BMS) was reduced deliverability and reduced angiographic visibility (16). The use of alloys (see earlier) addressed these limitations while allowing for thin struts (17,18). Thus, currently available BMS are generally made of chromium alloys with strut thicknesses of ~80 μm.

Despite serial changes in coronary bare-metal stent design, to include changes in metallic composition, lower-profile stent struts, improved flexibility/deliverability, and enhancements to radial/longitudinal strength, BMS continue to demonstrate high restenosis rates, often approaching 20% to 40% at 6 to 12 months in clinical trials (19). As a result, coronary restenosis led to investigation into a multitude of anti-restenotic therapies (see Figure 15.2), ultimately leading to the development of drug-eluting stents (DESs).

DES Overview

DESs were designed specifically to reduce the neointimal hyperplasia associated with early coronary stents. By inhibiting cellular proliferation with local delivery of substances designed to inhibit cellular proliferation, a drug-eluting stent can result in a marked reduction in angiographic restenosis and TLR.

Modern DESs are composed of three key components: the stent, the antiproliferative agent, and the drug carrier, as illustrated in Figure 15.3. For each DES variety, a detailed description is beyond the overview of this text, but a general knowledge of these components is highly recommended. The majority of current, commercially available DESs utilize alloys and have thin struts.

While a variety of anti-restenotic agents have been developed, the two most clinically utilized classes of agents have been the sirolimus family of drugs and paclitaxel. Briefly, sirolimus, also known as rapamycin (and its analogues including zotarolimus, everolimus, biolimus A9, novolimus, and amphilimus, among others), inhibits the mammalian target of rapamycin (mTOR) protein, preventing

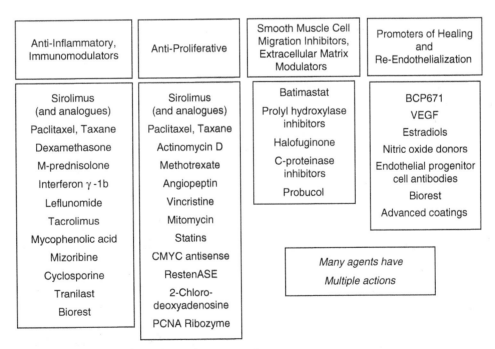

FIGURE 15.2 Potential agents to reduce restenosis.
PCNA, proliferating cell nuclear antigen; VEGF, vascular endothelial growth factor.

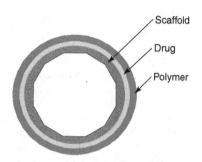

FIGURE 15.3 Components of drug-eluting stents. Modern drug-eluting stents are composed of three key components: the stent, the antiproliferative agent, and the polymer/carrier.

cell cycle progression from the G1 to S phase (20,21). On the other hand, paclitaxel stabilizes microtubule formation: At doses seen in coronary stents, it affects the G0–G1 and G1–S phases, resulting in cytostasis without cell death (22,23).

Regarding drug carriers, early DES development experienced considerable difficulty in predictably delivering a specific dose of active drug in a controlled manner (24). Thus, a drug carrier needed to be developed to allow for a more precise local delivery of the anti-restenotic agent to the vessel wall. While the polymer is instrumental in regulating the pharmacokinetics of drug delivery to the arterial wall, modification of the polymer may diminish some of the inflammatory reactions seen in these platforms (25–27). These observations led to the subsequent development of more biocompatible polymers, biodegradable polymers, and even polymer-free drug-eluting stent platforms, (see Second-Generation Drug-Eluting Stents for more details).

First-Generation, Drug-Eluting Stents

Sirolimus-Eluting Stents (SES)

The prototype antiproliferative DES was the sirolimus-eluting Cypher (Cypher, Cordis) stent. This platform incorporated the following: a thick-strut, 316L, stainless-steel, closed-cell, slotted-tube scaffold; non-erodible polymer coatings that were adherent to both the luminal and abluminal surfaces of the stent; and sirolimus as the antiproliferative agent. This design allowed for a "slow release" of sirolimus, whereby approximately 80% of the sirolimus was released within the first month after stent implantation. After initial evaluation with the first-in-man (FIM) study and RAVEL trials, which demonstrated suppression of neointimal hyperplasia (resulting in marked improvement in late loss) (28–30), the SIRIUS trial was conducted as a randomized comparison between the Cypher stent and the analogous bare-metal platform. The primary endpoint of TVF (a composite of death, MI, or TVR at 9 months) was significantly lower among sirolimus-eluting stent patients (8.6% vs. 21.0%, p < 0.001), results largely driven by reduction in TVR attributable to decreased rates of neointimal hyperplasia and late loss (31). Longer-term follow-up analyses demonstrated sustained reductions in clinical restenosis endpoints with similar rates of death, MI, and stent thrombosis compared with BMS (32,33). Due to the availability of newer stent platforms and designs, this stent is no longer commercially available.

Paclitaxel-Eluting Stents (PES)

The Taxus (Boston Scientific, Natick, MA) PES became commercially available soon after the Cypher stent. These stents utilized paclitaxel contained within a non-erodible polymer. By adjusting the ratio of paclitaxel to polymer, drug-release kinetics could be altered to

allow for slower drug elution, of which the SR formulation results in approximately 8% paclitaxel elution in 30 days. While the majority of early clinical trial data was based on the Express open-cell slotted-tube stainless-steel stent platform (PES[E]), serial iterations of Taxus stent design have incorporated different stent designs, including the Liberte stent (a thinner strut open-cell stainless steel design) and the Element stent (a platinum–chromium–based stent). The PES(E) has been studied in numerous randomized trials and observational analyses, resulting in reductions in measures of angiographic and clinical restenosis endpoints compared with BMS (34).

Comparisons among First-Generation Drug-Eluting Stents

A series of comparisons between the first two approved devices (the SES and PES) have been conducted to determine if superiority could be established for a particular DES. In summary, evidence from these trials seem to indicated similar clinical performance with a decreased rate of neointimal hyperplasia in the SES-treated patients. In a meta-analysis including 16 randomized trials involving 8,695 patients comparing the SES with PES, the SES was found to significantly reduce TLR (HR 0.74; 95% CI 0.63–0.87; p < 0.001) and stent thrombosis (HR 0.66; 95% CI 0.46–0.94; p = 0.02) without a statistical difference in the risk for death or MI (35). In two randomized clinical trials involving up to 10 years of long-term follow-up, the rate of definite stent thrombosis at 10 years were very similar at 5.6% (36,37). Commonly-accepted definitions of stent thrombosis classification is provided in Table 15.3.

Second-Generation Drug-Eluting Stents

Despite the demonstrated efficacy of the SES and PES platforms, adverse vessel responses to these first-generation stents were observed, which included delayed reendothelialization, hypersensitivity and eosinophilic inflammatory reactions, and, importantly, late stent thrombosis. Two studies reported an increase in mortality with the first-generation DES compared with the BMS (38,39), resulting in a significant decrease in the clinical use of DES (40). While many potential mechanisms may contribute to stent thrombosis, summarized in Table 15.4, these findings led to additional modifications in stent design. As a

---

TABLE 15.3 Academic Research Consortium (ARC) Definition of Stent Thrombosis Summarized

Definite stent thrombosis

Angiographic or pathologic evidence of thrombus that originates within or 5 mm adjacent to the stent, and clinical evidence of an acute coronary syndrome within a 48-hour time window

Probable stent thrombosis

Unexplained death within the first 30 days after stent implantation
Target vessel infarction without angiographic confirmation

Possible stent thrombosis

Unexplained death beyond 30 days after the procedure

Stent thrombosis timing

Acute stent thrombosis: 0–24 hours after stent implantation
Subacute stent thrombosis: >24 hours to 30 days after stent implantation
Late stent thrombosis: >30 days to 1 year after stent implantation
Very late stent thrombosis: >1 year after stent implantation

TABLE 15.4 Potential Mechanisms of Stent Thrombosis

Patient	Premature discontinuation of dual antiplatelet therapy
	Smoking
	Diabetes
	Chronic kidney disease
	Acute coronary syndrome presentation
	High post-treatment platelet reactivity
	Early post-implantation surgical procedures
Lesion	Diffuse coronary artery disease with long-stented segment
	Small vessel disease
	Bifurcation disease
	Thrombus containing lesions
	Significant inflow or outflow lesions proximal or distal to the stented segment
Stent	Stent underexpansion
	Edge dissection
	Poor endothelialization
	Thick stent struts
	Strut fracture
	Hypersensitivity/inflammatory reactions to specific DES components (e.g. some polymers)
	Late malapposition
	Neo-atherosclerosis with plaque rupture

DES, drug-eluting stents.

result, serial refinements to the stent platform, polymer composition, pharmacologic agent, and its elution kinetics have been implemented in order to address the safety issues while maintaining efficacy.

Zotarolimus-Eluting Stents (ZES)

Although initially developed contemporaneously with first-generation stents, the Endeavor (ZES[E], Medtronic, Santa Rosa, CA) stent incorporated zotarolimus, a lipophilic sirolimus derivative that would prevent rapid release in to the circulation and favor direct crossing of cell membranes to inhibit neointimal proliferation. Nevertheless, the release rates of zotarolimus from Endeavor (90% within 7 days, 100% within 30 days) were higher than those observed with prior drug-eluting stents (41). In addition, Endeavor incorporated a biocompatible polymer called phosphorylcholine and a flexible, low-profile cobalt–chromium stent. Clinical trials comparing the ZES with SES and/or PES demonstrated lesser neointimal suppression with the Endeavor ZES (i.e., more neointimal proliferation) compared with either the SES or PES, resulting in lesser performance of this stent with respect to angiographically measured trial endpoints (42). An interesting observation from these trials is the similar rates of TLR among the various DES in patients receiving clinical (as opposed to routine angiographic) follow-up. Patients undergoing routine angiographic follow-up had increased rates of revascularization, a concept previously termed the "oculostenotic reflex" (43). Although angiographic efficacy was lower with the Endeavor stent, it had very low rates of late adverse events, including very late stent thrombosis, cardiac death, or MI (44). In fact, the PROTECT trial comparing safety endpoints of the Endeavor stent with the Cypher SES platform demonstrated reduced rates of stent thrombosis (1.6% of E-ZES vs. 2.6% of C-SES patients [HR 0.63 (95% CI 0.46–0.85), p = 0.003] and a composite outcome of all-cause death or large MI (HR 0.84 [95% CI 0.71–0.98], p = 0.024) (45).

An updated version of a zotarolimus-eluting stent, the Resolute Integrity (Medtronic), incorporates an updated and more deliverable cobalt-alloy platform (Integrity) and employs a different biocompatible polymer (BioLinx tripolymer coating) designed to slow the elution of zotarolimus (60% elution by 30 days, 100% by 180 days). In a single-arm trial, these modifications resulted in reduced rates of restenosis than those seen with the prior ZES(E) or BMS (46). Furthermore, this platform has been studied in a series of trials comparing angiographic and clinical outcomes with everolimus-eluting stents (everolimus-eluting stents are discussed in the next section). In summary, although slight differences in angiographic and clinical outcomes may exist, the Resolute platform seems to demonstrate similar overall safety and efficacy to the EES platforms (47,48).

Everolimus-Eluting Stents (EES)

The EES (Xience, Abbott Vascular, Santa Clara, CA; also Promus, Boston Scientific, Natick, MA) is another next-generation stent incorporating a sirolimus derivative called everolimus, combined with a durable biocompatible polymer coated onto a low-profile cobalt–chromium (Xience) or platinum–chromium (Promus Element/Premier) stent. The release kinetics of EES are similar to that seen with SES (approximately 80% release of the drug at 30 days, 100% after 120 days). The EES polymer has been demonstrated to be non-inflammatory in porcine experiments, with the additional property of resisting platelet and thrombus deposition in blood-contact applications (49). Furthermore, EESs demonstrate more rapid functional re-endothelialization compared with SESs, PESs, or ZESs (26). The EES has been studied in multiple randomized clinical trials comparing the device to BMS, PES, SES, and ZES platforms. Comparisons of the EES with PES demonstrate marked differences, best demonstrated by the SPIRIT IV and COMPARE trials. In SPIRIT IV, the EES demonstrated significant reductions in target lesion failure (TLF), stent thrombosis (0.3% vs. 1.1%, p = 0.0008), MI (1.9% vs. 3.1%, p = 0.02), and TLR (2.3% vs. 4.5%, p = 0.0008) (50). Longer-term follow-up at 3 years demonstrated sustained reductions in TLF, MI, and stent thrombosis (51). Furthermore, both all-cause mortality (3.2% vs. 5.1%, p = 0.02) and death or MI (5.9% vs. 9.1%, p = 0.001) were reduced with the EES compared with the PES. Similarly, in COMPARE, event rates were lower with the EES compared to the PES, driven by reductions in stent thrombosis, MI, and TLR (52). On the other hand, when the EES was compared with the SES, smaller differences have been observed, possibly with the exception of the ESSENCE-DIABETES trial, in which the EES was associated with lower rates of angiographic late loss and binary restenosis in diabetic patients at 8 months without differences in clinical outcomes (53).

One notable attribute of the EES is the very low rates of stent thrombosis observed in both clinical trials and observational studies. Of note, several recent studies suggest a lower rate of definite/probable stent thrombosis with EES compared with BMS (54–56).

Additional modifications of stent technology continue to develop. As an example, the Synergy stent (Boston Scientific) incorporates a thin-strut platinum chromium everolimus-eluting stent with a bioresorbable polymer, which enables complete polymer absorption to occur by 4 months after implantation. In a 5-year follow-up of the EVOLVE trial, these modifications appear to result in no probable/definite stent thrombosis events and a low rate of TLF at 5.5% (57).

Biolimus A9-Eluting Stents (BES)

Biolimus A9, a semi-synthetic sirolimus analogue with enhanced lipophilicity, has been incorporated into two clinically available stent platforms that utilize a fully biodegradable abluminal polymer (poly-L-lactic acid [PLLA]), which is co-released with biolimus A9 and converted to carbon dioxide and water via the Krebs cycle over a 6- to 9-month period (58). The BioMatrix (Biosensors International, Switzerland) stent and Nobori DES (Terumo Medical Corporation, Japan) utilize a stainless-steel platform. While initial results comparing the BES to SES demonstrate similar results of primary endpoints, longer-term follow-up of up to 5 years suggests decreased rates of very late stent thrombosis (59). The recently released non-inferiority NEXT trial comparing the biodegradable polymer BES to the durable polymer EES demonstrated similar safety and efficacy outcomes 3 years after stent implantation (60).

As an alternative stent design utilizing Biolimus A9, the Bio-Freedom drug-coated stent is a polymer- and carrier-free stent. In a randomized trial comparing this platform with BMS in a population of high-bleeding-risk patients utilizing 30 days of dual antiplatelet therapy, the BioFreedom BES outperformed its comparable BMS platform with regard to both safety (composite of cardiac death, MI,

and stent thrombosis) and efficacy (clinically driven TLR) at 1 year, with findings preserved at 2-year follow-up (61). These findings further support the use of modern DES in high-bleeding-risk patients.

Hybrid Sirolimus Eluting Stents

Additional novel stent designs have incorporated drug delivery with a bioresorbable polymer coupled with a durable protective stent coating. One such stent platform is the Orsiro (Biotronik) stent, which uses a hybrid of active (sirolimus with bioabsorbable polymer matrix PLLA) and passive coatings (silicon carbide sealant) on a 60-μm strut platform. Conceptually, this allows for controlled drug release, followed by bioabsorption of the polymer, leaving a sealed stent to reduce interaction with the tissue or blood with the metallic surface of the stent. Initial comparative studies of this platform compared with the durable-polymer EES demonstrate comparable safety and efficacy at 2 years (62).

TABLE 15.5 Overview Classification of Drug-Eluting Stents

GENERATION	DRUG	POLYMER	STENT	STRUT THICKNESS (μm)
Early Bare Metal				
Wall Stent	n/a	n/a	Self-expanding	80–100
Gianturco-Roubin	n/a	n/a	Wire coil	127
Palmaz-Schatz	n/a	n/a	Slotted tube with articulating bridge	70
First				
Cypher	Sirolimus	Biostable mix of poly-*n*-butyl methacrylate (PBMA) and polyethylene-vinyl acetate	Bx Velocity	140
Taxus Express	Paclitaxel	Styrene-isobutylene-styrene (SIBS)	Express	132
Taxus Liberté	Paclitaxel	SIBS	Liberté	97
Taxus Element	Paclitaxel	SIBS	Element (platinum–chromium)	81
Second				
Endeavor	Zotarolimus	Phosphorylcholine	Driver (cobalt alloy)	91
Xience	Everolimus	PBMA and PVDF-HF	Multi-Link Vision/8 (cobalt–chromium)	81
Promus	Everolimus	PBMA and PVDF-HFP	Platinum–chromium	81
Resolute	Zotarolimus	Biolinx polymer	Integrity (cobalt alloy)	91
Absorbable Polymer or Polymer-Free				
Synergy	Everolimus	Abluminal poly-(D,L-lactide-co-glycolide) (bioabsorbable)	Platinum–chromium	74
Biomatrix	Biolimus A9	Abluminal poly-L-lactic acid (bioabsorbable)	Juno (stainless steel)	120
Nobori	Biolumus A9	Abluminal poly-L-lactic acid (bioabsorbable)	S-stent	120
BioFreedom	Biolimus A9	n/a	Gazelle (stainless steel)	120
Orsiro	Sirolimus	Abluminal poly-L-lactic acid (bioabsorbable)	PK Papyrus (cobalt–chromium)	60 (2.25–3.0 mm); 80 (3.5–4.0 mm)
Ultimaster	Sirolimus	Poly (D,L-lactide-co-caprolactone) (bioabsorbable)	Cobalt–chromium	80

PVDF-HF, polyvinylidene fluoride-hydrogen fluoride; PVDF-HFP, poly vinylidene fluoride-co-hexafluoropropylene.

Bioabsorbable Drug-Eluting Stents

Several bioabsorbable DESs are currently undergoing evaluation, and in 2016, the first FDA-approved bioabsorbable stent, the Absorb Bioresorbable Vascular Scaffold System (BVS-EES, Abbott Vascular, Santa Clara, CA) became commercially available. This device is a polymeric bioabsorbable scaffold constructed of PLLA, with a thin mixture of poly-D, L-lactic acid (PDLLA) that serves as the drug carrier for everolimus. Similar to EES and SES, everolimus is 80% eluted at 30 days. While initial data regarding safety and efficacy are promising, as demonstrated by a low MACE rate, recently released clinical trial data suggest a small residual long-term risk for very late scaffold thrombosis (63–65). Implantation technique and correct sizing is essential for this first iteration of a bioabsorbable scaffold. Adequate lesion preparation, intravascular imaging to accurately determine vessel diameter, and post-dilation after implantation may reduce the risk of scaffold thrombosis (66).

CONCLUSIONS

Considerable improvements in coronary intervention over the past three decades have led to remarkable progress in the treatment of coronary disease. While balloon angioplasty enabled coronary interventions to become possible, abrupt vessel closure and restenosis remained problematic. The development of the BMS largely addressed acute vessel closure, but restenosis rates, albeit improved, were still clinically significant. The development of first-generation, DES dramatically reduced the rates of restenosis and subsequent revascularization, but challenges with stent deliverability and adverse vessel reactions leading to stent thrombosis have led to serial improvements involving the pharmacologic agent, drug polymer, and stent design. These changes have further improved the safety, efficacy, and clinical utility of these newer stent platforms, becoming the preferred modality for most lesion and patient subsets. More recent changes have focused on continued improvements in drug platforms and polymers, to include the development of dissolving polymers, bioresorbable vascular scaffolds, and polymer-free DES. Although early experience with these improvements has been favorable, continued follow-up and evaluation of these newer developments are needed to continue to assess long-term efficacy and safety.

Key Points

- Compared with balloon angioplasty, BMSs result in a larger acute gain and larger late loss, but maintain a larger net gain.

- Compared with balloon angioplasty, BMSs reduce the rates of acute vessel closure. Restenosis rates remain problematic, occurring in 20% to 40% of cases.

- DES are composed of three key components: the stent, the antiproliferative agent, and the drug carrier, all of which can impact clinical and angiographic results.

- Compared with the BMS, first-generation DES demonstrate a 55% reduction in TVR, largely attributable to reduced rates of in-stent late loss, resulting in reduced angiographic and clinical restenosis.

- Compared with the BMS, first-generation DESs have similar mortality or MI rates (67). Concerns regarding late/very late stent thrombosis resulted in prolonged duration of dual antiplatelet therapy and development of newer stent platforms.

- In comparing first-generation DESs, the SES is superior to the PES in terms of TVR and stent thrombosis. There is no difference in death or MI rates.

- Second-generation DESs, including durable polymer ZESs and EESs, are safer and more effective than first-generation DESs.

- Second-generation DESs demonstrate similar MACE compared with BMSs.

- Several recent trials demonstrate a lower rate of definite/probable stent thrombosis with second-generation DESs compared with BMSs.

- Second-generation DESs are superior to BMSs in various complex lesion subsets, including chronic total occlusions, saphenous vein grafts, diabetic patients, and acute MI.

- Most clinically available second-generation DESs demonstrate similar safety and efficacy.

- The improved safety profile of second-generation DESs has allowed for progressive reductions in recommended duration of dual antiplatelet therapy, best demonstrated in low-risk patients and those with elevated bleeding risks.

- Multiple lesion, patient, and procedural factors influence restenosis and TLR following DES implantation. These are summarized in **Table 15.5**.

- Initial studies suggest that first-generation biodegradable vascular scaffolds are feasible; nevertheless, there may be residual risks of very late thrombosis compared with second-generation DESs, which may be reduced by improved implantation techniques and/or improved scaffold technology.

References

1. Popma JJ, Califf RM, Topol EJ. Clinical trials of restenosis after coronary angioplasty. *Circulation.* 1991;84(3):1426–1436.
2. Kuntz RE, et al. Novel approach to the analysis of restenosis after the use of three new coronary devices. *J Am Coll Cardiol.* 1992;19(7):1493–1499.
3. Schatz RA. A view of vascular stents. *Circulation.* 1989;79(2):445–457.
4. Sigwart U, et al. Intravascular stents to prevent occlusion and restenosis after transluminal angioplasty. *N Engl J Med.* 1987;316(12):701–706.
5. Serruys PW, et al. Angiographic follow-up after placement of a self-expanding coronary-artery stent. *N Engl J Med.* 1991;324(1):13–17.
6. George BS, et al. Multicenter investigation of coronary stenting to treat acute or threatened closure after percutaneous transluminal coronary angioplasty: clinical and angiographic outcomes. *J Am Coll Cardiol.* 1993;22(1):135–143.
7. MacIsaac AI, et al. Comparison of three coronary stents: clinical and angiographic outcome after elective placement in 134 consecutive patients. *Cathet Cardiovasc Diagn.* 1994;33(3):199–204.
8. Fischman DL, et al. A randomized comparison of coronary-stent placement and balloon angioplasty in the treatment of coronary artery disease. Stent Restenosis Study Investigators. *N Engl J Med.* 1994;331(8):496–501.
9. Serruys PW, et al. A comparison of balloon-expandable-stent implantation with balloon angioplasty in patients with coronary artery disease. Benestent Study Group. *N Engl J Med.* 1994;331(8):489–495.
10. Yamaji K, et al. Very long-term (15 to 20 years) clinical and angiographic outcome after coronary bare metal stent implantation. *Circ Cardiovasc Interv.* 2010;3(5):468–475.

11. Cutlip DE, et al. Beyond restenosis: five-year clinical outcomes from second-generation coronary stent trials. *Circulation.* 2004;110(10):1226–1230.

12. Garasic JM, et al. Stent and artery geometry determine intimal thickening independent of arterial injury. *Circulation.* 2000;101(7):812–818.

13. Rogers C, Edelman ER. Endovascular stent design dictates experimental restenosis and thrombosis. *Circulation.* 1995;91(12):2995–3001.

14. Colombo A, Stankovic G, Moses JW. Selection of coronary stents. *J Am Coll Cardiol.* 2002;40(6):1021–1033.

15. Kastrati A, et al. Intracoronary stenting and angiographic results: strut thickness effect on restenosis outcome (ISAR-STEREO) trial. *Circulation.* 2001;103(23):2816–2821.

16. Pache J, et al. Intracoronary stenting and angiographic results: strut thickness effect on restenosis outcome (ISAR-STEREO-2) trial. *J Am Coll Cardiol.* 2003;41(8):1283–1288.

17. Mani G, et al. Coronary stents: a materials perspective. *Biomaterials.* 2007;28(9):1689–1710.

18. Menown IB, et al. The platinum chromium element stent platform: from alloy, to design, to clinical practice. *Adv Ther.* 2010;27(3):129–141.

19. Cutlip DE, et al. Clinical restenosis after coronary stenting: perspectives from multicenter clinical trials. *J Am Coll Cardiol.* 2002;40(12):2082–2089.

20. Singh K, Sun S, Vezina C. Rapamycin (AY-22,989), a new antifungal antibiotic. IV. Mechanism of action. *J Antibiot (Tokyo).* 1979;32(6):630–645.

21. Kelly PA, et al. Sirolimus, a new, potent immunosuppressive agent. *Pharmacotherapy.* 1997;17(6):1148–1156.

22. Horwitz SB, et al. Taxol: mechanisms of action and resistance. *Ann N Y Acad Sci.* 1986;466:733–744.

23. Wall ME, Wani MC. Camptothecin and taxol: discovery to clinic—thirteenth Bruce F. Cain Memorial Award Lecture. *Cancer Res.* 1995;55(4):753–760.

24. Lansky AJ, et al. Non-polymer-based paclitaxel-coated coronary stents for the treatment of patients with de novo coronary lesions: angiographic follow-up of the DELIVER clinical trial. *Circulation.* 2004;109(16):1948–1954.

25. Virmani R, et al. Localized hypersensitivity and late coronary thrombosis secondary to a sirolimus-eluting stent: should we be cautious? *Circulation.* 2004;109(6):701–705.

26. Joner M, et al. Endothelial cell recovery between comparator polymer-based drug-eluting stents. *J Am Coll Cardiol.* 2008;52(5):333–342.

27. Nakazawa G, et al. Coronary responses and differential mechanisms of late stent thrombosis attributed to first-generation sirolimus- and paclitaxel-eluting stents. *J Am Coll Cardiol.* 2011;57(4):390–398.

28. Morice MC, et al. A randomized comparison of a sirolimus-eluting stent with a standard stent for coronary revascularization. *N Engl J Med.* 2002;346(23):1773–1780.

29. Sousa JE, et al. Four-year angiographic and intravascular ultrasound follow-up of patients treated with sirolimus-eluting stents. *Circulation.* 2005;111(18):2326–2329.

30. Morice MC, et al. Long-term clinical outcomes with sirolimus-eluting coronary stents: five-year results of the RAVEL trial. *J Am Coll Cardiol.* 2007;50(14):1299–1304.

31. Moses JW, et al. Sirolimus-eluting stents versus standard stents in patients with stenosis in a native coronary artery. *N Engl J Med.* 2003;349(14):1315–1323.

32. Caixeta A, et al. 5-year clinical outcomes after sirolimus-eluting stent implantation insights from a patient-level pooled analysis of 4 randomized trials comparing sirolimus-eluting stents with bare-metal stents. *J Am Coll Cardiol.* 2009;54(10):894–902.

33. Weisz G, et al. Five-year follow-up after sirolimus-eluting stent implantation results of the SIRIUS (sirolimus-eluting stent in de-novo native coronary lesions) trial. *J Am Coll Cardiol.* 2009;53(17):1488–1497.

34. Stone GW, et al. A polymer-based, paclitaxel-eluting stent in patients with coronary artery disease. *N Engl J Med.* 2004;350(3):221–231.

35. Schomig A, et al. A meta-analysis of 16 randomized trials of sirolimus-eluting stents versus paclitaxel-eluting stents in patients with coronary artery disease. *J Am Coll Cardiol.* 2007;50(14):1373–1380.

36. Galloe AM, et al. 10-year clinical outcome after randomization to treatment by sirolimus- or paclitaxel-eluting coronary stents. *J Am Coll Cardiol.* 2017;69(6):616–624.

37. Yamaji K, et al. Ten-year clinical outcomes of first-generation drug-eluting stents: the Sirolimus-Eluting vs. Paclitaxel-Eluting Stents for Coronary Revascularization (SIRTAX) VERY LATE trial. *Eur Heart J.* 2016;37(45):3386–3395.

38. Camenzind E, Steg PG, Wijns W. Stent thrombosis late after implantation of first-generation drug-eluting stents: a cause for concern. *Circulation.* 2007;115(11):1440–1455; discussion 1455.

39. Pfisterer M, et al. Late clinical events after clopidogrel discontinuation may limit the benefit of drug-eluting stents: an observational study of drug-eluting versus bare-metal stents. *J Am Coll Cardiol.* 2006;48(12):2584–2591.

40. Krone RJ, et al. Acceptance, panic, and partial recovery: the pattern of usage of drug-eluting stents after introduction in the U.S. (a report from the American College of Cardiology/National Cardiovascular Data Registry). *JACC Cardiovasc Interv.* 2010;3(9):902–910.

41. Burke SE, Kuntz RE, Schwartz LB. Zotarolimus (ABT-578) eluting stents. *Adv Drug Deliv Rev.* 2006;58(3):437–446.

42. Kandzari DE, et al. Comparison of zotarolimus-eluting and sirolimus-eluting stents in patients with native coronary artery disease: a randomized controlled trial. *J Am Coll Cardiol.* 2006;48(12):2440–2447.

43. Pinto DS, et al. Impact of routine angiographic follow-up on the clinical benefits of paclitaxel-eluting stents: results from the TAXUS-IV trial. *J Am Coll Cardiol.* 2006;48(1):32–36.

44. Kandzari DE, et al. Final 5-year outcomes from the Endeavor zotarolimus-eluting stent clinical trial program: comparison of safety and efficacy with first-generation drug-eluting and bare-metal stents. *JACC Cardiovasc Interv.* 2013;6(5):504–512.

45. Wijns W, et al. Endeavour zotarolimus-eluting stent reduces stent thrombosis and improves clinical outcomes compared with cypher sirolimus-eluting stent: 4-year results of the PROTECT randomized trial. *Eur Heart J.* 2014;35(40):2812–2820.

46. Meredith IT, et al. Long-term clinical outcomes with the next-generation Resolute Stent System: a report of the two-year follow-up from the RESOLUTE clinical trial. *EuroInterv.* 2010;5(6):692–697.

47. Serruys PW, et al. Comparison of zotarolimus-eluting and everolimus-eluting coronary stents. *N Engl J Med.* 2010;363(2):136–146.

48. von Birgelen C, et al. A randomized controlled trial in second-generation zotarolimus-eluting Resolute stents versus everolimus-eluting Xience V stents in real-world patients: the TWENTE trial. *J Am Coll Cardiol.* 2012;59(15):1350–1361.

49. Kolandaivelu K, et al. Stent thrombogenicity early in high-risk interventional settings is driven by stent design and deployment and protected by polymer-drug coatings. *Circulation.* 2011;123(13):1400–1409.

50. Stone GW, et al. Everolimus-eluting versus paclitaxel-eluting stents in coronary artery disease. *N Engl J Med.* 2010;362(18):1663–1674.

51. Brener SJ, et al. Everolimus-eluting stents in patients undergoing percutaneous coronary intervention: final 3-year results of the clinical evaluation of the XIENCE V everolimus eluting coronary stent system in the treatment of subjects with de novo native coronary artery lesions trial. *Am Heart J.* 2013;166(6):1035–1042.

52. Smits PC, et al. Final 5-year follow-up of a randomized controlled trial of everolimus- and paclitaxel-eluting stents for coronary revascularization in daily practice: the COMPARE trial (a trial of everolimus-eluting stents and paclitaxel stents for coronary revascularization in daily practice). *JACC Cardiovasc Interv.* 2015;8(9):1157–1165.

53. Kim WJ, et al. Randomized comparison of everolimus-eluting stent versus sirolimus-eluting stent implantation for de novo coronary artery disease in patients with diabetes mellitus (ESSENCE-DIABETES): results from the ESSENCE-DIABETES trial. *Circulation.* 2011;124(8):886–92.

54. Sabate M, et al. Clinical outcomes in patients with ST-segment elevation myocardial infarction treated with everolimus-eluting stents versus bare-metal stents (EXAMINATION): 5-year results of a randomised trial. *Lancet.* 2016;387(10016):357–366.

55. Palmerini T, et al. Long-term safety of drug-eluting and bare-metal stents: evidence from a comprehensive network meta-analysis. *J Am Coll Cardiol.* 2015;65(23):2496–2507.

56. Bonaa KH, et al. Drug-eluting or bare-metal stents for coronary artery disease. *N Engl J Med.* 2016;375(13):1242–1252.

57. Kereiakes DJ, et al. Efficacy and safety of a novel bioabsorbable polymer-coated, everolimus-eluting coronary stent: the EVOLVE II Randomized Trial. *Circ Cardiovasc Interv.* 2015;8(4). pii: e002372.

58. Grube E, Buellesfeld L. BioMatrix biolimus A9-eluting coronary stent: a next-generation drug-eluting stent for coronary artery disease. *Expert Rev Med Devices.* 2006;3(6):731–741.

59. Ghione M, et al. Five-year outcomes of chronic total occlusion treatment with a biolimus A9-eluting biodegradable polymer stent versus a sirolimus-eluting permanent polymer stent in the LEADERS all-comers trial. *Cardiol J.* 2016;23(6):626–636.

60. Natsuaki M, et al. Final 3-year outcome of a randomized trial comparing second-generation drug-eluting stents using either biodegradable polymer or durable polymer: NOBORI biolimus-eluting versus XIENCE/PROMUS everolimus-eluting stent trial. *Circ Cardiovasc Interv.* 2015;8(10). pii: e002817.

61. Garot P, et al. 2-year outcomes of high bleeding risk patients after polymer-free drug-coated stents. *J Am Coll Cardiol.* 2017;69(2):162–171.

62. Zbinden R, et al. Ultrathin strut biodegradable polymer sirolimus-eluting stent versus durable-polymer everolimus-eluting stent for percutaneous coronary revascularization: 2-year results of the BIOSCIENCE trial. *J Am Heart Assoc.* 2016;5(3):e003255.

63. Chevalier B, et al. Randomised comparison of a bioresorbable everolimus-eluting scaffold with a metallic everolimus-eluting stent for ischaemic heart disease caused by de novo native coronary artery lesions: the 2-year clinical outcomes of the ABSORB II trial. *EuroInterv.* 2016;12(9):1102–1107.

64. Rizik DG, et al. Bioresorbable vascular scaffolds for the treatment of coronary artery disease: what have we learned from randomized-controlled clinical trials? *Coron Artery Dis.* 2017;28(1):77–89.

65. Toyota T, et al. Very late scaffold thrombosis of bioresorbable vascular scaffold: systematic review and a meta-analysis. *JACC Cardiovasc Interv.* 2017;10(1):27–37.

66. Sotomi Y, et al. Possible mechanical causes of scaffold thrombosis: insights from case reports with intracoronary imaging. *EuroInterv.* 2017;12(14):1747–1756.

67. Kirtane AJ, et al. Safety and efficacy of drug-eluting and bare metal stents: comprehensive meta-analysis of randomized trials and observational studies. *Circulation.* 2009;119(25):3198–3206.

16

Elective Percutaneous Coronary Intervention for Stable Coronary Artery Disease and Silent Myocardial Ischemia

Ronan Margey, MD, MRCPI, FSCAI, FACC, Douglas E. Drachman, MD, FSCAI, FACC, and Katherine Yu, MD

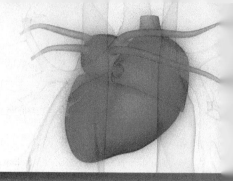

Coronary artery disease (CAD) remains the leading cause of mortality in most industrialized countries (1). The World Health Organization estimated that 7.4 million global deaths occurred due to CAD in 2015, and that the number may exceed 11 million by 2020 as the world population continues to age (2). Despite these staggering figures, the age-standardized mortality related to CAD has fallen by more than 40% over the past two decades. Half of the decline is attributed to improved primary preventive strategies, in concert with better early detection and reduction of major CAD risk factors; the other half is attributed to advances in medical and interventional therapies, particularly those related to the management of patients with acute coronary syndromes (ACSs) (3).

CAD results from the progressive formation of atherosclerotic plaque in the vessel wall (4,5). Mechanisms such as vascular inflammation, endothelial dysfunction, intraplaque hemorrhage, and plaque rupture may contribute to endoluminal disruption, with consequent arterial thrombosis and acute occlusion (1,6). The spectrum of clinical syndromes related to coronary atherosclerosis may be highly variable, depending on the location and degree of vessel stenosis and the potentially dynamic influence of plaque disruption and degree of vascular occlusion. Along this spectrum, CAD may be clinically inapparent, with asymptomatic ("silent") episodes of myocardial ischemia, or may produce symptomatic ischemic syndromes, including stable reproducible myocardial ischemia (characterized by angina pectoris), unstable myocardial ischemia (unstable angina), acute myocardial infarction (MI), congestive heart failure, arrhythmia, or sudden death.

The main therapeutic objectives for patients with CAD are to relieve anginal symptoms and to prevent adverse cardiovascular events. Medical treatment strategies may reduce the biologic activity within coronary plaques—so-called "plaque stabilization"—thereby reducing plaque formation and preventing future ischemic events by staving off plaque rupture. Medical therapies may also reduce myocardial oxygen and energy requirements, attenuating symptoms in the context of fixed coronary stenoses. Revascularization by either percutaneous coronary intervention (PCI) or coronary artery bypass grafting (CABG) surgery may improve myocardial perfusion in the context of flow-limiting coronary stenoses, thus reducing ischemia and the associated clinical manifestations.

Several large-scale, randomized clinical trials have demonstrated that compared with medical therapy, an "early invasive" approach with PCI may reduce adverse cardiovascular events—including death and recurrent MI—in patients who present with unstable, ACSs (7,8). In comparison, the outcomes of applying an "early invasive" approach to patients with chronic stable angina nevertheless remain far less clearly defined, and remain a topic of considerable controversy (9,10). On the one hand, it is not presently possible to identify which coronary stenoses may ultimately become "vulnerable" and cause adverse future events; and the presence of ischemia itself may confer long-term risk. On the other hand, PCI carries inherent, albeit small, risk. In chronic, stable coronary syndromes, it is difficult to calculate the "trade-off" point where the risk of performing PCI is

offset by future benefit from reducing the associated ischemia or the risk that the lesion may one day become unstable.

These limitations having been noted, it remains that the majority of elective PCI procedures—more than 400,000 annually in the United States—are performed for patients who present with chronic stable angina (11). Of these patients, fewer than 10% have documentation of myocardial ischemia with noninvasive testing, and only 44% are documented to have received an adequate trial of optimal medical therapy (OMT) prior to PCI (12,13).

Recent clinical trials and meta-analyses have demonstrated superior improvements in symptom control and quality of life with PCI compared with medical therapy in patients with chronic stable angina (14,15). Most have failed to demonstrate improvement in survival or reduction in MI with PCI compared with medical therapy, however (16). Although the mortality associated with unstable coronary syndromes has declined in recent years, the mortality from stable CAD remains unchanged (2). Increasingly, evidence suggests that not all angiographically significant coronary stenoses cause ischemia, and that the approach of performing PCI for all angiographically significant lesions may, on balance, lead to greater adverse outcomes and the lack of benefit of PCI over medical therapy (17–19).

In this chapter, we will review the epidemiology, pathophysiology, and prognosis of symptomatic and silent myocardial ischemia (SMI). With the perspective of contemporary practice, which emphasizes cost-effectiveness and appropriate use of medical therapies and intervention, we will provide review and future perspective on the roles of optimal medical and revascularization strategies for managing patients with stable CAD and SMI.

DEFINITION, EPIDEMIOLOGY, AND PROGNOSIS OF STABLE CAD AND SMI

Chronic Stable Angina

The diagnosis of angina pectoris is derived from the clinical history, classically described as exertional chest pain, relieved with rest or following administration of sublingual nitroglycerin. Chronic stable angina refers to the clinical syndrome in which the frequency and severity of angina is consistently provoked by a predictable amount of physical exertion or emotional stress over time (6,10).

Of the estimated 17 million individuals in the United States with CAD, approximately 10 million report angina pectoris. The prevalence is higher in men and increases with age 10-fold between the ages of 50 and 70. Chronic stable angina is the cardinal manifestation in more than half of patients newly identified to have CAD, and confers a substantially higher mortality than the average population, increasing with age (1). Population-based data from the Framingham Heart Study, predating the widespread adoption of antiplatelet therapy, β-blockers, and aggressive risk-factor modification, identified an annual mortality of 4% in patients with chronic stable angina (6).

The CLARIFY (prospeCtive observational LongitudinAl RegIstry oF patients with stable coronarY artery disease) registry enrolled 32,105 patients with stable CAD. After a median follow-up of 2 years, those with angina at baseline had a higher event rate than those without angina, regardless of the underlying ischemia, as measured by noninvasive testing (20).

Silent Myocardial Ischemia

Silent (asymptomatic) myocardial ischemia (SMI) is defined as objective evidence of myocardial ischemia in the absence of angina or angina equivalents (20). The clinical scenario was first described in the 1970s, and has subsequently been recognized as an important indicator of adverse prognosis (21).

SMI may be identified in individuals who develop signs of ischemia in the absence of symptoms during exercise or pharmaceutical stress testing. SMI was traditionally diagnosed using ambulatory electrocardiography (EKG) monitoring.

Cohn et al. (22) proposed a classification schema for asymptomatic myocardial ischemia: (a) type I SMI, describing asymptomatic individuals with CAD but no history of prior MI; (b) type II SMI, describing asymptomatic individuals with a history of prior MI; and (c) type III SMI, describing individuals with both symptomatic and asymptomatic episodes of ischemia (23).

SMI is common in the general population, described in 3% of the overall population older than 60 years and in 10% of those over 70 (24). In one of the earliest studies of exercise testing, 1,390 men in the U.S. Air Force were evaluated: 111 had abnormal findings, of whom 34 (2.5% of the original population tested) were found to have coronary artery lesions of >50% stenosis (22,23). Thaulow et al. evaluated 2,014 Norwegian male office workers with stress testing, and confirmed the presence of significant coronary lesions at angiography in 2.7% of the study population (25). In the Framingham Heart Study, 5,127 asymptomatic patients were followed up for 30 years, where 35% of females and 28% of males developed EKG evidence consistent with MI (22,24). Kral et al. studied the impact of silent ischemia over 25 years in asymptomatic patients with a positive family history of CAD: 28% of male siblings with a positive myocardial perfusion study (MPS) developed clinically manifest CAD compared with 12% of those with a negative MPS, with a mean time of 8 years between detection of silent ischemia to the first cardiovascular event (26).

Silent ischemia is a common finding in patients with traditional cardiac risk factors. In one study, 15% of patients with mild to moderate hypertension without symptoms or signs of CAD were found to have asymptomatic ST-segment depression during ambulatory EKG or exercise testing (27). In asymptomatic individuals with type II diabetes mellitus, 12% were identified to have abnormalities on exercise stress testing, with half of this 12% having abnormal myocardial perfusion studies (28). In individuals with diabetes plus at least one other CAD risk factor but no overt symptoms, 33% had evidence of silent ischemia.

In patients with documented CAD, episodes of silent ischemia occur frequently, despite apparent symptom control with medication. The presence of these asymptomatic episodes is associated with an increased risk of death and MI. On balance, asymptomatic ischemia occurs more frequently than symptomatic ischemia in patients with stable CAD (29–32). **Figure 16.1** highlights the *ischemic cascade* that results from the reduction of coronary blood flow because of coronary stenosis, or the relative imbalance of myocardial oxygen demand compared with delivery in the context of flow-limiting stenosis. The diagram highlights the concept that symptoms of

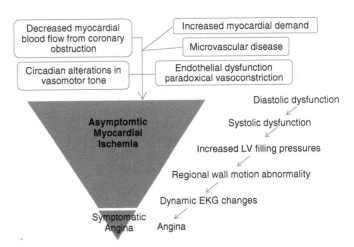

FIGURE 16.1   The iceberg effect of the ischemic cascade: the burden of asymptomatic myocardial ischemia and the tip of the iceberg, symptomatic angina.

angina represent the final manifestation of ischemia, with substantial asymptomatic hemodynamic and electromechanical consequences occurring well before the onset of chest pain. Using ambulatory EKG monitoring, 50% of individuals with stable CAD were found to have asymptomatic ST-segment depression. Additionally, more than 50% of patients monitored with telemetry during admission for unstable angina are found to have asymptomatic episodes of ischemic ST-segment changes. Sudden cardiac death comprises 18% of all primary clinical presentations with CAD; and more than 50% of sudden deaths occur without an antecedent history of CAD. As many as 40% of patients with stable angina treated with one or more antianginal medications, and 30% to 40% of patients after MI, have episodes of asymptomatic ischemia (22,24,30).

The presence of asymptomatic ischemia confers an elevated risk of adverse cardiovascular events. In the Multiple Risk Factor Intervention Trial (MRFIT) of over 12,000 asymptomatic middle-aged men with two or more CAD risk factors, the presence of ischemia during exercise testing was highly predictive of future cardiac death (relative risk [RR]: 3.4) (23,33). In the Lipid Research Clinic Primary Prevention Trial (LRCPPT) of greater than 6,000 males without prior CAD, asymptomatic ischemia on submaximal exercise testing was associated with a significantly greater age-adjusted cardiovascular mortality (34). In patients with established CAD identified at an index presentation with MI or unstable angina, 30% to 40% are subsequently found to have evidence for SMI, which is associated with a higher rate of future cardiovascular events and death (31).

The presence of SMI also confers a higher risk of adverse cardiovascular events in patients with documented CAD and chronic stable angina. In the Asymptomatic Cardiac Ischemia Pilot (ACIP) Study, the 1-year composite rate of death, MI, and hospital admission was 13% in 558 patients with SMI (35). The Coronary Artery Surgery Study (CASS) included 880 patients with documented CAD, and found that the 7-year incidence of MI and death was greatest in those with asymptomatic ischemia on exercise testing (26%) compared with 23% in patients with symptomatic ischemia on exercise testing and 2% in patients with no demonstrable ischemia (36).

More recent studies suggest that the identification of SMI during ambulatory EKG monitoring is a stronger predictor of future adverse events than ischemia found on exercise testing. In one study, 12.5-month follow-up of 86 patients with stable CAD and ischemia on exercise testing found a correlation between the number of

ST-segment depression events on ambulatory EKG monitoring with the duration of exercise, time to onset of ST-segment depression, and the depth of ST-segment depression at stress testing. Following multivariate adjustment, however, only ST-segment depression on ambulatory monitoring significantly predicted adverse future events. In another study, the presence of SMI during ambulatory monitoring was a more powerful predictor of mortality than exercise duration, age, prior MI, hypertension, diabetes, or smoking status in asymptomatic patients with CAD on antianginal therapy (24,29,31,32). *The most important factors in determining outcome in patients with CAD are the presence and extent of ischemia (37,38).*

PATHOPHYSIOLOGY OF SYMPTOMATIC ANGINA PECTORIS AND SMI

Myocardial ischemia is caused by an imbalance between myocardial oxygen requirements or demands and myocardial oxygen supply (5). The most important determinants of myocardial oxygen demand are heart rate, wall stress or tension, and contractility, which are influenced by activity and sympathetic tone. Myocardial oxygen supply is primarily increased by augmenting coronary blood flow.

When coronary stenosis is severe, coronary blood flow may be limited, particularly at times of increased demand, and results in ischemia. In the presence of vascular inflammation and endothelial dysfunction, exercise may provoke paradoxical vasoconstriction, rather than vasodilatation of the coronary arteries, further reducing myocardial perfusion. In cases of critical stenosis, coronary blood flow and myocardial oxygen supply may be so reduced as to cause ischemia even at rest or with vasoconstriction from elevated sympathetic tone. At a microvascular and cellular level, adaptive mechanisms, such as intracellular signaling with adenosine, increase myocardial capillary dilatation, reduce flow resistance, and optimize oxygen extraction. Because coronary blood flow is maximal in diastole, the perfusion gradient across the myocardium may be influenced by changes in wall tension and left ventricular filling pressures. The left ventricular wall tension is greatest at the subendocardial surface, which therefore is typically the first site of ischemia (5,22).

The precise mechanisms that determine when myocardial ischemia is silent or symptomatic remain to be elucidated. Ambulatory EKG monitoring demonstrates the propensity for asymptomatic ischemia in the morning, suggesting that a circadian pattern of increased myocardial oxygen demand related to increased heart rate and blood pressure may provoke some asymptomatic ischemia. Circadian rhythms may also alter vasomotor tone, platelet activity, and in vivo fibrinolytic activity, with implications on myocardial perfusion (39,40). Heterogeneity in peripheral and central nervous neural processing and nociception has also been implicated in patients with asymptomatic, versus those with symptomatic, ischemia. The presence of autonomic neuropathy and increased endogenous endorphin levels have been proposed as mechanisms that enable episodes of asymptomatic ischemia (22,24).

At the most fundamental level, myocardial ischemia reflects the mismatch between supply of, and demand for, blood flow and oxygen, resulting in a stereotyped sequence of hemodynamic and electromechanical alterations, the final step of which is the development of symptomatic angina. Figure 16.1 describes this ischemic cascade, and highlights the numerous subclinical alterations that occur before the onset of chest pain. When coronary arterial supply is outstripped by demand, first diastolic, then systolic regional wall dysfunction results. As a consequence, left ventricle (LV) filling

pressures rise, worsening the regional wall abnormality. Following mechanical disruption of LV function, the EKG becomes abnormal. Only at this point will the patient begin to develop symptomatic angina. This physiologic cascade reflects the "iceberg" concept of symptomatic and asymptomatic angina: The ultimate manifestation of angina pectoris represents only the final culmination of events, or the tip of the iceberg, while the majority of ischemic manifestations occur silently beneath the surface of clinical detection.

MANAGEMENT OF STABLE CAD AND SMI

The main goals in managing patients with stable CAD include the relief of symptoms, resulting in freedom from angina and improved quality of life, and the reduction of future cardiovascular events and mortality, through coronary plaque stabilization and slowing the progression of atherosclerosis. Regardless of patient symptomatology, the reduction of residual ischemia is the most important determinant of future prognosis and outcomes.

Comprehensive management of stable CAD requires a multifaceted simultaneous approach:

1. Identify and treat any associated medical conditions that may worsen or precipitate angina, such as thyrotoxicosis or anemia.
2. Modify established CAD risk factors and commence secondary preventative medications.
3. Modify lifestyle factors.
4. Commence, titrate, and ensure compliance with antianginal pharmacotherapy.
5. Perform revascularization (PCI or CABG) for persistent symptoms, or substantial residual ischemia on medical therapy.

The preceding treatment strategies are further outlined in **Table 16.1**. The current American College of Cardiology/American Heart Association recommendations for pharmacotherapy of stable CAD are outlined in **Table 16.2**, and the lifestyle goals are outlined in detail in **Table 16.3** (9,10).

Over the past three decades, significant advances in the array of medications targeting secondary prevention and symptomatic treatment of CAD have resulted in dramatic improvements in survival among patients with stable CAD (3). In the Framingham Heart Study, prior to the widespread adoption of current medical therapy, the annual mortality from stable CAD was 4% (2). In comparison, patients receiving contemporary medical therapy for stable CAD (92% were taking platelet inhibitors, 62% β-blockers, and 58% lipid-lowering therapy) were evaluated in the EUROPA trial and had an annual risk of cardiovascular death or MI of 2.5% (41). Of the medical therapies available, aspirin, angiotensin converting enzyme (ACE) inhibitors, and lipid-lowering statin medications have been proven to reduce mortality and morbidity in patients with stable CAD and preserved left ventricular function. To avoid one death or MI, about 175 patients need to be treated with aspirin for 1 year (relative risk reduction: 23%); 120 patients with standard dose statin medications (relative risk reduction: 30%); and 200 patients with an ACE inhibitor (relative risk reduction: 20%) (1). The other medications, including long-acting nitrates, β-blockers, and calcium-channel antagonists, have been shown to improve symptomatology, exercise tolerance, and quality of life among patients with stable CAD, but their effect on survival has not been definitely established, with the exception of β-blockers in patients with stable CAD and impaired left ventricular function (1,10).

A detailed discussion of the pharmacodynamics, side effects, interactions, and contraindications of each of the medication groups just mentioned is beyond the scope of this chapter. We will briefly

TABLE 16.1 Medical Therapies for Chronic Stable Angina

MANAGEMENT STRATEGY	INTERVENTION
1. Treatment of associated conditions that may precipitate or worsen angina	1. Check for anemia 2. Check for thyrotoxicosis 3. Control tachyarrhythmias 4. Check for concomitant left ventricular failure or valvular heart disease 5. Check for cocaine use
2. Reduction of coronary risk factors	1. Blood pressure control 2. Smoking cessation 3. LDL cholesterol reduction 4. HDL cholesterol elevation 5. Diabetes control 6. Physical exercise 7. Inflammation reduction 8. ACE inhibitors
3. Lifestyle adjustments	1. Weight loss 2. Physical exercise 3. Stress reduction 4. Antioxidants and dietary supplements
4. Antianginal pharmacotherapy	1. Antiplatelet therapy 2. β-blocker therapy 3. Combination of β-blocker with calcium-channel antagonist or long-acting nitrates 4. Ranolazine 5. Nicorandil 6. Ivabradine 7. Fasudil 8. Metabolic agents—trimetazidine
5. Revascularization	1. Percutaneous coronary intervention (stenting) 2. Coronary artery bypass grafting

ACE, angiotensin-converting-enzyme; HDL, high-density lipoprotein; LDL, low-density lipoprotein.

outline the evidence supporting the antianginal efficacy of each of the major medication groups. Long-acting nitrates are highly effective antianginal agents, reducing the frequency and duration of ischemic episodes and producing total suppression of ischemia in 35% of patients (1,24). Side effects and medication intolerance, most commonly headaches, must be considered. β-blockers represent the cornerstone of antianginal therapy, reducing myocardial oxygen demand, heart rate with exercise, resting heart rate, blood pressure, circadian effects, and ventricular contractility. In pooled analyses, β-blockers reduce the frequency and duration of silent ischemic episodes by 59% and 69%, respectively, with total abolition of ischemia in 55% of patients. β-blockers are contra-indicated in patients with severe asthma or significant conduction system disease. Calcium-channel antagonists may be used as an alternative to β-blockers for patients with contraindications or side effects. In pooled analyses, the use of calcium-channel blockers results in a 46% reduction in frequency and a 36% reduction in the duration of ischemic episodes (1,22,42). Prior studies have examined the

use of combining antianginal medications for potential synergy. In the ACIP study, the combination of β-blocker and calcium-channel antagonist resulted in total ischemia suppression of 48% compared with the combination of calcium-channel antagonist and long-acting nitrate (total suppression 33%) (35). Current treatment guidelines recommend initial therapy with an antiplatelet agent and β-blocker, with subsequent addition of a long-acting nitrate if symptoms persist.

Calcium-channel antagonists are most commonly used in place of β-blockers, and addition of a second agent is recommended if symptoms persist. Numerous additional antianginal agents are available for use, but a detailed discussion of these agents is beyond the scope of this chapter. They are listed in Table 16.1.

WHAT CONSTITUTES OMT?

There is no uniform definition of OMT. OMT for stable CAD has evolved significantly over the last 30 years. Societal guidelines for secondary prevention therapy were not introduced until 1995, with most therapy prior to this targeted toward ACS patients. The earlier trials of medical therapy for stable angina used different drug preparations and combinations, and different drug dosages and titration schedules (35). The sole lifestyle modification targeted was smoking cessation. It was not until the early 2000s that a greater emphasis was placed on β-blocker therapy and ACE inhibitor use in most patients with coronary heart disease (10,41). Successive treatment guidelines have broadened the indications for cholesterol reduction therapy, with endorsement of progressively earlier initiation of statin therapy. The 2013 ACC/AHA Guidelines on the Treatment of Blood Cholesterol to Reduce Atherosclerotic Cardiovascular Risk (ASCVD) in Adults recommends high-intensity statin therapy for all men and women ≤75 years of age who have clinical ASCVD to maximally lower LDL (low-density lipoprotein), usually by an average of 50% (42). The use of LDL targets is no longer supported in these guidelines (43). Nevertheless, measuring LDL levels is still clinically useful because the 2016 Expert Consensus Decision Pathway on the Role of Non-Statin Therapies for LDL Cholesterol Lowering in the management of ASCVD Risk recommends the addition of non-statin therapy to be considered for an LDL level >100 mg/dL or for less than anticipated response to statins (<50% LDL reduction) (44). PCSK9 inhibitors are novel non-statin agents that dramatically reduce LDL levels for those who are statin intolerant or who have had a less than anticipated response to statins. The FOURIER trial enrolled 27,564 patients with CAD on moderate- to high-intensity statin therapy with a median LDL 92 mg/dL and then randomized them to receive the PCSK9 inhibitor evolocumab or placebo. Results showed that evolocumab reduced LDL by 59%, from a median of 92 to 30 mg/dL. The primary endpoint of a composite of MI, stroke, hospitalization for angina, revascularization, or cardiovascular (CV) death was reduced by 15%, and the number of CV death, MI, or stroke after the first year was reduced by 25% in the evolocumab group. These results suggest that patients may benefit from LDL target levels that are well below current targets (45).

Similarly, targets for blood pressure control have been serially reduced. Over time, a more significant emphasis has been placed on diet, exercise, weight control, diabetes management, and blood pressure control. The Systolic Blood Pressure Intervention Trial (SPRINT) evaluated 9,361 patients at high risk for cardiovascular events but without diabetes, and found that the risk of the primary composite outcome of MI, other ACS, stroke, heart failure, or death from cardiovascular causes was 25% lower in patients with a target systolic blood pressure (SBP) <120 mm Hg as compared to patients with target SBP <140 mm Hg (46). In light of the evolution of

TABLE 16.2 ACC/AHA Recommended Pharmacotherapy for Chronic Stable Angina

CLASS	INDICATION	LEVEL OF EVIDENCE
I (indicated)	1. Aspirin in the absence of C/I	A
	2. β-Blockers for all patients with normal LV function after MI or ACS for 3 years	B
	3. β-Blockers for all patients with LV systolic dysfunction (EF ≤40%) with heart failure or prior MI, unless C/I (limited to carvedilol, metoprolol succinate, or bisoprolol, which have been shown to reduce mortality risk)	A
	4. ACE inhibitor in all patients (or ARBs for patients who are intolerant of ACE inhibitors) with impaired LV systolic function, chronic kidney disease, hypertension, and/or diabetes	A
	5. Moderate or high dose of a statin therapy, in the absence of C/I or documented adverse effects	A
	6. Sublingual nitroglycerin for immediate relief of angina	B
	7. Calcium-channel antagonists or long-acting nitrates as initial therapy when β-blockers C/I	B
	8. Calcium-channel antagonists or long-acting nitrates in combination with β-blockers for persistent symptoms despite β-blocker titration (avoid short-acting dihydropyridine calcium-channel antagonists)	B
	9. Calcium-channel antagonists and long-acting nitrates in combination as a substitute for β-blockers if β-blocker therapy produces side effects	C
	10. Clopidogrel when aspirin is absolutely C/I	B
IIa (good evidence)	1. Long-acting nondihydropyridine calcium antagonists instead of β-blockers as initial therapy	B
	2. LDL cholesterol lowering therapy with bile acid sequestrants, niacin, or both for those patients who do not tolerate statins	B
	3. ACE inhibitor in patients with CAD and other vascular disease	B
	4. ARBs in other patients who are ACE-I intolerant	C
	5. Ranolazine as a substitute for β-blockers for symptom relief if initial treatment with β-blockers leads to unacceptable side effects, is ineffective, or C/I	B
	6. Ranolazine in combination with β-blockers for symptom relief when initial treatment with β-blockers is not successful	A
IIb (weak evidence)	1. Aspirin 75–162 mg daily and clopidogrel 75 mg daily in certain high-risk patients with stable CAD	B
	2. β-Blockers as chronic therapy for patients with coronary or other vascular disease	C
	3. Pharmacotherapy to achieve target HbA1c	A
III (not indicated)	1. Dipyridamole	B
	2. Chelation therapy	B

ACE, angiotensin-converting-enzyme; ACS, acute coronary syndrome; ARBs, angiotensin receptor blockers; CAD, coronary artery disease; HbA1c, glycosylated hemoglobin percentage; LDL, low-density lipoprotein; LV, left ventricular; MI, myocardial infarction.

TABLE 16.3 Specific Lifestyle Goals in Patients with Chronic Stable Angina

RISK FACTOR/STRATEGY	GOAL
Smoking	Complete cessation, counseling and medications if necessary
Blood pressure	<140/90 or <130/80 if CHF, chronic kidney disease, or diabetes
Lipid management	Dietary guidelines should include reduced intake of saturated fats (<7% of total calories), trans fatty acids (to <1% of total calories), and cholesterol (<200 mg/d)
Physical activity	30–60 minutes a day of moderate-intensity aerobic activity; minimum 5 days a week. Complementary resistance training ≥2 days a week is reasonable.
Weight management	BMI: 18.5–24.9 kg/m²
Diabetes	HbA1C as near normal as possible; <7% minimum
Alcohol	Women—one drink a day; men—one to two drinks a day, unless alcohol is C/I

BMI, body mass index; CHF, congestive heart failure; C/I, contra-indication; HbA1c, glycosylated hemoglobin percentage.

medical therapy over time, it is difficult to compare the findings of multiple studies of medical therapy versus revascularization from different eras, or even to extrapolate the findings of prior studies to current practice, as therapeutic options, targets, and management strategies have changed so dramatically.

Tables 16.2 and 16.3 outline the latest ACC/AHA treatment guidelines for chronic stable angina (10). Despite the publication of these guidelines, prescribing rates of "OMT" and patient compliance with medical therapy nevertheless remain poor. In 2011, Borden et al. reported an analysis of the patterns and intensity of OMT in patients undergoing PCI from the National Cardiovascular Data Registry (NCDR), demonstrating that fewer than half of patients undergoing PCI for stable CAD were receiving OMT (11). Similarly, Hannan et al. in 2012 reported that in the New York State Registry of Cardiac Catheterization and Intervention between 2003 and 2008, only 11% of patients with stable CAD were managed with medical therapy alone (47,48). In the recently published guideline regarding appropriate use criteria for coronary revascularization, particular emphasis was placed on maximizing medical antianginal therapy, including dose escalation of β-blockers and then adding calcium-channel antagonists or nitrates, prior to considering PCI (9,49).

The Clinical Outcomes Utilizing Revascularization and Aggressive Drug Evaluation (COURAGE) trial represents the largest comparison of optimal medical to PCI for stable CAD (50,51). In this study, OMT was defined to include antiplatelet therapy, anti-ischemic medical therapy with long-acting β-blocker, calcium-channel antagonists, and long-acting nitrates, alone or in combination, along with an ACE inhibitor or angiotensin receptor antagonist for secondary prevention. All patients received therapy to reduce LDL cholesterol to target 65 to 80 mg/dL, then to raise high-density lipoprotein (HDL) cholesterol and reduce triglyceride level. Medication compliance was higher in COURAGE than in any previous trial or in rates observed in clinical practice, likely reflecting the fact that medications were provided free of charge, and compliance was supervised and reinforced by a clinical research nurse over the duration of the study. Although exquisite adherence to medical therapy yielded outcomes similar to those in PCI, the COURAGE trial has not significantly altered rates of medical therapy prescription in daily practice. In an analysis of the NCDR registry, Borden et al. identified that the rate of OMT prescription before PCI was 43.5% before the publication of COURAGE, and then 44.7% following the trial's publication (11). The challenge of implementing truly OMT—by rates of physician prescription or by compliance of patients—may represent an inherent obstacle to the extrapolation of the COURAGE trial results to "real-world" practice.

REVASCULARIZATION IN STABLE CAD AND SMI—MORE THAN JUST SYMPTOM ALLEVIATION

The conventional goals of coronary revascularization, which stem from the relief of myocardial ischemia, include improvement in quality of life, freedom from angina, increased exercise capacity, a reduction of the need for antianginal medication, and improvement in prognosis when coupled with OMT. Described previously, the factor that has the greatest impact on prognosis in patients with CAD is the presence and extent of myocardial ischemia (37,38). Coronary revascularization, whether by PCI or by CABG surgery, more effectively relieves ischemia than does medical therapy alone (35).

The ACIP study was one of the earliest studies that examined the impact of coronary revascularization on SMI (35). Enrolled patients had evidence of SMI, an abnormal exercise test, stable angina, and a documented stenosis of >50% in one vessel; one-third were asymptomatic at the time of enrollment. Patients were randomized to treatment with revascularization versus medical therapy. The medical therapy group was divided into treatment with an angina-guided strategy (titration of medications to eliminate symptoms only) and an ischemia-guided group (titration of medications to eliminate SMI on ambulatory EKG monitoring). Revascularization was performed with either percutaneous transluminal coronary angioplasty (PTCA) or CABG. At 12 weeks, 55% of the individuals in the revascularization group had suppression of ischemia events, compared with 39% in the angina-guided and 41% in the ischemia-guided groups. There was a trend toward fewer cardiovascular events in those with greater reduction of ischemia. The secondary composite endpoint of death, MI, revascularization, or hospitalization for unstable angina at 1 and 2 years was lowest in the revascularization group.

In the Swiss Interventional Study on Silent Ischemia Type II (SWISSI II) trial, 201 patients with a recent MI history, SMI, and one- or two-vessel CAD were randomized to medical therapy or revascularization with PTCA and followed up for 10 years (52). Medical therapy consisted of aspirin, statin, ACE inhibitor if hypertensive, and β-blocker/calcium-channel antagonist, or a combination of drug therapy for persistent symptoms. In this study, patients who underwent revascularization had a lower rate of ischemia (11.6% vs. 28.9%, p = 0.03), improved left ventricular ejection fraction (LVEF), and an absolute reduction in the composite endpoint (death/MI/revascularization) of 6.3% per year compared with those treated with medical therapy.

In the nuclear perfusion substudy of the COURAGE trial, 314 patients underwent serial myocardial perfusion imaging after randomization to medical therapy or PCI. At the time of randomization, one-third of the patients had evidence of moderate-to-severe ischemia. PCI engendered a greater absolute reduction in myocardial ischemia (−2.7% vs. −0.5%, p < 0.0001) compared with medical therapy, and more patients exhibited a reduction in ischemia burden (33% vs. 19%, p = 0.0004), particularly those with moderate-to-severe ischemia (78% vs. 52%, p = 0.007) (53,54). Of importance, the reduction in ischemia was found to correlate strongly with reduction in subsequent risk of death or MI.

In addition to the randomized studies that examined the clinical impact of reducing myocardial ischemia, there have been a number of observational studies that have specifically evaluated the influence of revascularization on prognosis. In a study by Hachamovitch et al., 10,627 patients without previously identified CAD were found to have improvement in survival with revascularization than with medical therapy when moderate-to-severe ischemia was demonstrated (55). In two other observational studies, the benefit of revascularization also appears to be most significant in patients with impaired left ventricular function and viable myocardium, and in those with multivessel CAD (56,57).

Despite this body of clinical trial and observational study evidence supporting revascularization in patients with moderate-to-severe ischemia, impaired left ventricular function with viability and multivessel CAD, large-scale randomized trials of PCI versus medical therapy for stable CAD have failed to demonstrate a survival advantage or reduction in MI with PCI. There are a number of possible explanations for this. First, these early studies (just discussed), with the exception of the COURAGE nuclear substudy, involve suboptimal medical treatment regimens inappropriately favoring PCI. Second, revascularization in the early studies (not including the nuclear substudy of the COURAGE trial) consisted of balloon angioplasty alone or a combination of angioplasty and CABG as the method of choice. The PCI technique evolved to bare-metal and then to drug-eluting stents (DESs), rendering it difficult to extrapolate early trial data to contemporary practice. Third, although many trials—including COURAGE—were evaluated with an intention-to-treat design, there is considerable crossover from patients randomized to medical therapy who ultimately receive PCI, making it difficult to attribute the outcome to the designated therapeutic strategy. Lastly, the benefit that results from revascularization of ischemia-provoking coronary stenoses may be offset by procedural and long-term risk of PCI in lesions that may appear severe but do not cause myocardial ischemia. In this context, it is increasingly recognized that angiographic severity does not perfectly correlate with the hemodynamic—and therefore the ischemic—significance of coronary stenoses (17–19,58–61).

COMPARISON OF OMT AND REVASCULARIZATION

Table 16.4 summarizes 23 clinical studies comparing medical therapy and revascularization (CABG initially, PCI subsequently), spanning 30 years of practice and ranging in size from 60 to >9,000 patients (35,36,50,52,54,62–79).

Initial comparisons were made between available medical therapy and the only mode of revascularization in the late 1970s: CABG surgery. In the CASS, 780 patients with symptomatic CAD were randomized to treatment with medical therapy or CABG. The primary endpoint was the combined incidence of mortality and nonfatal MI. After a mean follow-up of 6 years, compared with medically treated patients, those who underwent CABG had similar rates of mortality and nonfatal MI, with no difference when stratified by history of prior MI or evaluation of LV function (36).

The Veterans Administration Cooperative Study of Surgery (VACSS) evaluated 686 patients who were randomized to medical therapy versus CABG plus medical therapy. Following randomization, subjects were stratified into low-, moderate-, and high-clinical-risk groups. The primary endpoint was all-cause mortality, and the secondary endpoints were MI and severity of angina. After a median follow-up of 16.8 years, survival rates were 33% in the medical therapy group compared with 30% in the CABG group. A survival advantage was noted in the CABG group at 7 years (77% vs. 70% for OMT), although the survival advantage diminished and was equal to that of OMT at 11 years. For subjects who had suffered a prior MI, CABG conferred a 35% reduction in mortality compared with OMT at 10 years (p < 0.001), although this advantage did not persist at 18 years. CABG was also associated with an early improvement in angina compared with OMT, but the benefit was neutralized by 5 years' post-randomization, likely reflecting the impact of graft failure (63).

The Surgical Treatment of Ischemic Heart Failure (STICH) surgical revascularization trial evaluated 1,212 patients with CAD and an EF ≤ 35%. Patients were randomly assigned to medical therapy alone or medical therapy plus CABG. There was no significant difference in the rate of death from any cause between medical therapy alone and medical therapy plus CABG after 5 years (41% in the OMT group vs. 35% in the CABG + OMT group; hazard ratio with CABG 0.86; 95% CI 0.72–1.04, p = 0.12), but the rates of death or hospitalization from cardiovascular causes was lower in the CABG group (80). The STICH Extension Study evaluated the effects of CABG in patients with ischemic cardiomyopathy after 10 years and found that the rates of death from any cause was lower by 16% in the CABG plus medical therapy group compared to the medical therapy only group. The rates of death from cardiovascular causes and death from any cause, or hospitalization from cardiovascular causes, were also significantly lower over 10 years among the patients who underwent CABG with medical therapy (81).

Although all subjects enrolled in these trials received medical therapy for symptom control irrespective of the treatment strategy at randomization, none of the studies had a clearly defined medical regimen, and medication dosages were not controlled. At the time of several of these trials, OMT did not include the focus on antiplatelet agents, ACE inhibitors, or statins, as is now widely accepted. The CASS and VACSS trials included nitrates and propranolol for anti-anginal therapy, so comparison of their outcomes with those with modern OMT may be limited.

Following the development of balloon angioplasty, studies emerged comparing PTCA with medical therapy. In the ACME (Angioplasty Compared to Medicine) trial, 212 patients with stable angina were randomized to PTCA or medical therapy (63–65). Medical therapy consisted of aspirin and a combination of β-blockers, nitrates, and calcium-channel antagonists titrated to eliminate angina. Primary endpoints included change in exercise tolerance, frequency of angina, and nitroglycerin use; and exercise stress nuclear testing was evaluated at baseline and 6 months post-randomization. Compared with medical therapy, PTCA improved exercise duration and reduced time to onset of angina and frequency of angina episodes. There was no statistical difference in the mortality or MI rates between the two groups, although the study was underpowered to assess this endpoint. In a pilot study (ACME 2), 101 patients with two-vessel CAD were evaluated using the same inclusion criteria, outcomes, and study protocol. No difference was identified between the PTCA and OMT groups with respect to any of the endpoints. Of note, medical therapy did not mandate the use of statins (65).

In the RITA 2 (second Randomized Intervention Treatment of Angina) trial, 1,018 patients with at least one-vessel CAD were randomized to OMT or PTCA with a median follow-up of 2.7 years (68). This trial did not exclude patients with low LVEF or totally occluded coronary arteries. The combined primary endpoint of death or nonfatal MI occurred in 3.3% of patients in the medical group versus 6.3% in the PTCA group. There was no difference in mortality between the two groups, although there were more nonfatal MIs in the PTCA group (4.2% vs. 2.0%), primarily driven by periprocedural MI. Symptom relief was greater following PTCA in patients with Canadian Cardiovascular Society (CCS) Class ≥2 angina, but this benefit was lost at 2-year follow-up.

Statin use was not mandated, and only 4% of patients screened were eligible for the trial. Ultimately, only 1.5% of those deemed eligible were randomized, again weakening the generalizability of the study's findings.

In the AVERT (Atorvastatin Versus Revascularization Treatment) trial, 341 patients referred for PTCA were randomized to receive aggressive lipid-lowering therapy with atorvastatin 80 mg daily or PTCA with usual medical care (69). The primary endpoint was occurrence of a first ischemic event (cardiac death, cardiac arrest, nonfatal MI, stroke, CABG, PCI, or hospitalization for angina). Of those in the medical therapy arm, 13% had an ischemic event compared with

21% in the PTCA group (p = 0.045). The authors concluded that aggressive lipid lowering with a statin is at least as effective as PTCA.

In the JSAP (Japanese Stable Angina Pectoris) trial, 384 patients were randomized to receive OMT or PCI plus medical therapy, with median 3.3-year follow-up and primary endpoints, including all-cause mortality, ACS, cerebrovascular accidents (CVAs), or emergency hospitalization (78). Patients in both groups received aspirin, β-blockers, ACE inhibitors, calcium-channel antagonists, and statins. There was no difference between the two groups regarding death, but the composite outcomes were improved with PCI (p = 0.045 for death, ACS, and CVA), and there was a higher incidence of ACS with medical therapy in follow-up.

In the MASS (Medicine, Angioplasty or Surgery Study) (70), 214 patients from a single center were randomized to medical treatment, PTCA, or CABG with an internal mammary artery conduit (70). Subjects were followed up for an average of 5 years, with a composite primary endpoint of cardiac death, MI, or refractory angina requiring revascularization. Medical therapy consisted of aspirin, β-blockers, calcium-channel antagonists, and nitrates. Those in the CABG group had significantly fewer events (3%) compared with those in the PTCA (24%) and OMT (17%) groups, with no statistically significant difference between the latter two. The majority of the benefit was because of superior reduction in angina. Both the CABG and PTCA groups had significantly higher percentages of patients free of angina compared with OMT (CABG 98%, PTCA 82%, OMT 32%). In the MASS II trial (74), 611 patients with at least two-vessel CAD were randomized to OMT, PCI, or CABG, and followed up for 1-year (74). Medical therapy consisted of aspirin, β-blockers, nitrates, and calcium-channel antagonists that were titrated, as well as ACE inhibitors and statins. With the same primary endpoint as the MASS, there was a significant difference between the three groups, with more events occurring in the PCI group than in the CABG and OMT groups. While there was no difference between the three groups regarding cardiac mortality, both the PCI and the CABG patients had significant improvement in angina compared with OMT patients, but did not differ when compared with each other because of higher rates of revascularization in the PCI group.

The largest study comparing OMT and revascularization was the BARI 2D (Bypass Angioplasty Revascularization Investigation 2 Diabetes) trial (79). A total of 2,368 type 2 diabetic patients with CAD on angiography were randomized in a 2 × 2 factorial design to OMT or prompt revascularization (PCI, one-third DESs, or CABG) and to insulin sensitization or insulin-provision therapy. Medical therapy included aspirin, β-blockers, ACE inhibitors, statins, and lifestyle modification. After randomization to the OMT and revascularization groups, patients in each group were further stratified into CABG or PCI groups. The primary endpoint was all-cause death, and the principal secondary endpoint was a composite of death, MI, or CVA. After an average follow-up of 5.3 years, the rate of death from any cause did not differ significantly between the revascularization and the OMT groups. Also, the rate of freedom from major cardiovascular events did not differ significantly between these two groups.

The largest trial comparing OMT and PCI was the COURAGE trial, in which 2,287 patients with at least single-vessel, stable CAD were randomized to receive PCI with OMT or OMT alone (50,54). Medical therapy was strictly defined as outlined earlier. The primary outcome was a composite of all-cause death or nonfatal MI. After a median follow-up of 4.6 years, the cumulative primary event rates were 19.0% in the PCI group and 18.5% in the OMT group (p = 0.62). For the prespecified composite outcome of death, nonfatal MI, CVA,

and the hospitalization for unstable angina, there were no differences between the PCI and OMT groups. Although not a prespecified endpoint, both groups experienced significant improvement in rates of angina. There was a statistically significant difference in favor of the PCI group for symptom relief through most of the follow-up period, but the rates equalized by 5 years. Also, there were eight prespecified subgroups, including age, sex, previous MI, diabetes, angiographic extent of CAD, and ejection fraction less than 50%, but there was no significant interaction between treatment and any subgroup variable.

In an extended survival analysis up to 15 years, there was no difference in survival between the initial strategy of PCI plus medical therapy and medical therapy alone (25% vs. 24%, adjusted hazard ratio 1.03; 95% CI 0.83–1.21; p = 0.76). Nevertheless, this analysis was limited by a large percentage of patients who were lost to follow-up (47%), an unknown amount of crossover to PCI, and unknown causes of death (82).

The nuclear substudy of COURAGE evaluated 314 patients who underwent serial myocardial perfusion computed tomography to evaluate the effect of each treatment strategy on ischemic burden (54). Mild ischemia was defined as <5% ischemic burden, and moderate-to-severe ischemia was ≥10% ischemic myocardium. The primary endpoint was ≥5% reduction in ischemic myocardium. At follow-up, there was a significant reduction in the amount of ischemia (p < 0.0001) as well as an increase in the number of patients exhibiting ischemia reduction (p = 0.0004) in the PCI group. Although the substudy was not powered to detect this, those patients who exhibited significant ischemia reduction had lower rates of death or MI.

The COURAGE trial represents the largest and most current comparison of PCI and OMT. Nevertheless, it has proven controversial among the interventional community. First, it represents a highly selected patient population, with <10% of all patients screened enrolled on the trial, raising issue over its applicability to the general stable CAD population. The majority of patients enrolled were mildly symptomatic, 43% having minimal or no angina to begin with. The expected MI rate used to calculate the study power was 21% at 3 years, but at 4.6 years, the actual MI rate was only 12% in the OMT group, suggesting that the study was underpowered to detect an MI difference between the groups. Most importantly, enrolling physicians were allowed to review the patient angiogram prior to study entry, leading to potential selection bias issues. Finally, over time, one-third of the OMT group crossed over to receive PCI, and 15.7% of the PCI group did not actually receive PCI or were lost to follow-up. The medical therapy regimen was intensively supervised, and medications were provided free of charge to study participants, resulting in medication adherence rates far above those seen in practice. Despite these issues, it represents the largest and best-performed trial comparing OMT with a strategy of PCI with bare-metal stents.

Several meta-analyses have attempted to draw together these disparate trials' designs and patient populations to definitely determine whether medical therapy is superior to PCI, and not surprisingly, their conclusions have been diverse. In 2008, Schomig et al. reported a 20% mortality decrease for patients with stable CAD undergoing PCI compared with OMT (83). In this meta-analysis, however, studies that enrolled patients following an acute MI were included. In 2012, Stergiopoulos and Brown reanalyzed eight randomized trials, including the largest studied, COURAGE and BARI-2D (16). In this analysis, there was no benefit for PCI over OMT regarding death, nonfatal MI, unplanned revascularization, or persistent angina. Finally, Bangalore et al. recently published a meta-analysis of 12 randomized trials,

TABLE 16.4 Clinical Studies of CABG and PCI for Stable Coronary Artery Disease

STUDY	YEAR	INCLUSION CRITERIA	EXCLUSION CRITERIA	NO. PATIENTS; REVASC./ OMT	REVASC. METHOD	PCI METHOD PTCA, BMS, DES	PER PROTOCOL REVASC. IN REVASC. GROUP	NON-PROTOCOL REVASC. IN OMT GROUP	CAD SEVERITY
CASS	1984	Stable CAD or s/p MI	LM or EF < 35%	390/390	CABG	N/A	92%	24%	1 V 27%; 2 V 40%; 3 V 74%
VA Co-op study	1984	Stable CAD with ischemia	ACS, CHF	332/354	CABG	N/A	94%	38%	N/A
ACME-1	1992	1 V CAD with ischemia or recent MI	ACS, prior PCI, MVD, EF < 30%	112/115	PCI	PTCA	96%	41%	1 V CAD
ACME-2	1997	1 V CAD with ischemia or recent MI	ACS, prior PCI, MVD, EF < 30%	51/50	PCI	PTCA	100%	40%	1 or 2 V CAD
DANAMI	1997–2007	CAD with ischemia or inducible post-MI ischemia	Refractory angina, prior revasc.	503/505	CABG (147) PCI (266)	PTCA	82%	20%	1 V, 2 V, and 3 V CAD
ACIP	1997	Silent ischemia	Recent ACS, CCS IV, CHF, LMD, PCI within 6 months, CABG within 3 months	192/366	CABG/PCI	PTCA	89%	29%	1 V, 2 V, and 3 V CAD
RITA-2	1997–2003	Stable angina	Prior revasc, recent ACS, LMD	504/515	PCI	BMS 9%	93%	35%	1 V 60%; 2 V 33%; 3 V 7%
AVERT	1999	Stable angina	Age > 80; recent ACS; 3 V CAD; LMD; EF < 40%	177/164	PCI	BMS 30%	94%	12%	1 V 56%; 2 V 44%
MASS I PCI	1999	CAD with ischemia	Prior revasc, LMD, MI, LV dysfunc.	72/72	PCI	PTCA	100%	17%	1 V CAD
MASS I CABG	1999	CAD with ischemia	Prior revasc, MI, LMD, or LV dysfunc.	70/72	CABG	N/A	100%	17%	1 V CAD
TIME	2001–2004	CAD with ischemia; age > 75	Recent MI	153/148	CABG/PCI	N/A	71%	42%	1 V, 2 V, and 3 V CAD
TOAT	2002	CAD s/p anterior MI	N/A	32/34	PCI	BMS 100%	100%	N/A	1 V CAD
ALKK	2003	CAD s/p MI	CCS III or IV; >70% stenosis in non IRA; CABG indicated	149/151	PCI	BMS 11%	93%	24%	1 V CAD

TABLE 16.4 Clinical Studies of CABG and PCI for Stable Coronary Artery Disease (*continued*)

AGE	FEMALE GENDER (%)	DIABETES (%)	FOLLOW-UP IN YEARS	PRIMARY EP	OVERALL DEATH—REVASC. GROUP	OVERALL DEATH—OMT GROUP	CARDIAC DEATH—REVASC. GROUP	CARDIAC DEATH—OMT GROUP	MI—REVASC. GROUP	MI—OMT GROUP
52	10%	9%	5	Death and MI	6.7%	8.7%	N/A	N/A	13.6%	11%
51	0%	15%	11.2	Death	42%	43%	N/A	N/A	N/A	N/A
63	N/A	18%	2.4	Death, MI, rehosp. and revasc.	13.9%	13.4%	N/A	N/A	12.2%	7.1%
N/A	N/A	N/A	3	Death, MI, rehosp. and revasc.	17.6%	20%	N/A	N/A	11.8%	12%
56	18%	35%	2.4	Death, MI, and rehosp. for ACS	3.6%	4.4%	N/A	N/A	5.6%	10.5%
61	14%	16%	2	Death; MI, rehosp. and revasc.	2.2%	5.5%	N/A	N/A	3.6%	4.9%
58	18%	9%	7	Death and MI	8.5%	8.4%	4.0%	4.7%	6.3%	4.5%
58	16%	27%	1.5	Cardiac death; cardiac arrest; MI; CVA; rehosp. and revasc.	0.6%	0.6%	0.6%	0.6%	2.8%	2.4%
56	42%	18%	5	Cardiac death; MI and rehosp.	8.3%	8.3%	5.6%	2.8%	5.6%	4.2%
58	42%	19%	5	Cardiac death; MI and rehosp.	2.9%	8.3%	2.9%	2.8%	4.3%	4.2%
80	42%	34%	4.1	Death, MI and ACS	29.4%	27%	20.9%	22.3%	11.8%	12.2%
59	20%	14%	1	LV end systolic volume	6.3%	2.9%	N/A	N/A	9.4%	2.9%
58	14%	16%	4.7	Death, MI, rehosp. and revasc.	4%	11.3%	2.7%	9.3%	6.7%	7.9%

(*continued*)

TABLE 16.4 Clinical Studies of CABG and PCI for Stable Coronary Artery Disease (*continued*)

STUDY	YEAR	INCLUSION CRITERIA	EXCLUSION CRITERIA	NO. PATIENTS; REVASC./OMT	REVASC. METHOD	PCI METHOD PTCA, BMS, DES	PER PROTOCOL REVASC. IN REVASC. GROUP	NON-PROTOCOL REVASC. IN OMT GROUP	CAD SEVERITY
MASS II PCI	2004–2007	*CAD with ischemia*	Prior revasc, ACS, EF < 40%, 1 V CAD, LMD	205/203	PCI	BMS 72%	95%	24%	2 V 42%; 3 V 58%
MASS II CABG	2004–2007	*CAD with ischemia*	Prior revasc, ACS, EF < 40%, 1 V CAD, LMD	203/203	CABG	N/A	95%	24%	2 V 42%; 3 V 58%
OAT	2006	*CAD s/p recent MI*	Severe CHF; 3 V CAD; LM	1,082/1,084	PCI	BMS 79%; DES 8%	100%	9%	1 V and 2 V CAD
INSPIRE	2006	*CAD with ischemia and s/p MI*	Cardiogenic shock; recurrent CP; ACS	104/101	CABG 27%; PCI 43%	BMS 94%	67%	26%	1 V and 2 V CAD; 33% 3 V CAD; 12% LMD
COURAGE	2007	*Stable CAD*	CCS IV; CHF; EF < 30%; LMD	1,149/1,138	PCI	BMS 91%; DES 9%	96%	33%	1 V 31%; 2 V 39%; 3 V 30%
SWISS II	2007	*CAD s/p MI*	N/A	96/105	PCI	N/A	100%	44%	1 V and 2 V CAD
Nishigaki	2008	*CAD with ischemia*	3 V CAD; CTO; ACS; EF < 50%; CKD	192/188	PCI	PTCA 15%; BMS 76%	N/A	N/A	1 V 68%; 2 V 32%
BARI 2D	2009	*Stable angina with DM*	Urgent revasc; LMD; CHF; liver failure; CKD	1,176/1,192	CABG (378) PCI (798)	PTCA 9%; BMS 56%; DES 35%	95%	42%	1 V and 2 V CAD; 31% 3 V CAD
COURAGE nuclear substudy	2008	*Stable CAD with >70% stenosis in single vessel, plus positive MPS for ischemia*	CCS IV; shock; CHF; EF < 30%; LMD or anatomy unsuitable for PCI	314 pts from 2,287 pts (159 PCI; 155 OMT)	PCI	N/A	93%	21%	1 V 24%–27%; 2 V 34%–45%; 3 V 32%–39%
NY Registry	2012	*Stable angina and/or >70% stenosis of 1 V*	LMD; CCS IV; VT; valvular disease; negative stress test; high-risk stress test; recent MI; shock; EF < 35%; CABG anatomy; revasc. within 6 months	8,486/1,100	PCI	PTCA 5%; BMS 24%; DES 71%	89%	N/A	1 V 69.9%; 2 V 25%; 2 V with prox. LAD or 3 V 5%

TABLE 16.4 Clinical Studies of CABG and PCI for Stable Coronary Artery Disease (*continued*)

AGE	FEMALE GENDER (%)	DIABETES (%)	FOLLOW-UP IN YEARS	PRIMARY EP	OVERALL DEATH— REVASC. GROUP	OVERALL DEATH— OMT GROUP	CARDIAC DEATH— REVASC. GROUP	CARDIAC DEATH— OMT GROUP	MI— REVASC. GROUP	MI— OMT GROUP
60	30%	32%	5	Death; Q wave MI; revasc.	15.5%	16.2%	11.6%	12.3%	11.2%	15.3%
60	32%	33%	1	Death; Q wave MI; revasc.	12.8%	16.2%	7.9%	12.3%	8.3%	15.3%
59	22%	21%	4	Death, MI and CHF	9.1%	9.4%	6.3%	5%	7%	5.3%
61	15%	33%	1	LV perfusion defect decrease	1.9%	1%	1.9%	1%	4.8%	6.9%
61	15%	33%	4.6	Death and MI	7.4%	8.3%	2%	2.2%	12.4%	11.2%
55	13%	11%	10.2	Cardiac death, MI and revasc.	6.3%	21%	3.1%	21%	11.5%	38.1%
64	25%	40%	3.25	Death; CVA; and rehosp.	2.9%	3.9%	N/A	N/A	N/A	N/A
62	30%	100%	5.3	Death, MI and CVA	11.7%	12.2%	N/A	N/A	N/A	N/A
62–64	10%–15%	40%–46%	3.6 after 18 month MPS	>5% reduction in ischemia; death and MI	N/A	N/A	N/A	N/A	N/A	N/A
65	34%	32.7%	4	Death; MI; readmission for AMI; revasc.	10.1%	14.5%	N/A	N/A	8%	11.3%

ACS, acute coronary syndrome; AMI, Acute myocardial infarction; BMS, bare-metal stent; CABG, coronary artery bypass grafting; CAD, coronary artery disease; CCS, Canadian Cardiovascular Society; CHF, congestive heart failure; CKD, chronic kidney disease; CP, chest pain; CTO, chronic total occlusion; CVA, cerebrovascular accident; DES, drug-eluting stent; EF, ejection fraction; EP, endpoint; IRA, infarct-related artery; LAD, left anterior descending; LMD, left main disease; LV, left ventricle; MI, myocardial infarction; N/A, not available; OMT, optimal medical therapy; PCI, percutaneous coronary intervention; PTCA, percutaneous transluminal coronary angioplasty; Prox., proximal; rehosp., rehospitalization; Revasc., revascularization; VT, ventricular tachycardia.

including 7,182 subjects, concluding that compared with OMT, PCI did not reduce the risk of mortality, cardiovascular death, nonfatal MI, or revascularization, but did provide superior relief of angina compared with OMT (14).

Although a review of the literature raises many controversies regarding the utility of PCI versus OMT in stable CAD, in routine clinical practice, ad hoc PCI for stable CAD remains commonplace. In 2008, 440,000 PCIs for stable CAD were performed in the United States, according to an analysis of the NCDR registry, and only 44% of the patients treated had adequate documentation of ischemia prior to PCI (11). Subsequent to the publication of the COURAGE trial, the rates of physician prescription of OMT were not improved. In an analysis of the NCDR registry before and after publication of COURAGE, OMT was prescribed prior to and following PCI in only 43.5% and 63.5%, respectively. Following the publication of COURAGE, OMT was prescribed in only 44.7% before PCI and 66.5% after PCI. Hannan et al. presented an analysis of PCI versus regular medical therapy in patients with stable CAD undergoing intervention in the New York State registry (47). Only 11% of patients received medical therapy alone for treatment of stable CAD, and there was no impact in the rate of PCI for stable CAD after the publication of the COURAGE trial compared with that before its publication.

The International Study of Comparative Health Effectiveness with Medical and Invasive Approaches (ISCHEMIA) trial is an ongoing, multicenter, randomized controlled trial evaluating whether an initial conservative strategy of OMT versus an invasive strategy with cardiac catheterization, followed by revascularization plus OMT for patients with SIHD and at least moderate ischemia seen on stress testing, reduces the rate of death from cardiovascular causes or MI.

Enrollment started in 2012 and has been slow, with approximately 4,300 enrolled patients in June 2017, with a target enrollment of approximately 8,000 patients.

While it is imperative that OMT is conscientiously implemented as the first-line treatment of stable CAD (**Fig. 16.2**), it is also important to consider when optimal revascularization may improve patients' outcomes.

WHAT CONSTITUTES OPTIMAL REVASCULARIZATION PCI TECHNIQUE

As outlined earlier and in the section to follow, many of the clinical studies that used to inform decision making about PCI versus medical therapy for stable CAD are based on the evaluation of outdated PCI techniques. For example, prior to 1997, the PCI technique used in these clinical studies was mostly balloon angioplasty alone (35). In the most widely quoted clinical trial comparing medical therapy with PCI, the COURAGE trial, 91% of patients undergoing PCI received bare-metal stents (50,51). In more contemporary trials and practice, however, it is well established that DESs are superior to bare-metal stents, because they are associated with lower rates of restenosis and the consequent need for repeat revascularization, especially in patients with diabetes. Compared with the first-generation DESs, second-generation DESs are associated with exceptionally low rates of late stent thrombosis and equivalent antirestenotic efficacy. In addition, periprocedural pharmacotherapy has evolved substantially over time, focusing on the upstream use of thienopyridines and intraprocedural direct thrombin inhibitors rather than heparin and

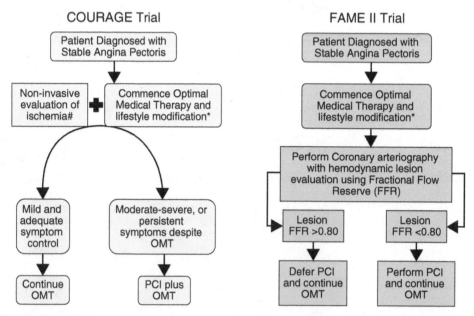

FIGURE 16.2 Treatment algorithm for patients with stable coronary artery disease after publication of the Courage Trial (2007) and possibly after publication of the FAME II Trial (2012). # In the Courage trial, 85% of the study population underwent noninvasive evaluation of ischemia. In practice, currently ~50% of stable CAD patients undergo noninvasive testing prior to catheterization. *OMT defined as antiplatelet therapy; cholesterol reduction/statin therapy with a LDL goal <100 mg/dL, or <70 mg/dL if prior MI/CVA/ diabetes; blood pressure control ACEI/ARB inhibitor if hypertensive / prior CVA / impaired LV function / chronic kidney disease or diabetic; combination antianginal therapy with either β-blocker / long-acting nitrate or calcium-channel antagonist / long-acting nitrate, titrated to symptom control or side effects / heart rate / blood pressure limits; smoking cessation; daily physical exercise and weight loss; diabetic control HbA₁C <7%. CAD, coronary artery disease; CVA, cerebrovascular accident; LDL, low-density lipoprotein; MI, myocardial infarction; OMT, optimal medical therapy; PCI, percutaneous coronary intervention.

glycoprotein IIb/IIIa inhibitors, resulting in lower rates of procedural bleeding complications, now recognized as a driver of future ischemic events, and lower rates of acute stent thrombosis. Transradial access for PCI continues to grow in popularity, with very low rates of vascular or bleeding complications. In a retrospective cohort study looking at data from the CathPCI Registry between 2007 and 2012, the proportion of radial PCI increased from 1.2% in 2007 to 16.1% in 2012, and accounted for 6.3% of the nearly 3 million procedures. Radial PCI was associated with lower risk of bleeding and vascular complications compared to transfemoral PCI and was consistent across subgroups of age, sex, and clinical presentation (84).

Perhaps the most important development, however, has been the recognition of the limitation of angiography in determining the functional significance or ischemia-causing potential of a coronary stenosis (17–19,58). Noninvasive testing often indicates the presence of ischemia in patients with multivessel CAD, but may fail to distinguish the specific territory or stenosis responsible. Moreover, in the case of balanced ischemia, noninvasive testing may not identify a perfusion abnormality, and may provide a false sense of security. The use of intracoronary pressure wire technology, permitting the evaluation of coronary fractional flow reserve (FFR), has emerged as an accurate and lesion-specific index that indicates whether a particular stenosis is responsible for downstream myocardial ischemia. Several recent clinical trials have shown that FFR-guided intervention may provide a sound basis for decision making in the catheterization laboratory, permitting selective intervention only on lesions responsible for ischemia (17–19,76).

In early trials, the measurement of FFR <0.75 was strongly correlated with a flow-limiting or ischemia-provoking stenosis; in more recent studies, particularly involving patients with multivessel CAD, the use of FFR <0.80 has been used to guide interventional therapy, although the FFR between 0.75 and 0.80 remains somewhat in a "gray zone," requiring tailored clinical decision making. Intervention may safely be deferred in favor of medical therapy for lesions with an FFR above 0.80. **Table 16.5** summarizes the clinical trial data supporting an ischemia-driven strategy of PCI revascularization (17–19,55,56,85,86).

In the DEFER study, 325 patients with a >50% coronary stenosis and a negative perfusion study within 2 months underwent angiography with measurement of FFR (18). If the FFR is <0.75, they underwent PCI. If the FFR is >0.75, the patients were randomized to either medical therapy alone ("Defer") or PCI. At 5 years of clinical follow-up, the risk of death or MI from a nonischemic (FFR >0.75) lesion was very low, and not altered by stenting. In contrast, ischemia-causing lesions were the most important predictor of death or MI in follow-up. The DEFER study established the safety of not performing PCI in a nonsignificant stenosis as identified by FFR.

Building on the findings of the DEFER study, the use of FFR in the evaluation of patients with multivessel disease was examined in the Fractional Flow Reserve versus Angiography for Multivessel Evaluation (FAME) trial (19). In FAME, 1,005 patients with at least two of three coronary vessels with a >50% stenosis were randomized to undergo FFR-guided revascularization of only ischemia-causing lesions versus angiographically guided PCI of all angiographically significant stenoses. The primary endpoint was a composite of death, MI, and revascularization at 2-year follow-up. The FFR-guided PCI had significantly fewer primary endpoint events, 17.9% overall versus 22.4% for the angiographically guided PCI group. The FAME study demonstrated that routine FFR assessment in patients with multivessel disease results in lower rates of stent use, and significantly reduces the composite endpoint of death, MI, and revascularization. In the lesions with FFR >0.80, deferral

of PCI appeared safe, resulting in a 2-year rate of MI of 0.2% and revascularization of 3.2% (19).

Both DEFER and FAME firmly establish the concept that stenoses that do not provoke ischemia may be safely treated with medications alone, and that a strategy of ischemia-guided PCI results in less stent use, and lower rates of death, MI, and revascularization (87). The FAME II trial examined whether FFR-guided PCI in addition to OMT would be superior to medical therapy alone (85). The study, which was halted prematurely by the data safety and monitoring board, had enrolled 1,220 patients with stable CAD and at least one coronary stenosis >50%. All patients received PCI using modern second-generation DES. The primary endpoint was a composite of death, MI, and unplanned hospitalization for revascularization. The study was halted early, because at less than 1-year of follow-up, FFR-guided PCI resulted in significantly fewer readmissions for urgent revascularization. At the time of termination, 4.3% of patients in the PCI plus OMT reached the primary endpoint compared with 12.7% for OMT alone. In patients with stable CAD and at least one functional significant lesion identified by FFR, PCI with DESs plus OMT decreased the rate of urgent revascularization as compared with best medical therapy alone. Patients with functionally nonsignificant lesions are best treated with OMT, regardless of the angiographic severity of the lesion. The findings of this study make a compelling argument for a hybrid strategy of OMT plus FFR-guided revascularization for patients with stable CAD and/or SMI. FAME 3 is a multicenter, randomized controlled trial that aims to compare FFR-guided PCI with new-generation DESs to CABG in patients with three-vessel CAD (88).

In a similar fashion, Park et al. reported the outcomes of a large >5,000-patient registry of stable CAD patients, comparing patients with an abnormal perfusion study with those with no perfusion study prior to PCI with DESs (86). In follow-up, the ischemia-guided cohort of 2,259 patients suffered the composite endpoint of death, MI, stroke, or revascularization in 17.4% of patients compared with the higher rate of 22.8% of patients in nonischemic-guided revascularization. This reduction in the primary endpoint in patients with ischemia-guided revascularization was primarily driven by a 34% reduction in urgent revascularizations. This further supports the concept of selective PCI for only those patients with an ischemia-causing stenosis.

By tailoring PCI to those lesions proven to be ischemia-invoking, the iatrogenic complications of PCI of nonsignificant stenoses are avoided. This includes vessel injury from guiding catheter or guide wire, vessel dissection, guide-wire perforation, restenosis, stent thrombosis, with no impact on overall mortality or future risk of cardiovascular events (see Fig. 16.2). This growing body of evidence supports the concept of functionally guided PCI revascularization of ischemic lesions in combination with OMT for stable CAD.

CONCLUSION

Stable CAD and SMI are common manifestations of coronary heart disease and are associated with substantial morbidity and mortality. The optimal management of patients with stable CAD and/or silent ischemia includes the introduction, titration, and adherence to combination medical therapy targeted to risk factor modification, lifestyle modification, secondary preventative medications, and antianginal medications. In patients with persistent symptoms or significant residual ischemia, revascularization is indicated. The use of FFR in an ischemia-guided approach to coronary revascularization, in combination with OMT, results in the best outcomes for patients with stable CAD.

TABLE 16.5 Benefit of Ischemia-Guided Revascularization with PCI and the Safety of Deferral of PCI in Non-Ischemia-Inducing Lesions

STUDY	YEAR	NUMBER OF PATIENTS	STUDY GROUPS	INCLUSION CRITERIA	EXCLUSION CRITERIA	PRIMARY EP	SECONDARY EP
DEFER	2007	325	FFR < 0.75–144 patients (reference group); FFR > 0.75 Deferred group (91 patients); FFR > 0.75 PCI performed group (90 patients)	>50% stenosis in epicardial coronary >2.5 mm in diameter; negative MPS within 2 months	Total occlusion; acute Q wave MI; unstable angina; vessel <2.5 mm in diameter	Freedom from CV events at 2 years; CV events, all-cause death, MI, CABG, PCI	Cardiac death; 5 year outcomes; CCS class change; antianginal medication use
FAME I	2009	1,005	Angio-guided PCI of all lesions; FFR-guided PCI of only lesions with FFR<0.8	MV CAD with stenosis >50% in at least 2 of 3 vessels; prior PCI; STEMI >5 days after event; NSTEMI <5 days if peak CK <1,000	LMD; prior CABG; cardiogenic shock; excessive tortuosity or calcified lesions; life expectancy <5 years; pregnancy; C/I to DES use	Composite of death, MI, revasc. at 1 year	Death; MI; Revasc; contrast volume use; CCS class; QoL score; antianginal medication use
FAME I	2010	1,005	Angio-guided PCI of all lesions; FFR-guided PCI of only lesions with FFR<0.8	MV CAD with stenosis >50% in at least two of three vessels; prior PCI; STEMI >5 days after event; NSTEMI <5 days if peak CK <1,000	LMD; prior CABG; cardiogenic shock; excessive tortuosity or calcified lesions; life expectancy <5 years; pregnancy; C/I to DES use	Composite of death, MI, revasc. at 2 year follow-up	Death; MI; revasc.; contrast volume use; CCS class; QoL score; antianginal medication use
FAME II	2012	1,220 when terminated; 888 patients with at least one lesion with FFR <0.8 randomized to OMT vs. OMT plus PCI; 332 enrolled in registry of patients with FFR >0.8	Stable CAD patients with FFR<0.8 randomized to OMT vs. FFR-guided PCI; FFR >0.8 treated with OMT and enrolled in registry	At least one stenosis with FFR <0.8;	LMD; prior CABG; cardiogenic shock; excessive tortuosity or calcified lesions; life expectancy <5 years; pregnancy; C/I to DES use	Composite EP of death, MI, and unplanned hospitalization for urgent revascularization in first 2 years	Death; MI; revascularization; CCS class; antianginal medication use; QoL
SJ Park JACC	2012	5,340	2,259 patients with MPS imaging within 1 year—used to define ischemia-guided revasc. group and non-ischemia-guided revasc. group.	All-comers	STEMI; cardiogenic shock	Composite MACCE—death, MI, CVA, revasc	Death; MI; CVA; revascularization

TABLE 16.5 Benefit of Ischemia-Guided Revascularization with PCI and the Safety of Deferral of PCI in Non-Ischemia-Inducing Lesions (*continued*)

PCI TYPE	FOLLOW-UP DURATION (YEAR)	PRIMARY EP%	DEATH%	MYOCARDIAL INFARCTION%	REVASCULARIZATION%	FREEDOM FROM ANGINA%	CONCLUSION
N/A	5 years	Defer group 23%; perform group 30%; reference group 27%	Defer 6.6%; perform 5.7%; reference 9%	Defer 0%; perform 5.5%; reference 9.7%	Defer 16.7%; perform 20.4%; reference 33.5%	Defer 67%; perform 57%; reference 72%	Risk of death or MI from non-ischemic lesion is very low and not altered by stenting; the most important prognostic factor for death or MI is ischemia demonstrated by FFR <0.75
96.9% DES use	1 year	Angio-guided 18.3% vs. FFR-guided 13.2%	Angio-guided 3% vs. FFR-guided 1.8%	Angio-guided 8.7% vs. FFR-guided 5.7%	Angio-guided 9.5% vs. FFR-guided 6.5%	Angio-guided 77.9% vs. FFR-guided 81.3%	Routine FFR assessment in patients with MV disease results in less stent use and significantly reduces the composite endpoint of death, MI, and revascularization
96.9% DES use	2 year	Angio-guided 22.4% vs. FFR-guided 17.9%	Angio-guided 3.8% vs. FFR-guided 2.6%	Angio-guided 9.9% vs. FFR-guided 6.1%	Angio-guided 12.7% vs. FFR-guided 10.6%	Angio-guided 76% vs. FFR-guided 80%	Routine FFR assessment in patients with MV disease results in less stent use and significantly reduces the composite endpoint of death, MI, and revascularization; for lesions deferred with FFR >0.8, 2-year rate of MI was 0.2% and revasc. 3.2%, indicated that deferral of intervention for non-ischemic lesions is safe
100% DES	1 year results	4.3% PCI plus OMT vs. 12.7% OMT alone; 3% in registry of nonsignificant lesions	0.2% PCI plus OMT vs. 0.7% OMT alone; 0 deaths in registry patients	3.4% PCI plus OMT vs. 3.2% OMT alone; 1.8% in registry patients	Any revascularization 3.1% PCI plus OMT vs. 19.5% for OMT alone; 3.6% in registry; non-urgent revascularization 1.6% PCI plus OMT vs. 8.6% OMT alone; 1.2% in registry	97.6% PCI plus OMT freedom from CCS II-IV angina at 1 year, 83.8% OMT alone; 85.8% in registry patients	In patients with stable CAD and at least one functional significant lesion identified by FFR, PCI with drug-eluting stents plus OMT as compared to best medical therapy alone decreased the rate of urgent revascularization. Patients with functionally nonsignificant lesions are best treated with optimal medical therapy, regardless of the angiographic severity of the lesion.
100% DES	5 year	Ischemia-guided PCI revasc. 17.4% vs. non-ischemia-guided PCI 22.8%	Ischemia-guided PCI death 6.4% vs. non-ischemia-guided PCI death 7.4%	Ischemia-guided PCI MI 0.9% vs. non–ischemia-guided PCI MI 1.2%	Ischemia-guided PCI revasc. 9.9% vs. non-ischemia-guided PCI revasc. 14.8%	N/A	Ischemia-guided revascularization by either PCI or CABG results in an overall 27% reduction in MACCE, driven largely by a 34% reduction in future revascularizations compared to non-ischemia-guided revascularization

ACS, acute coronary syndrome; BMS, bare-metal stent; CABG, coronary artery bypass grafting; CAD, coronary artery disease; CCS, Canadian Cardiovascular Society; CHF, congestive heart failure; CKD, chronic kidney disease; CP, chest pain; CTO, chronic total occlusion; CVA, cerebrovascular accident; DES, drug-eluting stent; EF, ejection fraction; EP, endpoint; FFR, fractional flow reserve; IRA, infarct-related artery; LMD, left main disease; LV, left ventricle; MI, myocardial infarction; N/A, not available; OMT, optimal medical therapy; PCI, percutaneous coronary intervention; PTCA, percutaneous transluminal coronary angioplasty; rehosp., rehospitalization; Revasc., revascularization; VT, ventricular tachycardia.

■ CAD represents the greatest cause of adult mortality in the United States, and affects over 17 million Americans, of whom 10 million suffer from chronic stable angina.

■ Episodes of SMI occur more commonly than symptomatic episodes, and are associated with worse prognoses.

■ Intensive lifestyle and risk-factor modification, combined with pharmacotherapy for secondary prevention and angina reduction, comprise the central focus of OMT for stable CAD.

■ PCSK9 inhibitors are novel non-statin agents that can dramatically lower LDL to levels well below conventional LDL targets.

■ The role of interventional therapy with PCI remains controversial in the management of patients with chronic stable angina and/or SMI.

■ The COURAGE trial concluded that PCI improves anginal symptoms in the short and medium term, but does not reduce mortality or future nonfatal MI compared with OMT in patients with chronic stable angina.

■ In addition to OMT, the use of FFR to target for PCI only the hemodynamically significant, ischemia-causing coronary lesions results in improvements in angina, reductions in urgent future PCI, and avoidance of potential complications associated with the treatment of nonsignificant coronary artery lesions, as published in the FAME I and FAME II trial.

■ The 8,000-patient, NIH-sponsored International Study of Co-operative Health Effectiveness with Medical and Invasive Approaches (ISCHEMIA) is enrolling patients with stable ischemic heart disease and at least moderate ischemia and randomizing to OMT versus cardiac catheterization with revascularization and OMT, and will provide further insight into the optimal management strategy for patients with stable coronary ischemia.

References

1. Simoons ML, Windecker S. Controversies in cardiovascular medicine: chronic stable coronary artery disease: drugs vs. revascularization. *Eur Heart J.* 2010;31(5):530–541. doi:10.1093/eurheartj/ehp605.
2. World Health Organization. *Cardiovascular Diseases Fact Sheet.* Geneva, Switzerland: World Health Organization. http://www.who.int/mediacentre/factsheets/fs317/en/. Updated May 2017.
3. Ford ES, et al. Explaining the decrease in U.S. deaths from coronary disease, 1980–2000. *N Engl J Med.* 2007;356(23):2388–2398. doi:10.1056/NEJMsa053935.
4. Falk E, Shah PK, Fuster V. Coronary plaque disruption. *Circulation.* 1995;92(3):657–671.
5. Fuster V, et al. The pathogenesis of coronary artery disease and the acute coronary syndromes (2). *N Engl J Med.* 1992;326(5):310–318. doi:10.1056/NEJM199201303260506.
6. Opie LH, Commerford PJ, Gersh BJ. Controversies in stable coronary artery disease. *Lancet.* 2006;367(9504):69–78. doi:1016/S0140-6736(06)67927-0.
7. Anderson JL, et al. ACC/AHA 2007 guidelines for the management of patients with unstable angina/non-ST-elevation myocardial infarction: a report of the American College of Cardiology/American Heart Association Task Force on Practice Guidelines (writing committee to revise the 2002 guidelines for the management of patients with unstable angina/non-ST-elevation myocardial infarction) developed in collaboration with the American College of Emergency Physicians, the Society for Cardiovascular Angiography and Interventions, and the Society of Thoracic Surgeons endorsed by the American Association of Cardiovascular and Pulmonary Rehabilitation and the Society for Academic Emergency Medicine. *J Am Coll Cardiol.* 2007;50(7):e1–e157. doi:10.1016/j.jacc.2007.02.013.
8. Kushner FG, et al. 2009 focused updates: ACC/AHA guidelines for the management of patients with ST-elevation myocardial infarction (updating the 2004 guideline and 2007 focused update) and ACC/AHA/SCAI guidelines on percutaneous coronary intervention (updating the 2005 guideline and 2007 focused update): a report of the American College of Cardiology Foundation/American Heart Association Task Force on Practice Guidelines. *Circulation.* 2009;120(22):2271–2306. doi:10.1161/CIRCULATIONAHA.109.192663.
9. Patel MR, et al. ACCF/SCAI/STS/AATS/AHA/ASNC 2009 appropriateness criteria for coronary revascularization: a report by the American college of Cardiology Foundation Appropriateness Criteria Task Force, Society for Cardiovascular Angiography and Interventions, Society of Thoracic Surgeons, American Association for Thoracic Surgery, American Heart Association, and the American Society of Nuclear Cardiology endorsed by the American Society of Echocardiography, the Heart Failure Society of America, and the Society of Cardiovascular Computed Tomography. *J Am Coll Cardiol.* 2009;53(6):530–553. doi:10.1016/j.jacc.2008.10.005.
10. Fihn SD, et al. 2012 ACCF/AHA/ACP/AATS/PCNA/SCAI/STS guideline for the diagnosis and management of patients with stable ischemic heart disease: a report of the American College of Cardiology Foundation/American Heart Association Task Force on Practice Guidelines, and the American College of Physicians, American Association for Thoracic Surgery, Preventive Cardiovascular Nurses Association, Society for Cardiovascular Angiography and Interventions, and Society of Thoracic Surgeons. *J Am Coll Cardiol.* 2012;60:e44–e164.
11. Borden WB, et al. Patterns and intensity of medical therapy in patients undergoing percutaneous coronary intervention. *JAMA.* 2011;305(18):1882–1889. doi:10.1001/jama.2011.601.
12. Lin GA, et al. Frequency of stress testing to document ischemia prior to elective percutaneous coronary intervention. *JAMA.* 2008;300(15):1765–1773. doi:10.1001/jama.300.15.1765.
13. Lin GA, Redberg RF. Use of stress testing prior to percutaneous coronary intervention in patients with stable coronary artery disease. *Expert Rev Cardiovasc Ther.* 2009;7(9):1061–1066. doi:10.1586/erc.09.94.
14. Pursnani S, et al. Percutaneous coronary intervention versus optimal medical therapy in stable coronary artery disease: a systematic review and meta-analysis of randomized clinical trials. *Circ Cardiovasc Interv.* 2012;5(4):476–490. doi:10.1161/CIRCINTERVENTIONS.112.970954.
15. Katritsis DG, Meier B. Percutaneous coronary intervention for stable coronary artery disease. *J Am Coll Cardiol.* 2008;52(11):889–893. doi:10.1016/j.jacc.2008.05.048.
16. Stergiopoulos K, Brown DL. Initial coronary stent implantation with medical therapy vs medical therapy alone for stable coronary artery disease: meta-analysis of randomized controlled trials. *Arch Intern Med.* 2012;172(4):312–319. doi:10.1001/archinternmed.2011.1484.
17. Pijls NH, Sels JW. Functional measurement of coronary stenosis. *J Am Coll Cardiol.* 2012;59(12):1045–1057. doi:10.1016/j.jacc.2011.09.077.
18. Pijls NH, et al. Percutaneous coronary intervention of functionally nonsignificant stenosis: 5-year follow-up of the DEFER study. *J Am Coll Cardiol.* 2007;49(21):2105–2111. doi:10.1016/j.jacc.2007.01.087.
19. Pijls NH, et al. Fractional flow reserve versus angiography for guiding percutaneous coronary intervention in patients with multivessel coronary artery disease: 2-year follow-up of the FAME (fractional flow reserve versus angiography for multivessel evaluation) study. *J Am Coll Cardiol.* 2010;56(3):177–184. doi:10.1016/j.jacc.2010.04.012.
20. Steg PG, et al. Prevalence of anginal symptoms and myocardial ischemia and their effect on clinical outcomes in outpatients with stable coronary artery disease: data from the International Observational CLARIFY Registry. *JAMA Intern Med.* 2014;174:1651–1659.
21. Schang SJ Jr, Pepine CJ. Transient asymptomatic S-T segment depression during daily activity. *Am J Cardiol.* 1977;39(3):396–402.

22. Cohn PF, Fox KM, Daly C. Silent myocardial ischemia. *Circulation.* 2003;108(10):1263–1277. doi:10.1161/01.CIR.0000088001.59265.EE.

23. Cohen JD. Abnormal electrocardiograms and cardiovascular risk: role of silent myocardial ischemia. Evidence from MRFIT. *Am J Cardiol.* 1992;70(16):14F–18F.

24. Conti CR, Bavry AA, Petersen JW. Silent ischemia: clinical relevance. *J Am Coll Cardiol.* 2012;59(5):435–441. doi:10.1016/j.jacc.2011.07.050.

25. Thaulow E, et al. Initial clinical presentation of cardiac disease in asymptomatic men with silent myocardial ischemia and angiographically documented coronary artery disease (the Oslo ischemia study). *Am J Cardiol.* 1993;72(9):629–633.

26. Kral BG, et al. Silent myocardial ischaemia and long-term coronary artery disease outcomes in apparently healthy people from families with early-onset ischaemic heart disease. *Eur Heart J.* 2011;32(22):2766–2772. doi:10.1093/eurheartj/ehr261.

27. Stramba-Badiale M, et al. Prevalence of episodes of ST-segment depression among mild-to-moderate hypertensive patients in northern Italy: the cardioscreening study. *J Hypertens.* 1998;16(5):681–688.

28. Milan study on atherosclerosis and diabetes (MiSAD) group. Prevalence of unrecognized silent myocardial ischemia and its association with atherosclerotic risk factors in noninsulin-dependent diabetes mellitus. *Am J Cardiol.* 1997;79(2):134–139.

29. Deedwania PC, Carbajal EV. Exercise test predictors of ambulatory silent ischemia during daily life in stable angina pectoris. *Am J Cardiol.* 1990;66(17):1151–1156.

30. Deedwania PC, Carbajal EV. Prevalence and patterns of silent myocardial ischemia during daily life in stable angina patients receiving conventional antianginal drug therapy. *Am J Cardiol.* 1990;65(16):1090–1096.

31. Deedwania PC, Carbajal EV. Silent ischemia during daily life is an independent predictor of mortality in stable angina. *Circulation.* 1990;81(3):748–756.

32. Deedwania PC, Nelson JR. Pathophysiology of silent myocardial ischemia during daily life. Hemodynamic evaluation by simultaneous electrocardiographic and blood pressure monitoring. *Circulation.* 1990;82(4):1296–1304.

33. Multiple risk factor intervention trial research group. Risk factor changes and mortality results. Multiple risk factor intervention trial research group. *JAMA.* 1982;248(12):1465–1477.

34. Gordon DJ, et al. Coronary risk factors and exercise test performance in asymptomatic hypercholesterolemic men: application of proportional hazards analysis. *Am J Epidemiol.* 1984;120(2):210–224.

35. Davies RF, et al. Asymptomatic cardiac ischemia pilot (ACIP) study two-year follow-up: outcomes of patients randomized to initial strategies of medical therapy versus revascularization. *Circulation.* 1997;95(8):2037–2043.

36. Weiner DA, et al. Prevalence and prognostic significance of silent and symptomatic ischemia after coronary bypass surgery: a report from the coronary artery surgery study (CASS) randomized population. *J Am Coll Cardiol.* 1991;18(2):343–348.

37. Shaw LJ, Iskandrian AE. Prognostic value of gated myocardial perfusion SPECT. *J Nucl Cardiol.* 2004;11(2):171–185. doi:10.1016/j.nuclcard.2003.12.004.

38. Metz LD, et al. The prognostic value of normal exercise myocardial perfusion imaging and exercise echocardiography: a meta-analysis. *J Am Coll Cardiol.* 2007;49(2):227–237. doi:10.1016/j.jacc.2006.08.048.

39. Yazdani S, et al. Percutaneous interventions alter the hemostatic profile of patients with unstable versus stable angina. *J Am Coll Cardiol.* 1997;30(5):1284–1287.

40. Worthley SG, et al. Arterial remodeling correlates positively with serological evidence of inflammation in patients with chronic stable angina pectoris. *J Invasive Cardiol.* 2006;18(1):28–31.

41. Fox KM. European trial on reduction of cardiac events with perindopril in stable coronary artery disease investigators. Efficacy of perindopril in reduction of cardiovascular events among patients with stable coronary artery disease: randomised, double-blind, placebo-controlled, multicentre trial (the EUROPA study). *Lancet.* 2003;362(9386):782–788.

42. Stone NJ, et al. 2013 ACC/AHA guideline on the treatment of blood cholesterol to reduce atherosclerotic cardiovascular risk in adults: a report of the American College of Cardiology/American Heart Association. *J Am Coll Cardiol.* 2013. Article. Circulation 2013.

43. Eid F, Boden WE. The evolving role of medical therapy for chronic stable angina. *Curr Cardiol Rep.* 2008;10(4):263–271.

44. Writing Committee, et al. 2016 ACC expert consensus decision pathway on the role of non-statin therapies for LDL-cholesterol lowering in the management of atherosclerotic cardiovascular disease risk: a report of the American College of Cardiology Task Force on Clinical Expert Consensus Documents. *J Am Coll Cardiol.* 2016;68:92–125.

45. Sabatine MS, et al. Evolocumab and clinical outcomes in patients with cardiovascular disease. *N Engl J Med.* 2017;376:1713–1722.

46. The SPRINT Research Group. A randomized trial of intensive versus standard blood-pressure control. *N Engl J Med.* 2015;373:2103–2116.

47. Hannan EL, et al. Comparative outcomes for patients who do and do not undergo percutaneous coronary intervention for stable coronary artery disease in New York. *Circulation.* 2012;125(15):1870–1879. doi:10.1161/CIRCULATIONAHA.111.071811.

48. Boden WE. Weighing the evidence for decision making about percutaneous coronary intervention in patients with stable coronary artery disease. *Circulation.* 2012;125(15):1827–1831. doi:10.1161/CIRCULATIONAHA.112.100669.

49. Blankenship JC, et al. Effect of percutaneous coronary intervention on quality of life: a consensus statement from the society for cardiovascular angiography and interventions. *Catheter Cardiovasc Interv.* 2013;81(2):243–259. doi:10.1002/ccd.24376.

50. Boden WE, et al. Optimal medical therapy with or without PCI for stable coronary disease. *N Engl J Med.* 2007;356(15):1503–1516. doi:10.1056/NEJMoa070829.

51. Boden WE, et al. Impact of optimal medical therapy with or without percutaneous coronary intervention on long-term cardiovascular end points in patients with stable coronary artery disease (from the COURAGE trial). *Am J Cardiol.* 2009;104(1):1–4. doi:10.1016/j.amjcard.2009.02.059.

52. Erne P, et al. Effects of percutaneous coronary interventions in silent ischemia after myocardial infarction: the SWISSI II randomized controlled trial. *JAMA.* 2007;297(18):1985–1991. doi:10.1001/jama.297.18.1985.

53. Shaw LJ, et al. Gated myocardial perfusion single photon emission computed tomography in the clinical outcomes utilizing revascularization and aggressive drug evaluation (COURAGE) trial, Veterans Administration Cooperative Study no. 424. *J Nucl Cardiol.* 2006;13(5):685–698. doi:10.1016/j.nuclcard.2006.06.134.

54. Shaw LJ, et al. Optimal medical therapy with or without percutaneous coronary intervention to reduce ischemic burden: results from the clinical outcomes utilizing revascularization and aggressive drug evaluation (COURAGE) trial nuclear substudy. *Circulation.* 2008;117(10):1283–1291. doi:10.1161/CIRCULATIONAHA.107.743963.

55. Hachamovitch R, et al. Comparison of the short-term survival benefit associated with revascularization compared with medical therapy in patients with no prior coronary artery disease undergoing stress myocardial perfusion single photon emission computed tomography. *Circulation.* 2003;107(23):2900–2907. doi:10.1161/01.CIR.0000072790.23090.41.

56. Allman KC, et al. Myocardial viability testing and impact of revascularization on prognosis in patients with coronary artery disease and left ventricular dysfunction: a meta-analysis. *J Am Coll Cardiol.* 2002;39(7):1151–1158.

57. Dzavik V, et al. Long-term survival in 11,661 patients with multivessel coronary artery disease in the era of stenting: a report from the Alberta Provincial Project for Outcome Assessment in Coronary Heart Disease (APPROACH) investigators. *Am Heart J.* 2001;142(1):119–126. doi:10.1067/mhj.2001.116072.

58. Fearon WF, et al. Rationale and design of the Fractional Flow Reserve versus Angiography for Multivessel Evaluation (FAME) study. *Am Heart J.* 2007;154(4):632–636. doi:10.1016/j.ahj.2007.06.012.

59. Heyndrickx GR. Is functional assessment necessary in patients with stable angina? *EuroIntervention.* 2010;6(suppl G):G101–G106. doi:10.4244/; 10.4244/.

60. Tonino PA, et al. Angiographic versus functional severity of coronary artery stenoses in the FAME study fractional flow reserve versus angiography in multivessel evaluation. *J Am Coll Cardiol.* 2010;55(25):2816–2821. doi:10.1016/j.jacc.2009.11.096.

61. Tonino PA, et al. Fractional flow reserve versus angiography for guiding percutaneous coronary intervention. *N Engl J Med.* 2009;360(3):213–224. doi:10.1056/NEJMoa0807611.

62. Peduzzi P, Kamina A, Detre K. Twenty-two-year follow-up in the VA cooperative study of coronary artery bypass surgery for stable angina. *Am J Cardiol.* 1998;81(12):1393–1399.

63. Hartigan PM, et al. Two- to three-year follow-up of patients with single-vessel coronary artery disease randomized to PTCA or medical therapy (results of a VA cooperative study). Veterans affairs cooperative studies program ACME investigators. Angioplasty compared to medicine. *Am J Cardiol*. 1998;82(12):1445–1450.

64. Parisi AF, Folland ED, Hartigan P. A comparison of angioplasty with medical therapy in the treatment of single-vessel coronary artery disease. Veterans affairs ACME investigators. *N Engl J Med*. 1992;326(1):10–16. doi:10.1056/NEJM199201023260102.

65. Folland ED, Hartigan PM, Parisi AF. Percutaneous transluminal coronary angioplasty versus medical therapy for stable angina pectoris: outcomes for patients with double-vessel versus single-vessel coronary artery disease in a veterans affairs cooperative randomized trial. Veterans affairs ACME investigators. *J Am Coll Cardiol*. 1997;29(7):1505–1511.

66. Madsen JK, et al. Danish multicenter randomized study of invasive versus conservative treatment in patients with inducible ischemia after thrombolysis in acute myocardial infarction (DANAMI). Danish trial in acute myocardial infarction. *Circulation*. 1997;96(3):748–755.

67. Henderson RA, et al. Seven-year outcome in the RITA-2 trial: coronary angioplasty versus medical therapy. *J Am Coll Cardiol*. 2003;42(7):1161–1170.

68. Pocock S. Coronary angioplasty versus medical therapy for angina: the second randomised intervention treatment of angina (RITA-2) trial. RITA-2 trial participants. *Lancet*. 1997;350(9076):461–468.

69. Pitt B, et al. Aggressive lipid-lowering therapy compared with angioplasty in stable coronary artery disease. Atorvastatin versus revascularization treatment investigators. *N Engl J Med*. 1999;341(2):70–76. doi:10.1056/NEJM199907083410202.

70. Hueb WA, et al. The medicine, angioplasty or surgery study (MASS): a prospective, randomized trial of medical therapy, balloon angioplasty or bypass surgery for single proximal left anterior descending artery stenoses. *J Am Coll Cardiol*. 1995;26(7):1600–1605. doi:10.1016/0735-1097(95)00384-3.

71. TIME investigators. Trial of invasive versus medical therapy in elderly patients with chronic symptomatic coronary-artery disease (TIME): a randomised trial. *Lancet*. 2001;358(9286):951–957. doi:10.1016/S0140-6736(01)06100-1.

72. Yousef ZR, et al. Late intervention after anterior myocardial infarction: effects on left ventricular size, function, quality of life, and exercise tolerance: results of the open artery trial (TOAT study). *J Am Coll Cardiol*. 2002;40(5):869–876.

73. Zeymer U, et al. Randomized comparison of percutaneous transluminal coronary angioplasty and medical therapy in stable survivors of acute myocardial infarction with single vessel disease: a study of the arbeitsgemeinschaft leitende kardiologische krankenhausarzte. *Circulation*. 2003;108(11):1324–1328. doi:10.1161/01.CIR.0000087605.09362.0E.

74. Pereira AC, et al. Clinical judgment and treatment options in stable multivessel coronary artery disease: results from the one-year follow-up of the MASS II (medicine, angioplasty, or surgery study II). *J Am Coll Cardiol*. 2006;48(5):948–953. doi:10.1016/j.jacc.2005.11.094.

75. Hochman JS, et al. Coronary intervention for persistent occlusion after myocardial infarction. *N Engl J Med*. 2006;355(23):2395–2407. doi:10.1056/NEJMoa066139.

76. Hochman JS, et al. Long-term effects of percutaneous coronary intervention of the totally occluded infarct-related artery in the subacute phase after myocardial infarction. *Circulation*. 2011;124(21):2320–2328. doi:10.1161/CIRCULATIONAHA.111.041749.

77. Mahmarian JJ, et al. An initial strategy of intensive medical therapy is comparable to that of coronary revascularization for suppression of scintigraphic ischemia in high-risk but stable survivors of acute myocardial infarction. *J Am Coll Cardiol*. 2006;48(12):2458–2467. doi:10.1016/j.jacc.2006.07.068.

78. Nishigaki K, et al. Percutaneous coronary intervention plus medical therapy reduces the incidence of acute coronary syndrome more effectively than initial medical therapy only among patients with low-risk coronary artery disease a randomized, comparative, multicenter study. *JACC Cardiovasc Interv*. 2008;1(5):469–479. doi:10.1016/j.jcin.2008.08.002.

79. BARI 2D Study Group, et al. A randomized trial of therapies for type 2 diabetes and coronary artery disease. *N Engl J Med*. 2009;360(24):2503–2515. doi:10.1056/NEJMoa0805796.

80. Velazquez EJ, et al. Coronary-artery bypass surgery in patients with left ventricular dysfunction. *N Engl J Med*. 2011;364:1607–1616.

81. Velazquez EJ, et al. Coronary artery bypass surgery in patients with ischemic cardiomyopathy. *N Engl J Med*. 2016;374:1511–1520.

82. Sedlis SP, et al. Effect of PCI on long-term survival in patients with stable ischemic heart disease. *N Engl J Med*. 2015;373:1937–1946.

83. Schomig A, et al. A meta-analysis of 17 randomized trials of a percutaneous coronary intervention-based strategy in patients with stable coronary artery disease. *J Am Coll Cardiol*. 2008;52(11):894–904. doi:10.1016/j.jacc.2008.05.051.

84. Feldman DN, et al. Adoption of radial access and comparison of outcomes to femoral access in percutaneous coronary intervention: an updated report from the National Cardiovascular Data Registry (2007–2012). *Circulation*. 2013;127:2295–2306.

85. Fearon WF, et al. Economic evaluation of fractional flow reserve-guided percutaneous coronary intervention in patients with multivessel disease. *Circulation*. 2010;122(24):2545–2550. doi:10.1161/CIRCULATIONAHA.109.925396.

86. De Bruyne B, et al. Fractional flow reserve-guided PCI versus medical therapy in stable coronary disease. *N Engl J Med*. 2012;367(11):991–1001. doi:10.1056/NEJMoa1205361.

87. Kim YH, et al. Impact of ischemia-guided revascularization with myocardial perfusion imaging for patients with multivessel coronary disease. *J Am Coll Cardiol*. 2012;60(3):181–190. doi:10.1016/j.jacc.2012.02.061.

88. Zimmermann FM, et al. Rationale and design of the Fractional flow reserve versus Angiography for Multivessel Evaluation (FAME) 3 trial: a comparison of fractional flow reserve-guided percutaneous coronary intervention and coronary artery bypass graft surgery in patients with multivessel coronary artery disease. *Am Heart J*. 2015;170:619–626.

17 Acute Coronary Syndromes

Arnold H. Seto, MD, MPA, FSCAI, FACC

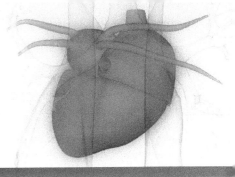

Acute coronary syndromes (ACSs) include unstable angina (UA), non-ST segment elevation myocardial infarction (NSTEMI), and ST-segment elevation myocardial infarction (STEMI) (Fig. 17.1). Patients presenting with chest pain without persistent ST-elevation are typically admitted to the hospital with the diagnosis of non-ST-elevation ACS (NSTE-ACS), and are later classified into UA or NSTEMI on the basis of cardiac biomarkers.

Patients with ACS constitute the vast majority of patients (>80%) who will require percutaneous coronary intervention (PCI). With the publication of the COURAGE trial and increasing scrutiny from payers, the use of PCI for stable angina is increasingly reserved for medically refractory symptoms (1).

EPIDEMIOLOGY

In the US, there are at least 625,000 hospital admissions for ACS annually. UA/NSTEMI patients constitute approximately 66% to 77% of the total. The incidence of STEMI has decreased significantly in the past decade, likely due to decreased smoking rates and improved medical therapy (esp. statins) (2).

The acute in-hospital mortality of STEMI (7%) is higher than for NSTE-ACS (3%–5%), but equalizes by 6 months. Longer-term follow-up demonstrates that NSTE-ACS has a higher mortality than STEMI. This is explained by different patient profiles: NSTE-ACS patients, on average, tend to be older and have more comorbidities, such as diabetes and renal failure, whereas STEMI patients tend to be younger smokers.

PATHOLOGY

ACSs result from coronary artery obstruction causing myocardial ischemia and subsequent myocardial necrosis. Acute coronary artery obstruction typically results from thrombosis of a ruptured coronary plaque, with or without concomitant vasoconstriction. In contrast to the previous conception that coronary artery disease (CAD) is a slowly progressive disease, the current understanding (see Chapter 1) is that of a stuttering inflammatory process of repeated plaque rupture and healing on top of a lipid core. Abrupt thrombotic occlusion can thus occur with plaques that are not obstructive at baseline, although plaques that are already obstructive are more likely to be metabolically active and lead to clinical syndromes.

Coronary thrombosis involves endothelial dysfunction and disruption, platelet activation, and circulating coagulation proteins. The platelet is a central actor and regulates the process of thrombosis (see

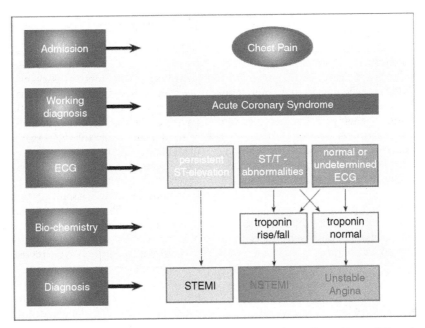

FIGURE 17.1 Spectrum of ACS. ACS, acute coronary syndrome (From: Hamm CW, et al. ESC guidelines for the management of acute coronary syndromes in patients presenting without persistent ST-segment elevation: the task force for the management of acute coronary syndromes (ACS) in patients presenting without persistent ST-segment elevation of the European Society of Cardiology (ESC). *Eur Heart J.* 2011;32:2999–3054.)

Chapter 3). When endothelial cells are injured, thrombosis begins with rapid adhesion of platelets to the site of injury. Within seconds, the platelets are activated, degranulate, and recruit additional platelets to the developing thrombus. The secretory granules release adenosine diphosphate (ADP) which stimulates further platelet activation, and thrombin, which initiates the coagulation system. Thromboxane is generated from the platelet phospholipase A2, and has an additional effect on platelet activation. Ultimately, glycoprotein IIb/IIIa receptors on the platelet are activated. Glycoprotein IIb/IIIa receptors bind to fibrinogen, cross-linking platelets together. Repetitive platelet activation and fibrinogen cross linking brings about platelet aggregation, which can then lead to occlusive thrombus formation. Although there are multiple pathways to platelet activation, the platelet GP IIb/IIIa receptor is the final common pathway in platelet aggregation that would lead to NSTEMI.

When plaque rupture results in complete (100%) thrombotic occlusion and is sustained, the myocardial infarction (MI) that results is typically transmural and associated with ST-segment elevation. Without reperfusion, a transmural infarction classically results in a Q-wave on ECG. With subtotal (99% or less) or temporary occlusion, the presentation may be either UA or NSTEMI, depending upon the degree and duration of ischemia. When ischemia is sufficient to cause myonecrosis detectable by serum biomarkers, NSTEMI is diagnosed. With the use of high-sensitivity troponin assays, patients that would have formerly been categorized as UA (based on negative creatine kinase) are increasingly diagnosed as NSTEMI.

Other less common causes of ACS include spontaneous coronary dissection, spasm (Prinzmetal's angina, cocaine), inflammatory arteritis, trauma, and thromboembolism. These rare causes should be considered in patients lacking coronary artery disease risk factors. For instance, a younger peripartum woman with chest pain and ECG changes may be more likely to have spasm or coronary dissection than atherosclerotic disease.

CLINICAL PRESENTATION

The clinical presentation of ACS classically includes substernal chest discomfort associated with diaphoresis and dyspnea. This sensation may variably be described as pressure or sharp pain depending on the patient. The chest discomfort may radiate to the left arm, but also to the shoulder, neck, or jaw. Relief of chest pain with nitroglycerin, and exacerbation of the chest pain with manual pressure, may point toward a noncardiac cause for chest pain, but these signs are insufficiently reliable for clinical diagnosis.

Atypical presentations occur frequently, particularly among diabetics and women. Dyspnea, epigastric pain, nausea, syncope, or unexplained tachycardia may be the only symptoms to suggest a cardiac pathology.

Physical examination of the ACS patients is often unremarkable. Signs of left ventricular dysfunction (rales, third heart sound, hypotension, jugular venous distention) or cardiogenic shock (cold clammy extremities, tachycardia) may be present in patients with extensive MI or prior injury.

INITIAL DIAGNOSIS

Patients with chest pain require prompt triage and risk assessment in an emergency room. An electrocardiography (ECG) should be immediately performed on presentation. Serial ECGs are recommended for patients with nondiagnostic ECGs or those who continue to be symptomatic. Comparison with prior ECGs can be extremely valuable, particularly in patients with baseline abnormalities such as hypertrophy or early repolarization. ECGs should be reviewed for ST-segment elevation (≥1 mm in two contiguous leads) or new left bundle branch block, which may indicate acute STEMI. Isolated ST-segment depression in right precordial leads (V1–V3) with tall R-waves may indicate a true posterior infarction, which should also be treated as a STEMI. NSTE-ACS may present as ST-segment depression, T-wave inversions, or be electrically silent. Dynamic ST-segment or T-wave changes increase the specificity of the ECG for ACS.

The history, physical, and ECG are sufficient to diagnose ACS in less than half of cases. Cardiac biomarkers should thus be drawn on all patients with suspected ACS. Biomarkers may not be elevated in the first 4 hours after the onset of symptoms, thus serial biomarkers should be drawn at 6- or 8-hour intervals. The preferred cardiac biomarker is the troponin assay (cTnI or cTnT), which has a very high (>95%) sensitivity for myocardial injury. Ultra high-sensitivity (>99%) troponin assays are increasingly becoming available and may reduce the time to diagnosis of ACS (3). Abnormal troponin levels connote an increased risk for major adverse cardiac events and death, with higher concentrations indicating progressively elevated risk (4). The specificity of the cardiac troponin for ACS is reported to be very high (>95%) when used in patients with chest pain. Nevertheless, when used in a broader patient population than that of clinical trials, the test is frequently abnormal for reasons besides ACS, and there may still be a role for less-sensitive (but more specific) markers such as creatine kinase-MB (CK-MB). For instance, following PCI, troponin assays are overly sensitive to clinically silent periprocedural necrosis, and do not carry the same prognostic value as elevations in CK-MB (5).

B-type natriuretic peptide (BNP) is increasingly used as a cardiac biomarker. Elevated levels may reflect either acquired or preexisting left ventricular dysfunction and are associated with an increased risk of complications (4).

IS IT ACS?

Although not typically the subject of board examination questions, the diagnosis of ACS is commonly misapplied clinically. With the use of high-sensitivity troponin assays as the preferred cardiac marker, one of the most common consultations received by the interventional cardiologist is for the positive troponin, which in the absence of chest pain or ECG changes is often due to demand ischemia, heart failure, or renal failure rather than ACS (6). The third universal definition of MI (Table 17.1) includes patients with positive biomarkers with either ischemic symptoms, ECG changes of ischemia or infarction, or echocardiographic evidence of infarction. This definition includes infarctions due to ACS, supply/demand imbalance, sudden cardiac death, PCI complications, or post-CABG (7). The terminology is thus muddled, in that a patient may have a MI without having an ACS, particularly when nondiagnostic symptoms (esp. dyspnea, hypotension) and ECG (T-wave inversions) are present. Changes in the concentration of troponin may be helpful in differentiating acute from chronic causes of myocardial damage, with a rise of 20% typically being used as a criterion for an acute injury, especially in patients with renal failure, heart failure, or left ventricular hypertrophy (8).

Antithrombotic therapies and PCI are beneficial only for patients with primary acute thrombotic coronary events. An incorrect diagnosis will be, at best, a distraction from the underlying illness, and at worst will be a therapeutic misadventure that will result in hemorrhagic or vascular complications. Caution is advisable when symptoms or

TABLE 17.1 Classification of Different Types of Myocardial Infarction

Type 1: Spontaneous Myocardial Infarction

Spontaneous myocardial infarction related to atherosclerotic plaque rupture, ulceration, assuring, erosion, or dissection with resulting intraluminal thrombus in one or more of the coronary arteries leading to decreased myocardial blood flow or distal platelet emboli with ensuing myocyte necrosis. The patient may have underlying severe CAD but on occasion non-obstructive or no CAD.

Type 2: Myocardial Infarction Secondary to an Ischemic Imbalance

In instances of myocardial injury with necrosis where a condition other than CAD contributes to an imbalance between myocardial oxygen supply and/or demand—e.g., coronary endothelial dysfunction, coronary artery spasm, coronary embolism, tachy-/brady-arrhythmias, anemia, respiratory failure, hypotension, and hypertension with or without LVH.

Type 3: Myocardial Infarction Resulting in Death when Biomarker Values are Unavailable

Cardiac death with symptoms suggestive of myocardial ischemia and presumed new ischemic ECG changes or new LBBB, but death occurring before blood samples could be obtained, before cardiac biomarker could rise, or in rare cases where cardiac biomarkers were not collected.

Type 4a: Myocardial Infarction Related to Percutaneous Coronary Intervention (PCI)

Myocardial infarction associated with PCI is arbitrarily defined by elevation of cTn values >5× 99th percentile URL in patients with normal baseline values (<99th percentile URL) or a rise of cTn values >20% if the baseline values are elevated and are stable or falling. In addition, either (i) symptoms suggestive of myocardial ischemia, or (ii) new ischemic ECG changes or new LBBB, or (iii) angiographic loss of patency of a major coronary artery or a side branch or persistent slow- or no-flow or embolization, or (iv) imaging demonstration of new loss of viable myocardium or new regional wall motion abnormality are required.

Type 4b: Myocardial Infarction Related to Stent Thrombosis

Myocardial infarction associated with stent thrombosis is detected by coronary angiography or autopsy in the setting of myocardial ischemia and with a rise and/or fall of cardiac biomarkers values with at least one value above the 99th percentile URL.

Type 5: Myocardial Infarction Related to Coronary Artery Bypass Grafting (CABG)

Myocardial infarction associated with CABG is arbitrarily defined by elevation cardiac biomarker values >10× 99th percentile URL in patients with normal baseline cTn values (<99th percentile URL). In addition, either (i) new pathological Q waves or new LBBB, or (ii) angiographic documented new graft or new native coronary artery occlusion, or (iii) imaging evidence of new loss of viable myocardium or new regional wall motion abnormality.

CAD, coronary artery disease; ECG, electrocardiography; LBBB, left bundle branch block; LVH, left ventricular hypertrophy; URL, upper reference limit.
Adapted from: Thygesen K, et al. Third universal definition of myocardial infarction. *J Am Coll Cardiol.* 2012;60:1581–1598.

ECG evidence of ACS are absent, or when clear alternative causes of troponin elevation are present.

INITIAL MEDICAL MANAGEMENT

ACC/AHA Guidelines for the management of UA/NSTEMI were updated in complete form in 2014 (9). A thorough review of these guidelines is suggested for board preparation.

Anti-ischemic Therapies

Anti-ischemic therapies reduce myocardial oxygen demand or increase myocardial oxygen supply. Recommended anti-ischemic therapies are listed in **Table 17.2**. Nonpharmacologic therapies include bed rest and supplemental oxygen. Nitroglycerin can cause coronary vasodilatation and increase myocardial blood flow. β-blockers and calcium-channel blockers reduce myocardial demand by reducing heart rate, contractility, and afterload. β-blockers should not be administered for patients with shock, heart failure, or heart block. Morphine is reserved for angina refractory to nitroglycerin, but by relieving pain and anxiety this also reduces myocardial oxygen demand.

Risk Stratification

Early risk stratification for ischemic complications is critical to form a management strategy for the heterogeneous NSTE-ACS population. A focused history and physical, a prompt EKG, and cardiac biomarkers (as described previously) will help distinguish UA and NSTEMI from noncardiac chest pain. Patients with a normal EKG and cardiac biomarkers can be safely sent for noninvasive stress testing for further risk assessment.

For those with UA/NSTEMI, risk-stratification models such as the thrombolysis in myocardial infarction (TIMI) or Global Registry of Acute Coronary Events (GRACE) risk score should be used to further identify those patients at high risk for cardiovascular death, recurrent MI, or urgent revascularization (**Fig. 17.2**, **Table 17.3**). The TIMI risk score is simpler to remember, but has a less discriminating power. Patients at low risk for cardiac events (TIMI score <3, GRACE score <108) are candidates for a conservative approach, whereas patients with a moderate or high score are best treated with an invasive approach (see below) (10,11).

TABLE 17.2 Recommended Anti-ischemic Therapies

Class Ia

1. Bed rest with continuous ECG monitoring
2. Supplemental oxygen in patients with respiratory distress or hypoxemia
3. Nitroglycerin for ischemic symptoms, heart failure, or hypertension
4. Oral β-blockers for patients without shock, heart failure, or heart block
5. ACE-inhibitors or angiotensin receptor blockers within 24 hours in patients with left ventricular dysfunction

Class IIa

6. Morphine for chest discomfort refractory to nitroglycerin
7. Intravenous β-blockers for patients without contraindications

ACE, angiotensin converting enzyme; ECG, electrocardiography.

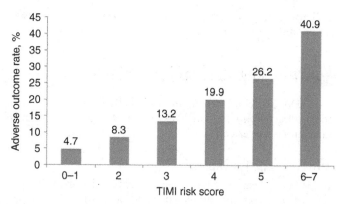

FIGURE 17.2 TIMI risk score in UA/NSTEMI. Adverse outcome: all-cause mortality, new or recurrent MI, or severe recurrent ischemia requiring urgent revascularization through 14 days after randomization, %. TIMI, thrombolysis in myocardial infarction. (Reprinted from: Anderson JL, et al. ACC/AHA 2007 guidelines for the management of patients with unstable angina/non-ST-elevation myocardial infarction: a report of the American College of Cardiology/American Heart Association Task Force on Practice Guidelines (Writing Committee to revise the 2002 guidelines for the management of patients with unstable angina/non-ST-elevation myocardial infarction) developed in collaboration with the American College of Emergency Physicians, the Society for Cardiovascular Angiography and Interventions, and the Society of Thoracic Surgeons endorsed by the American Association of Cardiovascular and Pulmonary Rehabilitation and the Society for Academic Emergency Medicine. *J Am Coll Cardiol.* 2007;50(7):e1–e157, with permission.)

Risk stratification of bleeding risks is recommended to guide the choice of pharmacology, strategy, and access site. Bleeding, especially major bleeding requiring blood transfusion, has been strongly correlated with adverse outcomes in ACS including mortality. The cause of this correlation remains to be determined, but likely includes the need to discontinue beneficial antithrombotic medications when bleeding occurs, along with an overlap of the risks of bleeding with risks of overall mortality. Blood transfusions may themselves exhibit an immunosuppressant effect that leads to complications.

A patient at high risk of bleeding might be more likely to benefit from a strategy of bivalirudin or radial access, or a conservative approach with fondaparinux. Another patient with a large NSTEMI and low bleeding risk might benefit from a triple antiplatelet strategy of aspirin, clopidogrel, and glycoprotein inhibitors.

Multiple scoring systems have been developed, with common risk factors including female gender, advanced age, renal insufficiency, diabetes, shock, baseline anemia, and extremes of weight (12). Most of these have been primarily validated when using femoral access, with potentially less validity when a radial access approach is chosen. All of the risk stratification tools are now readily available online or using portable electronic applications.

EARLY INVASIVE VERSUS CONSERVATIVE APPROACH

Multiple randomized controlled trials have compared a strategy of a routine invasive approach (angiography and revascularization) to a conservative approach (medical management with angiography only for recurrent angina, high-risk stress test findings, or hemodynamic compromise). The preponderance of the evidence favors the

TABLE 17.3 TIMI and GRACE Risk Score Components

TIMI RISK SCORE	
RISK SCORE COMPONENTS	
Age >65	Two anginal events in prior 24 hours
≥3 CAD risk factors	Use of aspirin in prior 7 days
Prior coronary stenosis of >50% ST-segment deviation on presentation	Elevated serum biomarkers

RISK SCORE	RISK OF DEATH, MI, OR URGENT REVASCULARIZATION
0–1	4.7%
2	8.3%
3	13.2%
4	19.9%
5	26.2%
6–7	40.9%

GRACE RISK SCORE	
VARIABLE	**ODDS RATIO**
Older age	1.7/10 year
Killip class	2.0/class
Systolic BP	1.4/20 mm Hg ↑
ST-segment deviation	2.4
Cardiac arrest during presentation	4.3
Serum creatinine level	1.2/1-mg/dL ↑
Positive initial cardiac biomarkers	1.6
Heart rate	1.3/30-beat/min ↑

BP, blood pressure; CAD, coronary artery disease; MI, myocardial infarction; TIMI, thrombolysis in myocardial ischemia.
Adapted from: Eagle KA, et al. A validated prediction model for all forms of acute coronary syndrome: estimating the risk of 6-month postdischarge death in an international registry. *JAMA.* 2004;291:2727–2733.

routine invasive approach for patients at moderate-to-high risk of cardiac complications from ACS, with low-risk patients having less benefit. The most definitive trials have included the FRISC2, TACTICS-TIMI 18, and RITA-3 trials. A meta-analysis of seven trials demonstrated a reduction in all-cause mortality (RR 0.75, 95% CI 0.63–0.90), recurrent MI (RR 0.83, 95% CI 0.72–0.96), and recurrent unstable angina (RR 0.69, 95% CI 0.65–0.74) (Fig. 17.3) with a routine invasive approach compared with a conservative approach (13).

The TIMI and GRACE scores generally stratify patients adequately; nevertheless, other conditions not included in the model place patients at higher risk for cardiac events. Renal insufficiency, diabetes, and left ventricular dysfunction are conditions that would generally lead to favoring routine revascularization over conservative management. Low-risk patients (especially women with negative biomarkers) and those with comorbidities that make them high risk for bleeding complications may be among the few patients where a conservative strategy is superior.

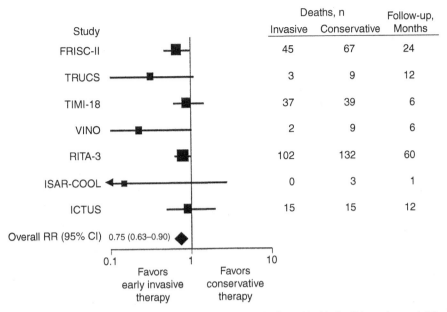

Study	Deaths, n		Follow-up, Months
	Invasive	Conservative	
FRISC-II	45	67	24
TRUCS	3	9	12
TIMI-18	37	39	6
VINO	2	9	6
RITA-3	102	132	60
ISAR-COOL	0	3	1
ICTUS	15	15	12
Overall RR (95% CI)	0.75 (0.63–0.90)		

FIGURE 17.3   Randomized trials of early invasive therapy for ACS. CL, confidence interval; RR, relative risk. (From: Bavry AA, et al. Benefit of early invasive therapy in acute coronary syndromes: a meta-analysis of contemporary randomized clinical trials. *J Am Coll Cardiol.* 2006;48:1319–1325, reprinted with permission from Elsevier.)

TIMING OF PCI

The optimal timing of angiography and PCI has been extensively studied. Patients at high risk— including those with heart failure, refractory angina, and hemodynamic instability—should be taken emergently to the catheterization laboratory for evaluation. Previously, it was suggested that a short period of medical management or "cooling off" of an acute infarction could lead to increased safety for PCI, but no benefit was seen from delaying PCI in the ISAR-COOL trial (14). The large TIMACS (15) trial demonstrated that an early invasive strategy (within the first 24 hours of presentation) compared with a delayed invasive strategy (>36 hours) was associated with a significant reduction in refractory ischemia, and a trend toward MACE reduction (9.6% vs. 11.6%, p = 0.15), particularly in the highest-risk patients. Unlike in acute STEMI, there may be little demonstrable benefit in NSTEMI of immediate revascularization (<2 hours) compared with deferral until the next working day (<24 hours), although a recent trial (RIDDLE-NSTEMI [16]) suggested that immediate revascularization effectively reduced reinfarction during the pre-catheterization period.

CORONARY ARTERY BYPASS SURGERY (CABG)

There have been no randomized trials comparing PCI and CABG specifically in patients with ACS. In general, the preferred revascularization technique is made in a similar fashion as in stable CAD. Nevertheless, where there is a clear thrombotic culprit lesion, PCI may be preferable even in the presence of multivessel CAD. A staged PCI or CABG can subsequently be performed when the patient has stabilized. Alternatively, calculation of the angiographic SYNTAX score can guide whether CABG would be advantageous for the patient. P2Y$_{12}$ inhibitors should be discontinued for 5 days prior to urgent CABG.

The proportion of ACS patients requiring CABG sometime during their initial hospitalization is on the order of 10%, with less than only 2% requiring emergency surgery. Although guidelines recommend preloading of clopidogrel or ticagrelor before PCI for ACS, the benefit of preloading remains debatable and may be limited to clopidogrel due to its slower onset of action. In current clinical practice only 40% of ACS patients are preloaded, primarily due to concerns of delaying bypass surgery when needed (17).

ANTIPLATELET THERAPIES

Aspirin

Aspirin (acetylsalicylic acid) irreversibly binds and inhibits platelet cyclo-oxygenase type 1 (COX-1), inhibiting thromboxane A2 formation for the lifetime of the platelet (7 days). Because it provides relatively weak platelet inhibition, it is considered safe for nearly every patient with potential ACS, often in conjunction with other agents. It should be administered as soon as possible after presentation, and continued indefinitely (Class I recommendation, LOE A). For more rapid absorption, a loading dose of 162 to 325 mg of plain (not enteric-coated) aspirin is recommended to be chewed and swallowed. A subsequent daily dose of 75 to 100 mg was recently shown to be as effective as 325 mg with fewer gastrointestinal reactions (CURRENT-OASIS 7) (18). Aspirin should be continued indefinitely following PCI. Non-steroidal anti-inflammatory drugs such as ibuprofen interfere with the antiplatelet effects of aspirin, have been associated with increased cardiovascular risk, and should be discontinued on hospital admission.

ADP Receptor Antagonists

The oral P2Y$_{12}$ inhibitors ticlopidine, clopidogrel, prasugrel, and ticagrelor inhibit ADP-induced amplification of platelet aggregation. Dual antiplatelet therapy with aspirin and either an ADP-receptor antagonist or a glycoprotein IIb/IIIa inhibitor is recommended for all patients with ACS at medium to high risk or in whom an invasive strategy is planned.

Ticlopidine was the first agent in this class tested in ACS, but was associated with serious hematologic reactions, including agranulocytosis and thrombotic thrombocytopenic purpura (TTP). Although used until recently for patients with allergic reactions to clopidogrel, ticlopidine has no remaining role with the availability of the newer agents prasugrel and ticagrelor.

Clopidogrel

Clopidogrel is a thienopyridine prodrug whose active metabolite irreversibly binds and inhibits the ADP receptor $P2Y_{12}$. It has an onset of action of 2 to 4 hours, with a 600-mg loading dose having more rapid onset than the 300-mg dose and generally preferred. A 75-mg maintenance dose is recommended for 12 months after PCI for ACS.

Clopidogrel is indicated for patients allergic to aspirin, and for most patients as a second antiplatelet agent. Due to its prolonged effect on platelet activity, it should be discontinued for 5 days prior to major surgery, especially cardiac surgery.

The landmark CURE trial demonstrated that a 300-mg dose of clopidogrel, followed by a daily 75-mg dose added to aspirin, reduced the risk of cardiovascular death, MI, or stroke from 11.4% to 9.3% (RR 0.80, $p < 0.001$) in patients with NSTE-ACS. Within the CURE trial, only 20% of patients received PCI (PCI-CURE), but the benefits of clopidogrel were more pronounced in this group (RR 0.70, $p = 0.03$) (19).

Due to its delayed onset of action, clopidogrel should be given on presentation to obtain maximal platelet inhibition at the time of PCI, although this is a subject of debate (as noted earlier).

Clopidogrel requires a two-step hepatic conversion to its active metabolite. Its clinical effect on platelet aggregation is highly variable among individual patients, due in part to variations in the cytochrome P450 system, especially CYP2C19. Patients who are poor metabolizers of clopidogrel are at increased risk for ischemic events, however, and the use of genetic testing to identify and treat such patients has not yet been found to be effective in reducing thrombotic risk.

Clopidogrel and aspirin increase the risk of gastrointestinal bleeding. Although in vivo studies have demonstrated an inhibition of clopidogrel metabolism with omeprazole, this has not been shown to have a clinical effect in the COGENT (20) study, and has not been shown with other agents. Due to the risk of bleeding, patients with prior gastrointestinal bleeding should be treated with a non-omeprazole proton-pump inhibitor.

Prasugrel

Prasugrel is a thienopyridine prodrug whose metabolite irreversibly inhibits the ADP receptor. Similar to clopidogrel, it requires a two-step metabolism, but one step is rapidly mediated by serum esterases. As a result, Prasugrel exhibits a high degree of platelet inhibition regardless of CYP inhibitors or variants. Its onset of action is rapid at 30 minutes, perhaps explaining why the ACCOAST trial demonstrated no benefit to up-front or preloaded prasugrel compared with prasugrel administered following PCI (21). The duration of effect of prasugrel is longer than clopidogrel at 5 to 10 days, and thus should be discontinued 7 days prior to major surgery.

The TRITON-TIMI 38 trial randomized 13,608 patients with ACS (74% NSTE-ACS) to either prasugrel (60-mg loading dose and 10-mg maintenance dose) or clopidogrel (300-mg loading and 75-mg daily). Among patients with NSTE-ACS undergoing PCI, prasugrel was administered only after diagnostic angiography. The primary efficacy endpoint of cardiovascular death, MI, or stroke occurred

in 9.9% of patients on prasugrel versus 12.1% of patients taking clopidogrel (HR 0.81, $p < 0.001$), mainly driven by recurrent MI. Nevertheless, the rate of major bleeding was increased with prasugrel from 1.8% to 2.4% (HR 1.32, $p = 0.03$), including fatal bleeding and CABG-related bleeding. Patients with a history of stroke or transient ischemic attack, patients older than 75 years of age, and patients with low body weight (<60 kg) had a higher risk of bleeding and no net benefit with prasugrel over clopidogrel (22).

Ticagrelor

Ticagrelor is a newer ADP-receptor antagonist called a cyclopentyl triazolo pyrimidine. It binds reversibly to the $P2Y_{12}$ receptor and has a half-life of 12 hours. Ticagrelor requires no metabolism for activity, exhibits a rapid onset of action, and high levels of platelet inhibition. Based on its shorter half-life and reversible inhibition, ticagrelor may be held for as little as 1 to 3 days prior to CABG, although 5 days are still preferred. Given its short half-life, ticagrelor must be administered twice daily. There is up to a 15% rate of dyspnea and an increase in bradycardia with ticagrelor, which may be confusing and complicating symptoms following MI.

The PLATO trial randomized 18,624 patients with ACS (11067 NSTE-ACS) to clopidogrel (300 mg/75 mg) or ticagrelor (180-mg loading with 90-mg twice daily maintenance). Patients receiving PCI were given an additional 300-mg load of clopidogrel, or 90-mg ticagrelor if PCI occurred >24 hours after the initial loading dose. Major adverse cardiovascular events were reduced from 11.7% in the clopidogrel group to 9.8% in the ticagrelor group (HR 0.84, $p < 0.001$). This benefit to ticagrelor appeared to result without any difference in the rates of major bleeding from clopidogrel (11.2% vs. 11.6%, $p = 0.43$). Finally, ticagrelor was found to have an overall mortality benefit compared with clopidogrel (4.7% vs. 9.7% $p < 0.01$) which was driven by reductions in cardiovascular death (23). As a result, ticagrelor has become the oral antiplatelet agent of choice in many laboratories, with the caveat of a higher cost and higher rates of intolerance in some patients.

GLYCOPROTEIN IIb/IIIa INHIBITORS (GP IIb/IIIa)

The intravenous glycoprotein IIb/IIIa inhibitors (GPI) abciximab, eptifibatide, and tirofiban all inhibit the final pathway of platelet aggregation: the binding of the platelet to fibrinogen. These agents exhibit high levels (>90%) of platelet inhibition, causing reduced ischemic complications (~9% relative risk reduction) but also increased risks of bleeding in patients with ACS (24).

The majority of the trials of these agents (EPIC, EPILOG, PURSUIT, PRISM) were conducted prior to the availability of clopidogrel, putting their ischemic benefits in the current era of dual-antiplatelet therapy with aspirin and clopidogrel in question.

The administration and pharmacology of the GPIs are reviewed in Chapter 3. Key points include the risk of thrombocytopenia (0.5%–5.6%) with their use, which may be especially profound with repeated use of the monoclonal antibody abciximab. Eptifibatide and tirofiban have a relatively short half-life of ~2 hours, making CABG safe 6 hours after administration. Abciximab has a prolonged effect of 48 hours, requiring platelet transfusion in the case of excessive bleeding.

GPI have primarily demonstrated a benefit in patients treated with an invasive approach; patients managed conservatively with a dual-antiplatelet regimen of aspirin and clopidogrel may not benefit from the approach. The benefits of GP IIb/IIIa inhibition is highest in those patients with elevated TIMI-risk scores (>4), especially those with positive troponin assays. It is reasonable to delay the administration of GP IIb/IIIa agents until the time of PCI, because the benefit of "upstream" treatment is nearly balanced by an increased risk of bleeding.

The use of GPIs has decreased with the availability of bivalirudin and more potent oral antiplatelet agents. Nevertheless, in those patients who do not receive a loading dose of clopidogrel prior to PCI, there may be inadequate platelet inhibition during stenting, and GP IIb/IIIa inhibition has a Class IIa recommendation. ACS, especially STEMI, is associated with high levels of platelet activation and a delayed onset of action of all of the oral $P2Y_{12}$ inhibitors. This increases the risk of acute stent thrombosis, especially when bivalirudin is used. Intravenous GPIs may effectively "bridge" the patient with dual antiplatelet inhibition until the oral agents take effect, a strategy that has demonstrated benefit with cangrelor.

Cangrelor

Cangrelor is an intravenous (IV), direct-acting ADP inhibitor that is both rapidly acting and rapidly reversible. The plasma half-life of cangrelor is 3 to 5 minutes, and platelet function normalizes within 1 to 2 hours of discontinuation of the drug, which may be useful when coronary anatomy is unknown and pre-treatment with dual antiplatelet therapy has not occurred. Cangrelor was compared against a 600-mg loading dose of clopidogrel given immediately before or after PCI in the recent CHAMPION-PHOENIX trial (25). This demonstrated a reduction in the primary ischemic endpoint (4.7% vs. 5.9%, p = 0.005) with an increase in minor bleeding such as small hematomas.

Cangrelor inhibits binding of clopidogrel and prasugrel metabolites to the $P2Y_{12}$ receptor. The package insert recommends that cangrelor be discontinued prior to administration of clopidogrel or prasugrel, making cangrelor less helpful in bridging to these oral antiplatelet agents. The binding of ticagrelor is unaffected by cangrelor.

Cangrelor was not compared against a strategy of pre-treatment with clopidogrel, or against prasugrel, ticagrelor, or GPIs. With its unique pharmacokinetic properties and safety profile, cangrelor may have a niche role for bridging off of other oral antiplatelet agents or as a safer alternative to GPIs.

ANTITHROMBOTIC THERAPIES

Unfractionated Heparin

Unfractionated heparin (UFH) is a mixture of polysaccharide molecules, one-third of which contain the key pentasaccharide sequence that binds to antithrombin. Antithrombin is then activated to inhibit factor Xa and thrombin. Due to variability in various heparin preparations, and protein binding, monitoring of the anticoagulant effect is necessary, with a goal of an activated partial thromboplastin time (aPTT) of 50 to 75 seconds, or 1.5 to 2.5 the upper limit of normal. For PCI, anticoagulation is measured using the whole blood activated clotting time (ACT), with a goal of 250 to 350 seconds, or 200 to 250 seconds if using a GPI. Typical bolus intravenous (IV) UFH doses in the catheterization laboratory are 70 to 100 IU/kg, or 50 to 60 IU/kg with GPI inhibitors. Repeated ACT measurements should be made with prolonged procedures. Continued anticoagulation following a successful PCI procedure has been associated with an increased risk of bleeding without ischemic benefits, and is not recommended.

Low Molecular Weight Heparins

The low molecular weight heparins (LMWH) (enoxaparin, tinzaparin, dalteparin) are heparin derivatives with a more consistent dose–response relationship than UFH. Like UFH, LMWH binds to antithrombin, causing inhibition of factor Xa and thrombin. Due to improved subcutaneous absorption, LMWH can be administered either subcutaneously (SQ) or by IV. Monitoring LMWH effects is considered unnecessary except for extremely obese patients, or those with renal insufficiency (CrCl <30 mL/min). The ACT assay does not reliably measure LMWH effect; the anti-factor Xa assay is preferred but is not routinely available on a rapid basis.

Enoxaparin is the best studied among the LMWH for ACS. The therapeutic dose is 1 mg/kg SQ every 12 hours, or 0.75 to 1 mg/kg IV for elective PCI where no other anticoagulant has been given. To optimize anti-Xa activity for PCI, an additional IV booster dose of 0.3 mg/kg is given if PCI is performed 8 to 12 hours after the prior SQ dose, particularly if fewer than three previous SQ doses have been received by the patient. Switching from one anticoagulant strategy to another (i.e. LMWH to UFH) is associated with increased bleeding risk and is discouraged.

Early studies comparing LMWH to UFH in ACS have demonstrated a reduction of MI (10.1% vs. 11%) without increases in bleeding. Nevertheless, many of these trials were performed without an invasive approach, putting the benefit in question. The more recent large SYNERGY trial of 9,978 patients undergoing PCI for NSTE-ACS demonstrated equivalent efficacy between enoxaparin and UFH (14% vs. 14.5%, p = NS) with more TIMI-major bleeding events (9.1% vs. 7.6%, p = 0.008), possibly due to switching of anticoagulation strategies (26).

Overall, LMWH is considered equivalent to UFH for ACS and PCI. Its advantages include the lack of monitoring, ease of administration, and lower risk of heparin-induced thrombocytopenia. The lack of monitoring can be a double-edged sword, because the inability to assess the adequacy of anticoagulation at the time of PCI may be perceived as a risk. LMWH has primarily been used in ACS in Europe and Canada, with a much lower market share than in the US.

Fondaparinux

The heparinoid fondaparinux is a synthetic pentasaccharide that is derived from the binding regions of UFH and LWH. It inhibits factor Xa with antithrombin at high potency, with a SQ dose of 2.5 mg daily. Compared with LMWH, the use of fondaparinux demonstrated non-inferiority for ischemic complications in the OASIS-5 trial, but decreased major bleeding from 4.1% to 2.2% (HR 0.52, p < 0.001). Major bleeding was associated with mortality, which was reduced with fondaparinux (2.9% vs. 3.5%, p = 0.02) (27). Unexpected episodes of catheter thrombosis were noted with fondaparinux (0.9% vs. 0.4%) but can be avoided with a standard bolus (85 IU/kg, or 60 IU/kg with GPI) of UFH at the time of PCI.

Fondaparinux carries a Class I recommendation for anticoagulation for ACS, but with a lower level of evidence than UFH, LMWH, and bivalirudin. Despite its mortality benefit in the OASIS-5 trial, fondaparinux has not been widely accepted by practicing interventionalists due to the small risk of catheter thrombosis. Nevertheless, it is the preferred agent for patients when a conservative, noninvasive approach is selected.

Bivalirudin

Bivalirudin is a direct thrombin inhibitor that does not require antithrombin as a cofactor. It inhibits both free thrombin and fibrin-bound thrombin, which may increase its efficacy in ACS. The drug generates a predictable anticoagulant effect that can be measured with the aPTT and ACT, but where repeated measurement is not required. Bivalirudin is given as an IV bolus of 0.75 mg/kg, with an infusion of 1.75 mg/kg/hr. It is excreted by the kidney, and the infusion must be dose-adjusted in renal insufficiency.

The ACUITY trial was a randomized, open-label trial of 13,819 patients with ACS planned for an invasive strategy. Patients were randomized to heparin with GPI, bivalirudin with GPI, or bivalirudin alone strategies, in a background of aspirin and clopidogrel loading. There was no significant difference among any of the groups with respect to a composite ischemia endpoint. Nevertheless, the bivalirudin alone strategy demonstrated a reduction in ACUITY-defined major bleeding (3.0% vs. 5.7%, RR 0.53, p < 0.001). The net clinical outcome (i.e., the risk of major adverse cardiac events added to the risk of major bleeding) was thus reduced from 11.7% to 10.1% with bivalirudin when compared to heparin with GPI. Crossover from heparin to bivalirudin did not result in excess bleeding, and may have had a beneficial effect on ischemia (28).

Because 40% of patients in the ACUITY did not end up having positive biomarkers and receiving PCI, the ISAR-REACT 4 trial tested 1,721 patients with NSTEMI receiving PCI, to either UFH with GPI, or bivalirudin alone. The trial also used a more rigorous definition of major bleeding than the ACUITY trial. Nevertheless, the ISAR-REACT 4 trial demonstrated similar results: equivalent ischemic efficacy of bivalirudin compared with UFH + GPI, but with decreased major bleeding (2.6% vs. 4.6%, p = 0.02) (29).

Finally, in the MATRIX trial, 7,213 ACS patients were randomized to bivalirudin (with or without an extended infusion) or heparin with selective GPI. There were no significant differences between the two groups in terms of MACE or net adverse clinical events, including bleeding. The risk of stent thrombosis was higher with bivalirudin. Continuation of the bivalirudin infusion after PCI did not change the results (30).

Overall, and as described in several meta-analyses, bivalirudin is equivalent to heparin in terms of ischemic MACE, with a reduction in bleeding risk due in part to differential GPI use, but at the cost of an increased risk of acute stent thrombosis.

Post-procedure Care

Optimal care following revascularization should include referral for cardiac rehabilitation, smoking cessation assistance, and medical management of heart failure, arrhythmias, and risk factors. Dual antiplatelet therapy should be continued for 12 months after ACS, with the more potent $P2Y_{12}$ antagonists prasugrel or ticagrelor preferred. Antithrombotic treatment beyond dual antiplatelet therapy (DAPT) is available for selected patients at high-risk for recurrent events, with some benefit demonstrated for low-dose rivaroxaban and the new PAR-1 antagonist vorapaxar, but at the cost of increased bleeding.

CONCLUSIONS

PCI is a highly proven revascularization strategy for ACSs. The benefit of PCI is greatest for those patients at moderate to high risk for cardiac complications, and for those who receive PCI early (<24 hours). Early risk stratification, preferably with a quantitative scoring system such as the TIMI or GRACE score, is the key guide to selecting a management strategy. An expanding array of antithrombotic agents—such as bivalirudin, prasugrel, and ticagrelor—give the informed interventionalist the ability to adjust each patient's regimen in accordance with their clinical presentation, ischemic risk, and bleeding profile.

Key Points

- History, physical exam, and ECG are essential for rapid diagnosis of ACS.

- Elevated cardiac biomarkers are highly sensitive for myocardial damage.

- Noncoronary causes for troponin elevation should be considered when the history and ECG are not consistent with ACS.

- Early risk stratification of ischemic and bleeding risks is critical to subsequent management decisions.

- Moderate- and high-risk patients benefit from an early invasive approach, preferably with revascularization within the first 24 hours.

- Aspirin should be administered to all ACS patients without an allergy.

- Dual antiplatelet inhibition with an ADP-receptor antagonist is indicated for all patients with ACS.

- Prasugrel and ticagrelor have superior and more consistent platelet inhibition than clopidogrel.

- GPI benefit patients with an early invasive approach but increase bleeding.

- UFH with a goal ACT of 250 to 300 seconds provides adequate anticoagulation for PCI.

- Low-molecular-weight heparin is an alternative to heparin, but is associated with increased bleeding if switching to UFH occurs.

- Fondaparinux reduces bleeding and mortality in ACS, and may be preferable for conservatively managed patients.

- Bivalirudin reduces bleeding compared with unfractionated heparin + glycoprotein inhibitors, without increased ischemic complications when used with a dual antiplatelet regimen.

References

1. Ahmed B, et al. Recent changes in practice of elective percutaneous coronary intervention for stable angina. *Circ Cardiovasc Qual Outcomes.* 2011;4(3):300–305.
2. Mozaffarian D, et al. Heart disease and stroke statistics—2016 update: a report from the American Heart Association. *Circulation.* 2015;133:e38–e360.
3. Reichlin T, et al. Early diagnosis of myocardial infarction with sensitive cardiac troponin assays. *N Engl J Med.* 2009;361(9):858–867.
4. Eggers KM, et al. Prognostic value of biomarkers during and after non-ST-segment elevation acute coronary syndrome. *J Am Coll Cardiol.* 2009;54(4):357–364.
5. Moussa ID, et al. Consideration of a new definition of clinically relevant myocardial infarction after coronary revascularization: an expert consensus document from the Society for Cardiovascular Angiography and Intervention (SCAI). *J Am Coll Cardiol.* 2013;62(17):1563–1570.
6. Newby LK, et al. ACCF 2012 expert consensus document on practical clinical considerations in the interpretation of troponin elevations: a report of the American College of Cardiology Foundation task force on Clinical Expert Consensus Documents. *J Am Coll Cardiol.* 2012;60(23):2427–2463.
7. Thygesen K, et al. Third universal definition of myocardial infarction. *J Am Coll Cardiol.* 2012;60:1581–1598.

8. Wu AH, et al. National Academy of Clinical Biochemistry laboratory medicine practice guidelines: use of cardiac troponin and B-type natriuretic peptide or N-terminal proB-type natriuretic peptide for etiologies other than acute coronary syndromes and heart failure. *Clin Chem.* 2007;53(12):2086–2096.

9. Amsterdam EA, et al. 2014 AHA/ACC guideline for the management of patients with non-ST-elevation acute coronary syndromes: a report of the American College of Cardiology/American Heart Association Task Force on practice guidelines. *J Am Coll Cardiol.* 2014;64(24):e139–e228.

10. Antman EM, et al. The TIMI risk score for unstable angina/non-ST elevation MI: a method for prognostication and therapeutic decision making. *JAMA.* 2000;284(7):835–842.

11. Fox KA, et al. Prediction of risk of death and myocardial infarction in the six months after presentation with acute coronary syndrome: prospective multinational observational study (GRACE). *BMJ.* 2006;333(7578):1091.

12. Rao SV, et al. An updated bleeding model to predict the risk of post-procedure bleeding among patients undergoing percutaneous coronary intervention: a report using an expanded bleeding definition from the National Cardiovascular Data Registry CathPCI Registry. *JACC Cardiovasc Interv.* 2013;6(9):897–904.

13. Bavry AA, et al. Benefit of early invasive therapy in acute coronary syndromes: a meta-analysis of contemporary randomized clinical trials. *J Am Coll Cardiol.* 2006;48(7):1319–1325.

14. Neumann FJ, et al. Evaluation of prolonged antithrombotic pretreatment ('cooling-off' strategy) before intervention in patients with unstable coronary syndromes: a randomized controlled trial. *JAMA.* 2003;290:1593–1599.

15. Mehta SR, et al. Early versus delayed invasive intervention in acute coronary syndromes. *N Engl J Med.* 2009;360:2165–2175.

16. Milosevic A, et al. Immediate versus delayed invasive intervention for non-STEMI patients: the RIDDLE-NSTEMI study. *JACC Cardiovasc Interv.* 2016;9(6):541–549.

17. Fan W, et al. Trends in P2Y12 inhibitor use in patients referred for invasive evaluation of coronary artery disease in contemporary US practice. *Am J Cardiol.* 2016;117(9):1439–1443.

18. Mehta SR, et al. Double-dose versus standard-dose clopidogrel and high-dose versus low-dose aspirin in individuals undergoing percutaneous coronary intervention for acute coronary syndromes (CURRENT-OASIS 7): a randomised factorial trial. *Lancet.* 2010;376(9748):1233–1243.

19. Yusuf S, et al. Effects of clopidogrel in addition to aspirin in patients with acute coronary syndromes without ST-segment elevation. *N Engl J Med.* 2001;345:494–502.

20. Bhatt DL, et al. Clopidogrel with or without omeprazole in coronary artery disease. *N Engl J Med.* 2010;363(20):1909–1917.

21. Montalescot G, et al. Pretreatment with prasugrel in non-ST-segment elevation acute coronary syndromes. *N Engl J Med.* 2013;369(11):999–1010.

22. Wiviott SD, et al. Prasugrel versus clopidogrel in patients with acute coronary syndromes. *N Engl J Med.* 2007;357(20):2001–2015.

23. Wallentin L, et al. Ticagrelor versus clopidogrel in patients with acute coronary syndromes. *N Engl J Med.* 2009;361(11):1045–1057.

24. Roffi M, et al. Platelet glycoprotein IIb/IIIa inhibition in acute coronary syndromes. Gradient of benefit related to the revascularisation strategy. *Eur Heart J.* 2002;23:1441–1448.

25. Bhatt DL, et al. Effect of platelet inhibition with cangrelor during PCI on ischemic events. *N Engl J Med.* 2013;368(14):1303–1313.

26. Ferguson JJ, et al. Enoxaparin vs unfractionated heparin in high-risk patients with non-ST-segment elevation acute coronary syndromes managed with an intended early invasive strategy: primary results of the SYNERGY randomized trial. *JAMA.* 2004;292:45–54.

27. Yusuf S, et al. Comparison of fondaparinux and enoxaparin in acute coronary syndromes. *N Engl J Med.* 2006;354:1464–1476.

28. Stone GW, et al. Bivalirudin for patients with acute coronary syndromes. *N Engl J Med.* 2006;355:2203–2216.

29. Kastrati A, et al. Abciximab and heparin versus bivalirudin for non-ST-elevation myocardial infarction. *N Engl J Med.* 2011;365(21):1980–1989.

30. Valgimigli M, et al. Bivalirudin or unfractionated heparin in acute coronary syndromes. *N Engl J Med.* 2015;373(11):997–1009.

18

STEMI Intervention:
Emphasis on Guidelines

Khalil Ibrahim, MD and Julie M. Miller, MD, FSCAI,

FACC, FAHA

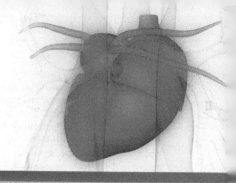

The treatment of ST-elevation myocardial infarction (STEMI) has evolved substantially over the last 10 years in the United States. To capture the important aspects and changes in management, specific and separate guidelines for STEMI were published first in 1990. A comprehensive understanding and integration of both STEMI and percutaneous coronary intervention (PCI) guidelines, as well as systems-of-care issues, reperfusion choices (pharmacologic or mechanical reperfusion), risk stratification, adjunctive medical therapies, technical issues related to PCI, and post-reperfusion management is required for the care of these complex patients. This chapter focuses on acute intervention for STEMI, as well as related adjunctive medical therapies, with a focus on guidelines. Detailed review of adjunctive medical therapies (including anticoagulants, thrombolytics, and platelet-inhibitor agents) are covered elsewhere.

Primary Interventions

PCI versus Thrombolytic Therapy

In patients presenting with STEMI, there are three choices for acute revascularization: primary PCI, fibrinolytic therapy, and acute surgical reperfusion (used rarely). Major factors in choosing the initial reperfusion approach include the resources available (PCI availability, systems of care, time to treatment), risks of therapy (medical and procedural), patient characteristics (onset of symptoms, ischemic time, presentation status, comorbidities), and anticipated benefits of the reperfusion-specific strategy (1). Importantly, no one approach is superior in all regions, clinical settings, or patients. Nevertheless, all patients should undergo rapid evaluation for reperfusion therapy and have a reperfusion strategy implemented promptly. Compared with fibrinolytic therapy, primary PCI is able to achieve higher rates of thrombolysis in myocardial infarction (TIMI) grade 3 flow and infarct artery patency, and lower rates of reinfarction, recurrent ischemia, intracranial hemorrhage, and death in randomized clinical trials (2).

Despite its limitations, the widespread availability and ease of administration of fibrinolytic therapy makes it a viable choice for reperfusion therapy when PCI is not rapidly available (Table 18.1). It should be noted that the efficacy of thrombolysis is diminished significantly as the duration from symptom onset to presentation increased; the greatest benefit is conferred in those patients presenting within 3 hours of symptom onset, reasonable benefit is seen within 12 hours, and unclear benefit >12 to 24 hours after symptoms. Furthermore, there are a number of absolute and relative contraindications to thrombolytic therapy (see Table 18.2). Thrombolytic therapy can fail to open the infarct-related artery (IRA) in nearly one-fifth of cases, and when reperfusion is achieved, re-occlusion of the artery can occur in approximately 20%. Given the risks, contraindications (relative and absolute), and overall effectiveness, the current guidelines emphasize the superiority of a PCI-based approach when reasonably available, and recommend consideration of fibrinolytic therapy only when patients present to

non-PCI hospitals and cannot likely receive PCI in <120 minutes due to unavoidable delays.

PCI is associated with an estimated 25% relative risk (RR) reduction (odds ratio of 0.75) 1-year mortality (2) compared with thrombolytic therapy in randomized trials. In the United States, use of primary PCI has increased dramatically; it is used more than four times as frequently as thrombolytic therapy. (Thrombolytic therapy remains a viable option in cases where PCI is not practical or there is significant reperfusion delay.) This is partly because PCI can achieve higher rates of IRA TIMI grade 3 flow and superior outcomes compared with thrombolytics, and because of the increased access to PCI services within the community, including improved systems of care.

Relationship between Time of Ischemia, Myocardial Salvage, and Survival

Benefits of reperfusion therapy are time-dependent. As time from symptom onset (artery occlusion) to reperfusion increases, the myocardium available to salvage decreases, which raises the risk of mortality (1,2). The greatest myocardial salvage and mortality benefit from reperfusion therapy comes within the first few hours of therapy (Fig. 18.1). Many modifying factors may influence the absolute time periods of salvage ability (collaterals, intermittent occlusion, myocardial oxygen consumption, ischemic preconditioning, persistence of residual blood flow, recruitment of collaterals, hibernating). Time-independent benefits of opening the artery have also been suggested to exist, and include improving infarct healing, electrical stability, and reducing reinfarction.

Current guidelines recommend a systems' goal of 90 minutes or less from the first medical contact to balloon angioplasty for hospitals that perform primary PCI. A number of variables may

TABLE 18.1 Indications for Fibrinolytic Therapy When There Is a >120-minute Delay from FMC to Primary PCI

	COR	LOE
Ischemic symptoms < 12 hours	I	A
Evidence of ongoing ischemia 12–24 hours after symptom onset and a large area of myocardium at risk or hemodynamic instability	IIa	C
ST depression, except if true posterior (inferobasal) MI is suspected or when associated with ST elevation in lead AVR	III: harm	B

AVR, augmented vector right. COR, class of recommendation; FMC, first medical contact; LOE, level of evidence; MI, myocardial infarction; PCI, percutaneous coronary intervention.
Modified from: O'Gara PT, et al. 2013 ACCF/AHA guideline for the management of ST-elevation myocardial infarction. *Circulation*. 2013;127(4):e362–e425, with permission.

TABLE 18.2 Contraindications for Thrombolysis Use in STEMI[a]

Absolute Contraindications

- Any prior ICH
- Known structural cerebral vascular lesions (e.g., AVM)
- Known malignant intracranial neoplasm (primary or metastatic)
- Ischemic stroke within 3 months EXCEPT acute ischemic stroke within 3 hours
- Suspected aortic dissection
- Active bleeding or bleeding diathesis (excluding menses)
- Significant closed head or facial trauma within 3 months
- Intracranial or intraspinal surgery within 2 months
- Severe uncontrolled hypertension (unresponsive to emergency therapy)
- For streptokinase, prior treatment within the previous 6 months

Relative Contraindications

- History of chronic, severe, poorly controlled hypertension
- Severe uncontrolled hypertension or presentation (SBP >180 mm Hg or DBP >110 mm Hg)
- History of ischemic stroke prior to 3 months, dementia, or known intracranial pathology not covered in contraindications
- Traumatic or prolonged (>10 minutes) CPR
- Major surgery (<3 weeks)
- Recent (within 2–4 weeks) internal bleeding
- Noncompressible vascular punctures
- For streptokinase/anistreplase: prior exposure (more than 5 days ago) or prior allergic reaction to these agents
- Pregnancy
- Active peptic ulcer
- Current use of anticoagulants: the higher the INR, the higher the risk of bleeding

[a]Viewed as advisory for clinical decision making and may not be all-inclusive or definitive.
AVM, arteriovenous malformation; CPR, cardiopulmonary resuscitation; DBP, diastolic blood pressure; ICH, intracranial hemorrhage; SBP, systolic blood pressure.
Modified from: O'Gara PT, et al. 2013 ACCF/AHA guideline for the management of ST-elevation myocardial infarction. *Circulation.* 2013;127(4):e362–e425, with permission.

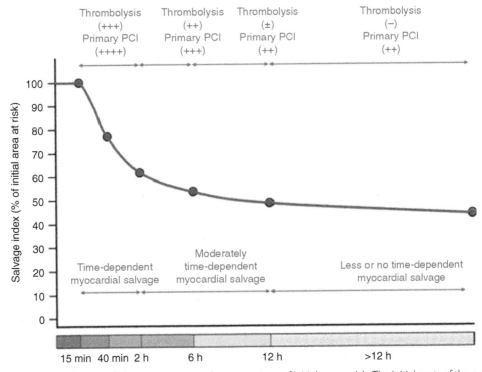

FIGURE 18.1 Time dependency of myocardial salvage expressed as percentage of initial area at risk. The initial parts of the curve up to 2 hours were reconstructed based on the experimental studies. For the first 15 minutes after coronary occlusion, myocardial necrosis is not observed. At 40 minutes after coronary occlusion, myocardial cell death develops rapidly, and the myocardial necrosis is confluent. After this point, progression to necrosis is slowed considerably. The other parts of the curve showing myocardial salvage from 2 to >12 hours from the symptom onset are reconstructed according to the data of scintigraphic studies in patients with acute myocardial infarction. Efficacy of reperfusion is expressed as follows: ++++, very effective; +++, effective; ++, moderately effective; ±, uncertainly effective; −, not effective. PCI, percutaneous coronary intervention. (From: Schömig A, Ndrepepa G, Kastrati A. Late myocardial salvage: time to recognize its reality in the reperfusion therapy of acute myocardial infarction. *Eur Heart J.* 2006;27:1900–1907, with permission.)

influence the total time of reperfusion with primary PCI. These include prehospital variables (symptom onset to first medical contact, prehospital transport, prehospital notification, emergency medical service (EMS)-administered therapies) and in-hospital factors (diagnosis time, patient variables, cath lab staffing, and procedural time). Symptom-onset-to-balloon time and door-to-balloon time are significantly correlated with mortality following primary PCI (3–5). Earlier reperfusion reduces mortality, particularly in those patients presenting early after symptoms onset (<2 hours). Delays in therapy affect mortality benefit to a greater degree in patients who are at higher risk (large territory at risk, anterior infarcts, congestive heart failure [CHF], advanced age, and renal insufficiency).

Data from National Cardiovascular Data Registry (NCDR) demonstrated a continuous relationship between in-hospital mortality and balloon time, including times below 90 minutes and above 90 minutes, suggesting any delay (even when time is <90 minutes) is associated with an increased mortality risk, as shown in **Figure 18.2** (4). Similarly, system delays (first medical contact to wire, including prehospital, transfer, and in-hospital delays) have been shown to be independently associated with worse long-term mortality, with each hour of delay associated with a 10% increase in the risk of death (5,6).

Figure 18.3 and **Table 18.3** summarize current recommendations regarding the triage, treatment, and transfer of patients presenting with STEMI.

Only in the rarest of circumstances, such as when there is a known and anticipated significant PCI delay (>120 minutes), should thrombolytics be considered in patients presenting to hospitals with PCI capability (e.g., catheterization lab not working or available; or staff not available to perform PCI). **Tables 18.4** and **18.5**

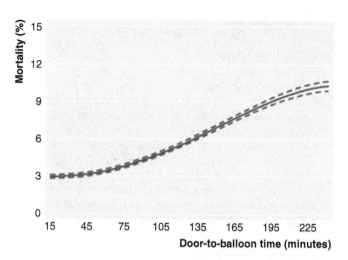

FIGURE 18.2 Adjusted in-hospital mortality as a function of door-to-balloon time. Median D2B time was 83 minutes, with 4.6% mortality. Longer door-to-balloon times were associated with a higher adjusted risk of mortality in hospital in a continuous nonlinear fashion (30 minutes = 3.0%, 60 minutes = 3.5%, 90 minutes = 4.3%, 120 minutes = 5.6%, 150 minutes = 7.0%, 180 minutes = 8.4%, p < 0.001). A reduction in door-to-balloon time from 90 to 60 minutes was associated with 0.8% lower mortality, and a reduction from 60 to 30 minutes with a 0.5% lower mortality. Data were from 43,801 STEMI patients undergoing primary PCI in NCDR (2005–2006). NCDR, national cardiovascular data registry; PCI, percutaneous coronary intervention; STEMI, ST-elevation myocardial infarction. (Modified from: Rathore SS, et al. Association of door-to-balloon time and mortality in patients admitted to hospital with ST elevation myocardial infarction: national cohort study. *BMJ.* 2009;338:b1807, with permission.)

TABLE 18.3 **Triage and Transfer Decisions for Reperfusion: Recommendations for STEMI Systems of Care**

Class I

1. All communities should create and maintain a regional system of STEMI care that includes assessment and continuous quality improvement of EMS and hospital-based activities.[a] Performance can be facilitated by participating in programs such as Mission: Lifeline and the D2B Alliance (LOE B).
   - Destination protocols to STEMI Receiving CTR
   - Transfer protocols for patients who arrive at STEMI Referral CTR and are primary PCI candidates, and/or are fibrinolytic ineligible and/or in cardiogenic shock (STEMI Referral Centers)
2. Performance of a 12-lead ECG by EMS personnel at the site of first medical contact (FMC) is recommended in patients with symptoms consistent with STEMI (LOE: B).
3. Reperfusion therapy should be administered to all eligible patients with STEMI with symptom onset within the prior 12 hours (LOE: A).
4. Primary PCI is the recommended method of reperfusion when it can be performed in a timely fashion by experienced operators (LOE: A).
5. EMS transport directly to a PCI-capable hospital for primary PCI is the recommended triage strategy for patients with STEMI, with an ideal FMC-to-device time system goal of 90 minutes or less[b] (LOE: B).
6. Immediate transfer to a PCI-capable hospital for primary PCI is the recommended triage strategy for patients with STEMI who initially arrive at or are transported to a non-PCI-capable hospital, with an FMC-to-device time system goal of 120 minutes or less[b] (LOE: B).
7. In the absence of contraindications, fibrinolytic therapy should be administered to patients with STEMI at non-PCI-capable hospitals when the anticipated FMC-to-device time at a PCI-capable hospital exceeds 120 minutes because of unavoidable delays (LOE: B).
8. When fibrinolytic therapy is indicated or chosen as the primary reperfusion strategy, it should be administered within 30 minutes of hospital arrival[b] (LOE: B).

Class IIa

1. Reperfusion therapy is reasonable for patients with STEMI and symptom onset within the prior 12–24 hours who have clinical and/or ECG evidence of ongoing ischemia. Primary PCI is the preferred strategy in this population (LOE: B).

[a]Ensure streamlined care paths that focus on primary PCI as the first-choice treatment for STEMI. Protocols for triage, diagnosis, and cardiac catheterization lab activation should be established within the primary PCI-capable hospitals (STEMI Receiving Centers), Process for prehospital identification and activation.
[b]The proposed time windows are system goals. For any individual patient, every effort should be made to provide reperfusion therapy as rapidly as possible.
ECG, electrocardiography; EMS, emergency medical services; LOE, level of evidence; PCI, percutaneous coronary intervention; STEMI, ST-elevation myocardial infarction.
Modified from: O'Gara PT, et al. 2013 ACCF/AHA guideline for the management of ST-elevation myocardial infarction. *Circulation.* 2013;127(4):e362–e425.

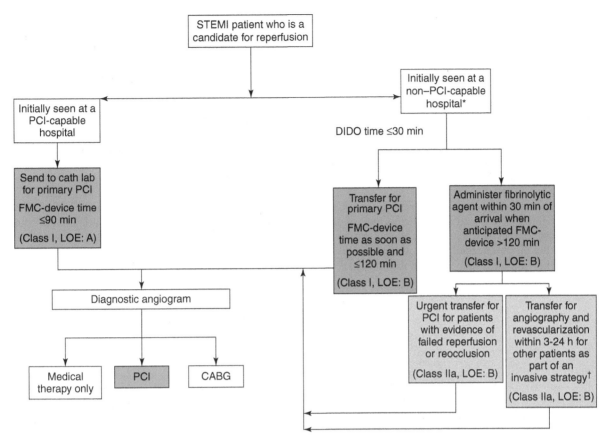

FIGURE 18.3 Guideline recommendations for triage and transfer for PCI in STEMI. Reperfusion therapy for patients with STEMI. The bold arrows and boxes are the preferred strategies. Performance of PCI is dictated by an anatomically appropriate culprit stenosis. *Patients with cardiogenic shock or severe heart failure initially seen at a non-PCI-capable hospital should be transferred for cardiac catheterization and revascularization as soon as possible, irrespective of time delay from MI onset (Class I, LOE: B). †Angiography and revascularization should not be performed within the first 2 to 3 hours after administration of fibrinolytic therapy. CABG indicates coronary artery bypass graft; DIDO, door-in–door-out; FMC, first medical contact; LOE, level of evidence; MI, myocardial infarction; PCI, percutaneous coronary intervention; and STEMI, ST-elevation myocardial infarction. (From: O'Gara PT, et al. 2013 ACCF/AHA guideline for the management of ST-elevation myocardial infarction. *Circulation.* 2013;127(4):e362–e425, with permission.)

summarize guidelines for coronary angiography and indications for PCI in STEMI patients.

TABLE 18.4 Indications for Coronary Angiography in ST-Segment Elevation Myocardial Infarction for Patients Who Were Managed with Fibrinolytic Therapy or Who Did Not Receive Reperfusion Therapy

INDICATIONS	COR	LOE
Severe heart failure or cardiogenic shock (if suitable revascularization candidate)	I	B
Intermediate- or high-risk findings on pre-discharge non-invasive ischemia testing	I	B
Spontaneous or easily provoked myocardial ischemia	I	C
Failed reperfusion or reocclusion after fibrinolytic therapy	IIa	B
Stable patients after successful fibrinolysis, before discharge and ideally between 3 and 24 hours	IIa	B

COR, class of recommendation; LOE, level of evidence.
Modified from: O'Gara PT, et al. 2013 ACCF/AHA guideline for the management of ST-elevation myocardial infarction: a report of the American College of Cardiology Foundation/American Heart Association Task Force on Practice Guidelines. *Circulation.* 2013;127(4):e362–e425, with permission.

Hospitals without PCI Capability

Less than half of US hospitals are capable of performing primary PCI. Nevertheless, nearly three-fourth of the population lives within 1 hour of a PCI-capable hospital (7). To reduce hospital treatment delays and maximize access to primary PCI, major efforts have focused on improving health systems of care for STEMI, including the continuum of care from EMS activation to transfer to PCI-capable facilities. An important focus of Mission Lifeline and the Door-to-Balloon Alliance is to increase the number of patients with timely access to primary PCI. For STEMI patients presenting to hospitals without primary PCI capability, the decision to use fibrinolytic therapy or transfer the patient to another facility for primary PCI must be made first. In general, a hospital without primary PCI capability should have an established treatment plan designating which primary reperfusion strategy it will generally use. The choice of this initial STEMI treatment should be based on a predetermined, institution-specific plan set in the context of the communities' system of available care (Table 18.3). If the referring hospital and the receiving PCI hospital have established a protocol that can minimize transfer delays, then transfer for primary PCI is generally recommended. Primary PCI performed within 120 minutes (<120 minutes from first medical contact to device) should be the systems' goal for these inter-hospital transfer patients (8,9). For hospitals without such a plan, or in cases where timely transfer to a PCI center is not possible, fibrinolytics should be the default therapy of choice, if the patient is eligible.

Note that primary PCI, irrespective of time delay, is indicated in patients with STEMI who develop severe heart failure (HF) or cardiogenic shock and are suitable candidates for revascularization as soon as possible (Class I, LOE B) (10). In addition, immediate transfer of patients from non-PCI hospitals to PCI-capable facilities following fibrinolysis is recommended as part of a "pharmacoinvasive" approach in high-risk patients. For these reasons, all hospitals without PCI should have an established transfer mechanism for STEMI patients.

The 2013 STREAM trial randomized 1,892 patients with symptom onset within 3 hours of medical contact who could not undergo primary PCI within 1 hour to primary PCI or fibrinolysis and then transfer to a PCI-capable hospital and found no significant difference in the primary endpoint of death from any cause, CHF, shock, or reinfarction at 30 days, although the fibrinolysis group had increased intracranial hemorrhage (11). This trial further supports the notion that prompt fibrinolysis should be administered when primary PCI is not able to be performed in a timely fashion.

Surgical and Nonsurgical Hospitals for Primary PCI

Nearly all states in the US now allow PCI (either primary and/or elective) at hospitals without on-site surgery (12). The 2011 guidelines now consider primary PCI without on-site surgery as a Class IIa recommendation. Nevertheless, primary PCI without surgical backup should not be performed at institutions without a proven plan for rapid transport to a cardiac surgery hospital or without appropriate hemodynamic support capability for transfer (Class III: harm). Despite an increase in the number of centers performing PCI (more often done in areas already with PCI programs), it has not substantially improved the access to PCI services for patients.

It is important to recognize that volume–outcome relationships exist (on both institutional and operator levels), but may be modified by experience. Overall, the ideal total procedural institutional volume is >400 PCIs/year (Class I), although volumes of 200 to 400 PCIs/year are acceptable (Class IIa). Specifically, for primary PCI, the lowest in-hospital mortality threshold was at institutions performing >36 per year (1,13). Therefore, Class I indications for primary PCI include performance at high-volume centers (>400 cases/year), ideally >36 primary PCIs/year. Previously, the 2011 Guidelines recommended individual operator volumes were ≥75 PCIs yearly, with at least 11 being primary (Class I), although a recent consensus statement endorses a lower annual PCI volume threshold of 50 PCIs for an individual operator. Primary PCI is not recommended (Class III—no benefit) at low-volume hospitals (<200/year) by low-volume operators (<50/year). **Table 18.6** lists the guidelines for operator and hospital volume. **Table 18.7** lists recommendations for PCI without on-site surgery.

Indications for Primary PCI (of the Infarct Artery)

Nearly all STEMI patients presenting within 12 hours of symptom onset (with either clinical or electrocardiographic evidence of ongoing ischemia, or with ongoing symptoms) are candidates for primary PCI (including those with true posterior infarcts, or other equivocal electrocardiography [ECG] findings and with a newly occluded artery in a clinical setting consistent with STEMI) (see ECG Criteria for STEMI section below).

Only in patients in whom the risk of revascularization outweighs benefit, or when the patient or designee does not agree to the procedure, would cath and PCI be considered inappropriate. The greatest mortality benefit of primary PCI is in patients who present early or are at highest risk; for example, with cardiogenic shock, an absolute 9% reduction in 30-day mortality was observed with PCI than with medical stabilization (14). Primary PCI is also clearly indicated for patients presenting within 12 to 24 hours of symptom onset and there is ongoing ischemia. Recent guidelines recognize that there is an indication for primary PCI in asymptomatic patients presenting between 12 and 24 hours after symptom onset and who are at higher risk (Class IIb) (2).

Coronary angiography and PCI are also indicated in patients presenting with severe HF or cardiogenic shock, regardless of presentation time from myocardial infarction (MI) symptom onset (Class I, LOE: B).

Table 18.5 summarizes the current guidelines for coronary angiography and for primary PCI.

ECG Criteria for STEMI

ECG evidence of acute MI is defined by the Task Force for the Universal Definition of Myocardial Infarction as new ST elevation at the J point in at least two contiguous leads of 2 mm (0.2 mV) in men or 1.5 mm (0.15 mV) in women in leads V2–V3 and/or of 1.0 mm (0.1 mV) in other contiguous chest leads or the limb leads. In addition, ST depression in ≥2 precordial leads (V1–V4) may indicate transmural posterior injury; multilead ST depression with coexistent ST elevation in lead aVR has been described in patients with left main or proximal left anterior descending artery occlusion. New or presumably new left bundle branch block (LBBB) has been considered a STEMI equivalent; nevertheless, it should not be considered a STEMI equivalent in isolation. If doubt persists based on ECG findings that are difficult to interpret, invasive angiography may be required to guide therapy.

TABLE 18.5 Indications for PCI in STEMI

INDICATIONS	COR	LOE
Primary PCI[a]		
STEMI symptoms within 12 hours	I	A
Severe heart failure or cardiogenic shock irrespective of time delay from MI onset	I	B
Contraindications to fibrinolytic therapy with ischemic symptoms <12 hours	I	B
Evidence of ongoing ischemia between 12 and 24 hours after symptom onset	IIa	B
Non-infarct-artery PCI at the time of primary PCI in patients without hemodynamic compromise	IIb[b]	B
Delayed PCI of a totally occluded infarct artery >24 hours after STEMI in stable patients	III: no benefit	B

[a]Systems goal of performing primary PCI within 90 minutes of first medical contact when the patient presents to a hospital with PCI capability (Class I; LOE: B) and within 120 minutes when the patient presents to a hospital without PCI capability (Class I; LOE: B).
[b]Updated recommendation from the 2015 ACC/AHA/SCAI focused update on primary PCI for Patients with STEMI.
COR, class of recommendation; LOE, level of evidence; PCI, percutaneous coronary intervention; and STEMI, ST-segment elevation.
Modified from: O'Gara PT, et al. 2013 ACCF/AHA guideline for the management of ST-elevation myocardial infarction. *Circulation.* 2013;127(4):e362–e425, with permission.

TABLE 18.6 PCI with or without On-Site Surgery: Recommendations

INDICATIONS	COR
Class I: PCI with On-site Surgery	
Elective or urgent PCI should be performed by: Operators with acceptable volumes (>75/year operator volume) and at High-volume institutions (>400 cases/year) with on-site surgery	I
Primary PCI should be performed by: Operators with volume >75/year, ideally >11 primary PCIs/year with on-site surgery, and Ideally, high-volume hospitals (>400 cases/year) and >36 primary PCIs/year	I
Elective/urgent should be performed by operators and institutions whose current risk-adjusted outcomes statistic are comparable to those reported in contemporary national data registries.	I
Class II: PCI with On-site Surgery	
It is reasonable that operators with acceptable volume (>75[a] PCI procedures per year) perform elective/urgent PCI at low-volume centers (200–400 PCI procedures per year) with on-site cardiac surgery.	IIa
It is reasonable that low-volume operators (<75[a] PCI procedures per year) perform elective/urgent PCI at high-volume centers (>400 PCI procedures per year) with on-site cardiac surgery. Ideally, at an institution with >600 PCIs/year, mentored relationship.	IIa
The benefit of primary PCI for STEMI patients eligible for fibrinolysis when performed by an operator who performs <75[a] procedures/year (or <11 PCIs for STEMI per year) is not well established.	IIb
Class II: PCI without On-site Surgical Backup	
Primary PCI is reasonable provided that appropriate planning for program development has been accomplished, including: Operation of lab 24 h/d, 365 d/y Experienced operator >75[a] PCIs/year; ideally >11 primary PCIs/year Hemodynamic support (IABP) and well-equipped Proven transport plans to surgical center Limited to STEMI or LBBB new Door-to-balloon (or first medical contact) goal 90 minutes Hospital >36 primary PCIs/year	IIa
Class III: Without On-site Surgery or Limited Volume	
Primary (or elective) PCI should not be performed in hospitals without on-site cardiac surgery capabilities without: A proven plan for rapid transport to a cardiac surgery hospital; or Without appropriate hemodynamic support capability for transfer	III: harm
It is not recommended that elective/urgent PCI be performed by low-volume operators (<75[a] procedures per year) at low-volume centers (200–400 procedures/year) with or without on-site cardiac surgery.	III: no benefit
An institution with a volume of fewer than 200 procedures/year, unless in a region that is underserved because of geography, should carefully consider whether it should continue to offer this service.	III: no benefit
Elective PCI should not be performed in institutions without on-site cardiac surgery[a] (might be considered under 2011 PCI guidelines)	IIb[b]
The benefit of primary PCI for STEMI patients eligible for fibrinolysis when performed by an operator who performs fewer than 75[a] procedures per year (11 PCIs for STEMI/year) is not well-established.	IIb

[a]The 2013 update of the clinical competence statement on coronary artery interventional procedures (*J Am Coll Cardiol.* 2013;62(4)) updated the recommendation for individual physician volume to 50 PCIs per year, averaged over a 2-year period.
[b]CLASS IIb (LOE B). Elective PCI might be considered, provided that appropriate planning for program development has been accomplished and rigorous clinical and angiographic criteria are used for proper patient selection.
IABP, indicates intra-aortic balloon pump; LBBB, left bundle branch block; LOE, level of evidence; PCI, percutaneous coronary intervention; STEMI, ST-segment elevation myocardial infarction.
Modified from: Levine GN, et al. *Circulation.* 2011;124(23):e574–e651; Harold JG, et al. ACCF/AHA/SCAI 2013 update of the clinical competence statement on coronary artery interventional procedures. *Catheter Cardiovasc Interv.* 2013;82(2):E69–E111, with permission.

PCI Following Fibrinolysis

From the available data and expert opinion, the 2013 ACC/AHA STEMI emphasize that fibrinolysis should be generally limited to hospitals without on-site PCI and when there is an anticipated delay to performing primary PCI beyond 120 minutes of first medical contact.

In these cases, guidelines make the following recommendations regarding fibrinolysis:

1. STEMI (ST-elevation ≥0.1 mV in at least two contiguous precordial leads or at least two adjacent limb leads), onset of ischemic symptoms <12 hours (Class I);

TABLE 18.7 PCI without On-site Surgery: Recommendations for Case Selection

2014 SCAI EXPERT CONSENSUS DOCUMENT REQUIREMENTS FOR PRIMARY PCI AND EMERGENCY AORTOCORONARY BYPASS SURGERY AT HOSPITALS WITHOUT ON-SITE CARDIAC SURGERY

Avoid Intervention in Patients with:

>50% diameter stenosis of left main artery proximal to infarct-related lesion, especially if the area in jeopardy is relatively small and overall LV function is not severely impaired

Long, calcified, or severely angulated target lesions at high risk for PCI failure with TIMI flow grade 3 present during initial diagnostic angiography

Lesions in other than the infarct artery (unless they appeared to be flow limiting in patients with hemodynamic instability or ongoing symptoms)

Lesions with TIMI flow grade 3 in patients with left main or three-vessel disease where bypass surgery is likely a superior revascularization strategy compared with PCI

Culprit lesions in more distal branches jeopardizing only a modest amount of myocardium when there is more proximal disease that could be worsened by attempted intervention

Chronic total occlusion

Transfer Emergently for Coronary Bypass Surgery Patients with:

High-grade left main or three-vessel coronary disease with clinical or hemodynamic instability after successful or unsuccessful PCI of an occluded vessel and preferably with IABP support

Failed or unstable PCI result and ongoing ischemia, with IABP support during transfer

IABP, indicates intra-aortic balloon pump; LV, left ventricular; PCI, percutaneous coronary intervention; SCAI, society for cardiovascular angiography and interventions; TIMI, thrombolysis in myocardial infarction.
Adapted from: Dehmer GJ, et al. SCAI/ACC/AHA expert consensus document. *Catheter Cardiovasc Interv.* 2014;84(2):169–187, with permission.

2. STEMI, PCI not available, clinical and/or ECG evidence of ongoing ischemia within 12 to 24 hours of symptom onset and large area of myocardium at risk or hemodynamic instability (Class IIa).

PCI can be performed in a number of different scenarios following fibrinolysis. Changes in PCI availability, evolution of triage and transfer capabilities, and the research in pharmacologic therapy have allowed the evolution of a number of terms in parallel, including "facilitated PCI," "rescue PCI," and "pharmacoinvasive PCI." These strategies are summarized in Table 18.8.

Rescue PCI (PCI after Fibrinolytic Failure)

Thrombolysis fails to completely reperfuse the IRA in 30% to 40% of STEMI patients. After early recognition of thrombolysis failure, immediate PCI (called "rescue angioplasty") has been shown to reduce recurrent MI, repeat revascularization, and improve event-free survival (15,16). Failed fibrinolysis can be recognized by (a) ongoing symptoms or (b) failure of electrocardiographic evidence of reperfusion. ECG evidence of failed reperfusion is most easily made by <50% ST-segment resolution 90 minutes after initiation of therapy in the lead showing the greatest degree of ST-segment

TABLE 18.8 Definitions of PCI

Primary PCI

PCI used as the primary reperfusion method in patients with STEMI.

Rescue Angioplasty

PCI following the use of fibrinolysis for STEMI, when based on evidence of failed reperfusion by fibrinolysis. Generally, this requires time for fibrinolysis (60–90 minutes) to allow time for reperfusion and assessment of reperfusion to determine the need for PCI.

Facilitated Angioplasty

A strategy of planned immediate PCI after administration of an initial pharmacologic regimen intended to improve coronary patency before the emergency PCI procedure. A strategy upstream use of a pharmacologic therapy to "facilitate" primary PCI.

Early Routine Angioplasty/Pharmacoinvasive Approach

Immediate referral for PCI (following initial fibrinolytic therapy). Performed within several hours after fibrinolytic administration, regardless of whether or not clinical or electrocardiographic evidence of ongoing myocardial injury is present. Generally applies to patients presenting to hospitals without primary PCI who cannot undergo timely primary PCI. Sometimes referred to as "delayed" PCI, or as "immediate" PCI after administration of fibrinolysis at non-PCI-capable facilities.

Delayed Angioplasty in STEMI

The angioplasty is delayed, either due to delays from transport to a PCI facility or the choice of initial fibrinolysis for reperfusion.

PCI, percutaneous coronary intervention; STEMI, ST-segment elevation myocardial infarction.

elevation 60 to 80 ms following the J point at presentation. Chest pain is not a requirement of failed reperfusion.

Rescue PCI is a better alternative than conservative therapy or repeat fibrinolysis for treatment of failed reperfusion (14,17). A meta-analysis of eight randomized trials of rescue PCI compared with conservative management in patients with failed fibrinolytic therapy for STEMI showed that rescue PCI was associated with no significant reduction (but favorable trend) in all-cause mortality, but with significant risk reductions in HF and reinfarction compared with conservative treatment. Rescue PCI was also associated with an increased risk of stroke and minor bleeding.

Facilitated Angioplasty

Facilitated PCI is a strategy of initial upstream thrombolytic therapy to "facilitate" coronary reperfusion prior to immediate (within 2–3 hours) PCI for STEMI. The "Facilitated PCI" term is no longer used in current guidelines. Multiple regimens have been studied in clinical trials. Pharmacologic regimens have included full-dose or reduced-dose fibrinolytic therapy, and the combination of a glycoprotein (GP) IIb/IIIa inhibitor with a reduced-dose fibrinolytic agent (e.g., a fibrinolytic dose typically reduced 50%), and GP IIb/IIIa inhibitors alone.

Facilitated PCI is not beneficial compared with primary PCI. The ASSENT-4 study compared up-front full-dose tenecteplase followed by PCI with primary PCI. The study was prematurely terminated because of an increased in-hospital mortality with the facilitated approach (6.5% vs. 3.4%; p < 0.01) (18). On the basis of these data, facilitated PCI is not recommended.

Fibrinolysis Followed by PCI (Pharmacoinvasive Approach): Non-PCI Hospitals

Thrombolysis at a non-PCI hospital, followed by transfer and catheterization with or without PCI at a PCI center 3 to 24 hours after fibrinolysis is called a "pharmacoinvasive approach" or "delayed PCI," and should not be confused with "facilitated PCI," a strategy that has not been shown to be beneficial and which may be harmful.

Current guidelines (Class IIa) recommend the transfer of high-risk patients who receive fibrinolytic therapy as primary reperfusion therapy at a non-PCI-capable facility to a PCI-capable facility as soon as possible, where PCI can be performed either when needed or as a pharmacoinvasive strategy. Recommendations are primarily based on the two largest studies, CARESS and TRANSFER-AMI (19,20) (Figs. 18.4 and 18.5). Transfer of all patients, regardless of risk, who receive fibrinolytic therapy as primary reperfusion therapy at non-PCI-capable facilities may also be considered (Class IIb) for transfer as soon as possible to a PCI-capable facility, where PCI can be performed when needed or as part of a pharmacoinvasive strategy. Bleeding risk is an obvious concern when performing PCI after fibrinolytics; nevertheless, improvements in equipment and adjunctive pharmacotherapies have improved success rates, while keeping bleeding risks low. TRANSFER-AMI and a large meta-analysis have not observed a significantly increased risk of TIMI major bleeding (19–21), although minor bleeding is increased.

PCI for Late-Arriving STEMI Patients

The OAT (Occluded Artery Trial) (22) tested the hypothesis that routine PCI for total occlusion 3 to 28 days after MI would reduce the composite of death, reinfarction, or Class IV HF in otherwise stable patients. The minimal time from symptom onset to angiography in patients with a total occlusion of the IRA (TIMI grade 0 or 1) was just over 24 hours. Important exclusion criteria were NYHA Class III or IV HF, rest angina, renal impairment, left main or three-vessel disease, clinical instability, or severe inducible ischemia on stress testing. The 4-year cumulative endpoint was 17% in the PCI group and 16% in the medical therapy group (HR 1.16; 95% CI 0.92–1.45; p = 0.2). Reinfarction rates tended to be higher in the PCI group, which may have attenuated any benefit in left ventricular (LV) remodeling. TOSCA-2 (Total Occlusion Study of Canada) (23), an angiographic sub-study of OAT, demonstrated high success rates of IRA reperfusion, but no significant benefit. These studies demonstrate that elective PCI of an occluded infarct artery 1 to 28 days after MI in stable patients with single- or double-vessel disease had no incremental benefit beyond optimal medical therapy (aspirin, β-blockers, angiotensin converting enzyme [ACE] inhibitors, and statins) in preserving LV function and preventing subsequent cardiovascular events. It should be noted that delayed PCI of the infarct artery is indicated in patients who become unstable because of the development of cardiogenic shock, acute severe HF, or unstable postinfarction angina. Delayed PCI can also be performed in patients who did not receive reperfusion therapy but who did demonstrate significant residual ischemia during hospitalization. The DANAMI trial (24) evaluated the benefit of angioplasty in patients with residual ischemia following fibrinolysis. A total of 1,008 patients with inducible ischemia after fibrinolytic therapy for a first acute myocardial infarction (AMI) were randomized to conservative care or to catheterization followed by revascularization with balloon angioplasty or coronary artery bypass grafting (CABG) surgery. At 2.4 years follow-up (median), mortality was 4% in the invasive treatment group and 4% in the conservative treatment group (p = NS). Invasive treatment was

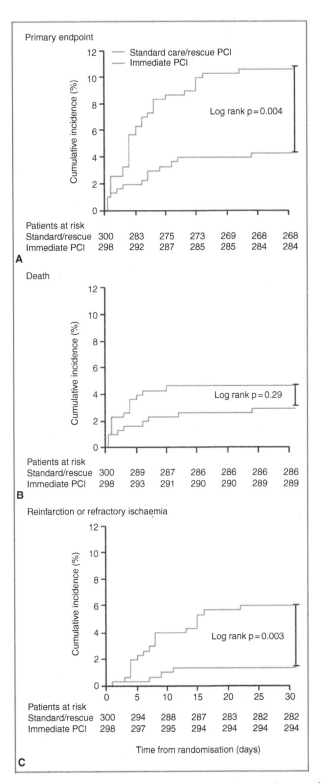

FIGURE 18.4 Results from the CARESS-in-AMI study: immediate transfer for PCI versus standard medical therapy with transfer as needed for rescue PCI, following fibrinolysis in STEMI patients presenting to hospitals without PCI capability. Shown are Kaplan–Meier event curves for the primary outcome (with 95%, CI) **(A)**, for death **(B)**, and for reinfarction, refractory ischaemia, or both **(C)**. Primary outcome was a composite of death, reinfarction, or refractory ischaemia at 30 days. PCI, percutaneous coronary intervention; STEMI, ST-elevation myocardial infarction. (From: Di Mario C, et al. Immediate angioplasty versus standard therapy with rescue angioplasty after thrombolysis in the Combined Abciximab REteplase Stent Study in Acute Myocardial Infarction (CARESS-in-AMI): an open, prospective, randomised, multicentre trial. *Lancet.* 2008;371:559–568, with permission.)

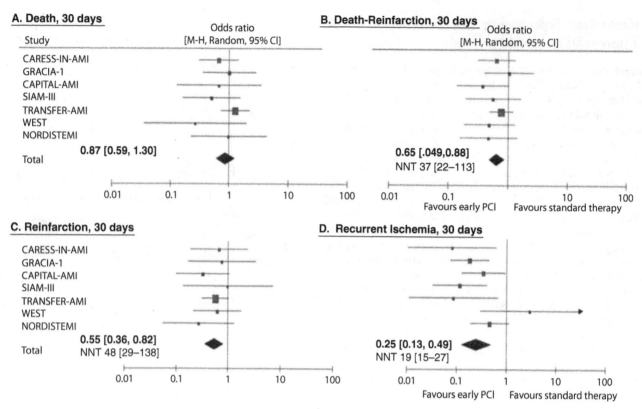

FIGURE 18.5 Meta-analysis of rescue PCI versus conservative therapy. Efficacy endpoints for rescue PCI versus conservative therapy. Clinical end points at 30 days for **(A)** death, **(B)** death and reinfarction, **(C)** reinfarction and **(D)** recurrent ischemia. CI, confidence interval; MERLIN, Middlesbrough Early Revascularization to Limit Infarction trial; NNT, number needed to treat; PCI, percutaneous coronary intervention; REACT, Rescue Angioplasty versus Conservative Treatment or Repeat Thrombolysis trial; RESCUE, Randomized Comparison of Rescue Angioplasty with Conservative Management of Patients with Early Failure of Thrombolysis for Acute Anterior Myocardial Infarction trial; RR, relative risk; TAMI, Thrombolysis and Angioplasty in Myocardial Infarction study. (From: Borgia, Francesco, et al. "Early routine percutaneous coronary intervention after fibrinolysis vs. standard therapy in ST-segment elevation myocardial infarction: a meta-analysis." *European heart journal* 31.17 (2010): 2156-2169.)

associated with a lower incidence of reinfarction (5.6% vs. 10.5%; p = 0.0038) and a lower incidence of admission for unstable angina (17.9% vs. 29.5%; p < 0.00001). The primary endpoint (composite endpoint of death, reinfarction, or readmission for unstable angina) was 15.4% and 29.5% at 1 year, 23.5% and 36.6% at 2 years, and 31.7% and 44.0% at 4 years (p = < 0.00001) in the invasive and conservative treatment groups, respectively. The study supports the use of delayed or elective PCI in patients, following thrombolysis with inducible ischemia (Class IIa). Patients with objective evidence of recurrent MI or spontaneous or provocable ischemia during recovery from STEMI are also suitable candidates (Class I).

PCI can be beneficial when performed hours, days, or weeks after successful fibrinolytic therapy, by reducing unstable angina, reinfarction, and long-term mortality. PCI of a hemodynamically significant stenosis >24 hours after STEMI in a patent infarct artery, as part of a revascularization strategy, has been shown to improve contemporary outcomes (25). In a large Danish registry of over 20,000 STEMI patients, early revascularization (within 14 days) in individuals with AMI was associated with a substantial reduction in 1-year mortality (26). A summary of indications for PCI in patients who were managed with fibrinolytics or who did not receive reperfusion therapy is listed in **Table 18.9**.

Management of Spontaneous Reperfusion

Not infrequently, a patient is brought to the catheterization lab, and diagnostic angiography demonstrates a reperfused vessel with

adequate flow (TIMI 3 flow). If the patient is asymptomatic and there is no evidence of ongoing ischemia, CHF, or instability, then there is a window for careful decision regarding the approach to revascularization. Where anatomy potentially is better suited for CABG, terminating the procedure after the completion of diagnostic coronary angiography may be reasonable. PCI in an effort to improve survival should not be performed in stable patients with significant (>50% diameter stenosis) unprotected left main coronary artery disease (CAD) who have unfavorable anatomy for PCI and who are good candidates for CABG (Class III, LOE: B). Nevertheless, PCI is reasonable in patients with acute STEMI when an unprotected left main coronary artery is the culprit lesion, distal coronary flow is less than TIMI grade 3, and PCI can be performed more rapidly and safely than CABG (Class IIa, LOE: C).

Emergency CABG Surgery for STEMI

Emergency CABG surgery, either as a primary reperfusion strategy in STEMI or following primary PCI, is rarely needed. The overall need for emergency CABG for all PCI procedures (elective and primary PCI) is ~0.4%. Indications for emergency CABG in the setting of STEMI are listed in **Table 18.10**. Note that in patients presenting with three-vessel disease but with an occluded culprit artery with ongoing ischemia, PCI of the IRA should be performed if feasible. In this setting, consideration of balloon-only (with or without thrombectomy) may avoid the need for a thienopyridine during the perioperative period. Obviously, if emergent surgical

TABLE 18.9 Indications for PCI of an Infarct Artery in Patients Who Were Managed with Fibrinolytic Therapy or Who Did Not Receive Reperfusion Therapy

	COR	LOE
Cardiogenic shock or acute severe HF	I	B
Intermediate- or high-risk findings on pre-discharge non-invasive ischemia testing	I	C
Spontaneous or easily provoked myocardial ischemia	I	C
Patients with evidence of failed reperfusion or reocclusion after fibrinolytic therapy (as soon as possible)	IIa	B
Stable[a] patients after successful fibrinolysis, ideally between 3 and 24 hours	IIa	B
Stable[a] patients >24 hours after successful fibrinolysis	IIb	B
Delayed PCI of a totally occluded infarct artery >24 hours after STEMI in stable patients	III: no benefit	B

[a]Although individual circumstances will vary, clinical stability is defined by the absence of low output, hypotension, persistent tachycardia, apparent shock, high-grade ventricular or symptomatic supraventricular tachyarrhythmias, and spontaneous recurrent ischemia.
COR, class of recommendation; HF, heart failure; LOE, level of evidence; PCI, percutaneous coronary intervention; and STEMI, ST-elevation myocardial infarction.
From: O'Gara PT, et al. 2013 ACCF/AHA guideline for the management of ST-elevation myocardial infarction. *Circulation.* 2013;127(4):e362–e425.

TABLE 18.10 Emergency CABG Indications in STEMI

INDICATIONS	COR	LOE
Class I		
Emergency or urgent CABG in patients with STEMI should be undertaken in the following circumstances:		
Patients with STEMI and coronary anatomy not amenable to PCI who have ongoing or recurrent ischemia, cardiogenic shock, severe HF, or other high-risk features.	I	B
At the time of operative repair of mechanical defects.	I	B
Class IIa		
The use of mechanical circulatory support is reasonable in patients with STEMI who are hemodynamically unstable and require urgent CABG.	IIa	B
Class IIb		
Emergency CABG within 6 hours of onset may be considered in patients with STEMI who do not have cardiogenic shock and are not candidates for PCI or fibrinolytic therapy.	IIb	C

The 2011 PCI guidelines do provide for consideration of PCI of the LM in STEMI: In patients with acute STEMI when an unprotected left main coronary artery is the culprit lesion, a decision needs to be made balancing the delay in surgery with the potential to perform PCI. Emergency PCI in this setting may be reasonable if distal coronary flow is less than TIMI grade 3, and PCI can be performed more rapidly and safely than CABG (class IIa, 2011 guidelines).
CABG, coronary artery bypass grafting; COR, class of recommendation; HF, heart failure; LOE, level of evidence; PCI, percutaneous coronary intervention; STEMI, ST-segment elevation myocardial infarction.
Adapted from: O'Gara PT, et al. 2013 ACCF/AHA guideline for the management of ST-elevation myocardial infarction: a report of the American College of Cardiology Foundation/American Heart Association Task Force on Practice Guidelines. *Circulation.* 2013;127(4): e362–e425, with permission.

management is required for other reasons (ventricular septal defect [VSD], postinfarction mechanical issues, or rupture), the patient should go immediately for CABG, without delay for PCI.

The 2011 PCI guidelines do provide for consideration of PCI of the left main in STEMI. In patients with acute STEMI, when an unprotected left main coronary artery is the culprit lesion, the decision is to balance the delay in surgery by performing PCI. In this setting, emergency PCI may be reasonable if distal coronary flow is less than TIMI grade 3 and PCI can be performed more rapidly and safely than CABG (Class IIa).

PCI of the Non-infarct Vessel during PCI in STEMI

A substantial number of patients (40%–60%) presenting with STEMI have multivessel disease with a significant stenosis in at least one non-IRA, which presents the operator with several PCI options, including: (1) primary PCI of the culprit vessel only, with PCI of non-culprit arteries only for high-risk features; (2) multivessel PCI at the time of primary PCI; (3) primary PCI followed by staged PCI of the non-culprit vessels. The previous 2013 STEMI guidelines did not recommend PCI of non-culprit vessels at the time of primary PCI in the setting of STEMI and gave a class III (harmful) recommendation based on previous studies, including a large meta-analysis that showed worse mortality when performing multivessel PCI and concern for increased procedural complications, longer procedure time leading to increased contrast nephropathy, and increased risk of stent thrombosis (27,28). Nevertheless,

more recent studies, including several randomized control studies, have demonstrated multivessel PCI at the time of primary PCI or staged may be safe and beneficial. The PRAMI trial (n = 465) (29) showed that patients undergoing multivessel PCI had a lower composite endpoint of cardiac death, nonfatal MI, or refractory angina compared to culprit PCI only (9% vs. 22%; HR 0.35, 95% CI 0.21–0.58; p < 0.001) (see **Fig. 18.6**). Similarly, the CvLPRIT trial (n = 296) (30) demonstrated a lower composite outcome of death, reinfarction, HF, and ischemia-driven revascularization at 12 months in multivessel PCI during index hospitalization compared to culprit only PCI (10% vs. 21%; HR 0.49, 95% CI 0.24–0.84; p = 0.009). The DANAMI 3 PRIMULTI (n = 627) (31) compared multivessel PCI guided by angiography and fractional flow reserve occurring before discharge versus culprit artery only PCI and found the composite primary outcome of all-cause mortality, nonfatal MI, or ischemia-driven revascularization of non-culprit artery occurred in 13% of multivessel PCI versus 22% of culprit artery only PCI (HR 0.56; 95% CI 0.38–0.83; p = 0.004). See **Table 18.11** for a summary of these three studies. Based on these new findings the prior Class III (harm) recommendation for multivessel primary PCI from the 2013 STEMI guideline was upgraded to a Class IIb recommendation in the most recent 2015 updated guideline; however, the guideline committee emphasized in the document that the change in recommendation does not mean they are endorsing routine performance of multivessel PCI in all STEMI patients, rather

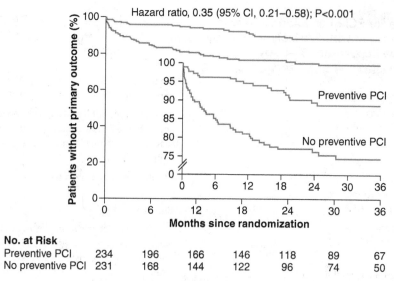

FIGURE 18.6   The primary outcome was a composite of death from cardiac causes, nonfatal myocardial infarction, or refractory angina. The inset graph shows the same data on a larger scale. All patients in the trial underwent infarct-artery PCI immediately before randomization. PCI, percutaneous coronary intervention. (From: Wald DS, et al. Randomized trial of preventive angioplasty in myocardial infarction. Randomized trial of preventive angioplasty in myocardial infarction. *N Engl J Med.* 2013;369(12):1115–1123, with permission.)

it can be considered, and the operator should integrate the full clinical picture, including lesion complexity and risk of contrast nephropathy, to determine the optimal approach.

In summary, the data on multivessel PCI during STEMI is mixed, but recent randomized controlled trials (RCT) have suggested benefits either at the time of primary PCI or staged during the index hospitalization, which has resulted in an upgraded recommendation in the latest 2015 STEMI guideline update to Class IIb from Class III, meaning multivessel PCI may be considered either at the time of primary PCI or as a planned staged procedure in selected patients with STEMI and multivessel disease who are hemodynamically stable.

Balloon Angioplasty Alone versus Stenting in Primary PCI

Stents produce superior outcome results compared with balloon angioplasty results alone. The reocclusion rate following percutaneous transluminal coronary angioplasty (PTCA) is 15% versus 5% with stenting (32).

Primary stenting reduces the risk of target vessel revascularization (TVR), and reinfarction when compared with balloon angioplasty alone. Randomized clinical trials, and numerous comprehensive meta-analyses (32,33) have demonstrated a significant mortality

TABLE 18.11   Summary of Multi-PCI trials

	CVLPRIT			PRIMULTI			PRAMI		
Non-IRA lesion criteria	>70% DS or >50% DS in two views			>50% DS and FFR <0.80 or >90% DS			>50% DS		
Randomization for non-IRA lesions	Immediate or staged complete revascularization (angio-guided) within index admission vs. culprit only			Staged complete revascularization (FFR-guided) within index admission vs. culprit only			Immediate complete revascularization (angio-guided) vs. culprit only		
1° endpoint	D, MI, HF, Ischemia-driven revascularization at 1 year			D, MI, ischemia-driven revascularization at 1 year			D, MI or refractory angina		
Results	MV PCI	Culprit-only	p	MV PCI	Culprit-only	p	MV PCI	Culprit-only	p
1° endpoint	10%	21%	0.009	13%	22%	0.004	8.9%	22.9%	<0.001
Death	1%	4%	0.14	5%	4%	0.43	1.7%	4.3%	0.07
Reinfarction	1%	3%	0.39	5%	5%	0.87	3%	8.6%	0.009
Heart failure	3%	6%	0.14	–	–	–	–	–	
Revascularization	5%	8%	0.20	5%	17%	17%	6.8%	19.9	<0.001

D, death; DS, diameter stenosis; FFR, fractional flow reserve; HF, heart failure; IRA, infarct-related artery; MI, myocardial infarction; MV PCI, multi-vessel PCI.

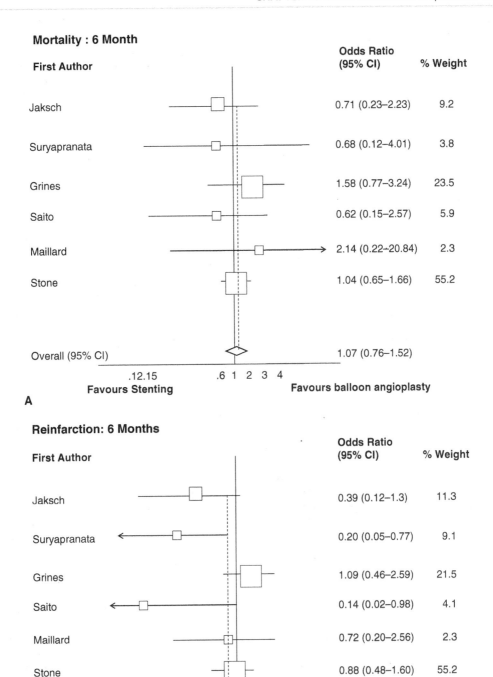

FIGURE 18.7 Bare-metal stenting versus balloon angioplasty for STEMI. Meta-analysis results (6 months) comparing patients with myocardial infarction who were treated with primary stenting versus balloon angioplasty. **A:** Odds ratios for mortality. **B:** Odds ratio for reinfarction.

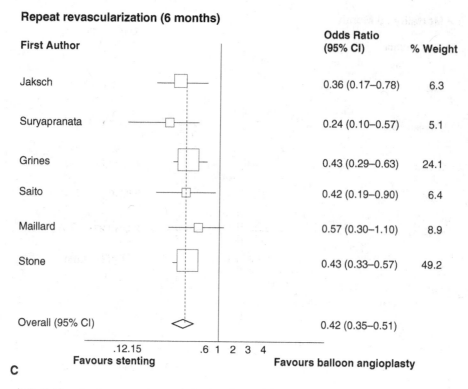

Repeat revascularization (6 months)

First Author	Odds Ratio (95% CI)	% Weight
Jaksch	0.36 (0.17–0.78)	6.3
Suryapranata	0.24 (0.10–0.57)	5.1
Grines	0.43 (0.29–0.63)	24.1
Saito	0.42 (0.19–0.90)	6.4
Maillard	0.57 (0.30–1.10)	8.9
Stone	0.43 (0.33–0.57)	49.2
Overall (95% CI)	0.42 (0.35–0.51)	

.12.15   .6 1 2 3 4
Favours stenting   **Favours balloon angioplasty**

C

FIGURE 18.7 (continued) **C:** Odds ratios for repeat revascularization. CI, confidence interval; STEMI, ST-elevation myocardial infarction. (From: Nordmann AJ, et al. Clinical outcomes of primary stenting versus balloon angioplasty in patients with myocardial infarction: a meta-analysis of randomized controlled trials. *Am J Med.* 2004;116:253–262, with permission.)

reduction with stenting compared with balloon angioplasty alone in STEMI (**Fig. 18.7**). Stenting significantly reduces the incidence of overall major adverse cardiac events (MACE) (OR 0.49 [0.40–0.59]), primarily driven by a significant reduction in TVR (OR 0.44 [0.36–0.54]) with a nonsignificant trend toward a decrease in reinfarction (32).

Drug-Eluting Stents versus Bare-Metal Stents during Primary PCI

Stent placement in a highly thrombogenic milieu of the infarct-related artery may predispose to acute or late-stent thrombosis. Because the risk of stent thrombosis caused by bare-metal stents (BMSs) is greatest within the first 30 days after implantation, the use of thienopyridine (in addition to aspirin) is necessary for a minimum of 30 days. When BMSs are placed in the setting of STEMI, 1 year of dual antiplatelet therapy (DAPT) is recommended (Class I indication) based on the acute coronary syndrome. Aspirin should be continued indefinitely.

Drug-eluting stents (DESs), compared with BMSs, significantly reduce intimal proliferation, restenosis, and the need for TVR. In the acute setting of STEMI, controversy still exists regarding safety, and so DES placement should not be routine.

The safety of DES in STEMI has been studied in registries, RCT, and meta-analysis, with the general conclusion that DES do not significantly reduce mortality, but the benefit of DES lies with the reduction of restenosis (target lesion revascularization [TLR] and TVR). Stent thrombosis is still a concern.

Data from large STEMI registries have had conflicting findings regarding the mortality associated with DES compared with BMS when used for STEMI. The GRACE registry on 5,093 patients with STEMI showed propensity and risk-adjusted mortality that was similar between BMS and DES up to 6 months for DES compared, but late post-discharge mortality was higher in DES patients from 6 months to 2 years (HR 4.90; p = 0.01) or from 1 to 2 years (HR: 7.06; p = 0.02) (32). In contrast, a registry for Massachusetts State data, including 7,217 patients with STEMI, described in a matched-paired analysis that the 2-year risk-adjusted mortality was lower for patients who received a DES compared with those who received a BMS among patients with MI with ST-segment elevation (8.5% vs. 11.6%; p = 0.008) (33).

The HORIZONS-AMI study randomized (in a 3:1 ratio) 3,006 patients presenting with ST-segment elevation MI to receive paclitaxel-eluting stents or otherwise identical BMSs. The trial showed that placement of a paclitaxel-eluting stent rather than a BMS reduced the 1-year rates of ischemia-driven repeat target lesion (4.5% vs. 7.5%; HR 0.59; 95% CI 0.43–0.83; p = 0.002), TVR (5.8% vs. 8.7%; HR 0.65; 95% CI 0.48–0.89; p = 0.006), with no significant difference in rates of the composite safety endpoint (stent thrombosis, reinfarction, stroke, or death) (34). Patients had similar 12-month rates of death and stent thrombosis. The rate of 13-month angiographic binary restenosis was significantly decreased by DES compared with BMS (10.0% vs. 22.9%; HR 0.44; 95% CI 0.33–0.57; p < 0.001) (**Table 18.12**). Results at 3 years demonstrated that the use of paclitaxel-eluting stents significantly reduced the 3-year rates of ischemia-driven TLR from 15.1% to 9.4% (40% relative reduction) (**Fig. 18.8** and **Table 18.13**) (34).

The HORIZONS-AMI study also showed that patients who had a combination of risk factors associated with restenosis—insulin-dependent diabetes, small vessel size (≤3.0 mm), and long lesion length (≥30 mm)—benefited from DES rather than BMS for reducing TVR and angiographic restenosis. Patients without these risk factors had no benefit in terms of 1-year TLR with the use of DESs compared with BMSs (**Fig. 18.9**).

In summary, the benefit of DESs compared with BMSs in STEMI cases is for reducing restenosis and the need for repeat intervention (target vessel and target lesion). DESs do not reduce incidence of death or recurrent MI. Stent thrombosis does not appear to be increased with DESs over BMSs in randomized trials, although it remains a concern (see the discussion in the following section) in the real-world setting.

Risk of Stent Thrombosis in DESs for STEMI

The general risk of stent thrombosis is higher in STEMI patients than in elective PCI (with both BMSs and DESs). Although stent thrombosis rates in STEMI trials are higher than in trials of elective PCI (estimated 1-year risk is 3%–4% for STEMI vs. 0.5%–1.2% for elective setting), the rates of stent thrombosis do not appear to be higher with DES than with BMS in STEMI. Other lesion and patient subsets also have higher rates of thrombosis: smaller arteries (<2.5 mm diameter), longer lesions, bifurcations, and diabetics. These risk factors predict both stent thrombosis and restenosis. The greatest risk of stent thrombosis is within the first 30 days with BMS, and within the first year with DES, but ongoing incremental risk is observed.

The greatest risk for DES thrombosis is early discontinuation of DAPT associated with stent thrombosis rehospitalization and death (35–38). For example, in the Premier Registry, a surprisingly high number of DES-treated MI patients (13.6%) stopped their thienopyridine within 30 days. Patients who stopped this therapy by 30 days were more likely to die during the next year (7.5% vs. 0.7%; p < 0.0001; adjusted HR 9.0; 95% CI 1.3–60.6) or to be rehospitalized (23% vs. 14%; p = 0.08; adjusted HR >1.5; 95% CI 0.78–3.0) (37).

Adjunctive Therapies for Primary PCI

Management of Thrombus in STEMI

Previously, there was great enthusiasm for use of routine manual aspiration thrombectomy in the setting of STEMI, especially after

TABLE 18.12 Drug-Eluting Stents Compared with Bare-Metal Stents: 1- and 3-Year Results from the HORIZONS-AMI Study

	DES PACLITAXEL-ELUTING STENTS (%)	BMS	P	HAZARD RATIO (95% CI)
Ischemia-Driven Target Lesion Revascularization				
1 year	4.5	7.5	0.002	0.59 (0.43–0.83)
3 years	9.4	15.1	<0.0001	0.60 (0.48–0.76)
Ischemia-Driven Target Vessel Revascularization				
1 year	5.8	8.7	0.006	0.65 (0.48–0.89)
3 years	12.4	17	0.0003	
Death				
1 year	3.5	3.5	0.98	
3 years	5.6	6.6	0.31	
Reinfarction				
1 year	3.7	4.5	0.31	
3 years	7.0	6.6	0.77	
Death or Reinfarction				
1 year	6.8	7.0	0.83	
3 years	11.8	11.5	0.88	
Stroke				
1 year	1.0	0.7	0.39	
3 years	1.6	1.4	0.70	
Stent Thrombosis (Definite or Probable)				
1 year	3.2	3.4	0.77	
3 years	4.8	4.3	0.63	1.10 (0.74–1.65)
Safety MACE (Death, Reinfarction, Stroke, and Stent Thrombosis)				
1 year	8.1	8.0	0.92	1.02 (0.76–1.36)
3 years	13.6	12.9	0.66	

Results for 1-year differ in stent thrombosis, TLR from NEJM.
BMS, bare-metal stent; DES, drug-eluting stent; MACE, major adverse cardiac events; TLR, target lesion revascularization.
Data taken from: Stone GW, et al. Paclitaxel-eluting stents versus bare-metal stents in acute myocardial infarction. *N Engl J Med.* 2009;360:1946–1959; Stone GW, et al. Heparin plus a glycoprotein IIb/IIIa inhibitor versus bivalirudin monotherapy and paclitaxel-eluting stents versus bare-metal stents in acute myocardial infarction (HORIZONS-AMI): final 3-year results from a multicentre, randomised controlled trial. *Lancet.* 2011;377(9784):2193–2204, with permission.

TABLE 18.13 Meta-analysis of Drug-Eluting Compared with Bare-Metal Stent Use during Primary PCI: Long-Term (>3 years) Follow-up of Major Randomized Clinical Trials

TRIAL	DEATH OR (95% CI)	TVR OR (95% CI)	STENT THROMBOSIS[a]
Dedication	1.73 (0.97–3.08)	0.40 (0.25–0.64)	0.90 (0.36–2.24)
Paseo	0.65 (0.29–1.49)	0.24 (0.11–0.54)	0.49 (0.07–3.57)
Strategy	1.19 (0.54–2.62)	0.33 (0.14–0.75)	0.86 (0.28–2.66)
Sesami	0.61 (0.20–1.92)	0.46 (0.23–0.92)	1.00 (0.37–2.73)
Mission	0.69 (0.25–1.85)	0.54 (0.27–1.09)	1.69 (0.40–7.20)
Typhoon	0.61 (0.27–1.36)	0.49 (0.30–0.80)	0.92 (0.42–2.00)
Passion	0.75 (0.45–1.27)	0.73 (0.42–1.26)	1.19 (0.52–2.69)
Meta-analysis	0.89 (0.64–1.24)	0.46 (0.36–0.58)	0.99 (0.68–1.45)

[a]Definition of stent thrombosis differed among studies.
PCI, percutaneous coronary intervention; TVR, target vessel revascularization.
Modified from: Ziada KM, Charnigo R, Moliterno DJ. Long-term follow-up of drug-eluting stents placed in the setting of ST-segment elevation myocardial infarction. *JACC Cardiovasc Interv.* 2011;4(1):39–41, with permission.

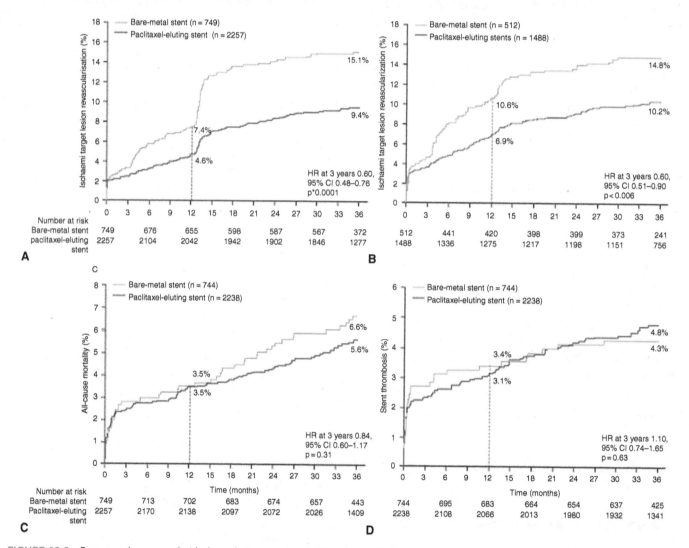

FIGURE 18.8 Bare-metal compared with drug-eluting stenting during primary PCI for STEMI in the HORIZONS-AMI study. Shown are the time-to-event curves for 3 years for major bleeding not related to coronary artery bypass graft surgery **(A)**, cardiac mortality **(B)**, reinfarction **(C)**, and definite or probable stent thrombosis **(D)** in patients randomized to heparin plus a GPI or bivalirudin monotherapy. GPI, glycoprotein IIb/IIIa inhibitor; HR, hazard ratio; PCI, percutaneous coronary intervention; STEMI, ST-elevation myocardial infarction. The vertical dotted line shows the 1-year event rate. One-year rates are also displayed. Also, see **Table 18.12.** (From: Stone GW, et al. Heparin plus a glycoprotein IIb/IIIa inhibitor versus bivalirudin monotherapy and paclitaxel-eluting stents versus bare-metal stents in acute myocardial infarction (HORIZONS-AMI): final 3-year results from a multicentre, randomised controlled trial. *Lancet.* 2011;377(9784):2193–2204, with permission.)

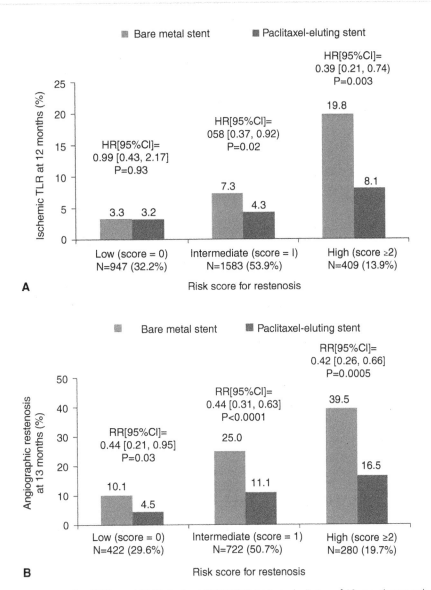

FIGURE 18.9 Risk for restenosis comparing DESs and BMSs in the HORIZONS-AMI study. Rates of 12-month target-lesion revascularization (TLR) and 13-month angiographic restenosis. **A:** Rates of 12-month ischemic TLR and **B:** 13-month angiographic restenosis in patients randomly allocated to paclitaxel-eluting stents (*red bars*) or to bare-metal stents (*blue bars*), according to the risk strata for restenosis. BMSs, bare-metal stents; CI, confidence interval; DESs, drug-eluting stents; HR, hazard ratio; RR, relative risk; RVD, reference vessel diameter. Low-, intermediate-, and high-risk groups for restenosis were created using three variables (one point each): (a) RVD <3.0 mm, (b) lesion length >30 mm, and (c) insulin-treated diabetes. Patients with 0, 1, and >2 of these three risk factors were defined as being at low, intermediate, or high risk for TLR and restenosis, respectively. (From: Stone, et al. Selection criteria for drug-eluting versus bare-metal stents and the impact of routine angiographic follow-up: 2-year insights from the HORIZONS-AMI (Harmonizing Outcomes With Revascularization and Stents in Acute Myocardial Infarction) trial. *J Am Coll Cardiol.* 2010;56:1597–1604, with permission.)

the results of the TAPAS trial (39,40) came out in 2008. TAPAS was a large single-center study that randomized 1,071 STEMI patients to aspiration thrombectomy prior to primary PCI versus primary PCI only and demonstrated that aspiration thrombectomy provided improved TVR with improved myocardial blush and ST-segment resolution, as well as lower mortality in those with better myocardial blush grade and ST segment resolution. In this setting, aspiration thrombectomy had a Class IIa recommendation in the 2013 STEMI guidelines, but subsequent negative trials resulted in a change in the guidelines. The TASTE trial (n = 7,244) (30,31) was a large RCT published in 2013 comparing routine aspiration thrombectomy before primary PCI to primary PCI only and showed no difference in 30 days, as well as 1 year, in death, hospitalization for recurrent MI, stent thrombosis, TVR, or MACE between the two

groups (**Fig. 18.10**) (62). Another large RCT comparing manual thrombectomy versus PCI alone in STEMI was the TOTAL trial (n = 10,732) (41). Published in 2015, it showed similar results to TASTE, with no difference in the primary outcome of death from cardiovascular causes, recurrent MI, cardiogenic shock, or NYHA class IV HF within 180 days. TOTAL also showed an increased risk of stroke within 30 days in patients receiving manual thrombectomy (0.7% vs. 0.3%, HR 2.06; 95% CI 1.13–3.75; p = 0.02) (63). Finally, an updated meta-analysis (42) was performed, which included the new trials mentioned earlier and found no significant reduction in death, reinfarction, or stent thrombosis with routine aspiration thrombectomy prior to primary PCI. In addition, the study showed a small but nonsignificant increase risk of stroke in patients receiving aspiration thrombectomy. With this newly available data, the 2015

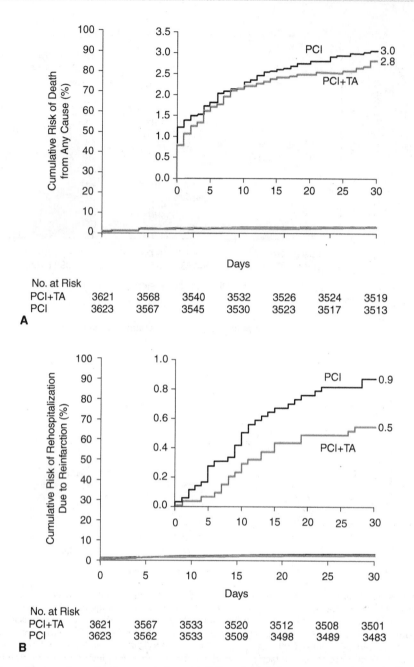

FIGURE 18.10 Kaplan–Meier curves are shown for the cumulative probability of death from any cause **(A)** and of hospitalization due to reinfarction **(B)** up to 30 days after PCI only (PCI) or after PCI with thrombus aspiration (PCI + TA). The insets show the same data on an enlarged y axis. PCI, percutaneous coronary interventions. (From: Fröbert O, et al. Thrombus aspiration during ST-segment elevation myocardial infarction. N Engl J Med. 2013;369(17):1587–1597, with permission.)

STEMI guideline changed the prior Class IIa recommendation for aspiration thrombectomy in STEMI patients. Now, routine aspiration thrombectomy before primary PCI is *not* recommended (Class III; no benefit, LOE A). Selective or bailout thrombectomy has a Class IIb recommendation and can be considered, but its usefulness is not well-established.

Rheolytic thrombectomy removes thrombus by using high-velocity saline jets around the catheter tip that entrain thrombus toward the inflow windows. Routine rheolytic thrombectomy for acute MI has not consistently been demonstrated to improve outcomes. In early meta-analysis of rheolytic therapy involving small studies and one larger study (AIMI study), it was associated with increased mortality risk

(43). No clinical benefit for routine (i.e., all cases, not those selected by thrombus burden) rheolytic thrombectomy (AngioJet device, Boston Scientific, Marlborough MA) has been demonstrated in primary PCI, and routine use is not recommended in current guidelines. Selective use in cases of large thrombus burden may be beneficial.

Three principal categories of embolic protection devices devices exist: proximal occlusive devices, distal occlusive devices, and filter-based systems. Embolic protection devices have been clearly demonstrated to be advantageous during saphenous vein graft (SVG) interventions. Nevertheless, their effectiveness during primary PCI in native coronary arteries has not been shown in randomized clinical trials (neutral effect) (44).

Pharmacologic Therapies

Parenteral Anticoagulants

This group includes unfractionated heparin (UFH), direct thrombin inhibitors such as bivalirudin, and fondaparinux (a direct factor Xa inhibitor). A number of trials have evaluated the safety and efficacy of parenteral anticoagulants in the setting of primary PCI for STEMI. The HERO-1 (45) and HERO-2 trials (46), comparing bivalirudin with heparin among STEMI patients receiving aspirin and streptokinase, showed higher coronary patency rates at 90 to 120 minutes, and had sustained coronary patency at 3 days among bivalirudin recipients. In order to further investigate the efficacy of bivalirudin in the setting of STEMI, the HORIZONS-AMI trial was performed and published in 2008 (47). This pivotal trial prospectively compared UFH in combination with a GP IIb/IIIa inhibitor with bivalirudin (primarily as monotherapy although with provisional abciximab or double-bolus eptifibatide), among 3,600 patients. The primary endpoint of composite major bleeding plus MACE (death, reinfarction, TVR for ischemia, and stroke) within 30 days was lower among bivalirudin recipients (9% vs. 12%), largely because of lower rates of major bleeding both at 30 days (5% vs. 8.4%) and at 1 year

(6% vs. 9%) (Fig. 18.11). There was no significant difference in MACE alone (5.5% vs. 5.5%). There was a significant absolute 1% increased rate of stent thrombosis within the first 24 hours with the use of bivalirudin (1.3% vs. 0.3%, p < 0.001), but there was no significant difference between the two groups beyond this period. Finally, cardiac mortality (1.8% vs. 2.9%) and all-cause mortality (2.1% vs. 3.1%) rates were both significantly lower in the bivalirudin group. At 3 years, bivalirudin had lower rates of all-cause mortality (5.9% vs. 7.7%, HR 0.75 [0.58–0.97]; p = 0.03), cardiac mortality (2.9% vs. 5.1%, HR 0.56 [0.40–0.80]; p = 0.001), reinfarction, and major bleeding (not related to bypass graft surgery), with no significant differences in ischemia-driven TVR, stent thrombosis, or composite adverse events (MACE 21.9% vs. 21.8%, p = 0.95) (48).

Two subsequent clinical trials did not find superiority of bivalirudin compared with heparin. The HEAT-PPCI study was a randomized, single-center study comparing heparin to bivalirudin (similar use of GP IIb/IIIa inhibitors in both groups at 13% and 15%) (49). The primary efficacy outcome (composite of all-cause mortality, cerebrovascular accident, reinfarction, or unplanned TLR at 28 days) occurred in 8.7% in the bivalirudin group and 5.7% in the heparin group (absolute risk difference 3.0%; RR 1.52, 95% CI 1.09–2.13, p = 0.01). Notably, the rates of acute stent thrombosis were 3.4%

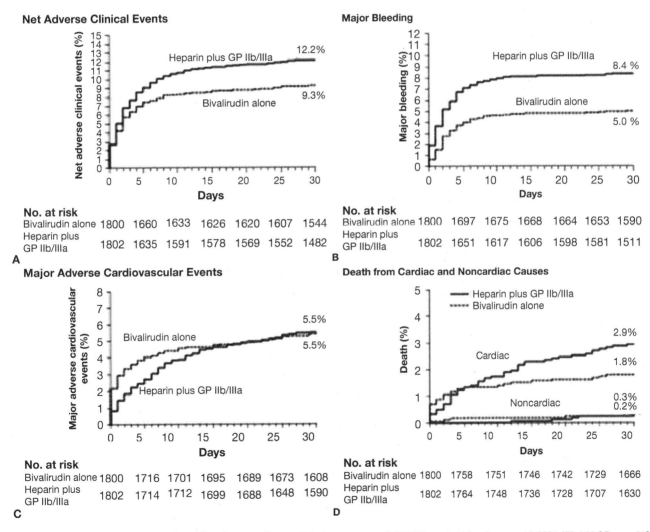

FIGURE 18.11 Time-to-event through 30 days for net adverse clinical events, p = 0.006 **(A)**, major bleeding, p < 0.0001 **(B)**, MACE, p = NS **(C)**, and death from cardiac causes, p = 0.03, **(D)**. GP, glycoprotein; MACE, major adverse cardiac events. (Reproduced from: Stone GW, et al. Bivalirudin during primary PCI in acute myocardial infarction. *N Engl J Med.* 2008;358(21):2218–2230, with permission.)

versus 0.9% (p = 0.001), and acute stent thrombosis 2.9% versus 0.9% (p = 0.007), and reinfarction 2.7% versus 0.9%, (p = 0.004), favoring the use of heparin. There was no difference in major bleeding (BARC 3–5) at 3.5% versus 3.1% (p = 0.59).

The MATRIX trial also demonstrated no significant difference in outcomes or net adverse clinical events with heparin (and discretionary use of GP IIb/IIIa inhibitors) versus bivalirudin in 7,213 acute coronary syndrome patients (over one-half were STEMI). Neither MACE (10.3% and 10.9%, respectively, p = 0.44) or net adverse clinical events (NACE) (composite of major bleeding or MACE) were different (NACE 11.2% and 12.4%; p = 0.12). The rate of definite stent thrombosis was significantly higher in the bivalirudin group than in the heparin group. Post-PCI bivalirudin infusion, as compared with no infusion, did not significantly decrease the rate of urgent TVR, definite stent thrombosis, or net adverse clinical events (11.0% and 11.9%, respectively; RR, 0.91; 95% CI, 0.74–1.11; p = 0.34). Nevertheless, bivalirudin was associated with a lower rate of death from any cause than was heparin (1.7% vs. 2.3%; rate ratio, 0.71; 95% CI 0.51–0.99; p = 0.04), cardiac death (1.5% vs. 2.2%; p = 0.03), and major bleeding (BARC 3 or 5) (1.4% vs. 2.5%; p < 0.001) (50). In summary, controversy still exists regarding the use of bivalirudin versus heparin, but bleeding does seem to be reduced and stent thrombosis increased with the use of bivalirudin.

TABLE 18.14 2013 ACC/AHA STEMI Guideline Recommendations for Antithrombotic Therapy for Primary PCI

RECOMMENDATIONS	COR	LOE
Antiplatelet Therapy		
Aspirin		
162–325 mg load before procedure	I	B
81–325 mg daily maintenance dose (indefinite)[a]	I	A
81 mg daily is the preferred maintenance dose[a]	IIa	B
P2Y$_{12}$ Inhibitors		
Loading doses		
Clopidogrel: 600 mg as early as possible or at time of PCI	I	B
Prasugrel: 60 mg as early as possible or at time of PCI	I	B
Ticagrelor: 180 mg as early as possible or at time of PCI	I	B
Maintenance Doses		
Clopidogrel: 75 mg daily	I	B
Prasugrel: 10 mg daily	I	B
Ticagrelor: 90 mg twice a day[a]	I	B
Patients with STEMI with prior stroke or TIA: prasugrel	III: harm	B
IV GP IIb/IIIa Receptor Antagonist in Conjunction with UFH or Bivalirudin in Selected Patients		
Abciximab: 0.25 mg/kg IV bolus, then 0.125 µg/kg/min (maximum 10 µg/min)	IIa	A
Tirofiban (high-dose bolus) 25 µg/kg IV bolus, then 0.15 µg/kg/min	IIa	B
• In patients with CrCl <30 mL/min, reduce infusion by 50%		
Eptifibatide: (double bolus): 180 µg/kg IV bolus, then 2 µg/kg/min; a second 180 µg/kg bolus is administered 10 minutes after the bolus	IIa	B
• In patients with CrCl <50 mL/min, reduce infusion by 50%		
• Avoid in patients on hemodialysis		
Pre-catheterization laboratory administration of IV GP IIb/IIIa receptor antagonist	IIb	B
Intracoronary abciximab 0.25 mg/kg bolus	IIb	B
Anticoagulant Therapy		
UFH:		
• With GP IIb/IIIa receptor antagonist planned: 50–70 U/kg IV bolus to achieve therapeutic ACT (200–250 seconds)	I	C
• With no GP IIb/IIIa receptor antagonist planned: 70–100 U/kg bolus to achieve therapeutic ACT (250–300 seconds)	I	C
Bivalirudin: 0.75 mg/kg IV bolus, then 1.75 mg/kg/h infusion with or without prior treatment with UFH. An additional bolus of 0.3 mg/kg may be given if needed.	I	B
• Reduce infusion to 1 mg/kg/h with estimated CrCl <30 mL/min		
• Referred over UFH with GP IIb/IIIa receptor antagonist in patients at high risk of bleeding	IIa	B
Fondaparinux: not recommended as sole anticoagulant for primary PCI	III: harm	B

[a]The recommended maintenance dose of aspirin to be used with ticagrelor is 81 mg daily.

ACT, activated clotting time; COR, class of recommendation; GP, glycoprotein; LOE, level of evidence; PCI, percutaneous coronary intervention; STEMI, ST-segment elevation myocardial infarction; UFH, unfractionated heparin.

Modified from: O'Gara PT, et al. 2013 ACCF/AHA guideline for the management of ST-elevation myocardial infarction. *Circulation.* 2013;127(4):e362–e425, with permission.

Finally, fondaparinux was compared with UFH in the OASIS-6 trial (51). Importantly, patients who received fondaparinux and underwent primary PCI had a significantly higher risk of guiding-catheter thrombosis (0 vs. 22, p < 0.001) and coronary complications such as abrupt closure, new angiographic thrombus, catheter thrombus, no reflow, dissection, or perforation (225 vs. 270, p = 0.04). Thus, the latest guidelines recommend against the use of fondaparinux as the sole anticoagulant during PCI (Class III indication, ACC/AHA 2007 STEMI Guidelines Focused Update). **Table 18.14** shows the current recommendations regarding anticoagulation therapy during PCI for STEMI.

Antiplatelet Agents in Primary PCI

Oral and parenteral antiplatelet agents play a crucial role as adjunctive therapies in primary PCI for STEMI. The basic mechanisms of the various agents are summarized in **Figure 18.12** (52) and are discussed in detail in Chapter 3. The following agents will be discussed in this section: GP IIb/IIIa inhibitors (eptifibatide, abciximab, tirofiban), thienopyridines (clopidogrel, prasugrel), aspirin, and ticagrelor.

Only a few trials have studied GP IIb/IIIa inhibitors in conjunction with oral antiplatelet therapies. The BRAVE-3 trial studied 800 patients pretreated with 600 mg of clopidogrel randomly assigned to either abciximab or placebo prior to PCI (53). At 30 days, the composite of death, recurrent MI, stroke, or urgent revascularization of the infarct-related artery was not significantly different. There was also no difference in infarct size or major bleeding.

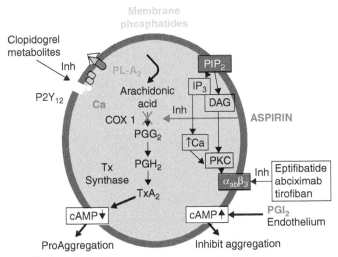

FIGURE 18.12 Activation of phospholipase A2 liberates arachidonic acid (AA) from the cell membrane. AA then metabolizes to thromboxane A2 (TxA2) by cyclooxygenase (COX), which is inhibited by aspirin (AS). TxA2 is a potent platelet agonist and vasoconstrictor. When ADP is released from activated platelets, it binds to the P2Y$_{12}$ receptor of circulating platelets which initiates platelet aggregation and amplification. Clopidogrel, prasugrel, and ticlopidine all irreversibly bind the P2Y$_{12}$ receptor, thereby preventing ADP. Ticagrelor, in contrast, is a reversible P2Y$_{12}$ receptor inhibitor. Inosine diphosphate (IP2) is released after activation of the P2Y$_{12}$ receptor. IP2 is phosphorylated to IP3. The release of both IP3 and diacylglycerol leads to activation of protein kinase C (PKC) and to the eventual activation of GP IIb/IIIa, which permits its binding to fibrinogen, the final step in platelet activation and aggregation. ADP, adenosine diphosphate; GP, glycoprotein. (Redrawn from: Dupont AG, Gabriel DA, Cohen MG. Antiplatelet therapies and the role of antiplatelet resistance in acute coronary syndrome. *Thromb Res.* 2009;124(1):6–13, with permission.)

The On-TIME 2 study randomized 491 patients to tirofiban versus placebo prior to primary PCI. All patients received IV heparin bolus, aspirin, and 600-mg clopidogrel prior to randomization (54). Tirofiban recipients had improved ST-segment resolution before and after PCI; nevertheless, there were no significant differences in TIMI grade 3 coronary flow, major or minor bleeding rates, or in death, recurrent MI, or urgent TVR. A meta-analysis by Gurm et al. (55) compared abciximab with small molecule GP IIb/IIIa inhibitors (eptifibatide or tirofiban). There were no differences in 30-day mortality (1.9% small molecule vs. 2.3% abciximab, p = NS) or in reinfarction rates (1.3% vs. 1.2%, p = NS). Rates of TVR were identical (1.7%) for both groups. Both major and minor bleeding rates were similar for both groups. Finally, one study, FINESSE, investigated the issue of timing of a GP IIb/IIIa antagonist administration (56). This double-blind, placebo-controlled study randomized 2,453 patients to pre-PCI treatment with half-dose fibrinolysis plus abciximab, pre-PCI abciximab alone, and abciximab during the time of PCI. The primary endpoint was a composite of all-cause death, ventricular function >48 hours after randomization, cardiogenic shock, and CHF during the first 90 days of randomization. The trial showed no benefit (including mortality) with pre-PCI abciximab compared with abciximab at the time of PCI. Based on the preceding studies, among others, the guideline writing committee concluded that the various GP IIb/IIIa antagonists have similar efficacy and that in the setting of DAPT, it is reasonable to start treatment with GP IIb/IIIa antagonists at the time of primary PCI (with or without stenting) in selected patients such as those with large thrombus burden (Class IIa indication).

The TRITON-TIMI 38 trial evaluated the safety and efficacy of the most recent member of the thienopyridine family, prasugrel (57). This double-blinded study randomized 13,600 acute coronary syndrome patients to prasugrel (loading dose 60 mg followed by 10 mg daily) versus clopidogrel (loading dose 300 mg followed by 75 mg daily) for 6 to 15 months. Twenty-six percent of patients in the TRITON-TIMI 38 trial presented with STEMI. In the overall cohort, the primary efficacy endpoint of death from cardiovascular causes, nonfatal MI, or nonfatal stroke was seen in 12.1% of clopidogrel patients and in 9.9% of prasugrel patients (p < 0.001); there was a significant benefit of prasugrel seen in the STEMI subset as well. The benefit of prasugrel in the primary efficacy endpoint was seen within the first 24 hours of randomization and persisted through 15 months of follow-up (**Fig. 18.13**). The difference in the primary endpoint was largely due to the reduction in MI among prasugrel recipients (7.4% vs. 9.7%, p < 0.001). Subgroups of patients also had a significant benefit with prasugrel, and this included diabetics and patients receiving GP IIb/IIIa inhibitors. Rates of stent thrombosis (definite or probable) were also reduced in the prasugrel group (1.1% vs. 2.4%, p < 0.001). These improved efficacy outcomes, but did come at a price with respect to safety endpoints. Major bleeding was seen in 2.4% of prasugrel patients compared with 1.8% seen in the clopidogrel group, and life-threatening bleeding, including both fatal and nonfatal bleeding rates, was also higher among prasugrel recipients. Three groups in particular were found not to have a net clinical benefit from prasugrel: patients with a prior transient ischemic attack (TIA) or stroke, patients weighing <60 kg, and patients >75 years of age. Patients with prior TIA or stroke were in fact found to have net harm from prasugrel. Based on these data, the US Food and Drug Administration (FDA) declared prasugrel to be contraindicated in these patients (57).

Finally, no up-to-date discussion on antiplatelet therapies for STEMI would be complete without mention of ticagrelor, a reversible

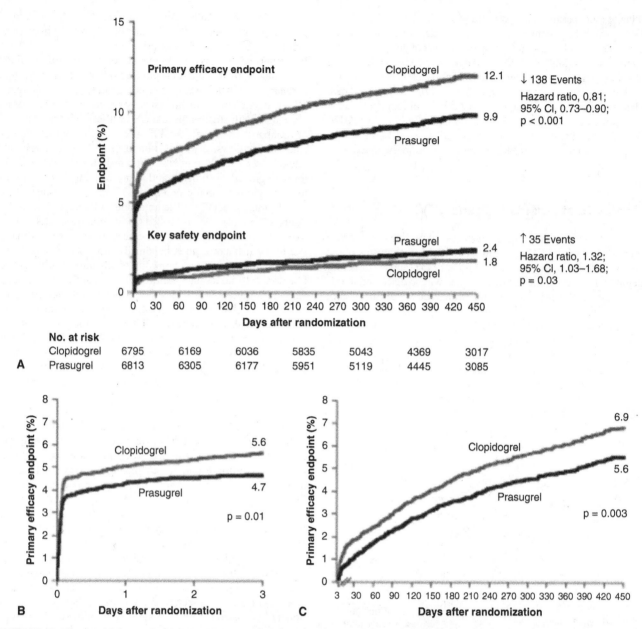

FIGURE 18.13 Kaplan–Meier survival curves comparing clopidogrel and prasugrel. Panel A shows data for the primary efficacy end point (death from cardiovascular causes, nonfatal myocardial infarction [MI], or nonfatal stroke) (top) and for the key safety end point (Thrombolysis in Myocardial Infarction [TIMI] major bleeding not related to coronary-artery bypass grafting) (bottom) during the full follow-up period. The hazard ratio for prasugrel, as compared with clopidogrel, for the primary efficacy end point at 30 days was 0.77 (95% confidence interval [CI], 0.67 to 0.88; P>0.001) and at 90 days was 0.80 (95% CI, 0.71 to 0.90; P<0.001). Data for the primary efficacy end point are also shown from the time of randomization to day 3 (Panel B) and from 3 days to 15 months, with all end points occurring before day 3 censored (Panel C). In Panel C, the number at risk includes all patients who were alive (regardless of whether a nonfatal event had occurred during the first 3 days after randomization) and had not withdrawn consent for follow-up. The P values in Panel A for the primary efficacy end point were calculated with the use of the Gehan–Wilcoxon test; all other P values were calculated with the use of the log-rank test. (Reproduced from: Wiviott SD, et al. Prasugrel versus clopidogrel in patients with acute coronary syndromes. *N Engl J Med.* 2007;357(20):2001–2015, with permission.)

P2Y$_{12}$ inhibitor. This medication was recently tested in the PLATO trial, which randomized 18,600 patients with the acute coronary syndrome to either clopidogrel (300-mg or 600-mg loading dose, followed by 75 mg daily) or ticagrelor (180-mg loading dose, followed by 90 mg twice daily) (58). A total of 38% of patients presented with STEMI. The primary endpoint of death from vascular causes or cerebrovascular causes, or death from an unknown cause, was seen in 9.8% in the ticagrelor group versus 11.7% in the clopidogrel group (p < 0.001), with the difference in treatment effect being apparent within the first 30 days of therapy. Furthermore,

the composite of all-cause death, MI, or stroke was also reduced in the ticagrelor group (10.2% vs. 12.3%, p < 0.001). Rates of stent thrombosis were also lower among those who received ticagrelor (1.3% vs. 1.9%, p = 0.009). The rates of major bleeding and TIMI major bleeding were also similar between the two groups. Although intracranial bleeding episodes were more common among ticagrelor recipients, there were no significant differences in the rates of stroke, including hemorrhagic stroke. Based on the PLATO trial, ticagrelor was FDA-approved for patients with acute coronary syndromes as of July 2011. Table 18.14 includes the latest ACC/AHA guideline

TABLE 18.15 Recommendations for DAPT in ACS Patients from the 2016 ACC/AHA Focused Update on DAPT Duration in ACS Patients

RECOMMENDATIONS FOR DURATION OF DAPT IN PATIENTS WITH ACS TREATED WITH FIBRINOLYTIC THERAPY		
RECOMMENDATION	COR	LOE
In patients with STEMI treated with DAPT in conjunction with fibrinolytic therapy, P2Y$_{12}$ inhibitor therapy (clopidogrel) should be continued for a minimum of 14 days (level of evidence: A) and ideally at least 12 months (level of evidence: C).	I	A C
In patients treated with DAPT, a daily aspirin dose of 81 mg (range, 75–100 mg) is recommended.	I	B
In patients with STEMI treated with fibrinolytic therapy who have tolerated DAPT without bleeding complications and who are not at high bleeding risk (e.g., prior bleeding on DAPT, coagulopathy, oral anticoagulant use), continuation of DAPT for longer than 12 months may be reasonable	IIb	A
Recommendations for Duration of DAPT in Patients with ACS Treated with PCI		
In patients with ACS treated with DAPT after BMS or DES implantation, P2Y$_{12}$ inhibitor therapy (clopidogrel, prasugrel, or ticagrelor) should be given for at least 12 months.	I	B
In patients treated with DAPT, a daily aspirin dose of 81 mg (range, 75–100 mg) is recommended.	I	B
In patients with ACS treated with DAPT after coronary stent implantation, it is reasonable to use ticagrelor in preference to clopidogrel for maintenance P2Y$_{12}$ inhibitor therapy.	IIa	B
In patients with ACS treated with DAPT after coronary stent implantation, who are not at high risk for bleeding complications and who do not have a history of stroke or TIA, it is reasonable to choose prasugrel over clopidogrel for maintenance P2Y$_{12}$ inhibitor therapy.	IIa	B
In patients with ACS treated with coronary stent implantation who have tolerated DAPT without bleeding complications and who are not at high bleeding risk (e.g., prior bleeding on DAPT, coagulopathy, oral anticoagulant use), continuation of DAPT for longer than 12 months may be reasonable.	IIb	A
In patients with ACS treated with DAPT after DES implantation who develop a high risk of bleeding (e.g., treatment with oral anticoagulant therapy), are at high risk of severe bleeding complications (e.g., major intracranial surgery), or develop significant overt bleeding, discontinuation of P2Y$_{12}$ therapy after 6 months may be reasonable.	IIb	C
Prasugrel should not be administered to patients with a prior history of stroke or TIA.	III: harm	B

ACS, acute coronary syndrome; BMS, bare-metal stent; DAPT, dual antiplatelet therapy; DESs, drug-eluting stents; PCI, percutaneous coronary intervention; STEMI, ST-elevation myocardial infarction; TIA, transient ischemic attack.
Modified from: Levine GN, et al. 2016 ACC/AHA guideline focused update on duration of dual antiplatelet therapy in patients with coronary artery disease. *J Am Coll Cardiol.* 2016;68(10):1082.

recommendations for antithrombotic therapy at the time of PCI based on the preceding data.

In 2016, the ACC/AHA released a focused guideline update on duration of DAPT in patients with CAD (59). The recommendations are summarized in Table 18.15.

Adjunctive Antithrombotics to Support Reperfusion with Fibrinolytic Therapy

Therapy

Fibrinolytic therapy (fibrin-specific agents preferred—see Chapter 4) requires the concurrent use of adjunctive antiplatelet and/or anticoagulant therapies to optimize the effectiveness of reperfusion and prevent reocclusion. Further details regarding anticoagulation, fibrinolysis, and antiplatelet therapy can be found in Chapters 3 and 4.

Adjunctive Anticoagulant Therapy with Fibrinolysis

A number of anticoagulants now have proven efficacy when used concurrently with fibrinolysis agents with class I indications for use with fibrinolysis. These include UFH, enoxaparin, and fondaparinux. Anticoagulant therapy is generally recommended for

a minimum of 48 hours, and preferably for the duration of the index hospitalization, up to 8 days or until revascularization. It is important for the interventionalist performing early or rescue PCI in patients treated with fibrinolytics to be aware of the anticoagulant used, and make changes if necessary during PCI (see Chapter 4). Specifically, fondaparinux should not be used as the sole anticoagulant during PCI. For Enoxaparin, additional intravenous dose may be required in subsequent PCI.

Antiplatelet Agents in STEMI Treated with Fibrinolysis

The beneficial effects of aspirin are well established. The evidence in favor of the use of thienopyridines in addition to aspirin in the setting of STEMI treated with fibrinolysis is also compelling. The COMMIT-CCS-2 study randomized 45,852 patients in China to clopidogrel, 75 mg daily (treatment was to continue until discharge or up to 4 weeks in hospital), with no loading dose versus placebo in addition to aspirin (162 mg/day). Use of clopidogrel produced a highly significant 9% (CI 3–14) reduction in death, reinfarction, or stroke (2,121 [9.2%] clopidogrel vs. 2,310 [10.1%] placebo; p = 0.002), and a significant 7% reduction in any death (1,726 [7.5%] vs. 1,845 [8.1%]; p = 0.03). There was no significant increase risk of major bleeding (60).

In addition, in 1,863 patients <75 years of age undergoing PCI after mandatory angiography in the CLARITY-TIMI 28 trial to either clopidogrel (300-mg oral loading dose followed by 75 mg daily) or placebo (61), the primary efficacy endpoint was a composite of an occluded infarct-related artery (defined TIMI flow grade of 0 or 1) on angiography or death or recurrent MI before angiography. This totaled 21.7% in the placebo group and 15.0% in the clopidogrel group, representing a 36% reduction in the odds of the endpoint with clopidogrel. The primary 30-day outcome of the composite of cardiovascular death, recurrent MI, or stroke from PCI to 30 days post-randomization was seen in 3.6% in the clopidogrel group versus 6.2% in the placebo group (p = 0.008). Pre-treatment with clopidogrel additionally reduced the incidence of MI or stroke prior to PCI (4.0% vs. 6.2%, p = 0.03), with no significant difference in both major and minor bleeding risks. Hence, current dosing recommendations are 75 mg/day for 14 days (Class I), with a 300-mg load if patients are <75 years of age. Duration is daily 75 mg for 14 days (Class I) up to one year (Class IIa).

Despite its widespread use as a comparator for newer P2Y$_{12}$ antagonists, clopidogrel has not been rigorously compared against placebo in STEMI patients treated with primary PCI (as opposed to fibrinolytics).

Key Points

- Time-independent benefits of opening the artery have also been suggested to exist, which include improving infarct healing, electrical stability, and reducing in reinfarction.

- Compared with fibrinolytic therapy, primary PCI is able to achieve higher rates of TIMI grade 3 flow and infarct artery patency, and lower rates of reinfarction, recurrent ischemia, intracranial hemorrhage, and death in randomized clinical trials.

- Current guidelines recommend a systems goal of 90 minutes or less from the first medical contact to balloon angioplasty for hospitals that perform primary PCI.

- Primary PCI without surgical backup should not be performed at institutions without a proven plan for rapid transport to a cardiac surgery hospital or without appropriate hemodynamic support capability for transfer.

- Primary PCI is indicated for patients presenting within 12 to 24 hours of symptom onset and ongoing ischemia. There is an indication for primary PCI in 12 to 24 hours with either clinical or electrocardiographic evidence of ongoing myocardial injury.

- Facilitated PCI is not beneficial compared with primary PCI.

- Current guidelines recommend the transfer of high-risk patients who receive fibrinolytic therapy as primary reperfusion therapy at a non-PCI-capable facility to a PCI-capable facility as soon as possible, where either PCI can be performed.

- PCI is reasonable in patients with acute STEMI when an unprotected left main coronary artery is the culprit lesion, distal coronary flow is less than TIMI grade 3, and PCI can be performed more rapidly and safely than CABG.

- PCI in a non-infarct artery at the time of primary PCI or staged during the same hospitalization has been shown to have benefits in more recent trials and now has a Class IIb recommendation and can be considered at the time of primary PCI.

- Compared with BMSs in STEMI cases, DESs reduce restenosis and the need for repeat intervention (target vessel and target lesion). DESs do not reduce the incidence of death or recurrent MI. Stent thrombosis does not appear to be increased with DESs over BMSs in randomized trials.

- Regarding routine aspiration thrombectomy, more recent trials have demonstrated no benefit in the setting of STEMI and it now has a Class III (harm) recommendation. Bailout or selective thrombectomy has a Class IIb recommendation and can be considered.

- Meta-analyses have not demonstrated a consistent clinical benefit to the use rheolytic thrombectomy (mechanical thrombectomy) or embolic protection devices in STEMI.

- For patients undergoing primary PCI for STEMI, anticoagulation with either UFH or bivalirudin should be given in order to reach a therapeutic activating clotting time. Both anticoagulants have proven beneficial in the setting of STEMI; however, bivalirudin has been shown to be associated with less major bleeding both at 30 days and at 1 year.

- Compared with clopidogrel, prasugrel has been found to have reduced rates of death from cardiovascular causes, nonfatal MI, or nonfatal stroke. Nevertheless, patients >75 years, prior stroke, or <60 kg should avoid prasugrel, in particular, patients with a prior TIA or cerebrovascular accident.

References

1. O'Gara, et al. 2013 ACCF/AHA guideline for the management of ST-elevation myocardial infarction. *Circulation.* 2013;127(4):e362–e425.
2. Keeley EC, Boura JA, Grines CL. Primary angioplasty versus intravenous thrombolytic therapy for acute myocardial infarction: a quantitative review of 23 randomized trials. *Lancet.* 2003;361:13–20.
3. Brodie BR, et al. Door-to-balloon time with primary percutaneous coronary intervention for acute myocardial infarction impacts late cardiac mortality in high-risk patients and patients presenting early after the onset of symptoms. *J Am Coll Cardiol.* 2006;47:289–295.
4. Rathore SS, et al. Association of door-to-balloon time and mortality in patients admitted to hospital with ST elevation myocardial infarction: national cohort study. *BMJ.* 2009;338:b1807.
5. Terkelsen CJ, et al. System delay and mortality among patients with STEMI treated with primary percutaneous coronary intervention. *JAMA.* 2010;304(7):763–771.
6. Blankenship JC, et al. Door-to-balloon times under 90 min can be routinely achieved for patients transferred for ST-segment elevation myocardial infarction percutaneous coronary intervention in a rural setting. *J Am Coll Cardiol.* 2011;57:272–279.
7. Concannon TW, et al. A percutaneous coronary intervention lab in every hospital? *Circ Cardiovasc Qual Outcomes.* 2012;5(1):14–20.
8. Henry TD, et al. A regional system to provide timely access to percutaneous coronary intervention for ST-elevation myocardial infarction. *Circulation.* 2007;116:721–728.
9. Dehmer GJ, et al. The current status and future direction of percutaneous coronary intervention without on-site surgical backup: an expert consensus document from the Society for Cardiovascular Angiography and Interventions. *Catheter Cardiovasc Interv.* 2007;69:471–478.
10. Hochman JS, et al. Early revascularization in acute myocardial infarction complicated by cardiogenic shock. SHOCK investigators. Should we emergently revascularize occluded coronaries for cardiogenic shock. *N Engl J Med.* 1999;341:625–634.
11. Armstrong PW, et al. Fibrinolysis or primary PCI in ST-segment elevation myocardial infarction. *N Engl J Med.* 2013;368(15):1379–1387.
12. Dehmer GJ, et al. SCAI/ACC/AHA expert consensus document. *Catheter Cardiovasc Interv.* 2014;84(2):169–187.

13. Harold JG, et al. ACCF/AHA/SCAI 2013 update of the clinical competence statement on coronary artery interventional procedures. *Catheter Cardiovasc Interv.* 2013;82(2):E69–E111.

14. Sutton AG, et al. A randomized trial of rescue angioplasty versus a conservative approach for failed fibrinolysis in ST-segment elevation myocardial infarction: the Middlesbrough Early Revascularization to Limit INfarction (MERLIN) trial. *J Am Coll Cardiol.* 2004;44:287–296.

15. Gershlick AH, et al. Rescue angioplasty after failed thrombolytic therapy for acute myocardial infarction. *N Engl J Med.* 2005;353:2758–2768.

16. Wijeysundera HC, et al. Rescue angioplasty or repeat fibrinolysis after failed fibrinolytic therapy for ST-segment myocardial infarction: a meta-analysis of randomized trials. *J Am Coll Cardiol.* 2007;49:422–430.

17. Keeley EC, Boura JA, Grines CL. Comparison of primary and facilitated percutaneous coronary interventions for ST-elevation myocardial infarction: quantitative review of randomized trials. *Lancet.* 2006;367:579–588.

18. Assessment of the Safety and Efficacy of a New Treatment Strategy with Percutaneous Coronary Intervention (ASSENT-4 PCI) investigators. Primary versus tenecteplase-facilitated percutaneous coronary intervention in patients with ST-segment elevation acute myocardial infarction (ASSENT-4 PCI): randomized trial. *Lancet.* 2006;367:569–578.

19. Cantor WJ, et al. Routine early angioplasty after fibrinolysis for acute myocardial infarction. *N Engl J Med.* 2009;360:2705–2718.

20. Di Mario C, et al. Immediate angioplasty versus standard therapy with rescue angioplasty after thrombolysis in the Combined Abciximab REteplase Stent Study in Acute Myocardial Infarction (CARESS-in-AMI): an open, prospective, randomised, multicentre trial. *Lancet.* 2008;371:559–568.

21. Borgia F, et al. Early routine percutaneous coronary intervention after fibrinolysis vs standard therapy in ST-segment elevation myocardial infarction: a meta-analysis. *Eur Heart J.* 2010;31:2156–2169.

22. Hochman JS, et al. Coronary intervention for persistent occlusion after myocardial infarction. *N Engl J Med.* 2006;355:2395–2407.

23. Dzavik V, et al. Randomized trial of percutaneous coronary intervention for subacute infarct-related coronary artery occlusion to achieve long-term patency and improve ventricular function: the Total Occlusion Study of Canada (TOSCA) 2 trial. *Circulation.* 2006;114:2449–2457.

24. Madsen JK, et al. Danish multicenter randomized study of invasive versus conservative treatment in patients with inducible ischemia after thrombolysis in acute myocardial infarction (DANAMI). DANish trial in Acute Myocardial Infarction. *Circulation.* 1997;96:748–755.

25. Zeymer U, et al. Randomized comparison of percutaneous transluminal coronary angioplasty and medical therapy in stable survivors of acute myocardial infarction with single vessel disease: a study of the Arbeitsgemeinschaft Leitende Kardiologische Krankenhausarzte. *Circulation.* 2003;108:1324–1328.

26. Stenestrand U, Wallentin L. Early revascularization and 1-year survival in 14-day survivors of acute myocardial infarction: a prospective cohort study. *Lancet.* 2002;359:1805–1811.

27. Vlaar PJ, et al. Culprit vessel only versus multivessel and staged percutaneous coronary intervention for multivessel disease in patients presenting with ST-segment elevation myocardial infarction: a pairwise and network meta-analysis. *J Am Coll Cardiol.* 2011;58:692–703.

28. Kornowski R, et al. Prognostic impact of staged versus "one-time" multivessel percutaneous interventions in acute myocardial infarction: analysis from the HORIZONS-AMI trial. *J Am Coll Cardiol.* 2011;58:704–711.

29. Wald DS, et al. Randomized trial of preventive angioplasty in myocardial infarction. *N Engl J Med.* 2013;369:1115–1123.

30. Gershlick AH, et al. Randomized trial of complete versus lesion-only revascularization in patients undergoing primary percutaneous coronary intervention for STEMI and multivessel disease: the CvLPRIT trial. *J Am Coll Cardiol.* 2015;65:963–972.

31. Engstrøm T, et al. Complete revascularisation versus treatment of the culprit lesion only in patients with ST-segment elevation myocardial infarction and multivessel disease (DANAMI 3-PRIMULTI): an open-label, randomised controlled trial. *Lancet.* 2015;386:665–671.

32. Zhu MM, et al. Primary stent implantation compared with primary balloon angioplasty for acute myocardial infarction: a meta-analysis of randomized clinical trials. *Am J Cardiol.* 2001;88(3):297–301.

33. Nordmann AJ, et al. Clinical outcomes of primary stenting versus balloon angioplasty in patients with myocardial infarction: a meta-analysis of randomized controlled trials. *Am J Med.* 2004;116:253–262.

34. Stone GW, et al. Paclitaxel-eluting stents versus bare-metal stents in acute myocardial infarction. *N Engl J Med.* 2009;360:1946–1959.

35. Ziada KM, Charnigo R, Moliterno DJ. Long-term follow-up of drug-eluting stents placed in the setting of ST-segment elevation myocardial infarction. *JACC Cardiovasc Interv.* 2011;4(1):39–41.

36. Brar SS, et al. Use of drug-eluting stents in acute myocardial infarction: a systematic review and meta-analysis [review]. *J Am Coll Cardiol.* 2009;53(18):1677–1689.

37. Grines CL, et al. Prevention of premature discontinuation of dual antiplatelet therapy in patients with coronary artery stents: a science advisory from the American Heart Association, American College of Cardiology, Society for Cardiovascular Angiography and Interventions, American College of Surgeons, and American Dental Association, with representation from the American College of Physicians. *J Am Coll Cardiol.* 2007;49(6):734–739.

38. Spertus JA, et al. Prevalence, predictors, and outcomes of premature discontinuation of thienopyridine therapy after drug-eluting stent placement: results from the PREMIER registry. *Circulation.* 2006;113(24):2803–2809.

39. Svilaas T, et al. Thrombus aspiration during primary percutaneous coronary intervention. *N Engl J Med.* 2008;358(6):557–567.

40. Vlaar PJ, et al. Cardiac death and reinfarction after 1 year in the Thrombus Aspiration during Percutaneous coronary intervention in Acute myocardial infarction Study (TAPAS): a 1-year follow-up study. *Lancet.* 2008;371:1915–1920.

41. Lagerqvist B, et al. Outcomes 1 year after thrombus aspiration for myocardial infarction. *N Engl J Med.* 2014;371:1111–1120.

42. Elgendy IY, et al. Is aspiration thrombectomy beneficial in patients undergoing primary percutaneous coronary intervention? Meta-analysis of randomized trials. *Circ Cardiovasc Interv.* 2015;8:e002258.

43. Ali A, et al. Rheolytic thrombectomy with percutaneous coronary intervention for infarct size reduction in acute myocardial infarction: 30-day results from a multicenter randomized study. *J Am Coll Cardiol.* 2006;48(2):244–252.

44. Bavry AA, Kumbhani DJ, Bhatt DL. Role of adjunctive thrombectomy and embolic protection devices in acute myocardial infarction: a comprehensive meta-analysis of randomized trials. *Eur Heart J.* 2008;29:2989–3001.

45. White HD, et al. Randomized, double-blind comparison of hirulog versus heparin in patients receiving streptokinase and aspirin for acute myocardial infarction (HERO). Hirulog Early Reperfusion/Occlusion (HERO) Trial Investigators. *Circulation.* 1997;96:2155–2161.

46. White HD, on behalf of the Hirulog and Early Reperfusion or Occlusion (HERO-2) Trial Investigators. Thrombin-specific anticoagulation with bivalirudin versus heparin in patients receiving fibrinolytic therapy for acute myocardial infarction: the HERO-2 randomised trial. *Lancet.* 2001;358:1855–1863.

47. Stone GW, et al. Bivalirudin during primary PCI in acute myocardial infarction. *N Engl J Med.* 2008;358(21):2218–2230.

48. Stone GW, et al. Heparin plus a glycoprotein IIb/IIIa inhibitor versus bivalirudin monotherapy and paclitaxel-eluting stents versus bare-metal stents in acute myocardial infarction (HORIZONS-AMI): final 3-year results from a multicentre, randomised controlled trial. *Lancet.* 2011;377(9784):2193–2204.

49. Shahzad A, et al. Unfractionated heparin versus bivalirudin in primary percutaneous coronary intervention (HEAT-PPCI): an open-label, single centre, randomised controlled trial. *Lancet.* 2014;384(9957):1849–1858.

50. Valgimigli M, et al. Bivalirudin or unfractionated heparin in acute coronary syndromes. *N Engl J Med.* 2015;373(11):997–1009.

51. Yusuf S, et al. Effects of fondaparinux on mortality and reinfarction in patients with acute ST-segment elevation myocardial infarction: the OASIS-6 randomized trial. *JAMA.* 2006;295(13):1519–1530.

52. Dupont AG, Gabriel DA, Cohen MG. Antiplatelet therapies and the role of antiplatelet resistance in acute coronary syndrome. *Thromb Res.* 2009;124(1):6–13.

53. Mehilli J, et al. Abciximab in patients with acute ST-segment elevation myocardial infarction undergoing primary percutaneous coronary intervention after clopidogrel loading: a randomized double-blind trial. *Circulation.* 2009;119(14):1933–1940.

54. Van't Hof AW, et al. Prehospital initiation of tirofiban in patients with ST-elevation myocardial infarction undergoing primary angioplasty (On-TIME 2): a multicentre, double-blind, randomised controlled trial. *Lancet.* 2008;372:537–546.

55. Gurm HS, et al. A comparison of abciximab and small molecule glycoprotein IIb/IIIa inhibitors in patients undergoing primary percutaneous coronary intervention: a meta-analysis of contemporary randomized controlled trials. *Circ Cardiovasc Interv.* 2009;2(3):230–236.

56. Ellis SG, et al. Facilitated PCI in patients with ST-elevation myocardial infarction. *N Engl J Med.* 2008;358(21):2205–2217.

57. Wiviott SD, et al. Prasugrel versus clopidogrel in patients with acute coronary syndromes. *N Engl J Med.* 2007;357(20):2001–2015.

58. Wallentin L, et al. Ticagrelor versus clopidogrel in patients with acute coronary syndromes. *N Engl J Med.* 2009;361(11):1045–1057.

59. Levine GN, et al. 2016 ACC/AHA guideline focused update on duration of dual antiplatelet therapy in patients with coronary artery disease. *J Am Coll Cardiol.* 2016;68(10):1082.

60. Chen ZM, et al. Addition of clopidogrel to aspirin in 45,852 patients with acute myocardial infarction: randomised placebo-controlled trial. *Lancet.* 2005;366(9497):1607–1621.

61. Sabatine MS, et al. Effect of clopidogrel pretreatment before percutaneous coronary intervention in patients with ST-elevation myocardial infarction treated with fibrinolytics: the PCI-CLARITY study. *JAMA.* 2005;294(10):1224–1232.

62. Fröbert O, et al. Thrombus aspiration during ST-segment elevation myocardial infarction. *N Engl J Med.* 2013;369:1587–1597.

63. Jolly SS, et al. Randomized trial of primary PCI with or without routine manual thrombectomy. *N Engl J Med.* 2015;372:1389–1398.

19

High-Risk Percutaneous Coronary Intervention, Cardiogenic Shock, and Acute Mechanical Circulatory Support Devices

Daniel H. Steinberg, MD, FSCAI and Navin K. Kapur, MD

With the clinical and technologic advances seen over the past two decades, interventional cardiology has undoubtedly evolved. The dividing lines between what could traditionally be accomplished only through surgery and what can now be described as standard of care in the catheterization laboratory continue to blur. Accordingly, the risk profile of patients referred to percutaneous coronary intervention (PCI) has evolved, and the level of acuity has intensified. Additionally, the management of cardiogenic shock (CS) has evolved with the advent of hemodynamic support devices, many of which can be inserted percutaneously. PCI-related risk, the nature and hemodynamics of CS, and the relative merits of hemodynamic support in the management of both has become increasingly relevant and important over the past few years. This chapter serves to review high-risk PCI and CS, and outline the support devices utilized in the catheterization laboratory.

HIGH-RISK PCI

While no PCI is truly free of procedural complication, the spectrum of patients and lesions treated by PCI is associated with a wide range of risk. Advances in technology and the advent of hemodynamic support has enhanced our ability to treat more complex and higher-risk patient subsets. Understanding the clinical and anatomic features associated with elevated procedural risk is paramount to ensuring optimal case management and patient outcomes. With appropriate preparation and anticipation, adjunct procedural strategies can be employed to mitigate risk and optimize care.

DEFINING RISK

PCI-related risk is associated with both clinical and anatomic features. From the clinical perspective, patient presentation, along with baseline characteristics such as age, gender, diabetes, prior myocardial infarction (MI), left ventricular (LV) dysfunction, peripheral artery disease, and renal insufficiency, have all been associated with increased risk of complications, including death, MI, stroke, and stent thrombosis (1). Importantly, many of these factors are not modifiable—these are inherent to the patient and cannot be improved prior to the procedure. Conversely, some preprocedural characteristics such as renal function or volume status can be medically optimized prior to PCI, and an effort to mitigate risk should logically focus on optimization where possible.

Anatomically, numerous factors have been associated with an increased risk of procedural failure and/or complications. These factors include left main (LM) stenosis, bifurcation disease, saphenous vein graft stenosis, ostial stenosis, heavily calcified lesions, and chronic total occlusions (1). Recognizing the inherent risk associated with each lesion, especially in the context of clinical risk factors, allows for appropriate planning of treatment strategy and adjunct equipment. Specific strategies to treat these types of lesions are covered elsewhere in this text.

Assessing Risk

Incorporating patient presentation, baseline characteristics and relevant anatomy, a subjective assessment of risk is a basic component of any interventional procedure. To help objectify this process, multiple risk calculators have been developed and validated. Two of the best validated and commonly used calculators are the Mayo Clinic Risk Score and the New York State PCI Database. The Mayo Clinic Risk Score was originally derived from 7,457 patients undergoing PCI at a single center (2). It was reiterated in 2007 and validated with data collected by the NCDR Cath PCI Registry of over 300,000 patients undergoing PCI between 2004 and 2006 (Fig. 19.1) (3). The New York State PCI Database analyzed 45,000 PCI procedures in 2002 and identified nine factors associated with an increased risk of adverse events, assigning weighted integer scores to each variable (4). Both the Mayo Clinic and NY State risk scores continue to accurately predict in-hospital mortality in the current era (5).

Anatomic risk scores have also been developed. The *SYNTAX score* was developed as part of a trial comparing PCI to coronary artery bypass surgery in patients with LM or multivessel disease (6). Based upon anatomic factors for each lesion, an overall score is derived to depict complexity of the interventional procedure. Divided by tertiles, the SYNTAX score has been shown to predict death, MI, stroke, and/or repeat revascularization at 1 year (7). Importantly, the SYNTAX score does not predict in-hospital outcomes, and the score lacks any clinical modifiers of risk. The SYNTAX II score was developed to incorporate both the anatomic SYNTAX score and clinical predictors of risk such as age, gender, ejection fraction, renal function, and the presence of peripheral or chronic lung disease to predict in hospital and mortality for both PCI and coronary artery bypass grafting (CABG). The SYNTAX II score predictive accuracy on 4-year mortality was validated in an analysis of 1,480 patients enrolled in two studies comparing PCI and CABG for multivessel or LM coronary disease (8). While no single calculator will capture every variable, these calculators all serve to provide a conceptual framework upon which to gauge periprocedural risk.

While high-risk PCI applies to a wide spectrum of clinical and anatomic scenarios, an important subset relates to the potential for hemodynamic collapse and CS. Patients undergoing PCI targeting an unprotected LM coronary artery or a last remaining conduit, especially in the setting of complex disease and reduced ejection fraction, are at particularly high risk. The remainder of this chapter focuses on this subset of high-risk PCI and CS, including the use of circulatory support devices for the management of both.

CARDIOGENIC SHOCK

CS is a major cause of global morbidity and mortality. CS most commonly occurs after an acute myocardial infarction (AMI) or in patients with advanced heart failure (HF). Shock from any cause is characterized by tissue hypoperfusion leading to end-organ damage, and CS is defined as tissue hypoperfusion secondary to cardiac failure despite adequate circulatory volume and LV filling pressure.

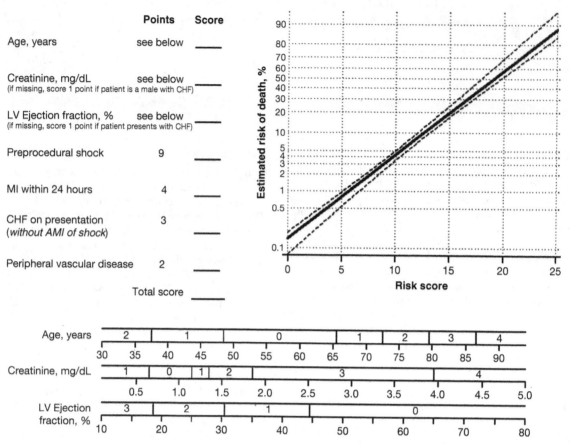

FIGURE 19.1   Mayo Clinic risk calculator. AMI, acute myocardial infarction; CHF, congestive heart failure; LV, left ventricular; MI, myocardial infarction.

Hemodynamic criteria for CS include the following: a systolic blood pressure <90 mm Hg for >30 minutes or a fall in mean arterial blood pressure greater than 30 mm Hg below baseline with a cardiac index (CI) of <1.8 L/min/m² without hemodynamic support or <2.2 L/min/m² with support and a pulmonary capillary wedge pressure (PCWP) >15 mm Hg (9–11).

CAUSES OF CARDIOGENIC SHOCK

A wide range of conditions can lead to CS (**Table 19.1**). CS can develop in the setting of AMI, and can occur after both ST-elevation myocardial infarction (STEMI) and non–ST-elevation myocardial infarction (NSTEMI), either as a manifestation of primary pump failure or as a mechanical complication. While thrombotic coronary artery occlusion is often well-tolerated, approximately 5% to 8% of AMI patients develop clinical manifestations of hemodynamic collapse (12). Early preclinical studies suggest that approximately 40% of the myocardium must be involved in an AMI to cause CS) (13), and risk factors include occlusion of the left anterior descending (LAD) artery, age over 65, hypertension, prior infarction, or multivessel disease (14). Mortality associated with CS after AMI is high, with in-hospital mortality approaching 60% in multiple studies (15).

TABLE 19.1 Causes of Cardiogenic Shock

ISCHEMIC	NONISCHEMIC	NONCARDIAC
Acute myocardial infarction	Chronic systolic heart failure	Severe sepsis
Pump failure	Myocarditis	Subarachnoid hemorrhage
Right ventricular infarction	Hypertrophic cardiomyopathy	Hypothyroidism
Post–myocardial infarction complications	Valvular heart disease	
Arrhythmia	Myocardial contusion	
Papillary muscle rupture	Stress cardiomyopathy	
Ventricular septal rupture	Arrhythmia	
Free wall rupture/tamponade		

Post-myocardial mechanical complications (acute mitral regurgitation, papillary muscle rupture, ventricular septal rupture, and free wall rupture) are important and clinically dramatic events that can lead to CS. In the revascularization era, these events are fortunately rare, with papillary muscle rupture and ventricular septal or free wall rupture collectively occurring in only about 1% of cases. Risk factors include female gender and absence of coronary artery disease, suggesting the relevance of "at risk" myocardium and the importance of collateral circulation in chronic disease. When it does occur, papillary muscle rupture most commonly involves the posteromedial papillary muscle because it receives a singular blood supply from the dominant coronary vessel supplying the posterior descending artery (16). It manifests as acute, severe mitral regurgitation and heart failure. Septal rupture occurs within subtended territory from the infarcted related artery (anteroapical with left anterior descending [LAD] occlusion, or posterobasal with right coronary artery [RCA] occlusion) and presents as acute heart failure from a left–right shunt (17,18). Free wall rupture can occur anywhere within subtended territory and manifests most commonly as pulseless electrical activity and tamponade (19,20).

While CS following AMI is typically related to left-sided heart failure, right ventricular (RV) myocardial infarction (RVMI) can also lead to CS, and it is associated with a high risk of morbidity and mortality, ventricular fibrillation, and high-grade AV-conduction block (21,22). As the RV receives blood from acute marginal branches of the RCA and the posterior descending artery, RVMI occurs most commonly after acute proximal right coronary occlusion, but can occur after occlusion of a dominant circumflex artery) (23,24). RV ischemia leads to RV systolic failure and reduced LV preload. As RV pressure and volume overload develop, the interventricular septum shifts toward the LV cavity, further reducing LV stroke volume. Hemodynamic indices of RV failure in AMI include measurements of RV stroke work (RVSW), right atrial to PCWP (RA:PCWP) ratio of >0.8, and pulmonary artery pulse pressure (25). In the SHOCK registry, isolated RV failure accounted for 49 (5.3%) of the 933 patients with myocardial dysfunction as the primary mechanism underlying CS (26).

CS in the absence of AMI occurs most commonly in the presence of advanced HF. In the United States alone, over 7 million individuals suffer from HF. As a manifestation of acutely decompensated HF, CS is included among several HF classification systems (Table 19.2) (27). The New York Heart Association (NYHA) classifies HF severity based on symptoms. CS is categorized as a manifestation of NYHA Class IV heart failure (HF). For patients with advanced HF (NYHA Class III or IV), the Interagency Registry for Mechanically Assisted Circulatory Support (INTERMACS) has defined seven clinical profiles before implantation of a LV assist device (LVAD) (28). CS is identified by INTERMACS profiles 1 and 2, where patients may be "crashing" despite aggressive therapy or "sliding fast on inotropes," respectively. Both INTERMACS 1 and 2 subjects may be considered for temporary circulatory support as a bridge to recovery, surgical LVAD, or cardiac transplantation.

Primary valvular heart disease is another important cause of CS. Endocarditis, mitral valve prolapse, chordal rupture, or aortic dissection extending to the aortic annulus may cause CS secondary to valve failure (29–33). Patients with chronic valve disease, including aortic/mitral stenosis, may also develop CS secondary to progressive LV failure or arrhythmias (34).

HEMODYNAMICS OF CARDIOGENIC SHOCK

As defined earlier, CS is characterized by sustained hypotension, low cardiac output, and impaired tissue perfusion despite adequate intravascular volume. Cardiac function is best represented by the pressure–volume (PV) loop. Each PV loop represents one cardiac cycle (Fig. 19.2A) (35).

The PV loop can be modulated in various ways (Fig. 19.2B–D). Increasing preload will increase SV without changing E_{max} or E_a. Vasopressors designed to increase afterload will increase E_a, which may reduce stroke volume, without affecting E_{max}. Inotropes will primarily increase E_{max}, while decreasing E_a. These approaches increase cardiac stroke work and myocardial oxygen demand, which may propagate myocardial ischemia.

In the setting of an AMI, E_{max} and stroke volume may be reduced, while E_a increases to compensate for hypotension (Fig. 19.3A) (36,37). Without treatment, cardiac function worsens and significant reductions in E_{max} and stroke volume are observed, which contribute to both systemic hypotension and progressively increasing LV end-diastolic volume (LVEDV). Increased systemic vascular resistance (SVR) is reflected as an increase in E_a. As CS progresses, the PV loop becomes smaller and shifts to the right of the PV plane (Fig. 19.3B). The goal of therapy in the setting of CS is to increase contractility, improve stroke volume, and reduce intracardiac volume overload while maintaining an adequate mean arterial pressure (MAP) to support end-organ tissue perfusion.

Changes in afterload are variable in CS. Reduced cardiac output activates the sympathetic nervous system, which increases SVR

TABLE 19.2 Classifications of Heart Failure and Cardiogenic Shock

ACC/AHA STAGE	NYHA	INTERMACS	TERMINOLOGY
D	IV	I	"Crash and burn," emergent mechanical support
D	IV	II	Intravenous inotropes, may need mechanical support
D	IV	III	Stable, but inotrope-dependent
D	IV (ambulatory)	IV	Resting symptoms, oral therapy, peak VO$_2$ <12 L/min
D	IV (ambulatory)	V	ADL is severely limited, peak VO$_2$ <12 L/min
D	III	VI	ADL is possible but limited
D	III	VII	Advanced Class III symptoms
C	I–III	–	Structural disease, current or past symptoms
B	I	–	Structural disease, no symptoms
A	I	–	At risk, no structural disease or symptoms

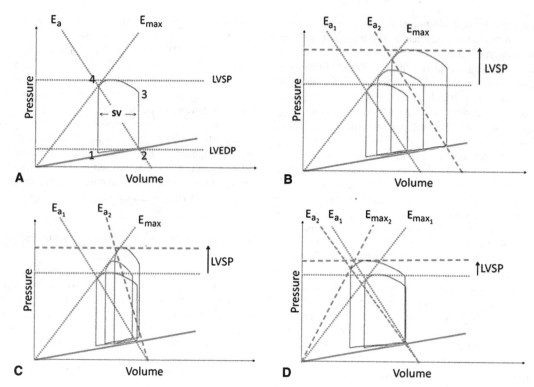

FIGURE 19.2   PV loops. **(A)** Normal pressure volume (PV) loop. The impact of **(B)** increased LV preload (volume resuscitation), **(C)** increased LV afterload (vasopressors), **(D)** increased LV contractility (inotropes).

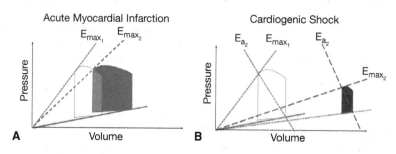

FIGURE 19.3   PV loops in AMI and cardiogenic shock. Cardiac hemodynamics in AMI **(A)** and cardiogenic shock **(B)**. AMI, acutemyocardial infarctio; PV, pressure–volume.

through adrenergic agonists, including norepinephrine and epinephrine. Nevertheless, measured SVR in the setting of CS can often be normal or low. In the SHOCK trial, nearly 20% of subjects with CS had signs of systemic inflammatory response syndrome (SIRS), as defined by fever, leukocytosis, and low SVR (38,39). A postulated mechanism for low SVR in these CS subjects was the activation of inducible nitric oxide synthase (iNOS) by inflammatory mediators, thereby leading to systemic vasodilatation.

MANAGEMENT OF CARDIOGENIC SHOCK

Diagnosis and Initial Stabilization

Early diagnosis is essential for successful management of CS. Rapid bedside assessment of signs and symptoms include hypotension, tachycardia, oliguria, change in mental status, hypoxia, cyanosis, and cold or clammy skin. Rales suggestive of pulmonary edema

may not be consistently present in CS. Initial diagnostic testing includes electrocardiography to diagnose AMI or arrhythmia. Bedside echocardiography can rapidly define cardiac etiologies for CS, including primary systolic failure, tamponade, valvular insufficiency, valvular stenoses, or septal/free wall rupture. Pulmonary artery (PA) catheterization may help discriminate noncardiac from cardiac causes of shock and help define the underlying cause of cardiac failure, including LV failure, RV failure, cardiac tamponade, severe mitral regurgitation, and ventricular septal defects. PA catheterization provides critical information, including intracardiac filling pressures, screening oximetry, and quantification of cardiac output. ACC/AHA guidelines identify PA catheterization as a Class I recommendation when echocardiography is not available for patients with refractory hypotension, suspected AMI, or mechanical complications secondary to AMI (40). PA catheterization is a Class IIA recommendation for hemodynamic monitoring in patients requiring inotropic/vasopressor support or for patients with refractory hypoperfusion.

The goal of initial treatment for CS includes maintenance of tissue perfusion, which includes both maintaining MAP and oxygenation. Early mechanical ventilation should be considered in patients with persistent hypoxemia despite supplemental oxygen. Volume resuscitation should be attempted to maintain MAP in subjects without evidence of overt volume overload (elevated jugular venous pressure or pulmonary congestion). In the setting of symptomatic bradycardia, transvenous pacing may be required to enhance cardiac output.

Pharmacologic Therapy

Pharmacologic support with inotropes or vasopressors is recommended for individuals not responsive to volume resuscitation or in the setting of decompensated HF. Each pharmacologic agent provides a unique profile of hemodynamic support (Table 19.3) (41). First-line agents for blood pressure support include escalating doses of dopamine, norepinephrine, or epinephrine. High-dose dopamine, norepinephrine, or epinephrine will stimulate both α- and β-adrenergic receptors, thereby providing primarily vasopressor and minimal inotropic support. Inotropes such as dobutamine and milrinone should be initiated in individuals with primary cardiac failure. Both agents will provide β-receptor agonism by stimulating the receptor directly or promoting accumulation of cyclic adenosine monophosphate (cAMP), respectively.

Through inotropic and vasopressor support, these pharmacologic agents serve to increase cardiac output and maintain a MAP to sustain vital organ perfusion. Disadvantages of inotropes include increased risk for ventricular arrhythmia, increased myocardial oxygen demand and increased stroke work. These all can lead to myocardial ischemia—especially in the setting of obstructive coronary artery disease (42). Inotropes may also promote systemic hypotension and may require use of concomitant vasopressors to sustain blood pressure while enhancing cardiac output. While maintaining central MAP, vasopressor agents may lead to peripheral vasoconstriction and related complications. In cases of refractory shock despite pharmacologic support, mechanical assist devices may be considered.

Revascularization

In the setting of AMI and CS, early revascularization (ER) via PCI or coronary artery bypass grafting (CABG) improves survival compared with medical therapy, including fibrinolysis. In the Global Utilization of Streptokinase to Open occluded arteries study (GUSTO-I) evaluating 2,972 patients with shock in the setting of AMI randomized to PCI or fibrinolysis. Thirty-day mortality was significantly reduced in patients treated with PCI compared with fibrinolysis (30%–40% vs. 60%, respectively) (43). This observation has been confirmed in several follow-up studies, and multivariate logistic regression analyses of these studies demonstrated that an invasive strategy was independently associated with reduced mortality (12,44–46).

The SHOCK trial randomized 302 patients with STEMI complicated by CS to emergent revascularization ER within 6 hours via coronary angioplasty (64%), or CABG (36%), or intensive medical therapy (including thrombolytics) and delayed (≥54 hours) revascularization if clinically and angiographically appropriate (47). While there was a difference in the primary endpoint of 30-day survival between ER and optimal medical therapy (OMT) (53% vs. 44%), it did not reach statistical significance (95% CI: 0.96–1.53; p = 0.109). Nevertheless, at 6 months, 1 year, and 6 years, absolute survival was significantly better after ER compared with OMT (48). No significant survival difference was observed in subjects undergoing coronary angioplasty compared with CABG. Of note, although there was a suggestion of increased mortality in the 56 patients over age 75 who were enrolled in the SHOCK trial, several studies have since demonstrated improved survival with ER in elderly patients presenting with AMI and CS (49,50).

Circulatory Support Devices

Mechanistically, the goals of hemodynamic support devices are to improve oxygen delivery to the vital organs, improve cardiac output, decrease LV oxygen demand and increase coronary flow. Indications for mechanical cardiac support (MCS) can range from short-term protection during a PCI procedure to indefinite term support in

TABLE 19.3 Pharmacologic Agents in Cardiogenic Shock

AGENT	GENERAL MECHANISM	RECEPTORS				DOSE RANGE	OVERALL EFFECT	CAUTIONS
		α-1	β-1	β-2	DA			
Phenylephrine	Pure α	+++	0	0	0	Up to 180 µg/min	= to ↑ CO ↑ SVR	Caution with high SVR
Norepinephrine	α-1, some β-1	+++	++	0	0	Up to 350 µg/min	↑ CO ↑ SVR	Reflex bradycardia
Epinephrine	β-1 at low doses, increasing α-1 and β-2 with higher doses	+++	+++	++	0	Up to 0.5 µg/kg/min	↑ CO, ↓ SVR at low dose ↑ SVR at high dose	May induce vasospasm
Dopamine	Low dose—DA Mid doses—β-2 High doses—α-1	0 + ++	+ + ++	0 0 0	++ ++ ++	0.5–2 µg/kg/min 2–10 µg/kg/min 10–20 µg/kg/min	↑ CO at all doses ↑ SVR at higher doses	Arrhythmogenic
Dobutamine	β-1, β-2 at low doses, some α-1 with higher doses	+	+++	++	0	Up to 40 µg/kg/min	↑ CO ↓ SVR	Arrhythmogenic
Milrinone	Nonadrenergic PDE inhibitor, but similar effects as dobutamine	PDE inhibitor				Up to 0.5 µg/min	↑ CO ↓ SVR	Hypotension, thiocyanate poisoning

CO, cardiac output; PDE, phosphodiesterase; SVR, systemic vascular resistance.

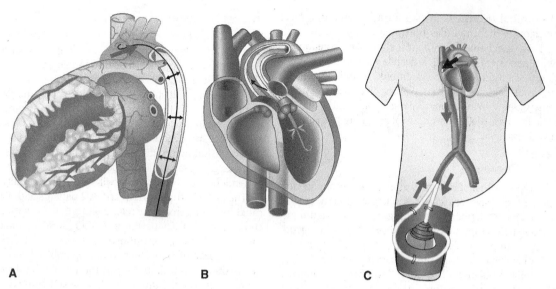

FIGURE 19.4 **Percutaneous support devices.** Percutaneous mechanical support devices **(A)** IABP, **(B)** Impella, **(C)** Tandem Heart. IABP, intra-aortic balloon pumping.

fulminant CS. Currently available options for LV support include the intra-aortic balloon pump (IABP), Impella 2.5, CP and 5.0 (Abiomed, Danvers, MA), TandemHeart (Cardiac Assist, Pittsburgh, PA), and extracorporeal membrane oxygenation (ECMO). Right-sided support devices include the Impella RP and ProtekDuo (Cardiac Assist, Pittsburgh, PA). Each device (**Fig. 19.4**) has a role in the management of high-risk PCI or CS, and their relative characteristics are discussed in the following text. .

As noted earlier, a subset of high-risk PCI relates to the potential for hemodynamic collapse and CS, including unprotected LM and last remaining conduit in patients with reduced ejection fractions. In these patients, it is important to have hemodynamic support available. In fact, it can be argued the prophylactic support may even be of benefit.

For those in CS related from any cause, mechanical support devices are often beneficial. These devices allow for adequate distal tissue perfusion while allowing the heart time to recover from a transient insult or serving as a bridge to more definitive therapy (revascularization, durable LV assist, or transplantation). In these cases, the underlying cause of shock, stability of the system, degree of support necessary, and expected time course to definitive outcome are important in choosing the appropriate device.

INTRA-AORTIC BALLOON PUMP

An IABP is a balloon catheter placed percutaneously, most commonly through the femoral artery, into the descending aorta distal to the left subclavian artery. The IABP is connected to a pump console. Helium inflation and deflation is gated to the electrocardiogram (ECG) or aortic pressure-tracing and serves to enhance coronary perfusion during diastole by displacing blood volume within the descending aorta, and augment cardiac output via pressure sink in the aorta during systole. The primary effects of IABP support are to: (a) increase coronary perfusion, (b) reduce LV afterload, (c) increase LV SV, and (d) reduce LV end-diastolic pressure (**Fig. 19.5A**) (51). The degree of hemodynamic support afforded by an IABP is dictated by the size of the IABP, which ranges between 34 and 50 mL.

While intuitively attractive in high-risk PCI, the routine use of the IABP is not without controversy. The Balloon pump assisted Coronary Intervention Study (BCIS-1) evaluated routine intra-aortic balloon

pumping (IABP) support versus no routine support in 301 patients undergoing HR-PCI (52). While there was no difference in major adverse cardiovascular and cerebrovascular endpoints at 28 days (15.2% routine vs. 16.0% no routine IABP), there were significantly fewer major procedural complications in those who received routine IABP. The Counterpulsation to Reduce Infarct Size Pre-PCI Acute MI (CRISP-AMI) trial was a multicenter, prospective, randomized to 337 patients with acute ST-segment elevation MI without shock undergoing planned primary PCI to either IABP support prior to PCI (n = 161) or primary PCI without IABP (n = 176), The primary endpoint was infarct size, measured by cardiac magnetic resonance imaging. Mean infarct size was not significantly different between the groups (42.1% vs. 37.5%); nevertheless, a trend toward reduced 6-month mortality was observed in the patients receiving up-front IABP (53).

In patients with AMI and CS, IABP was associated with a significant reduction in mortality from 67% to 49% in the NRMI-2 database (46). Similarly, in the Shock Registry, this combination was also associated with a significant reduction of mortality from 63% to 47% (54). This survival benefit may relate to several factors, including improved delivery of drugs to the site of occlusion, improved penetration into the thrombus, or rapid reversal of hypotension.

Though an IABP can improve vital organ perfusion, the increase in cardiac output is modest and estimated at about 1 L/min. Additionally, the IABP depends on cardiac performance to function appropriately. For high-risk PCI and CS, this support may not prove adequate, and more aggressive mechanical support is necessary. The primary goal of a pLVAD is to reduce native LV SV, thereby reducing LV stroke work, while maintaining systemic perfusion.

IMPELLA

The Impella is an axial flow device placed in retrograde fashion across the aortic valve that directly unloads the left ventricle and directs blood flow into the proximal aorta. The primary hemodynamic effect of the Impella is to reduce native LV SV and LVEDP (55). The Impella is available in three forms (2.5, CP and 5.0), providing an estimated 2.5, 3.5, or 5.0 L/min of flow. The 2.5 and CP can be inserted percutaneously either as a standalone device or through

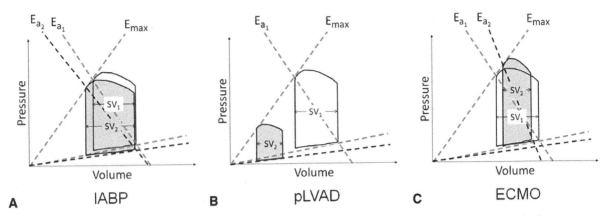

FIGURE 19.5 Hemodynamics of IABP, Impella/Tandem, VA ECMO. PV loops after treatment with **(A)** intra-aortic balloon counter-pulsation, **(B)** percutaneous LV assist devices: Impella and TandemHeart, or **(C)** veno-arterial extra-corporeal membrane oxygenation.

a 12- to 14-French sheath respectively, while the 5.0 is generally placed by surgical cutdown.

For patients undergoing high-risk PCI, Impella may have some advantage over the IABP. The PROTECT II trial was a randomized trial comparing the Impella 2.5 to the IABP in 448 patients with LV ejections fraction <35% undergoing non-emergent PCI to either unprotected LM or a last patent coronary vessel (or ejection fraction <30% with three vessel coronary disease). Approximately two-thirds of patients had NYHA Class III or IV systolic heart failure symptoms, with an average ejection fraction of less than 25% and similarly high PCI risk (New York, Mayo, and SYNTAX) scores. The Impella was associated with improved hemodynamic support measured by cardiac power output. In the intention to treat population, the primary endpoint of 30-day major adverse cardiac events (MACE) was similar between the two groups (35.1% Impella vs. 40.1% IABP, p = 0.227), but a trend toward the reduction of MACE with Impella was noted at 90 days (40.6% Impella vs. 49.3% IABP, p = 0.066) (56).

The US-Pella registry analyzed 154 patients with AMI and CS who underwent revascularization with mechanical support via an Impella 2.5. In 38 patients, no hemodynamic support was provided during the PCI, and the Impella was placed following the procedure. In 53 patients, an IABP was placed prior to the PCI, and an Impella was placed following the procedure. In the remaining 63 patients, the Impella was placed prior to revascularization. Respective survival rates were 41% for the patients not receiving support, 42.3% for those under IABP support during PCI, and 62.1% for those with Impella support prior to the procedure (57). These results imply utility of early Impella placement in patients with AMI and CS.

For patients with CS complicating AMI, non-randomized trials have compared the Impella 2.5 to IABP with no significant survival benefit demonstrated. The lack of difference was largely attributed to the fact the 2.5 L/min of support was inadequate for CS. The IMPella versus IABP Reduces mortality in STEMI patients treated with primary PCI in Severe cardiogenic SHOCK (IMPRESS in Severe Shock) trial compared Impella CP to IABP in 48 patients with a primary endpoint of 30-day mortality. All patients underwent primary PCI, and the two devices were associated with similar mortality rates at both 30 days (46% Impella vs. 50% IABP, p = 0.92) and 6 months (50% vs. 50%, p = 0.92) (58).

For patients with isolated right-sided failure or biventricular failure, the Impella RP provides support via right atrium (RA) to

PA configuration. The device is inserted through 22 French access in the right femoral vein, and it is generally guided to the left PA. With appropriate placement, it bypasses the RV by taking blood from the right atrial and pumping it through to the PA. It is capable of up to 5 L/min. The device has a humanitarian device exemption.

TANDEMHEART

The TandemHeart is a centrifugal continuous flow pump that can generate between 3.5 and 5.0 L/min of flow. It is typically configured from the left atrium-to-femoral artery (LA-FA), drawing oxygenated blood from the LA and circulating it back to the common femoral artery, effectively bypassing the native LV. This original device requires a trans-septal puncture for LV support, and configurations now exist to provide pure ECMO through inferior vena cava inflow, oxygenation, and femoral artery outflow, as well as RV support via cannula placement in the RA and PA with or without an oxygenation.

As with the Impella device, the primary hemodynamic effect of the TandemHeart device is to reduce native LV SV and LVEDP (Fig. 19.5B) (55,59). Compared to IABP in CS, these devices are associated with higher CI, MAP, and lower PCWP in a meta-analysis of three trials involving 100 patients, 40 of whom were treated with the TandemHeart device (60). Nevertheless, despite improved hemodynamic profiles in CS, no difference in 30-day mortality was observed across the studies in this analysis, and patients treated with TandemHeart experienced an increase in bleeding complications. Future studies are required to determine the clinical utility of percutaneous ventricular assist devices (pVADs) in CS.

Potential complications associated with pMCS devices include peripheral vascular obstruction and ischemia, bleeding, infection, and stroke. IABP-specific complications include the following: malposition resulting in subclavian, mesenteric, or renal arterial obstruction; aortic dissection; and air or plaque embolism. Complications associated with the Impella 2.5 LP device include ventricular arrhythmias and hemolysis, while complications specific to the TandemHeart device include the risk of left atrial perforation during trans-septal cannula insertion, cannula migration (antegrade or retrograde), and the potential for interatrial shunting after device removal.

EXTRACORPOREAL MEMBRANE OXYGENATION

For individuals with cardiorespiratory or biventricular failure, ECMO can be considered. Specifically, veno-arterial ECMO is performed by pumping blood from the venous system into the arterial system using a centrifugal pump attached to an external oxygenator. Multiple ECMO pump devices are in commercial production, and ECMO can be rapidly initiated by percutaneous cannulation. While providing peripheral support by circulating oxygenated blood into the arterial system, ECMO effectively decreases LV SV by decreasing preload to the LV. As a result, increased afterload has been observed with ECMO due to retrograde flow through the arterial system (**Fig. 19.5C**) (61). For patients with severe LV dysfunction, "venting" the LV with an Impella may provide adequate decompression while maintaining sufficient systemic support through ECMO. This strategy may lead to improved survival compared to veno-arterial ECMO alone. In a propensity matched study of 63 patients with CS, the 42 pateints receiving veno-arterial ECMO alone had a significantly lower in-hospital survival rate compared to the 21 patients receiving veno-arterial ECMO and Impella support (20% vs. 53%, p < 0.01). Further study is clearly required, but the results of this study suggest that LV decompression is an important component in the management of CS (62).

CONCLUSIONS

The clinical and hemodynamic profiles of patients presenting to the catheterization laboratory have come to include increasingly complex, high-risk and high-acuity situations. From high-risk PCI to CS, the various characteristics, physiology, and treatment modalities continue to develop and evolve. Over the next decade, new advances and emerging clinical evidence will further shape the approaches to high-risk PCI and CS.

Key Points

- Hemodynamic criteria for CS include a systolic blood pressure <90 mm Hg for >30 minutes or a fall in mean arterial blood pressure greater than 30 mm Hg below baseline with a CI of <1.8 L/min/m^2 without hemodynamic support or <2.2 L/min/m^2 with support and a PCWP >15 mm Hg.

- Postmyocardial infarction complications leading to CS include acute mitral regurgitation, ventricular septal rupture, ventricular free wall rupture, and RV failure.

- The goal of initial treatment for CS includes maintenance of tissue perfusion, which includes maintaining both MAP and oxygenation. CS refractory to volume resuscitation or that associated with decompensated HF may require escalating doses of dopamine, norepinephrine, or epinephrine. Hypotension and ventricular arrhythmias may occur with initiation of inotropes such as dobutamine and milrinone.

- ER was associated with a statistically significant difference in survival compared with OMT after 6 months, 1 year, and 6 years of follow-up in the SHOCK trial.

- Percutaneous mechanical support options for CS include IABP, Impella axial flow pumps, the TandemHeart centrifugal flow pump, or ECMO.

- The ACC/AHA definition of a "successful" PCI can be classified into three categories: angiographic, procedural, and clinical success. Each of these should be carefully considered when approaching a high-risk coronary intervention.

- Clinical variables of risk predict clinical outcomes, while anatomic lesion characteristics predict angiographic success.

- The ACC/AHA and SCAI lesion classification systems remain highly relevant in the modern era for grading the likelihood of technical success.

- The Mayo Clinic Clinical Scoring system demonstrates a high predictive value for identifying complications associated with PCI.

- The overall goals of percutaneous mechanical support devices are to: (a) maintain vital organ perfusion, (b) improve native cardiac output by reducing intracardiac filling pressures, (c) reduce LV volumes, wall stress, and myocardial oxygen consumption, and (d) augment coronary perfusion during high-risk PCI.

- Based on emerging data and experience, the updated PCI guidelines have recently incorporated hemodynamic support devices as an adjunct to HR-PCI in select cases, as a Class IIB recommendation.

References

1. Fihn SD, et al. 2012 ACCF/AHA/ACP/AATS/PCNA/SCAI/STS guideline for the diagnosis and management of patients with stable ischemic heart disease: a report of the American College of Cardiology Foundation/American Heart Association Task Force on practice guidelines, and the American College of Physicians, American Association for Thoracic Surgery, Preventive Cardiovascular Nurses Association, Society for Cardiovascular Angiography and Interventions, and Society of Thoracic Surgeons. *J Am Coll Cardiol.* 2012;60:e44–e164.
2. Singh M, et al. Bedside estimation of risk from percutaneous coronary intervention: the new Mayo Clinic risk scores. *Mayo Clin Proc.* 2007;82:701–708.
3. Singh M, et al. Validation of the Mayo clinic risk score for in-hospital mortality after percutaneous coronary interventions using the national cardiovascular data registry. *Circ Cardiovasc Interv.* 2008;1:36–44.
4. Wu C, et al. A risk score to predict in-hospital mortality for percutaneous coronary interventions. *J Am Coll Cardiol.* 2006;47:654–660.
5. Brener SJ, et al. Precision and accuracy of risk scores for in-hospital death after percutaneous coronary intervention in the current era. *Catheter Cardiovasc Interv.* 2010;75:153–157.
6. Sianos G, et al. The SYNTAX score: an angiographic tool grading the complexity of coronary artery disease. *EuroIntervention.* 2005;1:219–227.
7. Serruys PW, et al. Percutaneous coronary intervention versus coronary-artery bypass grafting for severe coronary artery disease. *N Engl J Med.* 2009;360:961–972.
8. Sotomi Y, et al. Individual long-term mortality prediction following either coronary stenting or bypass surgery in patients with multivessel and/or unprotected left main disease: an external validation of the SYNTAX Score II Model in the 1,480 patients of the BEST and PRECOMBAT randomized controlled trials. *JACC Cardiovasc Interv.* 2016;9:1564–1572.
9. Antonelli M, et al. Hemodynamic monitoring in shock and implications for management. International Consensus Conference, Paris, France, 27–28 April 2006. *Intensive Care Med.* 2007;33:575–590.
10. Reynolds HR, Hochman JS. Cardiogenic shock: current concepts and improving outcomes. *Circulation.* 2008;117:686–697.
11. Topalian S, Ginsberg F, Parrillo JE. Cardiogenic shock. *Crit Care Med.* 2008;36:S66–S74.
12. Goldberg RJ, et al. Temporal trends in cardiogenic shock complicating acute myocardial infarction. *N Engl J Med.* 1999;340:1162–1168.
13. Alonso DR, et al. Pathophysiology of cardiogenic shock. Quantification of myocardial necrosis, clinical, pathologic and electrocardiographic correlations. *Circulation.* 1973;48:588–596.
14. Lindholm MG, et al. Cardiogenic shock complicating acute myocardial infarction; prognostic impact of early and late shock development. *Eur Heart J.* 2003;24:258–265.

15. Babaev A, et al. Trends in management and outcomes of patients with acute myocardial infarction complicated by cardiogenic shock. *JAMA*. 2005;294:448–454.

16. Barbour DJ, Roberts WC. Rupture of a left ventricular papillary muscle during acute myocardial infarction: analysis of 22 necropsy patients. *J Am Coll Cardiol*. 1986;8:558–565.

17. Radford MJ, et al. Ventricular septal rupture: a review of clinical and physiologic features and an analysis of survival. *Circulation*. 1981;64:545–553.

18. Moore CA, et al. Postinfarction ventricular septal rupture: the importance of location of infarction and right ventricular function in determining survival. *Circulation*. 1986;74:45–55.

19. Shapira I, et al. Cardiac rupture in patients with acute myocardial infarction. *Chest*. 1987;92:219–223.

20. Mann JM, Roberts WC. Rupture of the left ventricular free wall during acute myocardial infarction: analysis of 138 necropsy patients and comparison with 50 necropsy patients with acute myocardial infarction without rupture. *Am J Cardiol*. 1988;62:847–859.

21. Chockalingam A, et al. Right ventricular myocardial infarction: presentation and acute outcomes. *Angiology*. 2005;56:371–376.

22. Engstrom AE, et al. Right ventricular dysfunction is an independent predictor for mortality in ST-elevation myocardial infarction patients presenting with cardiogenic shock on admission. *Eur J Heart Fail*. 2010;12:276–282.

23. Verani MS, et al. Effect of coronary artery recanalization on right ventricular function in patients with acute myocardial infarction. *J Am Coll Cardiol*. 1985;5:1029–1035.

24. Andersen HR, Falk E, Nielsen D. Right ventricular infarction: frequency, size and topography in coronary heart disease: a prospective study comprising 107 consecutive autopsies from a coronary care unit. *J Am Coll Cardiol*. 1987;10:1223–1232.

25. Dell'Italia LJ, et al. Right ventricular infarction: identification by hemodynamic measurements before and after volume loading and correlation with noninvasive techniques. *J Am Coll Cardiol*. 1984;4:931–939.

26. Jacobs AK, et al. Cardiogenic shock caused by right ventricular infarction: a report from the SHOCK registry. *J Am Coll Cardiol*. 2003;41:1273–1279.

27. Yancy CW, et al. 2013 ACCF/AHA guideline for the management of heart failure: a report of the American College of Cardiology Foundation/American Heart Association Task Force on Practice Guidelines. *J Am Coll Cardiol*. 2013;62:e147–e239.

28. Stevenson LW, et al. INTERMACS profiles of advanced heart failure: the current picture. *J Heart Lung Transplant*. 2009;28:535–541.

29. Erbel R. Role of transesophageal echocardiography in dissection of the aorta and evaluation of degenerative aortic disease. *Cardiol Clin*. 1993;11:461–473.

30. Tiong IY, et al. Bacterial endocarditis and functional mitral stenosis: a report of two cases and brief literature review. *Chest*. 2002;122:2259–2262.

31. Brizzio ME, Zapolanski A. Acute mitral regurgitation requiring urgent surgery because of chordae ruptures after extreme physical exercise: case report. *Heart Surg Forum*. 2008;11:E255–E256.

32. Yuan SM. Clinical significance of mitral leaflet flail. *Cardiol J*. 2009;16:151–156.

33. Wang A. Recent progress in the understanding of infective endocarditis. *Curr Treat Options Cardiovasc Med*. 2011;13:586–594.

34. Nishimura RA, et al. 2014 AHA/ACC guideline for the management of patients with valvular heart disease: executive summary: a report of the American College of Cardiology/American Heart Association Task Force on Practice Guidelines. *J Am Coll Cardiol*. 2014;63:2438–2488.

35. Burkhoff D, Mirsky I, Suga H. Assessment of systolic and diastolic ventricular properties via pressure-volume analysis: a guide for clinical, translational, and basic researchers. *Am J Physiol Heart Circ Physiol*. 2005;289:H501–H512.

36. Shioura KM, Geenen DL, Goldspink PH. Assessment of cardiac function with the pressure-volume conductance system following myocardial infarction in mice. *Am J Physiol Heart Circ Physiol*. 2007;293:H2870–H2877.

37. Remmelink M, et al. Acute left ventricular dynamic effects of primary percutaneous coronary intervention from occlusion to reperfusion. *J Am Coll Cardiol*. 2009;53:1498–1502.

38. Hochman JS. Cardiogenic shock complicating acute myocardial infarction: expanding the paradigm. *Circulation*. 2003;107:2998–3002.

39. Kohsaka S, et al. Systemic inflammatory response syndrome after acute myocardial infarction complicated by cardiogenic shock. *Arch Intern Med*. 2005;165:1643–1650.

40. O'Gara PT, et al. 2013 ACCF/AHA guideline for the management of ST-elevation myocardial infarction: a report of the American College of Cardiology Foundation/American Heart Association Task Force on Practice Guidelines. *J Am Coll Cardiol*. 2013;61:e78–e140.

41. Mann HJ, Nolan PE Jr. Update on the management of cardiogenic shock. *Curr Opin Crit Care*. 2006;12:431–436.

42. Petersen JW, Felker GM. Inotropes in the management of acute heart failure. *Crit Care Med*. 2008;36:S106–S111.

43. Anderson RD, et al. Use of intraaortic balloon counterpulsation in patients presenting with cardiogenic shock: observations from the GUSTO-I study. Global utilization of streptokinase and TPA for occluded coronary arteries. *J Am Coll Cardiol*. 1997;30:708–715.

44. Hasdai D, et al. Frequency and clinical outcome of cardiogenic shock during acute myocardial infarction among patients receiving reteplase or alteplase. Results from GUSTO-III. Global use of strategies to open occluded coronary arteries. *Eur Heart J*. 1999;20:128–135.

45. Edep ME, Brown DL. Effect of early revascularization on mortality from cardiogenic shock complicating acute myocardial infarction in California. *Am J Cardiol*. 2000;85:1185–1188.

46. Goldberg RJ, et al. Recent magnitude of and temporal trends (1994–1997) in the incidence and hospital death rates of cardiogenic shock complicating acute myocardial infarction: the second national registry of myocardial infarction. *Am Heart J*. 2001;141:65–72.

47. Hochman JS, et al. Early revascularization in acute myocardial infarction complicated by cardiogenic shock. SHOCK investigators. Should we emergently revascularize occluded coronaries for cardiogenic shock. *N Engl J Med* 1999;341:625–634.

48. Hochman JS, et al. One-year survival following early revascularization for cardiogenic shock. *JAMA*. 2001;285:190–192.

49. Dauerman HL, et al. Outcomes of percutaneous coronary intervention among elderly patients in cardiogenic shock: a multicenter, decade-long experience. *J Invasive Cardiol*. 2003;15:380–384.

50. Prasad A, et al. Outcomes of elderly patients with cardiogenic shock treated with early percutaneous revascularization. *Am Heart J*. 2004;147:1066–1070.

51. Kawaguchi O, et al. Ventriculoarterial coupling with intra-aortic balloon pump in acute ischemic heart failure. *J Thorac Cardiovasc Surg*. 1999;117:164–171.

52. Perera D, et al. Elective intra-aortic balloon counterpulsation during high-risk percutaneous coronary intervention: a randomized controlled trial. *JAMA*. 2010;304:867–874.

53. Patel MR, et al. Intra-aortic balloon counterpulsation and infarct size in patients with acute anterior myocardial infarction without shock: the CRISP AMI randomized trial. *JAMA*. 2011;306:1329–1337.

54. Holmes DR Jr, et al. Cardiogenic shock in patients with acute ischemic syndromes with and without ST-segment elevation. *Circulation*. 1999;100:2067–2073.

55. Valgimigli M, et al. Left ventricular unloading and concomitant total cardiac output increase by the use of percutaneous Impella Recover LP 2.5 assist device during high-risk coronary intervention. *Catheter Cardiovasc Interv*. 2005;65:263–267.

56. O'Neill WW, et al. A prospective, randomized clinical trial of hemodynamic support with Impella 2.5 versus intra-aortic balloon pump in patients undergoing high-risk percutaneous coronary intervention: the PROTECT II study. *Circulation*. 2012;126:1717–1727.

57. O'Neill WW, et al. The current use of Impella 2.5 in acute myocardial infarction complicated by cardiogenic shock: results from the USpella Registry. *J Interv Cardiol*. 2014;27:1–11.

58. Ouweneel DM, et al. Percutaneous mechanical circulatory support versus intra-aortic balloon pump in cardiogenic shock after acute myocardial infarction. *J Am Coll Cardiol*. 2017;69:278–287.

59. Goldstein AH, Pacella JJ, Clark RE. Predictable reduction in left ventricular stroke work and oxygen utilization with an implantable centrifugal pump. *Ann Thorac Surg*. 1994;58:1018–1024.

60. Cheng JM, et al. Percutaneous left ventricular assist devices vs. intra-aortic balloon pump counterpulsation for treatment of cardiogenic shock: a meta-analysis of controlled trials. *Eur Heart J*. 2009;30:2102–2108.

61. Kawashima D, et al. Left ventricular mechanical support with Impella provides more ventricular unloading in heart failure than extracorporeal membrane oxygenation. *ASAIO J*. 2011;57:169–176.

62. Pappalardo F, et al. Concomitant implantation of Impella® on top of veno-arterial extracorporeal membrane oxygenation may improve survival of patients with cardiogenic shock. *Eur J Heart Fail*. 2017;19(3):404–412.

Multivessel Percutaneous Coronary Interventions

Creighton W. Don, MD, MS, PhD, FSCAI and

Sandeep Krishnan, MD, RPVI

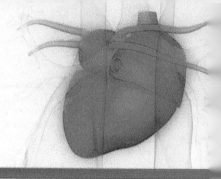

Coronary artery bypass graft surgery (CABG) has been the standard of care for revascularization of patients with complex multivessel coronary artery disease (CAD) since its introduction in 1968 (1). When percutaneous coronary intervention (PCI) was introduced in 1977 (2), it was thought to be appropriate only for patients with single-vessel disease, but as operator ability and device technologies have advanced, the use of PCI has expanded to treat patients with increasingly complex diseases, such as multivessel and left main coronary disease. This chapter focuses on the data and guidelines supporting multivessel PCI, compared to bypass surgery, among patients with appropriate indications of revascularization.

Approximately 40% to 60% of patients undergoing percutaneous revascularization have multivessel CAD, defined as ≥70% stenosis in ≥2 coronary arteries or involving the left main (3). As many as 30% to 40% of patients with multivessel disease and class I indications for CABG undergo PCI (4,5). The utilization of PCI in patients with multivessel disease may be partially explained by data supporting early invasive strategies in patients with acute coronary syndromes (5), patient comorbidities that preclude surgical candidacy (6), or patient and operator preference. Importantly, technical advancements in PCI and recent studies comparing PCI with CABG may justify multivessel interventions as an option for some patients.

Improvements in stent design, guide catheters, coronary wires, and debulking technologies, along with emerging techniques and dedicated equipment for treating chronic total occlusions (CTO) and bifurcation lesions, have improved the procedural success of PCI in patients with complex disease, making multivessel PCI more feasible from a technical standpoint. Additionally, the availability of percutaneous ventricular assist devices (pVAD) have allowed longer and more difficult procedures to be performed in high-risk patients (7). Improved image quality and lower radiation from newer fluoroscopy equipment with digital image processing have also reduced the radiation exposure of patients undergoing multivessel PCI. Finally, the emergence of more effective and safer anticoagulants, antiplatelet therapies, and lipid-lowering agents has made a major contribution to improved outcomes in patients undergoing multivessel coronary interventions.

Concomitantly, however, the outcomes of medical therapy alone have also improved significantly, and there are scarce data supporting improved survival with revascularization, compared with optimal medical therapy (8). Improved patient comfort and long- and short-term operative morbidity of CABG have also improved with shorter pump times, off-pump procedures, complete arterial revascularization, and minimally invasive approaches (9). In the current era, the decision to perform multivessel coronary interventions often requires the thoughtful decision making of an interdisciplinary heart team to consider myriad clinical trial data, assess myocardial viability and ischemia, as well as potential restenosis rates, and consider patients' surgical risks, all of which rarely presents a simple or unambiguous choice.

Clinical Trials and Guidelines: CABG Versus Multivessel PCI

The rapidly changing techniques and technology of coronary interventions present a challenge in interpreting long-term outcomes of clinical trials evaluating multivessel PCI. The results of the studies comparing angioplasty with CABG were soon eclipsed by the ubiquitous use of coronary stents, while the studies performed in the stent era have evaluated outmoded technologies as thinner, open-cell, and drug-eluting stents (DESs) were introduced that have improved deliverability and reduced restenosis. The second- and third-generation DESs with polymer and stent design modifications further reduce restenosis rates (10), making interpretation of older studies difficult.

CABG versus Angioplasty

In the Bypass Angioplasty Revascularization Investigation (BARI) study comparing CABG with percutaneous transluminal coronary angioplasty (PTCA)—balloon angioplasty—70% of patients randomized to PTCA underwent multivessel interventions. While there was no difference in the primary outcome of death or myocardial infarction (MI) at 5 years, the need for repeat revascularization was dramatically higher in the PTCA group. There was a significant survival advantage for diabetic patients undergoing CABG who received a left internal mammary artery (LIMA) graft, but none for the nondiabetic group or those with multivessel disease (11). Among those with multivessel disease randomized to PTCA, patients who had successful complete percutaneous multi-lesion revascularization had the lowest death and MI rates, compared with those in whom multivessel PTCA was unsuccessful or not attempted (12). A meta-analysis of trials comparing multivessel angioplasty with CABG reinforced these results, demonstrating similar outcomes between these two revascularization strategies in nondiabetics, but a survival benefit of CABG among diabetics (13).

CABG versus Bare-Metal Stents

Multivessel PCI studies performed in the bare-metal stent (BMS) era produced similar results, with only a modest reduction in repeat revascularization rates compared with CABG (Table 20.1). The 5-year death and MI outcomes were equivalent to CABG in the major studies in which bare-metal stents were used in the PCI arm, with the exception of the Surgery or Stent (SOS) study, in which mortality was significantly higher at 2 years for patients undergoing PCI. Although there was an unequal distribution of diabetics in the PCI group, further adjustment in the SOS study did not change the higher observed mortality at 2 years and subsequent time points (14). A recent meta-analysis of the ARTS, ERACI II, MASS II, and SOS studies, which compared bare-metal stenting to CABG, found no significant differences between the two strategies in death, MI,

TABLE 20.1 Studies Comparing Multivessel Percutaneous Coronary Intervention with Coronary Artery Bypass Grafting

STUDY	N	FOLLOW-UP	PRIMARY OUTCOME	PCI	CABG	p-VALUE	NOTES
Angioplasty							
BARI[a]	1,829	5-year	Death	13.7%	10.7%	0.19	Significant survival benefit of CABG among diabetics
			Death or MI	21.3%	19.6%	0.84	
			Revascularization	54.0%	8.0%	<0.01	
CABRI[b]	1,054	4-year	Death	10.9%	7.4%	0.09	No difference among diabetics
ERACI[c]	127	3-year	Death	9.5%	4.7%	0.50	No difference among diabetics
			MI	7.8%	7.8%	0.80	
			Revascularization	37.0%	6.3%	<0.01	
Bare-Metal Stents							
ARTS[d]	1,205	5-year	Death	8.0%	7.6%	0.83	No difference among diabetics
			Death, stroke, MI	18.2%	14.9%	0.14	
			Revascularization	30.3%	8.8%	<0.01	
ERACI II[e]	450	5-year	Death	7.1%	11.5%	0.18	Trend for benefit of PCI among nondiabetics
			Death or MI	2.7%	6.0%	0.15	
			Revascularization	28.5%	7.6%	<0.01	
MASS II[f]	611	5-year	Death	15.5%	12.8%	0.82	No difference among diabetics
			MI	11.2%	8.3%	0.78	
			Revascularization	32.2%	3.5%	0.02	
SOS[g]	988	2-year	Death	4.5%	1.6%	0.01	No difference among diabetics
			Death or MI	9.4%	9.8%	0.80	
			Revascularization	20.7%	6.0%	<0.01	
Drug-Eluting Stents							
SYNTAX[h]	1,800	3-year	Death	8.6%	6.7%	0.13	Reduced revascularization among diabetics
			Stroke	2.0%	3.4%	0.07	
			Death, stroke, MI	14.1%	12.0%	0.21	
			Revascularization	21.0%	11.0%	<0.01	
SYNTAX 5 year[i]	1,676	5-year	Death	13.9%	11.4%	0.10	No difference at 5 years in MACCE rates in patients with LM disease
			Stroke	2.4%	3.7%	0.09	
			Death, stroke, MI	20.8%	16.7%	0.03	
			Revascularization	25.9%	13.7%	<0.01	
CARDia[j]	510	1-year	Death	3.2%	3.2%	0.97	No difference for DES
			Death, MI, stroke	13.0%	10.5%	0.39	
			Death, MI, stroke, revascularization	19.3%	11.3%	0.02	
EXCEL[k]	1,905	3-year	Death, stroke, MI @ 30 days	4.9%	4.9%	0.008	No difference for EES vs. CABG
			Death, MI, stroke @ 3 years	15.4%	14.7%	0.98	
			Death, MI, stroke, revascularization @ 3 years	23.1%	19.1%	0.10	

[a]The bypass angioplasty revascularization investigation (BARI) investigators. Comparison of coronary bypass surgery with angioplasty in patients with multivessel disease. N Engl J Med. 1996;335:217–225.
[b]Kurbaan AS, et al. Difference in the mortality of the cabri diabetic and nondiabetic populations and its relation to coronary artery disease and the revascularization mode. Am J Cardiol. 2001;87:947–950, A943.
[c]Rodriguez A, et al. Three-year follow-up of the argentine randomized trial of percutaneous transluminal coronary angioplasty versus coronary artery bypass surgery in multivessel disease (ERACI). J Am Coll Cardiol. 1996;27:1178–1184.
[d]Serruys PW, et al. Five-year outcomes after coronary stenting versus bypass surgery for the treatment of multivessel disease: the final analysis of the arterial revascularization therapies study (ARTS) randomized trial. J Am Coll Cardiol. 2005;46:575–581.
[e]Rodriguez AE, et al. Five-year follow-up of the argentine randomized trial of coronary angioplasty with stenting versus coronary bypass surgery in patients with multiple vessel disease (ERACI II). J Am Coll Cardiol. 2005;46:582–588.
[f]Hueb W, et al. Five-year follow-up of the Medicine, Angioplasty, or Surgery Study (MASS II): a randomized controlled clinical trial of 3 therapeutic strategies for multivessel coronary artery disease. Circulation. 2007;115:1082–1089.

CABG, coronary artery bypass graft surgery; DES, drug-eluting stent; LM, left main; MACCE, major adverse cardiac and cerebrovascular event; MI, myocardial infarction; PCI, percutaneous coronary intervention.

or stroke. There was no heterogeneity in treatment in any of the subgroups, including diabetics and patients with left-ventricular dysfunction (15). Repeat revascularization was the primary driver behind differences in the composite outcome in all of these studies. Revascularization rates at 5 years following PCI was 20% to 30% in these studies, many times higher than the 3% to 8% rates for CABG, although an improvement from the 54% revascularization rate for PTCA in the BARI study (Table 20.1).

CABG versus DESs

Given that repeat revascularization was the primary driver for differences between PCI and CABG in these studies, the introduction of DES was expected to narrow the gap for multivessel PCI. The ERACI III (16) and the ARTS II (17) registries followed patients who underwent nonblinded multivessel PCI using first-generation paclitaxel and sirolimus-eluting stents. The event rates in the ARTS II registry more closely approximated the CABG outcomes of the original study (5-year major adverse cardiac events, including repeat revascularization 27.5% for PCI vs. 21.1% for CABG, p = 0.02, compared with 41.5% for BMS, p < 0.01), although the rates were statistically higher in the PCI groups. A similar finding was reported among patients in the ERACI III registry, where patients with multivessel PCI with DES had a much lower repeat revascularization rate, similar to the CABG patients in ERACI II. An analysis of the New York cardiac surgery and PCI reporting system, however, found a persistently high level of repeat revascularization among patients with multivessel disease initially treated with PCI compared with CABG, even among patients receiving DES (18).

The CARDia study randomized patients to PCI or CABG among 510 patients with multivessel CAD. Mortality, MI, and stroke at 1 year were equivalent, but revascularization was higher in the PCI group. Among patients who received DESs, however, the composite outcome and repeat revascularization were equivalent to CABG (12.4% vs. 11.6%, p = 0.82) (19).

The Synergy between Percutaneous Coronary Intervention with Taxus and Cardiac Surgery (SYNTAX) clinical trial is the largest study to date comparing stenting to surgery. The study randomized 1,800 patients with left main and/or three-vessel coronary disease to CABG or PCI using paclitaxel DESs with the intent of achieving complete revascularization (20). Operators were allowed to be aggressive in treating chronically occluded vessels, long lesions, bifurcations, and unprotected left main disease. Minimally invasive CABG was not permitted. Reflecting this aggressive approach, in the PCI group 63% had a bifurcation or trifurcation treated, 39.5% had left main disease, 33% of patients had more than 100 mm of stents placed, and, on average, 3.6 ± 1.6 lesions were treated and 4.6 ± 2.3 stents were implanted per patient. Despite this, complete revascularization was not performed in many patients, although this was achieved in a greater proportion of CABG patients, 63.2% versus 56.7% (p < 0.01). While the study was designed as a non-inferiority trial, at 12 months, death from any cause, stroke, MI, or repeat revascularization was lower among CABG patients (12.4%) than the PCI group (17.8%, p < 0.01). This endpoint was almost entirely explained by

revascularization because the rate of death, stroke, or MI was 7.7% for CABG versus 7.6% for PCI, p = 0.98. There were over three times as many strokes in the CABG group (2.2% vs. 0.6%, p < 0.01), while all-cause death and MI were not statistically different.

At 3-year follow-up, the death, stroke, and MI rates remained similar between the two groups. The early difference in stroke was no longer present. The revascularization rates continued to be twice as high in the PCI group (Table 20.1) (21). Five-year results of the SYNTAX trial were reported in 2013. Of the original 1,800 patients enrolled, 897 were assigned to CABG and 903 to PCI. Eight hundred and five (89.7%) patients in the CABG group and 871 (96.5%) in the PCI group completed 5 years' follow-up. Kaplan–Meier estimates of major adverse cardiac and cerebrovascular event (MACCE) rates were 26.9% for the CABG group versus 37.3% in the PCI group (p < 0.0001). The rates of all-cause mortality and stroke, however, were not significantly different between groups. Patients with left main disease did not demonstrate a difference in MACCE at 5 years between CABG and PCI; however, among the patients with three-vessel disease, MACCE rates were more than 50% higher at 5 years in those patients undergoing PCI (24.2% in the CABG group vs. 37.5% in the PCI group; p < 0.0001), explained almost entirely by clinically driven revascularization (22). There were important lower-risk subsets, with anatomic SYNTAX scores ≤22 in which PCI was equivalent to CABG, discussed in greater detail in the section "Lesion Related Factors: Coronary Anatomy."

A meta-analysis of six trials comparing multivessel PCI with DES to CABG reinforced these results (**Fig. 20.1**). Compared to CABG, at 1 year PCI was associated with a significantly higher incidence of revascularization (RR = 2.31; 95% CI [1.80–2.96]; p < 0.01), lower incidence of stroke (RR = 0.35; 95% CI [0.19–0.62]; p < 0.01), and no difference in death (RR = 1.02; 95% CI [0.77–1.36]; p = 0.88) or MI (RR = 1.16; 95% CI [0.72–1.88]; p = 0.53). At 5 years, PCI was associated with a higher incidence of death (RR = 1.3; 95% CI [1.10–1.54]; p < 0.01) and MI (RR = 2.21; 95% CI [1.75–2.79]; p < 0.01). While the higher incidence of MI with PCI was noticed in both diabetic and non-diabetics, death was increased primarily in diabetic patients (23).

Almost all CABG patients in these studies received an internal mammary artery (IMA) graft, and several patients had bilateral internal mammary grafts and full arterial revascularization, which helps to explain the lower need for repeat revascularization, because vein graft failure is as high as 40% in the first 18 months following CABG (24). Therefore, despite improvements in the techniques and outcomes of PCI, CABG remains preferred in surgically eligible patients with multivessel and left main disease owing to its relatively lower revascularization rates.

Guidelines

The American College of Cardiology Foundation/American Heart Association/Society for Cardiac Angiography and Interventions (ACCF/AHA/SCAI) practice guideline for percutaneous coronary intervention recommends CABG for patients with three-vessel CAD (Class I), or two-vessel disease with proximal left anterior descending

gBooth J, et al. Randomized, controlled trial of coronary artery bypass surgery versus percutaneous coronary intervention in patients with multivessel coronary artery disease: six-year follow-up from the Stent Or Surgery trial (SOS). *Circulation.* 2008;118:381–388.

hSerruys PW, et al. Percutaneous coronary intervention versus coronary-artery bypass grafting for severe coronary artery disease. *N Engl J Med.* 2009;360:961–972.

iMohr FW, et al. Coronary artery bypass graft surgery versus percutaneous coronary intervention in patients with three-vessel disease and left main coronary disease: 5-year follow-up of the randomised, clinical SYNTAX trial. *Lancet.* 2013;381:629.

jKapur A, et al. Randomized comparison of percutaneous coronary intervention with coronary artery bypass grafting in diabetic patients. 1-year results of the CARDia (Coronary Artery Revascularization in Diabetes) trial. *J Am Coll Cardiol.* 2010;55:432–440.

kStone GW, et al. Everolimus-eluting stents or bypass surgery for left main coronary artery disease. *N Engl J Med.* 2016;375:2223–2235.

A – Death

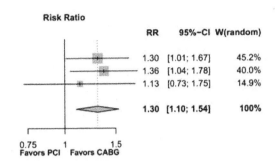

B – MI

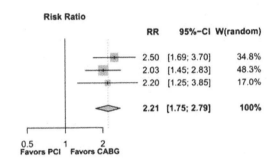

C – Stroke

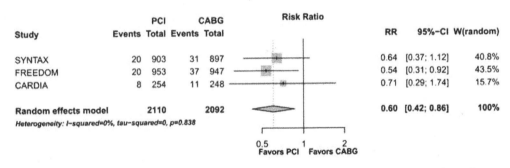

FIGURE 20.1 Meta-analysis of SYNTAX, FREEDOM, and CARDIA 5-year outcomes. CABG, coronary artery bypass graft surgery. (From: Fanari Z, et al. Comparison of percutaneous coronary intervention with drug eluting stents versus coronary artery bypass grafting in patients with multivessel coronary artery disease: meta-analysis of six randomized controlled trials. *Cardiovasc Revasc Med.* 2015;16(2):70–77.)

(LAD) disease (Class I). In both of these circumstances, PCI is given a Class IIB recommendation (**Table 20.2**) (25). Generally, either PCI or CABG can be chosen for treating symptomatic two-vessel disease not involving the proximal LAD (Class IIA); however, there are several patient, anatomic, and functional considerations that influence the choice of one procedure over the other (25).

The focused update on management of stable ischemic heart disease emphasized a preference for CABG over PCI in diabetics with two- or three-vessel disease (Class I) (26). This document recognized that patients with low SYNTAX scores ≤22 may have outcomes similar to CABG, but did not offer specific recommendations for

clinical practice. In the ACC/AATS/AHA/ASE/ASNC/SCAI/SCCT/STS 2017 appropriate use criteria for coronary revascularization, patients with three-vessel disease, with low CAD complexity and SYNTAX scores ≤22, PCI or CABG is considered appropriate, but for SYNTAX scores ≥22, CABG is preferred and PCI "may be appropriate" (**Table 20.3**) (27).

The 2014 European Society of Cardiology/European Association of Cardio-Thoracic Surgery (ESC/EACTS) guidelines on myocardial revascularization give a Class I recommendation for PCI in patients with three-vessel disease and a SYNTAX score of ≤22 (Class I), but a Class III for three-vessel disease with SYNTAX scores >22 (28).

TABLE 20.2 ACCF/AHA/SCAI Guidelines for PCI and CABG in Patients with Multivessel Coronary Artery Disease

CLINICAL SETTING	CABG	PCI
Unprotected Left Main Stenosis ≥50%		
No surgical contraindication and unfavorable anatomy for PCI	I	III
High-risk surgical patients (STS ≥5%), with ostial or trunk lesion, and SYNTAX score ≤22	I	IIA
Unstable angina/NSTEMI in nonsurgical candidates where left main is the culprit lesion	I	IIA
ST-elevation MI where left main is the culprit lesion	I	IIA
High-risk surgical patients (STS >2%) and SYNTAX score <33	I	IIB
Multivessel Disease		
3-vessel disease	I	IIB
Symptomatic 2-vessel disease (with proximal LAD)	I	IIB
Symptomatic 2-vessel disease (without proximal LAD)	IIA	IIB
Diabetics with multivessel coronary artery disease, especially if a left internal mammary graft will be anastomosed to the LAD	I	
2- or 3-vessel disease and prior CABG	IIB	IIA
Hybrid coronary revascularization (LIMA to LAD, and PCI of non-LAD vessels) if one or more of the following apply: 1. Limitations to traditional CABG 2. Lack of graft conduits 3. LAD unfavorable for PCI	IIA	IIA
Bifurcation Lesions		
Provisional stenting: small side branch with mild/moderate disease		IA
Bifurcation stenting: large side branch with disease		IIA

CABG, coronary artery bypass graft surgery; LAD, left anterior descending; LIMA, left internal mammary artery; PCI, percutaneous coronary intervention; STS, Society of Thoracic Surgeons.

Adapted from: Levine GN, et al. 2011 ACCF/AHA/SCAI guideline for percutaneous coronary intervention: executive summary: a report of the American College of Cardiology Foundation/American Heart Association Task Force on practice guidelines and the Society for Cardiovascular Angiography and Interventions. *Circulation.* 2011;124:2574–2609; Fihn SD, et al. 2014 ACC/AHA/AATS/PCNA/SCAI/STS focused update of the guideline for the diagnosis and management of patients with stable ischemic heart disease: a report of the American College of Cardiology/American Heart Association Task Force on Practice Guidelines, and the American Association for Thoracic Surgery, Preventive Cardiovascular Nurses Association, Society for Cardiovascular Angiography and Interventions, and Society of Thoracic Surgeons. *Circulation.* 2014;130:1749–1767.

Hybrid Approaches

Surgical and percutaneous revascularization strategies are far from mutually exclusive—with the growth of minimally invasive bypass techniques, hybrid approaches may be beneficial for specific patient subgroups. Hybrid coronary revascularization combines minimally invasive grafting of the IMA to the LAD artery with PCI of the remaining lesions to shorten recovery time, decrease the morbidity associated with CABG surgery, and take advantage of the superior longevity of the mammary graft.

A large retrospective study comparing 308 patients undergoing hybrid revascularization to 8,254 patients undergoing conventional single or bilateral IMA CABG showed no survival and 30-day MACCE rates were comparable. In-hospital complications and blood transfusions were lower after hybrid revascularization, and hospital stays were shorter (29). Small prospective and registry studies have shown similar, but mixed results (30–33). The POL-MIDES (HYBRID) study randomized 200 patients with multivessel disease involving the LAD to conventional CABG or hybrid coronary revascularization with PCI and a LIMA-LAD. There were six patients in the hybrid arm that crossed over to conventional surgery and two who were unable to complete PCI. In-hospital outcomes, including lengths of stay, were equivalent. MACCE at 1 year occurred in 10.2% for hybrid CABG-PCI and 7.8% for CABG (p = 0.54). There was a higher 1-year total vessel patency among patients who underwent hybrid revascularization compared to conventional CABG (90% vs. 81%, p = 0.01).

Several meta-analyses comparing hybrid coronary revascularization to CABG have been published (34–36) which showed equivalent outcomes of hospital and 1-year death, MI, stroke, atrial fibrillation, and renal failure. Hybrid revascularization was associated with fewer transfusions, shorter lengths of stay in the intensive care unit and hospital (36), and faster return to work (37). It was noted, however, that among patients treated with hybrid coronary revascularization, there was a higher rate of repeat revascularization (37).

Although hybrid revascularization is not superior to conventional CABG, a hybrid approach utilizing a surgical LIMA to LAD and PCI of non-LAD vessels is reasonable if there are limitations to surgery, lack of graft conduits, or a LAD unfavorable for PCI (Class IIA) (25).

Patient Comorbidities and the Heart Team

Age, diabetes, renal dysfunction, liver disease, chronic obstructive pulmonary disease, prior stroke, burden of vascular disease, and reduced LV function are among the major clinical factors that must be weighed in considering whether a patient can undergo CABG surgery. The patients enrolled in the clinical trials described previously were required to be reasonable CABG candidates, and so were at comparatively low risk for major perioperative complications.

The Society of Thoracic Surgeons (STS) risk model for perioperative morbidity and mortality and the European System for Cardiac Operative Risk Evaluation (euroSCORE) can help risk stratify the patient, and provide a starting point for discussions among the cardiologists, surgeons, patient, and family (38,39). These models provide some estimation of risk for CABG, valvular, and other thoracic surgeries by taking into account comorbidities such as age, diabetes, renal function, left ventricular (LV) dysfunction, chronic obstructive pulmonary disease, and prior open-heart procedures. These models are by no means perfect and tend to underestimate risk due to significant unaccounted conditions such as prior chest radiation, hepatic dysfunction, or pulmonary hypertension.

For the individual patient, physicians must also weigh the risks of future repeat revascularization associated with PCI against the immediate risks of CABG, which may not fit within the scope of patients treated in clinical trials. Hence, a collaborative approach to decision making between interventional cardiologists, cardiac surgeons, and the patient's general cardiologist is recommended. For patients with left main disease, three-vessel disease, or two-vessel disease involving the LAD in whom optimal revascularization strategy is not straightforward, a multidisciplinary "Heart Team" should evaluate the technical feasibility, risks, and benefits of PCI and CABG, followed by discussion with the patient about treatment options. The 2014

TABLE 20.3 ACC/AATS/AHA/ASE/ASNC/SCAI/SCCT/STS 2017 Appropriate Use Criteria for Coronary Revascularization in Patients with Stable Ischemic Heart Disease (Patients with Ischemic Symptoms on ≥2 Antianginals)

	CABG	PCI
Two-vessel CAD with proximal LAD stenosis	Appropriate	Appropriate
Three-vessel CAD with low CAD complexity (focal stenoses, SYNTAX score ≤22)	Appropriate	Appropriate
Three-vessel CAD with intermediate to high CAD complexity (SYNTAX score >22)	Appropriate	May be appropriate
Isolated left main disease (ostial/midshaft)	Appropriate	Appropriate
Left main stenosis (ostial/midshaft) with low CAD burden (one to two additional vessels, SYNTAX score ≤22)	Appropriate	Appropriate
Left main stenosis (bifurcation) with low CAD burden (one to two additional vessels, SYNTAX score ≤22)	Appropriate	May be appropriate
Left main stenosis (bifurcation) and additional CAD with intermediate to high CAD burden (SYNTAX score >22)	Appropriate	Rarely appropriate
Non-culprit lesion in ACS for symptomatic ischemia, FFR <0.80, or positive stress test	Appropriate	Appropriate

ACS, acute coronary syndrome; CABG, coronary artery bypass graft surgery; CAD, coronary artery disease; FFR, fractional flow reserve; PCI, percutaneous coronary intervention.

From: Patel MR, et al. ACC/AATS/AHA/ASE/ASNC/SCAI/SCCT/STS 2017 appropriate use criteria for coronary revascularization in patients with stable ischemic heart disease: a report of the American College of Cardiology Appropriate Use Criteria Task Force, American Association for Thoracic Surgery, American Heart Association, American Society of Echocardiography, American Society of Nuclear Cardiology, Society for Cardiovascular Angiography and Interventions, Society of Cardiovascular Computed Tomography, and Society of Thoracic Surgeons. *J Am Coll Cardiol.* 2017;69(17):2212–2241; Patel MR. ACC/AATS/AHA/ASE/ASNC/SCAI/SCCT/STS 2016 appropriate use criteria for coronary revascularization in patients with acute coronary syndromes: a report of the American College of Cardiology Appropriate Use Criteria Task Force, American Association for Thoracic Surgery, American Heart Association, American Society of Echocardiography, American Society of Nuclear Cardiology, Society for Cardiovascular Angiography and Interventions, Society of Cardiovascular Computed Tomography, and the Society of Thoracic Surgeons. *J Am Coll Cardiol.* 2016;69(5):570–591.

update to the stable ischemic heart disease guidelines makes the "Heart Team approach to revascularization in patients with diabetes mellitus and complex multivessel CAD" a Class I recommendation (26). Stable patients with diagnostic angiograms demonstrating complex multivessel disease should be taken off the table to allow for a thorough discussion of surgical, percutaneous options, and medical options among the Heart Team (38).

Advanced Age

Beyond being a risk factor for CAD and comorbidities in general, advanced age is an important predictor of outcome following PCI, and more so following CABG surgery. In the National Heart Lung and Blood Institute (NHLBI) dynamic registry, patients of advanced age (>80 years old) were twice as likely to have three-vessel CAD compared with younger (<65 years) patients (38% vs. 20%), and were more likely to have calcified arteries (40% vs. 20%) and undergo multivessel PCI (40% vs. 30%) (40). Many clinical trials have excluded patients >75 years old, so trial data should be cautiously extrapolated to the elderly population. Although CABG surgery can be safely performed in selected octogenarians, such patients are at particularly high risk for in-hospital mortality and postoperative complications (41). In both the STS and the euroSCORE models, age is strongly weighted in calculating risk, particularly in patients >80 (42). Thus, percutaneous revascularization may be a preferable approach even for the elderly with multivessel disease and other comorbidities.

Nevertheless, elderly patients have more procedural complications and poor long-term outcomes after PCI compared with younger patients. Several contemporary retrospective studies of PCI in patients >80 years old, with approximately one-third undergoing multivessel interventions, found a significant graded association of age with increased in-hospital mortality, contrast-induced nephropathy, transfusion requirements, stroke, and vascular complications (43–45). Much of the in-hospital morbidity was associated with acute coronary syndromes,

however, because the in-hospital event rates in stable patients was as low as 1.34% in patients >90 years (43). There also appears to be a temporal trend toward decreased complications over time (44). A retrospective study comparing CABG to multivessel PCI in patients >85 years of age found that CABG mortality was higher in the first 2 years, associated with patients having prior stroke, pre-existing congestive heart failure (CHF), and chronic obstructive pulmonary disease (46).

LV Dysfunction and Viability

Reduced LV function is an independent predictor of worse outcomes in patients undergoing percutaneous or surgical revascularization. Several older studies have demonstrated improved survival and LV function following CABG, among patients with mild to moderate systolic dysfunction (47). In the STICH trial, patients with symptomatic ischemia from multivessel CAD and LV ejection fractions (EF) <35% did not have improved survival with CABG compared with medical therapy at 5 years, although the composite outcome of death and re-hospitalization favored CABG (48). The STICH Extension Study (STICHES), however, demonstrated lower cardiovascular and all-cause mortality and composite outcome for CABG at 10 years (58.9% vs. 66.1%, hazard ratio 0.84 [95% CI, 0.73–0.97]; p = 0.02) (49).

In a similar fashion, the PROTECT II study showed that there may be some benefit to complete revascularization in patients with reduced LV function. In this study, 452 symptomatic patients with complex three-vessel disease or unprotected left main CAD and severely depressed left ventricular function (EF ≤35%) were randomized to ventricular support using an intra-aortic balloon pump or Impella 2.5 device during non-emergent high-risk PCI (50).

In a sub-study of PROTECT II, among patients with quantitative echocardiography (LV volumes and biplane EF), Daubert et al. assessed the extent and predictors of reverse LV remodeling, defined as improved systolic function with an absolute increase in EF

≥5%. Reverse LV remodeling occurred more frequently in patients with more extensive revascularization (odds ratio, 7.52; 95% CI [1.31–43.25]) and was associated with significantly fewer major adverse events (composite of death/MI stroke/transient ischemic attack): 9.7% versus 24.2% (p < 0.01). There was also a greater reduction in New York Heart Association Class III/IV heart failure among reverse LV remodelers (51).

Diabetes

Diabetic patients represent 20% to 25% of patients undergoing revascularization, and they are more likely to have diffuse CAD, multivessel involvement, and LV dysfunction (52). The mortality rate of diabetics following PCI is almost twice as high as that of nondiabetics (53). The BARI trial compared PCI with CABG in the management of patients with multivessel disease and found a survival advantage with surgical revascularization among diabetic patients (11). Five-year survival for diabetics assigned to PTCA was 65.5% compared with 80.6% for those assigned to CABG. The survival benefit was evident in patients who had at least one IMA used as a conduit. This finding was not corroborated by several smaller randomized studies published since BARI. ARTS (54), MASS II (55), ERACI/ERACI II (56,57), and SOS (14) studies of PCI versus CABG showed statistically equivalent outcomes in their diabetic subsets (Fig. 20.1).

Among diabetics in the SYNTAX trial, the composite major adverse cardiac, cerebrovascular, and revascularization event rate was significantly higher for patients receiving PCI (46.5% in the PCI group vs. 29.0% in the CABG group; p < 0.01).

The FREEDOM trial (Future Revascularization Evaluation in Patients with Diabetes Mellitus: Optimal Management of Multivessel Disease) is a multicenter, prospective randomized trial comparing CABG with PCI stenting using sirolimus-eluting stents in diabetic patients with multivessel disease. The trial followed patients out to a minimum of 2 years, with all patients required to be on goal-directed medical therapy for CAD. These results parallel that of the 5-year SYNTAX diabetic subset. Patients in the CABG group had significantly lower rates of the composite endpoint of all-cause death, cerebrovascular accident, or MI compared with patients in the first-generation DES group (18.7% in the CABG group vs. 26.6% in the PCI group; p < 0.01). As in the SYNTAX study, among patients with SYNTAX scores ≤22, however, the FREEDOM trial reported no difference between treatment groups for the composite endpoint. There was a mortality benefit associated with CABG in patients with SYNTAX scores of 23–32, but this was not the case for patients with SYNTAX scores of 33 or higher. The reason for this difference in outcomes is unclear, but might be related to statistical power, because less than 20% of patients in the FREEDOM trial had a SYNTAX score of 33 or higher (58).

Based on the findings of the FREEDOM, BARI, and SYNTAX studies, the 2014 ACC/AHA/AATS/PCNA/SCAI/STS update on revascularization for stable ischemic CAD changed the recommendation for CABG among diabetic patients with multivessel disease to a Class I indication (25). PCI is reasonable in diabetics with low complexity disease, and may be appropriate when there are limitations with surgery (Table 20.2). The 2014 ESC/EACTS guidelines recommend CABG over PCI as a Class IA indication in diabetic patients with stable multivessel CAD and an acceptable surgical risk. Nevertheless, in patients with stable multivessel CAD but with lower SYNTAX scores (≤22), PCI could be considered as an alternative to CABG as a Class IIA recommendation (28).

Functional Testing, Ischemic Burden, and Viability

Functional stress testing can help risk-stratify patients with multivessel coronary disease and identify patients who might likely benefit from revascularization. In addition to ascertaining the significance of individual coronary stenosis, stress testing can help quantify the percentage of ischemic myocardium and identify nonviable regions. A clinical or functional assessment of ischemia should factor into the collaborative risk benefit discussion between patient and the heart team regarding the relative merits of medical therapy, PCI, and CABG.

The number of ischemic territories identified by stress testing is associated with worse prognosis (59) and a retrospective study showed that patients with ischemia in >10% of the myocardium who undergo revascularization have a lower mortality than similarly matched patients who are medically treated. Among patients with ≤10% ischemia of the myocardium, revascularization did not confer a clear benefit in this study (**Fig. 20.2**) (60). The finding that patients with larger ischemic territories benefited the most from revascularization persisted after adjustment for common risk factors.

Although a substudy of the STICH trial did not demonstrate a benefit of revascularization associated with viable myocardium, a meta-analysis of patients with LV dysfunction showed that the benefit of revascularization was achieved only in patients with documented myocardial viability (61). Additionally, viability itself is a marker of survival benefit regardless of revascularization (62), and would inform the collaborative decision making regarding risks and benefits of multivessel revascularization.

Coronary anatomy alone does not always give an accurate assessment of the amount of myocardium at risk. Revascularization of nondominant branches, small vessels, distal vessels, or vessels supplying primarily infarcted territory are unlikely to confer the same benefits on patients as observed in clinical trials of multivessel PCI. Visual assessment of coronary stenosis severity can be inaccurate for determining the hemodynamic significance of atherosclerotic disease (63). A recent study by Nam et al. demonstrated that the

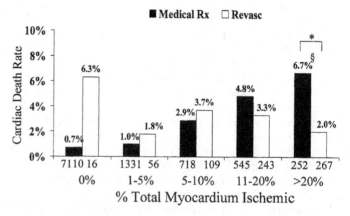

FIGURE 20.2 Cardiac death rates in patients undergoing revascularization versus medical therapy stratified by amount of inducible ischemia. (From: Hachamovitch GN, et al. Comparison of the short-term survival benefit associated with revascularization compared with medical therapy in patients with no prior coronary artery disease undergoing stress myocardial perfusion single photon emission computed tomography. *Circulation.* 2003;107:2900–2907.)

use of coronary fractional flow reserve (FFR) changed the severity assessment of atherosclerotic lesions based on anatomy alone, which led to reclassification of angiographic SYNTAX scores to a lower risk group for 32% of patients. The combination of the functional assessment and anatomical SYNTAX score was a better predictor of major adverse cardiac events at 1 year than the SYNTAX score alone (64).

Functional assessments of lesions may help to better classify the severity and ischemic burden of a patient's coronary anatomy, which will help determine whether a patient truly has multivessel disease, left main, or LAD involvement, which directly impacts whether medical therapy, PCI, or CABG is preferred.

Complete or Incomplete Revascularization

The magnitude of ischemia reduction by PCI appears to be associated with improved patient outcomes, while selective or partial revascularization, limited by anatomical or technical complexity, or operator error, is associated with worse mortality and cardiovascular outcomes (65,66). In this light, successful multivessel revascularization potentially has a greater positive impact on patients than revascularization on patients with single-vessel disease.

The concept of complete cardiac revascularization for patients with multivessel disease has been of ongoing interest in interventional cardiology. In older surgical studies, 68% to 78% of patients with complete revascularization were asymptomatic, whereas only 42% to 58% of patients with incomplete revascularization were asymptomatic (67–69). In the BARI trial, patients who had surgical revascularization were more likely to be free of angina at 5 years, and the need for repeat revascularization was substantially greater in the ICR angioplasty arm (11).

The Clinical Outcomes Utilizing Revascularization and Aggressive Drug Evaluation (COURAGE) trial nuclear sub-study evaluated the effectiveness of PCI for reducing ischemia, compared with optimal medical therapy. Baseline and post-randomization nuclear stress perfusion imaging were obtained in a subset of patients in the main trial (70). Among those undergoing PCI, the reduction in ischemic myocardium was greater than medical therapy (−2.7% vs. −0.5%, p < 0.01). More patients in the PCI group met the primary endpoint criteria of a significant ≥5% reduction in ischemia (33% vs. 19%, p < 0.01). Although the sub-study was not powered to evaluate the interaction of treatment and ischemia reduction on outcomes, patients who had a larger reduction in ischemia had better outcomes.

A subanalysis of the PROTECT II reported that extensive revascularization was associated with an increased likelihood of improvement in LV function and 90-day clinical outcomes than those who had limited revascularization (51). Similar findings were reported in the SYNTAX trial. In the PCI cohort (n = 903), the baseline and residual SYNTAX scores were calculated. Subjects with a residual SYNTAX score of 0 were defined as having undergone complete revascularization. Five-year clinical outcomes were stratified by tertiles of the residual SYNTAX score: >0 to 4, >4 to 8, and >8. The mean baseline and residual SYNTAX scores were 28.4 ± 11.5 and 4.5 ± 6.9, respectively. The residual SYNTAX score was distributed as follows: 0 (n = 386, 42.7%); >0 to 4 (n = 184, 20.4%), >4 to 8 (n = 167, 18.5%), >8 (n = 153, 16.9%) (**Fig. 20.3**). A progressively higher residual SYNTAX Score was shown to be a surrogate marker of increasing clinical comorbidity and anatomic complexity. Subjects with complete revascularization and residual SYNTAX scores ≤8 had a comparable 5-year mortality (0, 8.5%; >0–4, 8.7%; >4–8, 11.4%; p = 0.60). A residual SYNTAX score >8 was associated with 35.3% all-cause mortality at 5 years (p <0. 01). Similar results were found in the predefined diabetic and left main subgroups (71).

A recent meta-analysis buttresses these findings. There were 35 studies, totaling 89,883 patients, that compared 45,417 (50.5%) patients who received complete revascularization and 44,466 (49.5%) with incomplete revascularization. Incomplete revascularization was more common after PCI than after CABG (56% vs. 25%; p < 0.01). Complete revascularization was associated with lower long-term mortality (RR 0.71, 95% CI 0.65–0.77; p < 0.01), MI (RR 0.78, 95% CI 0.68–0.90; p < 0.01), and repeat coronary revascularization (RR 0.74, 95% CI 0.65–0.83; p < 0.01). The mortality benefit associated with complete revascularization was consistent across studies irrespective of revascularization modality (CABG: RR 0.70, 95% CI 0.61–0.80; p < 0.01; and PCI: RR 0.72, 95% CI 0.64–0.81; p < 0.01). Consistent with the prior studies,

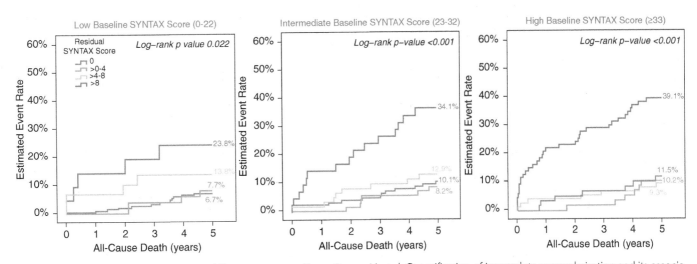

FIGURE 20.3   Residual SYNTAX score and 5-year outcomes. (From: Farooq V, et al. Quantification of incomplete revascularization and its association with five-year mortality in the synergy between percutaneous coronary intervention with taxus and cardiac surgery (SYNTAX) trial validation of the residual SYNTAX score. *Circulation.* 2013;128:141–151.)

the authors concluded CR is achieved more commonly with CABG than with PCI (72).

This non-randomized data taken from post-hoc analyses should be interpreted cautiously, because the findings may be confounded by the fact that patients with incomplete revascularization may have more complex and advanced atherosclerosis, which may lead to treatment and selection bias, and which itself may be a marker for patients with greater comorbidities.

Nevertheless, patients who have the greatest reduction in ischemic territory are the ones who benefit the most clinically, supporting the view that multivessel interventions potentially have a greater impact on improving patient outcomes than simple single-vessel interventions. This question is being directly addressed in the currently ongoing multicenter International Study of Comparative Health Effectiveness with Medical and Invasive Approaches (ISCHEMIA) study, which compares revascularization to optimal medical therapy in patients with moderate to severe ischemia.

Acute Coronary Syndromes (ACS)

Multivessel CAD is a key predictor of increased mortality and reduced global LV systolic function after ST-elevation MI (STEMI) or non-STEMI (NSTEMI). Almost half of patients presenting with an acute MI have multivessel disease, which is associated with worse procedural and in-hospital outcomes compared with patients with single-vessel disease (73,74). A study of patients with acute MI treated with PTCA demonstrated a 3-fold higher mortality rate (7.5% vs. 2.5% p < 0.01) and reinfarction rate (3.2% vs. 0.6% p = 0.02) at 30-day follow-up in patients with multivessel disease as compared to those with single-vessel disease (75).

The early studies of multivessel PCI at the time of ACS were unfavorable. A retrospective study of 820 patients treated with primary angioplasty for AMI found that among patients with multivessel disease, those undergoing multivessel PCI had higher rates of reinfarction (13.0% vs. 2.8%, p < 0.01), revascularization (25% vs. 15%, p = 0.01), and major cardiac complications (40% vs. 28%, p < 0.01). Multivessel PCI was an independent predictor of increased periprocedural MIs and overall major adverse outcomes at 1 year (75,76). A subanalysis of patients with multivessel disease in the APEX-AMI trial of pexelizumab or placebo in acute MI found a 2-fold higher rate of death and composite death, heart failure, and shock in patients who had multivessel PCI compared with those who had PCI of the infarct-related artery only (77). In TARGET (do Tirofiban and Reopro Give similar Efficacy Trial), patients with NSTE-ACS undergoing multivessel revascularization had similar 1-year mortality and target vessel revascularization (TVR) at 1 year compared with patients undergoing single-vessel revascularization. The multivessel revascularization group did have a higher rate of periprocedural MI (HR 1.47; 95% CI 1.12–1.92; p < 0.01) (78).

On the other hand, recent studies have suggested that because PCI techniques and technology have improved, complete revascularization at the time of ACS may be a preferable strategy.

Small, non-blinded studies and registries have shown multivessel PCI at the time of culprit-lesion PCI to be safe, without any differences in mortality or MI at 1 year (79–81). Likewise, Brener et al. demonstrated the safety and efficacy of multivessel PCI compared with culprit-lesion only PCI among patients with ACS and microvascular dysfunction (MVD) from the TACTICS-TIMI 18 (Treat Angina with aggrastat and determine Cost of Therapy with an Invasive or Conservative Strategy-Thrombolysis in MI 18) trial (82). The

group of patients who underwent multivessel PCI had similar rates for mortality and MI at 30 days and 6 months compared with the culprit-lesion-only group; however, they had a significantly lower rate of subsequent revascularization at 6 months (1.5% vs. 6.3%, p = 0.04).

In a substudy of 2,686 patients with ACS undergoing PCI enrolled in the ACUITY (Acute Catheterization and Urgent Intervention Triage Strategy) trial, the impact of residual SYNTAX scores was assessed. Following PCI, 40.4% of patients had complete revascularization, 19.5% had residual SYNTAX scores between 0 and 2, 21.5% between 2 and 8, and 18.7% >8. The 30-day and 1-year rates of ischemic events were significantly higher in the incomplete revascularization group, especially those with high rSS. Residual SYNTAX score remained an independent predictor of all ischemic outcomes at 1 year, including all-cause mortality after adjustment for patient comorbidities (HR 1.05, 95% CI 1.02–1.09, p < 0.01) (83).

The trial that heralded a tidal wave of change in the complete revascularization debate was the single-blind, randomized Preventive Angioplasty in Acute Myocardial Infarction (PRAMI) trial. Four hundred and sixty-five consecutive patients with acute STEMI and multivessel coronary disease detected at the time of emergency PCI were enrolled at five coronary care centers, excluding those patients in cardiogenic shock or with high-risk lesions (CTO or stenoses of the left main stem or ostia of both the LAD and circumflex arteries). After the completion of PCI in the infarct artery, eligible patients were randomly assigned to undergo PCI in non-infarct arteries with more than 50% stenosis, or no further intervention.

During a mean follow-up of 23 months, the primary outcome of cardiac death, nonfatal MI, or refractory angina occurred in 21 patients assigned to preventive PCI and in 53 patients assigned to infarct artery–only PCI (HR for preventive-PCI, 0.35; 95% CI, 0.21–0.58; p < 0.01). Hazard ratios for the three components of the primary outcome were significant: HR 0.34 (95% CI, 0.11–1.08) for cardiac death, 0.32 (95% CI, 0.13–0.75) for nonfatal MI, and 0.35 (95% CI, 0.18–0.69) for refractory angina (84).

A meta-analysis of six registry studies of over 5,000 patients found no significant difference in MI and mortality between multivessel PCI and culprit vessel PCI, but multivessel PCI may decrease long-term MACCE (OR, 0.69; 95% CI 0.51–0.93; p = 0.02) and unplanned revascularization (OR, 0.64; 95% CI 0.45–93; p = 0.02) compared with culprit vessel PCI (85).

Patients with cardiogenic shock during or shortly following STEMI may be a unique subgroup that derives particular benefit from complete revascularization during index PCI. In the SHOCK trial among patients with a ≥5% reduction in ischemia, there was a significantly lower 30-day mortality (41.4%–56.8% p = 0.01) and event-free survival at 5 years (86.6% vs. 75.3%, p = 0.03). This benefit was even more pronounced for patients with >10% ischemia of total myocardium at baseline. The patients with no residual ischemia had no events at 5 years (Fig. 20.3) (86).

Multivessel revascularization may be useful if ischemia is due to disease in the non-culprit artery caused by a compensatory hypercontractile response in non-culprit territory in the setting of an acute MI. In light of this recent data, the 2015 ACC/AHA/SCAI focused update on primary PCI committee assigned a new Class IIB recommendation for considering multivessel PCI in selected hemodynamically stable patients with significant non-infarct artery stenosis (28, 87). The 2016 ACCF/AHA/SCAI appropriate use criteria deem multivessel revascularization of a non-culprit artery appropriate in the setting of clinically apparent ischemia, or ischemia demonstrated by non-invasive stress testing or FFR of the nonculprit vessel (27).

Lesion-Related Factors

In addition to factors such as ischemic burden and patient characteristics described earlier, the decision on how to manage a patient with multivessel coronary disease must take into account anatomical features, including lesion complexity, presence of left main disease, bifurcation lesions, CTO, and target vessel location and diameter. Not only are such features relevant to technical feasibility, but they also have valuable prognostic value that informs the choice of revascularization strategy. Complete anatomical revascularization may not be the objective in all patients with multivessel disease, while for others adequate revascularization of multiple major coronary arteries may be necessary to realize comparable reductions in ischemia and angina, or improvements in LV function associated with surgical revascularization. The 2017 ACCF/AHA/SCAI appropriateness criteria endorse using anatomical data, as well as symptoms status and non-invasive testing data, to guide decisions regarding revascularization method (Table 20.3) (88).

Coronary Anatomy

Coronary anatomy is a crucial factor affecting the decision to choose CABG or PCI. Compared with patients with single-vessel CAD, patients with multivessel disease are more likely to require complex procedures owing to anatomical reasons such as calcified lesions, CTO, extreme tortuosity and angulation, and diffusely diseased and smaller vessels. These anatomic and procedural variables are related not only to the technical feasibility of PCI, but also to the long-term outcomes of PCI, which will help estimate the relative benefit of CABG or PCI.

The traditional lesion classification schemes, such as the ACC/AHA ABC lesion classification, or more recently the SCAI modification for non-C and high-C lesions, have long provided a general rule of thumb for estimating PCI success and long-term patient outcomes (38,89,90), but provide information only with regard to single vessels and do not account for complexity based on multivessel disease and global ischemic burden. Furthermore, the terms "multivessel" or "three-vessel disease" define a very heterogeneous group of patients, ranging from patients with small severely diseased last-remaining conduits, left main disease, trifurcation stenosis, or chronically occluded arteries, to patients with single focal stenoses in two to three large arteries. There are several angiographic CAD scoring systems available, but the SYNTAX score in particular has gained traction in classifying the heterogeneous populations in clinical trials of multivessel disease, and in risk-stratifying patients in clinical practice. The SYNTAX score gives various weights to the number, location, length, tortuosity, calcification, and percent diameter reduction of all stenosis, in addition to other anatomic characteristics such as angulation, total occlusion, bifurcations, trifurcation, and calcification. Each lesion is given a score, and a total of 12 lesions can be counted. Non-lesion characteristics, such as diffuse disease, can contribute to the score (91). Although scores can theoretically range from 0 to the 100s, clinically meaningful SYNTAX scores fall into the tertiles described by Serruys et al., as low ($\leq$22), intermediate (23–32), and high ($\geq$33), which have prognostic value regarding long-term major cardiovascular outcomes (92). The performance

of this anatomical score may be even stronger when age, creatinine clearance, LV ejection fraction, and diabetes are also added into the model (93).

In a subanalysis of the SYNTAX trial, CABG and PCI performed equally for patients with low SYNTAX scores. Even among diabetic patients there was no benefit for CABG over PCI for those with low SYNTAX scores (94). In patients with three-vessel disease and left main involvement who had intermediate and high SYNTAX scores, however, there was a significant benefit with CABG (Fig. 20.4) (92). Smaller lesion diameter and longer lesion length, diffuse disease, and CTO are associated with higher rates of in-stent restenosis and repeat revascularization (95). Also, PCI success is associated with the complexity of coronary anatomy (96). It follows that patients with smaller, more diffuse, and complicated disease are at higher risk for restenosis and residual ischemia, and need to undergo subsequent revascularization; therefore, such patients may have better outcomes with CABG.

EXCEL trial randomly assigned 1,905 eligible patients with left main CAD of low or intermediate anatomical complexity (SYNTAX scores <33) to undergo PCI or CABG. This trial demonstrated non-inferiority of PCI with regard to death, MI, or stroke (15.4% for PCI vs. 14.7% for CABG, HR, 1.00; 95% CI, 0.79–1.26; p = 0.98 for superiority). Ischemia-driven revascularization, however, was higher among those undergoing PCI (12.6% vs. 7.5%, HR 1.72, 95% CI 1.27–2.33, p < 0.01) (97).

PCI can be considered for high-risk surgical patients (STS $\geq$5%) with multivessel CAD including ostial or mid-trunk left-main stenosis, but with SYNTAX scores <22 (Class IIA), or intermediate to higher surgical risk (STS >2%) and SYNTAX <33 (Class IIB) (Table 20.3).

Bifurcation Lesions

Patients with significant atherosclerosis of a major artery and a large side branch may have myocardium at risk and long-term outcomes similar to patients with traditionally defined multivessel disease. The presence of a bifurcation lesion of major arteries is also associated with increased procedural complexity and worse clinical outcomes (98, 99), as well as higher SYNTAX scores, which also may affect the risk stratification of patients undergoing multivessel intervention (92).

Multiple studies have demonstrated an equivalence of provisional stenting (stenting the side branch only if it develops significant stenosis or becomes occluded) with true bifurcation stenting, and in some series have reported lower rates of restenosis and adverse outcomes with provisional stenting (98–100). Provisional stenting is given a Class IA recommendation, and up-front bifurcation stenting is considered a Class IIA recommendation (Table 20.2). If a major side branch becomes severely stenotic, or occludes completely after the main branch is treated, it appears reasonable to treat the side branch in order to minimize ischemia and myocardial damage (101). Otherwise, if the side branch remains patent with TIMI 3 flow or an FFR >0.8 (38,39), current consensus opinion is that it does not need to be treated. Similar outcomes have been reported with a similar PCI strategy for left main bifurcation disease (102).

In light of this, the presence of bifurcation disease in multivessel CAD should factor into the risk-benefit discussion with regard to choice of revascularization strategy, because it may increase the complexity and potential risk for PCI, the long-term risk for restenosis.

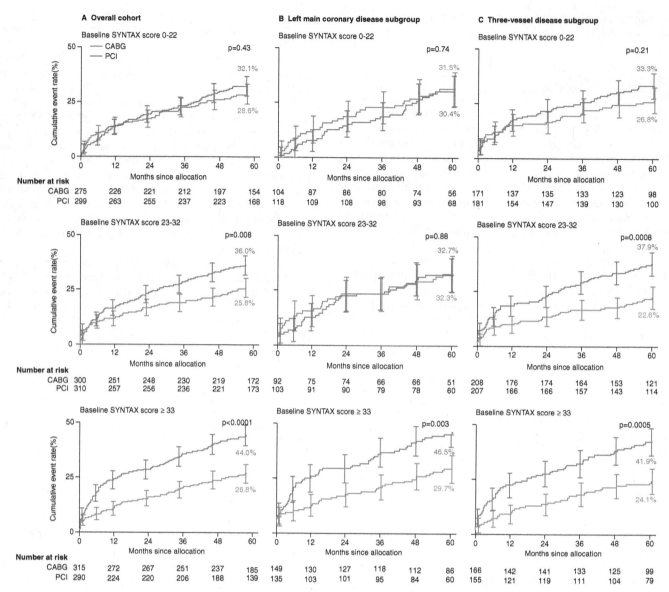

FIGURE 20.4 Death, stroke, or MI in patients randomized to CABG or PCI, in the overall **(A)**, left main **(B)**, and three-vessel disease subgroups **(C)**, stratified by SYNTAX score. CABG, coronary artery bypass graft surgery; PCI, percutaneous coronary intervention. (From: Mohr FW, et al. Coronary artery bypass graft surgery versus percutaneous coronary intervention in patients with three-vessel disease and left main coronary disease: 5-year follow-up of the randomised, clinical SYNTAX trial. *Lancet.* 2013;381:629–638.)

Summary

The decision to perform multivessel PCI is not binary, nor is it easily reduced to simple algorithms, but must weigh complex clinical, anatomic, and technical variables, along with a patient's surgical risk factors, in the context of an evidence-based landscape that is constantly changing. Stenting of more than one coronary artery in the same setting remains the small minority of PCIs performed in the United States, estimated at only 12% of procedures performed (103). In general, patients with multivessel disease undergoing PCI are more likely to have an intervention upon a "culprit" vessel, while patients undergoing CABG will generally undergo complete revascularization. Therefore, the choice of CABG over PCI may be influenced by the clinical necessity of complete revascularization for a particular patient. Myocardial viability, extent of ischemia, and LV function are invaluable for determining the targets and extent of revascularization.

Key Points

- Multivessel revascularization should be guided by the extent of symptomatic, clinically significant ischemia refractory to optimal medical therapy.

- CABG is preferred for diabetics with complex multivessel CAD due to improved survival over PCI (Class I).

- PCI for isolated left main disease or low complexity multivessel disease with SYNTAX scores (<22) is appropriate, with outcomes similar to CABG.

- Revascularization of non-infarct-related arteries during acute coronary syndromes is *appropriate* in the presence of symptomatic ischemia, FFR <0.80, or a positive stress test.

- A *heart team* approach is recommended for making decisions about revascularization of patients with multivessel CAD (Class I).

References

1. Favaloro RG. Saphenous vein autograft replacement of severe segmental coronary artery occlusion: operative technique. *Ann Thorac Surg.* 1968;5:334–339.

2. Gruntzig AR, Senning A, Siegenthaler WE. Nonoperative dilatation of coronary-artery stenosis: percutaneous transluminal coronary angioplasty. *N Engl J Med.* 1979;301:61–68.

3. Anderson HV, et al. A contemporary overview of percutaneous coronary interventions. The American College of Cardiology-National Cardiovascular Data Registry (ACC-NCDR). *J Am Coll Cardiol.* 2002;39:1096–1103.

4. Frutkin AD, et al. Drug-eluting stents and the use of percutaneous coronary intervention among patients with class I indications for coronary artery bypass surgery undergoing index revascularization: analysis from the NCDR (National Cardiovascular Data Registry). *JACC Cardiovasc Interv.* 2009;2:614–621.

5. Gogo PB Jr, et al. Changes in patterns of coronary revascularization strategies for patients with acute coronary syndromes (from the CRUSADE Quality Improvement Initiative). *Am J Cardiol.* 2007;99:1222–1226.

6. Mokadam NA, et al. Prevalence and procedural outcomes of percutaneous coronary intervention and coronary artery bypass grafting in patients with diabetes and multivessel coronary artery disease. *J Card Surg.* 2011;26:1–8.

7. Sjauw KD, et al. Supported high-risk percutaneous coronary intervention with the Impella 2.5 device the Europella registry. *J Am Coll Cardiol.* 2009;54:2430–2434.

8. Boden WE, et al. Optimal medical therapy with or without PCI for stable coronary disease. *N Engl J Med.* 2007;356:1503–1516.

9. Tarakji KG, et al. Temporal onset, risk factors, and outcomes associated with stroke after coronary artery bypass grafting. *JAMA.* 2011;305:381–390.

10. Stone GW, et al. Comparison of an everolimus-eluting stent and a paclitaxel-eluting stent in patients with coronary artery disease: a randomized trial. *JAMA.* 2008;299:1903–1913.

11. The Bypass Angioplasty Revascularization Investigation (BARI) Investigators. Comparison of coronary bypass surgery with angioplasty in patients with multivessel disease. *N Engl J Med.* 1996;335:217–225.

12. Kip KE, et al. Influence of pre-PTCA strategy and initial PTCA result in patients with multivessel disease: the Bypass Angioplasty Revascularization Investigation (BARI). *Circulation.* 1999;100:910–917.

13. Hlatky MA, et al. Coronary artery bypass surgery compared with percutaneous coronary interventions for multivessel disease: a collaborative analysis of individual patient data from ten randomised trials. *Lancet.* 2009;373:1190–1197.

14. Booth J, et al. Randomized, controlled trial of coronary artery bypass surgery versus percutaneous coronary intervention in patients with multivessel coronary artery disease: six-year follow-up from the Stent or Surgery Trial (SoS). *Circulation.* 2008;118:381–388.

15. Daemen J, et al. Long-term safety and efficacy of percutaneous coronary intervention with stenting and coronary artery bypass surgery for multivessel coronary artery disease: a meta-analysis with 5-year patient-level data from the ARTS, ERACI-II, MASS-II, and SoS trials. *Circulation.* 2008;118:1146–1154.

16. Rodriguez AE, et al. Revascularization strategies of coronary multiple vessel disease in the drug eluting stent era: one year follow-up results of the ERACI III trial. *EuroIntervention.* 2006;2:53–60.

17. Serruys PW, et al. 5-year clinical outcomes of the ARTS II (Arterial Revascularization Therapies Study II) of the sirolimus-eluting stent in the treatment of patients with multivessel de novo coronary artery lesions. *J Am Coll Cardiol.* 2010;55:1093–1101.

18. Hannan EL, et al. Drug-eluting stents vs. coronary-artery bypass grafting in multivessel coronary disease. *N Engl J Med.* 2008;358:331–341.

19. Kapur A, et al. Randomized comparison of percutaneous coronary intervention with coronary artery bypass grafting in diabetic patients. 1-year results of the CARDia (Coronary Artery Revascularization in Diabetes) trial. *J Am Coll Cardiol.* 2010;55:432–440.

20. Serruys PW, et al. Percutaneous coronary intervention versus coronary-artery bypass grafting for severe coronary artery disease. *N Engl J Med.* 2009;360:961–972.

21. Kappetein AP, et al. Comparison of coronary bypass surgery with drug-eluting stenting for the treatment of left main and/or three-vessel disease: 3-year follow-up of the SYNTAX trial. *Eur Heart J.* 2011;32:2125–2134.

22. Mohr FW, et al. Coronary artery bypass graft surgery versus percutaneous coronary intervention in patients with three-vessel disease and left main coronary disease: 5-year follow-up of the randomised, clinical SYNTAX trial. *Lancet.* 2013;381:629–638.

23. Fanari Z, et al. Comparison of percutaneous coronary intervention with drug eluting stents versus coronary artery bypass grafting in patients with multivessel coronary artery disease: meta-analysis of six randomized controlled trials. *Cardiovasc Revasc Med.* 2015;16:70–77.

24. Halabi AR, et al. Relation of early saphenous vein graft failure to outcomes following coronary artery bypass surgery. *Am J Cardiol.* 2005;96:1254–1259.

25. Levine GN, et al. 2011 ACCF/AHA/SCAI guideline for percutaneous coronary intervention: executive summary: a report of the American College of Cardiology Foundation/American Heart Association Task Force on Practice Guidelines and the Society for Cardiovascular Angiography and Interventions. *Circulation.* 2011;124:2574–2609.

26. Fihn SD, et al. 2014 ACC/AHA/AATS/PCNA/SCAI/STS focused update of the guideline for the diagnosis and management of patients with stable ischemic heart disease: a report of the American College of Cardiology/American Heart Association Task Force on Practice Guidelines, and the American Association for Thoracic Surgery, Preventive Cardiovascular Nurses Association, Society for Cardiovascular Angiography and Interventions, and Society of Thoracic Surgeons. *Circulation.* 2014;130:1749–1767.

27. Patel MR, et al. ACC/AATS/AHA/ASE/ASNC/SCAI/SCCT/STS 2016 appropriate use criteria for coronary revascularization in patients with acute coronary syndromes: a report of the American College of Cardiology Appropriate Use Criteria Task Force, American Association for Thoracic Surgery, American Heart Association, American Society of Echocardiography, American Society of Nuclear Cardiology, Society for Cardiovascular Angiography and Interventions, Society of Cardiovascular Computed Tomography, and the Society of Thoracic Surgeons. *J Am Coll Cardiol.* 2017;69:570–591.

28. Authors/Task Force members, et al. 2014 ESC/EACTS guidelines on myocardial revascularization: the Task Force on Myocardial Revascularization of the European Society of Cardiology (ESC) and the European Association for Cardio-Thoracic Surgery (EACTS) developed with the special contribution of the European Association of Percutaneous Cardiovascular Interventions (EAPCI). *Eur Heart J.* 2014;35:2541–2619.

29. Rosenblum JM, et al. Hybrid coronary revascularization versus coronary artery bypass surgery with bilateral or single internal mammary artery grafts. *J Thorac Cardiovasc Surg.* 2016;151:1081–1089.

30. Holzhey DM, et al. Minimally invasive hybrid coronary artery revascularization. *Ann Thorac Surg.* 2008;86:1856–1860.

31. Hu S, et al. Simultaneous hybrid revascularization versus off-pump coronary artery bypass for multivessel coronary artery disease. *Ann Thorac Surg.* 2011;91:432–438.

32. Reicher B, et al. Simultaneous "hybrid" percutaneous coronary intervention and minimally invasive surgical bypass grafting: feasibility, safety, and clinical outcomes. *Am Heart J.* 2008;155:661–667.

33. Zhao DX, et al. Routine intraoperative completion angiography after coronary artery bypass grafting and 1-stop hybrid revascularization results from a fully integrated hybrid catheterization laboratory/operating room. *J Am Coll Cardiol.* 2009;53:232–241.

34. Hu FB, Cui LQ. Short-term clinical outcomes after hybrid coronary revascularization versus off-pump coronary artery bypass for the treatment of multivessel or left main coronary artery disease: a meta-analysis. *Coron Artery Dis.* 2015;26:526–534.

35. Fan MK, et al. Clinical outcomes of revascularization strategies for patients with MVD/LMCA disease: a systematic review and network meta-analysis. *Medicine (Baltimore).* 2015;94:e1745.

36. Zhu P, et al. Hybrid coronary revascularization versus coronary artery bypass grafting for multivessel coronary artery disease: systematic review and meta-analysis. *J Cardiothorac Surg.* 2015;10:63.

37. Harskamp RE, et al. Clinical outcomes after hybrid coronary revascularization versus coronary artery bypass surgery: a meta-analysis of 1,190 patients. *Am Heart J.* 2014;167:585–592.

38. Ahn JM, et al. Functional assessment of jailed side branches in coronary bifurcation lesions using fractional flow reserve. *JACC Cardiovasc Interv.* 2012;5:155–161.

39. Koo BK, et al. Physiological evaluation of the provisional side-branch intervention strategy for bifurcation lesions using fractional flow reserve. *Eur Heart J.* 2008;29:726–732.

40. Cohen HA, et al. Impact of age on procedural and 1-year outcome in percutaneous transluminal coronary angioplasty: a report from the NHLBI Dynamic Registry. *Am Heart J.* 2003;146:513–519.

41. Baskett R, et al. Outcomes in octogenarians undergoing coronary artery bypass grafting. *CMAJ.* 2005;172:1183–1186.

42. Toumpoulis IK, et al. EuroSCORE predicts long-term mortality after heart valve surgery. *Ann Thorac Surg.* 2005;79:1902–1908.

43. Thomas MP, et al. Outcome of contemporary percutaneous coronary intervention in the elderly and the very elderly: insights from the Blue Cross Blue Shield of Michigan Cardiovascular Consortium. *Clin Cardiol.* 2011;34:549–554.

44. Singh M, et al. Trends in the association between age and in-hospital mortality after percutaneous coronary intervention: National Cardiovascular Data Registry experience. *Circ Cardiovasc Interv.* 2009;2:20–26.

45. Appleby CE, et al. In-hospital outcomes of very elderly patients (85 years and older) undergoing percutaneous coronary intervention. *Catheter Cardiovasc Interv.* 2011;77:634–641.

46. Sheridan BC, et al. Three-year outcomes of multivessel revascularization in very elderly acute coronary syndrome patients. *Ann Thorac Surg.* 2010;89:1889–1894; discussion 1894–1895.

47. Yusuf S, et al. Effect of coronary artery bypass graft surgery on survival: overview of 10-year results from randomised trials by the Coronary Artery Bypass Graft Surgery Trialists Collaboration. *Lancet.* 1994;344:563–570.

48. Velazquez EJ, et al. Coronary-artery bypass surgery in patients with left ventricular dysfunction. *N Engl J Med.* 2011;364:1607–1616.

49. Velazquez EJ, et al. Coronary-artery bypass surgery in patients with ischemic cardiomyopathy. *N Engl J Med.* 2016;374:1511–1520.

50. O'Neill WW, et al. A prospective, randomized clinical trial of hemodynamic support with Impella 2.5 versus intra-aortic balloon pump in patients undergoing high-risk percutaneous coronary intervention: the PROTECT II study. *Circulation.* 2012;126:1717–1727.

51. Daubert MA, et al. High-risk percutaneous coronary intervention is associated with reverse left ventricular remodeling and improved outcomes in patients with coronary artery disease and reduced ejection fraction. *Am Heart J.* 2015;170:550–558.

52. Ammann P, et al. Coronary anatomy and left ventricular ejection fraction in patients with type 2 diabetes admitted for elective coronary angiography. *Catheter Cardiovasc Interv.* 2004;62:432–438.

53. Laskey WK, et al. Comparison of in-hospital and one-year outcomes in patients with and without diabetes mellitus undergoing percutaneous catheter intervention (from the National Heart, Lung, and Blood Institute Dynamic Registry). *Am J Cardiol.* 2002;90:1062–1067.

54. Serruys PW, et al. Five-year outcomes after coronary stenting versus bypass surgery for the treatment of multivessel disease: the final analysis of the Arterial Revascularization Therapies Study (ARTS) randomized trial. *J Am Coll Cardiol.* 2005;46:575–581.

55. Hueb W, et al. Five-year follow-up of the Medicine, Angioplasty, or Surgery Study (MASS II): a randomized controlled clinical trial of 3 therapeutic strategies for multivessel coronary artery disease. *Circulation.* 2007;115:1082–1089.

56. Rodriguez A, et al. Three-year follow-up of the argentine randomized trial of percutaneous transluminal coronary angioplasty versus coronary artery bypass surgery in multivessel disease (ERACI). *J Am Coll Cardiol.* 1996;27:1178–1184.

57. Rodriguez AE, et al. Five-year follow-up of the argentine randomized trial of coronary angioplasty with stenting versus coronary bypass surgery in patients with multiple vessel disease (ERACI II). *J Am Coll Cardiol.* 2005;46:582–588.

58. Farkouh ME, et al. Strategies for multivessel revascularization in patients with diabetes. *N Engl J Med.* 2012;367:2375–2384.

59. Bourque JM, Beller GA. Stress myocardial perfusion imaging for assessing prognosis: an update. *JACC Cardiovasc Imaging.* 2011;4:1305–1319.

60. Hachamovitch R, et al. Comparison of the short-term survival benefit associated with revascularization compared with medical therapy in patients with no prior coronary artery disease undergoing stress myocardial perfusion single photon emission computed tomography. *Circulation.* 2003;107:2900–2907.

61. Allman KC, et al. Myocardial viability testing and impact of revascularization on prognosis in patients with coronary artery disease and left ventricular dysfunction: a meta-analysis. *J Am Coll Cardiol.* 2002;39:1151–1158.

62. Bonow RO, et al. Myocardial viability and survival in ischemic left ventricular dysfunction. *N Engl J Med.* 2011;364:1617–1625.

63. Tonino PA, et al. Angiographic versus functional severity of coronary artery stenoses in the FAME study fractional flow reserve versus angiography in multivessel evaluation. *J Am Coll Cardiol.* 2010;55:2816–2821.

64. Nam CW, et al. Functional SYNTAX score for risk assessment in multivessel coronary artery disease. *J Am Coll Cardiol.* 2011;58:1211–1218.

65. Lehmann R, et al. Complete revascularization in patients undergoing multivessel PCI is an independent predictor of improved long-term survival. *J Interv Cardiol.* 2010;23:256–263.

66. Tamburino C, et al. Complete versus incomplete revascularization in patients with multivessel disease undergoing percutaneous coronary intervention with drug-eluting stents. *Catheter Cardiovasc Interv.* 2008;72:448–456.

67. Cukingnan RA, et al. Influence of complete coronary revascularization on relief of angina. *J Thorac Cardiovasc Surg.* 1980;79:188–193.

68. Lawrie GM, et al. The influence of residual disease after coronary bypass on the 5-year survival rate of 1274 men with coronary artery disease. *Circulation.* 1982;66:717–723.

69. Lavee J, et al. Does complete revascularization by the conventional method truly provide the best possible results? Analysis of results and comparison with revascularization of infarct-prone segments (systematic segmental myocardial revascularization): the Sheba Study. *J Thorac Cardiovasc Surg.* 1986;92:279–290.

70. Shaw LJ, et al. Optimal medical therapy with or without percutaneous coronary intervention to reduce ischemic burden: results from the Clinical Outcomes Utilizing Revascularization and Aggressive Drug Evaluation (COURAGE) trial nuclear substudy. *Circulation.* 2008;117:1283–1291.

71. Farooq V, et al. Quantification of incomplete revascularization and its association with five-year mortality in the synergy between percutaneous coronary intervention with taxus and cardiac surgery (SYNTAX) trial validation of the residual SYNTAX score. *Circulation.* 2013;128:141–151.

72. Garcia S, et al. Outcomes after complete versus incomplete revascularization of patients with multivessel coronary artery disease: a meta-analysis of 89,883 patients enrolled in randomized clinical trials and observational studies. *J Am Coll Cardiol.* 2013;62:1421–1431.

73. Bates ER, et al. PCI strategies in patients with ST-segment elevation myocardial infarction and multivessel coronary artery disease. *J Am Coll Cardiol.* 2016;68:1066–1081.

74. Park DW, et al. Extent, location, and clinical significance of non-infarct-related coronary artery disease among patients with ST-elevation myocardial infarction. *JAMA.* 2014;312:2019–2027.

75. Corpus RA, et al. Multivessel percutaneous coronary intervention in patients with multivessel disease and acute myocardial infarction. *Am Heart J.* 2004;148:493–500.

76. Meliga E, et al. Early angio-guided complete revascularization versus culprit vessel PCI followed by ischemia-guided staged PCI in STEMI patients with multivessel disease. *J Interv Cardiol.* 2011;24:535–541.

77. Toma M, et al. Non-culprit coronary artery percutaneous coronary intervention during acute ST-segment elevation myocardial infarction: insights from the APEX-AMI trial. *Eur Heart J.* 2010;31:1701–1707.

78. Shishehbor MH, et al. Outcome of multivessel coronary intervention in the contemporary percutaneous revascularization era. *Am J Cardiol.* 2006;97:1585–1590.

79. Chen LY, et al. In-hospital and long-term outcomes of multivessel percutaneous coronary revascularization after acute myocardial infarction. *Am J Cardiol.* 2005;95:349–354.

80. Politi L, et al. A randomised trial of target-vessel versus multi-vessel revascularisation in ST-elevation myocardial infarction: major adverse cardiac events during long-term follow-up. *Heart.* 2010;96:662–667.

81. Hannan EL, et al. Culprit vessel percutaneous coronary intervention versus multivessel and staged percutaneous coronary intervention for ST-segment elevation myocardial infarction patients with multivessel disease. *JACC Cardiovasc Interv.* 2010;3:22–31.

82. Brener SJ, et al. Efficacy and safety of multivessel percutaneous revascularization and tirofiban therapy in patients with acute coronary syndromes. *Am J Cardiol.* 2002;90:631–633.

83. Genereux P, et al. Quantification and impact of untreated coronary artery disease after percutaneous coronary intervention: the residual SYNTAX (Synergy Between PCI with Taxus and Cardiac Surgery) score. *J Am Coll Cardiol.* 2012;59:2165–2174.

84. Wald DS, et al. Randomized trial of preventive angioplasty in myocardial infarction. *N Engl J Med.* 2013;369:1115–1123.

85. Qiao Y, et al. A comparison of multivessel and culprit vessel percutaneous coronary intervention in non-ST-segment elevation acute coronary syndrome patients with multivessel disease: a meta-analysis. *EuroIntervention.* 2015;11:525–532.

86. Hochman JS, et al. Early revascularization in acute myocardial infarction complicated by cardiogenic shock. SHOCK Investigators. Should we emergently revascularize occluded coronaries for cardiogenic shock. *N Engl J Med.* 1999;341:625–634.

87. Levine GN, et al. 2015 ACC/AHA/SCAI focused update on primary percutaneous coronary intervention for patients with ST-elevation myocardial infarction: an update of the 2011 ACCF/AHA/SCAI guideline for percutaneous coronary intervention and the 2013 ACCF/AHA guideline for the management of ST-elevation myocardial infarction. *J Am Coll Cardiol.* 2016;67:1235–1250.

88. Patel MR, et al. ACC/AATS/AHA/ASE/ASNC/SCAI/SCCT/STS 2017 appropriate use criteria for coronary revascularization in patients with stable ischemic heart disease: a report of the American College of Cardiology Appropriate Use Criteria Task Force, American Association for Thoracic Surgery, American Heart Association, American Society of Echocardiography, American Society of Nuclear Cardiology, Society for Cardiovascular Angiography and Interventions, Society of Cardiovascular Computed Tomography, and Society of Thoracic Surgeons. *J Am Coll Cardiol.* 2017;69:2212–2241.

89. Ellis SG, et al. Coronary morphologic and clinical determinants of procedural outcome with angioplasty for multivessel coronary disease. Implications for patient selection. Multivessel Angioplasty Prognosis Study Group. *Circulation.* 1990;82:1193–1202.

90. Krone RJ, et al. A simplified lesion classification for predicting success and complications of coronary angioplasty. Registry Committee of the Society for Cardiac Angiography and Intervention. *Am J Cardiol.* 2000;85:1179–1184.

91. Sianos G, et al. The SYNTAX score: an angiographic tool grading the complexity of coronary artery disease. *EuroIntervention.* 2005;1:219–227.

92. Serruys PW, et al. Assessment of the SYNTAX score in the Syntax study. *EuroIntervention.* 2009;5:50–56.

93. Garg S, et al. A new tool for the risk stratification of patients with complex coronary artery disease: the Clinical SYNTAX score. *Circ Cardiovasc Interv.* 2010;3:317–326.

94. Mack MJ, et al. Bypass versus drug-eluting stents at three years in SYNTAX patients with diabetes mellitus or metabolic syndrome. *Ann Thorac Surg.* 2011;92:2140–2146.

95. Habara S, et al. The impact of lesion length and vessel size on outcomes after sirolimus-eluting stent implantation for in-stent restenosis. *Heart.* 2008;94:1162–1165.

96. Ragosta M, et al. Prevalence of unfavorable angiographic characteristics for percutaneous intervention in patients with unprotected left main coronary artery disease. *Catheter Cardiovasc Interv.* 2006;68:357–362.

97. Stone GW, et al. Everolimus-eluting stents or bypass surgery for left main coronary artery disease. *N Engl J Med.* 2016;375:2223–2235.

98. Al Suwaidi J, et al. Immediate and long-term outcome of intracoronary stent implantation for true bifurcation lesions. *J Am Coll Cardiol.* 2000;35:929–936.

99. Yamashita T, et al. Bifurcation lesions: two stents versus one stent—immediate and follow-up results. *J Am Coll Cardiol.* 2000;35:1145–1151.

100. Latib A, Colombo A. Bifurcation disease: what do we know, what should we do? *JACC Cardiovasc Interv.* 2008;1:218–226.

101. Chaudhry EC, et al. Percutaneous coronary intervention for major bifurcation lesions using the simple approach: risk of myocardial infarction. *J Thromb Thrombolysis.* 2007;24:7–13.

102. Kim WJ, et al. Comparison of single- versus two-stent techniques in treatment of unprotected left main coronary bifurcation disease. *Catheter Cardiovasc Interv.* 2011;77:775–782.

103. Riley RF, et al. Trends in coronary revascularization in the United States from 2001 to 2009: recent declines in percutaneous coronary intervention volumes. *Circ Cardiovasc Qual Outcomes.* 2011;4:193–197.

21 Bifurcation Lesions and Intervention

Alaa S. Ayyoub, MD and Michael S. Levy, MD, MPH

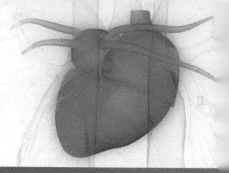

Introduction

Bifurcation coronary intervention has long been one of the most intriguing, challenging, and controversial aspects of the percutaneous coronary intervention (PCI) era. This was noted in the literature as early as the 1970s when Meier and Gruentzig published on this topic and were dismayed at the rate of side-branch occlusion and dissection that resulted in this group of coronary lesions (1). In clinical practice, bifurcation lesions are thought to represent approximately 20% of coronary interventions (2). Prior to the stent era, there was general concern because there were no modalities that adequately dealt with dissection or abrupt closure of either a main-branch or a side-branch vessel. In addition, studies had shown that this lesion subset met with a lower rate of success and a higher rate of restenosis compared with lesions that did not involve bifurcations (3). With the advent of stents, operators were given new tools to tackle this problem. Early evidence showed that stenting improved outcomes in this group of patients (4). Nevertheless, despite these advances, coronary bifurcation interventions yield lower procedural success rates and increased rates of long-term adverse cardiac events (5).

Initial improvement over angioplasty alone was seen with the advent of bare-metal stents (BMSs), but studies still demonstrated a high rate of restenosis (especially at the side-branch ostium) and side-branch occlusion with these particular stents (4,6). Studies from this era cite side-branch occlusion rates as high as 19% (7) and rates of side-branch stenoses of 27% (8), once a main-branch stent was initially deployed. Drug-eluting stents (DESs) appeared to be successful tools to deal with restenosis, and further studies demonstrated the benefit of DESs in dealing with restenosis and, in turn, target lesion revascularization (TLR) and target vessel revascularization (TVR) in this subset of coronary lesions (9–11). Early studies with DESs suggested that DESs were preferable to BMSs in this lesion subset (12), and that sirolimus conferred benefits over paclitaxel stents.

Still, much controversy remains concerning this topic. A number of trials dedicated specifically to bifurcation stenting have been completed over the last several years, providing further evidence within this field to help inform clinical decision making. Nevertheless, as multiple classification schemes, multiple techniques, and even new stent technology (including stents specifically designed for bifurcation lesions) are created, it is becoming more and more apparent that this subset of lesions is a heterogeneous group. Not all bifurcations are created equal, and because of this it is necessary to review the literature on the topic, including the classification schemes and seminal trials, along with advice from the current guidelines, in order to provide a balanced treatment of this topic, as well as some potential approaches for dealing with this patient population in clinical practice.

Pathophysiologic Considerations in Bifurcation Lesions

Research has sought to examine what determines plaque distribution within coronary artery bifurcations. It is believed that the local flow pattern and endothelial shear stress are conducive to plaque development. Areas of low and oscillatory endothelial shear stress, which is non-uniform, can lead to plaque accumulation. This is typically seen in the lateral walls of the main vessel and side branch. Conversely, high uniform shear stress is exhibited at the carinal level, and these areas are not as likely to exhibit plaque formation (13).

With the advent of angioplasty and stent technology, further tools were created to help tackle these complex lesions. Nevertheless, the challenge is that these lesions are more prone to restenosis than nonbifurcation lesions. Two different mechanisms are proposed: neointimal formation and elastic recoil. When stenting has been performed, the most common reason for lumen loss over time is neointimal formation. This is felt to account for 90% of the restenotic process. Nevertheless, in balloon-only angioplasty, the major mechanism of restenosis for balloon angioplasty is from elastic recoil and late vessel shrinkage, with neointimal formation accounting for less than 30% of the restenotic mechanism (14,15).

Additionally, as research progressed within this field, it was found that not all side-branch lesions require intervention. An important study by Koo et al. examined the hemodynamic significance of these lesions. They performed FFR (fractional flow reserve) in a subset of coronary side-branch bifurcation lesions that had been "jailed" after bifurcation stenting. They found that, of those lesions they examined that were of 90% severity or greater, only 14 out of 25 had FFR values <0.75, demonstrating the fact that angiography is imperfect in being able to predict the actual hemodynamic importance of residual side-branch lesions. Further, these data suggest that stable lesions that are less than 90% angiographically may be lesions that can be left alone after bifurcation stenting, provided they have thrombolysis in myocardial infarction (TIMI) 3 flow (16).

Bifurcation Classifications

It is important to accurately define what constitutes a bifurcation lesion, because the failure to do so has caused much of the controversy and uncertainty involving the trials that have attempted to study this topic. In 2007, a consensus group proposed the following definition: a bifurcation was "a coronary artery narrowing occurring adjacent to, and/or involving, the origin of a significant side branch" (17). A significant side branch is defined by this group as a "branch that you do not want to lose in the global context of a particular patient (symptoms, location of ischemia, branch responsible for symptoms or ischemia, viability, collateralizing vessel, left ventricular function. . .)."

Once the definition of a bifurcation lesion is established, the next important question is: What defines the main branch and the side branch? Louvard et al. (17) propose two approaches. The first they term the "nosologic approach," where the left anterior descending (LAD), Circumflex, and posterior descending artery, regardless of their size, are always considered the main branch. The second approach they propose relates to quantitative coronary angiography, where the main branch is the largest distal branch and the side branch is smaller.

There are currently seven major classification schemes for bifurcation lesions (18). The most commonly used, both in clinical practice and in the trial literature, is the Medina classification (19) (see **Fig. 21.1**), likely due to its ease of use. The Medina classification system is based on three number binary notations. Its focus is primarily on lesion location, assigning a value of 1 or 0 based on the presence or absence of a lesion. A lesion is defined angiographically for this classification as being significant if it has a 50% or greater diameter stenosis. It then examines three positions: the main branch *proximal* to the side branch, the main branch *distal* to the side branch, and the *side branch* itself. As an example, a bifurcation that involved lesions in the main branch proximal to the side branch, as well as the side branch itself, would be coded as a 1,0,1 (see **Figs. 21.2** to **21.5** for further examples).

The main limitation to this classification system is that there is no way to stratify the overall prognostic importance of the side branch. As an example, it has been demonstrated that side-branch occlusion is more common in a long side branch lesion as compared with a short one (20). Further, as pointed out by Colombo et al., the more important issue is the plaque burden surrounding the bifurcation and the angle of the side branch in relation to the main branch. As Colombo states, bifurcations that are more Y-shaped and have angles <70° make wire access to the side branch more favorable, but also create a greater risk of plaque shift into the side branch. Nevertheless, those lesions that are more T-shaped, with an angle >70°, can be tougher to wire, but the overall risk of plaque shift is lower (21). Additional studies reiterate the issue of the side-branch angle being an overall predictor of procedural success and outcomes (22).

To date, all classification schemes have difficulty giving full clinical importance to the different issues surrounding side-branch lesions. These include issues such as angle and length, as mentioned earlier, in addition to how big the side branch is and what importance it holds to a particular territory (both myocardial size and how it provides collaterals) (18).

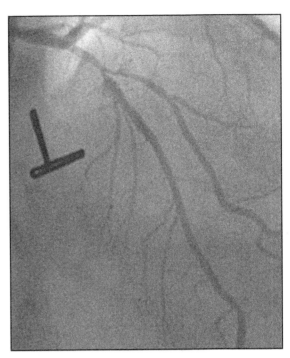

FIGURE 21.2 Medina classification 1,1,1, in which the proximal and distal main branch, as well as the side branch, are involved in the lesion. (Image courtesy of Dr. Issam Moussa.)

Separate from the classification scheme is the fact that the concept of a "true bifurcation" according to the Medina classification used in many trials is either: 1,1,1; 1,0,1; or 0,1,1. Nevertheless, not all trials were this strict in the lesions they included. Additionally, long side-branch lesions were often not included in the trials.

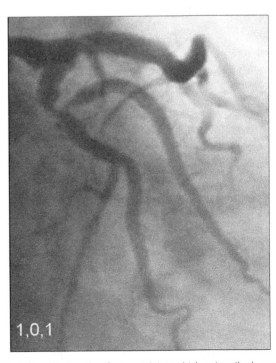

FIGURE 21.3 Medina classification 1,0,1, in which, primarily, the proximal main branch and side branch are involved in the lesion. (Image courtesy of Dr. Issam Moussa.)

Medina	1,1,1	1,1,0	1,0,1	0,1,1	1,0,0	0,1,0	0,0,1
Duke (modified)	D	C	F	G	A	B	E
Sanborn	I	-	-	III	IV	II	IV
Lefevre	1	2	-	4	3	4a	4b
Safian	IA	IB	IIA	IIIA	IIB	IIIB	IV
Movahed	L	S	2	1m	1s	V	T
Staico-Feres	3	2A	2B	2C	1A	1B	1C

FIGURE 21.1 Bifurcation classifications. (Courtesy of Dr. Issam Moussa.)

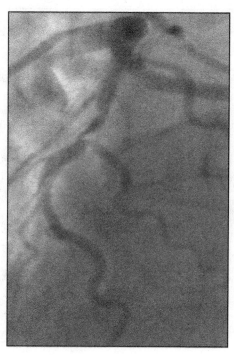

FIGURE 21.4 An additional example of Medina Classification 1,0,1. (Image courtesy of Dr. Issam Moussa.)

Stenting Methods

Some of the stenting strategies outlined in the following text have come in and out favor as the outcomes of new trials are taken into account. New-generation DESs are recommended for bifurcation treatment. Many trials have compared the use of one versus two DESs in non-left main bifurcations. The majority of randomized trials comparing the one-stent with the two-stent techniques have shown no advantage of implanting two stents regardless of stent type (9,10,23–25). A meta-analysis of these randomized trials

demonstrated that both treatment strategies resulted in similar outcomes in terms of the risk of cardiac death, TLR, and stent thrombosis. Nevertheless, the rate of periprocedural myocardial infarction (MI) was significantly higher in the complex versus simple strategies, and showed a lower rate of death, MI, and TVR in favor of the single-stent strategy. The results from the Nordic IV and the EBC TWO (European Bifurcation Club 2) trials showed no difference between provisional and two-stent techniques with regard to major adverse cardiac events (MACE) (26–29).

Provisional Stenting

With the current evidence, provisional stenting (PS) should be considered the primary strategy if anatomically feasible. The main vessel is stented first, and the side branch is treated in cases of significant flow limitation. FFR guided assessment of the side branch can be considered in cases of uncertainty of the residual side-branch lesion (16). As a general rule, the most difficult branch is wired first. A second wire is then passed while trying to avoid wire entanglement. Wiring the side branch allows for access to the side branch, opens the bifurcation angle, and reduces the risk of side-branch occlusion. The side-branch wire will also serve as an anatomic marker if the side branch becomes occluded during stent implantation (26).

V Stenting

A method where two stents are deployed simultaneously in both a main branch and a side branch such that the stents touch at their proximal portions forming a "carina" (30) (**Fig. 21.6**).

Simultaneous Kissing Stents

Simultaneous kissing stents (SKSs) is a process similar to V stenting, except that the proximal stents hang back into the main vessel >5 mm or more (30). Some operators also refer to this as the "double barrel" technique, especially when this is performed in left-main bifurcation stenting (**Fig. 21.7**). The advantage of both the V and the SKS techniques is that neither branch access is lost, and no "recrossing" is required.

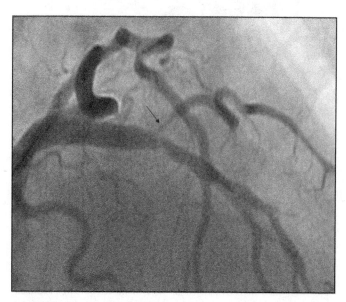

FIGURE 21.5 Medina classification 0,1,1, in which, primarily, the side branch and distal main branch are involved in the lesion.

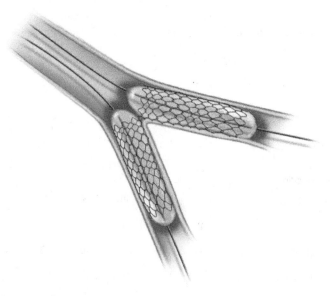

FIGURE 21.6 V stenting. In this technique, two stents are deployed simultaneously, creating a "carina" at the site of the bifurcation. (Image courtesy of Alice McKinney.)

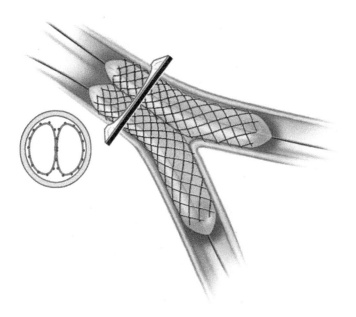

FIGURE 21.7 SKS (Simultaneous Kissing Stents). In this technique, both stents are deployed simultaneously, but a portion of the stents in the proximal main branch overlap. (Diagram courtesy of Alice McKinney, Mayo Clinic.)

Crush

This technique involves stenting the side branch first, with some degree of proximal stent hanging from the side branch into the main branch. The next step is deploying the main-branch stent, which "crushes" the proximal side branch stent to the artery wall. The "mini" crush is the same procedure, but with less of the proximal side-branch stent hanging into the main branch. Advantages include the fact that both branches will remain patent, and the ostium of the side branch will be covered (31) (Figure 21.9).

Reverse Crush

In this technique, a main-branch stent is deployed in the setting of provisional side-branch stenting. Then, when it is realized that the side branch requires stenting, a stent is positioned in the side branch. A balloon is placed in the main branch, and the side-branch stent is then pulled back 2 to 3 mm across the ostium and deployed. The side-branch stent balloon is removed, and the main-branch balloon is deployed at high atmospheres.

Step Crush

The side branch is stented first, with a stent placed 2 to 3 mm across the ostium. A balloon in the main vessel is positioned prior to side-branch stent deployment. The side-branch stent is deployed, and the stent balloon is removed. Then, the main-branch balloon is inflated at high atmospheres. Next, the main-branch stent is deployed.

T Stent

In this technique (Figure 21.8), a stent is placed in the side branch and positioned right at the ostium with no protrusion into the main branch. A balloon in the main branch is helpful in positioning the side-branch balloon. After side-branch deployment, a stent is placed in the main branch. The "modified" T stent involves positioning of

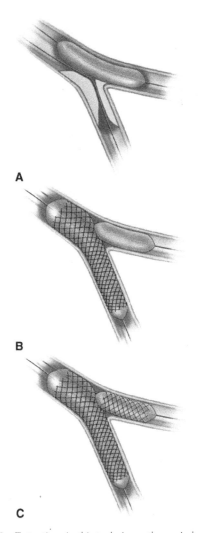

FIGURE 21.8 T-stenting. In this technique, the main branch and side branch are both wired. Diagram **A** shows the side branch being ballooned first. Diagram **B** shows a stent being deployed in the main branch. The side branch is rewired through the main-branch stent strut. Sometimes a balloon in the side branch can help estimate where the side branch stent will be placed. Diagram **C** shows a stent being deployed in the side branch. A final "kissing balloon" inflation (in which balloons are deployed simultaneously in both stents) is performed. (Diagrams courtesy of Alice McKinney, Mayo Clinic.)

the side branch and main-branch stents simultaneously. Then, the side-branch stent is deployed first and equipment removed before deploying the main-branch stent.

Culotte

In this technique, two stents are used to create "pants legs" (Figure 21.10). First, both branches are individually predilated. Next, a stent is deployed across the side branch with the proximal portion positioned into the main branch. Then, the main branch is rewired through the first stent and predilated. Next, a stent is positioned through the first stent into the main branch. The final step is to perform kissing balloon. This allows for excellent coverage of the side-branch ostium.

T and Protrusion (TAP)

This technique consists of several steps. The first step involves stenting the main branch while jailing the guide wire in the side

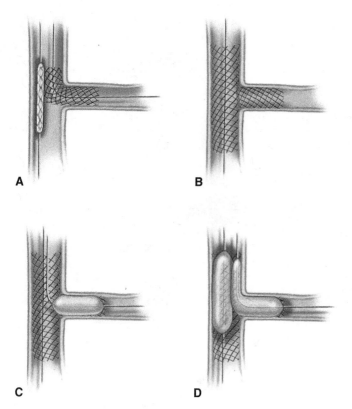

FIGURE 21.9 Crush stenting. In this technique, the main branch and side branch are wired. Diagram **A** shows two stents being brought into the lesion. The side-branch stent is deployed first and the balloon is removed. Diagram **B** shows the main-branch stent being deployed and "crushing" the overlapping portion of the side-branch stent. Diagram **C** shows the side branch being rewired and then being ballooned. Diagram **D** shows a final "kissing balloon" inflation. (Diagrams courtesy of Alice McKinney, Mayo Clinic.)

branch. Next, the side branch is rewired, and then kissing balloon is performed. Next, a stent is placed in the side branch and a balloon is kept in the main branch. The side branch stent is pulled back just enough to cover the ostium. The stent is then deployed. Next, the stent balloon is pulled back slightly into the main branch. Finally, kissing balloon is performed with the side-branch and main-branch balloons.

Double Kiss Crush II

In the Double Kiss (DK), the side branch is stented, followed by a balloon inflation in the main branch (balloon crush). Kissing balloons in the side and main branch are then performed. Next, the main vessel is stented, before a final kissing inflation is performed (32).

Y Stent and Skirt Stent Techniques

These techniques (30) are currently of historical value, but are worth mentioning because more and more research is being committed to the creation of a "true" bifurcation stent. The Y stent is a technique in which a stent is placed in both the main branch and in the side branch, and then a final stent is placed in the main branch proximal to the prior two stents. Nevertheless, this final stent is crimped onto a double balloon in order to cover the proximal ends of the prior stents. Currently, there are experimental stents, which can replicate this method.

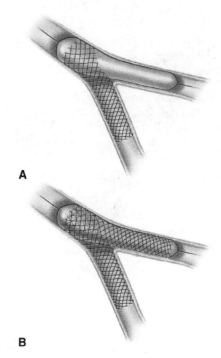

FIGURE 21.10 Culottes stenting. In this technique, the main-branch and side-branch vessels are wired. Diagram **A** shows the main-branch stent deployed and the side-branch stent rewired and ballooned. Diagram **B** shows the side-branch stent being deployed in a "pants leg" type fashion with proximal overlap. As a final step, the main branch would be rewired and the final "kissing balloon" would be performed. (Diagrams courtesy of Alice McKinney, Mayo Clinic.)

The EBC proposed a new classification to help describe and further define the preceding techniques. It is referred to as the Main, Across, Distal, Side (MADS) classification. It regroups the preceding strategies into generalized approaches. For example, Main stands for Main proximal first, which represents approaches in which the proximal main-branch stent is deployed first. This previously would have required the "skirt" approach, but can now be done with dedicated bifurcation stents. A represents Main ACROSS side first. This encompasses several of the crush, TAP, and culotte techniques. D is for Distal first; examples being the V stenting and SKS approaches. Finally, S represents side branch first, with several crush and mini-crush examples (17).

Technology Considerations

Stent Design

It is currently felt that an open-celled stent is more favorable toward bifurcation lesions in terms of gaining and maintaining wire access, compared with the older designs. TAXUS Liberté, XIENCE, and Resolute stents are some examples of more current open-celled designs.

Drug-Eluting Balloons

Because it remains difficult to adequately cover (and sometimes access) the side-branch ostium, one could hypothesize the theoretical advantage of drug-eluting balloons in ballooning the side-branch ostium to help prevent restenosis (33).

Bifurcation Stents

As mentioned earlier, there is currently much interest in creating a stent specifically designed for the bifurcation lesion. Several of these are currently being investigated. There are currently four available dedicated stents: the BIOSS (Bifurcation Optimization Stent System), the Stentys (STENTYS), the Axxess stent (Biosensors International), and the Tryton stent (Tryton Medical) (34).

Bio-resorbable Scaffold (BRS)

The idea of a scaffold that could cover the ostium of a side branch and then gradually disappear over time, restoring patency in the side branch, seems promising. This would be especially useful in situations where one is forced to place a stent in the side branch, and not simply balloon it (35). Nevertheless, there is limited technology available for current use. Further, the strut thickness of the current Absorb BRS (Abbott Vascular) stent technology could potentially increase the risk of side branch occlusion. (36–38) Due to this limitation, the only conformations that can be recommended with current available technology are T-stenting with two BRSs or one BRS in the main branch and one DES in the side branch.

Intravascular Imaging Techniques

The use of intravascular ultrasound (IVUS) and optical coherence tomography (OCT) can provide important information before and after stent deployment. Plaque configuration, including side branch involvement, can be better delineated allowing for the selection of the most appropriate stenting strategy. In some cases, this may reduce the necessity for a two-stent strategy, thereby improving outcomes. Pre-stent intravascular imaging provides information regarding vessel sizing and identification of calcium; whereas post-stenting these modalities can be used to evaluate stent expansion, edge dissection, or stent malapposition. OCT can also be a useful tool to aid in recrossing a jailed side branch via the distal struts to allow for more favorable stent positioning against the side branch ostium.

Nevertheless, despite the additional anatomic understanding offered by the use of intravascular imaging, current evidence does not demonstrate improved outcomes, with the exception of left main stenting (26). The Main Compare Study showed that not using IVUS was associated with a higher mortality rate. Thus, imaging of the left main prior to left main bifurcation stenting is strongly recommended (39).

Important Clinical Trials

The following are several seminal trials in this field.

NORDIC Bifurcation Study 2006 (40)

This was a multicenter, European trial that randomized 413 patients to a provisional (or simple) approach to stenting of bifurcation lesions, versus a complex (or routine) stenting approach. Sirolimus stents were utilized in this population. In this trial, complex bifurcation stenting strategies were left to the individual operators. The primary endpoint was MACE defined as cardiac death, MI, TVR, and stent thrombosis at 6 months. Follow-up was achieved in all patients, and 8-month angiograms were scheduled. MACE was the same at 6 months (3.4% in MV and SB, vs. 2.9% SB). In the dual stent group, there were longer procedure times, more fluoroscopy and

radiation dose, and higher biomarker rises. Only 74% (307/413) had angiographic follow-up at 8 months.

The side branch was provisionally stented in 4.3% of the simple strategy group and in 95.1% of the complex strategy group. In the PS group, the side branch was dilated through the main vessel stent in 32% of the procedures. In the complex group, the crush technique was used in 50%, the culotte technique was used in 21%, and others (mostly T-stent technique) in 29%. A final kissing balloon dilatation was performed in 32% of the PS group and in 74% of the complex strategy group. Procedure time, fluoroscopy time, and contrast volume were significantly in favor of simple strategy. Further, there was no difference in restenosis rates between the two groups at 8-month follow-up with respect to the main branch. Nevertheless, there was an increased rate of side-branch restenosis in the PS group compared with the complex strategy group: simple 19.2% versus 10.9% complex (p = 0.041).

Overall, the authors suggest the "simple strategy" due to the issues with longer procedure and increased biomarkers. They note that even though biomarkers were elevated in the complex group, this did not translate into an increased MACE rate at 6 months. The authors also note that this was not a blinded study. There was no ischemia testing, so it is unclear how these strategies would have reduced ischemia.

Bifurcations Bad Krozingen 2008 (23)

This was a non-blinded, single-center trial that examined routine versus provisional T-stenting of side-branch lesions to determine the effect on restenosis. Two hundred and two patients with de novo bifurcation lesions were randomized to routine versus provisional T-stenting. Sirolimus DESs were used. The primary endpoint was percent diameter stenosis on angiographic follow-up at 9 months. Secondary endpoints assessed 1- and 2-year incidence of death and MI.

Post-PCI patients were recommended lifelong aspirin and also plavix for a minimum of 6 months. An angiographic core lab was used in this study. About 18.8% of patients in the provisional group received a stent. Note is made of no difference between procedural times, contrast, or fluoroscopy between the groups. Overall, there was no difference in TLR and freedom from death or MI. Death, MI, and stent thrombosis were approximately 3%, which was consistent with DES use at the time of the trial. The authors noted that, within their study population, acute gain was better with routine stenting, but late loss was better with PS. Angiographic follow-up was achieved in 95% of patients. Overall, this trial showed no difference in angiographic restenosis between the two groups. It also showed no difference in TVR.

CACTUS 2009 (41)

This trial examined whether elective crush stenting would be better than provisional T-stenting. Three hundred and fifty patients were randomized at 12 European centers. Sirolimus stents were used. The primary angiographic endpoint was in-segment restenosis rate. The primary clinical endpoint was occurrence of MACE (cardiac death, MI, TVR) at 6 and 12 months. Overall, there was a similar angiographic rate of recurrence in both groups. Side-branch stenting in the provisional group occurred in 31% of lesions. MACE was similar in both groups: simple 15% versus 15.8% crush group. The authors concluded that a single-stent strategy was sufficient, with the comment that 30% of provisional stents would require a side-branch stent. In the trial, predilation was mandatory in the main vessel and side branch in all cases, as was final kissing balloon inflation. Provisional T-stenting in the side branch was permitted if there was either: (a) a residual stenosis of greater than 50%, (b) a dissection of at least type B, or (c) TIMI flow less than 3. An independent core lab was part of this study. Full follow-up was achieved in all patients. Plavix or ticlid were continued for at least 6 months. By Medina classification, 94% of lesions were labeled as "true" bifurcations.

There was no difference in overall clinical outcomes. Additionally, there was no difference in in-segment restenosis between the two groups. More side-branch stenting was done than in other trials before it in the provisional group. The authors attribute this to less strict criteria with respect to side branches, and state that, in comparison with other trials, CACTUS had a higher rate of "true" side-branch lesions. They note that the trial had higher event rates compared to contemporary studies, and hypothesized that this was due to a lack of emphasis on a "two-step" final kissing inflation.

British Bifurcation Coronary Study: Old, New, and Evolving Strategies (BBC ONE) 2010 (25)

This was a randomized multicenter trial conducted in the UK, which examined a simple versus complex PCI strategy for bifurcation lesions. TAXUS DESs were used. The simple arm consisted of main-vessel stenting with provisional side-branch kissing balloon or T-stenting. In the complex arm, both vessels were stented with either a culotte or crush strategy, followed by a mandatory attempt at kissing balloon. Five hundred patients were randomized, with 82% having "true" bifurcation lesions—defined as stenosis of at least 50% in each branch. Baseline characteristics were balanced between the groups. The complex group had larger sheath French size and more glycoprotein 2B/3A use than the simple strategy group. Final kissing was successfully achieved in 95% of those attempted in the simple strategy group versus 85% in the complex group (p = 0.01). An intention to treat analysis was used. Within the complex strategy group, the culotte group had more successful kissing balloon compared with crush techniques (89% vs. 72%). The majority of kissing balloon failure was due to unsuccessful attempts at wiring the side branch. The primary endpoint was a composite of death, MI, and target vessel failure at 9 months. This was achieved in 8% of the simple arm versus 15.2% in the complex group (HR 2.02, 95% CI 1.17–3.47, p = 0.009). MI occurred in 3.6% simple versus 11.2% complex group (p = 0.001), and in-hospital MACE was seen in 2% simple versus 8% complex group (p = 0.002). Although target vessel failure was similar between the groups, more patients in the complex group underwent coronary artery bypass grafting (CABG). Procedure time, fluoroscopy time, radiation dose, and amount of coronary equipment used were significantly less in the simple strategy group. The authors felt that the in-hospital and 9-month MACE rates were driven primarily by MI. They concluded that a provisional (simple) strategy should be the preferred approach in bifurcation lesions.

This study did not have angiographic follow-up, which the authors said was intentional so that operators would not be obliged to aim for "angiographic perfection." Along with this is the criticism that an angiographic core lab was not employed in this study.

Nordic Baltic Bifurcation Study III 2010 (42)

This trial randomized 477 patients to a one-stent technique with or without kissing balloon in the side branch. The results showed that kissing balloon in the side branch did not make a difference for a 6-month composite endpoint of MACE (which included cardiac death, index lesion MI, TLR, and stent thrombosis). Additionally,

procedure times and fluoroscopy times were significantly longer. Further, more contrast was used with the kissing balloon technique. These results suggest that if TIMI 3 flow is achieved, the side branch could be left alone in the setting of a one-stent technique. Nevertheless, criticism of this study emphasized its small size and questioned its applicability in the setting where a side-branch stent would be required.

Several of the early trials put a particular emphasis on kissing balloon in the setting of a two-stent technique. Additionally, there is evidence that certain bifurcation stenting strategies (such as the crush technique) benefit greatly from a final kissing balloon inflation.

DK CRUSH II 2011 (32)

This trial was designed as a response to some of the earlier bifurcation stenting trials and the criticism that the criteria used were too selective. The authors touted this as a trial designed to mimic the real world. The authors deliberately chose "unselected patients" because it was felt that the original trials showing PS was better were very selective in the patients and lesions chosen for enrollment.

In this trial, 370 patients enrolled, and all were considered "true" bifurcation lesions according to the Medina classification. For this trial, a very specific technique was used, as described earlier. Aspirin and clopidogrel were continued for at least 12 months in the patient groups. The Medina classification fell into two groups (as opposed to BBC One, in which all classifications were represented): 1,1,1 (83.8% in the DK group and 77.8% in the PS group) and 0,1,1 (16.2% DK and 22.2% PS). The LAD-diagonal was the most common lesion type, representing approximately 60% of cases in both arms. A total of 28.6% of patients in the PS arm did receive side-branch stenting. Final kissing was performed in 100% of cases in the DK group and 79.5% in the PS group. Unsatisfactory kissing was found in 8.1% of patients in the DK group and 25.4% in the PS group. The primary endpoint was the occurrence of MACE at 12 months (this included cardiac death, MI, or TVR). Secondary angiographic endpoints were restenosis in the MV and SB at 8 months.

At 8-month follow-up, there was more restenosis seen in the main vessel of the PS group, as compared with the DK group (9.7% vs. 3.8%, p = 0.036), and also in the side branch of PS compared with DK groups (22.2% vs. 4.9%, p ≤ 0.001).

TLR was more common in the PS group—13% versus 4.3%—and TVR was also more common in the PS group—14.6% versus 6.5%. Overall, MACE rates were not statistically different between the groups, but there was a trend toward lower rates in the DK group: PS 17.3% versus 10.3% (p = 0.070).

NORDIC IV (28)

The aim of the NORDIC IV study was to compare PS and two-stent techniques for the treatment of true coronary bifurcation lesions involving a large side branch. The study enrolled 450 patients who were randomized to either PS or the two-stent technique. With both arms, specific interventional techniques were prescribed. The strategy in the "provisional group" required two wires, predilatation, stenting of the main vessel and kissing balloons if TIMI flow < III or >75% disease in the ostial side branch; and the T- or culotte stenting technique if there was residual poor flow in the side branch after kissing balloons. The "two stent" strategy allowed for culotte, T-stenting, or mini-crush techniques, along with final kissing balloon dilatation.

Procedure and fluoroscopy times were significantly longer in the two-stent cohort, as was the contrast volume used. There was no significant difference in post-procedural MI (as defined by creatine kinase-MB (CK-MB) >3x UPL), MACE, death, stent thrombosis, TLR, TVR, or angina at 6 months. Longer and more complex procedures in the two-stent group did not translate into more procedural MIs.

EBC TWO (29)

The aim of this study was to compare an up-front two-stent technique for bifurcation lesions with significant ostial side-branch disease. The study randomized symptomatic patients with large-caliber bifurcation lesions with side branches >2.5 mm and significant ostial disease >5 mm to either a provisional T-stent strategy or a dual-stent culotte technique. Two hundred patients were randomized in 20 European centers. The clinical presentations were stable coronary disease (69%) and acute coronary syndromes (31%). Procedural success (provisional 97% and culotte 94%) and kissing balloon inflation (provisional 95% and culotte 98%) were high. Sixteen percent of patients in the provisional group underwent T-stenting. The primary endpoint (a composite of death, MI, and TVR at 12 months) occurred in 7.7% of the provisional T-stent group versus 10.3% of the culotte group (hazard ratio, 1.02; 95% CI, 0.78–1.34; P = 0.53). Procedure time, x-ray dose, and cost all favored the simpler procedure. The authors concluded that when treating complex coronary bifurcation lesions with large side branches, there is no difference between a provisional T-stent strategy and a systematic two-stent culotte strategy in a composite endpoint of death, MI, and TVR at 12 months.

Current Bifurcation Stenting Guidelines (43)

As of the most recent 2011 PCI Guidelines, an expert consensus review of the literature has created the following recommendations when approaching bifurcation lesions:

CLASS I:1. Provisional side-branch stenting should be the initial approach in patients with bifurcation lesions when the side branch is not large and has only mild or moderate focal disease at the ostium. (Level of Evidence: A)

CLASS IIa:1. It is reasonable to use elective double stenting in patients with complex bifurcation morphology involving a large side branch where the risk of side-branch occlusion is high and the likelihood of successful side-branch reaccess is low. (Level of Evidence: B)

Summary

Bifurcation lesions remain a challenging subset of coronary lesions. Much discussion, debate, and research continue in this field with regard to best practices. Clinical trial data continue to assist in decision making in this arena. Further, the guidelines have evolved to reflect current evidence. New technology may help revolutionize this field further in the coming years.

Key Points

- Bifurcations lesions occur at areas of low shear stress that lead to plaque accumulation.
- Restenosis with stenting is mainly due to neointimal formation.
- Restenosis with balloon-only angioplasty is mainly due to elastic recoil.

- "Pinched" side branches with TIMI 3 flow and <90% stenosis may be hemodynamically insignificant lesions.
- The Medina classification is the most widely used system in providing anatomical descriptions of bifurcation lesions.
- No classification scheme adequately describes the important clinical issues surrounding side-branches lesions.
- Numerous bifurcation techniques are available.
- Understanding the nomenclature is important in interpreting the current trial literature.
- Future technology may change the landscape of bifurcation stenting practice.
- The current body of literature suggests that main-branch stenting with provisional side-branch stenting is the preferred strategy.

References

1. Meier B, et al. Risk of side branch occlusion during coronary angioplasty. *Am J Cardiol.* 1984;53:10–14.
2. Tsuchida K, et al. The clinical outcome of percutaneous treatment of bifurcation lesions in multivessel coronary artery disease with the sirolimus-eluting stent: insights from the Arterial Revascularization Therapies Study part II (ARTS II). *Eur Heart J.* 2007;28(4):433–442.
3. Al Suwaidi J, et al. Immediate and long-term outcome of intracoronary stent implantation for true bifurcation lesions. *J Am Coll Cardiol.* 2000;35:929–936.
4. Al Suwaidi J, et al. Immediate and one-year outcome in patients with coronary bifurcation lesions in the modern era (NHLBI dynamic registry). *Am J Cardiol.* 2001;87:1139–1144.
5. Steigen TK, et al. Randomized study on simple versus complex stenting of coronary artery bifurcation lesions: the Nordic bifurcation study. *Circulation* 2006;114:1955–61.
6. Sheiban I, et al. Immediate and long-term results of "T" stenting for bifurcation coronary lesions. *Am J Cardiol.* 2000;85:1141–1144.
7. Aliabadi D, et al. Incidence and angiographic predictors of side branch occlusion following high-pressure intracoronary-stenting. *Am J Cardiol.* 1997;80:994–997.
8. Bhargava B, et al. Clinical outcomes of compromised side branch (stent jail) after coronary stenting with the NIR stent. *Catheter Cardiovasc Interv.* 2001;54:295–300.
9. Colombo A, et al. Randomized study to evaluate sirolimus-eluting stents implanted at coronary bifurcation lesions. *Circulation.* 2004;109:1244–1249.
10. Pan M, et al. Rapamycin-eluting stents for the treatment of bifurcated coronary lesions: a randomized comparison of a simple versus complex strategy. *Am Heart J.* 2004;148: 857–864.
11. Di Mario C, et al. Predictors of restenosis after treatment of bifurcational lesions with paclitaxel eluting stents: a multicenter prospective registry of 150 consecutive patients. *Catheter Cardiovasc Interv.* 2007;69:416–424.
12. Thuesen L, et al. Comparison of sirolimus-eluting and bare metal stents in coronary bifurcation lesions: sub-group analysis of the Stenting Coronary Arteries in Non-Stress/Benestent Disease Trial (SCANDSTENT). *Am Heart J.* 2006;152:1140–1145.
13. Chatzizisis YS, et al. Prediction of the localization of high-risk coronary atherosclerotic plaques on the basis of low endothelial shear stress: an intravascular ultrasound and histopathology natural history study. *Circulation* 2008;117:993–1002.)
14. Mintz GS, Popma JJ, Pichard AD. Arterial remodeling after coronary angioplasty: a serial intravascular ultrasound study. *Circulation.* 1996;94:35–43.
15. Hoffmann R, et al. Chronic arterial responses to stent implantation: a serial intravascular ultrasound analysis of Palmaz-Schatz stents in native coronary arteries. *J Am Coll Cardiol.* 1996;28:1134–1139.

16. Koo BK, et al. Physiologic evaluation of jailed side branch lesions using fractional flow reserve. *J Am Coll Cardiol.* 2005;46:633–637.

17. Louvard Y, et al. Classification of coronary artery bifurcation lesions and treatments: time for a consensus! *Catheter Cardiovasc Interv.* 2008;71(2):175–183.

18. Moussa ID. Coronary artery bifurcation interventions: the disconnect between randomized clinical trials and patient centered decision-making. *Catheter Cardiovasc Interv.* 2011;77:537–545.

19. Medina A, Suárez de Lezo J, Pan M. A new classification of coronary bifurcation lesions. *Rev Esp Cardiol.* 2006;59(2):183.

20. Furukawa E, et al. Intravascular ultrasound predictors of side branch occlusion in bifurcation lesions after percutaneous coronary intervention. *Circ J.* 2005;69(3):325–330.

21. Iakovou I, Ge L, Colombo A. Contemporary stent treatment of coronary bifurcations. *J Am Coll Cardiol.* 2005;46(8):1446–1455.

22. Dzavik V, et al. Predictors of long-term outcome after crush stenting of coronary bifurcation lesions: importance of the bifurcation angle. *Am Heart J.* 2006;152(4):762–769.

23. Ferenc M, et al. Randomized trial on routine vs. provisional T-stenting in the treatment of de novo coronary bifurcation lesions. *Eur Heart J.* 2008;29:2859–2867.

24. Colombo A, et al. Randomized study of the crush technique versus provisional side-branch stenting in true coronary bifurcations: the CACTUS (Coronary Bifurcations: Application of the Crushing Technique Using Sirolimus-Eluting Stents) Study. *Circulation.* 2009;119:71–78.

25. Hildick-Smith D, et al. Randomized trial of simple versus complex drug eluting stenting for bifurcation lesions: the British Bifurcation Coronary Study: old, new, and evolving strategies. *Circulation.* 2010;121:1235–1243.

26. Sawaya FJ, et al. Contemporary approach to coronary bifurcation lesion treatment. *JACC Cardiovasc Interv.* 2016;9(18):1861–1878. doi:10.1016/j.jcin.2016.06.056.

27. Behan MW, et al. Simple or complex stenting for bifurcation coronary lesions: a patient-level pooled-analysis of the Nordic Bifurcation Study and the British Bifurcation Coronary Study. *Circ Cardiovasc Interv.* 2011;4: 57–64.

28. Kumsars IHN, et al. Randomized comparison of provisional side-branch stenting versus a 2-stent strategy for treatment of true coronary bifurcation lesions involving a large side branch. 2-year results in the Nordic-Baltic Bifurcation Study IV. Presented at: EuroPCR; May 21, 2015; Paris, France.

29. Hildick-Smith D, et al. A European bifurcation coronary study: a randomized comparison of provisional T-stenting versus a systematic 2-stent strategy in large caliber true bifurcations. Presented at: EuroPCR; May 21, 2015; Paris, France.

30. Iakovou I, Ge L, Colombo A. Contemporary stent treatment of coronary bifurcations. *J Am Coll Cardiol.* 2005;46(8):1446–1455.

31. Ge L, et al. Clinical and angiographic outcome after implantation of drug-eluting stents in bifurcation lesions with the crush stent technique: importance of final kissing balloon post-dilation. *J Am Coll Cardiol.* 2005;46:613–620.

32. Chen SL, et al. A randomized clinical study comparing double kissing crush with provisional stenting for treatment of coronary bifurcation lesions results from the DKCRUSH-II (Double Kissing Crush versus Provisional Stenting Technique for Treatment of Coronary Bifurcation Lesions) Trial. *J Am Coll Cardiol.* 2011;57(8):914–920.

33. Fanggiday JC, et al. Safety and efficacy of drug-eluting balloons in percutaneous treatment of bifurcation lesions: the DEBIUT (drug-eluting balloon in bifurcation Utrecht) registry. *Catheter Cardiovasc Interv.* 2008;71(5):629–635.

34. Latib A, Colombo A, Sangiorgi GM. Bifurcation stenting: current strategies and new devices. *Heart.* 2009;95(6):495–504.

35. Garg S, et al. The outcome of bifurcation lesion stenting using a biolimus-eluting stent with a bio-degradable polymer compared to a sirolimus-eluting stent with a durable polymer. *EuroIntervention.* 2011;6(8):928–935.

36. Kawamoto H, et al. Bioresorbable scaffolds for the management of coronary bifurcation lesions. *J Am Coll Cardiol Intv.* 2016;9:989–1000.

37. Kraak RP, et al. The future of BRS in bifurcations. *EuroIntervention* 2015;11 Suppl V:V188–92.

38. Ormiston J, et al. Bioresorbable scaffolds on the bench. *EuroIntervention.* 2015;11 Suppl V:V166–9.

39. Park SJ, et al. Impact of intravascular ultrasound guidance on long-term mortality in stenting for unprotected left main coronary artery stenosis. *Circulation: Cardiovascular Interventions.* 2009; 2(3):167 LP-177.

40. Steigen TK, et al. Randomized study on simple versus complex stenting of coronary artery bifurcation lesions: the Nordic bifurcation study. *Circulation.* 2006;114:1955–1961.

41. Colombo A, et al. Randomized study of the crush technique versus provisional side-branch stenting in true coronary bifurcations: the CACTUS (Coronary bifurcations: Application of the Crushing Technique Using Sirolimus-Eluting Stents) study. *Circulation.* 2009;119(1):71.

42. Niemelä M, et al. Randomized comparison of final kissing balloon dilatation versus no final kissing balloon dilatation in patients with coronary bifurcation lesions treated with main vessel stenting: the Nordic-Baltic Bifurcation Study III. *Circulation.* 2011;123(1):79–86.

43. Levine GN, et al. 2011 ACCF/AHA/SCAI Guideline for percutaneous coronary intervention. A report of the American College of Cardiology Foundation/American Heart Association Task Force on Practice Guidelines and the Society for Cardiovascular Angiography and Interventions. *J Am Coll Cardiol.* 2011;58(24):e44–e122.

22

Small Vessel and Diffuse Disease

Mladen I. Vidovich, MD, FSCAI, FACC

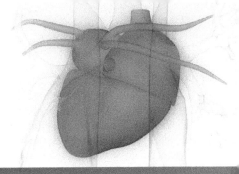

Percutaneous coronary intervention (PCI) in small vessels (SVs) remains one of the most challenging aspects of current interventional practice. Along with diabetes mellitus and diffuse coronary artery disease, SV PCI has traditionally been associated with increased restenosis rate, reduced success rates, overall increased complication rates, higher target lesion revascularization (TLR), and consequently increased major adverse cardiac event (MACE) rates (1–4). Similar to percutaneous revascularization, in-hospital mortality after coronary artery bypass grafting (CABG) is higher in patients with small coronary arteries (5).

The issue of SV PCI has undergone substantial change since the advent of angioplasty and can be generally divided into three phases: percutaneous transluminal coronary angioplasty (PTCA), bare-metal stenting (BMS), and contemporary drug-eluting stenting (DES). In addition, current approaches to SV disease will be discussed: bioabsorbable vascular scaffolds (BVSs) and bioabsorbable polymer metallic stents. While drug-eluting balloons (DEBs) have been used extensively outside the United States in SVs and diffuse disease, they are currently not approved by the US Food and Drug Administration for coronary artery use.

Definition

Currently, there is no accepted definition for "SVs." While most interventionalists would agree that vessel size <2.5 mm represents a SV, numerous trials have used vessel sizes <2.75 mm and up to <3.0 mm to define "SV" size. Some authors have reported vessels of <2.25 mm in diameter as "very small vessels."

Historically, SV PCI was performed in approximately 30% to 50% of interventions (2,6); however, contemporary "all-comers" clinical trials have enrolled a substantially higher proportion of patients with SV disease. These trials include broader patient populations with a high percentage of "off-label use" and may be more representative of patients and lesions encountered in everyday clinical practice. Both in the Resolute All-comers trial, which compared the everolimus-eluting stent (EES) with the zotarolimus-eluting stent (ZES) platforms, and in the LEADERS trial (biolimus platform), almost 68% of patients had reference vessel diameters of ≥2.75 mm (7,8). Thus, such a large proportion of SV PCI represents an important clinical and economic consideration. The availability of modern, thin-strut DESs in 2.25-mm diameter sizes has facilitated the continued search for solutions for PCI in ever-smaller vessels. This is well illustrated with the XIENCE Nano trial that enrolled patients with lesions in vessels between 2.25 and 2.5 mm in size (9). It is clear that, as the PCI and stent technology advance, our definition of what a "small vessel" represents will continue to evolve.

Balloon Angioplasty Versus BMS

After the initial success of PTCA in large vessels, it was quickly recognized that PTCA for SVs disease was associated with considerable difficulties, particularly frequent restenosis requiring repeat interventions. SV size had been previously identified as an independent risk factor contributing to vessel restenosis (2). Because the amount of neointimal hyperplasia is largely independent of vessel size (10), the late loss is similar in small and large vessels (11). Conversely to late loss, which is the absolute measure of restenosis, relative measures of restenosis, such as percent diameter stenosis, are directly dependent on vessel size. In SVs, the acute gain achieved is much smaller than in large vessels. As a result, the net lumen gain is less, which results in a higher rate of restenosis (12) (Fig. 22.1).

After studies performed in large vessels (>3.0 mm) demonstrated that the BMS was superior to PTCA regarding restenosis, interest and research among interventionalists gradually shifted to SVs.

In an initial study, BMS PCI in large vessels (>3.0 mm) was compared with SVs (<3.0 mm) and demonstrated higher restenosis in the SV group (32.6% vs. 19.9%, p < 0.0001). A conceptually very important finding was that the late loss was similar in the two groups (SVs, 1.11 ± 0.85 mm vs. large vessels, 1.05 ± 0.91 mm, p = NS). Predictors of

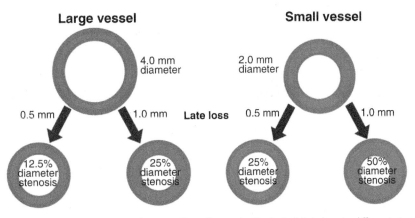

FIGURE 22.1 Impact of late loss on diameter stenosis in large and small vessels. Equivalent late loss in different sized vessels causes significantly different percent diameter stenosis.

freedom from restenosis were a larger post-procedure minimal stent cross-sectional area (OR 1.190, p = 0.0001) and shorter lesions (OR 1.037, p = 0.01). At 1-year follow-up, patients with SVs also had a lower rate of event-free survival (63% vs. 71.3%, p = 0.007) (3).

Subsequently, numerous trials were performed to determine the role of stent placement in SVs when compared with balloon angioplasty alone. Major findings of some of the representative trials are summarized in **Table 22.1** (13–17).

The accumulated knowledge gained from those studies is well summarized in two major meta-analyses performed at that time. The meta-analysis by Agostoni et al. included 4,383 patients from 13 trials with reference vessel size <3.0 mm. One of the most important findings was that neither death (OR 0.81, 95% CI, 0.48–1.36) nor myocardial infarction (MI) (OR 0.80, 95% CI 0.58–1.11) were different between the BMS and PTCA groups. Nevertheless, major adverse cardiac events (MACE) (OR 0.71, 95% CI 0.57–0.90) were favoring the BMS stenting approach (17.6%) compared with the PTCA strategy (22.7%). Decreased MACE were driven mainly by reduced repeat revascularization (OR 0.76, 95% CI 0.61–0.95). Notably, in further analyses, *optimal* PTCA had similar MACE-to-BMS stenting (OR 0.84, 95% CI 0.63–1.12) while *suboptimal* PTCA was associated with significantly worse MACE than BMS (OR 0.53, 95% CI 0.37–0.76, p < 0.001) (18).

The meta-analysis by Moreno et al. included 3,541 patients from 11 studies. SVs were similarly defined as <3 mm in diameter. The restenosis rate across those studies was 25.8% for BMS stenting and 34.2% in patients allocated to the PTCA strategy (RR 0.77, 95% CI 0.65–0.92, p = 0.003). Patients receiving BMS had lower MACE rates (15.0% vs. 21.8%, RR 0.70, 95% CI 0.57–0.87, p = 0.002) and less target vessel revascularizations (TVR) (12.5% vs. 17.0%, RR 0.75, 95% CI 0.61–0.91, p = 0.004). There were no differences in death or MI. The overall conclusion was that elective BMS stenting was superior to provisional stenting (19).

Strut Thickness and BMS

The ISAR-STEREO-2 trial was an initial study performed in large vessels comparing two different BMS platforms—a thin-strut stent (50 μm) with a thick-strut stent (140 μm)—and a significant decrease was found in angiographic restenosis in the thin-strut group (17.9%) when compared with the thick-strut group (31.4%) (RR 0.57, 95% CI 0.39–0.84, p < 0.001), with no difference in death and MI at 1 year (20). This was further confirmed in an analysis that encompassed several stent platforms. In this analysis, thin-strut stents were defined as having a strut thickness <100 μm. Restenosis was significantly lower in the thin-strut group (28.5%) compared with the thick-strut

group (36.6%) (21). Somewhat discordant with these and subsequent studies investigating the effect of strut thickness on outcomes, a large meta-analysis did not demonstrate any association between strut thickness and restenosis reduction, likely due to smaller differences in strut thickness among the trials (19).

Importantly, when a thick-strut DES (Cypher 140 μm, sirolimus-eluting stent) was compared with a thin-strut BMS (BeStent 76 μm), angiographic restenosis rate was 8.3% for the Cypher stent and 25.5% for the BeStent (p < 0.001), further underlining the importance of anti-proliferative therapies in SVs and the high risk of these lesions even when treated with a thin-strut BMS (22).

Heparin Stent Coating with BMS in Small Vessels

Before the introduction of contemporary anti-proliferative stent technologies, attempts were made to study the effect of heparin coating in the prevention of restenosis and stent thrombosis. COAST was a randomized trial in which PTCA was compared with uncoated BMSs and with BMSs with a heparin coating in SVs ranging from 2.0 to 2.6 mm. Restenosis rates were found to be similar (32%, 25%, and 30%, respectively) with similar stent thrombosis rates (1.0% for PTCA and 0.5% for BMSs or heparin-coated BMSs) (23).

Cilostazol and BMS in Small Vessels

Given the overall high rates of restenosis associated with BMSs in SVs, additional efforts in providing systemic pharmacologic therapy have yielded somewhat positive results. Subgroup analysis of 316 patients with vessel diameter <2.75 mm in the CREST trial demonstrated that restenosis in the group that received cilostazol 100 mg twice daily in addition to dual antiplatelet therapy with aspirin and clopidogrel had lower restenosis rates compared with the traditional arm (23.6% vs. 35.2%, RR 0.67, 95% CI 0.47–0.95). Nonetheless, these rates remained significantly higher than those that could be achieved with DESs (24).

IVUS and BMS in Small Vessels

Because the acute gain is less in SVs, use of intravascular ultrasound (IVUS) and IVUS-guided stent postdilation would be expected to improve outcomes in SV PCI. This hypothesis was tested in a for a while that retrospectively analyzed patients who underwent SV PCI (reference diameter <2.75 mm) with IVUS-guidance. Based on final IVUS lumen areas, two groups were identified and prospectively followed, ≥6.0 mm^2 and >6.0 mm^2 lumen area groups. TLR was significantly lower in the larger lumen group (39% vs. 26%, p = 0.01) and MACE non-significantly reduced (44% vs. 34%, p = 0.07). Death

TABLE 22.1 Representative Trials of BMS versus PTCA in Small Vessel Disease

TRIAL	RVD (mm)	STRUT THICKNESS (μm)	RESTENOSIS (%)		MACE (%)		TVR (%)	
			PTCA	BMS	PTCA	BMS	PTCA	BMS
ISAR-SMART (13) N = 404	2.0–2.8	50.0	37.4	35.7	19.0	23.0	16.5	20.1
BESMART (14) N = 381	<3.0	85.0	47.0	21.0	33.7	18.8	27.1	15.3
SISA (15) N = 351	2.3–2.9	85.0	32.9	28.0	22.0	18.3	20.3	17.8
SISCA (16) N = 145	2.1–3.0	85.0	18.8	9.7	23.9	9.5	22.5	9.5
COAST (23) N = 588	2.0–2.6	90.0	32.2	27.2	15.4	11.7	14.4	10.7
Park et al. (17) N = 120	<3.0	100.0	30.9	35.7	8.3	5.0	5.0	3.3

BMS, bare-metal stent; MACE, major adverse cardiac events; PTCA, percutaneous transluminal coronary angioplasty; RVD, reference vessel diameter; TVR, target vessel revascularization.

and MI were similar. A final IVUS cross-sectional area of ≥ 6.0 mm^2 was independently associated with higher TLR (OR 1.84, 95% CI 1.23–2.51, p = 0.01) (25).

Stent Thrombosis and BMS SV PCI

A large study that included a very broad population of unselected and consecutive patients offered an early understanding of factors associated with stent thrombosis in SV PCI (4). In this study, average vessel size was 2.6 mm and 30-day stent thrombosis was 4.2%. Residual dissection (OR 5.38), reduced left ventricular (LV) function (OR 3.08), and acute coronary syndrome (OR 2.53) were some of the factors associated with thrombotic events. Similarly, a pooled analysis in 2001 using aspirin and ticlopidine demonstrated that final minimal lumen diameter within the stent (OR, 0.4; 95% CI, 0.2–0.7/1 mm) was associated with increased risk of stent thrombosis (26).

Nowadays, the findings of these studies are of somewhat historical interest because contemporary dual antiplatelet therapy and devices were not used at that time, contributing to the high observed rates of stent thrombosis.

Balloon Angioplasty and Adjunctive Devices

Before the introduction of DESs, research had focused on alternative strategies to reduce high rates of restenosis in SVs. Interestingly, as early as 1993, a landmark study recognized that late outcome after PTCA, BMSs, and directional atherectomy depended mainly on the *immediate results* and not on the *procedure per se* used to obtain the results (27). Although not specifically describing SV use, this important concept was confirmed in a large meta-analysis in 2004 (28). To test whether these adjunctive devices were a possible solution to high MACE rates in SVs, and to test the hypothesis about whether reduction of plaque burden was beneficial in SVs, several trials focusing on those devices were performed.

Rotational Atherectomy in SV Disease

The value of rotational atherectomy compared with PTCA in SVs (mean reference diameter 2.46 mm) was reported in the DART trial. Target vessel failure (composite of death, Q-wave MI, and clinically driven revascularization) was similar in the rotational atherectomy and PTCA groups (30.5% vs. 31.2%). Both acute gain (rotablation 0.86 mm vs. PTCA 0.88 mm) and late loss were similar (rotablation 0.49 mm vs. PTCA 0.56 mm) (29).

Cutting Balloon in SV Disease

Similarly, the use of cutting balloon in SVs was investigated in a large randomized trial (mean reference diameter 2.86 mm). This study demonstrated essentially equivalent six-month binary angiographic restenosis in the cutting balloon group (31.4%) compared with the PTCA group (30.4%). There were statistically more perforations (0.8% vs. 0%) and higher rates of MI, death, and total MACE in the cutting balloon group (4.7% vs. 2.4%), however (30).

Despite the overall equivalence between PTCA and these adjunctive techniques, these trials demonstrated that their use remains safe and equally effective in lesions subsets that are more amenable to rotational atherectomy (e.g., heavily calcified lesions) or cutting balloon use (e.g., fibrotic lesions prone to recoil or "watermelon seeding effect").

In summary, the two large meta-analyses and subsequent specialized trials had solidified our understanding on the impact of BMS PCI and outcomes of PTCA in SVs. Compared with today's DESs, restenosis rates were high, albeit lower, with BMS stenting. It is important to emphasize that even in today's practice, where modern medical therapy has been shown to be extremely important in the treatment of coronary artery disease (31), optimal PTCA may in certain clinical scenarios offer quite satisfactory results compared with BMSs. SV coronary stenting with BMSs reduces the restenosis rate with subsequently fewer MACE. The reduced MACE is driven mainly by reduced target vessel revascularization. There is no difference in MI and death. BMSs with thinner stent struts are associated with lower restenosis rates.

First-Generation DESs
SIROLIMUS-ELUTING STENTS

The SIRIUS 2.25 trial was a small nonrandomized study that used propensity-matched PTCA and BMS historical controls, yet it easily demonstrated a remarkable reduction in 6-month TLR with sirolimus-eluting stent (SES) (4.0%) versus the Bx Velocity BMS (15.0%). In-lesion binary restenosis was similarly reduced to 16.9% in the SES group compared with the 30.6% to 45.9% range in the historical BMS controls (32).

Subsequently, in a randomized prospective fashion, the SES-SMART trial compared SES versus BMS in vessels with mean vessel diameter of 2.2 mm. The binary in-segment restenosis after 8 months was 53.1% in the BMS group and 9.8% in the SES group (RR, 0.18; 95% CI 0.10–0.32; p < 0.001). Similarly, MACE was significantly reduced in the SES group, 9.3%, versus 31.3% in the BMS group (RR, 0.30; 95% CI 0.15–0.55; p < 0.001), mainly because of a reduction in TLR (7% vs. 21.1%) and MI (1.6% vs. 7.8%) (33).

PACLITAXEL-ELUTING STENTS

In the large TAXUS V trial, stents of 2.25 mm in diameter were used in almost 18% of patients, with a mean SV diameter of only 2.08 mm. The 2.25-mm paclitaxel-eluting stents (PESs) significantly reduced in-stent restenosis to 24.7% compared with 44.7% with the BMS. Nine-month MACE were similarly lower with PESs (18.9%) compared with 26.9% with BMSs. Nonetheless, after 9 months, non-Q wave MI was non-significantly higher in the PES (5.7%) group compared with the BMS (2.2%). In comparison, in the whole trial, which also included large vessels, overall PES restenosis rates were lower at 15.4% for the PES platform compared with 39.6% for the BMS (34).

HEAD-TO-HEAD FIRST-GENERATION DES COMPARISON

The SIRTAX trial was a prospective and randomized trial that directly compared the two first-generation DESs. A subgroup analysis of the SIRTAX trial focused on SVs defined as ≥ 2.75 mm and found that at 2 years SESs significantly reduced MACE by 55% compared with PESs (10.4% vs. 21.4%, p < 0.004). This was driven mainly by lower TLR (6.0% vs. 17.7%, p = 0.001). Death, cardiac death, stent thrombosis, and MI at 2 years were similar between SESs and PESs (35).

In a recent network meta-analysis, that compared balloon angioplasty, BMSs, DEBs, PESs, and SESs, the aforementioned findings were confirmed, suggesting the best clinical and angiographic outcomes were with early-generation SESs, followed by PESs, DEBs, BMSs, and balloon angioplasty (36).

As illustrated by these early DES trials, the first-generation DES PCI in SVs represented a major breakthrough, with a remarkable reduction in restenosis and a dramatic improvement in MACE and TLR.

Second- and Third-Generation DESs

Although the reduction in restenosis was remarkable with the introduction of first-generation DES in SV PCI, it was clearly apparent that these types of lesions continued to present a formidable challenge for interventional cardiology. The restenosis and MACE rates remained higher than those observed in large-vessel PCI. As the volume of PCIs continued to grow, more complex patients and lesions were being treated. As a result, small-vessel disease currently comprises an ever-larger proportion of interventions in daily practice. Further refinement in the polymer composition and design, reduction in stent strut thickness and overall stent design advances, as well as improvements in delivery balloons, have yielded improved angiographic and clinical results with the currently available second- and third-generation DESs.

EVEROLIMUS-ELUTING STENTS

The EES, a second-generation stent, was compared with the PES, a first-generation stent, in the large prospective randomized SPIRIT IV trial. Target vessel failure was significantly reduced with the EES (3.9%) compared with the PES (6.8%) in the group with reference vessel diameter ≥2.75 mm (RR 0.57, 95% CI 0.35–0.91). Remarkably, the second-generation EES reduced the overall rates of stent thrombosis by nearly 75% (37). An additional study focusing on the impact of lesion length and vessel size pooled results from the SPIRIT and COMPARE families of trials. Large vessels were compared with higher-risk lesions involving long or SVs (but not both) and long lesions (LLs) in SVs. At 2 years, MACE was non-significantly different between EESs and PESs in the large vessel group (4.8% vs. 7.0%, p = 0.11); however, both in the *LL or SV group* EESs had lower MACE compared with PESs (6.6% vs. 11.2%, p <0.01) and in the *long and SV group* (9.1% vs. 12.7%, p = 0.008). Furthermore, MI, TLR, and stent thrombosis were also lower with EESs (38). Therefore, high-risk SV lesions particularly benefited from the use of a second-generation stent platform.

The pooled, patient-level analysis of SPIRIT II and SPIRIT III trials specifically investigating SVs (<2.765 mm reference vessel diameter) demonstrated significantly reduced MACE with EES compared with PES (5.2% vs. 10.7%, p = 0.037). Taking into consideration the previously well-known findings from the TAXUS V trial (34), a very important finding of the SPIRIT II and III trials was that reduction in MACE was driven mainly by reduced non-Q-wave MIs (1.6% vs. 5.0%) and TLR (3.0% vs. 6.0%). Such findings in SV lesions and their high-risk features further stressed the importance of strut thickness, polymer formulation, and choice of antiproliferative drugs on PCI outcomes (39).

In a 643-patient study, the SES was compared to the EES in SV disease (defined as stent size ≤2.5 mm) and showed no difference in 1-year MACE (EES, 9.1% vs. SES 8.6%, p = 0.83). There was no stent thrombosis in the EES group and 1.2% in the SES group (p = 0.17). This trial re-demonstrated that despite a newer stent design, SV disease remained a treatment challenge (40).

ZOTAROLIMUS-ELUTING STENTS

The ENDEAVOR IV Trial compared the second-generation ZES (Endeavor) with the PES. The ZES is a cobalt-alloy stent with a phosphorylcholine drug carrier for the active drug zotarolimus. In the subgroup with the reference vessel diameter <2.5 mm, TVR was non-significantly lower with this second-generation ZES (7.9% vs. 10.3%, RR 0.76, 95% CI: 0.44–1.33). Overall, this trial demonstrated similar clinical safety and efficacy between ZES and PES (41).

A third-generation ZES (Endeavor Resolute) was compared with second-generation EES in the Resolute All Comers Trial. A different polymer, BioLinx, was used to elute the antiproliferative drug zotarolimus. In this "real-world" trial, 70% of interventions had at least one vessel that was ≥2.75 mm in size. In the prespecified subgroup analysis, lesions ≥2.75 mm had a *near-equivalent* primary endpoint of target lesion failure at 1 year (OR 1.01, 95% CI 0.69–1.48) when compared with the EES. The overall TLF was 8.2 for ZES and 8.3% for EES (7).

DIFFERENT POLYMERS AND DESs

In the RESOLUTE-US trial, the third-generation ZES (Endeavor Resolute) was compared with historical controls obtained with the second-generation ZES (Endeavor). This is a unique trial that compared the direct influence of a different polymer (phosphorylcholine with Endeavor vs. BioLinx for Endeavor Resolute) and its differential drug-eluting performance employing the same stent platform. In the 2.25 mm vessel group, the 12-month target lesion failure was 4.8%, which met the prespecified non-inferiority endpoint (42).

Reduced Strut Thickness, Metallurgy, and DESs

The TAXUS ATLAS SV was a nonrandomized trial that specifically compared a thin-strut 2.25-mm PES with historical controls of the thick-strut first-generation PES (43). Both stents had the same polymer coating containing 1 μg/mm² of paclitaxel in a slow-release formulation, and both were stainless-steel stents. The only difference was comparing the thin-strut stent (97 μm) with the thick-strut stent (132 μm). Unlike the RESOLUTE-US trial, which compared the same stent and the same drug delivered on a different polymer, the TAXUS ATLAS SV trial compared identical polymer, drug dosage, and elution kinetics on different strut-thickness stent platforms. The thin-strut stainless-steel stent significantly reduced 9-month angiographic restenosis (18.5% vs. 32.7%, p = 0.0219) and 12-month TLR (6.1% vs. 16.9%, p = 0.0039). The importance of this trial is that these findings were concordant with previous data obtained with the thin-strut BMS, suggesting that thinner struts were associated with better outcomes. This confirms the concept that even with antiproliferative agents, strut thickness plays a central role in SV PCI outcomes.

The PERSEUS SV trial compared the even thinner-strut platinum–chromium stent (81 μm) with historical BMS controls. Both had the same paclitaxel-eluting polymer coatings. The platinum–chromium PES (TAXUS Element) was superior to the Express BMS for late loss (0.38 ± 0.51 mm vs. 0.80 ± 0.53 mm, respectively; p < 0.001), and TLF (7.3%) was significantly less than the 19.5% with the BMS (p < 0.001). There were no differences in mortality, MI, or stent thrombosis observed during 12 months of follow-up (44).

Somewhat similar to the PERSEUS SV trial, the single-arm, open-label XIENCE Nano trial studied a cobalt–chromium EES in SVs (reference vessel diameter ≥2.25 mm and <2.5 mm). The 1-year target lesion failure was 8.1%, cardiac death 1.5%, and the clinically indicated TLR 5.1% (9).

The RESOLUTE-US, TAXUS ATLAS SV, and XIENCE Nano trials are prime examples of how continued research and development of the drug-delivery polymers and stent designs continue to incrementally improve angiographic and clinical outcomes.

Bioabsorbable Polymer DESs

The SYNERGY stent is a thin-strut (74–81 μm) platinum–chromium stent with an ultrathin (4 μm) abluminal bioabsorbable polymer. Although the EVOLVE II trial did not specifically address SV disease, the mean vessel size was 2.6 mm and nearly a quarter of the vessels were <2.25 mm in diameter. The stent was compared to the Promus Element Plus (81–86 μm strut thickness), given its 7.8-μm thick conformal durable polymer. Target lesion failure was non-inferior at 12 months, 6.7% for Synergy, and 6.5% for Promus Element Plus (45).

Lastly, BIO-RESORT was a three-arm, randomized, non-inferiority trial that compared the Synergy bioresorbable polymer thin-strut stent with the Orsinor sirolimus-eluting cobalt–chromium stent and the Resolute Integrity stent in an all-comer design. At 1 year, there was no difference in the composite primary endpoint with equal rates of stent thrombosis (0.3%). The mean vessel size overall was 2.76 mm, and there was no difference in stent outcome among the three stents in the SVs subgroup defined as <2.75 mm (46).

Contemporary Outcomes in SV PCI in the United States

A study of the NHLBI Dynamic Registry, describing contemporary United States practice patients with small coronary arteries demonstrated that patients treated with DESs had significantly lower rates of repeat revascularization and MACE (HR 0.59, 95% CI 0.42–0.83, p = 0.002) at 1 year compared with those treated with BMSs. The risks of death and MI were similar. Lesions treated with DESs tended to be longer (16.7 mm vs. 13.1 mm, p < 0.001) and vessel sizes smaller (2.6 mm vs. 2.7 mm, p < 0.001). Furthermore, underscoring the impact of widespread adoption of DESs in the United States, the use of DESs in high-risk SV lesions was associated with lower 1-year CABG and repeat PCI rates (47).

Cilostazol and DESs

Whether further improvement in angiographic and clinical outcomes can be achieved with an oral agent was tested in the DECLARE-DIABETES trial. High-risk diabetic patients were treated with SESs and PESs and randomized to receive standard DAPT or triple antiplatelet therapy (aspirin, clopidogrel, and cilostazol). Cilostazol was administered as a 200-mg oral loading dose, followed by 100 mg orally twice daily for 6 months. Six-month in-segment restenosis was lowered with the addition of cilostazol (8.0% vs. 15.6%, p = 0.033%), as was the 9-month TLR (2.5% vs. 7.0%, p = 0.034). Although this trial did not specifically describe SV disease, the mean reference diameter was quite representative at 2.8 mm (48).

Stent Thrombosis and DES SV PCI

There is conflicting data in the literature regarding the issue of impact of SV disease as an *independent* risk factor for stent thrombosis (ST) (49). The most important cause for this incongruence in the literature is that ST is a complex phenomenon and is associated with numerous covariates that include patient comorbidities (e.g., diabetes, renal insufficiency), lesion characteristics (e.g., small vessel, LL, bifurcation disease), device types (e.g., polymer type, strut thickness, anti-proliferative drug), and DAPT considerations (e.g., various drugs, compliance, DAPT duration) (50).

As a result, there has been great difficulty in the literature to associate SVs PCI *per se* with increased rates of stent thrombosis, while stent length and diabetes have. Although many retrospective analyses have adjusted for multiple patient and lesion characteristics, it remains difficult to separate small and long vessel disease from co-morbid diabetes because they frequently tend to occur simultaneously (51,52).

Another important study that deserves special mention is that at the beginning of the DES era, it was observed that stent thrombosis was associated with small minimum stent size at the end of PCI. Small minimum stent area, in turn, is most commonly associated with stent underexpansion and small vessel size. As such, this IVUS study elegantly summarizes the difficulty in separating the aforementioned factors coexisting with SV that may contribute to stent thrombosis (53).

The following is a brief review of several important studies that have addressed the issue of ST in SV.

A meta-analysis that pooled 12 trials and included 3,182 patients demonstrated that SV size *did not appear* to be associated with higher risk for definite or probable stent thrombosis when comparing DES (2.1%) to BMS (2.4%) (OR 0.63, 95% CI 0.34–1.17) (54). In contrast, another study demonstrated association of small vessel size with stent thrombosis (OR 0.11/mm increase, 95% CI 0.01–0.73, p = 0.021) (55).

Different DES platforms may be associated with different stent thrombosis rates. A large European first-generation stent analysis did not demonstrate an increased risk of early (adjusted HR 0.66, 95% CI 0.35–1.24) or late-stent thrombosis (adjusted HR 0.82, 95% CI 0.33–2.06) associated with stent diameter. Nevertheless, while early stent thrombosis was similar with the SES (1.1%) and PES (1.3%), late stent thrombosis was somewhat more frequent with the PES (1.8%) than with the SES (1.4%) (p = 0.031) (56).

Further refinements achieved with second-generation stents have yielded lower rates of stent thrombosis in the SV PCI. Interestingly, in the large vessel group, stent thrombosis rates were comparable (EES 0.6% vs. PES 0.2%, p = 0.29), while in small and long vessels, EES performed significantly better (EES 0.5% vs. PES 1.9%) (38).

In a recent analysis of the XIENCE V trial, SV (<2.5 mm) was not shown to contribute to stent thrombosis. DAPT interruption, renal insufficiency, and stent length were associated with increased ST (57).

An additional study, with pooled data from SPIRIT III and SPIRIT IV showed that, for larger vessels (≥2.5 mm), PESs had s higher stent thrombosis compared to smaller vessels (≤2.5 mm) (0.4% vs. 0.1%). EES, nevertheless, had overall lower and equal ST rates in large and SV (0.1% vs. 0.1%) (58).

Therefore, there is a clear indication that with continued improvement in the stent platforms stent thrombosis rates continue to decrease and that different antiproliferative agents, polymers, and stent platforms are associated with different stent thrombosis rates. Based on the current favorable reduction in overall stent thrombosis, it is likely that more intense platelet inhibition with prasugrel or ticagrelor may further reduce stent thrombosis in SVs (59,60).

Late Loss with Various DES Platforms

Whether late loss is an adequate surrogate marker of subsequent TLR and clinical events has been a matter of significant debate (11,61). Nonetheless, in a large analysis of 11 randomized controlled trials, in-stent and in-segment late loss and percent diameter stenosis were found to reliably estimate TLR for both the DES and BMS. As would be predicted, late loss as a surrogate marker was dependent on vessel size, while percent diameter stenosis was not (12). The late loss with different DES platforms is shown in Figure 22.2. MACE rates associated with different DES platforms are shown in Figure 22.3.

BVS in SV PCI

The use of ABSORB BVS in SVs (<2.5 mm) compared to large vessels (≥2.5 mm) reported no difference in late lumen loss at 2-year follow-up (0.29 ± 0.16 mm vs. 0.25 ± 0.22 mm, p = 0.4391). The 2-year MACE was similar (7.3% vs. 6.7%, p = 1.0). This was a small study (101 patients) and it should be noted that a 3.0-mm ABSORB stent was implanted in SVs because the 2.5-mm platform was not available at that time. There was no BVS thrombosis reported (62).

In the ABSORB III trial, target-lesion failure (TLF) was investigated in a subgroup analysis. The vessels <2.63 mm had a TLF RR of 1.27 (95% CI 0.82–1.94), whereas the vessels ≥2.63 mm had RR of 1.34 (0.73–2.44), and the difference in RR was nonsignificant (p = 0.90). The overall trial findings were non-inferior compared to the XIENCE CoCr EES. Scaffold thrombosis was higher in the small-vessel group (<2.65 mm), and was 2.3% versus 0.9% in the

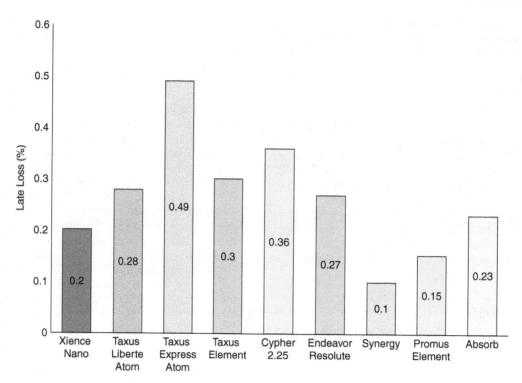

FIGURE 22.2 Comparison of in-stent late loss with different drug-eluting stent platforms. Note that the late loss data are from different clinical trials that have enrolled different patient populations and may not be directly comparable. (From: Serruys PW, et al. Comparison of zotarolimus-eluting and everolimus-eluting coronary stents. *N Engl J Med*. 2010;363:136–146; Cannon LA, et al. Cardiovascular outcomes following rotational atherectomy: a UK multicentre experience. *Catheter Cardiovasc Interv*. 2012;80(4):546–553; Moses JW, et al. Safety and efficacy of the 2.25-mm sirolimus-eluting Bx Velocity stent in the treatment of patients with de novo native coronary artery lesions: the SIRIUS 2.25 trial. *Am J Cardiol*. 2006;98:1455–1460; Stone GW, et al. Comparison of a polymer-based paclitaxel-eluting stent with a bare metal stent in patients with complex coronary artery disease: a randomized controlled trial. *JAMA*. 2005;294:1215–1223; Turco MA, et al. Reduced risk of restenosis in small vessels and reduced risk of myocardial infarction in long lesions with the new thin-strut TAXUS Liberté stent: 1-year results from the TAXUS ATLAS program. *JACC Cardiovasc Interv*. 2008;1:699–709; Cannon LA, et al. A prospective evaluation of the safety and efficacy of TAXUS Element paclitaxel-eluting coronary stent implantation for the treatment of de novo coronary artery lesions in small vessels: the PERSEUS Small Vessel trial. *EuroIntervention*. 2011;6:920–927; Meredith IT, et al. Primary endpoint results of the EVOLVE trial: a randomized evaluation of a novel bioabsorbable polymer-coated, everolimus-eluting coronary stent. *J Am Coll Cardiol*. 2012;59:1362–1370; Diletti R, et al. Clinical and intravascular imaging outcomes at 1 and 2 years after implantation of absorb everolimus eluting bioresorbable vascular scaffolds in small vessels. Late lumen enlargement: does bioresorption matter with small vessel size? Insight from the ABSORB cohort B trial. *Heart*. 2013;99:98–105; Kereiakes DJ, et al. Efficacy and safety of a novel bioabsorbable polymer-coated, everolimus-eluting coronary stent: the EVOLVE II randomized trial. *Circ Cardiovasc Interv*. 2015;8(4). pii: e002372 with permission.)

XIENCE group, RR was 2.65 (95% CI, 0.77–9.07), but likely did not reach statistical significance due to the small sample size in this subgroup analysis. In contrast, scaffold thrombosis in the large vessel group (>2.65 mm) was 0.8% versus 0.6% in the XIENCE group (RR 1.28, 98% CI 0.25–6.54) (63).

The small BVS-Save Registry, which retrospectively analyzed 121 patients with BVS PCI in vessels <2.75 mm found MACE of 9.0%. The BVS thrombosis rate was 1.5% (64).

Lastly, a large all-comer European study investigated predictors of BVS thrombosis. BVS thrombosis was strongly associated with a low post-procedural minimal lumen diameter (MLD) and reference vessel diameter (RVD) (both p < 0.0001). The risk of BVS thrombosis was particularly prominent with post-procedural MLD (<2.4 mm) in SVs. One of the most important findings of this study is that the change in BVS implantation strategy, namely aggressive pre- and post-dilation, resulted in a significant reduction in BVS thrombosis (3.3%–1.0%) (65).

In summary, these contemporary trials indicate that challenges with the treatment of SV disease remain after the introduction of BVS. These studies strongly suggest there is a connection between vessel size and scaffold thrombosis.

IVUS and OCT in DES SV PCI

Consistent with previous IVUS findings, a small study investigating association of Optical Coherence Tomography (OCT) and restenosis found that, in SVs, the minimum stent area of 3.5 mm² adequately predicted 9-month in-stent restenosis (66).

FFR SV PCI

The use of fractional flow reserve (FFR) has been associated with improved outcomes in PCIs in a wide variety of lesions and vessel sizes (67). Of particular interest is the use of FFR in SV disease. In a study where SV was defined as lesions <3 mm, patients treated with FFR-guided PCI had significantly lower MACE (HR, 0.458; 95% CI, 0.310–0.679; p < 0.001), but not mortality (HR, 0.684; 95% CI, 0.355–1.316; p = 0.255). Procedure costs were lower in the FFR group (68).

Diffuse Disease

Similar to SV disease, diffuse disease, also frequently referred to as "LL," has been associated with worse outcomes when compared with

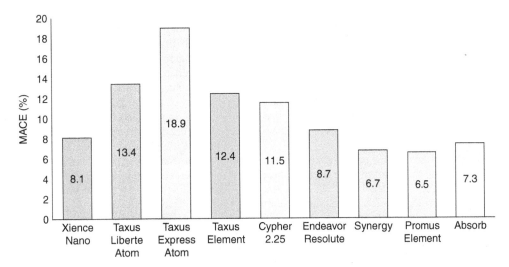

FIGURE 22.3 Comparison of Major Adverse Cardiac Events (MACE) with different drug-eluting stent platforms. Note that the MACE data sources are from different clinical trials that have enrolled different patient populations and may not be directly comparable. (From: Serruys PW, et al. Comparison of zotarolimus-eluting and everolimus-eluting coronary stents. *N Engl J Med.* 2010;363:136–146; Cannon LA, et al. Cardiovascular outcomes following rotational atherectomy: a UK multicentre experience. *Catheter Cardiovasc Interv.* 2012;80(4):546–553; Moses JW, et al. Safety and efficacy of the 2.25-mm sirolimus-eluting Bx Velocity stent in the treatment of patients with de novo native coronary artery lesions: the SIRIUS 2.25 trial. *Am J Cardiol.* 2006;98:1455–1460; Stone GW, et al. Comparison of a polymer-based paclitaxel-eluting stent with a bare metal stent in patients with complex coronary artery disease: a randomized controlled trial. *JAMA.* 2005;294:1215–1223; Turco MA, et al. Reduced risk of restenosis in small vessels and reduced risk of myocardial infarction in long lesions with the new thin-strut TAXUS Liberté stent: 1-year results from the TAXUS ATLAS program. *JACC Cardiovasc Interv.* 2008;1:699–709; Cannon LA, et al. A prospective evaluation of the safety and efficacy of TAXUS Element paclitaxel-eluting coronary stent implantation for the treatment of de novo coronary artery lesions in small vessels: the PERSEUS Small Vessel trial. *EuroIntervention.* 2011;6:920–927; Meredith IT, et al. Primary endpoint results of the EVOLVE trial: a randomized evaluation of a novel bioabsorbable polymer-coated, everolimus-eluting coronary stent. *J Am Coll Cardiol.* 2012;59:1362–1370; Diletti R, et al. Clinical and intravascular imaging outcomes at 1 and 2 years after implantation of absorb everolimus eluting bioresorbable vascular scaffolds in small vessels. Late lumen enlargement: does bioresorption matter with small vessel size? Insight from the ABSORB cohort B trial. *Heart.* 2013;99:98–105; Kereiakes DJ, et al. Efficacy and safety of a novel bioabsorbable polymer-coated, everolimus-eluting coronary stent: the EVOLVE II randomized trial. *Circ Cardiovasc Interv.* 2015;8(4). pii: e002372, with permission.)

shorter lesions and lesions in larger vessels. Both diffuse disease and SV disease are frequently seen in diabetic populations (69).

Definition

The traditional ACC/AHA definition from the PTCA era classified lesions >20 mm in length as Type C lesions with an anticipated success rate of <60% (70). With the advances in stenting technology and adjunctive pharmacology, the definition has undergone significant modification, and a contemporary definition, developed for the SYNTAX trial, defines a "diffuse disease/SV" category when "75% length of the segment distal to the lesion has a vessel diameter of <2 mm irrespective of absence of disease at that distal segment" (71). Hence, from the standpoint of nomenclature, "diffuse disease" is different from "multivessel" disease because diffuse disease refers to LL in one specific vessel. As previously shown, the shift in overall perception regarding "SVs" has similarly changed for "diffuse disease," with current clinical PCI practice addressing ever-longer lesions than in the PTCA era.

Diffuse Disease and Bare-Metal Stents

In the era of BMS, it was quickly recognized that stent length predicted stent restenosis. In a classic study that examined three groups: lesions ≤20 mm, lesions >20 mm but ≤35 mm, and lesions ≥35 mm, restenosis was 23.9%, 34.6%, and 47.2%, respectively. Most interestingly, the rates of subacute stent thrombosis were similar at 0.4%, 0.4%, and 1.2% (72).

It is quite important to consider the impact of lesion coverage during BMS on PCI outcome. Excess stent length beyond the lesion itself increases restenosis risk independently of lesion length (for each 10-mm excess stent length, TLR increased by an odds ratio of 1.12) (73).

As both of those trials demonstrate, BMS in LSs was associated with very high rates of restenosis and a high penalty for excessive lesion coverage.

Diffuse Disease and DESs

FIRST-GENERATION DESs

TAXUS VI compared the PES with BMS, specifically focusing on long and complex coronary lesions. The mean lesion length was 20.6 mm. At 5-year follow-up, TLR was lower in the PES group (14.6%) compared with the BMS group (21.4%) (p = 0.0325). Stent thrombosis rates were equivalent at 0.9% with no difference in death and MACE (74).

A study that investigated outcome with SES in both LL and SV disease was E-SIRIUS. It is noteworthy to stress that in this early DES trial, specifically addressing "LL," mean lesion length would have been considered short by today's standard of 15 mm. Binary restenosis was markedly reduced with SES compared with BMS controls (5.9% vs. 42.3%, p = 0.0001), with a resulting reduction in MACE (8.0% vs. 22.6%, p = 0.0002) (75).

Finally, in a head-to-head comparison between the SES and PES in LLs, the SES was associated with lower late loss (0.09 mm) compared with the PES (0.45 mm), and lower TLR at 9 months (2.4%) versus the PES (7.2%). Rates of death or MI were not different, however. The average lesion in this trial was significantly higher: 34 mm (76).

SECOND- AND THIRD-GENERATION STENTS

Although the outcomes with first-generation DESs clearly presented a major advancement, compared with BMSs, by reducing the profound impact that lesion length had on restenosis, TLR and MACE still remained higher than with shorter lesions.

The EES was compared with the PES in a pooled analysis of the SPIRIT and COMPARE trials, and three groups were studied: short lesions in large vessels, LL or SVs, and finally LLs in SVs. Two-year MACE were similar in the lower-risk group comprising short lesions in large vessels (4.8% vs. 7.0%, p = 0.11). Nevertheless, the EES outperformed the SES in the high-risk groups: lower MACE in the LL or SV group (6.6% vs. 11.2%, p < 0.01) and in the LL in SV group (9.1% vs. 12.7%). EES had lower MACE compared with the PES, regardless of lesion length or reference vessel diameter. Stent thrombosis was low and similar: 0.5%, 0.8%, and 0.9%, respectively (38).

In the TAXUS ATLAS LL trial, the 38-mm thin-strut stainless-steel PES was compared with historical controls, which included the overlapping thick-strut PES. The 38-mm PES significantly reduced the risk of 12-month MI compared with TAXUS Express (1.4% vs. 6.5%, p = 0.0246). Restenosis rates were similar, however. In the LVs of the TAXUS ATLAS trial, stent strut thickness did not appear to be associated with better outcomes (43).

The third-generation ZES had equivalent target lesion failure in LLs (defined as >18 mm) compared to the second-generation EESs in the Resolute All-Comers trial (OR 0.86, 95% CI 0.44–1.67, p = 0.74) (7).

A large, contemporary pooled analysis of 13,266 patients receiving XIENCE EESs, two groups were compared: very LSs (≥35 mm) and control (>24 to <35 mm). The mean lesion length in the very LS group was 47.1 mm. There was no difference in target lesion failure, MACE, nor stent thrombosis at 1 year (77). This trial is important because it shows that improvement in stent technology has resulted in better outcomes in LL.

Stent Overlap

It is estimated that stent overlap occurs in approximately 10% of PCIs. The reasons for this are multifold and are mainly due to LLs, incomplete lesion coverage, or technical issues, such as edge dissections (78).

BMS overlap is associated with higher 12-month MACE compared with the single-stent approach (31.5% vs. 18.1%, p < 0.01) mainly due to high TLR (28.2% vs. 16.8%, p < 0.01). Late-stent thrombosis (0.4%) was similar, with somewhat higher periprocedural MI (3.4% vs. 0.9%, p = 0.03). Average stent length in the overlap group was 28 mm compared to 18 mm in the single-stent group (79).

The same study investigated outcomes with SES stent overlap. Overlapped SES lesions were, on average, 28 mm long, and single-stented lesions were 18 mm long. There was no difference in MACE between the two groups (7.4% SES overlap vs. 6.7% single SES). TLR were comparable between the overall and the non-overlap groups (4.7% vs. 3.3%, p = 0.30), as was periprocedural MI (2.1% vs. 1.6%, p = 0.61). The findings of this study are important because they indicate that a strategy of overlapping SES was safe overall in regard to restenosis and TLR reduction without an increase in periprocedural MI (59).

Divergent to these findings, a subanalysis of the SIRTAX trial demonstrated increased MACE, TLR, and composite of death or MI

in the overlapping stent group when compared with single-stent and multiple-stent groups (78).

Although these two trials demonstrate incongruous outcomes with a first-generation DES, they have significant limitations because reasons for stent overlap were various and frequently associated with higher-risk patient characteristics. Multiple unmeasured confounders could have accounted for the observed differences and differing outcomes. Nonetheless, modern second- and third-generation stents have more deliverable characteristics and are available in longer stent lengths, reducing the need for stent overlap because of the presence of LL. The outcome for overlapping stents in the Resolute All-Comers trial was equivalent between third-generation ZESs and second-generation EESs (7).

In a small retrospective multicenter analysis, heterogeneous stent overlap (indicating the overlapping of different stent types), when used in LLs, was found to be associated with similar safety and efficacy outcomes. Second-generation stent overlap was similarly found to be safe and effective (80).

"Full-Metal Jacket" and Very Long Lesions (>60 mm)

In a small study, very long SES stent lengths were studied. Mean stent length was 61 mm, with an average of 2.7 SESs per lesion. The results were somewhat encouraging, with TLR of 4.2% and death of 2.1% at 320 days. Interestingly, no documented stent thrombosis was reported (81). The "full-metal jacket" strategy with DESs was studied in another trial, with a maximum continuous stent length of 78 mm. TLR was high at 23.4%, with cardiac death at 3.6%. Stent thrombosis was equally elevated at 2.6%—of the 17 cases, 5 were acute, 2 subacute, 6 late, and 4 very late (82).

Long-term outcomes of "full-metal jacket" stenting were investigated in a retrospective study with 357 patients. The follow-up was 8 years, and 90.5% of the patients were alive at the end of the observation period. Stent thrombosis occurred in 12 patients. LV dysfunction, stent length >80 mm were major predictors of MACE (83).

These trials suggest that further improvements in stent technology and adjunctive pharmacology are needed to address very LLs ("full-metal jacket") that very frequently may involve chronic total occlusions.

IVUS, OCT, and DESs in Long Lesions

In a recent randomized, multicenter study with second-generation EESs and DESs, the use of IVUS (IVUS-XPL) resulted in lower risk of ischemia-driven TLR (HR, 0.51, 95% CI 0.28–0.91). Death and TLR-related MI were not significantly different. While this study primarily focused on LLs, the mean vessel size was small: 2.85 in the angiography group and 2.89 in the IVUS-guided PCI group. The stented length was 39.2 mm and 39.3 mm, respectively (84).

Stent Thrombosis and Long Lesions

Risk factors for stent thrombosis appear to differ according to the time of stent thrombosis occurrence. In a comprehensive 5-year analysis of the j-Cypher registry, with an average stent length per lesion of 30 mm, early and late stent thromboses were not associated with stent lengths >28 mm. Nevertheless, stent length was a risk factor for very-late stent thrombosis (HR 1.58, CI 1.04–2.41, p = 0.03). Importantly, stent thrombosis occurred without attenuation up to 5 years after SES implantation at a rate of 0.26% per annum (52).

Whether second-generation stents improve very-late stent thrombosis was reported in the Bern-Rotterdam Cohort Study. Average stent lengths were for EES 33 mm, SES 34 mm, and PES 39 mm. During a 4-year follow-up, EES had the lowest incidence rate of definite stent thrombosis (1.4 incidence rate/100 patient-years). Stent thrombosis rates were statistically significantly higher for SESs (2.9) and highest for PESs (4.4 incidence rate/patient-years). The lower rates of stent thrombosis with EESs were most evident beyond the first year and were associated with lower cardiac death and MI when compared with PESs (HR: 0.65, 95% CI 0.56–0.75, p < 0.0001) (85).

EES stent thrombosis is associated with increased stent length. Per each 10 mm length, the HR was increased by 1.30 (95% CI 1.16–1.47, p < 0.001) (57).

Intensive antiplatelet inhibition with prasugrel compared with clopidogrel has been shown to significantly reduce stent thrombosis with both BMSs (1.27% vs. 2.41%) and DESs (0.84% vs. 2.31%). These findings hold true for both LLs >20 mm and those ≥20 mm (risk reduction of 53% and 52%, respectively) (59).

Similarly, patients with a planned interventional strategy in the PLATO trial who received ticagrelor compared with clopidogrel had lower definite stent thrombosis rates (1.3% vs. 2.0%; HR 0.64; 95% CI 0.46–0.88, p = 0.0054) (60). Therefore, it appears that newer stent platforms and more intense antiplatelet medications significantly reduce the rates of stent thrombosis in long vessels. Long-vessel PCI remains a risk factor for very-late stent thrombosis.

Bioabsorbable Stents in LL

Because the longest BVS available in the US was 28 mm long, treatment of LL required overlapping stents. The impact of overlapping BVSs was retrospectively studied in a large European registry (GHOST-EU). Among 1,477 patients, 320 (21.7%) had overlapping BVS placed with a total scaffold length of 61.2 ± 26.8 mm. Imaging was used more frequently in the overlapping BVS group (e.g., IVUS 32% and OCT 26% vs. 10% and 10%, respectively, in the no-overlap group). Stent thrombosis was similar between the groups (1-year overlap 1.9% vs. no-overlap 2.1%, p = 1.0). The 1-year patient-oriented composite endpoints (death, MI, revascularization) were similar (18.4% overlap vs. 18.2% non-overlap, p = 636) (86).

Conclusions

The majority of contemporary PCIs are performed in SVs and/or LLs underscoring the large clinical and economic impact. Second- and third-generation DESs have improved TLR and MACE compared with PTCA and BMS. Current rates of stent thrombosis appear to be decreasing, likely as a result of improved DES technology and newer antiplatelet drugs. MACE and TLR in small and long vessels remain higher than in large vessels; addressing this issue will require further technologic and pharmacologic advances. Outcomes in SVs and/or LLs with BVS, bioabsorbable polymer stents, and drug-coated balloons (not approved in US) will require further research.

Key Points

BMSs in SVs

■ MACE and TLR are reduced with BMSs.

■ PTCA and BMSs have similar death and MI rates.

Specific Considerations

■ Thin-strut stents are preferred.

■ The IVUS-guided approach may improve TLR.

■ Rotablation and cutting balloons are safe but do not reduce restenosis/MACE.

■ Cilostazol may further reduce restenosis.

DESs versus BMSs

■ DESs presented a major breakthrough in the search to prevent high restenosis and MACE rates encountered in SV PCI.

■ DESs and the modification of vascular biology provided indispensable evolutionary progress in the treatment of SV disease. Most DES platforms had initially been tested in large vessels, but various sub-studies subsequently focused on SV disease.

DESs in SVs

■ DESs are superior to BMSs.

■ DESs reduce MACE and TLR.

■ Second- and third-generation DESs improve outcomes compared with first-generation DESs.

■ Second-generation DESs have lower stent thrombosis compared with first-generation DESs.

Specific Considerations

■ Thin-strut stents are generally preferred.

■ Cilostazol may further reduce restenosis.

■ Antiproliferative drugs, polymers, and stent design all influence outcomes.

Diffuse Disease and LLs

■ BMS restenosis rates in LLs are excessively high.

■ DESs are superior to BMSs in LL.

■ LLs are risk factors for stent thrombosis.

■ Overlapping DESs may be associated with worse outcomes.

■ Second-generation DESs lower restenosis, MACE, and stent thrombosis compared with first-generation DESs.

■ "Full-metal jacket" PCI is associated with high MACE.

■ BVS and bioabsorbable polymer stents require further study in SV and LL.

References

1. Saucedo JF, et al. Relation of coronary artery size to one-year clinical events after new device angioplasty of native coronary arteries (a New Approach to Coronary Intervention [NACI] Registry Report). *Am J Cardiol.* 2000;85(2):166–171.

2. Schunkert H, Harrell L, Palacios IF. Implications of small reference vessel diameter in patients undergoing percutaneous coronary revascularization. *J Am Coll Cardiol.* 1999;34(1):40–48.

3. Akiyama T, et al. Angiographic and clinical outcome following coronary stenting of small vessels: a comparison with coronary stenting of large vessels. *J Am Coll Cardiol.* 1998;32(6):1610–1618.

4. Hausleiter J, et al. Predictive factors for early cardiac events and angiographic restenosis after coronary stent placement in small coronary arteries. *J Am Coll Cardiol.* 2002;40(5):882–889.

5. O'Connor NJ, et al. Effect of coronary artery diameter in patients undergoing coronary bypass surgery. Northern New England Cardiovascular Disease Study Group. *Circulation.* 1996;93(4):652–655.

6. Lau KW, Hung JS, Sigwart U. The current status of stent placement in small coronary arteries < 3.0 mm in diameter. *J Invasive Cardiol.* 2004;16(8):411–416.

7. Serruys PW, et al. Comparison of zotarolimus-eluting and everolimus-eluting coronary stents. *N Engl J Med.* 2010;363(2):136–146.

8. Windecker S, et al. Biolimus-eluting stent with biodegradable polymer versus sirolimus-eluting stent with durable polymer for coronary revascularisation (LEADERS): a randomised non-inferiority trial. *Lancet.* 2008;372(9644):1163–1173.

9. Cannon LA, et al. The XIENCE nano everolimus eluting coronary stent system for the treatment of small coronary arteries: the SPIRIT Small Vessel trial. *Catheter Cardiovasc Interv.* 2012;80(4):546–553.

10. Hoffmann R, et al. Intimal hyperplasia thickness at follow-up is independent of stent size: a serial intravascular ultrasound study. *Am J Cardiol.* 1998;82(10):1168–1172.

11. Mauri L, Orav EJ, Kuntz RE. Late loss in lumen diameter and binary restenosis for drug-eluting stent comparison. *Circulation.* 2005;111(25):3435–3442.

12. Pocock SJ, et al. Angiographic surrogate end points in drug-eluting stent trials: a systematic evaluation based on individual patient data from 11 randomized, controlled trials. *J Am Coll Cardiol.* 2008;51(1):23–32.

13. Kastrati A, et al. A randomized trial comparing stenting with balloon angioplasty in small vessels in patients with symptomatic coronary artery disease. ISAR-SMART Study Investigators. Intracoronary stenting or angioplasty for restenosis reduction in small arteries. *Circulation.* 2000;102(21):2593–2598.

14. Koning R, et al. Stent placement compared with balloon angioplasty for small coronary arteries: in-hospital and 6-month clinical and angiographic results. *Circulation.* 2001;104(14):1604–1608.

15. Doucet S, et al. Stent placement to prevent restenosis after angioplasty in small coronary arteries. *Circulation.* 2001;104(17):2029–2033.

16. Moer R, et al. Stenting in small coronary arteries (SISCA) trial. A randomized comparison between balloon angioplasty and the heparin-coated beStent. *J Am Coll Cardiol.* 2001;38(6):1598–1603.

17. Park SW, et al. Randomized comparison of coronary stenting with optimal balloon angioplasty for treatment of lesions in small coronary arteries. *Eur Heart J.* 2000;21(21):1785–1789.

18. Agostoni P, et al. Is bare-metal stenting superior to balloon angioplasty for small vessel coronary artery disease? Evidence from a meta-analysis of randomized trials. *Eur Heart J.* 2005;26(9):881–889.

19. Moreno R, et al. Coronary stenting versus balloon angioplasty in small vessels: a meta-analysis from 11 randomized studies. *J Am Coll Cardiol.* 2004;43(11):1964–1972.

20. Pache J, et al. Intracoronary stenting and angiographic results: strut thickness effect on restenosis outcome (ISAR-STEREO-2) trial. *J Am Coll Cardiol.* 2003;41(8):1283–1288.

21. Briguori C, et al. In-stent restenosis in small coronary arteries: impact of strut thickness. *J Am Coll Cardiol.* 2002;40(3):403–409.

22. Pache J, et al. Drug-eluting stents compared with thin-strut bare stents for the reduction of restenosis: a prospective, randomized trial. *Eur Heart J.* 2005;26(13):1262–1268.

23. Haude M, et al. Heparin-coated stent placement for the treatment of stenoses in small coronary arteries of symptomatic patients. *Circulation.* 2003;107(9):1265–1270.

24. Douglas JS Jr, et al. Coronary stent restenosis in patients treated with cilostazol. *Circulation.* 2005;112(18):2826–2832.

25. Iakovou I, et al. Optimal final lumen area and predictors of target lesion revascularization after stent implantation in small coronary arteries. *Am J Cardiol.* 2003;92(10):1171–1176.

26. Cutlip DE, et al. Stent thrombosis in the modern era: a pooled analysis of multicenter coronary stent clinical trials. *Circulation.* 2001;103(15):1967–1971.

27. Kuntz RE, et al. Generalized model of restenosis after conventional balloon angioplasty, stenting and directional atherectomy. *J Am Coll Cardiol.* 1993;21(1):15–25.

28. Bittl JA, et al. Meta-analysis of randomized trials of percutaneous transluminal coronary angioplasty versus atherectomy, cutting balloon atherotomy, or laser angioplasty. *J Am Coll Cardiol.* 2004;43(6):936–942.

29. Mauri L, et al. Comparison of rotational atherectomy with conventional balloon angioplasty in the prevention of restenosis of small coronary arteries: results of the Dilatation vs Ablation Revascularization Trial Targeting Restenosis (DART). *Am Heart J.* 2003;145(5):847–854.

30. Mauri L, et al. Cutting balloon angioplasty for the prevention of restenosis: results of the cutting balloon global randomized trial. *Am J Cardiol.* 2002;90(10):1079–1083.

31. Boden WE, et al. Optimal medical therapy with or without PCI for stable coronary disease. *N Engl J Med.* 2007;356(15):1503–1516.

32. Moses JW, et al. Safety and efficacy of the 2.25-mm sirolimus-eluting Bx Velocity stent in the treatment of patients with de novo native coronary artery lesions: the SIRIUS 2.25 trial. *Am J Cardiol.* 2006;98(11):1455–1460.

33. Ardissino D, et al. Sirolimus-eluting vs uncoated stents for prevention of restenosis in small coronary arteries: a randomized trial. *JAMA.* 2004;292(22):2727–2734.

34. Stone GW, et al. Comparison of a polymer-based paclitaxel-eluting stent with a bare metal stent in patients with complex coronary artery disease. *JAMA.* 2005;294(10):1215–1223.

35. Togni M, et al. Impact of vessel size on outcome after implantation of sirolimus-eluting and paclitaxel-eluting stents: a subgroup analysis of the SIRTAX trial. *J Am Coll Cardiol.* 2007;50(12):1123–1131.

36. Siontis GC, et al. Percutaneous coronary interventions for the treatment of stenoses in small coronary arteries: a network meta-analysis. *JACC Cardiovasc Interv.* 2016;9(13):1324–1334.

37. Stone GW, et al. Everolimus-eluting versus paclitaxel-eluting stents in coronary artery disease. *N Engl J Med.* 2010;362(18):1663–1674.

38. Claessen BE, et al. Impact of lesion length and vessel size on clinical outcomes after percutaneous coronary intervention with everolimus- versus paclitaxel-eluting stents pooled analysis from the SPIRIT (clinical evaluation of the XIENCE V everolimus eluting coronary stent system) and COMPARE (second-generation everolimus-eluting and paclitaxel-eluting stents in real-life practice) randomized trials. *JACC Cardiovasc Interv.* 2011;4(11):1209–1215.

39. Bartorelli AL, et al. An everolimus-eluting stent versus a paclitaxel-eluting stent in small vessel coronary artery disease: a pooled analysis from SPIRIT II and SPIRIT III trials. *Catheter Cardiovasc Interv.* 2010;76(1):60–66.

40. Kitabata H, et al. Comparison of long-term outcomes between everolimus-eluting and sirolimus-eluting stents in small vessels. *Am J Cardiol.* 2013;111(7):973–978.

41. Leon MB, et al. A randomized comparison of the ENDEAVOR zotarolimus-eluting stent versus the TAXUS paclitaxel-eluting stent in de novo native coronary lesions 12-month outcomes from the ENDEAVOR IV trial. *J Am Coll Cardiol.* 2010;55(6):543–554.

42. Yeung AC, et al. Clinical evaluation of the Resolute zotarolimus-eluting coronary stent system in the treatment of de novo lesions in native coronary arteries: the RESOLUTE US clinical trial. *J Am Coll Cardiol.* 2011;57(17):1778–1783.

43. Turco MA, et al. Reduced risk of restenosis in small vessels and reduced risk of myocardial infarction in long lesions with the new thin-strut TAXUS Liberte stent: 1-year results from the TAXUS ATLAS program. *JACC Cardiovasc Interv.* 2008;1(6):699–709.

44. Cannon LA, et al. A prospective evaluation of the safety and efficacy of TAXUS Element paclitaxel-eluting coronary stent implantation for the treatment of de novo coronary artery lesions in small vessels: the PERSEUS Small Vessel trial. *EuroIntervention.* 2011;6(8):920–927, 1–2.

45. Kereiakes DJ, et al. Efficacy and safety of a novel bioabsorbable polymer-coated, everolimus-eluting coronary stent: the EVOLVE II randomized trial. *Circ Cardiovasc Interv.* 2015;8(4). pii: e002372.

46. von Birgelen C, et al. Very thin strut biodegradable polymer everolimus-eluting and sirolimus-eluting stents versus durable polymer zotarolimus-eluting stents in allcomers with coronary artery disease (BIO-RESORT): a three-arm, randomised, non-inferiority trial. *Lancet.* 2016;388(10060):2607–2617.

47. Parikh SV, et al. Outcomes of small coronary artery stenting with bare-metal stents vs. drug-eluting stents: results from the NHLBI dynamic registry. *Catheter Cardiovasc Interv.* 2014;83(2):192–200.

48. Lee SW, et al. Drug-eluting stenting followed by cilostazol treatment reduces late restenosis in patients with diabetes mellitus the DECLARE-DIABETES trial (a randomized comparison of triple antiplatelet therapy with dual antiplatelet therapy after drug-eluting stent implantation in diabetic patients). *J Am Coll Cardiol.* 2008;51(12):1181–1187.

49. Baran KW, et al. A clinical risk score for prediction of stent thrombosis. *Am J Cardiol.* 2008;102(5):541–545.

50. Holmes DR Jr, et al. Thrombosis and drug-eluting stents: an objective appraisal. *J Am Coll Cardiol.* 2007;50(2):109–118.

51. Iakovou I, et al. Incidence, predictors, and outcome of thrombosis after successful implantation of drug-eluting stents. *JAMA.* 2005;293(17):2126–2130.

52. Kimura T, et al. Very late stent thrombosis and late target lesion revascularization after sirolimus-eluting stent implantation: five-year outcome of the j-Cypher registry. *Circulation.* 2012;125(4):584–591.

53. Okabe T, et al. Intravascular ultrasound parameters associated with stent thrombosis after drug-eluting stent deployment. *Am J Cardiol.* 2007;100(4):615–620.

54. Cortese B, et al. Drug-eluting stents perform better than bare metal stents in small coronary vessels: a meta-analysis of randomised and observational clinical studies with mid-term follow up. *Int J Cardiol.* 2012;161(2):73–82.

55. Biondi-Zoccai GG, et al. Validation of predictors of intraprocedural stent thrombosis in the drug-eluting stent era. *Am J Cardiol.* 2005;95(12):1466–1468.

56. Daemen J, et al. Early and late coronary stent thrombosis of sirolimus-eluting and paclitaxel-eluting stents in routine clinical practice: data from a large two-institutional cohort study. *Lancet.* 2007;369(9562):667–678.

57. Naidu SS, et al. Contemporary incidence and predictors of stent thrombosis and other major adverse cardiac events in the year after XIENCE V implantation: results from the 8,061-patient XIENCE V United States study. *JACC Cardiovasc Interv.* 2012;5(6):626–635.

58. Ito H, et al. Performance of everolimus-eluting versus paclitaxel-eluting coronary stents in small vessels: results from the SPIRIT III and SPIRIT IV clinical trials. *J Interv Cardiol.* 2011;24(6):505–513.

59. Wiviott SD, et al. Intensive oral antiplatelet therapy for reduction of ischaemic events including stent thrombosis in patients with acute coronary syndromes treated with percutaneous coronary intervention and stenting in the TRITON-TIMI 38 trial: a subanalysis of a randomised trial. *Lancet.* 2008;371(9621):1353–1363.

60. Cannon CP, et al. Comparison of ticagrelor with clopidogrel in patients with a planned invasive strategy for acute coronary syndromes (PLATO): a randomised double-blind study. *Lancet.* 2010;375(9711):283–293.

61. Ellis SG, et al. Relationship between angiographic late loss and target lesion revascularization after coronary stent implantation: analysis from the TAXUS-IV trial. *J Am Coll Cardiol.* 2005;45(8):1193–1200.

62. Diletti R, et al. Clinical and intravascular imaging outcomes at 1 and 2 years after implantation of absorb everolimus eluting bioresorbable vascular scaffolds in small vessels. Late lumen enlargement: does bioresorption matter with small vessel size? Insight from the ABSORB cohort B trial. *Heart.* 2013;99(2):98–105.

63. Ellis SG, et al. Everolimus-eluting bioresorbable scaffolds for coronary artery disease. *N Engl J Med.* 2015;373(20):1905–1915.

64. Latini RA, et al. Bioresorbable vascular scaffolds for small vessels coronary disease: the BVS-save registry. *Catheter Cardiovasc Interv.* 2016;88(3):380–387.

65. Puricel S, et al. Bioresorbable coronary scaffold thrombosis: multicenter comprehensive analysis of clinical presentation, mechanisms, and predictors. *J Am Coll Cardiol.* 2016;67(8):921–931.

66. Matsuo Y, et al. Optimal threshold of postintervention minimum stent area to predict in-stent restenosis in small coronary arteries: an optical coherence tomography analysis. *Catheter Cardiovasc Interv.* 2016;87(1):E9–E14.

67. Tonino PA, et al. Fractional flow reserve versus angiography for guiding percutaneous coronary intervention. *N Engl J Med.* 2009;360(3):213–224.

68. Puymirat E, et al. Long-term clinical outcome after fractional flow reserve-guided percutaneous coronary revascularization in patients with small-vessel disease. *Circ Cardiovasc Interv.* 2012;5(1):62–68.

69. Ledru F, et al. New diagnostic criteria for diabetes and coronary artery disease: insights from an angiographic study. *J Am Coll Cardiol.* 2001;37(6):1543–1550.

70. Ryan TJ, et al. Guidelines for percutaneous transluminal coronary angioplasty. A report of the American College of Cardiology/American Heart Association Task Force on Assessment of Diagnostic and Therapeutic Cardiovascular Procedures (Subcommittee on Percutaneous Transluminal Coronary Angioplasty). *Circulation.* 1988;78(2):486–502.

71. Sianos G, et al. The SYNTAX Score: an angiographic tool grading the complexity of coronary artery disease. *EuroIntervention.* 2005;1(2):219–227.

72. Kobayashi Y, et al. Stented segment length as an independent predictor of restenosis. *J Am Coll Cardiol.* 1999;34(3):651–659.

73. Mauri L, et al. Effects of stent length and lesion length on coronary restenosis. *Am J Cardiol.* 2004;93(11):1340–1346, A5.

74. Grube E, et al. TAXUS VI final 5-year results: a multicentre, randomised trial comparing polymer-based moderate-release paclitaxel-eluting stent with a bare metal stent for treatment of long, complex coronary artery lesions. *EuroIntervention.* 2009;4(5):572–577.

75. Schofer J, et al. Sirolimus-eluting stents for treatment of patients with long atherosclerotic lesions in small coronary arteries: double-blind, randomised controlled trial (E-SIRIUS). *Lancet.* 2003;362(9390):1093–1099.

76. Kim YH, et al. Sirolimus-eluting stent versus paclitaxel-eluting stent for patients with long coronary artery disease. *Circulation.* 2006;114(20):2148–2153.

77. Bouras G, et al. Clinical outcomes after PCI treatment of very long lesions with the XIENCE V everolimus eluting stent; pooled analysis from the SPIRIT and XIENCE V USA prospective multicenter trials. *Catheter Cardiovasc Interv.* 2017;89(6):984–991.

78. Raber L, et al. Impact of stent overlap on angiographic and long-term clinical outcome in patients undergoing drug-eluting stent implantation. *J Am Coll Cardiol.* 2010;55(12):1178–1188.

79. Kereiakes DJ, et al. Periprocedural and late consequences of overlapping Cypher sirolimus-eluting stents: pooled analysis of five clinical trials. *J Am Coll Cardiol.* 2006;48(1):21–31.

80. Her SH, et al. Long-term clinical outcomes of overlapping heterogeneous drug-eluting stents compared with homogeneous drug-eluting stents. *Heart.* 2011;97(18):1501–1506.

81. Degertekin M, et al. Very long sirolimus-eluting stent implantation for de novo coronary lesions. *Am J Cardiol.* 2004;93(7):826–829.

82. Sharp AS, et al. Long-term follow up on a large cohort of "full-metal jacket" percutaneous coronary intervention procedures. *Circ Cardiovasc Interv.* 2009;2(5):416–422.

83. Lee CW, et al. Long-term (8 year) outcomes and predictors of major adverse cardiac events after full metal jacket drug-eluting stent implantation. *Catheter Cardiovasc Interv.* 2014;84(3):361–365.

84. Hong SJ, et al. Effect of intravascular ultrasound-guided vs angiography-guided everolimus-eluting stent implantation: the IVUS-XPL randomized clinical trial. *JAMA.* 2015;314(20):2155–2163.

85. Raber L, et al. Very late coronary stent thrombosis of a newer generation everolimus-eluting stent compared with early generation drug-eluting stents: a prospective cohort study. *Circulation.* 2012;125(9):1110–1121.

86. Ortega-Paz L, et al. Impact of overlapping on 1-year clinical outcomes in patients undergoing everolimus-eluting bioresorbable scaffolds implantation in routine clinical practice: Insights from the European multicenter GHOST-EU registry. *Catheter Cardiovasc Interv.* 2017;89(5):812–818.

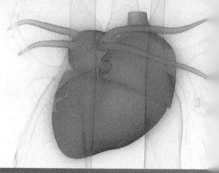

23 Left Mainstem Intervention

Michael S. Lee, MD, MPH, FSCAI, FACC and

Gopi Manthripragada, MD

Guidelines

Advances in the understanding and performance of unprotected left main coronary artery (ULMCA) intervention have allowed interventional cardiologists to perform percutaneous coronary intervention (PCI) in patients who otherwise would undergo coronary artery bypass grafting (CABG). The prevalence of left main coronary disease is approximately 4% of patients undergoing coronary angiography (1). The primary advantage of surgical revascularization is a decreased rate of repeat revascularization with the remainder of clinical endpoints, such as mortality, being equivocal up to 3 years (2–4). This has made ULMCA PCI an attractive option for some patients, particularly those with low- and intermediate-risk coronary anatomy (5), with the optimal strategy being devised by a multidisciplinary team of specialists in concert with patient preference. The 2011 ACCF/AHA/SCAI Guidelines for PCI support percutaneous revascularization in patients with favorable anatomic conditions (isolated ostial and shaft disease, and the absence of multivessel disease), low risk of procedure-related complications, and/or clinical conditions associated with high surgical risk (Class IIA, level of evidence (LOE) B) (Fig. 23.1) (6). The 2014 focused update on the guidelines for stable ischemic heart disease noted that major clinical outcomes in selected patients with ULMCA disease were similar with CABG and PCI at 1- to 2-year follow-up (7).

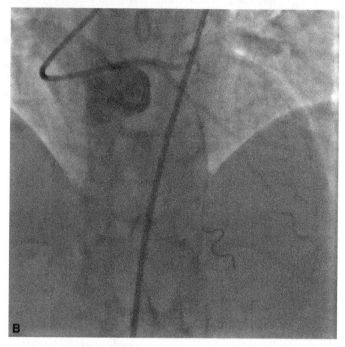

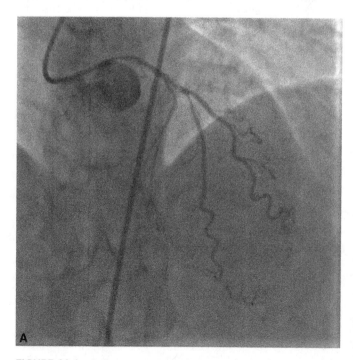

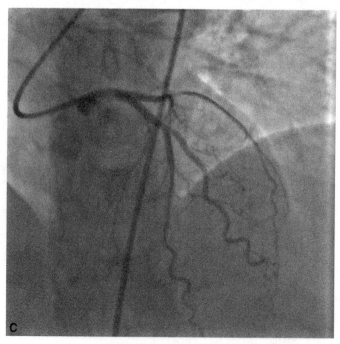

FIGURE 23.1 **A:** A coronary angiogram reveals significant disease at the ostium of the ULMCA. **B:** In the cranial view, the proximal portion of the stent should be positioned such that the stent covers the inferior lip of the left main ostium. **C:** Final angiography demonstrates a satisfactory post-intervention result after stenting of a short left main, left anterior descending, and proximal circumflex coronary arteries. ULMCA, unprotected left main coronary artery.

Pre-procedural Considerations

A comprehensive assessment of clinical and anatomic factors is critical to the success of ULMCA PCI. Low-risk clinical predictors include younger age, preserved left ventricular ejection fraction, normal renal function, and an elective, as opposed to an urgent or emergent, procedure (8). Low-risk anatomical predictors include isolated ostial or shaft disease, lack of severe coronary artery calcification, and the absence of multivessel disease (9). Distal bifurcation lesions are associated with disease within the left anterior descending and circumflex coronary arteries on pathologic and intravascular ultrasound (IVUS) studies (10), and usually require a two-stent strategy. Distal bifurcation disease is associated with significantly higher rates of repeat revascularization and overall major adverse cardiac events (MACE) compared with ostial or shaft lesions (Fig. 23.2) (11,12).

The Synergy between PCI with Taxus and Cardiac Surgery (SYNTAX) Trial was a large, multicenter trial that randomized 1,800 patients with either three-vessel or ULMCA disease to PCI with first-generation paclitaxel-eluting stents or CABG. A heart team, comprised of a cardiac surgeon and an interventional cardiologist, concluded that equivalent anatomic revascularization could be attained with either approach. Pre-procedure characteristics were similar (5). At 1 year, the rate of revascularization was significantly higher in the PCI group (13.5% vs. 5.9%, p <0.001), while the stroke rate was higher in the surgical group (2.2% vs. 0.6%, p = 0.003).

Due to variation in risk based on clinical and anatomic factors, predictive models have been developed to help determine the optimal revascularization strategy that is tailored to a specific patient.

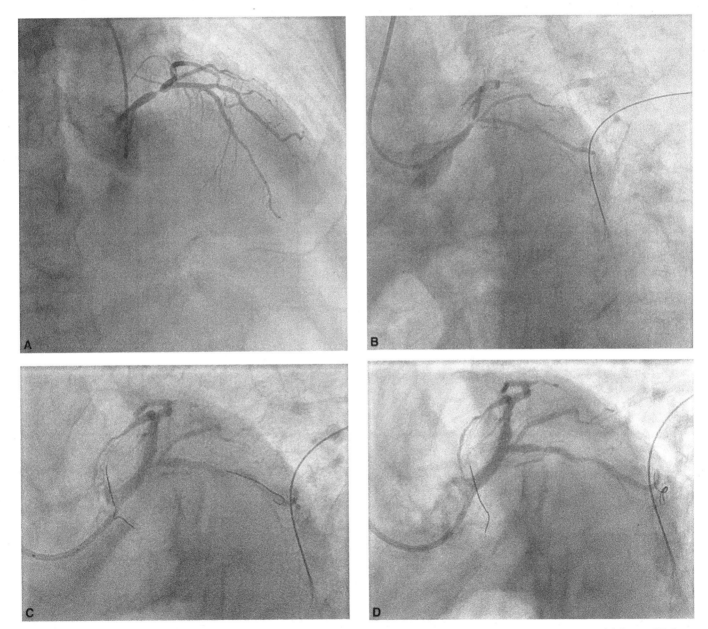

FIGURE 23.2   A: Coronary angiography reveals severe ULMCA disease involving the distal bifurcation in a patient presenting with left main ST elevation myocardial infarction (STEMI). **B:** Distal left main disease in a patient presenting with anterior ST elevation, with a LAO caudal view demonstrating involvement of the ostial left anterior descending and circumflex coronary arteries, as well as a high rising obtuse marginal branch. **C:** Stenting of the main vessel with residual severe stenosis of the ostial left circumflex. **D:** Final angiography after kissing balloon inflation and proximal optimization technique (POT). LAO, left anterior oblique; ULMCA, unprotected left main coronary artery.

Models include clinical, angiographic, or procedural variables with some including a combination of all three. The SYNTAX score stratifies patients into tertiles of low, medium, and high risk based on an angiographic score (13). Outcomes between CABG and PCI in ULMCA disease for low- (SYNTAX score 0–22) and medium- (23–32) risk patients show clinical equipoise, while outcomes in high-risk (>32) patients favored CABG (13,14). Major adverse cardiovascular events (MACE) rates increase with the number of vessels intervened upon during PCI, with the most recent guidelines giving ULMCA PCI in intermediate-risk-score patients a IIA indication (6).

In the Premier of Randomized Comparison of Bypass Surgery Versus Angioplasty Using Sirolimus-Eluting Stent in Patients With Left Main Coronary Artery Disease (PRECOMBAT) trial of 600 patients with ULMCA disease, the composite endpoint of death, myocardial infarction (MI), or stroke at 2 years was similar in patients treated with drug-eluting stents (DESs) compared with CABG (4.4% vs. 4.7%, p = 0.83). As has been demonstrated in other trials, ischemia-driven target vessel revascularization was required more often in the patients treated with PCI (9.0% vs. 4.2%, p = 0.02) (15). At 5-year follow-up, equipoise in the composite endpoint persisted (8.4% vs. 9.6%, p = 0.66), while ischemia-driven target vessel revascularization continued to occur more frequently in the PCI group (11.4% vs. 5.5%, p = 0.012) (16).

In the Everolimus-Eluting Stents or Bypass Surgery for Left Main Coronary Artery Disease (EXCEL) trial, 1,905 patients with SYNTAX scores ≤32, the composite endpoint of death, MI, or stroke at 3 years occurred in 15.4% of patients treated with PCI and 14.7% of patients in the CABG group (p = 0.02 for non-inferiority, p = 0.98 for superiority) (17). The secondary endpoint of death, stroke, MI, or ischemia-driven revascularization at 3 years occurred in 23.1% of the PCI group and 19.1% in the CABG group (p = 0.01 for non-inferiority, p = 0.10 for superiority).

Procedural Strategies and Techniques

Candidacy for dual antiplatelet therapy (DAPT) is imperative in those being considered for ULMCA PCI. Because target lesion revascularization is the most common adverse outcome of ULMCA PCI when compared with CABG, DES should be the default stent choice (18,19). Exceptions to this tenet are increased bleeding risk, large left main diameter (≥5 mm), or impending surgery, with studies showing favorable comparisons of bare-metal stents (BMSs) to CABG (20). In the absence of large clinical trials addressing ideal duration of DAPT after ULMCA PCI, both aspirin and a $P2Y_{12}$ inhibitor should be continued for at least 1-year after PCI, as long as there are no contraindications. Clinical trials suggest equipoise regarding the choice of DESs (21,22). Clinical features that might merit consideration for advanced hemodynamic support include left ventricular dysfunction (ejection fraction <25%), hemodynamic or arrhythmic instability (Fig. 23.3), occlusion of a dominant right or left circumflex coronary artery, or the need for atherectomy (Fig. 23.3) (7).

Lesion assessment by angiography alone is frequently insufficient, with IVUS and fractional flow reserve (FFR) each providing imperative information (**Table 23.1**) (23,24). FFR values ≥0.80 have been associated with similar outcomes between CABG and medical therapy, and as such, intervention may safely be deferred. Minimal luminal area (MLA) on IVUS less than 6 mm^2, and in some studies <4.8 mm^2, suggests significant ULMCA disease and remains a valuable adjunctive tool to FFR and angiography (24),

and is of particular importance post-procedure following distal left main bifurcation stenting.

Distal bifurcation disease accounts for two-thirds of ULMCA lesions, and is associated with a higher risk of target lesion revascularization due to frequent restenosis at the ostium of the left circumflex coronary artery. The provisional stenting approach is the preferred approach in bifurcation disease, and FFR of the non-stented vessel can guide the need for a second stent (25,26). When a two-stent strategy is required, the T and protrusion (TAP) technique, simultaneous kissing stents, crush technique, and culotte technique are reasonable options to treat distal bifurcation disease with choice of technique based on the angle of the bifurcation, size of the side branch vessel, and operator experience. The proximal optimization technique (POT) involving postdilation of the main-vessel stent is recommended.

IVUS of the ULMCA is informative pre-procedure, providing data on plaque burden, morphology, and vessel size, and is critical post-procedure in evaluating stent expansion, ostial coverage, and assessment of the ostium of the left circumflex artery if a two-stent strategy is utilized (24). IVUS can also be used to assess the MLA of the left circumflex artery and determine whether subsequent intervention is needed. Approximately 30% of ULMCA lesions are ostial or mid-shaft lesions and portend a favorable outcome. Adequate coverage of the ostium without unnecessary protrusion of stent struts into the aorta is preferable because significant protrusion would make repeat selective engagement of the LMCA challenging (27). Shallow left anterior oblique (LAO), LAO cranial, or anteroposterior (AP) cranial views allow the delineation of the superior and inferior lip of the left main ostium and ensure adequate ostial coverage (**Fig. 23.4**) (7).

The use of biodegradable polymer stents in ULMCA PCI is not recommended at this time, based on the results of the percutaneous coronary angioplasty versus CABG in treatment of unprotected left main stenosis (NOBLE) trial, which randomized 1,182 patients to either CABG or Biolimus DES (28). The primary outcome composite of death, MI, stroke, and repeat revascularization was 28.9% for the PCI arm versus 19.1% for the CABG arm (p = 0.0066), with significant differences in non-procedural MI and repeat revascularization.

Post-Revascularization Issues and Follow-up

Elective angiography after ULMCA PCI without a change in clinical status may lead to unnecessary revascularization and has not been shown to be of benefit (29). Routine angiography in this setting has been ascribed a Class III indication (contraindicated) in the most recent clinical guidelines (6). The incidence of in-stent restenosis following ULMCA PCI with DES is approximately 10% at 2 years (16). Non-invasive assessment of ischemia at 6 months and annually thereafter is a reasonable approach, barring recurrence of anginal symptoms (7). Computed tomography coronary angiography may be of benefit, particularly with larger-diameter stents, but may be of limited use with narrower diameter or multiple stents due to artifact (30). Intermediate angiographic restenosis should be evaluated with FFR, and if significant, the mechanism (incomplete stent expansion or lesion coverage) should be assessed with IVUS (31) prior to intervention. Treatment modalities include angioplasty alone, alternate DES placement, or CABG. In patients undergoing repeat revascularization with either PCI or CABG, observational studies have demonstrated very low rates of MACE compared with medical therapy alone (16).

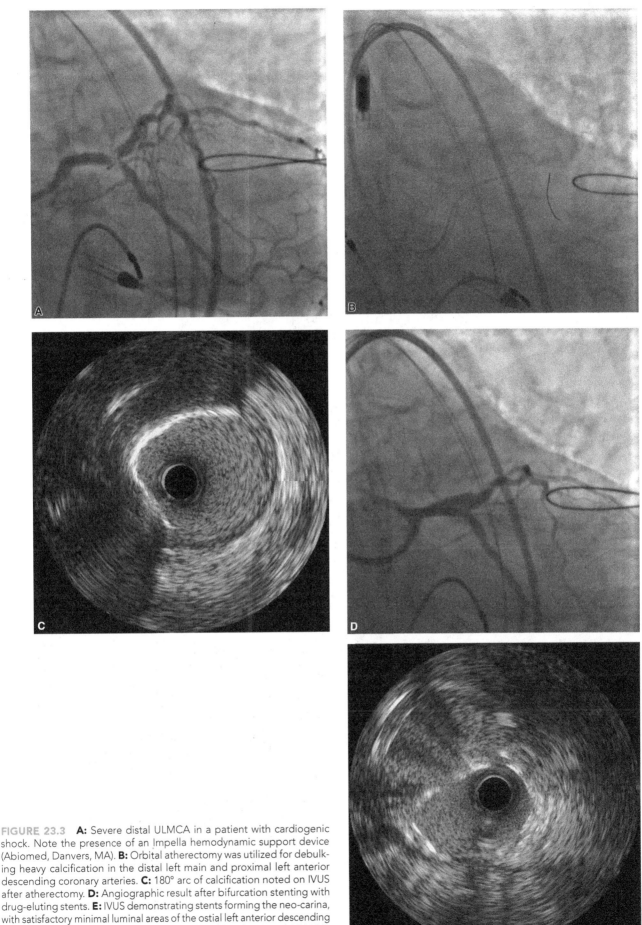

FIGURE 23.3 **A:** Severe distal ULMCA in a patient with cardiogenic shock. Note the presence of an Impella hemodynamic support device (Abiomed, Danvers, MA). **B:** Orbital atherectomy was utilized for debulking heavy calcification in the distal left main and proximal left anterior descending coronary arteries. **C:** 180° arc of calcification noted on IVUS after atherectomy. **D:** Angiographic result after bifurcation stenting with drug-eluting stents. **E:** IVUS demonstrating stents forming the neo-carina, with satisfactory minimal luminal areas of the ostial left anterior descending and circumflex coronary arteries. IVUS, intravascular ultrasound; ULMCA, unprotected left main coronary artery.

TABLE 23.1 Comparison between IVUS and FFR for Assessment of ULMCA Disease

	IVUS	FFR
Type of lesion assessment	Anatomic	Hemodynamic
Abnormal value	MLA <6.0 mm^2	<0.80
Characterization of plaque morphology	Yes	No
Characterization of plaque distribution	Yes	No
Stent diameter and length sizing	Yes	No
Post-PCI stent expansion	Yes	No
Post-PCI stent apposition	Yes	No
Post-PCI side-branch compromise	Yes	Yes
Post-PCI dissection	Yes	No

FFR, fractional flow reserve; IVUS, intravascular ultrasound; MLA, minimal luminal area; PCI, percutaneous coronary intervention; ULMCA, unprotected left main coronary artery.

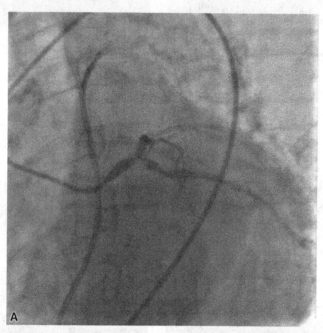

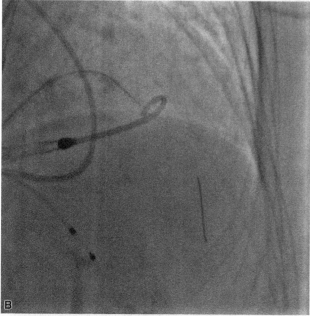

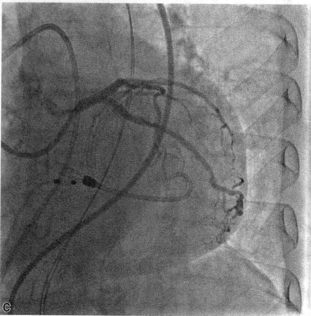

FIGURE 23.4   A: Coronary angiography reveals a significant distal ULMCA stenosis. **B:** Orbital atherectomy being performed with hemodynamic support (*black arrow*). **C:** Final angiography demonstrates excellent results. ULMCA, unprotected left main coronary artery

Summary

ULMCA PCI is a viable revascularization strategy for a significant subset of patients with ULMCA disease. The EXCEL and NOBLE trials yielded differing results with respect to non-inferiority of ULMCA PCI to CABG, and reiterated the need for a multidisciplinary heart team guiding the patient in decision making (IC Recommendation). Liberal use of FFR in diagnosing indeterminate ULMCA disease, and IVUS in executing planning and post-stent optimization are imperative.

Key Points

- ULMCA PCI is a reasonable alternative to CABG in low-risk patients (SYNTAX scores ≤22) or in those with prohibitive surgical risk (≥5% based on STS scores [IIA, LOE B]).

- ULMCA PCI may also be reasonable in intermediate risk patients (SYNTAX ≤32) as determined by the heart team.

- ULMCA PCI is reasonable in UA/NSTEMI if the patient is not a surgical candidate.

- Ostial and shaft lesions in the absence of multivessel disease may be percutaneously intervened upon (IIA, LOE B).

- The SYNTAX score (http://www.syntaxscore.com) is a useful tool that helps differentiate between low, intermediate, and high-risk patients on the basis of anatomic features, with the latter deriving the highest benefit from CABG.

- DES should be used for ULMCA PCI whenever possible, with longer-term DAPT (at least 1 year).

- A single-stent provisional strategy should be the default approach to bifurcation lesions, with care taken to optimize the ostium of the left circumflex because it is the most frequent restenotic site.

- When treating ostial LM stenoses, LAO or AP cranial views are helpful in determining stent positioning and avoiding unnecessary protrusion of struts in the aorta.

- FFR and IVUS are critical in assessing indeterminate LM stenoses, and to obtaining a satisfactory result when stenting is performed. FFR can help guide the need for a second stent in distal left main PCI.

- Routine angiography after ULMCA PCI is contraindicated.

- Restenosis may be addressed with either repeat PCI or CABG, with low MACE rates when compared with medical therapy.

References

1. Ragosta M, et al. Prevalence of unfavorable angiographic characteristics for percutaneous intervention in patients with unprotected left main coronary artery disease. *Catheter Cardiovasc Interv.* 2006;68:357–362.
2. Caracciolo EA, et al. Comparison of surgical and medical group survival in patients with left main equivalent coronary artery disease. Long-term CASS experience. *Circulation.* 1995;91(9):2335–2344.
3. Javaid A, et al. Outcomes of coronary artery bypass grafting versus percutaneous coronary intervention with drug-eluting stents for patients with multi-vessel coronary artery disease. *Circulation.* 2007;116(suppl):I200–I206.
4. Park DW, et al. Long-term mortality after percutaneous coronary intervention with drug-eluting stent implantation versus coronary artery bypass surgery for the treatment of multivessel coronary artery disease. *Circulation.* 2008;117:2079–2086.
5. Serruys PW, et al. Percutaneous coronary intervention versus coronary-artery bypass grafting for severe coronary artery disease. *N Engl J Med.* 2009;360:961–972.
6. Levine GN, et al. 2011 ACCF/AHA/SCAI guideline for percutaneous coronary intervention: a report of the American College of Cardiology Foundation/American Heart Association Task Force on Practice Guidelines and the Society for Cardiovascular Angiography and Interventions. *J Am Coll Cardiol.* 2011;58:e44–e122.
7. Fihn SD, et al. 2014 ACC/AHA/AATS/PCNA/SCAI/STS focused update of the guideline for the diagnosis and management of patients with stable ischemic heart disease. A report of the American College of Cardiology/American Heart Association Task Force on Practice Guidelines, and the American Association for Thoracic Surgery, Preventive Cardiovascular Nurses Association, Society for Cardiovascular Angiography and Interventions, and Society of Thoracic Surgeons. *Circulation.* 2014;130:1749–1767.
8. Lee MS, et al. Percutaneous coronary intervention of unprotected left main coronary artery disease. *Catheter Cardiovasc Interv.* 2012;9(5):812–822.
9. Chieffo A, et al. Favorable long-term outcome after drug-eluting stent implantation in nonbifurcation lesions that involve unprotected left main coronary artery: a multicenter registry. *Circulation.* 2007;116:158–162.
10. Tamburino C, et al. Plaque distribution patterns in distal left main coronary artery to predict outcomes after stent implantation. *JACC Cardiovasc Interv.* 2010;3:624–631.
11. Biondi-Zoccai GG, et al. A collaborative systematic review and meta-analysis on 1,278 patients undergoing percutaneous drug-eluting stenting for unprotected left main coronary artery disease. *Am Heart J.* 2008;155:274–283.
12. Kim YH, et al. Impact of the extent of coronary artery disease on outcomes after revascularization for unprotected left main coronary artery stenosis. *J Am Coll Cardiol.* 2010;55:2544–2552.
13. Morice MC, et al. Outcomes in patients with de novo left main disease treated with either percutaneous coronary intervention using paclitaxel-eluting stents or coronary artery bypass graft treatment in the synergy between percutaneous coronary intervention with TAXUS and cardiac surgery (SYNTAX) trial. *Circulation.* 2010;121:2645–2653.
14. Sianos G, et al. The SYNTAX score: an angiographic tool grading the complexity of coronary artery disease. *EuroIntervention.* 2005;1:219–227.
15. Park SJ, et al. Randomized trial of stents versus bypass surgery for left main coronary artery disease. *N Engl J Med.* 2011;364:1718–1727.
16. Ahn JM, et al. Randomized trial of stents versus bypass surgery for left main coronary artery disease. 5-year outcomes of the PRECOMBAT study. *J Am Coll Cardiol.* 2015;65(20):2198–2206.
17. Stone GW, et al. Everolimus-eluting stents or bypass surgery for left main coronary artery disease. *N Engl J Med.* 2016;375:2223–2235.
18. Kim YH, et al. Revascularization for unprotected left main coronary artery stenosis: comparison of percutaneous coronary angioplasty versus surgical revascularization investigators. Longterm safety and effectiveness of unprotected left main coronary stenting with drug-eluting stents compared with bare-metal stents. *Circulation.* 2009;120:400–407.
19. Buszman PE, et al. Early and long-term results of unprotected left main coronary artery stenting. The LE MANS (left main coronary artery stenting) registry. *J Am Coll Cardiol.* 2009;54:1500–1511.
20. Park DW, et al. Long-term outcomes after stenting versus coronary artery bypass grafting for unprotected left main coronary artery disease: 10-year results of bare-metal stents and 5-year results of drug-eluting stents from the ASAN-MAIN (ASAN Medical Center-Left MAIN Revascularization) registry. *J Am Coll Cardiol.* 2010;56:1366–1375.
21. Lee JY, et al. Long-term clinical outcomes of sirolimus-versus paclitaxel-eluting stents for patients with unprotected left main coronary artery disease. *J Am Coll Cardiol.* 2009;54:853–859.

22. Meliga E, et al. Impact of drug-eluting stent selection on long-term clinical outcomes in patients treated for unprotected left main coronary artery disease: the sirolimus vs paclitaxel drug-eluting stent for left main registry (SPDELFT). *Int J Cardiol.* 2009;137:16–21.

23. Jasti V, et al. Correlations between fractional flow reserve and intravascular ultrasound in patients with ambiguous left main coronary artery stenosis. *Circulation.* 2004;110:2831–2836.

24. Puri R, et al. Optimizing outcomes during left main percutaneous coronary intervention with intravascular ultrasound and fractional flow reserve: the current state of evidence. *JACC Cardiovasc Interv.* 2012;5(7):697–707.

25. Koo BK. Physiologic evaluation of bifurcation lesions using fractional flow reserve. *J Interv Cardiol.* 2009;22:110–113.

26. Palmerini T, et al. Impact of bifurcation technique on 2-year clinical outcomes in 773 patients with distal unprotected left main coronary artery stenosis treated with drug-eluting stents. *Circ Cardiovasc Interv.* 2008;1:185–192.

27. Mehilli J, et al. LEFT-MAIN intracoronary stenting and angiographic results: drug-eluting stents for unprotected coronary left main lesions study investigators. Paclitaxel- versus sirolimus-eluting stents for unprotected left main coronary artery disease. *J Am Coll Cardiol.* 2009;53:1760–1768.

28. Makikallio T, et al. Percutaneous coronary angioplasty versus coronary artery bypass grafting in treatment of unprotected left main stenosis (NOBLE): a prospective, randomized, open-label, non-inferiority trial. *Lancet.* 2016;388:2743–2752.

29. Biondi-Zoccai GG, et al. Impact of routine angiographic follow-up after percutaneous coronary drug-eluting stenting for unprotected left main disease: the Turin registry. *Clin Res Cardiol.* 2010;99:235–242.

30. Gilard M, et al. Noninvasive assessment of left main coronary stent patency with 16-slice computed tomography. *Am J Cardiol.* 2005;95:110–112.

31. Koo BK, et al. Physiologic assessment of jailed side branch lesions using fractional flow reserve. *J Am Coll Cardiol.* 2005;46:633–637.

24

Bypass Graft Intervention and Embolic Protection

Emmanouil S. Brilakis, MD, PhD, FSCAI, FACC, FESC, FAHA, Mario Gössl, MD, FSCAI, Paul Sorajja, MD, FSCAI, FACC, FAHA, and Subhash Banerjee, MD, FSCAI, FACC, FAHA

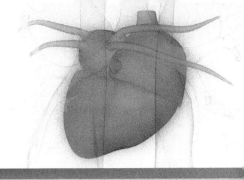

In the National Cardiovascular Data Registry (NCDR) registry, 17.5% of all percutaneous coronary interventions (PCI) are performed in patients with prior coronary artery bypass graft surgery (CABG) (1): 11% are performed in native coronary arteries, 6.1% in saphenous vein grafts (SVGs), 0.4% in arterial grafts, and 0.04% in both arterial grafts and SVGs (1). SVGs have high failure rates: 40% to 50% are occluded 10 years post-CABG (2). With longer time from CABG, proportionately more interventions are required in SVGs, which is consistent with the accelerated atherosclerotic process of these grafts. Intervention in bypass grafts is challenging because of (1) difficulties in graft localization and engagement; (2) high rates of periprocedural myocardial infarction due to distal embolization in SVGs; and (3) high restenosis rates. Prior CABG patients undergoing PCI of a native coronary artery have better outcomes compared with those undergoing bypass graft PCI (1,3), hence PCI of a native coronary artery is preferred over graft PCI if technically feasible.

Percutaneous revascularization is generally preferred over surgical revascularization in patients with prior CABG, given the higher risk of repeat CABG compared with first CABG and comparable post-procedural outcomes (4). Factors favoring repeat CABG include vessels unsuitable for PCI, multiple diseased bypass grafts, availability of the internal mammary artery (IMA) for grafting chronically occluded coronary arteries, and good distal targets for bypass graft placement (5). In contrast, factors favoring PCI over CABG include limited areas of ischemia-causing symptoms, suitable PCI targets, a patent graft to the left anterior descending artery, poor CABG targets, and comorbid conditions (5).

Bypass Graft Anatomy

Knowledge of bypass graft anatomy is critical for optimizing cardiac catheterization and interventions among prior CABG patients: When anatomy is not known, more contrast, fluoroscopy time, and catheters are needed to identify all patent grafts (6). Graft markers are very helpful for engaging bypass grafts, but are not used in most patients.

In patients with unknown CABG anatomy, performance of bilateral subclavian artery angiography can help assess whether one or both IMAs are utilized as grafts, and whether proximal subclavian artery stenosis is present, which could lead to subclavian steal (7). In some patients, aortography is performed, usually in the left anterior oblique projection to assist with graft localization.

Engagement of SVGs for angiography and/or PCI can be performed using either a femoral or radial approach; however, femoral access facilitates the procedure and is associated with lower utilization of contrast and radiation (8). The RADIAL Versus Femoral Access for Coronary Artery Bypass Graft Angiography and Intervention (RADIAL CABG) trial reported that diagnostic coronary angiography via radial access was associated with a higher mean contrast volume (142 ± 39 mL vs. 171 ± 72 mL, p < 0.01), longer procedure time (21.9 ± 6.8 minutes vs. 34.2 ± 14.7 minutes, p < 0.01), greater patient air kerma radiation exposure (1.08 ± 0.54 Gy vs. 1.29 ± 0.67 Gy,

p = 0.06), and higher operator radiation doses (first operator: 1.3 ± 1.0 mrem vs. 2.6 ± 1.7 mrem, p < 0.01), as compared with femoral access (9). When radial access is utilized and graft engagement is challenging, early conversion to femoral access should be considered (10).

If graft intervention is needed, obtaining adequate guide catheter support is critical. This can be accomplished by using larger-sized guide catheters (7 French or 8 French), supportive guide catheter shapes (such as Amplatz), or by employing deep graft intubation—for example, using a guide catheter extension (11). The multipurpose guide is most commonly used for SVGs to the right coronary/posterior descending artery, and the Amplatz left or left coronary bypass (LCB) for left-sided grafts.

Adjunctive Pharmacotherapy

A significant difference between native vessel and SVG PCI is that glycoprotein (GP) IIb/IIIa inhibitors are not beneficial in SVG PCI (12) and may be harmful (13). Hence, GP IIb/IIIa inhibitors should not be used in SVG interventions, with the possible exception of heavily thrombotic lesions, yet they are still frequently used (in 40% of SVG PCI in the US according to the NCDR) (14). The 2011 American College of Cardiology/American Heart Association (ACC/AHA) PCI guidelines state that "platelet GP IIb/IIIa inhibitors are not beneficial as adjunctive therapy during SVG PCI" (Class III, level of evidence B) (5).

Intragraft vasodilators, such as adenosine (15), nitroprusside (16), nicardipine (17), and verapamil (18), might also be useful in preventing no-reflow and periprocedural myocardial infarction during SVG interventions, and are often used due to low cost and risk, but they have not been proven to be effective in randomized-controlled trials.

Choice of Stents in SVGs

Several studies have compared various PCI techniques in SVGs (Table 24.1).

The Saphenous VEin De novo (SAVED) trial compared BMS implantation to balloon angioplasty. Although the study missed its primary angiographic endpoint (6-month binary angiographic restenosis), it demonstrated improved procedural success and lower incidence of the composite endpoint of death, myocardial infarction, and target vessel revascularization at 6 months (19). Similar results were observed in the Venestent trial (20), and stent implantation became the standard of care for the percutaneous treatment of SVG lesions.

Covered stents were subsequently developed and tested in SVGs in an attempt to reduce the rates of distal embolization and periprocedural myocardial infarction. Nevertheless, none of four randomized trials showed a decrease in the incidence of periprocedural myocardial infarction (21–23), and covered stents also had higher risk for subsequent myocardial infarction and thrombotic occlusion (23).

TABLE 24.1 Large Published Trials of Stenting for Saphenous Vein Graft Lesions

AUTHOR	YEAR	N	PRIMARY ENDPOINT	BARE-METAL STENT EVENT RATE (%)	OTHER GROUP EVENT RATE (%)	P
BMSs vs. Balloon Angioplasty						
SAVED (19)	1997	220	6-month angiographic restenosis	37	46	0.24
Venestent (20)	2003	150	6-month angiographic restenosis	19.1	32.8	0.069
BMSs vs. Covered Stents						
RECOVERS (21)	2003	301	6-month angiographic restenosis	24.8	24.2	0.237
STING (22)	2003	211	6-month angiographic restenosis	20	29	0.15
SYMBIOT III (41)	2006	700	8-month angiographic percent diameter stenosis	30.9	31.9	0.80
BARRICADE (23)	2011	243	8-month angiographic restenosis	28.4	31.8	0.63
BMSs vs. DESs						
RRISC	2006 (26)	75	6-month angiographic restenosis	32.6	13.6	0.031
	2007 (27)		MACE at 32 months	41	58	0.13
SOS	2009 (28)	80	12-month angiographic restenosis	51	9	<0.001
	2010 (29)	80	Target vessel failure at 35 months	72	34	0.001
ISAR-CABG (30)	2011	610	12-month composite of death, MI and TLR	22	15	0.02
BASKET-SAVAGE[a]	2016	173	12-month composite of cardiac death, MI, and TVR	17.9	2.3	<0.001
DIVA[b]	2017	597	12-month composite of cardiac death, target vessel MI, and TLR	19%	17%	0.67

[a]Presented at the 2016 European Society of Cardiology meeting.
[b]Presented at the 2017 European Society of Cardiology meeting
BARRICADE, Barrier Approach to Restenosis: Restrict Intima to Curtail Adverse Events Trial; BASKET-SAVAGE, Study to Test the Efficacy and Safety of Drug Eluting vs. Bare-Metal Stents for Saphenous Vein Graft Interventions; BMS, bare metal stent; DES, drug-eluting stent; ISAR-CABG, Is Drug-Eluting-Stenting Associated with Improved Results in Coronary Artery Bypass Grafts? Trial; MACE, major adverse cardiac events; MI, myocardial infarction; RECOVERS, European multicenter Randomized Evaluation of polytetrafluoroethylene COVERed stent in Saphenous vein grafts Trial; RRISC, Reduction of Restenosis In Saphenous vein grafts with Cypher sirolimus-eluting stent Trial; SAVED, Saphenous Vein De Novo Trial; SOS, Stenting Of Saphenous vein grafts Trial; STING, Stents IN Grafts Trial; SYMBIOT III, A Prospective, Randomized Trial of a Self-Expanding PTFE Stent Graft During SVG Intervention; TLR, target lesion revascularization; TVR, target vessel revascularization.

As a result, covered stents are currently used in SVGs only for the treatment of perforations. Newer micro-mesh-coated stents are currently being developed in an effort to prevent distal embolization, but have undergone limited clinical evaluation (24,25).

Whether drug-eluting stents (DESs) provide better outcomes in SVGs has been controversial for several years. Three published and two presented prospective, randomized-controlled trials have compared DES with bare-metal stents (BMS) in SVG lesions (Table 24.1).

The Reduction of Restenosis In Saphenous vein grafts with Cypher sirolimus-eluting stent trial (RRISC) compared a sirolimus-eluting stent (Cypher, Cordis, Warren, NJ) with a BMS of similar design in 75 patients (26,27) and reported lower rates of angiographic restenosis and lower incidence of target lesion revascularization at 6 months. Nevertheless, at during long-term follow-up (median: 32 months), mortality was higher in the SES group (29% vs. 0%, p = 0.001) and there was no reduction with DES in the incidence of target vessel revascularization (27). The RRISC study raised concerns about the long-term safety of DES in SVGs, but these results have not been replicated in subsequent studies, and it is highly unusual for patients undergoing SVG PCI with BMSs to have 0% mortality for nearly 3 years (mortality during the first-year post–SVG PCI is approximately 5% in most series).

The Stenting Of Saphenous Vein Grafts trial (SOS) compared a paclitaxel-eluting stent (PES, Taxus, Boston Scientific, Natick, MA) with a similar BMS in 80 patients and reported angiographic and clinical benefit with DESs during early and long-term follow-up (28,29).

Both the RRISC and SOS trials had a primary angiographic endpoint and were underpowered for clinical events. The "Is Drug-Eluting-Stenting Associated with Improved Results in Coronary Artery Bypass Grafts?" (ISAR-CABG) study is the largest randomized controlled-trial performed to date in SVGs and demonstrated that implantation of first-generation DESs (sirolimus-eluting and paclitaxel-eluting) significantly reduced the incidence of target lesion revascularization (7% vs. 13%, p = 0.01) compared with BMSs, without significant differences in the incidence of all-cause death (5% vs. 5%, p = 0.83), myocardial infarction (5% vs. 6%, p = 0.27), and definite of probable stent thrombosis (1% vs. 1%, p = 0.99) (30). The Basel Kosten Effektivitäts Trial—SAphenous Venous Graft Angioplasty Using GP IIa/IIIb Receptor Inhibitors and Drug-Eluting Stents (**BASKET-SAVAGE**, n = 173) trial (presented at the 2016 European Society of Cardiology meeting) revealed a lower incidence of major adverse cardiac events with the Taxus DES, compared with BMS at 12 months (2.3% vs. 17.9%, p < 0.001) and 3 years (12.4% vs. 29.8%, p = 0.0012), driven mainly by lower target vessel revascularization in the DES group (19.1% vs. 4.5% at 3 years). The Drug-Eluting Stents vs. Bare Metal Stents In Saphenous Vein Graft Angioplasty (DIVA) Trial (presented at the 2017 European Society of Cardiology meeting) showed similar incidence of target vessel failure with DES (88% second generation) and BMS both at 12 months and during long-term follow-up (median 2.7 years). In contrast to ISAR-CABG DIVA used blinding and did not have routine angiographic follow-up.

In summary, mainly based on the results of DIVA, BMS and DES have similar outcomes in de novo SVG lesions, making BMS preferred due to lower cost (5).

Embolic Protection Devices

SVG interventions may be complicated by distal embolization causing periprocedural myocardial infarction and no-reflow. Several strategies, both pharmacologic (GP IIb/IIIa inhibitors and vasodilators) and mechanical (covered stents and embolic protection devices (EPDs)) have been tested in an effort to prevent such complications, yet the only strategy proven to improve outcomes in a large randomized-controlled trial is use of EPDs, (**Fig. 24.1** and **Table 24.2**) (31).

The 2011 ACC/AHA PCI guidelines state that "EPDs should be used during SVG PCI when technically feasible" (class I indication, level of evidence B) (5). This recommendation is based on a single randomized-controlled trial, the Saphenous vein graft Angioplasty Free of Emboli Randomized (SAFER) trial (31), which used a distal occlusion balloon (GuardWire, Medtronic Vascular, Santa Rosa, CA, **Figs. 24.2** and **24.3**). In SAFER, the primary endpoint (a composite of death, myocardial infarction, emergency bypass, or target lesion revascularization by 30 days) was observed in 65 patients (16.5%) assigned to control versus 39 patients (9.6%) assigned to EPD (p = 0.004). This 42% relative reduction in major adverse cardiac

Embolic Protection Devices available in the US for SVG interventions in 2012

Device	Manufacturer	Approval date
Guardwire	Medtronic	6/2001
Filterwire	Boston Scientific	6/2003
Spider	ev3	6/2006

FIGURE 24.1 Embolic protection devices available in the US for SVG interventions in 2017. SVG, saphenous vein graft.

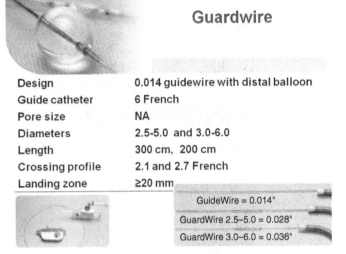

Guardwire

Design	0.014 guidewire with distal balloon
Guide catheter	6 French
Pore size	NA
Diameters	2.5-5.0 and 3.0-6.0
Length	300 cm, 200 cm
Crossing profile	2.1 and 2.7 French
Landing zone	≥20 mm

GuideWire = 0.014"
GuardWire 2.5–5.0 = 0.028"
GuardWire 3.0–6.0 = 0.036"

FIGURE 24.2 Description of the GuardWire (Medtronic Vascular, Santa Rosa, CA).

TABLE 24.2 Major Published Trials of Embolic Protection in SVGs

AUTHOR	YEAR	N	PRIMARY ENDPOINT			
EPD VS. NO EPD				**EPD EVENT RATE (%)**	**CONTROL GROUP EVENT RATE (%)**	**P SUPERIORITY**
SAFER (31)	2002	801	30-day composite of death, MI, emergency CABG, or TLR	(GuardWire) 9.6	16.5	0.004
EPD VS. ANOTHER EPD				**TEST EPD EVENT RATE (%)**	**CONTROL EPD EVENT RATE (%)**	**P NON-INFERIORITY**
FIRE (42)	2003	651	30-day composite of death, MI, or TVR	(FilterWire) 9.9	(GuardWire) 11.6	0.0008
SPIDER	2005	732	30-day composite of death, MI, urgent CABG, or TVR	(Spider) 9.1	(GuardWire 24% or FilterWire 76%) 8.4	0.012
PRIDE (43)	2005	631	30-day composite of cardiac death, MI, or TLR	(Triactiv) 11.2	(FilterWire) 10.1	0.02
CAPTIVE (44)	2006	652	30-day composite of death, MI, or TVR	(Cardioshield) 11.4	(GuardWire) 9.1	0.057
PROXIMAL (45)	2007	594	30-day composite of death, MI, or TVR	(Proxis) 9.2	(GuardWire 19% or FilterWire 81%) 10.0	0.006
AMETHYST (46)	2008	797	30-day composite of death, MI, or urgent repeat revascularization	(Interceptor Plus) 8.0	(GuardWire 72% or FilterWire 18%) 7.3	0.025

GuardWire, Medtronic Vascular, Santa Rosa, CA; FilterWire, Boston Scientific, Natick, MA; SPIDER, ev3, Plymouth, MN; Triactive, Kensey Nash Corp., Exton, PA; Cardioshield, MedNova, Galway; Proxis, St Jude Medical, Minneapolis, MN; Interceptor Plus, Medtronic Vascular.
AMETHYST, Assessment of the Medtronic AVE Interceptor Saphenous Vein Graft Filter System; CABG, coronary artery bypass graft surgery; CAPTIVE, CardioShield Application Protects during Transluminal Intervention of Vein grafts by reducing Emboli; EPD, embolic protection device; FIRE, FilterWire EX Randomized Evaluation; MI, myocardial infarction; PRIDE, Protection During Saphenous Vein Graft Intervention to Prevent Distal Embolization; PROXIMAL, Proximal Protection During Saphenous Vein Graft Intervention; SAFER, Saphenous vein graft Angioplasty Free of Emboli Randomized; SPIDER, Saphenous Vein Graft Protection In a Distal Embolic Protection Randomized Trial; TLR, target lesion revascularization; TVR, target vessel revascularization.

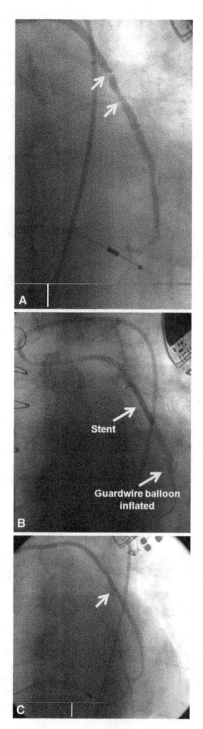

FIGURE 24.3 Saphenous vein graft intervention using the GuardWire (Medtronic Vascular, Santa Rosa, CA). Coronary angiography demonstrating a lesion in the body of the saphenous vein graft (*arrows*, **panel A**). A stent was implanted after inflation of the GuardWire balloon distally (**panel B**), with an excellent final angiographic result (**panel C**).

events was driven by a reduction in the incidence of myocardial infarction (8.6% vs. 14.7%, p = 0.008) and the "no-reflow" phenomenon (3% vs. 9%, p = 0.02).

Given the results of SAFER, subsequent EPD studies utilized a non-inferiority design, because it was not considered to be ethical to deny patients the benefits associated with EPD use (Table 24.2). Several devices

were shown to be non-inferior to the GuardWire (Table 24.2), yet only two of those are currently available in the US: the FilterWire, (Boston Scientific Natick MA, **Fig. 24.4**) and the Spider (ev3, Plymouth, MN, **Fig. 24.5**). A proximal occlusion device (Proxis, St Jude) was clinically available in the past, but production was discontinued in 2012.

The choice of EPD for a specific SVG lesion depends on lesion location: Ostial and proximal lesions can only be protected with a filter because use of distal occlusion balloons may result in embolic debris embolization in the aorta; body lesions can be protected with any device, whereas distal anastomotic lesions cannot be protected with any of the currently available devices (**Fig. 24.6**). Use of a filter requires the presence of an adequately long landing zone. EPDs may not be necessary for the treatment of SVG in-stent restenotic lesions because these fibrotic lesions are less likely to cause distal embolization and myocardial infarction (32). In spite of their demonstrated clinical benefit and class I guideline indication, EPDs are underutilized in SVG interventions: They were only used in 21% of SVG PCI in NCDR (33).

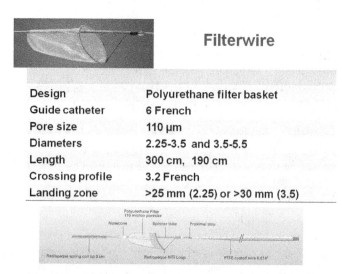

Filterwire

Design	Polyurethane filter basket
Guide catheter	6 French
Pore size	110 μm
Diameters	2.25-3.5 and 3.5-5.5
Length	300 cm, 190 cm
Crossing profile	3.2 French
Landing zone	>25 mm (2.25) or >30 mm (3.5)

FIGURE 24.4   Description of the FilterWire (Boston Scientific, Natick, MA).

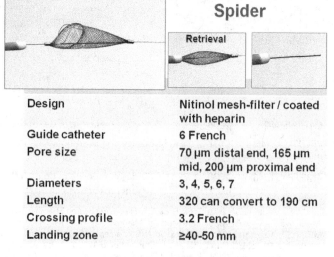

Spider

Design	Nitinol mesh-filter / coated with heparin
Guide catheter	6 French
Pore size	70 μm distal end, 165 μm mid, 200 μm proximal end
Diameters	3, 4, 5, 6, 7
Length	320 can convert to 190 cm
Crossing profile	3.2 French
Landing zone	≥40-50 mm

FIGURE 24.5   Description of the Spider (ev3, Plymouth, MN).

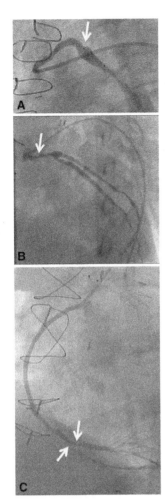

Intermediate SVG Lesions

Unlike native coronary arteries, SVG intermediate lesions have high rates of progression (38). Prophylactic stenting of such lesions was associated with a lower rate of SVG disease progression and a trend toward a lower incidence of major adverse cardiac events at 1-year follow-up compared with medical treatment alone in the Moderate *VEin Graft LEsion Stenting With the Taxus Stent and Intravascular Ultrasound* (VELETI) Pilot Trial (39). Nevertheless, the subsequent VELETI II study did not demonstrate benefit with prophylactic SVG stenting and was stopped prematurely for futility after randomizing 125 patients (40).

Arterial Grafts

PCI of arterial grafts is infrequent (1), especially for IMA grafts that have high long-term patency rates (2). PCI of IMA grafts is most commonly required at the distal anastomotic site and can be challenging due to (1) difficulty engaging the graft, especially in the presence of proximal subclavian artery tortuosity, (2) difficulty wiring and delivering equipment through the graft due to "pseudolesion" formation, and (3) difficulty reaching the target lesion, due to long graft length. Specialized catheters, such as the internal mammary VB (IM VB1) catheter, can facilitate IMA graft engagement, but occasionally using the ipsilateral radial access may be required. Using soft guide wires may decrease the risk for IMA kinking, and occasional use of shortened guide catheters may be required to allow balloon or stent delivery to a distal anastomotic lesion, or to a lesion in the native vessel distal to the IMA anastomosis.

FIGURE 24.6 Saphenous vein graft lesions in which an embolic protection device could not be used because of the large caliber of the graft (**panel A**), the lesion is proximal to a Y-graft bifurcation (**panel B**), or because of tis location at the distal SVG anastomosis (**panel C**).

Special Lesion Subsets

SVG Acute Occlusions

Acute SVG thrombosis is challenging to treat due to large thrombus burden, diffuse SVG degeneration, and high recurrent SVG failure rates (34). Aggressive use of thrombectomy and EPDs is often required to restore luminal patency, but even if acute recanalization is achieved, long-term SVG patency is low (34). Alternative revascularization approaches, such as PCI of the bypassed native coronary artery (35), may provide better outcomes (1,3), but these can be challenging procedures, requiring dedicated equipment and expertise (36).

SVG Chronic Total Occlusions

In the 2011 PCI guidelines, PCI is not recommended for chronic SVG occlusions (class III, level of evidence C) (5), because of low success and high restenosis rates: In a series of 34 patients undergoing SVG CTO PCI, procedural success was achieved in 23 patients (68%); during a median follow-up of 18 months, 68% developed in-stent restenosis; and 61% required target vessel revascularization (37).

Key Points

- SVG interventions currently account for approximately 6% of PCIs performed in the United States.

- GP IIb/IIIa inhibitors should not be used in SVG interventions.

- DESs are associated with similar clinical outcomes as bare metal stents in SVG lesions.

- EPDs should be used during SVG PCI when technically feasible.

- Three EPDs are available for clinical use in SVGs in the US in 2017: the GuardWire (Medtronic Vascular), FilterWire (Boston Scientific), and Spider (ev3).

References

1. Brilakis ES, et al. Percutaneous coronary intervention in native arteries versus bypass grafts in prior coronary artery bypass grafting patients a report from the national cardiovascular data registry. *JACC Cardiovasc Interv.* 2011;4:844–850.
2. Goldman S, et al. Long-term patency of saphenous vein and left internal mammary artery grafts after coronary artery bypass surgery results from a Department of Veterans Affairs Cooperative Study. *J Am Coll Cardiol.* 2004;44:2149–2156.

3. Brilakis ES, et al. Percutaneous coronary intervention in native coronary arteries versus bypass grafts in patients with prior coronary artery bypass graft surgery: insights from the Veterans Affairs Clinical Assessment, Reporting, and Tracking Program. *JACC Cardiovasc Interv*. 2016;9:884–893.

4. Morrison DA, et al. Percutaneous coronary intervention versus repeat bypass surgery for patients with medically refractory myocardial ischemia: AWESOME randomized trial and registry experience with post-CABG patients. *J Am Coll Cardiol*. 2002;40:1951–1954.

5. Levine GN, et al. 2011 ACCF/AHA/SCAI guideline for percutaneous coronary intervention. A report of the American College of Cardiology Foundation/American Heart Association Task Force on Practice Guidelines and the Society for Cardiovascular Angiography and Interventions. *J Am Coll Cardiol*. 2011;58:e44–e122.

6. Varghese I, et al. Impact on contrast, fluoroscopy, and catheter utilization from knowing the coronary artery bypass graft anatomy before diagnostic coronary angiography. *Am J Cardiol*. 2008;101:1729–1732.

7. Dimas B, et al. ST-segment elevation acute myocardial infarction due to severe hypotension and proximal left subclavian artery stenosis in a prior coronary artery bypass graft patient. *Cardiovasc Revasc Med*. 2009;10:191–194.

8. Rigattieri S, et al. Meta-analysis of radial versus femoral artery approach for coronary procedures in patients with previous coronary artery bypass grafting. *Am J Cardiol*. 2016;117:1248–1255.

9. Michael TT, et al. A randomized comparison of the transradial and transfemoral approaches for coronary artery bypass graft angiography and intervention: the RADIAL-CABG trial (RADIAL Versus Femoral Access for Coronary Artery Bypass Graft Angiography and Intervention). *JACC Cardiovasc Interv*. 2013;6:1138–1144.

10. Cooper L, Banerjee S, Brilakis ES. Crossover from radial to femoral access during a challenging percutaneous coronary intervention can make the difference between success and failure. *Cardiovasc Revasc Med*. 2010;11:266. e5–266.e8.

11. Farooq V, et al. The use of a guide catheter extension system as an aid during transradial percutaneous coronary intervention of coronary artery bypass grafts. *Catheter Cardiovasc Interv*. 2011;78:847–863.

12. Roffi M, et al. Lack of benefit from intravenous platelet glycoprotein IIb/IIIa receptor inhibition as adjunctive treatment for percutaneous interventions of aortocoronary bypass grafts: a pooled analysis of five randomized clinical trials. *Circulation*. 2002;106:3063–3067.

13. Coolong A, et al. Saphenous vein graft stenting and major adverse cardiac events: a predictive model derived from a pooled analysis of 3958 patients. *Circulation*. 2008;117:790–797.

14. Brilakis E, et al. Frequency and predictors of drug-eluting stent use in saphenous vein bypass graft percutaneous coronary interventions: a report from the American College of Cardiology National Cardiovascular Data CathPCI Registry. *JACC-Cardiovasc Interv*. 2010;3:1068–1073.

15. Sdringola S, et al. Adenosine use during aortocoronary vein graft interventions reverses but does not prevent the slow-no reflow phenomenon. *Catheter Cardiovasc Interv*. 2000;51:394–399.

16. Zoghbi GJ, et al. Pretreatment with nitroprusside for microcirculatory protection in saphenous vein graft interventions. *J Invasive Cardiol*. 2009;21:34–39.

17. Fischell TA, et al. "Pharmacologic" distal protection using prophylactic, intragraft nicardipine to prevent no-reflow and non-Q-wave myocardial infarction during elective saphenous vein graft intervention. *J Invasive Cardiol*. 2007;19:58–62.

18. Michaels AD, et al. Pretreatment with intragraft verapamil prior to percutaneous coronary intervention of saphenous vein graft lesions: results of the randomized, controlled vasodilator prevention on no-reflow (VAPOR) trial. *J Invasive Cardiol*. 2002;14:299–302.

19. Savage MP, et al. Stent placement compared with balloon angioplasty for obstructed coronary bypass grafts. Saphenous Vein De Novo Trial Investigators. *N Engl J Med*. 1997;337:740–747.

20. Hanekamp CE, et al. Randomized study to compare balloon angioplasty and elective stent implantation in venous bypass grafts: the Venestent study. *Catheter Cardiovasc Interv*. 2003;60:452–457.

21. Stankovic G, et al. Randomized evaluation of polytetrafluoroethylene-covered stent in saphenous vein grafts: the Randomized Evaluation of polytetrafluoroethylene COVERed stent in Saphenous vein grafts (RECOVERS) Trial. *Circulation*. 2003;108:37–42.

22. Schachinger V, et al. A randomized trial of polytetrafluoroethylene-membrane-covered stents compared with conventional stents in aortocoronary saphenous vein grafts. *J Am Coll Cardiol*. 2003;42:1360–1369.

23. Stone GW, et al. 5-year follow-up of polytetrafluoroethylene-covered stents compared with bare-metal stents in aortocoronary saphenous vein grafts the randomized BARRICADE (barrier approach to restenosis: restrict intima to curtail adverse events) trial. *JACC Cardiovasc Interv*. 2011;4:300–309.

24. Maia F, et al. Preliminary results of the INSPIRE trial with the novel MGuard stent system containing a protection net to prevent distal embolization. *Catheter Cardiovasc Interv*. 2010;76:86–92.

25. Abizaid A, et al. Use of a self-expanding super-elastic all-metal endoprosthesis; to treat degenerated SVG lesions: the SESAME first in man trial. *Catheter Cardiovasc Interv*. 2010;76:781–786.

26. Vermeersch P, et al. Randomized double-blind comparison of sirolimus-eluting stent versus bare-metal stent implantation in diseased saphenous vein grafts: six-month angiographic, intravascular ultrasound, and clinical follow-up of the RRISC Trial. *J Am Coll Cardiol*. 2006;48:2423–2431.

27. Vermeersch P, et al. Increased late mortality after sirolimus-eluting stents versus bare-metal stents in diseased saphenous vein grafts: results from the randomized DELAYED RRISC Trial. *J Am Coll Cardiol*. 2007;50:261–267.

28. Brilakis ES, et al. A randomized controlled trial of a paclitaxel-eluting stent versus a similar bare-metal stent in saphenous vein graft lesions the SOS (Stenting of Saphenous Vein Grafts) trial. *J Am Coll Cardiol*. 2009;53:919–928.

29. Brilakis ES, et al. Continued benefit from paclitaxel-eluting compared with bare-metal stent implantation in saphenous vein graft lesions during long-term follow-up of the SOS (Stenting of Saphenous Vein Grafts) trial. *JACC Cardiovasc Interv*. 2011;4:176–182.

30. Mehilli J, et al. Drug-eluting versus bare-metal stents in saphenous vein graft lesions (ISAR-CABG): a randomised controlled superiority trial. *Lancet*. 2011;378:1071–1078.

31. Baim DS, et al. Randomized trial of a distal embolic protection device during percutaneous intervention of saphenous vein aorto-coronary bypass grafts. *Circulation*. 2002;105:1285–1290.

32. Ashby DT, et al. Effect of percutaneous coronary interventions for in-stent restenosis in degenerated saphenous vein grafts without distal embolic protection. *J Am Coll Cardiol*. 2003;41:749–752.

33. Brennan JM, et al. Three-year outcomes associated with embolic protection in saphenous vein graft intervention: results in 49 325 senior patients in the Medicare-linked National Cardiovascular Data Registry CathPCI Registry. *Circ Cardiovasc Interv*. 2015;8:e001403.

34. Abdel-Karim AR, Banerjee S, Brilakis ES. Percutaneous intervention of acutely occluded saphenous vein grafts: contemporary techniques and outcomes. *J Invasive Cardiol*. 2010;22:253–257.

35. Nguyen-Trong PK, et al. Use of saphenous vein bypass grafts for retrograde recanalization of coronary chronic total occlusions: insights from a Multicenter Registry. *J Invasive Cardiol*. 2016;28:218–224.

36. Brilakis ES, Banerjee S, Lombardi WL. Retrograde recanalization of native coronary artery chronic occlusions via acutely occluded vein grafts. *Catheter Cardiovasc Interv*. 2010;75:109–113.

37. Al-Lamee R, et al. Clinical and angiographic outcomes after percutaneous recanalization of chronic total saphenous vein graft occlusion using modern techniques. *Am J Cardiol*. 2010;106:1721–1727.

38. Ellis SG, et al. Late myocardial ischemic events after saphenous vein graft intervention—importance of initially "nonsignificant" vein graft lesions. *Am J Cardiol*. 1997;79:1460–1464.

39. Rodes-Cabau J, et al. Comparison of plaque sealing with paclitaxel-eluting stents versus medical therapy for the treatment of moderate nonsignificant saphenous vein graft lesions. The moderate VEin Graft LEsion stenting with the Taxus stent and Intravascular Ultrasound (VELETI) Pilot Trial. *Circulation*. 2009;120:1978–1986.

40. Rodes-Cabau J, et al. Sealing intermediate nonobstructive coronary saphenous vein graft lesions with drug-eluting stents as a new approach to reducing cardiac events: a randomized controlled trial. *Circ Cardiovasc Interv*. 2016;9. pii: e004336.

41. Turco MA, et al. Pivotal, randomized U.S. study of the Symbiot™ covered stent system in patients with saphenous vein graft disease: eight-month angiographic and clinical results from the Symbiot III trial. *Catheter Cardiovasc Interv*. 2006;68:379–388.

42. Stone GW, et al. Randomized comparison of distal protection with a filter-based catheter and a balloon occlusion and aspiration system during percutaneous intervention of diseased saphenous vein aorto-coronary bypass grafts. *Circulation*. 2003;108:548–553.

43. Carrozza JP Jr, et al. Randomized evaluation of the TriActiv balloon-protection flush and extraction system for the treatment of saphenous vein graft disease. *J Am Coll Cardiol*. 2005;46:1677–1683.

44. Holmes DR, et al. Comparison of the CardioShield filter with the guardwire balloon in the prevention of embolisation during vein graft intervention: results from the CAPTIVE randomised trial. *EuroIntervention*. 2006;2:161–168.

45. Mauri L, et al. The PROXIMAL trial: proximal protection during saphenous vein graft intervention using the Proxis Embolic Protection System: a randomized, prospective, multicenter clinical trial. *J Am Coll Cardiol*. 2007;50:1442–1449.

46. Kereiakes DJ, et al. A novel filter-based distal embolic protection device for percutaneous intervention of saphenous vein graft lesions: results of the AMEthyst randomized controlled trial. *JACC Cardiovasc Interv*. 2008;1:248–257.

25

Complications of Coronary Intervention

Ryan A. Berg, MD, FSCAI, FACC and

Michael Lim, MD, FSCAI, FACC

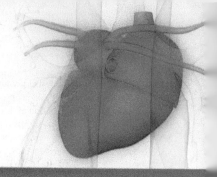

Understanding and addressing complications of percutaneous coronary intervention (PCI) is critical to the practice of interventional cardiology.

It is critical to appreciate and explain the possible complications of PCI to provide proper informed consent to the patient. It is also critical to be vigilant and to recognize potential complications at an early stage to try to reverse an adverse outcome, because the most common cause of all post-PCI deaths is from a procedural complication rather than from a preexisting cardiac condition (1).

Some of the complications are generic to all coronary angiography procedures, while others are specific to coronary intervention. Events such as death, myocardial infarction (MI), and bleeding occur at higher rates for interventional procedures because there is direct manipulation of the coronary arteries, often accompanied by prolonged procedural time, complexity, and the use of higher-intensity anticoagulation (**Tables 25.1** and **25.2**). Complications of PCI can occur at any step of the procedure, from the administration of sedation to transfer as the patient leaves the laboratory. The goal of this chapter is to incorporate the latest statistics and guidelines regarding the diagnosis and management of complications of PCI.

Mortality

Mortality is the most serious complication of PCI. The cause can be secondary to any of the other complications listed in this chapter. In-hospital mortality is very rare with diagnostic angiography (<0.1%), but the rate increases exponentially with the addition of coronary intervention. The mortality rate greatly varies, depending on the urgency of PCI, with a range of 0.2% in elective PCI to up to 66% in the highest-risk patients with ST-segment elevation myocardial infarction (STEMI) in myocardial shock (2,3).

The most comprehensive risk prediction tool for in-hospital mortality is the CathPCI registry. Version 4 was updated in 2009 to include extreme-risk patients, such as those with cardiogenic shock and preoperative cardiac arrest. Data from 1.2 million procedures were used to develop both a full (precatheterization and postcatheterization data) and a pre-catheterization-only risk prediction model for PCI in-hospital mortality. These models show that increasing clinical acuity is the strongest predictor of mortality. In the absence of cardiogenic shock, the risk of in-hospital mortality for elective, urgent, and emergent cases was 0.2%, 0.6%, and 2.3%, respectively. In the presence of transient shock but not salvage status, the risk of in-hospital mortality was 15.1%; with sustained shock or

TABLE 25.2 Complications Specific to PCI

COMPLICATION	EVENT RATE
No-reflow phenomenon	2%
Stent thrombosis	1%
Vessel perforation	0.4%
Stent embolization	0.4%–1.7%
Need for emergent bypass surgery	0.15%–0.3%
Wire fracture	<0.1% (case reports only)
Stent infection	<0.1% (case reports only)

PCI, percutaneous coronary intervention.

TABLE 25.1 Event Rates of Common Complications Diagnostic versus PCI

COMPLICATION	EVENT RATE DIAGNOSTIC PROCEDURE	EVENT RATE INTERVENTIONAL PROCEDURE
Death	0.1%	1.27%
Significant bleed	0.5%	5%–12%
AV fistula	0.75%	1.1%
Pseudoaneurysm	0.2%	1%–2%
Periprocedural MI (>3× ULN cardiac enzyme)	0.1%	16%–18%
Air embolism	0.1%–0.3%	0.1%–0.3%
Cerebrovascular accident	0.3%	0.3%
Ventricular fibrillation	0.4%	0.84%
Coronary dissection	0.06%	29%
Aortic dissection	<0.01%	0.02%
Infection/bacteremia	0.11%	0.64%
Anaphylactoid reaction to contrast	0.23%	0.23%
Cholesterol embolization	0.8%–1.4%	0.8%–1.4%

PCI, percutaneous coronary intervention.

salvage, the risk was 33.8%; and, with sustained shock and salvage, the risk was 65.9% (3).

Besides clinical acuity, higher age (especially >70 years), history of renal disease, history of cerebrovascular disease, history of peripheral arterial disease, history of chronic obstructive pulmonary disease (COPD), history of diabetes, history of heart failure, lower ejection fraction, cardiac arrest within 24 hours, having a STEMI, or BMI >30 kg were all independent predictors of mortality. After diagnostic catheterization, the full model also predicts higher mortality if there was recent (<30 days) in-stent thrombosis, proximal LAD disease, left main disease, multivessel disease, or a chronic total occlusion. These anatomic risks correlate to increased SYNTAX scores, another anatomic risk prediction model that can assess preoperative major adverse cardiac events when treating complicated coronary anatomy.

Complications of Vascular Access/Bleeding

The first part of any procedure begins with vascular access. The major complications are femoral artery pseudoaneurysm, arteriovenous fistula, and bleeding (including retroperitoneal hemorrhage). As seen in Table 25.1, the incidence of these complications is increased in procedures in which PCI is performed compared with that in a strictly diagnostic procedure (4). Specific discussion of each of these complications of vascular access is beyond the scope of this chapter (see Chapter 28).

While bleeding can be a complication of vascular access, it can be a general complication of PCI, and the current guidelines recommend as a class I indication that all patients should be evaluated for risk of bleeding for PCI given that periprocedural bleeding is a major risk factor for subsequent mortality (5). Risk scores/calculators can be used to assess the risk of bleeding with independent predictors, including advanced age, smaller body mass index, chronic kidney disease, baseline anemia, vascular access site (femoral vs. radial), sheath size, and the number and type of antiplatelet agents and anticoagulants used (see Chapters 3 and 4).

Complications of Atheroembolism (Stroke, Periprocedural MI, Cholesterol Embolization)

Advancing large-bore guiding catheters or even 6-Fr catheters across a diseased aorta (either abdominal or thoracic) heavily burdened with atherosclerotic plaques may cause thromboembolic events, resulting in peripheral ischemia, renal failure, or stroke. Peripheral atheroembolism with obstruction of small arteries and arterioles by cholesterol crystals is known as cholesterol embolization syndrome (CES). This is relatively rare (incidence of 0.75%–1.4%). Typically, this is diagnosed by one of three typical cutaneous signs: livedo reticularis, blue toe syndrome/trash foot, or frank digital gangrene, in addition to laboratory evidence of an elevated eosinophil count. In-hospital mortality is as high as 16% in those patients with definite CES, because multiorgan embolization can often lead to multiorgan failure (6).

Atheroembolisms can also obstruct the arteries of the brain, causing a cerebral vascular accident (CVA) or transient ischemic attack (TIA). The overall incidence of TIA or CVA is quite low after PCI (5). There are various multivariate predictors of in-hospital CVA (Table 25.3). The most common symptoms of a perioperative TIA or CVA are motor or speech deficits. In-hospital death can occur in up to 25% of those with a CVA, but increased mortality is not expected

TABLE 25.3 Independent Predictors of In-Hospital CVA

PREDICTOR OF CVA	ODDS RATIO
Thrombolytics prior to PCI	4.7
Creatinine clearance <40 mL/min	3.1
Urgent or emergent PCI	2.7
Unplanned intra-aortic balloon pump	2.3
IV heparin prior to PCI	1.9
Hypertension	1.9
Diabetes	1.8

CVA, cerebral vascular accident; PCI, percutaneous coronary intervention.
Adapted from: Dukkipati S, et al. Characteristics of cerebrovascular accidents after percutaneous coronary interventions. J Am Coll Cardiol. 2004;43(7):1161–1167, with permission.

with a TIA (7). Intravenous thrombolytic therapy is the treatment of choice if the stroke occurs within 4.5 hours of the procedure if there are no absolute contraindications to thrombolysis (8). For patients ineligible for intravenous thrombolytic therapy, neurointervention with intraarterial mechanical thrombectomy or intraarterial thrombolytic therapy can be given within 6 hours of onset or even as an adjunct in select patients with large vessel occlusions (especially in the proximal anterior circulation) that have already received intravenous thrombolytic therapy. Before intravenous thrombolytic therapy can be considered, typically a noncontrast CT scan is first done to rule out hemorrhagic stroke or hemorrhagic conversion of an ischemic stroke. In rare cases, if the stroke occurs and is recognized during the procedure in a hybrid room with appropriate personnel capable of cerebral angiography, consideration should be given for emergent cerebral angiography and intervention if an ischemic stroke with large arterial occlusion is found (9).

Intracoronary atheroembolism is one mechanism of periprocedural MI. Periprocedural MI is considered a major adverse cardiac event and a core measure in the recent SCAI quality assessment and improvement position statement (10). A meta-analysis of 15 observational studies found that periprocedural MIs were linked with worse in-hospital and long-term outcomes (11). According to the new universal definitions of MI, a PCI-related MI is the increase of biomarkers greater than three times the 99th percentile of the upper reference limit (12). While it is common (24%) to have some evidence of myonecrosis (any enzyme level above the upper limits of normal) after a percutaneous intervention, it is rarer (8%) to have a true periprocedural MI (13). Besides intracoronary atheroembolism, other causes of periprocedural MI include occluded side branches, no-reflow, vessel perforation, vasospasm, acute stent thrombosis, and dissection. The management of the periprocedural MI depends on its underlying cause.

Arterial Dissection

The guide catheter itself can cause coronary dissection with or without extension to the aortic root. More commonly, coronary dissection is caused by advancement of the coronary guide wire or by balloon inflation. Large visible dissections have been described in up to 30% of all angioplasty procedures (14). Previously, this was a significant risk factor for acute/abrupt vessel closure, which occurs rarely in the era of coronary stenting. The National Heart Lung and Blood Institute (NHLBI) classifications of coronary dissections are seen in **Table 25.4** (15). Types E and F may represent the additional complication of intracoronary thrombus.

Catheter-related dissection is a much rarer event, with a reported incidence of 0.06% (16). The mechanism of the dissection is likely because of mechanical trauma to the intima of the vessel (either normal or with plaque) from a catheter that is wedged into the wall rather than lying coaxial. A jet of contrast from an abnormally seated catheter might also cause or worsen a coronary dissection. Risk factors for catheter-induced coronary artery dissection include left main disease, use of Amplatz-shaped catheters, acute MI, extensive catheter manipulation, vigorous contrast injection, deep intubation of the catheter within the coronary artery (sometimes caused by deep inspiration by the patient), and variant anatomy of the coronary ostia (17).

Stenting the dissected area remains the standard of treatment. If a guide catheter-induced dissection is noticed, this should be fixed before the initial intended lesion that prompted the PCI. The rationale is that if the dissection is not fixed, it can propagate forward and cause abrupt vessel closure or propagate backward and cause aortic dissection.

The incidence of aortic dissection caused by catheter trauma is very rare, 0.02%. **Table 25.5** shows a classification scheme for extension of an aortic dissection (18). Almost all cases of retrograde extension of dissection are from the right coronary artery (RCA). Class I and II lesions have a good prognosis, and just require stenting of the coronary dissection with close clinical follow-up.

It is reasonable to follow the evolution of the dissection with imaging modalities (CT or TEE). If the patient remains stable over the next 24 to 48 hours of hospitalization, then he or she can be safely discharged without the expectation for further complication (18). To reduce the chance of extension, the systolic blood pressure must be optimally controlled. Nevertheless, antiplatelet therapy should not be suspended with a freshly placed coronary stent. Class III aortic dissections generally should be treated surgically and are associated with a much higher mortality rate. If surgery is not a possibility, then the entrance of the dissection in the coronary should be stented to avoid further propagation of the aortic dissection.

TABLE 25.4 Classification of Coronary Dissection

TYPE OF DISSECTION	DESCRIPTION
Type A	Luminal haziness
Type B	Linear dissection
Type C	Extraluminal contrast staining
Type D	Spiral dissection
Type E	Dissection with persistent filling defects
Type F	Dissection with total occlusion

TABLE 25.5 Classification of Coronary Dissection with Retrograde Extension into the Aortic Root

CLASSIFICATION	EXTENT OF AORTIC INVOLVEMENT IN THE DISSECTION
Class I	Involving the ipsilateral cusp
Class II	Involving cusp and extending up the aorta <40 mm
Class III	Involving cusp and extending up the aorta >40 mm

Contrast Media Reactions

Angiography with radiocontrast media is the first step to every intervention. The most severe contrast media reactions include anaphylactoid reactions and acute renal failure from contrast-induced nephropathy (CIN). Anaphylactoid reactions are rare, occurring in only 0.23% of procedures (19). The 2011 PCI guidelines (5) list two recommendations regarding anaphylactoid reactions.

1. It is a class I recommendation with patients with prior evidence of an anaphylactoid reaction to contrast media to receive appropriate steroid (60 mg prednisone night before and morning of procedure) and antihistamine prophylaxis (50 mg 1 hour prior) before repeat contrast administration.
2. It is a Class III recommendation (no benefit) in patients with a prior history of allergic reactions to shellfish or seafood to give prophylaxis for a contrast reaction as iodine does not mediate seafood, shellfish, or contrast media reactions.

To prevent acute renal failure from contrast induced nephropathy, the 2011 guidelines state:

1. It is recommended that patients be assessed for CIN before PCI.
2. Patients undergoing cardiac catheterization with contrast should receive adequate preparatory hydration (normal saline has been shown to be more ideal than ½ normal saline).
3. In patients with creatinine clearance <60 mL/min, the volume of contrast media should be minimized.

Air Embolism

With contrast administration, another potential complication is air embolization, which can be a cause of periprocedural MI or stroke. This is always an iatrogenic complication caused by failure to clear the air from the manifold system. Automatic injection systems have a lower rate of air embolism because of their air sensors, which prevent injection of air if detected in the system. Nevertheless, their air detection systems do not fully eliminate the incidence of air embolisms and should be considered another safety mechanism, not a replacement, for good technique of aspiration and visual inspection. Treatment of coronary air embolism consists of immediate initiation of 100% oxygen by facemask. The oxygen helps to minimize ischemia and to produce a diffusion gradient, which helps with reabsorption. If large air bubbles persist, the air can then be aspirated by various aspiration catheters. Further general complications of PCI that might occur at any time during the procedure include arrhythmias and the "no-reflow" phenomenon.

Arrhythmia

Arrhythmias can consist of tachycardia or bradycardia. Typically, the unstable tachycardias such as ventricular tachycardia or ventricular fibrillation are more commonly seen in the setting of an acute MI (up to 4%) compared with elective PCI (0.8%) (20,21). Bradycardia can be seen in the case of RCA occlusion, use of rotational atherectomy in the RCA, or use of rheolytic thrombectomy catheters. For treatment, adherence to standard Adult Cardiovascular Life Support (ACLS) protocols is recommended. In general, for unstable patients, it is always good practice to electrically cardiovert tachycardic arrhythmias. For unstable bradycardia, atropine can be given, and transcutaneous pacing can be initiated. These measures can buy some time to set up for temporary transvenous balloon flotation pacemaker placement. Transvenous pacemakers should be placed prophylactically for cases of rotational atherectomy in the RCA and in all cases of rheolytic thrombectomy. If transvenous pacing is not readily available, then guide wire pacing (hooking a negative lead to the guide wire and a positive lead to the patient) has been shown to be a viable alternative.

No-Reflow Phenomenon

An acute onset of TIMI 0 flow in a coronary vessel during PCI is known as abrupt vessel closure. It may be because of dissection, thrombus, spasm, or the "no-reflow" phenomenon. There can be some confusion in nomenclature because some authors only use the term "no-reflow" in conjunction with microembolization during primary PCI leading to microvascular obstruction or vasospasm, whereas others use the term loosely to describe the sudden absence of flow during any PCI procedure. Intravascular ultrasound is the gold standard to help discern the cause of no-reflow if not already obvious by clinical suspicion or angiographic appearance. If closure is caused by thrombus or new plaque rupture, then manual aspiration with an aspiration catheter is appropriate. Additional anticoagulation with glycoprotein IIb/IIIa inhibitors by either the intravenous or the intracoronary route should be started if there is no contraindication. Rechecking activated clotting time levels is prudent. Additional angioplasty and stenting might be necessary. If closure is because of dissection, then additional stenting is necessary. If closure is caused by severe spasm, then intracoronary nitroglycerin doses at a concentration of 100 μg/mL are given until the vasospasm is relieved.

Although intracoronary nitroglycerin can help relieve vasospasm, it has not been shown to be effective in relief of the no-reflow phenomenon from distal microembolization (22). The 2011 ACC PCI guidelines give a Class IIa recommendation for administration of an intracoronary vasodilator (specifically, adenosine, calcium-channel blocker, or nitroprusside) to treat PCI-related no-reflow that occurs during primary or elective PCI (5). Often, several grams of these agents given in small 100-μg intracoronary boluses will be necessary. No-reflow from embolization to the microvasculature is most commonly seen in interventions on saphenous vein grafts and in primary PCI for acute MIs. Prophylactic distal filters can help reduce the microembolic burden in saphenous vein graft interventions. In fact, embolic protection devices are considered a Class I indication in PCI of saphenous vein grafts when technically feasible. On the other hand, recent guidelines list glycoprotein IIb/IIIa inhibitors as a Class III recommendation in SVG interventions because they have shown no benefit (5). Initially, based on earlier studies, aspiration thrombectomy prior to primary PCI was initially a Class IIa recommendation in the 2011 PCI guidelines (5). Nevertheless, with additional evidence from larger trials, the 2015 focused update moved routine aspiration thrombectomy to a class III (no benefit) recommendation, with limited use in bailout scenarios as a class IIb recommendation (23).

Coronary Perforation

Finally, as seen in Table 25.2, there are more technically specific complications that can occur with the intracoronary use of wires and stents. These complications include coronary perforation, wire fracture, stent dislodgement with or without embolization, stent infection, and stent thrombosis. Nearly all of these complications are rare and may not be seen during a training fellowship. Coronary

perforation happens in 0.4% of PCI cases (24). Coronary perforation can be caused by a wire "exiting" the vessel or by a tear in the vessel from angioplasty or stenting or rotational atherectomy. **Table 25.6** shows the Ellis classification of coronary perforations (25).

Class I and II perforations are usually just managed conservatively without any specific treatment. They have a low incidence of tamponade (0.4% and 3.3%, respectively). Class III perforations, however, have a much higher rate of tamponade (45.7%) and a high mortality rate (21.2%) (24). As little as 100 mL of an acute pericardial effusion can cause chamber compression and hemodynamic collapse. To minimize the chance of wire exit, hydrophilic-tipped or stiff wires that are used to get through difficult lesions should be exchanged for typical workhorse wires with softer hydrophobic tips. Also, it is good practice to always have the tip of the wire in the radiographic plane of view at all times. If a distal perforation from a wire tip occurs, the initial step should be balloon tamponade of the vessel at the perforation site. Prolonged (several minutes) inflations with test deflations can be tried over an hour. If balloon tamponade is not successful, then consideration must be given for distal coil placement (26). Anticoagulation should *not* be immediately reversed with the wire and balloon in the vessel during the attempted perforation occlusion. Immediate reversal could lead to thrombosis throughout the whole vessel along the length of the wire or in recently stented segments, which could lead to a higher degree of mortality than the perforation itself (27,28). Reversal of anticoagulation should be reserved until the PCI equipment is removed from the coronary vessel. If a GP IIb–IIIa inhibitor is in use, it should be turned off during the case. Covered stents are not helpful at the site of distal wire perforations because of the tapered vessel size at its end. Nevertheless, if a branch of a main vessel is the one that is leaking, the whole branch can be excluded with a covered stent.

For larger perforations, a covered stent placement with a PTFE-covered stent is often the best choice of treatment. After every balloon inflation or atherectomy run, a puff of contrast should be given to assess the vessel for perforation. This will allow for immediate recognition of perforation, because delay in recognition could lead to cardiovascular collapse. If the perforation occurred after a balloon inflation or stent placement, the balloon should be immediately reintroduced and reinflated to stop further extravasation of blood into the pericardial space. At this point, if tamponade has occurred, a pericardial drain should be placed to relieve any tamponade, while more definitive measures to control the perforation are instituted. Again, if heparin is used, immediate reversal with heparin should not be done as long as equipment remains in the artery (27,28). Bivalirudin should be discontinued immediately as it will take up to 2 hours to decrease the anticoagulation status to a normal level. GP IIb–IIIa inhibitors should also be discontinued.

TABLE 25.6 Ellis Classification of Coronary Perforations

CLASS	DESCRIPTION
I	Extraluminal crater without extravasation
II	Pericardial or myocardial blush/staining without contrast jet extravasation
III	Perforation >1 mm in diameter with contrast streaming or cavity spilling

From: Ellis SG, et al. Increased coronary perforation in the new device era: incidence, classification, management, and outcome. *Circulation.* 1994;90:2725–2730, with permission.

Retained PCI Equipment Components

Rarely, fragments of interventional equipment may be broken and remain in a coronary artery. This may occur with guide-wire tips, fragments of various other catheters, or stents. These retained intravascular fragments carry the risk of coronary artery occlusion because of thrombus formation, distal embolization of clot, and vessel perforation.

Guide-wire fracture has an incidence of less than 0.1% according to very rare case reports in the literature compared with the number of interventions done worldwide. More cases of guide-wire fracture have been reported with the rotational atherectomy wires. There are multiple options to deal with a retained wire fragment. If the retained fragment is very small, it can be left in place and allowed to endothelialize, as a stent would. Nevertheless, a balloon should be used to position the fragment against the wall rather than intraluminally, which would be a risk for thrombosis. Dual antiplatelet therapy should be initiated for 1 month in this circumstance.

Alternatively, a stent can be deployed to trap the wire in place and avoid any possibility of further migration (29). If the wire fragment is very long and extends into the guiding catheter, then a balloon can be advanced to the end of the guide catheter and inflated, thereby trapping the wire against the side of the guide (30). At this point, the guide, balloon, and retained wire can be removed all at once. If a longer wire is retained but does not extend into the guide, then removal with a microsnare is the best choice (31). If a microsnare is not readily available, then using two new guide wires through one torquing device can create an effective helical snare to entrap the retained wire (32).

Stent dislodgement and embolization is much rarer with current-generation premounted balloons. Nevertheless, the incidence remains at ~0.36%, typically because of dislodgement in tortuous, calcified vessels (33). Management includes retrieval, deployment in place, or crushing against the wall of the vessel with a balloon or new stent. Ideally, retrieval should be tried first so you can avoid placing a stent in an unintended position. Mortality rates have been reported as high as 17% for stent embolizations that are unsuccessfully managed (usually requiring emergent surgery), but they are as low as 0.9% in patients who have successful retrieval of a stent (34). Retrieval methods are similar to those discussed with fractured wire retrieval. Microsnares or dual wires can be used to ensnare and remove the loose stent. Additional methods include advancing a small balloon over the same wire upon which the undeployed stent is sitting, inflating the balloon past the stent, and then pulling back the balloon, which should shift the free stent into the guide. If the stent is dislodged in a large proximal vessel, then consideration for retrieval with myocardial biopsy forceps can be considered as well. If retrieval is not possible, then "playing the stent where it lies" (i.e.,

deploying or crushing the stent at that site) is the best option. First, place a small balloon (similar to the stent length) over the wire and through the uninflated stent. Initially, this can be attempted with a small 1.5-mm balloon blown up to 1 to 2 atm; this might be enough to capture the stent and move the system as a whole to a more desirable spot (to the initial lesion or at least out of the left main). If it cannot be moved, then deploy the balloon at full atmospheres to dilate the stent as much as possible. A second deflated balloon equal to the vessel diameter can then be placed to assure adequate stent apposition. Rarely, a small-diameter balloon will not recross the stent. In this case, another stent is placed adjacent to the embolized stent and is used to crush the loose stent against the wall of the artery. In up to 50% of embolization cases, the stent might be embolized outside the coronary artery. In these situations, snares or forceps can be used to retrieve the stent if it can be visualized in the periphery (34). If it cannot be retrieved or even visualized, this is usually not a concern regarding adverse events, as reported by a large case series (33).

Stent Thrombosis

Stent thrombosis is a rare but devastating complication of PCI. Mortality rates are reported from 25% to 40% (35–37). Stent thrombosis is defined as acute (<24 hours), subacute (within 30 days), late (between 1 month and 1 year), or very late (>1 year). In an attempt to standardize the definition of stent thrombosis, the academic research consortium divided the criteria for stent thrombosis into definite, probable, or possible (**Table 25.7**) (38).

Both bare-metal stent and drug-eluting stent thromboses occur most commonly in the acute or subacute time frame. Drug-eluting stents, however, also have a higher risk of thrombosis in the late and very late period because of incomplete endothelialization of the target vessel. This risk was higher with first-generation drug-eluting stents. Therefore, dual antiplatelet therapy is crucial for at least 6 months to 1 year after drug-eluting stent implantation. Premature discontinuation of dual antiplatelet therapy is the greatest risk factor for stent thrombosis. Other risk factors are listed in **Table 25.8** (39).

Up to 29% of patients in whom antiplatelet therapy is discontinued prematurely are at risk of stent thrombosis (39). Because drug-eluting stents require a longer duration of dual antiplatelet therapy, it is crucial to decide before the diagnostic angiogram whether the patient is an appropriate candidate for long-term dual antiplatelet therapy.

Stent Infection

The rarest complication of PCI is stent infection. Less than 15 case reports of intracoronary stent infection are presented in the literature (40). Both drug-eluting stents and bare-metal stents have been

TABLE 25.7 Academic Research Consortium Criteria for Stent Thrombosis

DEFINITION	CRITERIA
Definite stent thrombosis	Angiographic confirmation of thrombus that originates inside or within 5 mm of the stent, which is associated with symptoms, ECG changes or biomarker elevation, or pathologic confirmation of stent thrombosis determined at autopsy or from tissue obtained following thrombectomy
Probable stent thrombosis	Unexplained death occurring within 30 days after the index procedure, or a myocardial infarction occurring at any time after the index procedure that was documented by ECG or imaging to occur in an area supplied by the stented vessel in the absence of angiographic confirmation of stent thrombosis or other culprit lesion
Possible stent thrombosis	Unexplained death occurring more than 30 days after the index procedure

TABLE 25.8 Risk Factors for Stent Thrombosis

Premature discontinuation of antiplatelet therapy

Renal failure

Bifurcation lesion

Left ventricular ejection fraction

Stent length

Adapted from: Lakovou I, et al. Incidence, predictors and outcome of thrombosis after successful implantation of drug-eluting stents. *JAMA.* 2005;293(17):2126–2130, with permission.

associated with stent infection. In some cases, mycotic aneurysms are formed at the site of stenting, but other cases just present with persistent bacteremia. *Staphylococcus aureus* is the most common microorganism implicated. Stent infection presents within 4 weeks after stent implantation with fever and bacteremia. Chest pain, ECG changes, and troponin elevation might be absent, so a high degree of suspicion must be raised for any fever occurring within 1 month of PCI. Diagnosis can be confirmed by angiography, CT, or MRI. Besides antibiotic therapy, most cases (>60%) will require surgery. In general, there is up to a 40% mortality rate with stent infection (41). Strict infection control measures must be adhered to in the catheterization laboratory to avoid bacteremia. Risk factors for bacteremia associated with cardiac catheterization are shown in **Table 25.9**.

Key Points

■ CES is rare, but if extensive, it can be associated with high mortality because of multiorgan showering/failure. Livedo reticularis is a common physical finding in this syndrome.

■ Periprocedural MI is currently defined as a biomarker increased greater than three times the 99th percentile of the upper reference limit.

■ Periprocedural MI has been associated with worse short-term and long-term prognosis.

■ Periprocedural CVA must be identified quickly. Acute thrombolysis or neurointervention must be considered depending on the timing of recognition of the stroke and/or exclusion criteria for thrombolytics.

■ Coronary dissection is extremely common with angioplasty, but usually easily fixed with stenting.

■ Limited aortic dissection from catheter trauma is usually well-tolerated and does not require surgery.

■ Extensive iatrogenic aortic dissections >40 mm in length generally require cardiothoracic surgery and are associated with a high mortality rate.

■ Reduce CIN with adequate hydration and decreased contrast use.

■ IV normal saline is the hydration fluid of choice. It has proven benefits compared with 1/2 normal saline.

■ Follow current ACLS protocols for arrhythmia questions that arise on boards.

TABLE 25.9 Risk Factors for Bacteremia after Cardiac Catheterization

Avoidable Risk Factors

Difficult vascular access

Multiple skin punctures

Repeated catheterization at the same vascular access site

Extended duration of the procedure

Use of multiple PTCA balloons

Deferred removal of the arterial sheath

Unavoidable Risk Factors

Presence of congestive heart failure

Patient's age >60 years

PTCA, percutaneous transluminal coronary angioplasty.
Adapted from: Kaufman BA, et al. Coronary stent infection: a rare but severe complication of percutaneous coronary intervention. *Swiss Med Weekly.* 2005;135:483–487, with permission.

■ Prophylactic transvenous pacing should be done in all cases of rheolytic thrombectomy (AngioJet).

■ Prophylactic transvenous pacing should be done in rotational atherectomy cases of the RCA.

■ Adenosine, nitroprusside, and calcium-channel blockers (verapamil was studied the most) are effective for the no-reflow phenomenon because of microembolization.

■ Nitroglycerine is *not* useful for the no-reflow phenomenon because of microembolization.

■ Intracoronary thrombectomy with thrombus aspiration devices (not rheolytic thrombectomy) has shown improved outcomes in primary PCI.

■ The initial treatment for any perforation is immediate balloon inflation.

■ Immediate pericardiocentesis should follow balloon inflation.

■ Covered stents are necessary for those perforations that aren't resolved by balloon inflation.

■ Immediate reversal of anticoagulation with PCI equipment in the artery can lead to acute thrombosis—wait until all equipment is out before reversal, if necessary.

■ Retained PCI equipment is a rare phenomenon.

■ Stent embolization can usually be resolved percutaneously.

■ The mortality rate is 25% to 40% with stent thrombosis.

■ Premature discontinuation of antiplatelet therapy causes up to a 29% incidence of stent thrombosis.

■ Compliance, risk of bleeding, and the need for upcoming surgery are all important factors when considering the use of bare-metal or drug-eluting stents.

■ Stent infection is very rare (only case reports).

■ Stent infection has up to a 40% mortality rate.

■ Most cases will require surgery in addition to antibiotic therapy.

References

1. Malenka DJ, et al. Cause of in-hospital death in 12,232 consecutive patients undergoing percutaneous transluminal coronary angioplasty. The Northern New England Cardiovascular Disease Study Group. *Am Heart J.* 1999;137(4, pt 1):632–638.

2. Peterson ED, et al. Contemporary mortality risk prediction for percutaneous coronary intervention: results from 588,398 procedures in the National Cardiovascular Data Registry. *J Am Coll Cardiol.* 2010;55:1923–1932.

3. Brennan JM, et al. Enhanced mortality risked prediction with a focus on high risk percutaneous coronary intervention. *JACC Cardiovasc Interv.* 2013;6(8):790–799.

4. Messina LM, et al. Clinical characteristics and surgical management of vascular complication in patients undergoing cardiac catheterization: interventional versus diagnostic procedures. *J Vasc Surg.* 1991;13:593–600.

5. Levine G, et al. ACCF/AHA/SCAI guideline for percutaneous coronary intervention: a report of the American College of Cardiology Foundation/American Heart Association Task Force on Practice Guidelines and the Society for Cardiovascular Angiography and Interventions. *J Am Coll Cardiol.* 2011;58:e44–e122.

6. Fukumoto Y, et al. The incidence and risk factors of cholesterol embolization syndrome, a complication of cardiac catheterization: a prospective study. *J Am Coll Cardiol.* 2003;42:211–216.

7. Dukkipati S, et al. Characteristics of cerebrovascular accidents after percutaneous coronary interventions. *J Am Coll Cardiol.* 2004;43(7):1161–1167.

8. Khatri P, et al. The safety and efficacy of thrombolysis for strokes after cardiac catheterization. *J Am Coll Cardiol.* 2008;51(9):906–911.

9. Hamon M, et al. Periprocedural stroke and cardiac catheterization. *Circulation.* 2008;118:678–683.

10. Bashore TM, et al. 2012 American College of Cardiology Foundation/Society for Cardiovascular Angiography and Interventions Expert Consensus Document on Cardiac Catheterization Laboratory Standards Update. *J Am Coll Cardiol.* 2012;59:2221–2305.

11. Testa L, et al. Myocardial infarction after percutaneous coronary intervention: a meta analysis of troponin elevation applying the new universal definition. *QJM.* 2009;102:369–378.

12. Thygesen K, Alpert JS, White HD. Universal definition of myocardial infarction. *Eur Heart J.* 2007;28:2525–2538.

13. Wang T, et al. Patterns of cardiac marker surveillance after percutaneous coronary intervention and implications for the use of periprocedural myocardial infarction as a quality metric: a report from the National Cardiovascular Data Registry (NCDR). *J Am Coll Cardiol.* 2008;51(21):2068–2074.

14. Brelau C, et al. In-hospital morbidity and mortality in patients undergoing elective coronary angioplasty. *Circulation.* 1985;72(5):1044–1052.

15. Huber M, et al. Use of a morphologic classification to predict clinical outcome after dissection from coronary angioplasty. *Am J Cardiol.* 1991;15(5):467–471.

16. Knight C, Stables R, Sigwart U. Emergency coronary artery stenting for coronary dissection complicating diagnostic cardiac catheterization. *Br Heart J.* 1995;74(8):199–201.

17. Boyle A, et al. Catheter-induced coronary artery dissection: risk factors, prevention, and management. *J Invasive Cardiol.* 2006;18(10):500–503.

18. Dunning DW, et al. Iatrogenic coronary artery dissections extending into and involving the aortic root. *Catheter Cardiovasc Interv.* 2000;51:387–393.

19. Goss JE, Chambers CE, Heupler FA. Systemic anaphylactoid reactions to iodinated contrast media during cardiac catheterization procedures: guidelines for prevention, diagnosis, and treatment. *Cathet Cardiovasc Diagn.* 1995;34(2):99–104.

20. Addala S, et al. Outcome of ventricular fibrillation developing during percutaneous coronary interventions in 19,497 patients without cardiogenic shock. *Am J Cardiol.* 2005;96(6):764–765.

21. Mehta R, et al. Sustained ventricular tachycardia or fibrillation in the cardiac catheterization laboratory among patients receiving primary percutaneous coronary intervention: incidence, predictors, and outcomes. *J Am Coll Cardiol.* 2004;43(10):1765–1772.

22. Werner GS, et al. Intracoronary Verapamil for reversal of no-reflow during coronary angioplasty for acute myocardial infarction. *Catheter Cardiovasc Interv.* 2002;57:444–451.

23. Levine GN, et al. 2015 ACC/AHA/SCAI focused update on primary percutaneous coronary intervention for patients with ST-elevation myocardial infarction. *J Am Coll Cardiol.* 2016;67(10):1235–1250.

24. Shimony A, et al. Coronary artery perforation during percutaneous coronary intervention: a systematic review and meta-analysis. *Can J Cardiol.* 2011;27(6):843–850.

25. Ellis SG, et al. Increased coronary perforation in the new device era: incidence, classification, management, and outcome. *Circulation.* 1994;90:2725–2730.

26. Pershad A, Yarkoni A, Biglari D. Management of distal coronary perforations. *J Invasive Cardiol.* 2008;20(6):E187–E191.

27. Cosgrave J, et al. Protamine usage following implantation of drug-eluting stents: a word of caution. *Catheter Cardiovasc Interv.* 2008;71:913–914.

28. Wilsmore B, Gunalingam B. Iatrogenic coronary arteriovenous fistula during percutaneous coronary intervention: unique insight into intra-procedural management. *J Interv Cardiol.* 2009;22:460–465.

29. Kilic H, Akdemir R, Bicer A. Rupture of guide wire during percutaneous transluminal coronary angioplasty, a case report. *Int J Cardiol.* 2008;128:e113–e114.

30. Patel T, et al. Broken guidewire fragment: a simplified retrieval technique. *Catheter Cardiovasc Interv.* 2000;51:483–486.

31. Gavlick K, Blankenship JC. Snare retrieval of the distal tip of a fractured rotational atherectomy guidewire: roping the steer by its horns. *J Invasive Cardiol.* 2005;17(12):E55–E58.

32. Gurley J, et al. Removal of retained intracoronary percutaneous transluminal coronary angioplasty equipment by a percutaneous twin guidewire method. *Cathet Cardiovasc Diagn.* 1990;19:251–256.

33. Dunning DW, et al. The long-term consequences of lost intracoronary stents. *J Interv Cardiol.* 2002;15:345–348.

34. Bolte J, et al. Incidence, management, and outcome of stent loss during intracoronary stenting. *Am J Cardiol.* 2001;88:565–567.

35. Spertus JA, et al. Prevalence, predictors, and outcomes of premature discontinuation of thienopyridine therapy after drug-eluting stent placement: results from the PREMIER registry. *Circulation.* 2006;113:2803–2809.

36. Pfisterer M, et al. Late clinical events after clopidogrel discontinuation may limit the benefit of drug-eluting stents. *J Am Coll Cardiol.* 2006;48:2584–2591.

37. Eisenstein EL, et al. Clopidogrel use and long-term clinical outcomes after drug-eluting stent implantation. *JAMA.* 2006;5:E1–E10.

38. Cutlip DE, et al. Clinical end points in coronary stent trials: a case for standardized definitions. *Circulation.* 2007;115(17):2344.

39. Iakovou I, et al. Incidence, predictors and outcome of thrombosis after successful implantation of drug-eluting stents. *JAMA.* 2005;293(17):2126–2130.

40. Viola GM, Darouiche RO. Cardiovascular implantable device infections. *Curr Infect Dis Rep.* 2011;12:333–342.

41. Kaufman BA, et al. Coronary stent infection: a rare but severe complication of percutaneous coronary intervention. *Swiss Med Weekly.* 2005;135:483–487.

Chronic Total Occlusion Percutaneous Coronary Intervention

Emmanouil S. Brilakis, MD, PhD, FSCAI, FACC, FESC, FAHA, M. Nicholas Burke, MD, FSCAI, FACC, and Subhash Banerjee, MD, FSCAI, FACC, FAHA

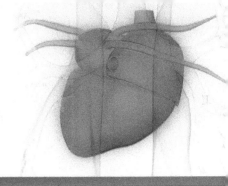

Definition and Prevalence

Coronary chronic total occlusions (CTOs) are defined as coronary lesions with Thrombolysis In Myocardial Infarction (TIMI) grade 0 flow of at least 3-months' duration. A coronary CTO is found in approximately *one in three patients* undergoing diagnostic coronary angiography (1–3).

When Should CTO PCI be Performed?

As in every patient with coronary artery disease, treatment of patients with coronary CTOs includes medical therapy (every patient should receive aspirin and a statin unless they have a contraindication) and possibly coronary revascularization, with either percutaneous coronary intervention (PCI) or coronary artery bypass graft surgery (CABG). CABG is generally preferred in patients with complex multivessel disease (especially patients with diabetes mellitus), whereas PCI is preferred in patients with simple multivessel disease, single-vessel disease, or prior CABG (Fig. 26.1) (4).

The decision on whether to perform CTO PCI depends on: (a) the anticipated benefit; (b) the estimated likelihood for success; and (c) the estimated risk.

a. **Anticipated benefits:** CTO PCI could provide several potential benefits, as follows:
   - **Improve quality of life**
     For patients with medically refractory angina caused by a CTO, successful CTO recanalization could reduce or eliminate the angina and the need for anti-anginal medications and improve exercise capacity (5,6). Bruckel et al. demonstrated that several patients with CTOs also suffer from undiagnosed major depression, and depressed patients derive the most benefit from successful CTO PCI through reduction of angina (7). The Drug-Eluting stent Implantation versus optimal Medical Treatment in patients with Chronic Total Occlusion (DECISION-CTO; NCT01078051 - presented at the 2017 American College of Cardiology meeting) randomized patients with coronary CTOs to optimal medical therapy alone or optimal therapy with CTO PCI. At 3 years, the primary endpoint of death, MI, stroke, or repeat revascularization occurred in 19% of the OMT vs. 21.4% of the CTO PCI group, suggesting non-inferiority of OMT and quality of life was also similar in the two groups. DECISION CTO, however, had several important limitations such as high prevalence of non-CTO lesions in both groups and high crossover from the medical therapy to the CTO PCI group that limit interpretation of the study findings. The Randomized Multicenter Trial to Evaluate the Utilization of Revascularization or Optimal Medical Therapy for the Treatment of Chronic Total Coronary Occlusions (EuroCTO; NCT01760083 - presented at the 2017 EuroPCR meeting) randomized patients to CTO PCI vs medical therapy alone and showed more improvement at 12 months in angina frequency in the CTO PCI group.

   - **Improve myocardial function**
     In patients with impaired myocardial contractility due to ischemia, CTO recanalization can improve myocardial function. Several studies using fractional flow reserve measurement after CTO crossing but before stent implantation showed that nearly all myocardial territories supplied by a CTO are ischemic, even when extensive collateral circulation is present (8). In patients with systolic heart failure, CTO revascularization was associated with improvement in left ventricular ejection fraction and improvement in New York Heart Association functional class, angina, and brain natriuretic peptide levels (9). Three-year follow-up after successful CTO PCI suggested a beneficial effect on left ventricular remodeling, as well as a tendency toward improvement in left ventricular ejection fraction (10). As anticipated, myocardial function only improved in patients with viable myocardium, with no benefit in patients with transmural scarring.

     In the Evaluating XIENCE and Left Ventricular Function in Percutaneous Coronary Intervention on Occlusions After ST-Elevation Myocardial Infarction (EXPLORE) trial, patients who underwent primary PCI for ST-segment elevation acute myocardial infarction (STEMI) and were found to have a concomitant CTO were randomized to CTO PCI or medical therapy alone within 7 days (11). Core laboratory adjudicated procedural success was 73%. At 4 months, left ventricular ejection fraction and left-ventricular end-diastolic volume were similar in the two study groups, although patients who underwent PCI of a left anterior descending artery CTO had significantly higher ejection fraction as compared with those treated with medical therapy alone.

   - **Improve long-term survival and tolerance of subsequent coronary events**
     The presence of a CTO has been independently associated with worse long-term outcomes in patients presenting with acute coronary syndromes (12). Moreover, presence of a CTO is one of the most common reasons for incomplete revascularization, which has in turn been associated with higher risk for subsequent major adverse cardiovascular events (13). Several observational studies and meta-analyses (6,14) have reported higher long-term survival after successful versus failed CTO PCI. Nevertheless, given the lack of prospective, randomized-controlled trials, the potential beneficial effect of CTO PCI on subsequent mortality remains unproven.

   - **Prevent arrhythmias**
     Nombela-Franco and colleagues showed that the presence of a CTO in patients with implanted cardioverter-defibrillators was associated with the higher risk for ventricular arrhythmias and

Revascularization Options For Patients With Coronary Total Occlusions

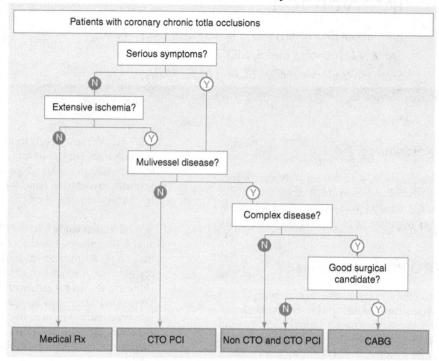

FIGURE 26.1 Revascularization options for patients with coronary chronic total occlusions. Algorithm for determining the need for coronary revascularization in patients with coronary chronic total occlusions, assuming expertise in both surgical and percutaneous coronary revascularization. Chronic total occlusion percutaneous coronary intervention (CTO PCI) and coronary artery bypass graft surgery are both treatment options, with coronary bypass graft surgery (CABG) preferred for patients with multivessel complex disease, and PCI (including CTO PCI) preferred for patients with simple multivessel or single-vessel disease. (Reproduced with permission from: Brilakis ES, Abdullah SM, Banerjee S. Who should undergo chronic total occlusion percutaneous coronary intervention?: the EXPLORation continues. *J Am Coll Cardiol.* 2016;68:1633–1636.)

TABLE 26.1 Comparison of Currently Available Scores for CTO PCI

	J-CTO (25)	CL (26)	PROGRESS-CTO (27)	ORA (21)
Number of variables	5	6	4	3
Number of cases	494	1,657	781	1,073
Overall success	88.6% (guide-wire crossing)	72.5% (procedural success)	92.9% (technical success)	91.9% (technical success)
Clinical				
Age ≥75 years				+
Prior CABG		+		
Prior MI		+		
Prior CTO PCI failure	+			
Angiographic				
Blunt stump	+	+	+[a]	
Ostial location				+
Severe calcification	+	+		
Severe tortuosity	+		+	
CTO length >20 mm	+	+		
CTO target vessel		+ (non-LAD)	+ (circumflex)	
Collaterals			+ (interventional)	+ (Rentrop <2)

[a]Proximal cap ambiguity.

CABG, coronary artery bypass graft surgery; CL, Clinical and Lesion-related score; CTO, chronic total occlusion; J-CTO, Multicenter CTO Registry in Japan score; LAD, left anterior descending artery; MI, myocardial infarction; ORA score, Ostial location, Rentrop <2, Age ≥75 years score; PCI, percutaneous coronary intervention; Progress-CTO, Prospective Global Registry for the Study of Chronic Total Occlusion Intervention score.

higher mortality (15), although a subsequent study failed to confirm these findings (16). Patients with refractory arrhythmias due to ischemia could benefit from CTO recanalization (17).

b. **Estimated likelihood of success:** In the past, published success rates of CTO PCI were approximately 70% to 80% (18). With development of novel equipment, techniques, and treatment strategies, CTO PCI success rates have significantly improved, with experienced centers around the world consistently achieving 85% to 90% success rates (19–23). Nevertheless, at less experienced centers, outcomes remain less favorable: In an analysis from National Cardiovascular Data Registry (NCDR), procedural success of CTO PCI between 2009 and 2013 was 59% (24).

In addition to operator experience, several angiographic characteristics can help predict the likelihood of success. Such parameters have been included in scores developed through various CTO PCI cohorts that can be used to estimate CTO PCI success rates (**Table 26.1**) (21,25–27). The first such score, the J-CTO score (Multicenter CTO Registry in Japan) uses five variables (occlusion length ≥20 mm, blunt stump, CTO calcification, CTO tortuosity, and prior failed attempt) to create a five-point score that predicts successful guidewire crossing within the first 30 minutes (**Fig. 26.2**)

(25). The Progress CTO score (Prospective Global Registry for the Study of Chronic Total Occlusion Intervention) uses four variables (proximal cap ambiguity, moderate/severe tortuosity, circumflex artery CTO, and absence of "interventional" collaterals) to create a four-point score that predicts technical success (**Fig. 26.3**) (27).

c. **Estimated risk:** CTO PCI carries increased risk for complications, as compared with less complex PCI. In NCDR, the risk for major adverse cardiac events (MACE) was 1.6% for CTO PCI versus 0.8% for non-CTO PCI ($p < 0.001$) (24). In the Prospective Global Registry for the Study of Chronic Total Occlusion Intervention (PROGRESS CTO), the risk for MACE was 2.8%, and was associated with age >65, occlusion length ≥23 mm, and use of the retrograde approach (28). Similar to the scores developed to determine the likelihood of procedural success, a score has been developed to predict the risk for MACE during CTO PCI (Progress-CTO Complications score) (**Fig. 26.4**) (28).

The importance of weighting the anticipated benefit and likelihood of success versus the estimated risk can help both the patient and physician choose a treatment strategy. This is reflected in the American College of Cardiology/American Heart Association/Society of Cardiovascular

J-CTO Score

494 native CTO lesions
Crossing within 30 minutes

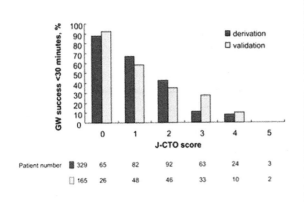

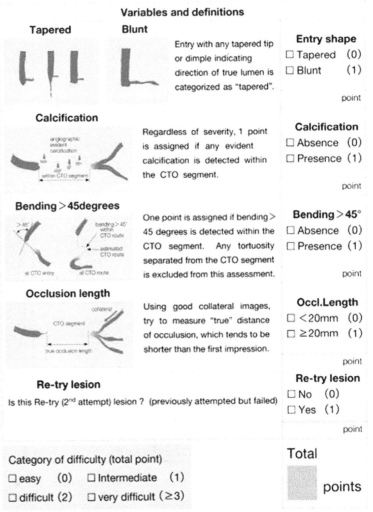

FIGURE 26.2   The J-CTO score. Description of the components of the J-CTO score that was developed to predict the likelihood of successful guide wire crossing of the occlusion within 30 minutes. CTO, chronic total occlusion. (Reproduced with permission from: Morino Y, et al. Predicting successful guide wire crossing through chronic total occlusion of native coronary lesions within 30 minutes: the J-CTO (Multicenter CTO Registry in Japan) score as a difficulty grading and time assessment tool. *JACC Cardiovasc Interv.* 2011;4:213–221.)

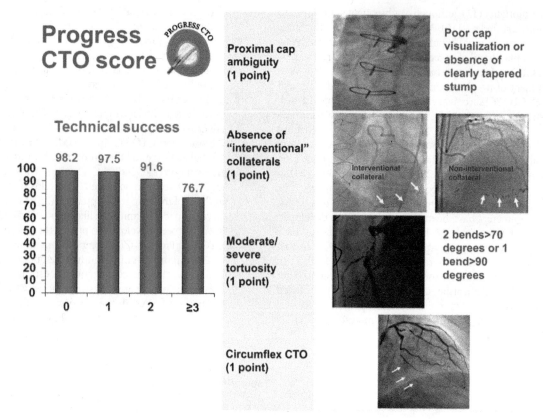

FIGURE 26.3 The Progress-CTO score. Description of the components of the Progress-CTO score that was developed to predict technical success of CTO PCI. CTO PCI, Chronic total occlusion percutaneous coronary intervention. (Reproduced with permission from: Christopoulos G, et al. Development and validation of a novel scoring system for predicting technical success of chronic total occlusion percutaneous coronary interventions: the PROGRESS CTO (Prospective Global Registry for the Study of Chronic Total Occlusion Intervention) Score. *JACC Cardiovasc Interv.* 2016;9:1–9.)

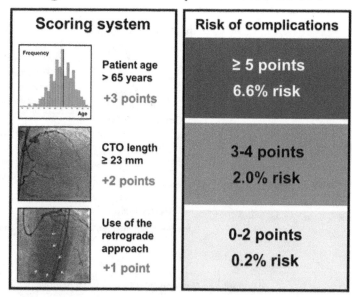

FIGURE 26.4 The Progress-CTO Complications score. Description of the components of the Progress-CTO Complications score that was developed to predict periprocedural complications during CTO PCI. Periprocedural complications included any of the following adverse events prior to hospital discharge: death, myocardial infarction, recurrent symptoms requiring urgent repeat target vessel revascularization with PCI or CABG, tamponade requiring either pericardiocentesis or surgery, and stroke. CABG, coronary artery bypass graft; CTO PCI, Chronic total occlusion percutaneous coronary intervention (Reproduced with permission from: Danek BA, et al. Development and validation of a scoring system for predicting periprocedural complications during percutaneous coronary interventions of chronic total occlusions: the Prospective Global Registry for the Study of Chronic Total Occlusion Intervention (PROGRESS CTO) complications score. *J Am Heart Assoc.* 2016;5. pii: e004272 [open access article].)

Angiography and Interventions guideline recommendation for CTO PCI: "PCI of a CTO in patients with appropriate clinical indications and suitable anatomy is reasonable when performed by operators with appropriate expertise" (class of recommendation IIa, level of evidence B) (29).

Procedural Planning and Equipment Selection for CTO PCI

Careful planning is critical for the success of CTO PCI. Unless there is an urgent indication, CTO PCI should not be performed at the same time as diagnostic angiography. Deferred CTO PCI: (a) allows detailed discussion with the patient and the family about the specific risks, goals, benefits, and alternatives of the procedure; (b) reduces radiation and contrast dose; and (c) allows in-depth review of the coronary angiogram.

Bifemoral access is used by most CTO PCI operators, although high success rates can be achieved using radial access (30); 8-French guide catheters provide strong support and allow liberal use of the trapping technique for equipment exchanges. AL1 is the most commonly used guide for the right coronary artery, and the XB 3.5 or EBU 3.75 for the left main. Anticoagulation is almost always achieved with unfractionated heparin because it can be reversed if a complication occurs. Careful attention to radiation dose is required throughout the procedure, and dedicated equipment, such as covered stents and coils, should be available to treat coronary perforations.

CTO PCI requires use of standard and specialized equipment that can be grouped into 10 categories (**Table 26.2**). An over-the-wire system should be used in all cases, ideally employing a microcatheter, such as the Corsair or Caravel (Asahi Intecc; Nagoya, Japan), Turnpike and Turnpike LP (Vascular Solutions; Minneapolis, MN), or Finecross (Terumo; Somerset, NJ). Use of a microcatheter facilitates

TABLE 26.2 Equipment Needed for CTO PCI

CATEGORY NO.	EQUIPMENT	MUST HAVE	GOOD TO HAVE
1.	Sheaths		45-cm long sheaths
2.	Guides	• XB/EBU 3.0, 3.5, 3.75, 4.0 • AL1, AL0.75 • JR4 • Y-connector with hemostatic valve (such as Co-pilot or Guardian) • Guide catheter extensions (Guideliner and Guidezilla)	• 90-cm long • Side hole guides, especially AL1
3.	Microcatheters	• Finecross (150 cm for retrograde—135 cm for antegrade) • Corsair or TurnPike (150 cm for retrograde—135 cm for antegrade) • Small (1.20, 1.25, or 1.5 mm diameter), 20-mm long, over-the-wire balloons of 145 cm or longer total length	• Venture • TwinPass • SuperCross • MultiCross and CenterCross (increase support)
4.	Guidewires[a]	Fielder XT, Fighter Confianza Pro 12 Pilot 200 Gaia 1, 2, and 3 Sion Fielder FC RG3 (for externalization)	Miracle 3 or 12
5.	Dissection/reentry equipment	CrossBoss catheter Stingray balloon and wire	
6.	Snares	Ensnare or Atrieve 18–30 mm or 27–45 mm	Amplatz Gooseneck snares
7.	Balloon "uncrossable-undilatable" lesion equipment	Small, 20-mm long, over-the-wire and rapid-exchange balloons Threader Turnpike Spiral or Gold Laser	Rotablator AngioSculpt Tornus
8.	Intravascular imaging	IVUS (any)	IVUS (solid state)
9.	Complication management	Covered stents Coils + delivery microcatheters (such as Renegade or Progreat) Pericardiocentesis tray	Pericardiocentesis tray
10.	Radiation protection		Radiation scatter shields x-ray machine with radiation-reduction protocols

[a]For radial operators, 300-cm wires are required because the trapping technique cannot be used through a 6-Fr guide catheter for trapping over-the-wire balloons, the CrossBoss catheter, and the Stingray balloon.
CTO, chronic total occlusion; PCI, percutaneous coronary intervention; IVUS, intravascular ultrasound.

guidewire exchanges and provides strong guidewire support. Some of the most commonly used guidewires for CTO PCI are the following:

1. Fielder XT (Asahi Intecc) or Fighter (Boston Scientific, Natick, MA), which are soft polymer-jacketed, tapered wires for initial antegrade crossing.
2. Gaia second and Confianza Pro 12 (Asahi Intecc), which are stiff tapered-tip, penetrating wires for subsequent attempts, if the course of the vessel is well understood.
3. Pilot 200 (Abbott Vascular; Santa Clara, CA), a polymer-jacketed and moderately stiff, non-tapered tip wire, when the course of the target lesion and vessel is not well understood.
4. Sion (hydrophilic, highly torquable soft guide wire with excellent shape retention, Asahi Intecc) or Fielder FC (polymer-jacketed soft wire, Asahi Intecc) for wiring collaterals during retrograde crossing attempts.
5. RG3 (Asahi Intecc) or R350 (Vascular Solutions), which are long (330- and 350-cm, respectively) guide wires designed for externalization when the retrograde approach is used.

Specialized dissection/reentry equipment includes the CrossBoss catheter and the Stingray system (Boston Scientific). Additional equipment includes low-profile balloons, laser, and rotational atherectomy for "balloon uncrossable" and "balloon undilatable" lesions. Use of intravascular ultrasonography can facilitate CTO crossing and stent optimization. The availability of covered stents and coils are important for treating perforations. Collecting all CTO PCI equipment in a single location (CTO cart) can facilitate access to the equipment and improve efficiency of the procedure.

CTO Crossing: The Hybrid Approach

Crossing the occlusion with a guide wire is the most challenging part of CTO PCI. CTO crossing techniques can be grouped into three categories: antegrade wire escalation (**Fig. 26.5**), antegrade dissection/reentry (**Fig. 26.6**), and the retrograde approach (**Fig. 26.7**). Antegrade wire escalation is the most commonly used technique; however, antegrade-dissection and reentry, as well as the retrograde approach, are especially important with more complex lesions (31). Selecting the starting and subsequent crossing strategies can be guided by the hybrid algorithm to CTO PCI (**Fig. 26.8**) (32). The key components of this algorithm are the following: (a)

upfront use of dual injection in nearly all cases, examining the four key angiographic characteristics described in the prior section; (b) selection of an initial crossing technique based on review of the angiogram; and (c) early change to another crossing technique if the initially selected technique fails to achieve progress. The hybrid approach has been associated with high success rates in various CTO PCI cohorts around the world (19,20,22,33).

Review of the Angiogram

Detailed review of the angiogram is critical for CTO PCI. Dual injection is performed by first injecting the donor vessel, followed by injection of the CTO target vessel 2 to 3 seconds later. Angiographic review focuses on four angiographic parameters: (a) proximal cap morphology (clear-cut or ambiguous); (b) length of the occlusion; (c) quality of the distal vessel size and presence of bifurcations; and (d) suitability of the collateral circulation for retrograde access (32).

a. **Proximal cap morphology:** If the beginning of the occlusion is unclear, additional angiographic projections may be needed, or occasionally, use of intravascular ultrasound or computed tomography. If proximal cap ambiguity cannot be resolved, a primary retrograde approach is recommended.
b. **Lesion length:** Longer (≥20-mm) lesions can be harder to cross (25).
c. **Distal vessel quality:** CTOs with small and diffusely diseased distal vessels may be difficult to cross due to difficulty reentering

Antegrade dissection/re-entry

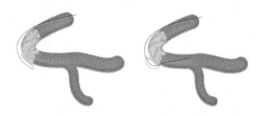

FIGURE 26.6   Illustration of antegrade dissection and reentry. (Reproduced with permission from: Brilakis ES, ed. *Manual of Coronary Chronic Total Occlusion Interventions. A Step-By-Step Approach.* Waltham, MA: Elsevier; 2013.)

Antegrade crossing

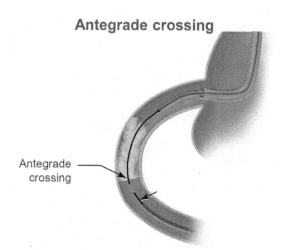

Antegrade crossing

FIGURE 26.5   Illustration Hof antegrade wire escalation. (Reproduced with permission from: Brilakis ES, ed. *Manual of Coronary Chronic Total Occlusion Interventions. A Step-By-Step Approach.* Waltham, MA: Elsevier; 2013.)

Retrograde crossing

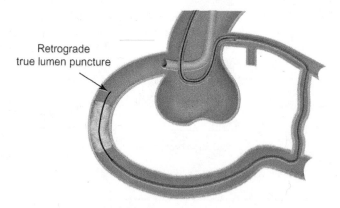

Retrograde true lumen puncture

FIGURE 26.7   Illustration of the retrograde approach. (Reproduced from: Brilakis ES, ed. *Manual of Coronary Chronic Total Occlusion Interventions. A Step-By-Step Approach.* Waltham, MA: Elsevier; 2013.)

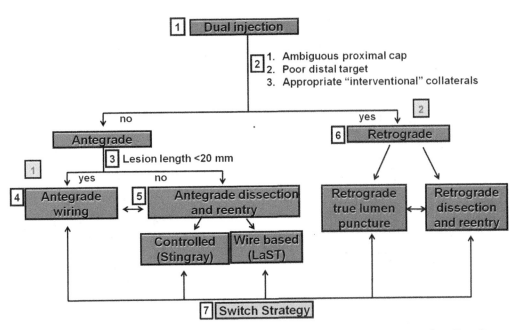

FIGURE 26.8 Overview of the hybrid CTO crossing algorithm. The algorithm starts with dual coronary injection (**box 1**) to allow assessment of several angiographic parameters (**box 2**), and allow selection of a primary antegrade (**boxes 3–5**) or primary retrograde (**box 6**) strategy. Strategy changes are made (**box 7**), depending on the progress of the case. CTO, chronic total occlusion; LAST, limited antegrade subintimal tracking. (Reproduced with permission from: Brilakis ES, et al. A percutaneous treatment algorithm for crossing coronary chronic total occlusions. *JACC Cardiovasc Interv.* 2012;5:367–379.)

into the distal true lumen in the case of subintimal guidewire entry. Failure to recanalize all major distal branches may result in incomplete revascularization and increased risk for periprocedural myocardial infarction.

d. **Collateral circulation:** The availability of collaterals suitable for the retrograde approach increases the likelihood of successful CTO crossing and revascularization. Septal collaterals or saphenous vein grafts are more commonly used for retrograde crossing, followed by epicardial collaterals.

Antegrade Wire Escalation

Antegrade wire escalation is the crossing technique of choice for short (<20-mm-long) occlusions and is performed by advancing guidewires of increasing stiffness through a microcatheter or over-the-wire balloon. Usually, a soft tapered-tip, polymer-jacketed guidewire (such as the Fielder XT or Fighter wire) is initially used, followed by a stiff polymer-jacketed wire (such as the Pilot 200) if the CTO course is unclear, or a stiff tapered-tip guide wire (such as the Gaia second wire) if the course of the CTO is clear. The wire is shaped through the introducer, aiming to create a 1-mm short and about 30° bend at the tip. In case of subintimal guidewire entry, a second guidewire can be advanced parallel to the first guidewire (parallel-wire technique), or the Stingray reentry system can be utilized to achieve distal true lumen entry.

Antegrade Dissection and Reentry

Antegrade dissection/reentry is usually recommended for long (≥20-mm) lesions approached in the antegrade direction. Antegrade dissection/reentry was initially described by Antonio Colombo, who advanced a knuckled polymer-jacketed guidewire until it spontaneously entered into the distal true lumen (subintimal tracking and reentry—STAR—technique) (34). Such extensive dissection/reentry techniques were, however, associated with high restenosis and reocclusion rates (35). As a result, limited dissection/reentry techniques are currently recommended (36).

Dissection can be achieved by advancing a knuckled, polymer-jacketed guidewire (usually the Fielder XT, Fighter, or Pilot 200) or by using the CrossBoss catheter (37). The CrossBoss catheter has a 1-mm round distal blunt tip and is advanced with rapid rotation using a torqueing device (fast-spin) technique (38). Although guidewires can be used for reentry, using the dedicated Stingray system is preferred so as to minimize the likelihood for subintimal hematoma formation that can hinder reentry. The Stingray system consists of a specially designed balloon and a guidewire. The Stingray balloon has a flat shape with two side exit ports, designed to self-orient one exit port toward the true lumen upon low-pressure (2–4 atm) inflation (37). The Stingray guidewire has a 20-cm distal radiopaque segment and a stiff (12 g) 0.009-inch tapered tip with a 0.0035-inch distal prong. Using fluoroscopic guidance, the Stingray wire is advanced through the side port of the Stingray balloon facing the distal true lumen until reentry is achieved.

The Retrograde Approach

In the retrograde approach, a guide wire is advanced via a collateral vessel or a bypass graft to the target vessel distal to the occlusion (39,40). This is achieved using specialized guidewires, such as the Sion wire (Asahi Intecc), and microcatheters, such as the Corsair, Caravel, Turnpike, and Turnpike LP. The CTO is then crossed either in the retrograde direction using a variety of specialized techniques, or the distal guide wire acts as a marker for antegrade crossing. Several techniques have been developed to facilitate retrograde crossing, such as the controlled antegrade and retrograde tracking and dissection (CART) and the reverse CART technique (41,42). The retrograde approach is especially important for crossing more complex CTOs (22,31).

Complications

CTO PCI complications can be classified according to timing (as acute and long-term), and according to location (cardiac coronary, cardiac non-coronary and non-cardiac) (**Fig. 26.9**) (18,43,44).

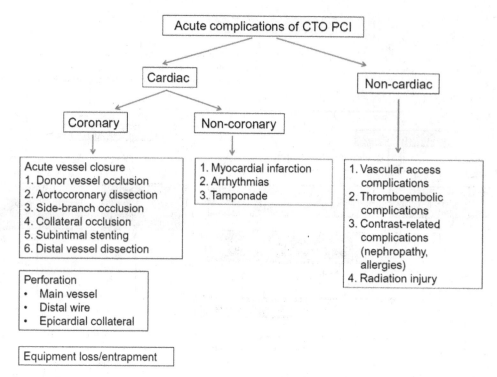

FIGURE 26.9 Classification of acute complications of CTO PCI. CTO PCI, chronic total occlusion percutaneous coronary interventions.

Acute coronary complications include acute vessel occlusion, perforation, and equipment loss or entrapment. Coronary perforation can be (a) main vessel perforation, (b) distal artery wire perforation, and (c) collateral vessel perforation, in either a septal or epicardial collateral. Covered stents are the treatment for main vessel perforations if bleeding cannot be stopped with prolonged balloon inflations. Coil and fat embolization (or occasionally, a covered stent) are usually used for distal vessel perforations (45,46). Collateral vessel perforation may require embolization from both sides to prevent continued bleeding through contralateral blood flow (47). Coronary perforation carries increased risk among prior CABG patients in whom pericardial adhesions could lead to loculated pericardial effusions, causing hemodynamic compromise, shock, and death (48). Perforation should be treated immediately upon identification, especially in prior CABG patients (49).

Non-coronary cardiac complications include tamponade (due to perforation), periprocedural myocardial infarction, and arrhythmias (that can result from compromising collateral blood flow). As with all cardiac catheterization procedures, non-cardiac acute complications can include vascular access complications, systemic thromboembolic complications, contrast allergic reactions, and radiation skin injury. Attention to radiation dose is critical to prevent patient exposure to high radiation doses. In most cases, the procedure should be stopped if CTO crossing has not been achieved after a radiation dose of 6 to 8 Gy has been administered.

Long-term complications of CTO PCI include in-stent restenosis, stent thrombosis, and coronary aneurysm formation. Although not supported by randomized data, prolonged (>12 months) dual antiplatelet therapy duration is frequently administered after CTO PCI.

Key Points

- CTO are commonly found during diagnostic coronary angiography.
- CTO PCI should be performed when the anticipated benefits exceed the potential risks.
- Potential benefits of CTO PCI include improved quality of life, improvement of left ventricular function, and decrease in the risk for arrhythmias.
- Complications, such as perforation, can occur during CTO PCI and require alertness and readiness to treat.
- Careful angiographic review is critical for planning CTO PCI.
- There are three major CTO crossing strategies: antegrade wire escalation, antegrade dissection/reentry, and retrograde. The hybrid algorithm provides guidance on initial and subsequent crossing strategy selection.

Disclosures:

Dr. Brilakis: consulting/speaker honoraria from Abbott Vascular, ACIST, Amgen, Asahi, CSI, Elsevier, GE Healthcare, Medicure, and Nitiloop; research support from Boston Scientific and Osprey. Board of Directors: Cardiovascular Innovations Foundation. Board of Trustees: Society of Cardiovascular Angiography and Interventions.

Dr. Burke: consulting/speaker honoraria from Abbott Vascular and Boston Scientific Dr. Banerjee: research grants from Gilead and The Medicines Company; has received institutional research grants from Boston Scientific and Merck; has received consultant and speaker honoraria from Covidien and Medtronic; has ownership in MDCARE Global (spouse); has intellectual property in HygeiaTel; spouse has received an educational grant from Boston Scientific.

References

1. Christofferson RD, et al. Effect of chronic total coronary occlusion on treatment strategy. *Am J Cardiol.* 2005;95:1088–1091.
2. Fefer P, et al. Current perspectives on coronary chronic total occlusions: the Canadian Multicenter Chronic Total Occlusions Registry. *J Am Coll Cardiol.* 2012;59:991–997.
3. Jeroudi OM, et al. Prevalence and management of coronary chronic total occlusions in a tertiary veterans affairs hospital. *Catheter Cardiovasc Interv.* 2014;84:637–643.
4. Brilakis ES, Abdullah SM, Banerjee S. Who should undergo chronic total occlusion percutaneous coronary intervention?: the EXPLORation continues. *J Am Coll Cardiol.* 2016;68:1633–1636.
5. Olivari Z, et al. Immediate results and one-year clinical outcome after percutaneous coronary interventions in chronic total occlusions: data from a multicenter, prospective, observational study (TOAST-GISE). *J Am Coll Cardiol.* 2003;41:1672–1678.
6. Christakopoulos GE, et al. Meta-analysis of clinical outcomes of patients who underwent percutaneous coronary interventions for chronic total occlusions. *Am J Cardiol.* 2015;115:1367–1375.
7. Bruckel JT, et al. Angina severity, depression, and response to percutaneous revascularization in patients with chronic total occlusion of coronary arteries. *J Invasive Cardiol.* 2016;28:44–51.
8. Sachdeva R, et al. The myocardium supplied by a chronic total occlusion is a persistently ischemic zone. *Catheter Cardiovasc Interv.* 2014;83:9–16.
9. Cardona M, et al. Benefits of chronic total coronary occlusion percutaneous intervention in patients with heart failure and reduced ejection fraction: insights from a cardiovascular magnetic resonance study. *J Cardiovasc Magn Reson.* 2016;18:78.
10. Kirschbaum SW, et al. Evaluation of left ventricular function three years after percutaneous recanalization of chronic total coronary occlusions. *Am J Cardiol.* 2008;101:179–185.
11. Henriques JP, et al. Percutaneous intervention for concurrent chronic total occlusions in patients with STEMI: the EXPLORE trial. *J Am Coll Cardiol.* 2016;68:1622–1632.
12. Claessen BE, et al. Evaluation of the effect of a concurrent chronic total occlusion on long-term mortality and left ventricular function in patients after primary percutaneous coronary intervention. *JACC Cardiovasc Interv.* 2009;2:1128–1134.
13. Garcia S, et al. Outcomes after complete versus incomplete revascularization of patients with multivessel coronary artery disease: a meta-analysis of 89,883 patients enrolled in randomized clinical trials and observational studies. *J Am Coll Cardiol.* 2013;62:1421–1431.
14. Hoebers LP, et al. Meta-analysis on the impact of percutaneous coronary intervention of chronic total occlusions on left ventricular function and clinical outcome. *Int J Cardiol.* 2015;187:90–96.
15. Nombela-Franco L, et al. Ventricular arrhythmias among implantable cardioverter-defibrillator recipients for primary prevention: impact of chronic total coronary occlusion (VACTO Primary Study). *Circ Arrhythm Electrophysiol.* 2012;5:147–154.
16. Raja V, et al. Impact of chronic total occlusions and coronary revascularization on all-cause mortality and the incidence of ventricular arrhythmias in patients with ischemic cardiomyopathy. *Am J Cardiol.* 2015;116:1358–1362.
17. Mixon TA. Ventricular tachycardic storm with a chronic total coronary artery occlusion treated with percutaneous coronary intervention. *Proc (Bayl Univ Med Cent).* 2015;28:196–199.
18. Patel VG, et al. Angiographic success and procedural complications in patients undergoing percutaneous coronary chronic total occlusion interventions: a weighted meta-analysis of 18,061 patients from 65 studies. *JACC Cardiovasc Interv.* 2013;6:128–136.
19. Christopoulos G, et al. Application and outcomes of a hybrid approach to chronic total occlusion percutaneous coronary intervention in a contemporary multicenter US registry. *Int J Cardiol.* 2015;198:222–228.
20. Maeremans J, et al. The hybrid algorithm for treating chronic total occlusions in Europe: the RECHARGE registry. *J Am Coll Cardiol.* 2016;68:1958–1970.
21. Galassi AR, et al. Percutaneous coronary revascularization for chronic total occlusions: a novel predictive score of technical failure using advanced technologies. *JACC Cardiovasc Interv.* 2016;9:911–922.
22. Wilson WM, et al. Hybrid approach improves success of chronic total occlusion angioplasty. *Heart.* 2016;102:1486–1493.
23. Habara M, et al. Comparison of percutaneous coronary intervention for chronic total occlusion outcome according to operator experience from the Japanese retrograde summit registry. *Catheter Cardiovasc Interv.* 2016;87:1027–1035.
24. Brilakis ES, et al. Procedural outcomes of chronic total occlusion percutaneous coronary intervention: a report from the NCDR (National Cardiovascular Data Registry). *JACC Cardiovasc Interv.* 2015;8:245–253.
25. Morino Y, et al. Predicting successful guidewire crossing through chronic total occlusion of native coronary lesions within 30 minutes: the J-CTO (Multicenter CTO Registry in Japan) score as a difficulty grading and time assessment tool. *JACC Cardiovasc Interv.* 2011;4:213–221.
26. Alessandrino G, et al. A clinical and angiographic scoring system to predict the probability of successful first-attempt percutaneous coronary intervention in patients with total chronic coronary occlusion. *JACC Cardiovasc Interv.* 2015;8:1540–1548.
27. Christopoulos G, et al. Development and validation of a novel scoring system for predicting technical success of chronic total occlusion percutaneous coronary interventions: the PROGRESS CTO (Prospective Global Registry for the Study of Chronic Total Occlusion Intervention) Score. *JACC Cardiovasc Interv.* 2016;9:1–9.
28. Danek BA, et al. Development and validation of a scoring system for predicting periprocedural complications during percutaneous coronary interventions of chronic total occlusions: the Prospective Global Registry for the Study of Chronic Total Occlusion Intervention (PROGRESS CTO) Complications Score. *J Am Heart Assoc.* 2016;5. pii: e004272.
29. Levine GN, et al. 2011 ACCF/AHA/SCAI guideline for percutaneous coronary intervention. a report of the American College of Cardiology Foundation/American Heart Association Task Force on Practice Guidelines and the Society for Cardiovascular Angiography and Interventions. *J Am Coll Cardiol.* 2011;58:e44–e122.
30. Alaswad K, et al. Transradial approach for coronary chronic total occlusion interventions: insights from a contemporary multicenter registry. *Catheter Cardiovasc Interv.* 2015;85:1123–1129.
31. Christopoulos G, et al. Clinical utility of the Japan-chronic total occlusion score in coronary chronic total occlusion interventions: results from a multicenter registry. *Circ Cardiovasc Interv.* 2015;8:e002171.
32. Brilakis ES, et al. A percutaneous treatment algorithm for crossing coronary chronic total occlusions. *JACC Cardiovasc Interv.* 2012;5:367–379.
33. Nombela-Franco L, et al. Validation of the J-chronic total occlusion score for chronic total occlusion percutaneous coronary intervention in an independent contemporary cohort. *Circ Cardiovasc Interv.* 2013;6:635–643.
34. Colombo A, et al. Treating chronic total occlusions using subintimal tracking and reentry: the STAR technique. *Catheter Cardiovasc Interv.* 2005;64:407–411; discussion 12.
35. Valenti R, et al. Predictors of reocclusion after successful drug-eluting stent-supported percutaneous coronary intervention of chronic total occlusion. *J Am Coll Cardiol.* 2013;61:545–550.
36. Mogabgab O, et al. Long-term outcomes with use of the CrossBoss and stingray coronary CTO crossing and re-entry devices. *J Invasive Cardiol.* 2013;25:579–585.
37. Michael TT, et al. Subintimal dissection/reentry strategies in coronary chronic total occlusion interventions. *Circ Cardiovasc Interv.* 2012;5:729–738.
38. Whitlow PL, et al. Use of a novel crossing and re-entry system in coronary chronic total occlusions that have failed standard crossing techniques: results of the FAST-CTOs (Facilitated Antegrade Steering Technique in Chronic Total Occlusions) trial. *JACC Cardiovasc Interv.* 2012;5:393–401.
39. Brilakis ES, et al. The retrograde approach to coronary artery chronic total occlusions: a practical approach. *Catheter Cardiovasc Interv.* 2012;79:3–19.
40. El Sabbagh A, et al. Angiographic success and procedural complications in patients undergoing retrograde percutaneous coronary chronic total

occlusion interventions: a weighted meta-analysis of 3,482 patients from 26 studies. *Int J Cardiol.* 2014;174:243–248.

41. Rathore S, et al. A novel modification of the retrograde approach for the recanalization of chronic total occlusion of the coronary arteries intravascular ultrasound-guided reverse controlled antegrade and retrograde tracking. *JACC Cardiovasc Interv.* 2010;3:155–164.

42. Surmely JF, et al. New concept for CTO recanalization using controlled antegrade and retrograde subintimal tracking: the CART technique. *J Invasive Cardiol.* 2006;18:334–338.

43. Brilakis ES, ed. *Manual of Coronary Chronic Total Occlusion Interventions. A Step-By-Step Approach.* Waltham, MA: Elsevier; 2013.

44. Brilakis ES, et al. Complications of chronic total occlusion angioplasty. *Interv Cardiol Clin.* 2012;1:373–389.

45. Shemisa K, Karatasakis A, Brilakis ES. Management of guidewire-induced distal coronary perforation using autologous fat particles versus coil embolization. *Catheter Cardiovasc Interv.* 2017;89:253–258.

46. Tarar MN, Christakopoulos GE, Brilakis ES. Successful management of a distal vessel perforation through a single 8-French guide catheter: combining balloon inflation for bleeding control with coil embolization. *Catheter Cardiovasc Interv.* 2015;86:412–416.

47. Kotsia AP, Brilakis ES, Karmpaliotis D. Thrombin injection for sealing epicardial collateral perforation during chronic total occlusion percutaneous coronary interventions. *J Invasive Cardiol.* 2014;26:E124–E126.

48. Aggarwal C, Varghese J, Uretsky BF. Left atrial inflow and outflow obstruction as a complication of retrograde approach for chronic total occlusion: report of a case and literature review of left atrial hematoma after percutaneous coronary intervention. *Catheter Cardiovasc Interv.* 2013;82:770–775.

49. Karatasakis A, Akhtar YN, Brilakis ES. Distal coronary perforation in patients with prior coronary artery bypass graft surgery: the importance of early treatment. *Cardiovasc Revasc Med.* 2016;17:412–417.

Vascular Access: Radial and Femoral Approaches

Beau M. Hawkins, MD, FACC, FSCAI and

Mazen S. Abu-Fadel, MD, FACC, FSCAI

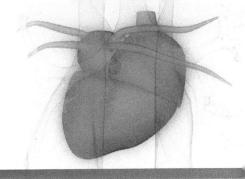

Few tasks are as important as arterial access in performing diagnostic and interventional catheterization procedures. The initial approach to all of these procedures requires vascular access into the arterial or venous circulation. Although access is just a means to an end, it remains one of the most challenging and life-threatening steps we perform. While the femoral artery has been the default access site in the United States for decades, owing to its large-caliber, compressible location and technical ease, there has been a significant uptake in radial artery approaches in recent years (1). Nonetheless, peripheral vascular and structural interventions are being increasingly performed by interventional cardiologists, and these procedures often necessitate femoral access due to the large-bore equipment required. As such, the modern interventionalist must practice meticulous access techniques, and master both femoral and radial approaches. This chapter reviews the technical aspects and complications of transradial and transfemoral procedures, and summates the important clinical trials comparing these two approaches in terms of percutaneous coronary intervention (PCI) outcomes.

Radial Artery Access

Anatomy

The brachial artery bifurcates near the antecubital space into radial and ulnar arteries. The radial artery runs laterally toward the thumb, while the ulnar artery passes medially as it approaches the hand. There are several variations of this anatomy, including radial-ulnar loops, brachial loops, stenotic lesions, excessive tortuosity, and anomalous origins of the radial artery (Fig. 27.1) (2). Although the "normal" anatomy is by far the most common, one must be aware of these common variations. After crossing the wrist joint, these arteries divide and form superficial and deep arches (3). The radial artery is relatively superficial even in the most obese patients and lies directly above the distal radius, which offers a reliable compressive surface.

Case Selection

A stepwise approach is an important aspect of developing experience with a particular technique. Performing transradial procedures is no different. Several features have been associated with procedural failure, including advanced age, short stature, and prior coronary artery bypass graft (CABG) surgery (4). Women are also known to have smaller radial arteries and are more prone to spasm (5,6).

While there is no definitive number of cases that ensures proficiency with the approach, some have suggested that after 50 cases (7) or 6 months (8), transradial interventions can be performed safely. There are some relative contraindications that may evolve as one's experience with the technique grows, while the only real "absolute" contraindication is an absent radial artery. Table 27.1 highlights some variables that should be considered when selecting transradial approaches for diagnostic and interventional coronary procedures.

Access Technique

The radial artery is usually accessed 1 to 2 cm proximal to the wrist joint with the hand in an extended, supinated position. The radial artery in this region is quite superficial and very compressible owing to the bony structures immediately posterior to this site of cannulation. The artery is accessed using either a true or modified Seldinger technique depending on operator preference. In the true Seldinger technique (9), an angiocatheter is advanced through the artery until blood cessation occurs. The angiocatheter is then withdrawn until blood flow reappears, and the vessel is then wired with standard sheath placement thereafter. A randomized trial demonstrated quicker access time, fewer arterial punctures, and similar bleeding complication rates when routinely employing the true, as opposed to the modified, Seldinger approach (10).

Recently, there has been growing interest in utilization of ultrasound to assist in accessing radial arteries. In the Radial Artery Access with Ultrasound trial (RAUST), ultrasound-guided radial access was shown to reduce the number of access attempts, increase first-pass access attempts, and reduce time to access compared to traditional access strategies (11).

Complications

A host of complications may occur during transradial procedures (Table 27.2). In general, due to the compressible nature of the radial artery, hematoma, if recognized early, can often be conservatively managed with compression (manual pressure, transradial bands, or blood pressure cuffs). Rarely, bleeding can be so advanced that compartment syndrome may develop. In such instances, surgical consultation may be necessary to minimize limb dysfunction and/ or loss. Radial artery spasm (RAS) and occlusion (RAO) are two unique complications associated with transradial procedures and are discussed in detail next.

RADIAL ARTERY SPASM

RAS continues to be a source of frustration for operators as they transition to radial access. The incidence of RAS decreases rapidly with experience, perhaps as a result of improved access technique and minimizing catheter manipulation (12). Despite this, it remains the most common cause of procedural failure. Predictors of spasm include younger age, female gender, diabetes, smaller wrist circumference, and lower body weight (5).

RAS refers to friction between the artery and wires or guide catheters, accompanied by a subjective feeling of pain. Pain from RAS increases vasomotor tone, resulting in further spasm. In current practice, careful puncture technique, an antispasmodic "cocktail," and hydrophilic-coated sheaths are the mainstays of RAS prevention (13).

Intra-arterial (IA) administration of antispasmodic medications has been shown to decrease the incidence of RAS (14,15). Calcium-channel blockers, nitrates, local anesthetics (e.g., lidocaine), and β-antagonists are the most common medications used

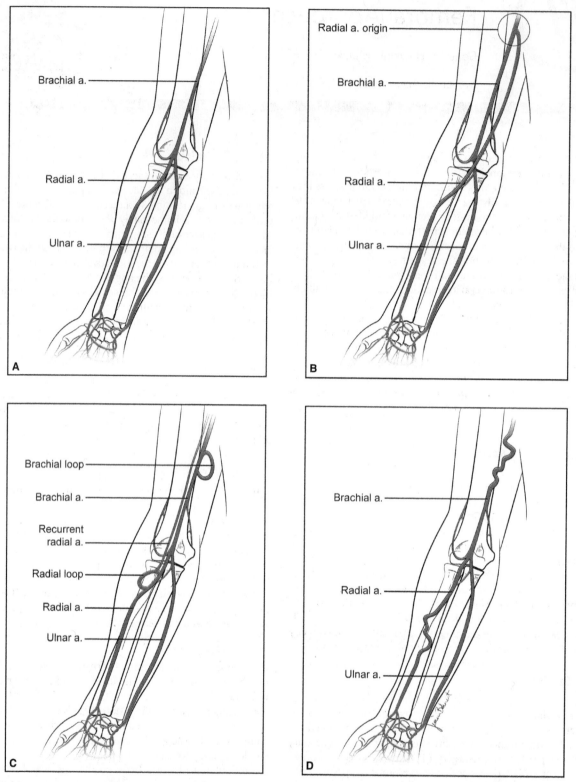

FIGURE 27.1 Common anatomical variations of upper extremity arterial circulation. **A:** Normal anatomy. **B:** High bifurcation of the radial artery. **C:** Arterial loops. **D:** Tortuosity .

for this purpose. While there is no consensus on the exact regimen or dose, the routine use of an antispasmodic "cocktail" containing a calcium-channel blocker with or without a nitrate is an effective strategy in decreasing the occurrence of RAS.

Sheath characteristics also influence RAS risk. Hydrophilic-coated sheaths have been shown to decrease the incidence of RAS and

improve patient comfort during sheath insertion and removal by lowering the friction between the sheath and radial artery wall (16,17). Regarding sheath length, it has been suggested that a longer sheath may protect the entire length of the radial artery from catheter and wire manipulation at the time of equipment exchanges (18). In contrast, others have reported that should spasm develop, a longer

TABLE 27.1 Considerations for Transradial Selection Stratified by Operator Experience

	BEGINNING OPERATOR/PROGRAM	EXPERIENCED OPERATOR/PROGRAM
Patient features	• Elderly • Prior CABG • Short stature • Dialysis fistula in ipsilateral arm • Extensive upper extremity trauma/burns	• Dialysis fistula in ipsilateral arm • Extensive upper extremity trauma/burns
Clinical scenarios	STEMI or unstable patients	NA
Angiographic or lesion-related	• Contralateral IMA graft • Need for large access sheath (>6 Fr in women, >7 Fr in men) • Inadequate guide support or engagement during diagnostic procedure • Sustained spasm or arm pain during diagnostic procedure	• Contralateral IMA graft • Need for large access sheath (>6 Fr in women, >7 Fr in men) • Sustained spasm or arm pain during diagnostic procedure

TABLE 27.2 Selected Complications Associated with Radial Artery Access

Hematoma

Compartment syndrome

Infection/abscess

Pseudoaneurysm

Hand ischemia

Artery avulsion

Radial artery spasm

Radial artery occlusion

sheath would prove more difficult to remove, and in very extreme cases may lead to avulsion of the radial artery (19). Rathore found no reduction in spasm with long (23 cm) versus short (13 cm) arterial sheaths. There was a higher rate of RAO at the 4- to 6-month follow-up visit in the long sheath group versus short (8.3% vs. 5.3%, respectively, p = 0.042) (5).

If clinically severe spasm does occur, it can often be treated successfully with repeated doses of IA vasodilators, local anesthetics, increased analgesia and sedation, and patience. In extreme cases, operators have successfully employed an axillary nerve block, deep sedation with propofol, or even general anesthesia to allow sheath removal (20). Care must be taken not to forcibly remove equipment should resistance occur, as this can cause transection or eversion endarterectomy of the adherent section of the radial artery (19).

RADIAL ARTERY OCCLUSION

RAO is a well-recognized complication of radial artery cannulation. In certain clinical contexts, such as prolonged hemodynamic monitoring in the perioperative period, rates of RAO have been reported to be as high as 25% (21). The incidence of RAO after transradial catheterization has been significantly lower, with some series demonstrating rates under 10% (22). RAO can be documented by an abnormal Barbeau's test (23), visible obstruction on two-dimensional ultrasound, or absence of Doppler flow signal distal to puncture site (24). The presence of a radial artery pulse does not rule out RAO, because retrograde flow via palmar arch collaterals can occur (25).

RAO is usually clinically silent, but clinically relevant instances of hand ischemia have been reported (26). Despite the uncommon occurrence of symptomatic RAO, preservation of radial patency is important to preserve access sites for future procedures. Predictors of RAO include low body weight, advanced age, female gender, degree of systemic anticoagulation, the hemostasis process, and a low radial artery diameter to sheath size ratio (27).

Anticoagulation is an effective means of reducing RAO risk. A recent best practices document recommends unfractionated heparin at doses of either 50 U/kg or 5,000 U for inpatients receiving diagnostic transradial procedures (27). Bivalirudin is recommended as an alternative for patients with heparin-induced thrombocytopenia. Unfractionated heparin can be administered either intravenously (IV) or through the arterial sheath (IA) with similar efficacy (28).

In addition to administering anticoagulation, maintaining flow through the radial artery during the hemostasis process is an important parameter in minimizing the incidence of RAO. In a prospective series, absence of blood flow during the hemostasis process significantly increased the risk of RAO (29). In light of this finding, Pancholy studied the concept of maintaining radial artery patency during the hemostasis process, a concept referred to as "patent hemostasis" (30). In this prospective, randomized study, the "patent hemostasis" group had lower rates of RAO than the conventional group at 24-hour follow-up (5% vs. 12%; p < 0.05) and after 30 days (1.8% vs. 7%; p < 0.05), respectively.

Femoral Artery Access

Femoral access remains the most widely used technique for angiography in the United States. Mastery of femoral access is critical for any interventionalist because it remains necessary for procedures requiring larger sheaths, and because transradial approaches are not feasible for many peripheral and structural interventions. The original percutaneous method of obtaining vascular access was pioneered by Seldinger in the 1950s (9). The original method involved performing a posterior wall stick with a needle and stilette, removal of the stilette, and withdrawal of the needle until blood exited the hub of the needle, followed by introduction of a wire into the vascular space. Over time, the technique for femoral artery access has been modified with emphasis on obtaining an anterior wall stick to help minimize potential complications arising from posterior wall access and/or injury. By contrast, radial artery access is most commonly achieved using a posterior wall approach. Traditionally, after local anesthesia with 1% lidocaine, an 18-gauge needle has been used to gain access, which can accommodate a 0.038-inch guide wire. More recently, micropuncture techniques have been popularized, which involve the use of small initial access needles and wires, <21 gauge, with upsizing catheters that ultimately allow placement of a standard guide wire and sheath.

The common femoral artery (CFA) is the continuation of the external iliac artery after it traverses the inguinal ligament. From there, the artery follows the medial side of the head and neck of the femur inferiorly and laterally before splitting into the superficial femoral artery and deep femoral artery. The CFA bifurcation may occur at any level along the course of the vessel. In a study that analyzed 972 femoral angiograms for the level of the CFA bifurcation, results showed that in 64.8% of patients the CFA bifurcation occurred below the inferior border of the head of the femur. In addition, the bifurcation was at or below the midline of the head of the femur in the same population in 98.5% of patients (31). Another important anatomic landmark is the take off and course of the inferior epigastric artery (IEA) and its relation to the arteriotomy site. The origin of the IEA arises from the external iliac, immediately above the inguinal ligament. It curves forward in the subperitoneal tissue, and then ascends obliquely along the medial margin of the abdominal inguinal ring and continues its course cranially. Patients demographics are of limited utility for predicting anatomic variants of the CFA bifurcation and the course of the IEA. The IEA origin has a more variable anatomical pattern, with high border surface area (BSA), male gender, and white race associated with a low IEA origin (32).

The ideal access site into the CFA should be below the most inferior point of the IEA and above the CFA bifurcation anterior to the femoral head (**Fig. 27.2**). As such, in the majority of patients, the ideal access site falls midway between the superior and inferior boarders of the head of the femur (33,34). Access sites below the CFA bifurcation or below the inferior border of the femoral head (whichever is higher), are associated with increased rates of pseudoaneurysms and hematomas, and limit the ultimate size of a sheath that can be used. Access sites above the most inferior deflection of the IEA are problematic in that the EIA is in a retroperitoneal location and can be associated with increased rates of bleeding, especially retroperitoneal hemorrhage (35,36). In addition to minimizing access

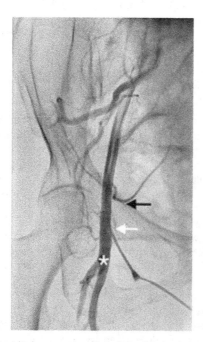

FIGURE 27.2   Ideal access site. Site of arteriotomy (*white arrow*) at the level of the mid femoral head, above the CFA bifurcation (*asterisk*) and below the most inferior border of the inferior epigastric artery (*black arrow*). CFA, common femoral artery.

site complications, CFA access through the anterior wall in an ideal location is necessary for optimal utilization of vascular closure devices.

Considerations Prior to CFA Access

Prior to attaining access, it is prudent to obtain a thorough history and physical and review all previous femoral angiograms available. Even though femoral access can be achieved on almost all patients, it should be reconsidered in patients who may have features that predispose them to an increased risk of femoral artery access complications. These considerations are presented in **Table 27.3**.

Techniques for CFA Access

The first step in obtaining access at any site is appropriate sedation and local anesthesia. Access is the most uncomfortable part of the procedure, thus sedation should be given 3 to 5 minutes prior to starting the procedure. Accessing the CFA in an ideal location may be accomplished more easily in patients with previous femoral angiography, where the relationship between the head of the femur, the CFA bifurcation, and the most inferior border of the IEA can be seen. In patients with no previous invasive or non-invasive femoral angiography, multiple methods have been described to assist the operator achieve in locating an ideal access site. Some of the techniques employed to guide femoral artery access include the use of anatomic landmarks, palpation of the strongest femoral pulse, fluoroscopy, and ultrasound. While all of the other techniques rely on extrapolating the relationship between the CFA and the head of the femur, only ultrasound allows visualization of the CFA and its bifurcation.

When originally described, fluoroscopy guided access (indirect fluoroscopy technique) involved placing a straight tip hemostat or radiopaque marker on the skin to mark the lower edge of the femoral head under fluoroscopy in the posterior–anterior projection. This was considered the skin entry level for retrograde femoral access. From that level, the needle would then be advanced at a 45° angle into the subcutaneous tissue toward the pulse until the needle crosses the anterior wall of the CFA. This technique was tested in a prospective randomized study against the use of bony anatomical landmarks. In this study, fluoroscopy guided access decreased arterial punctures below the femoral head especially in obese patients (3.3%

TABLE 27.3 Considerations Prior to CFA Access
• Patient preference
• Body habitus, especially severe obesity
• Inability to lay flat during or after the procedure
• Prior femoral access site complications
• Presence of a femoral bruit on exam
• Peripheral arterial disease of the lower extremities
• Prior bypass surgery, especially fem-fem bypass
• Prior radiation or surgery to the groin area
• Anticoagulation, bleeding and transfusion considerations
• Severe vessel tortuosity or aneurysmal dilatation
• Active infection in the groin area or skin breakdown
• Non-palpable femoral pulse
• Recent use of some vascular closure devices such as a collagen plug

CFA, common femoral artery.

vs. 6.4% in the traditional arm p = 0.03); however, fluoroscopy did not increase the percentage of patients with ideal arteriotomys in the CFA (31). It is now obvious that the skin entry site should vary depending on the amount of subcutaneous tissue between the skin and the CFA (Fig. 27.3).

Some operators use the direct fluoroscopy technique that goes multiple steps beyond the indirect technique that just locates the bottom of the femoral head. After fluoroscopically locating the inferior border of the femoral head, repeat fluoroscopy is performed after the needle (usually a micro-puncture needle) has been advanced into the subcutaneous tissue, but has not entered the CFA. This will help the operator guide the tip of the needle toward the middle of the femoral head to achieve an ideal puncture site (33,34). Under fluoroscopy, the transition between the micropuncture needle and its wire (needle/wire interface) will represent the site of entry into the CFA (Fig. 27.4). The micropuncture needle has been widely used anecdotally to obtain access into the CFA. Its use was mainly for smaller calcified arteries, or in coagulopathic patients in an attempt to decrease access site complications. More recently, the use of the micropuncture system has been more widely used despite having no data to show that it decreases vascular access site complications. As a matter of fact, a single-center study that evaluated complication rates between the micropuncture system and usual 18-gauge needle access into the CFA showed no difference in the overall complication rates but the risk of retroperitoneal bleed, even though small, was significantly higher in the micropuncture group due to wire migration (and perforation) into smaller pelvic arteries if not visualized while being advanced under fluoroscopy (37).

Fluoroscopy has multiple limitations when obtaining femoral artery access, mainly due to the anatomic variation in the CFA and its bifurcation. Ultrasound-guided access has emerged as an efficient and safe method to access the CFA. This technique offers

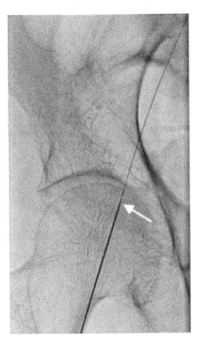

FIGURE 27.4 Fluoroscopy showing the interface or transition between the micropuncture needle and its 0.018-inch wire (*arrow*). This interface represents the site at which the needle entered the artery. In this case, the access was above the ideal position, so the needle/wire were removed and manual pressure was applied for 3 minutes to obtain hemostasis before reattempting access.

multiple advantages over fluoroscopy alone, including direct visualization of the CFA, needle advancement into a healthy part of the CFA through the anterior wall, prevention of accidental venous puncture, and a decrease in the radiation dose to both the patient and the operator. In the FAUST study—a multicenter randomized controlled trial—routine real-time US guidance improved CFA cannulation in patients with high CFA bifurcations. It also reduced the number of attempts to obtain access, decreased the total time to sheath insertion, and decreased the risk of venipuncture (11). In addition, the same study revealed that real-time ultrasound guidance significantly decreased the formation of groin hematomas (11). When using ultrasound-guided access, attempting to cannulate the CFA just above the bifurcation will generally avoid a high arteriotomy, and can be performed consistently with some practice. Nevertheless, this may lead to cannulating the artery below the femoral head in some patients with low CFA bifurcation, increasing the risk of access site complications. A combination of manual palpation of landmarks—or better fluoroscopy—to locate the inferior boarder of the femoral head prior to utilizing ultrasound-guided access will help resolve this possibility (38).

Irrespective of the technique used to obtain access into the CFA, it is important to obtain an access site angiogram at the beginning of the procedure to help risk stratify patients for possible complications. This can be achieved with a small volume of contrast. If the access site is below the femoral head or the CFA bifurcation, then considerations should be thought of prior to upsizing the sheath or giving anticoagulation for an intervention. Similarly, if the access site is above the lowest deflection of the IEA, the risk or retroperitoneal bleeding is increased and similar considerations should be taken (Fig. 27.5A and B). Femoral angiograms also help determine the appropriateness of using a vascular closure device at the end of the procedure based on the access site, size of the CFA, presence of site complications, and of peripheral vascular disease.

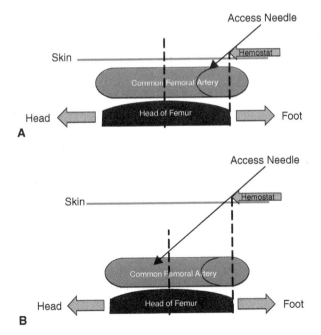

FIGURE 27.3 Illustration showing how the distance between the skin and the common femoral artery can affect the location of the arteriotomy even when the access needle is advanced at the same angle. In both illustrations **A** and **B**, the skin entry site is at the level of the inferior border of the femoral head (From: Abu-Fadel MS, ed. Common femoral artery access. In: *Arterial and Venous Access in the Cardiac Catheterization Lab.* 1st ed. New Brunswick, NJ: Rutgers University Press; 2016:1–20.)

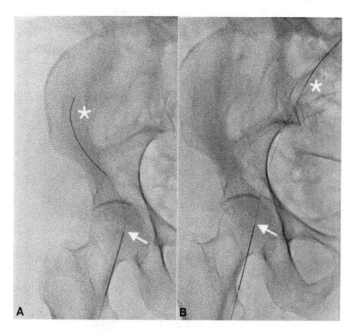

FIGURE 27.5   A: Fluoroscopy showing appropriate access using a micropuncture needle/wire at the level of the middle of the femoral head (*arrow*); however, the micropuncture wire traversed small pelvic arteries (*asterisk*), which may increase the risk of perforation and retroperitoneal bleeding. **B:** Redirecting the wire into the external iliac artery (*asterisk*) prior to dilating the access site and inserting the sheath into the common femoral artery.

Clinical Evidence—Radial Versus Femoral

In a large trial where patients were randomized by access site to either the femoral or the radial artery, the authors noted no difference in procedural success between approaches, while access-related complications were higher in the transfemoral group (3.71% vs. 0.58%, p = 0.0008). They did note a higher rate of access failure (3.5% vs. 0.2%, p < 0.0001) and radiation exposure (41.9 vs. 38.2 Gy cm², p = 0.034) among the radial patients in comparison with the femoral cohort (39). In terms of efficacy, Agostini et al. reported in a meta-analysis of 12 randomized trials that there was no difference in the rate of adverse cardiovascular events (2.1% vs. 2.4%; OR: 0.92; p = 0.7), despite a higher rate of procedural failure (7.2% vs. 2.4%; OR: 3.30; p < 0.001) between radial and femoral access strategies, respectively (40). In the National Cardiovascular Data Registry (NCDR), although the overall rate of transradial PCI was low (1.32%), there was a statistically significant lower risk of bleeding complications (OR 0.42; 95% CI 0.31–0.56) with similar procedural success (OR 1.02; 95% CI 0.92–1.12) (41).

Vorobcsuk et al. reviewed 12 prospective studies comprising 3,324 patients. Similar to prior studies of PCI, there was significantly less bleeding in the transradial group (p = 0.0001); however, they also noted a reduction in mortality (2.04% vs. 3.06%; OR 0.54; p = 0.01) among patients in the transradial as compared with the femoral group (42). In a subsequent analysis of only randomized trials of access sites for patients undergoing primary PCI, the radial approach was associated with lower mortality (OR 0.53; 95% CI 0.33–0.84) and reduced vascular complications (OR 0.35; 95% CI 0.24–0.53) compared to the femoral approach (43).

These observations have been corroborated in several large, modern, randomized trials. In the RIVAL trial, 7,021 patients with acute coronary syndromes were randomized to radial or femoral access. There was no difference in the overall composite primary endpoint of death, myocardial infarction, stroke, or major bleeding at 30 days. Nevertheless, among patients with STEMI, there was a benefit for radial over femoral access for the primary endpoint (p = 0.011), as well as for death (p = 0.001) (44). Most recently, in the MATRIX trial, a randomized study of 8,404 patients with acute coronary syndrome, patients in the radial arm had significant reductions in the primary endpoint of 30-day death, stroke, or bleeding (9.8% vs. 11.7%, p = 0.009). This benefit was driven by statistically significant reductions in death and bleeding (45).

Conclusion

The most common vascular access sites for angiography and interventions include the femoral and radial arteries. Best practice techniques differ for each vascular access site, and must be utilized to minimize difficulties and complications. The femoral artery remains an important access site, especially for peripheral and structural interventions. Knowledge of the anatomy and the course of the CFA, as well as the use of ultrasound guidance may facilitate better and safer femoral access and decrease complication rates. The use of the radial artery is increasing significantly in the United States and seems to provide a safer route for diagnostic and interventional procedures.

Key Points

- Several features are associated with transradial failure, including advanced age, short stature, and prior CABG surgery.
- Careful puncture technique, an antispasmodic "cocktail," and hydrophilic-coated sheaths are the mainstays of RAS prevention.
- Predictors of RAS include younger age, female gender, diabetes, smaller wrist circumference, and lower body weight.
- Predictors of RAO include low body weight, advanced age, female gender, degree of systemic anticoagulation, the hemostasis process, and low radial artery diameter to sheath size ratio.
- Anticoagulation and use of patent hemostasis are effective means to reduce risk of RAO.
- Most randomized trials have demonstrated that radial access is associated with less bleeding and vascular complications.
- Femoral access remains necessary for procedures requiring larger sheaths, and because transradial approaches are not feasible for many peripheral and structural interventions.
- The ideal access site into the CFA should be below the most inferior point of the IEA and above the CFA bifurcation anterior to the femoral head.
- Even though femoral access can be achieved on almost all patients, it should be reconsidered in patients who may have features that predispose them to an increased risk of femoral artery access complications.
- Fluoroscopy has multiple limitations when obtaining femoral artery access, mainly due to the anatomic variation in the CFA and its bifurcation.

■ Ultrasound guided access has emerged as an efficient and safe method to access the CFA and should be considered for all patients.

References

1. Bradley SM, et al. Change in hospital-level use of transradial percutaneous coronary intervention and periprocedural outcomes: insights from the national cardiovascular data registry. *Circ Cardiovasc Qual Outcomes.* 2014;7:550–559.

2. Norgaz T, Gorgulu S, Dagdelen S. Arterial anatomic variations and its influence on transradial coronary procedural outcome. *J Interv Cardiol.* 2012;25:418–424.

3. Ruengsakulrach P, et al. Surgical implications of variations in hand collateral circulation: anatomy revisited. *J Thorac Cardiovasc Surg.* 2001;122:682–686.

4. Dehghani P, et al. Mechanism and predictors of failed transradial approach for percutaneous coronary interventions. *JACC Cardiovasc Interv.* 2009;2:1057–1064.

5. Rathore S, et al. Impact of length and hydrophilic coating of the introducer sheath on radial artery spasm during transradial coronary intervention: a randomized study. *JACC Cardiovasc Interv.* 2010;3:475–483.

6. Saito S, et al. Influence of the ratio between radial artery inner diameter and sheath outer diameter on radial artery flow after transradial coronary intervention. *Catheter Cardiovasc Interv.* 1999;46:173–178.

7. Ball WT, et al. Characterization of operator learning curve for transradial coronary interventions. *Circ Cardiovasc Interv.* 2011;4:336–41.

8. Looi JL, Cave A, El-Jack S. Learning curve in transradial coronary angiography. *Am J Cardiol.* 2011;108:1092–1095.

9. Seldinger SI. Catheter replacement of the needle in percutaneous arteriography; a new technique. *Acta Radiol.* 1953;39:368–376.

10. Pancholy SB, Sanghvi KA, Patel TM. Radial artery access technique evaluation trial: randomized comparison of Seldinger versus modified Seldinger technique for arterial access for transradial catheterization. *Catheter Cardiovasc Interv.* 2012;80:288–291.

11. Seto AH, et al. Real-time ultrasound guidance facilitates transradial access: RAUST (Radial Artery access with Ultrasound Trial). *JACC Cardiovasc Interv.* 2015;8:283–291.

12. Goldberg SL, et al. Learning curve in the use of the radial artery as vascular access in the performance of percutaneous transluminal coronary angioplasty. *Cathet Cardiovasc Diagn.* 1998;44:147–152.

13. Kiemeneij F. Prevention and management of radial artery spasm. *J Invasive Cardiol.* 2006;18:159–160.

14. Coppola J, et al. Nitroglycerin, nitroprusside, or both, in preventing radial artery spasm during transradial artery catheterization. *J Invasive Cardiol.* 2006;18:155–158.

15. Kiemeneij F, et al. Evaluation of a spasmolytic cocktail to prevent radial artery spasm during coronary procedures. *Catheter Cardiovasc Interv.* 2003;58:281–284.

16. Koga S, et al. The use of a hydrophilic-coated catheter during transradial cardiac catheterization is associated with a low incidence of radial artery spasm. *Int J Cardiol.* 2004;96:255–258.

17. Dery JP, Simard S, Barbeau GR. Reduction of discomfort at sheath removal during transradial coronary procedures with the use of a hydrophilic-coated sheath. *Catheter Cardiovasc Interv.* 2001;54:289–294.

18. Caussin C, et al. Reduction in spasm with a long hydrophylic transradial sheath. *Catheter Cardiovasc Interv.* 2010;76:668–672.

19. Dieter RS, Akef A, Wolff M. Eversion endarterectomy complicating radial artery access for left heart catheterization. *Catheter Cardiovasc Interv.* 2003;58:478–480.

20. Pullakhandam NS, et al. Unusual complication of transradial catheterization. *Anesth Analg.* 2006;103:794–795.

21. Slogoff S, Keats AS, Arlund C. On the safety of radial artery cannulation. *Anesthesiology.* 1983;59:42–47.

22. Rathore S, et al. A randomized comparison of TR band and radistop hemostatic compression devices after transradial coronary intervention. *Catheter Cardiovasc Interv.* 2010;76:660–667.

23. Barbeau GR, et al. Evaluation of the ulnopalmar arterial arches with pulse oximetry and plethysmography: comparison with the Allen's test in 1010 patients. *Am Heart J.* 2004;147:489–493.

24. Stella PR, et al. Incidence and outcome of radial artery occlusion following transradial artery coronary angioplasty. *Cathet Cardiovasc Diagn.* 1997;40:156–158.

25. Greenwood MJ, et al. Vascular communications of the hand in patients being considered for transradial coronary angiography: is the Allen's test accurate? *J Am Coll Cardiol.* 2005;46:2013–2017.

26. Valentine RJ, Modrall JG, Clagett GP. Hand ischemia after radial artery cannulation. *J Am Coll Surg.* 2005;201:18–22.

27. Rao SV, et al. Best practices for transradial angiography and intervention: a consensus statement from the society for cardiovascular angiography and intervention's transradial working group. *Catheter Cardiovasc Interv.* 2014;83:228–236.

28. Pancholy SB. Comparison of the effect of intra-arterial versus intravenous heparin on radial artery occlusion after transradial catheterization. *Am J Cardiol.* 2009;104:1083–1085.

29. Sanmartin M, et al. Interruption of blood flow during compression and radial artery occlusion after transradial catheterization. *Catheter Cardiovasc Interv.* 2007;70:185–189.

30. Pancholy S, et al. Prevention of radial artery occlusion-patent hemostasis evaluation trial (PROPHET study): a randomized comparison of traditional versus patency documented hemostasis after transradial catheterization. *Catheter Cardiovasc Interv.* 2008;72:335–340.

31. Abu-Fadel MS, et al. Fluoroscopy vs. traditional guided femoral arterial access and the use of closure devices: a randomized controlled trial. *Catheter Cardiovasc Interv.* 2009;74(4):533–539.

32. Seto AH, et al. Defining the common femoral artery: Insights from the femoral arterial access with ultrasound trial. *Catheter Cardiovasc Interv.* 2017;89(7):1185–1192.

33. Cilingiroglu M, et al. Fluoroscopically-guided micropuncture femoral artery access for large-caliber sheath insertion. *J Invasive Cardiol.* 2011;23(4):157–161.

34. Abu-Fadel MS, ed. Common femoral artery access. In: *Arterial and Venous Access in the Cardiac Catheterization Lab.* 1st ed. New Brunswick, NJ: Rutgers University Press; 2016:1–20.

35. Sherev DA, Shaw RE, Brent BN. Angiographic predictors of femoral access site complications: implication for planned percutaneous coronary intervention. *Catheter Cardiovasc Interv.* 2005;65:196–202.

36. Tiroch KA, Matheny ME, Resnic FS. Quantitative impact of cardiovascular risk factors and vascular closure devices on the femoral artery after repeat cardiac catheterization. *Am Heart J.* 2010;159(1):125–130.

37. Ben-Dor I, et al. A novel, minimally invasive access technique versus standard 18-gauge needle set for femoral access. *Catheter Cardiovasc Interv.* 2012;79(7):1180–1185.

38. Seto AH, Patel, A. Ultrasound-guided arterial and venous access. In: Abu-Fadel MS, ed. *Arterial and Venous Access in the Cardiac Catheterization Lab.* 1st ed. New Brunswick, NJ: Rutgers University Press; 2016:117–151.

39. Brueck M, et al. A randomized comparison of transradial versus transfemoral approach for coronary angiography and angioplasty. *JACC Cardiovasc Interv.* 2009;2:1047–1054.

40. Agostoni P, et al. Radial versus femoral approach for percutaneous coronary diagnostic and interventional procedures; systematic overview and meta-analysis of randomized trials. *J Am Coll Cardiol.* 2004;44:349–356.

41. Rao SV, et al. Trends in the prevalence and outcomes of radial and femoral approaches to percutaneous coronary intervention: a report from the National Cardiovascular Data Registry. *JACC Cardiovasc Interv.* 2008;1:379–386.

42. Vorobcsuk A, et al. Transradial versus transfemoral percutaneous coronary intervention in acute myocardial infarction systematic overview and meta-analysis. *Am Heart J.* 2009;158:814–821.

43. Joyal D, et al. Meta-analysis of ten trials on the effectiveness of the radial versus the femoral approach in primary percutaneous coronary intervention. *Am J Cardiol.* 2012;109:813–818.

44. Jolly SS, et al. Radial versus femoral access for coronary angiography and intervention in patients with acute coronary syndromes (RIVAL): a randomised, parallel group, multicentre trial. *Lancet.* 2011;377:1409–1420.

45. Valgimigli M, et al. Radial versus femoral access in patients with acute coronary syndromes undergoing invasive management: a randomised multicentre trial. *Lancet.* 2015;385:2465–2476.

28 Vascular Access Site Management (Closure Devices and Complications)

Robert J. Applegate, MD, FACC, FAHA, MSCAI

Vascular access is required for all percutaneous endovascular procedures, and management of the access site is necessary at the completion of all of these procedures. Although access itself is simply a means to an end, unfortunate and potentially life-threatening complications can arrive at the access site independent of the outcomes of the actual endovascular procedure. Accordingly, it is crucial to the success of the endovascular procedure that optimal technique and best practices be employed when gaining vascular access and when obtaining hemostasis of the access site.

Femoral artery access and use of intravascular sheaths heralded the modern era of interventional cardiology, replacing cut down of the brachial artery as a predominant arterial access site. Because of its relative ease of access and size, accommodating most endovascular diagnostic and procedural devices, the femoral artery access site was preferred over brachial and radial access. The location of the common femoral artery (CFA) over the femoral head of the femur allows hemostasis to be achieved by manual compression using the femoral head as an anvil against which the femoral artery can be compressed. In the early 1990s, two interventional procedures—atherectomy and stents—severely challenged the safety and effectiveness of traditional manual compression. In response to the larger-bore arterial sheaths, as well as the intense anticoagulation regimen used with the first stents, vascular closure devices (VCDs) were developed and refined to accelerate the time to hemostasis and ambulation in the hopes of reducing vascular complications.

Indications and Guidelines for Use

VCDs have been FDA-approved since 1993 for use in closure of femoral artery access sites following diagnostic or interventional endovascular procedures. The safety and efficacy of these devices are optimized when used with a CFA access site, or when there is an appropriately sized landing zone (from 4 to 6 mm, varying by device type), and in the absence of severe access site atherosclerotic disease or calcification—although there are no clinical data specifically evaluating these standards (Table 28.1). In 2011, the ACCF/AHA/SCAI/PCI guideline update outlined several indications for vascular closure device use (Table 28.2) (1). Performing femoral angiography prior to use of a vascular closure device was given a Class I indication. A Class IIa recommendation was given for the use of VCDs for the purposes of achieving faster hemostasis and earlier ambulation compared with the use of manual compression. Nevertheless, the routine use of VCDs for the purpose of decreasing vascular complications including bleeding, received a Class III indication, no benefit. These latter two recommendations were based on existing clinical trial data comparing the safety and efficacy of VCDs to manual compression, showing that while VCDs consistently reduced time to hemostasis and ambulation compared to manual compression, they did not reduce the incidence of vascular complications (2–4).

There is general expert consensus that VCDs should not be routinely used in high sticks into the external iliac artery (above the common femoral artery angiographically demarcated by the inferior most border of the inferior epigastric artery), or in low sticks (i.e., below the bifurcation of the CFA into the profunda and superficial femoral arteries). In three independent registries, the use of a VCD was associated with a 1.4- to 2.3-fold higher odds ratio of a vascular complication in patients when it was used in the presence of a high stick, although in two of these studies the confidence intervals crossed 0 and were not statistically significant (5–7). Small registries have also evaluated the use of VCDs for brachial, axillary, antegrade femoral, and popliteal artery access (8). Nevertheless, the data are limited, and firm understanding of their safety and effectiveness in these alternative arterial access sites is lacking. Similarly, VCDs

---

TABLE 28.1 VCD Instructions for Use

Indications

- For use in closing and reducing time to hemostasis at the femoral artery puncture site for cardiac catheterization or interventional procedures.
- For use to allow ambulation as soon as possible after sheath removal.

Contraindications

- None

Warnings

- Do not use if the puncture site is at or distal to the common femoral artery bifurcation, or is proximal to the inguinal ligament.
- Do not use if there is posterior wall or multiple punctures.

Precautions

- Maintain sterility at all times during use of the devices.
- See specific device instructions.

VCD, vascular closure device.

TABLE 28.2 2011 ACCF/AHA/SCAI PCI Guidelines

Vascular Closure Devices: Recommendations

- Class I
  - Patients considered for vascular closure devices should undergo a femoral angiogram to ensure their anatomic suitability for deployment (level of evidence: C).
- Class IIa
  - The use of vascular closure devices is reasonable for the purposes of achieving faster hemostasis and earlier ambulation compared with the use of manual compression (level of evidence: B).
- Class III: NO BENEFIT
  - The routine use of vascular closure devices is not recommended for the purpose of decreasing vascular complications, including bleeding (level of evidence: B).

PCI, percutaneous coronary interventions.

have been used to close large venous access sites, but the data are extremely limited concerning the safety and efficacy of this procedure.

From the very outset of clinical introduction of VCDs, it was recognized that there was a learning curve associated with achieving optimal outcomes with these devices (9,10). Proficiency was dependent on both operator and institutional VCD and overall femoral artery experience, and also varied by device. Each currently available device has its own unique delivery system, and requires specific training on that device to achieve proficiency. In a recent study, Resnic et al. quantified the learning curve associated with use of the StarClose closure device from the National Cardiovascular Data Registry (NCDR) Cath/PCI registry (11). In 107,710 procedures with at least one VCD deployment, they found device success of 93% increasing to 97% at the end of the 2-year study period (2006–2007). They identified a triphasic learning curve: initial rapid learning from 0 to 22 cases followed by declining success rate in the next 23 to 50 cases with a final recovery to improved device success, requiring more than 50 cases (**Fig. 28.1**).

Infection Control

There were several case reports of early generation suture-based devices associated with access site infections (12). In hindsight, it was recognized that this most likely arose from the considerable tissue tract manipulation required for placement of these devices, as well as the "foreign body" left in the vessel itself. Nevertheless, and because of these reports, VCDs are discouraged in the presence of active local groin infections. Additionally, all of the device manufacturers strongly recommend complete re-prepping of the access site, as well as re-gloving of the operators, prior to the deployment of a VCD. Use of prophylactic antibiotics has been advocated by some in analogy to the recommendations for other minor surgical procedures involving manipulation of the vasculature within placement of in-dwelling devices such as pacemaker leads, but there are no clinical data to guide practice.

Re-Access After Use of VCD

The clinical scenario of having a VCD placed after a diagnostic procedure, and then needing to re-access that same access site is not uncommon. Nevertheless, there are only limited observational data suggesting that re-access is safe and effective. Applegate et al.

evaluated the safety of re-access in 181 patients following placement of an Angio-Seal device 1 day to 180 days after the initial VCD was placed, and observed three hematomas >5 cm as the only adverse outcome of this practice (13). Although other clinical data are lacking, re-access using other VCDs is commonly performed in routine practice.

Classification of VCDs

Currently, seven types of VCDs are FDA-approved for use in the United States (**Table 28.3**) (14). VCDs can be characterized by their mechanism of hemostasis, as well as whether or not there is any permanent intravascular element. The term "active approximation" is used to indicate that a mechanical seal of the opening of the arterial wall is achieved with the closure device. Active approximation devices include Angio-Seal, FISH, Perclose, and StarClose (**Fig. 28.2A**). The term "passive approximation" is used to indicate that hemostasis is achieved by tamponading the arterial access site just above the artery. Passive approximation devices include EXOSEAL, MYNX, and Vascade VCS (**Fig. 28.2B**). Passive approximation devices are also known as extravascular sealants because there is no intravascular element present at the completion of the closure. Each of the passive approximation devices utilize a vessel locator system using an intravascular identification system that is subsequently removed at completion of the closure. The Angio-Seal, FISH, and Perclose devices all have an intravascular component (with Angio-Seal and FISH bioresorbable), and at times the StarClose device may have a tine that is intravascular as well. Each manufacturer has guidelines for the puncture site size range of use for their device, although in clinical practice any of these devices can be used for sheath sizes up to 8 Fr in size. The lower limit of suitable vessel size for closure has not been rigorously studied, although it is generally accepted that vessels smaller than 4 to 5 mm are not optimal for VCD use.

Specific VCDs—Active Approximation

Angio-Seal

The Angio-Seal device (St. Jude Medical; St. Paul, MN) consists of an intraluminal polylactic-polyglycolic acid polymer anchor (2 × 11 mm) attached to a bioresorbable suture over which a collagen

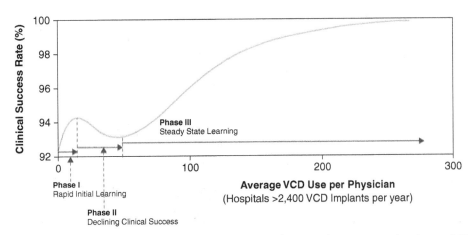

FIGURE 28.1 Graph of clinical success rate of use of the StarClose device as a function of average vascular closure device (VCD) use per physician. (Adapted from: Resnic FS, et al. Quantifying the learning curve in the use of a novel vascular closure device: an analysis of the NCDR (National Cardiovascular Data Registry) CathPCI registry. *JACC Cardiovasc Interv.* 2012;5(1):82–89.)

TABLE 28.3 Vascular Closure Devices FDA Approved 2017

CLOSURE DEVICE	TYPE	PRODUCTS	COMMENTS
Active Approximation Devices			
Angio-Seal	Bioresorbable intraluminal, anchor, suture, and collagen form arteriotomy sandwich	Evolution	Automated compaction
		STS Plus	Self-tightening suture
		VIP	V twist collagen
FISH	Small intestinal mucosa (SIS) plug pulled against vessel wall creates mechanical seal	CombiClose	Combined working sheath and closure device
		ControlClose	
Perclose	Suture-based "surgical" arterial wall closure	Perclose A-T	Braided suture with preformed knot
		ProGlide	Monofilament suture with preformed knot
		ProStar XL	Two braided and untied sutures
StarClose	Nitinol clip delivered onto vessel creates "purse string" closure	StarClose SE	Two major and four minor tissue tines
Passive Approximation Devices (Extravascular)			
EXOSEAL	Extravascular polyglycolic acid plug	EXOSEAL	Accurate extravascular placement
MYNX	Extravascular sealant	MYNX ACE	Seals arteriotomy and expands to fill tissue track
		MYNXGRIP	Active tissue adherence of sealant
Cardiva Catalyst	Collapsible disc with collagen patch (Vascade)	Cardiva Catalyst II	Collapsible disc with procoagulant material
		Cardiva Catalyst III	Additional thrombogenic material for anticoagulated patients
		Vascade	Collapsible disc with extravascular patch

plug is compressed against the external wall of the artery and is ultimately secured by a knot, forming an "arteriotomy sandwich" at the access site (Fig. 28.2A). The anchor is non-thrombogenic, and all of the components are bioresorbable, with chemically complete bioresorption occurring by 3 months. The device is introduced with its own delivery sheath and is available in 6 and 8 Fr sizes. The most recent iteration of the device, "Evolution" uses an automation tamping mechanism designed to optimize site closure.

FISH

The FISH device (Morris Innovative; Bloomington, IN) incorporates a sleeve of small intestinal mucosa (SIS) within the closure sheath (Fig. 28.2A). Hemostasis is attained immediately after sheath removal when the SIS is pulled up against the inner surface of the arterial wall at the access site and embedded into the arterial wall at the access site, secured by a bioresorbable extravascular plug. It is fully bioresorbable. The device can be either a standalone closure device (ControlClose) or a combination working sheath and closure device (CombiClose).

Perclose

The Perclose devices (Abbott Vascular; Redwood City, CA) ProGlide and ProStar both achieve percutaneous suture mediated closure in a fashion analogous to that obtained by direct surgical closure of a vessel. The ProGlide device deploys two sutures through the anterior wall of the artery, which is received by the footplate within the artery and then exteriorized (Fig. 28.2A). The device is then removed from the artery, leaving a pre-tied suture knot, with hemostasis achieved by tightening of the knot onto the surface of the artery. The 10-Fr

ProStar device requires tissue track manipulation to position the barrel of the receiving portion of the device with needles from inside the vessel wall into the receiving barrels, followed by exteriorization of the sutures. The sutures then are used to tie knots that are pushed down onto the artery's surface, achieving hemostasis. It is generally accepted that these devices can be used for ≤10 Fr or smaller sheath size closures. As will be discussed later, the devices can additionally be used for preclosure of large bore arteriotomies with more than one device.

StarClose

The StarClose device (Abbott Vascular; Redwood City, CA) delivers a nitinol clip to close the arteriotomy from the extravascular side to achieve hemostasis (Fig. 28.2A). The nitinol clip has two major and four minor tines that create a "purse string" type of closure at the surface of the arterial wall, with the tines secured within the arterial wall itself. The StarClose device is inserted over a wire through a sheath that comes with the device and which is specifically designed and required for use. A retractable anchor is used to ensure satisfactory positioning at the arteriotomy site, and then the clip is deployed on the exterior surface of the vessel.

Passive Approximation Devices

EXOSEAL

The EXOSEAL device (Cordis; Miami, FL) delivers an extravascular plug to the arteriotomy site. The plug consists of completely bioresorbable polyglycolic acid and achieves hemostasis by manual compression

Angio-Seal

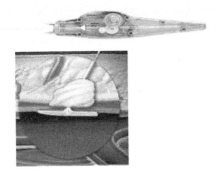

FISH

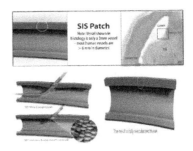

Perclose

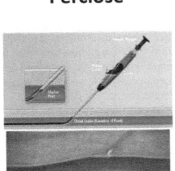

Starclose

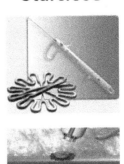
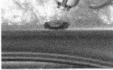

A

Passive approximation devices

Exoseal

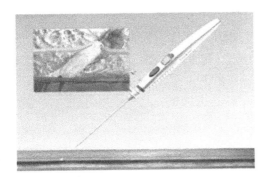

Mynx

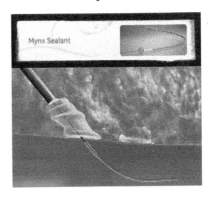

Vascade VCS

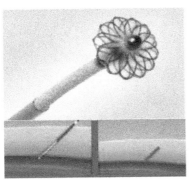

B

FIGURE 28.2   **A:** Cartoons of active approximation devices. **B:** Cartoon of passive approximation devices.

of the arteriotomy site under the femoral sheath (Fig. 28.2B). A vessel locator system prevents intravascular insertion of the plug, and allows very accurate placement of the plug.

MYNX

The MYNX VCD (Cordis; Miami, FL) utilizes an extravascular polyethylene glycol (PEG) sealant, which is completely bioresorbable, to achieve hemostasis. An intravascular balloon is pulled up against the inner surface of the artery through a delivery sheath, anchoring the device while the PEG plug is positioned on the exterior surface of the vessel (Fig. 28.2B). Within minutes, the plug hydrates and expands to form an extravascular seal above the vessel and within the tissue tract. MYNXGRIP was engineered to provide avid sealant adherence to tissue to prevent movement of the plug after deployment.

Vascade Vascular Closure System

The Vascade vascular closure system (Cardiva Medical Inc.; Santa Clara, CA) incorporates an extravascular collagen plug to the traditional Vascade footplate-facilitated manual compression system (Fig. 28.2B). After being put in place, the collagen plug is positioned in the track above the access site; the footplate is then removed, creating an external seal.

Clinical Evaluation of Safety and Efficacy of VCDs Since the Last SCAI Review

The first-generation VCDs, Angio-Seal and Perclose, as well as the VCDs most recently introduced into the market, have undergone a series of modifications designed to enhance their effectiveness and ease of use. Some of these modifications include the downsizing of devices, the streamlining of transitioning points into and out of the artery, simplifying and ensuring suture capture for the Perclose device,

and standardized device deployment techniques. As a reflection of these changes, the VCD deployment success rate increased from approximately 88% seen in the original randomized clinical trials to over 95% in the two most recent randomized trials, which are discussed in the next section.

Randomized Clinical Trials

ISAR CLOSURE compared the safety and efficacy of two closure devices, FemoSeal (St. Jude Medical; St Paul, MN) and EXOSEAL (Cordis; Miami, FL) to manual compression in patients undergoing transfemoral angiography (15). One thousand five hundred and nine patients received the FemoSeal device, 1,506 the EXOSEAL device, and 1,509 patients underwent manual compression. The primary endpoint of the study was access site complications at 30 days (Table 28.4). Overall rates of access site complications for VCDs was 6.9% compared to 7.9% for manual compression, p for non-inferiority <0.01. Nevertheless, rates of hematoma >5 cm were higher in the manual compression group (6.8%) compared to VCD (4.8%), p = 0.06. The authors concluded that, in patients undergoing transfemoral angiography, the use of VCDs were non-inferior to manual compression for overall vascular closure rates, although there were lower rates of hematoma >5 cm with VCD use.

The CLOSE UP Study compared the FemoSeal vascular closure device to manual compression in 1,001 patients undergoing diagnostic angiography (16). The primary endpoint was groin hematoma >5 cm which occurred in 2.2% of the Femoseal group compared to 6.7% of the manual compression group, p = 0.002 (Table 28.5). All major adverse vascular events at 14 days occurred in 0.6% of the Femoseal group, and 1.0% of the manual group, p = NS (Table 28.6). Similar to the ISAR CLOSURE Study, the authors concluded that, in patients undergoing diagnostic angiography via the femoral artery, use of a VCD resulted in similar overall rates of vascular complication, but lower rates of hematoma >5 cm.

TABLE 28.4 Outcomes at 30 Days

	NO. (%) OF PATIENTS			
	VASCULAR CLOSURE DEVICE (n = 3,015)	MANUAL COMPRESSION (n = 1,509)	DIFFERENCE IN PROPORTIONS, % (95% CI)	P VALUE
Vascular access site complications (primary endpoint)[a]	208 (6.9)	119 (7.9)	−1 (−2.7 to 0.7)	<0.001[b]
Hematoma ≥5 cm	145 (4.8)	102 (6.8)	−2 (−3.4 to −0.4)	0.006
Pseudoaneurysm	53 (1.8)	23 (1.5)	0.3 (−0.5 to 1.1)	0.56
Arteriovenous fistula	12 (0.4)	2 (0.1)	0.3 (−0.1 to 0.6)	0.13
Access site–related major bleeding[c]	3 (0.1)	3 (0.2)	−0.1 (−0.4 to 0.2)	0.39
Acute ipsilateral leg ischemia	0	0		
Need for vascular surgical or interventional treatment	0	0		
Local infection	1	0		0.48
Secondary Endpoints				
Time to hemostasis, median (IQR), min	1 (0.5 to 2.0)	10 (10 to 15)		<0.001
Repeat manual compression	53 (1.8)	10 (0.7)		0.003

[a]Primary endpoint defined as the composite of hematoma at least 5 cm in size, pseudoaneurysm, arteriovenous fistula, access site–related major bleeding, acute ipsilateral leg ischemia, need for vascular surgical or interventional treatment, or local infection.
[b]p value from the non-inferiority analysis.
[c]Based on criteria form REPLACE-2 (Randomized Evaluation in PCI Linking Angiomax to Reduced Clinical Events).
IQR, interquartile range; PCI, percutaneous coronary interventions.

TABLE 28.5 The Individual Components of Major Adverse Vascular Events (MAVE)

	MANUAL COMPRESSION (n = 500)	FEMOSEAL (n = 501)	p VALUE
Pseudoaneurysm	1 (0.2)	2 (0.4)	1.00
Infection	2 (0.4)	1 (0.2)	1.00
Need for vascular surgery	0 (0)	0 (0)	1.00
Major bleeding	2 (0.4)	0 (0)	0.50
Retroperitoneal bleeding	0 (0)	0 (0)	1.00

Values are n (%). Fisher's exact test was used.
Adapted from: Holm NR, et al. Randomised comparison of manual compression and FemoSeal™ vascular closure device for closure after femoral artery access coronary angiography: the CLOSure dEvices Used in everyday Practice (CLOSE-UP) study. *EuroIntervention*. 2014;9:183–190.

TABLE 28.6 Individual Rates of Haematoma >5 cm

	MANUAL COMPRESSION (n = 500)	FEMOSEAL (n = 501)	p VALUE
In-hospital (primary endpoint)	31 (6.2)	11 (2.2)	0.002
At 14 days (self-reporting)	38 (8.7)	29 (6.4)	0.20
14-day total (self-reporting)	38 (8.7)	29 (6.4)	0.20

Values are n (%). Fisher's exact test or chi-square test was used.
Adapted from: Holm NR, et al. Randomised comparison of manual compression and FemoSeal™ vascular closure device for closure after femoral artery access coronary angiography: the CLOSure dEvices Used in everyday Practice (CLOSE-UP) study. *EuroIntervention*. 2014;9:183–190.

A network meta-analysis of the safety of VCDs obtained from randomized clinical trials conducted from 1992 to 2014 has recently been published (17). They identified 40 randomized trials comprising 16,868 patients undergoing either diagnostic angiography or PCI from a transfemoral approach. Twenty eight of the trials were performed before 2005, while 12 of the trials were performed after 2005. The risk ratio for vascular complications of VCD compared to manual compression was 1.05 (95% CI, 0.83–1.32) for those studies before 2005, while the risk ratio was 0.64 (95% CI, 0.46–0.89) after 2005 (Fig. 28.3). The authors concluded that there was substantial heterogeneity in study design and outcomes among the studies. Despite this, there appeared to be a temporal trend toward lower rates of vascular complication with VCD use compared to manual compression after 2005, as opposed to those before 2005. Whether these results will change the guidelines outlining the indications for VCD use for improving safety remains to be determined.

Registries

Three very large contemporary registries merit mention. An instrumental variable analysis from the ACC NCDR Cath/PCI registry of cases performed between 2009 and 2013 identified 1,053,155 VCDs used during 2,056,585 PCIs (18). The overall absolute rate of vascular complication was 1.5%, with VCD use associated with a 0.4% absolute reduction in vascular complications (95% CI, 0.31–0.42); the number needed to treat to prevent one vascular complication: 250. The authors concluded that VCD use after PCI is associated with a significant but very small reduction in overall major bleeding compared to manual compression. The British Cardiovascular Intervention Society identified 271,845 patients undergoing PCI between 2006 and 2011 (19). They evaluated 30-day mortality stratified by VCD use or manual compression. VCD use was associated with 1.8% mortality at 30 days compared to 2.0% for manual compression, a hazard ratio of 0.91 (95% CI, 0.86–0.97, p < 0.01); after propensity score matching adjustment. The authors concluded that the use of a VCD was associated with a significant but small reduction in 30-day all-cause mortality. Finally, the Blue

Cross Blue Shield Cardiovascular Consortium of Michigan identified 85,048 PCIs occurring between 2007 and 2009 with VCD use in 28,528 (20). A vascular complication occurred in 1.9% of the overall study. After propensity score matching adjustment, the odds ratio of a vascular complication was 0.78 for VCD use compared to manual compression (95% CI, 0.67–0.90); p = 0.01. The odds ratio of transfusions for VCD use compared to manual compression was 0.85 (95% CI, 0.74–0.96), p = 0.011. The authors concluded that the use of a VCD was associated with a modest relative decrease in overall vascular complications and transfusions compared to manual compression, which was attenuated if glycoprotein IIb/IIIa inhibitors were used. They also noted that VCD use was associated with a small but significant relative increase in retroperitoneal bleeding compared to manual compression.

Head-to-Head Comparisons of VCD Types

There have been multiple small registries, and more than 10 randomized clinical trials, that have compared the safety and efficacy of one closure device to another (17). These studies have been limited by small study size and heterogeneity in study design and outcomes, weakening the strength of conclusions that can be reached from the comparisons. Current expert consensus opinion suggests that currently there are no definitive data showing that one device is superior to others with regard to safety and efficacy.

Clinical Utility of VCDs

With a growing emphasis on outpatient management of PCI patients, the use of VCDs to facilitate same-day PCI discharge has been evaluated in several small studies and found to be both safe and efficacious. Rao et al. evaluated clinical outcomes of 107,018 patients 65 years or older undergoing PCI from the ACC NCDR Cath/PCI registry (21). They identified 1,339 patients who underwent same-day PCI discharge, with femoral access used in 96% and VCD used in 65% of those patients. The authors found no difference in the rates of

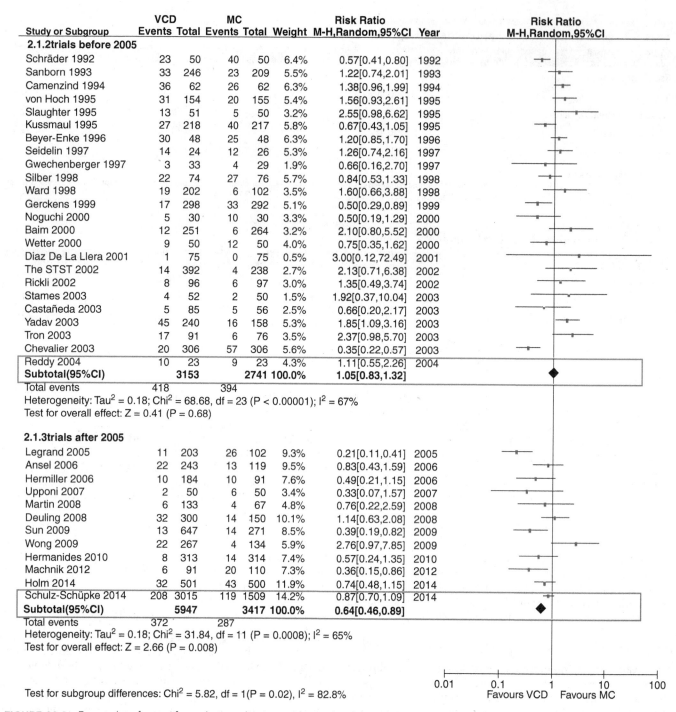

Study or Subgroup	VCD Events	Total	MC Events	Total	Weight	Risk Ratio M-H,Random,95%CI	Year
2.1.2 trials before 2005							
Schräder 1992	23	50	40	50	6.4%	0.57[0.41,0.80]	1992
Sanborn 1993	33	246	23	209	5.5%	1.22[0.74,2.01]	1993
Camenzind 1994	36	62	26	62	6.3%	1.38[0.96,1.99]	1994
von Hoch 1995	31	154	20	155	5.4%	1.56[0.93,2.61]	1995
Slaughter 1995	13	51	5	50	3.2%	2.55[0.98,6.62]	1995
Kussmaul 1995	27	218	40	217	5.8%	0.67[0.43,1.05]	1995
Beyer-Enke 1996	30	48	25	48	6.3%	1.20[0.85,1.70]	1996
Seidelin 1997	14	24	12	26	5.3%	1.26[0.74,2.16]	1997
Gwechenberger 1997	3	33	4	29	1.9%	0.66[0.16,2.70]	1997
Silber 1998	22	74	27	76	5.7%	0.84[0.53,1.33]	1998
Ward 1998	19	202	6	102	3.5%	1.60[0.66,3.88]	1998
Gerckens 1999	17	298	33	292	5.1%	0.50[0.29,0.89]	1999
Noguchi 2000	5	30	10	30	3.3%	0.50[0.19,1.29]	2000
Baim 2000	12	251	6	264	3.2%	2.10[0.80,5.52]	2000
Wetter 2000	9	50	12	50	4.0%	0.75[0.35,1.62]	2000
Diaz De La Llera 2001	1	75	0	75	0.5%	3.00[0.12,72.49]	2001
The STST 2002	14	392	4	238	2.7%	2.13[0.71,6.38]	2002
Rickli 2002	8	96	6	97	3.0%	1.35[0.49,3.74]	2002
Stames 2003	4	52	2	50	1.5%	1.92[0.37,10.04]	2003
Castañeda 2003	5	85	5	56	2.5%	0.66[0.20,2.17]	2003
Yadav 2003	45	240	16	158	5.3%	1.85[1.09,3.16]	2003
Tron 2003	17	91	6	76	3.5%	2.37[0.98,5.70]	2003
Chevalier 2003	20	306	57	306	5.6%	0.35[0.22,0.57]	2003
Reddy 2004	10	23	9	23	4.3%	1.11[0.55,2.26]	2004
Subtotal(95%CI)		**3153**		**2741**	**100.0%**	**1.05[0.83,1.32]**	
Total events	418		394				

Heterogeneity: Tau² = 0.18; Chi² = 68.68, df = 23 (P < 0.00001); I² = 67%
Test for overall effect: Z = 0.41 (P = 0.68)

Study or Subgroup	VCD Events	Total	MC Events	Total	Weight	Risk Ratio M-H,Random,95%CI	Year
2.1.3 trials after 2005							
Legrand 2005	11	203	26	102	9.3%	0.21[0.11,0.41]	2005
Ansel 2006	22	243	13	119	9.5%	0.83[0.43,1.59]	2006
Hermiller 2006	10	184	10	91	7.6%	0.49[0.21,1.15]	2006
Upponi 2007	2	50	6	50	3.4%	0.33[0.07,1.57]	2007
Martin 2008	6	133	4	67	4.8%	0.76[0.22,2.59]	2008
Deuling 2008	32	300	14	150	10.1%	1.14[0.63,2.08]	2008
Sun 2009	13	647	14	271	8.5%	0.39[0.19,0.82]	2009
Wong 2009	22	267	4	134	5.9%	2.76[0.97,7.85]	2009
Hermanides 2010	8	313	14	314	7.4%	0.57[0.24,1.35]	2010
Machnik 2012	6	91	20	110	7.3%	0.36[0.15,0.86]	2012
Holm 2014	32	501	43	500	11.9%	0.74[0.48,1.15]	2014
Schulz-Schüpke 2014	208	3015	119	1509	14.2%	0.87[0.70,1.09]	2014
Subtotal(95%CI)		**5947**		**3417**	**100.0%**	**0.64[0.46,0.89]**	
Total events	372		287				

Heterogeneity: Tau² = 0.18; Chi² = 31.84, df = 11 (P = 0.0008); I² = 65%
Test for overall effect: Z = 2.66 (P = 0.008)

Test for subgroup differences: Chi² = 5.82, df = 1(P = 0.02), I² = 82.8%

FIGURE 28.3 Forest plot of rates of vascular complications with vascular closure device (VCD) use or manual compression (MC) in studies before 2005 (*upper panel*) and after 2005 (*lower panel*). (Adapted from: Jiang J, et al. Network meta-analysis of randomized trials on the safety of vascular closure devices for femoral arterial puncture site haemostasis. *Sci Rep.* 2015;5:13761.)

death or re-hospitalization in the same-day discharge group 0.37% (95% CI, 0.16–0.87) versus overnight stay 0.5% (95% CI, 0.46–0.54, p = 0.51). Although use of transradial interventions has grown, principally because of the appeal of this access site for same-day PCI discharge, there are currently no conclusive data comparing outcomes of the radial artery to femoral artery access with VCD use on the safety and efficacy of these different access approaches.

The recent tremendous growth in the use of large-bore (i.e., >10 Fr) sheaths for both structural heart and endovascular procedures

has spurred interest in the percutaneous management of access sites. Currently, only the Perclose suture-based device allows preclosure of large-bore access sites. Preclosure is achieved by use of either one ProStar or two ProGlides through smaller procedural sheaths (typically, 6 Fr), with the sutures exteriorized but without tying the knots down to the surface of the artery. In the case of the use of two ProGlides, they are typically oriented 30° to 60° apart (on a clock face). At the end of the case, a number of strategies have been used to minimize bleeding while the preclosed sutures are tightened, allowing hemostasis. The preclosure technique, eliminating the need for surgical cut down, has allowed transition from general anesthesia to deep sedation and earlier ambulation of patients. The PEVAR trial (Percutaneous Access Versus Open Femoral Exposure for Endovascular Aortic Aneurysm Repair) compared clinical outcomes of 30 days using preclosure with ProGlide (n = 50), preclosure with ProStar (n = 51) or open femoral exposure (n = 101) (22). The primary endpoint of treatment success (composite of procedural technical success and absence of vascular complications) occurred in 88% of ProGlide patients, 78% of ProStar patients, and 78% of femoral exposure patients. ProGlide treatment success was non-inferior to femoral exposure, but ProStar was not non-inferior to femoral exposure.

Complications of VCDs

Both manual compression and VCD use can be associated with local access site complications, including hematoma formation, pseudoaneurysm, arterial venous fistulae, leg ischemia and occlusion, nerve injury, and infection and bleeding. The actual rates of vascular complications vary widely based on reporting methodology, time of assessment and definitions used (Table 28.7) (23). Hematoma >5 cm is far and away the most common access site complication. Nevertheless, major vascular complications occur in less than 1% of patients overall. The use of a VCD introduces several additional concerns following diagnostic angiography or intervention. Following an interventional procedure requiring systemic anticoagulation, failure of the device to achieve hemostasis can lead to immediate and potentially life-threatening bleeding. In those circumstances, failed closure has been associated with an increase of adverse vascular complications, including major vascular complications. In these circumstances, immediate hemostasis is needed with manual compression, and may require endovascular rescue, with contralateral access and a balloon or covered stent tamponade of the access site. While surgical closure is feasible, it is often impractical because of the time required to mobilize a surgical team. Use of a VCD may also be associated with embolization of device components. Embolization of an Angio-Seal anchor, intraluminal deployment of VasoSeal, and collagen thrombus from a DUETT device (the latter two are no longer clinically available) have all been reported and variably associated with morbidity. Additionally, all of the VCDs have been associated with local ischemic complications, although the mechanism leading to the ischemia differs for each of the different devices.

Local allergic reactions have also been reported after VCD use. The Angio-Seal device has a bovine collagen component that may elicit a localized inflammatory reaction manifesting as a small red bump at the access site. No specific management is usually necessary. Infections may also arise following VCD use. Fortunately, the overall incidence appears to be less than 0.1%. The organism responsible is generally *Staphylococcus aureus*, as would be expected from a skin source. There have been case fatalities associated with abscess formation in the subcutaneous base overlying the femoral artery associated with infectious arteritis itself.

Conclusions

Manual compression has been the gold standard for achieving hemostasis over 50 years. Nevertheless, limitations of manual compression including delayed time to hemostasis and ambulation, as well as patient discomfort, led to the development of VCDs. VCDs achieve hemostasis by both active and passive approximation at the access site, and require training and education to achieve competency in their use. Evaluation of the safety of first-generation VCDs revealed complication rates similar to those of manual compression, leading to a Class III 2011 PCI guideline for use of VCDs to reduce complications. Nonetheless, more recent randomized clinical trials and large registries suggest a decrease in rate of vascular complications with VCDs, which may lead to a modification of these recommendations. VCDs have been used clinically to achieve same-day discharge and allow percutaneous management of large-bore access sheaths using a preclosure technique. Access site complications, although infrequent, can be potentially life-threatening, and meticulous attention to detail is warranted to optimize the safe use of these devices.

Key Points

- Hemostasis of femoral artery access can be achieved with either manual compression or VCDs.

- VCDs reduce time to hemostasis and ambulation, but have not been shown to definitively reduce overall rates of vascular complications compared with manual compression, although two recent randomized trials (ISAR-CLOSURE and CLOSE UP) showed reduced rates of hematoma >5 cm with VCDs compared to manual compression.

- VCDs are classified as either active approximation (mechanical seal of the arterial wall) or passive approximation (external tamponade of the arterial access site).

- No VCD has been shown to be definitively more efficacious than another in reducing rates of vascular complications.

- Substantial improvements in the design of VCDs have improved deployment success and reduced failures.

- There is a significant learning curve associated with the use of VCDs, with a recent NCDR registry indicating "competence" after deployment of >50 VCDs.

- Vascular closure device use is optimal when used to close CFA access sites, avoiding both "high" (EIA access) and "low" (superficial) femoral or profunda femoral artery access.

- Specific vascular closure device complications—including embolization of the device, device-mediated leg ischemia, and access site infection—are uncommon, but potentially life-threatening.

TABLE 28.7 Vascular Closure Device Complications[a]

- Deployment failure with immediate bleeding (3.9%-6.7%)
- Leg ischemia and/or occlusion requiring surgery (0%-0.1%)
- Vessel dissection (not reported in studies)
- Bleeding including retroperitoneal hemorrhage (0.7%)
- Pseudoaneurysm (0.7%-1.6%)
- Arterio-venous fistulae (0.2%-0.3%)
- Hematoma (5.4%)
- Infection (0.2%-0.3%)
- Nerve injury (<0.1%)

[a]Abstracted from: Robertson L, et al. Vascular closure devices for femoral arterial puncture site hemostasis. *Cochrane Database Syst Rev.* 2016;3:CD009541. doi:10.1002/14651858.CD009541.pub2, for collagen-based, and suture-based device studies.

References

1. Levine GN, et al. 2011 ACCF/AHA/SCAI guideline for percutaneous coronary intervention: executive summary: a report of the American College of Cardiology Foundation/American Heart Association Task Force on Practice Guidelines and the Society for Cardiovascular Angiography and Interventions. *Circulation*. 2011;124:2574–2609.

2. Koreny M, et al. Arterial puncture closing devices compared with standard manual compression after cardiac catheterization: systematic review and meta-analysis. *JAMA*. 2004;291:350–357.

3. Nikolsky E, et al. Vascular complications associated with arteriotomy closure devices in patients undergoing percutaneous coronary procedures: a meta-analysis. *J Am Coll Cardiol*. 2004;44:1200–1209.

4. Biancari F, et al. Meta-analysis of randomized trials on the efficacy of vascular closure devices after diagnostic angiography and angioplasty. *Am Heart J*. 2010;159:518–531.

5. Ellis SG, et al. Correlates and outcomes of retroperitoneal hemorrhage complicating percutaneous coronary intervention. *Catheter Cardiovasc Interv*. 2006;67:541–545.

6. Farouque HM, et al. Risk factors for the development of retroperitoneal hematoma after percutaneous coronary intervention in the era of glycoprotein IIb/IIIa inhibitors and vascular closure devices. *J Am Coll Cardiol*. 2005;45:363–368.

7. Tiroch KA, Matheny ME, Resnic FS. Quantitative impact of cardiovascular risk factors and vascular closure devices on the femoral artery after repeat cardiac catheterization. *Am Heart J*. 2010;159:125–130.

8. Sheth RA, Ganguli S. Closure of alternative vascular sites, including axillary, brachial, popliteal, and surgical grafts. *Tech Vasc Interv Radiol*. 2015;18:113–121.

9. Balzer JO, et al. Postinterventional transcutaneous suture of femoral artery access sites in patients with peripheral arterial occlusive disease: a study of 930 patients. *Catheter Cardiovasc Interv*. 2001;53:174–181.

10. Warren BS, Warren SG, Miller SD. Predictors of complications and learning curve using the Angio-Seal closure device following interventional and diagnostic catheterization. *Catheter Cardiovasc Interv*. 1999;48:162–166.

11. Resnic FS, et al. Quantifying the learning curve in the use of a novel vascular closure device: an analysis of the NCDR (National Cardiovascular Data Registry) CathPCI registry. *JACC Cardiovasc Interv*. 2012;5:82–89.

12. Sohail MR, et al. Infectious complications of percutaneous vascular closure devices. *Mayo Clin Proc*. 2005;80:1011–1015.

13. Applegate RJ, et al. Restick following initial Angioseal use. *Catheter Cardiovasc Interv*. 2003;58:181–184.

14. 2017 Buyer's Guide: The sizes, specification, and unique characteristics of today's peripheral interventional devices. *Endovasc Today*. 2016;15:122–128.

15. Schulz-Schupke S, et al. Comparison of vascular closure devices vs. manual compression after femoral artery puncture: the ISAR-CLOSURE randomized clinical trial. *JAMA*. 2014;312:1981–1987.

16. Holm NR, et al. Randomised comparison of manual compression and FemoSeal™ vascular closure device for closure after femoral artery access coronary angiography: the CLOSure dEvices Used in everyday Practice (CLOSE-UP) study. *EuroIntervention*. 2014;9:183–190.

17. Jiang J, et al. Network meta-analysis of randomized trials on the safety of vascular closure devices for femoral arterial puncture site haemostasis. *Sci Rep*. 2015;5:13761.

18. Wimmer NJ, et al. Effectiveness of arterial closure devices for preventing complications with percutaneous coronary intervention: an instrumental variable analysis. *Circ Cardiovasc Interv*. 2016;9:e003464. doi:10.1161/CIRCINTERVENTIONS.115.003464.

19. Farooq V, et al. Relationship between femoral vascular closure devices and short-term mortality from 271,845 percutaneous coronary intervention procedrues performed in the United Kingdom between 2006 and 2011: a propensity score-corrected analysis from the British Cardiovascular Intervention Society. *Circ Cardiovasc Interv*. 2016;9:e003560. doi:10.1161/CIRCINTERVENTIONS.116.003560.

20. Gurm HS, et al. Comparative safety of vascular closure devices and manual closure among patients having percutaneous coronary intervention. *Ann Intern Med*. 2013;159:660–666.

21. Rao SV, et al. Prevalence and outcomes of same-day discharge after elective percutaneous coronary intervention among older patients. *JAMA*. 2011;306:1461–1467.

22. Nelson PR, et al. A multicenter, randomized, controlled trial of totally percutaneous access versus open femoral exposure for endovascular aortic aneurysm repair (the PEVAR trial). *J Vasc Surg*. 2014;59:1181–1194.

23. Robertson L, et al. Vascular closure devices for femoral arterial puncture site hemostasis. *Cochrane Database Syst Rev*. 2016;3:CD009541. doi:10.1002/14651858.CD009541.pub2.

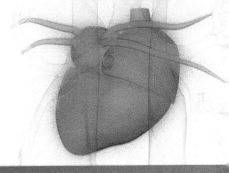

Women and Percutaneous Interventions

Binita Shah, MD, MS, FSCAI, FACC, Sasha Still, MD, and Molly Szerlip, MD, FSCAI, FACC, FACP

Cardiovascular disease (CVD) is highly prevalent and remains the leading cause of death in women (**Figs. 29.1** and **29.2**) (1). Despite improvement over the past 15 years, there remains a significant gap in the awareness, knowledge, and perceptions related to CVD in women (2). Note that, throughout this chapter, data will refer to *sex*, which classifies a person according to their reproductive organs and functions assigned by chromosomal complement, as opposed to *gender*, which refers to a person's self-representation as male or female.

Coronary Artery Disease

Characteristics at Time of Presentation

SYMPTOMS

Chest pain is the most common symptom in both women and men, and when a woman presents with classic angina symptoms, a misdiagnosis may lay in perception bias on the part of the patient and/or physician (2,3). Similarly, although a woman's cardiac presentation may be associated with less classic symptoms such as fatigue, dizziness, or palpitations, they do often present with the more classic associated symptoms of shortness of breath, nausea, and vomiting.

A multicenter, cross-sectional analysis of 619 patients presenting with ST-segment elevation myocardial infarction (STEMI), prodromal chest pain was noted in 35% of women compared to 51% of men (4). However, chest pain that seemed less likely to be definite angina was associated with a greater delay between symptom onset and the first electrocardiogram in women. In another single-center study of 217 patients presenting to the Emergency Department with an acute coronary syndrome (ACS), chest pain was the most frequently reported symptom in both sexes (5). After adjustment for age and diabetes, women were more likely than men to have associated nausea, vomiting, and indigestion-like symptoms. Overall, symptoms were more similar than different between the sexes, emphasizing the need to increase patient and physician awareness and limit unconscious bias.

Although younger women more often present with atypical presentations, a prospective cohort study of 1,015 patients <55 years of age hospitalized for ACS demonstrated that chest pain was still the most common symptom in both sexes (6). In fact, women were more likely to present without chest pain (19% vs. 14%) and also reported a greater number of symptoms than men without chest pain. The most common symptoms reported in patients without chest pain were weakness, feeling hot, shortness of breath, cold sweats, and left arm or shoulder pain. Some studies also suggest that women may experience their symptoms around the time of their menstrual period (7).

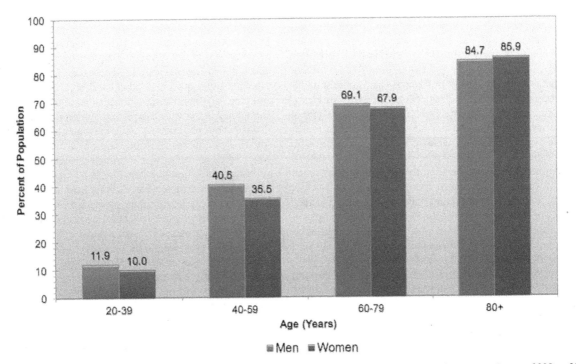

FIGURE 29.1 Prevalence of cardiovascular disease in adults by age and sex from the National Health and Nutrition Survey: 2009 to 2012. (From: National Center for Health Statistics and National Heart, Lung, and Blood Institute.)

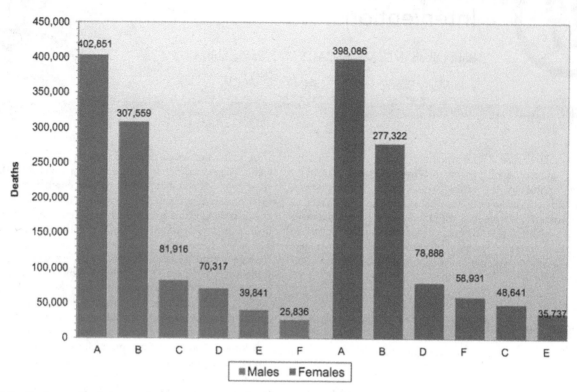

FIGURE 29.2 Cardiovascular disease and other major causes of death for all adults by sex in the United States in 2013. **(A)** cardiovascular diseases (International Classification of Diseases, 10th Revision codes I00–I99); **(B)** cancer (C00–C97); **(C)** accidents (V01–X59 and Y85–Y86); **(D)** chronic lower respiratory disease (J40–J47); **(E)** diabetes mellitus (E10–E14); **(F)** Alzheimer disease (G30). (From: National Center for Health Statistics and National Heart, Lung, and Blood Institute.)

DEMOGRAPHICS AND MEDICAL COMORBIDITIES

Although women are approximately 10 years older than men upon presentation with CVD, younger women who present with an myocardial infarction (MI) have a significantly worse outcome compared with age-matched men, and this disparity worsens with decreasing age. A retrospective analysis of 9,015 patients who underwent primary percutaneous coronary intervention (PCI) for MI in New York State demonstrated a significantly increased risk of in-hospital mortality in women than men under the age of 75 years (8). Similarly, in all-comers PCI population of 10,963 patients in the National Heart, Lung, and Blood Institute Dynamic Registry, the composite rate of death, MI, coronary artery bypass graft surgery (CABG), and repeat PCI at 1 year was significantly higher in women than men <50 years of age despite a similar rate of procedural success (9). Rate of CABG and repeat PCI remained significantly higher in young women compared with young men at 5 years follow-up.

Baseline factors, particularly traditional medical comorbidities, account for a substantial portion of the excess risk but do not explain it completely. Although an analysis of 16,771 patients with non-STEMI demonstrated that women present at an older age with more comorbidities, women underwent lower rates of PCI even after adjustment for the number of comorbidities (10). Women are also more likely to have comorbidities that are not considered traditional risk factors. The leading cause of death in patients with autoimmune disorders that predominately affect women, such as antiphospholipid syndrome and systemic lupus erythematosus, are accelerated atherosclerosis and CVD (11). In a study of people aged 25 to 54 years who died from ischemic heart disease in New York City, diabetes mellitus, systemic lupus erythematosus, and rheumatoid arthritis were more common in women than men,

while human immunodeficiency virus and cocaine use did not differ by sex (12).

Plaque Morphology

While most MIs are caused by plaque rupture, a significant number of MI presentations are due to underlying plaque erosion (Fig. 29.3). The precursor lesion of a ruptured plaque is the thin cap fibroatheroma, which is a plaque that has a lipid-rich core covered by a thin fibrous cap. Eroded plaques, on the other hand, are rich in smooth muscle cells and proteoglycans, and have no apparent injury except for a denuded endothelial lining with less plaque burden than ruptured plaques.

Plaque morphology may differ in women compared to men. Older studies demonstrate that plaque erosion occurs more often in younger women than men who died of sudden cardiac death, as well as smokers compared to non-smokers (13,14). More contemporary studies further demonstrate sex-based differences in plaque characteristics in younger compared to older patients presenting with MI. In 280 STEMI patients who underwent intravascular ultrasound evaluation prior to PCI, women were significantly older than men and had a significantly lower plaque burden, less fibro-fatty tissue, and more dense calcium then men (15). Women aged 66 to 75 years also had significantly more necrotic core than men; however, this disparity between sexes was not noted in patients >75 years. Similarly, in 697 patients presenting with ACS, intravascular ultrasound demonstrated significantly lower plaque volumes, fewer fibroatheromas, and more fibrotic plaques in women than men <65 years old, but no significant sex-based differences in older patients (16). In the Optical Coherence Tomography Assessment of Gender Diversity In Primary Angioplasty (OCTAVIA) study, 140 age-matched STEMI patients had no significant sex-based differences in the rate of plaque

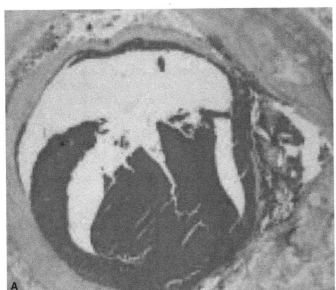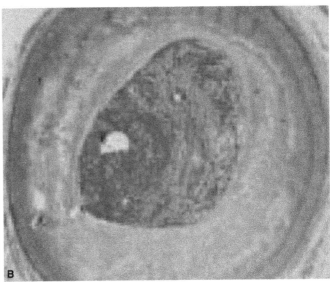

FIGURE 29.3   **(A)** Plaque rupture versus **(B)** plaque erosion. Plaque ruptures are defined as luminal thrombus in continuity with the necrotic core and an interrupted plaque cap, while plaque erosion is defined as thrombus in direct contact with fibrointimal plaque but with no continuity between the thrombus and the necrotic core. (Adapted from: Arbustini E, et al. Plaque erosion is a major substrate for coronary thrombosis in acute myocardial infarction. *Heart.* 1999;82:269–272.)

rupture versus nonrupture or eroded plaques when evaluated by optical coherence tomography (17).

Women often present with an MI but no evidence of obstructive disease on coronary angiography. In these patients, plaque disruption was often identifiable by intravascular ultrasound and present in plaques with lower plaque burden and more fibrous characteristics then elsewhere in the coronary arteries (18). The disrupted plaques did not occur in more eccentric or outwardly remodeled plaques than elsewhere in the coronary arteries.

Few studies have evaluated sex-based differences in stable coronary artery disease (CAD). In one analysis of 383 patients, there were no sex-based differences in plaque characteristics as assessed by optical coherence tomography with or without intravascular ultrasound or near infrared spectroscopy (19,20). Although plaque burden was significantly lower in the subset of women compared to men who underwent intravascular ultrasound assessment, there was no difference between the sexes after adjustment for age and other clinical risk factors.

Vascular Function

ENDOTHELIAL DYSFUNCTION

Vascular function plays a prominent role in ischemic heart disease in women. This may be due to variations in hormones (19,20). The Women's Ischemic Syndrome Evaluation (WISE) study evaluated 163 women with angina who underwent coronary angiography with reactivity assessment (21). Three quarters of the patients had a diameter stenosis <50% on quantitative coronary angiography, and about half of these patients had an abnormal response to acetylcholine. An abnormal response to acetylcholine, in turn, was an independent predictor of major adverse cardiovascular events (MACE) on a median follow-up of 48 months. In a multicenter registry of 1,429 patients with vasospastic angina, women were older, with a lower rate of tobacco use and obstructive CAD when compared to men (22). The rate of MACE-free survival was significantly lower in women <50 years of age compared to those >50 years of age, whereas the rate of MACE-free survival did not significantly differ by age among men.

SMOOTH MUSCLE DYSFUNCTION

Disorders related to smooth muscle dysfunction, such as Raynaud's phenomenon and migraine, are more common in women than men. Another analysis of the WISE study evaluated 189 women with baseline coronary flow reserve assessment after intracoronary adenosine, an agent that utilizes an endothelium-independent mechanism of vasodilation (23). In this subset, 80% of the patients did not have obstructive CAD, and low coronary flow reserve predicted MACE outcomes on a mean follow-up of 5.4 years independent of CAD severity.

INFLAMMATION

In addition to endothelial and smooth muscle dysfunction, inflammation may also alter the function of both the macro and microvasculature. As noted previously, women have a higher prevalence than men of autoimmune and vasculitis diseases, such as rheumatoid arthritis, systemic lupus erythematosus, and Takayasu's vasculitis. These inflammatory conditions are associated with accelerated atherosclerosis and abnormal myocardial perfusion imaging, as well as myocardial disease without underlying significant CAD (24–26). A study of patients with early chronic kidney disease and no history of ischemic heart disease demonstrated a higher prevalence of myocardial abnormalities on cardiac magnetic resonance imaging in patients with lupus or Wegener's granulomatosis than those without underlying vasculitis or autoimmune disease (26).

Spontaneous Coronary Artery Dissection

Spontaneous coronary artery dissection (SCAD) presents clinically similar to an MI, and is more common in women than men, particularly young women and women in the peripartum period (27,28). It remains unclear whether the underlying mechanism is a primary tear in the intima versus a primary medial hemorrhage (29). Potential predisposing factors include fibromuscular dysplasia, systemic inflammatory conditions, connective tissue disorders, hormonal therapy, and extrinsic stressors (30). SCAD can be classified by angiography in three ways (31). Type 1 is in the presence of arterial wall contrast staining with multiple radiolucent lumens. Type 2 is when there is an abrupt change in the caliber of the artery from normal to a smooth diffuse narrowing. Finally, type 3 is a focal short stenosis that has an angiographic appearance similar to atherosclerosis. Overall, the appearance of SCAD is a small-caliber but non-obstructive vessel, and when it does occur with obstruction, it can be mistaken for atherosclerosis if the index of suspicion is not high. Multiple coronary artery territories may also be involved (32).

There are limited data on management strategies. Consensus statements recommend β-blockade therapy to reduce arterial wall stress, and dual antiplatelet therapy (DAPT) to reduce thrombus in the false lumen. Nevertheless, more potent platelet inhibitors, such as glycoprotein (GP) IIb/IIIa inhibitors and thrombin inhibitors, such as heparin and thrombolytic therapy, are discouraged due to risk of propagation of the tear. Furthermore, an initial strategy of conservative management with observation of 3 to 5 days is preferred (33). PCI is associated with a high rate of technical failure and does not reduce the rate of recurrent SCAD or target vessel revascularization. Furthermore, with preserved flow, the artery heals spontaneously over a month's time, making the risks of PCI in these cases unacceptable (30). Only patients with ongoing or recurrent ischemia or hemodynamic instability should be considered for coronary revascularization. Nevertheless, CABG may be preferable over PCI because wiring, balloon inflation, or stent deployment can propagate the dissection further. If PCI is pursued, consideration should be made for use of meticulous technique, adjunctive intravascular ultrasound or optical coherence tomography imaging, and, for longer lesions, stenting of the distal edge and then the proximal edge before stenting the middle section to prevent propagation. More recently, a few successful cases have been reported with the use of undersized cutting balloons to fenestrate the medial hemorrhage and decompress the false lumen (34). An undersized balloon is used due to a theoretical risk of coronary perforation.

Ischemia without Obstructive CAD

The WISE study showed that women with symptoms of ischemia but without obstructive CAD on angiogram are at an increased risk for cardiovascular events compared with asymptomatic community-based women (35). The 5-year annualized adjusted rates for MACE were significantly higher in the WISE women with non-obstructive CAD (n = 222) compared to the WISE women with angiographically normal coronary arteries (n = 318) and the asymptomatic community-based women (n = 998) (16.0%, 7.9%, 2.4%; p ≥ 0.002).

Women with non-obstructive coronary arteries on angiography can also present with MI. In a report of 639 people aged 21 to 54 years who died of ischemic heart disease, women were more like to have non-obstructive disease and almost a quarter of them had pathologic evidence of MI (36). Several potential mechanisms include transient thrombosis with endogenous thrombolysis, distal embolization of microatherothrombotic debris, plaque disruption (rupture or ulceration) that does not lead to luminal occlusion, and Takotsubo cardiomyopathy, all of which may occur in both sexes (37).

Similar to the women with stable ischemic heart disease, women with MI in the setting of non-obstructive coronary arteries remains associated with a significant rate of MACE. In the Swedish Coronary Angiography and Angioplasty Registry (SCAAR) and the Register of Information and Knowledge about Swedish Heart Intensive Care Admissions (RIKS-HIA), patients with Takotsubo cardiomyopathy, an entity that predominantly affects women, was associated with a greater rate of cardiogenic shock than patients with non-STEMI (38). Patients with Takotsubo cardiomyopathy also had similar rates

of short- and long-term mortality when compared to both patients with non-STEMI and STEMI. The European Society of Cardiology working group on MI with non-obstructive CAD recommends evaluation with intracoronary nitroglycerin and possibly intracoronary imaging and/or coronary flow reserve measurements during invasive coronary angiography (39). The consensus statement also suggests the use of transesophageal echocardiogram to rule out cardioembolism and cardiac magnetic resonance imaging in the absence of obvious etiology.

Considerations during PCI
ANATOMICAL CONSIDERATIONS

Coronary anatomy differs between women and men. Hormones modify arterial size, and coronary arteries in women have smaller diameters than men, independent of body size and left ventricular mass (40). Furthermore, given the greater number of comorbidities in post-menopausal women than men, there is a higher likelihood of diffuse atherosclerosis in already small-caliber arteries, which may appear "normal" on angiography. Another sex-based anatomical disparity is the higher rate of arterial stiffness and calcification noted in women but not men (41).

These anatomic considerations may play a factor in the treatment of chronic total occlusions (CTO) in women. The Canadian Multicenter CTO Registry demonstrated a significantly lower number of women in the CTO versus non-CTO groups (42). In the CTO group, women were significantly older with more comorbidities. Although there were no differences in the rate of CTO PCI between women and men, there was a significantly lower rate of CABG in women than men, even after adjustment for differences in baseline characteristics. Outcomes after CTO PCI also differ by sex. In the United Kingdom CTO Database, women had a higher rate of coronary perforation, bleeding, and contrast-induced nephropathy (43). The investigators suggested technical considerations be made when it comes to selection of collateral, balloon size, and access site, as well as use of pre-hydration in women undergoing CTO PCI.

Women often present with calcified disease, which is another predictor of coronary perforation and adverse long-term outcomes (43,44). In the Evaluate the Safety and Efficacy of OAS in Treating Severely Calcified Coronary Lesions (ORBIT II) study, although the rate of stent delivery after orbital atherectomy did not differ by sex, the number of women who had a drug-eluting stent (DES) placed was lower than men (45,46). Furthermore, although there were no sex-based differences in short-term outcomes, women had significantly higher odds of severe dissection after atherectomy.

STENT TYPE

It would be expected that women should benefit from the use of DESs, given the presence of smaller-caliber arteries and more diffuse disease. The use of second-generation DESs increased over time in women undergoing PCI in the United States (47). Furthermore, the use of newer-generation DESs was associated with significantly lower rates of long-term MACE, including very late stent thrombosis, in women undergoing complex PCI in the Women in Innovations-DES collaboration (48). This benefit associated with newer-generation DESs was consistent across a spectrum of clinical presentations (49).

In comparisons between women and men, there were no differences in the benefit of DESs over bare-metal stents (BMSs) in long-term outcomes (50,51). A sex-based analysis of 2,132 patients receiving zotarolimus-eluting stents showed women and men had similar rates of long-term outcomes, and women actually had lower rates of target vessel revascularization and failure compared with men (52). A substudy of patients undergoing intravascular ultrasound further demonstrated female sex to be independently associated with decreased neointimal hyperplasia in patients treated with zotarolimus-eluting stents (53). Studies comparing women and men treated with everolimus-versus paclitaxel-eluting stents demonstrated that both women and men receiving everolimus-eluting stents had lower rates of long-term MACE than those receiving paclitaxel-eluting stents (54,55).

HEMODYNAMIC SUPPORT

Similar to the presentation of CAD, women who present with cardiogenic shock are older with more comorbidities and lower systolic and diastolic blood pressure (56). Furthermore, similar to the treatment for CAD with DESs, there are no sex-based differences in the effect of intra-aortic balloon pump treatment on outcomes in cardiogenic shock (56). Nevertheless, early initiation of mechanical circulatory support in acute MI complicated by cardiogenic shock was associated with significantly lower rates of in-hospital mortality in women compared to men, suggesting a benefit from greater hemodynamic support in this setting (57).

BLEEDING AND OTHER COMPLICATIONS

Major bleeding events are the most common non-cardiac complication of PCI, occurring in 2% to 4% of patients. Although there has been an overall decrease in vascular complications over the last 30 years, women still have a >2-fold risk of treatment-related bleeding over men following PCI (58). A study utilizing CathPCI Registry data demonstrated that women had an increase in rate of bleeding following PCI even when bleeding avoidance strategies are utilized (59). Older, age, smaller BMI, and the type of periprocedural antithrombotic therapy have been implicated. Nevertheless, a multi-registry study of 14,180 patients (60) comparing bleeding complications by gender found that despite matching for age, BMI, and type of antithrombotic therapy, the bleeding risk remained significantly higher in women (61). Increased susceptibility to mechanical-type vascular injury in women was suggested as a contributor to their increased bleeding risk (62). Shorter common femoral artery length and smaller vessel diameter may predispose women to increased bleeding from "high sticks" or catheter manipulation, although no study has confirmed the supposition (63). The Study of Access Site for Enhancement of PCI for Women (SAFE-PCI) is a multicenter randomised control trails (RCT) in which 1,787 women were randomized to radial or femoral access for angiography or PCI (64). Although there was a trend toward benefit, radial access did not significantly reduce bleeding or vascular complications in women undergoing PCI, which the authors ascribed to limited sample size. On the other hand, among women undergoing coronary catheterization or PCI, radial access decreased bleeding complications. The study was terminated early due to a lower-than-expected rate of bleeding complications.

STABLE CAD

Women and men differ in presentation and management of CAD, but it is unclear whether gender-specific differences translate to differences in clinical outcomes in stable CAD.

CLARIFY (ProspeCtive observational LongitudinAl RegIstry oF patients with stable CAD) is a prospective, multinational registry in 33,000 patients with stable CAD in 45 countries. One-year outcomes were analyzed in 30,977 outpatients with stable CAD (77.4% men, 22.6% women) (65). Women were older than men, had worse cardiovascular risk profiles, and more frequent angina, but were less likely to be receiving statins or β-blockers. Women were also less likely to have undergone both non-invasive testing and coronary

angiography. Furthermore, despite substantial differences in baseline characteristics, women and men had similar 1-year outcomes. Similar to previous published reports (66), women were also less likely to undergo revascularization with PCI or CABG. A subset analysis of the COURAGE trial evaluating sex-based differences in the outcomes of women and men randomized to PCI + optimal medical therapy (OMT) and OMT alone found there were no significant differences in the treatment effect on major outcomes (67). Although, women assigned to PCI + OMT showed greater benefit with a reduction in congestive heart failure (CHF) hospitalization and future revascularization.

NON ST-SEGMENT ELEVATION MI

There is continued debate as to whether a routine, early invasive versus conservative strategy is superior for the management of unstable angina and NSTEMI. The FRISC-II trial (n = 2,457, 30% women) was the first RCT to demonstrate a significant reduction in death and MI (RR 0.74, 95% CI 0.6–0.92) with early invasive (catheterization within 7 days) versus non-invasive treatment in patients with NSTEMI (68); however, these risk reductions were confined to their male cohorts at 1 year and persisted at 15-year follow-up (68,69). One subsequent RCT, RITA3 (n = 1,810, 38% women) exhibited similar beneficial effects for men undergoing early invasive versus non-invasive strategy (70). Furthermore, the OASIS 5 sub-study, which randomly assigned 184 women to a routine or selective invasive strategy, identified significantly more deaths after 1 year (HR 9.01, 95% CI 1.11–72.90) and higher rates of major bleeding at 30 days with the routine invasive strategy (71). A retrospective analysis of TACTICS-TIMI 18 data (n = 2,220, 34% women) found that the benefits of an early invasive strategy in women were the same as those seen in men after adjusting for baseline characteristics (72).

In 2008, a collaborative meta-analysis of eight RCTs was performed to examine the outcomes of an invasive approach for NSTEMI in women versus men (73). The authors concluded that the invasive strategy had comparable benefits for men and high-risk (biomarker-positive) women for reducing death, acute myocardial infarction (AMI), and re-hospitalization with ACS, and, furthermore, recommended a conservative approach to NSTEMI in low-risk women.

ST-SEGMENT ELEVATION MI

Historically, women experience higher mortality rates compared to men following STEMI, regardless of reperfusion modality. Sex-based differences in presentation, comorbid disease, pathophysiology, and treatment utilization contribute to this discrepancy in outcomes (74).

Guidelines recommend PCI as the preferred reperfusion modality in patients presenting with STEMI (75). Nevertheless, when logistic challenges preclude early PCI, fibrinolysis constitutes a viable option for reperfusion. Although the relative benefit of PCI to fibrinolysis for the treatment for STEMI in women and men is similar, women derive a larger absolute benefit from PCI (76). This is on account of the higher rate of intracranial hemorrhage and other adverse bleeding events experienced more often by women. Notwithstanding good outcomes following PCI, increased short- and long-term mortality is more prevalent among women. In a meta-analysis of 35 observational studies examining differences in mortality by sex in patients with STEMI treated with PCI, women were at higher risk for in-hospital mortality (RR 1.93; 95% CI, 1.75–2.14) and 1-year mortality (RR 1.58; 95% CI, 1.36–1.84) (77). Although associations were attenuated on adjusted analysis, the difference in in-hospital mortality (RR 1.48; 95% CI, 1.07–2.05) remained significant. Nevertheless, a multi-registry Italian study (n = 13,235 patients, 28% women) evaluating patients with STEMI treated with PCI, fibrinolysis, or no intervention demonstrated higher in-hospital mortality among women on adjusted analysis (78). Poorer cardiovascular risk profiles, higher bleeding rates, and greater incidences of cardiogenic shock among women have been implicated in these outcome disparities. Delayed or underutilized reperfusion strategies may also play a role.

Women of all age strata are less likely to undergo reperfusion and experience longer treatment delays for STEMI compared with age-matched males (78,79). Atypical symptoms may lead to delayed presentation, thus precluding acute reperfusion strategies. Additionally, lower revascularization rates may be explained by higher rates of major bleeding or higher frequency of alternative etiologies in women, such as Takotsubo cardiomyopathy, SCAD and coronary vasospasm.

Pharmacotherapy
ANTIPLATELET AGENTS

Gender influences on platelet biology were first reported over 40 years ago (80). Women have higher platelet counts (81), a higher number of cell surface antigens (GP Ib-IX-V and GP IIb/IIIa), and enhanced platelet reactivity and aggregability (80,82). There is conflicting evidence regarding the impact of menstrual-cycle hormones on sex-specific platelet function (83).

DAPT is a mainstay of treatment and prevention following coronary stent placement in patients with ACS to reduce thrombotic complications and atherosclerosis.

Gender-related divergences in cardioprotection afforded by anti-platelet agents have been identified. In women, ASA did not reduce the risk of major cardiovascular events but was shown to decrease the risk of ischemic stroke and increase the risk of bleeding (83). The TRITON-TIMI 38 comparing prasugrel versus clopidogrel in aspirin-treated ACS patients receiving PCI found higher absolute and relative risk reductions (2.4% vs. 1.6%; 21% vs. 12%) of major cardiovascular events in men compared to women (84). On the other hand, a separate analysis of PLATO data investigating the effect of ticagrelor on cardiovascular outcomes in women demonstrated that female sex was not associated with MACE when adjusting for baseline characteristics (85). Significant interaction between treatment and sex was also demonstrated in several trials evaluating the clinical efficacy of GP IIb/IIIa inhibitors in patients with ACS; however, the association was attenuated when adjusting for elevated troponin concentration (86).

Greater risk of major bleeding has been shown among women in studies evaluating anti-platelet agents in patients undergoing cardioprevention and in ACS (83,87). Bleeding site differences may relate to small-caliber vessels (61) or sex-specific vascular reactivity in women (88). Inappropriate dosing of GP IIb/IIIa inhibitors has also been implicated in their greater bleeding risk. In the CRUSADE trial, approximately 27% of patients treated with GP IIb/IIIa inhibitors received an excessive dose. Excess dosing was more common in women than men and in those >75 years of age (89).

DIRECT THROMBIN INHIBITORS

Bivalirudin is a direct thrombin inhibitor that is an effective alternative antithrombotic strategy during PCI. The REPLACE-2 trial demonstrated non-inferiority of bivalirudin + GP IIb/IIa inhibitors compared to heparin + GP IIa/IIa inhibitors in the suppression of ischemic endpoints (90). In a retrospective sex-based subgroup analysis (n = 6,010, 25.6% women), there was no difference in rates of death, MI, or revascularization in women compared to men (91). Nevertheless, women treated with bivalirudin + GP IIb/IIIa inhibitors

experienced significantly less major and minor bleeding compared to those who received heparin-based therapy.

In a subset analysis of the ACUITY trial (n = 13,819, 30.1% women) in which patients with NSTE-ACS were randomized to heparin + GP IIb/IIIa inhibitor, bivalirudin + GP IIb/IIIa inhibitor, or bivalirudin alone, women experienced similar event rates across all treatment arms and the lowest rates of bleeding with bivalirudin alone (92). The comparative efficacy of bivalirudin and its association with decreased bleeding rates has been confirmed in further study (93).

Sex-Related Disparities
PHYSICIAN AWARENESS AND REFERRAL

CVD is the leading cause of death among women worldwide, yet gender-related disparities in the prevention and treatment of ACS continue to be perceived. This so-called "gender gap" is multifactorial and represents a global misconception and underestimation of cardiovascular risk factors associated with the female sex.

Physicians underestimate the probability of CAD among women (94). In a study evaluating practice patterns of primary care physicians, OB-GYN, and cardiologists, intermediate risk women (as classified by Framingham ATII risk score) were significantly less likely to be assigned to a higher risk category than men by PCPs, with similar but nonsignificant trends for OB-GYNs and cardiologists (95). Another key observation of this study was that physicians' assessment of intermediate- or high-risk predicted recommendations for preventative intervention.

Gender-related discrepancy in treatment strategies has been observed. The unbalanced treatment dispersal may be due in part to the higher prevalence of atypical symptoms among women, leading to delayed diagnosis and precluding revascularization. The higher frequency of non-obstructive ACS among women may also play a role. Interestingly, in a multi-registry observational study evaluating sex-related differences in treatment patterns of physicians, the most commonly cited reason for not pursing angiography among males and females was that the patient was not of high enough risk (3).

REPRESENTATION OF WOMEN IN RESEARCH STUDIES

Historically, women have been underrepresented in clinical trials. In 1993, President Clinton signed the National Institute of Health's Revitalization Act of 1993, which legally required the inclusion of women and men to be consistent with known sex-related prevalence of a disease under investigation. An analysis of 76,148 patients with NSTE-ACS from 11 multinational, phase II RCTs conducted between 1994 and 2010 revealed an increase in the representation of women in CAD trials (33% vs. 25%), but no overall change in the enrollment of women relative to men in all the trials (96). Factors such as age, renal function limits, and comorbidities may have selected against women and led to low inclusion rates. Understanding gender-related differences is important to create and apply an individualized therapeutic approach and allows for generalizability of results.

Percutaneous Approach to Valvular Heart Disease

Transcatheter valve replacement is a novel therapeutic option for symptomatic aortic stenosis and severe mitral regurgitation in patients with a prohibitive surgical risk. Women undergoing either transfemoral aortic valve replacement (TAVR) and surgical aortic valve replacement (SAVR) tend to have lower rates of CAD and peripheral artery disease (PAD), and higher left ventricular ejection fraction (LVEF) (97,98) and smaller aortic annuli (20.9 ± 1.4 vs. 22.9 ± 1.7, p < 0.001), and require smaller bioprosthesis (23.9 ± 1.6 vs. 26.3 ± 1.5, p < 0.001) compared to men (99). Recent trials evaluating TAVR efficacy have demonstrated that females had higher short-, mid-, and long-term mortality compared to males (100–102). A PARTNER 1A subgroup analysis demonstrated a greater survival benefit with TAVR versus open surgery in women (98). Although men experienced lower procedural mortality with TAVR versus SAVR, mortality at 2 years was higher with TAVR. These differences are likely attributable to a poorer cardiovascular risk profile in men, which overtime overwhelms the initial benefit of TAVR; whereas in women, the initial benefit is sustained. Nevertheless, a Canadian study evaluating sex differences in mortality following TAVR determined that survival benefit among women persisted after adjustment for baseline characteristics, suggesting cardiovascular risk alone cannot explain differences in outcomes (99). While women appeared to benefit from TAVR, they also experienced more frequent strokes, vascular complications, and major bleeding.

Similarly, a study of 592 patients undergoing MitraClip therapy for severe mitral regurgitation found that female gender was associated with improved long-term survival, but failed to identify sex-specific differences in procedural success (103). Parallel findings have been reported in smaller series (104,105).

Percutaneous balloon mitral valvuloplasty (PMV) is a safe and effective therapy for rheumatic mitral stenosis (MS) and is associated with high procedural success rates, as well as good intermediate- and long-term outcomes (106,107). In a study evaluating the procedural success and clinical outcomes of patients undergoing PMV (n = 1,015, 83% women), women had lower procedural success rates, achieved smaller post-procedural mitral valve area (MVA), higher rates of post-procedure mitral regurgitation, and more frequent MV surgery on long-term follow-up compared to men (107). Nevertheless, procedural-related adverse events and long-term outcomes did not differ between the sexes. Mechanisms for these differences remain speculative, but authors suggest sex-based differences in anatomy and pathology may contribute.

Disease of the Carotids, Aorta, and Lower Extremities

One in five women who reach the age 55 develop a stroke during their remaining lifetime (108). Compared to men, women have a higher incidence of lifetime risk of stroke, post-stroke disability, and rates of institutionalization (109). Carotid endarterectomy (CEA) reduces the risk for stroke in selected patients with symptomatic internal carotid artery stenosis and, to a lesser extent, in those with asymptomatic carotid disease (110).

Women have a higher perioperative stroke rate and mortality compared to men following CEA (110). Carotid artery stenting (CAS) has emerged as an alternative to open CEA in select populations. A subgroup analysis of the Carotid Revascularization Endarterectomy versus Stenting Trial (CREST) noted a higher rate of periprocedural complications [stroke, AMI, death] following CAS as opposed to CEA, but no differences among men between treatment modalities (111).

Screening for abdominal aortic aneurysms (AAAs) in women is controversial given that the prevalence of AAA is approximately six times lower in women than men. The Society for Vascular Surgery practice guidelines recommend screening women >65 years old who have a history of smoking or a family history of AAA. Although

women are less likely to have AAAs, their AAAs are two to four times more likely to rupture than men (112).

Earlier studies suggested that peripheral vascular disease was more common in men, while recent reports suggest that the prevalence of PAD is at least equal among men and women (113), while the incidence of asymptomatic PAD tends to be higher in women compared to men (12.4% vs. 7.8%) (114). Only 10% of individuals have classic symptoms of intermittent claudication, whereas 50% experience atypical symptoms and the other 40% are asymptomatic (115). Men have higher rates of symptomatic PAD, and women have a higher overall prevalence when diagnosed with ankle-brachial index (ABI) (116). In fact, among patients referred for elective coronary angiography, women (as opposed to men) more frequently had an ABI <0.9 (117).

A study conducted by the Ankle Brachial Index Collaboration Group showed that the inclusion of the ABI in the calculation of the Framingham risk score increases the risk category, the effect being more dramatic for women (118). The use of ABI may improve the score's ability to classify women's risk more accurately. In regard to treatment, women are less often offered surgical revascularization (119). Later age at disease onset, smaller vessel size, and poorer surgical outcomes with both surgical and endovascular therapy have been proposed to contribute to these sex-based differences.

Secondary Prevention and Guidelines

Despite continued advances in the field, CVD remains the leading cause of death among women in the US. Evaluating temporal trends from 1994 to 2010, during index hospitalization and at discharge, the use of angiotensin-converting enzyme inhibitors/angiotensin II receptor blockers, thienopyridines, β-blockers, and lipid-lowering drugs have increased (96). Additionally, although significantly more men underwent coronary angiography, PCI, and CABG surgery, angiography and PCI increased among women over time.

The underutilization of therapies to reinforce cardioprotection is common. The American College of Cardiologists and American Heart Association class I medical therapies were given less frequently to women on admission and discharge (65,88). Furthermore, women are less likely to be discharged on β-blocks, angiotensin-converting enzyme inhibitors, aspirin, and GP IIb/IIIa inhibitors (97). Cardiac rehabilitation rates are also significantly lower among females compared to males.

Key Points

- Women have an excess mortality related to CVD compared to men, a trend that hasn't changed in nearly three decades.

- While obstructive atherosclerotic CAD remains a focus for interventional cardiologists, other causes of ischemic heart disease, such as endothelial dysfunction, coronary vasospasm, and microvascular disease, need to be considered in women, particularly in those who present with angina but have "normal appearing" coronary arteries on angiography.

- Current treatment of obstructive CAD with DESs achieves similar benefits in women and men, but certain technical considerations should be made for women undergoing PCI, given the underlying differences in anatomy and clinical profiles.

References

1. Mozaffarian D, et al. American Heart Association Statistics Committee; Stroke Statistics Subcommittee. Heart Disease and Stroke Statistics-2016 update: a report from the American Heart Association. *Circulation*. 2016;133:e38–360.

2. Mosca L, et al. Fifteen-year trends in awareness of heart disease in women: results of a 2012 American Heart Association national survey. *Circulation*. 2013;127:1254–1263, e1251–e1259.

3. Mosca L, et al. National study of physician awareness and adherence to cardiovascular disease prevention guidelines. *Circulation*. 2005;111:499–510.

4. von Eisenhart Rothe AF, et al. Sex specific impact of prodromal chest pain on pre-hospital delay time during an acute myocardial infarction: findings from the multicenter MEDEA study with 619 STEMI patients. *Int J Cardiol*. 2015;201:581–586.

5. Milner KA, et al. Gender differences in symptom presentation associated with coronary heart disease. *Am J Cardiol*. 1999;84:396–399.

6. Khan NA, et al. Sex differences in acute coronary syndrome symptom presentation in young patients. *JAMA Intern Med*. 2013;173:1863–1871.

7. Lloyd GW, et al. Does angina vary with the menstrual cycle in women with premenopausal coronary artery disease? *Heart*. 2000;84:189–192.

8. Berger JS, Brown DL. Gender-age interaction in early mortality following primary angioplasty for acute myocardial infarction. *Am J Cardiol*. 2006;98:1140–1143.

9. Epps KC, et al. Sex differences in outcomes following percutaneous coronary intervention according to age. *Circ Cardiovasc Qual Outcomes*. 2016;9:S16–S25.

10. Worrall-Carter L, et al. Impact of comorbidities and gender on the use of coronary interventions in patients with high-risk non-ST-segment elevation acute coronary syndrome. *Catheter Cardiovasc Interv*. 2016;87:E128–E36.

11. Asanuma Y, et al. Premature coronary artery atherosclerosis in systemic lupus erythematosus. *N Engl J Med*. 2003;349:2407–2415.

12. Quinones A, et al. Diabetes and ischemic heart disease death in people age 25–54: a multiple-cause-of-death analysis based on over 400 000 deaths from 1990 to 2008 in New York City. *Clin Cardiol*. 2015;38:114–120.

13. Burke AP, et al. Effect of risk factors on the mechanism of acute thrombosis and sudden coronary death in women. *Circulation*. 1998;97:2110–2116.

14. Arbustini E, et al. Plaque erosion is a major substrate for coronary thrombosis in acute myocardial infarction. *Heart*. 1999;82:269–272.

15. Ann SH, et al. Gender differences in plaque characteristics of culprit lesions in patients with ST elevation myocardial infarction. *Heart Vessels*. 2016;31:1767–1775.

16. Ruiz-García J, et al. Age- and gender-related changes in plaque composition in patients with acute coronary syndrome: the PROSPECT study. *EuroIntervention*. 2012;8:929–938.

17. Guagliumi G, et al. Mechanisms of atherothrombosis and vascular response to primary percutaneous coronary intervention in women versus men with acute myocardial infarction: results of the OCTAVIA study. *JACC Cardiovasc Interv*. 2014;7:958–968.

18. Iqbal SN, et al. Characteristics of plaque disruption by intravascular ultrasound in women presenting with myocardial infarction without obstructive coronary artery disease. *Am Heart J*. 2014;167:715–722.

19. Bharadwaj AS, et al. Multimodality intravascular imaging to evaluate sex differences in plaque morphology in stable CAD. *JACC Cardiovasc Imaging*. 2016;9:400–407.

20. Orshal JM, Khalil RA. Gender, sex hormones, and vascular tone. *Am J Physiol Regul Integr Comp Physiol*. 2004;286:R233–R249.

21. von Mering GO, et al. Abnormal coronary vasomotion as a prognostic indicator of cardiovascular events in women: results from the National Heart, Lung, and Blood Institute-Sponsored Women's Ischemia Syndrome Evaluation (WISE). *Circulation*. 2004;109:722–725.

22. Kawana A, et al. Gender differences in the clinical characteristics and outcomes of patients with vasospastic angina—a report from the Japanese Coronary Spasm Association. *Circ J*. 2013;77:1267–1274.

23. Pepine CJ, et al. Coronary microvascular reactivity to adenosine predicts adverse outcome in women evaluated for suspected ischemia results from the National Heart, Lung and Blood Institute WISE (Women's Ischemia Syndrome Evaluation) study. *J Am Coll Cardiol*. 2010;55:2825–2832.

24. Roman MJ, et al. Prevalence and correlates of accelerated atherosclerosis in systemic lupus erythematosus. *N Engl J Med*. 2003;349:2399–2406.

25. Bruce IN, et al. Single photon emission computed tomography dual isotope myocardial perfusion imaging in women with systemic lupus erythematosus. Prevalence and distribution of abnormalities. *J Rheumatol*. 2000;27(10):2372–2377.

26. Edwards NC, et al. Myocardial disease in systemic vasculitis and autoimmune disease detected by cardiovascular magnetic resonance. *Rheumatology (Oxford)*. 2007;46:1208–1209.

27. Nakashima T, et al. Prognostic impact of spontaneous coronary artery dissection in young female patients with acute myocardial infarction: a report from the Angina Pectoris-Myocardial Infarction Multicenter Investigators in Japan. *Int J Cardiol*. 2016;207:341–348.

28. Elkayam U, et al. Pregnancy-associated acute myocardial infarction: a review of contemporary experience in 150 cases between 2006 and 2011. *Circulation*. 2014;129:1695–1702.

29. Maehara A, et al. Intravascular ultrasound assessment of spontaneous coronary artery dissection. *Am J Cardiol*. 2002;89:466–468.

30. Saw J, et al. Spontaneous coronary artery dissection: association with predisposing arteriopathies and precipitating stressors and cardiovascular outcomes. *Circ Cardiovasc Interv*. 2014;7:645–655.

31. Saw J. Coronary angiogram classification of spontaneous coronary artery dissection. *Catheter Cardiovasc Interv*. 2014;84:1115–1122.

32. McGrath-Cadell L, et al. Outcomes of patients with spontaneous coronary artery dissection. *Open Heart*. 2016;3:e000491.

33. Tweet MS, et al. Spontaneous coronary artery dissection: revascularization versus conservative therapy. *Circ Cardiovasc Interv*. 2014;7:777–786.

34. Yumoto K, et al. Successful treatment of spontaneous coronary artery dissection with cutting balloon angioplasty as evaluated with optical coherence tomography. *JACC Cardiovasc Interv*. 2014;7:817–819.

35. Gulati M, et al. Adverse cardiovascular outcomes in women with non-obstructive coronary artery disease: a report from the Women's Ischemia Syndrome Evaluation Study and the St. James Women Take Heart Project. *Arch Intern Med*. 2009;169:843–850.

36. Smilowitz NR, et al. Women have less severe and extensive coronary atherosclerosis in fatal cases of ischemic heart disease: an autopsy study. *Am Heart J*. 2011;161:681–688.

37. Reynolds HR, et al. Mechanisms of myocardial infarction in women without angiographically obstructive coronary artery disease. *Circulation*. 2011;124:1414–1425.

38. Redfors B, et al. Mortality in Takotsubo syndrome is similar to mortality in myocardial infarction—a report from the SWEDEHEART registry. *Int J Cardiol*. 2015;185:282–289.

39. Agewall S, et al. ESC working group position paper on myocardial infarction with non-obstructive coronary arteries. *Eur Heart J*. 2017;38(3):143–153.

40. Hiteshi AK, et al. Gender differences in coronary artery diameter are not related to body habitus or left ventricular mass. *Clin Cardiol*. 2014;37:605–609.

41. De Angelis L, et al. Sex differences in age-related stiffening of the aorta in subjects with type 2 diabetes. *Hypertension*. 2004;44:67–71.

42. Wolff R, et al. Gender differences in the prevalence and treatment of coronary chronic total occlusions. *Catheter Cardiovasc Interv*. 2016;87:1063–1070.

43. Sharma V, et al. Comparison of characteristics and complications in men versus women undergoing chronic total occlusion percutaneous intervention. *Am J Cardiol*. 2017;119(4):535–541.

44. Giustino G, et al. Correlates and impact of coronary artery calcifications in women undergoing percutaneous coronary intervention with drug-eluting stents: from the Women in Innovation and Drug-Eluting Stents (WIN-DES) collaboration [abstract]. *JACC Cardiovasc Interv*. 2017;9(18):1890–1901.

45. Kim CY, et al. Gender differences in acute and 30-day outcomes after orbital atherectomy treatment of de novo, severely calcified coronary lesions. *Catheter Cardiovasc Interv*. 2016;87:671–677.

46. Chandrasekhar J, Mehran R. Orbital atherectomy for severely calcified lesions: more dissections in women but similar 30-day outcomes to men. *Catheter Cardiovasc Interv*. 2016;87:678–679.

47. Baber U, et al. Comparisons of the uptake and in-hospital outcomes associated with second-generation drug-eluting stents between men and women: results from the CathPCI Registry. *Coron Artery Dis*. 2016;27:442–448.

48. Giustino G, et al. Safety and efficacy of new-generation drug-eluting stents in women undergoing complex percutaneous coronary artery revascularization: from the WIN-DES collaborative patient-level pooled analysis. *JACC Cardiovasc Interv*. 2016;9:674–684.

49. Giustino G, et al. Impact of clinical presentation (stable angina pectoris vs unstable angina pectoris or non-ST-elevation myocardial infarction vs ST-elevation myocardial infarction) on long-term outcomes in women undergoing percutaneous coronary intervention with drug-eluting stents. *Am J Cardiol.* 2015;116:845–852.

50. Abbott JD, et al. Gender-based outcomes in percutaneous coronary intervention with drug-eluting stents (from the National Heart, Lung, and Blood Institute Dynamic Registry). *Am J Cardiol.* 2007;99:626–631.

51. Onuma Y, et al. Impact of sex on 3-year outcome after percutaneous coronary intervention using bare-metal and drug-eluting stents in previously untreated coronary artery disease: insights from the RESEARCH (Rapamycin-Eluting Stent Evaluated at Rotterdam Cardiology Hospital) and T-SEARCH (Taxus-Stent Evaluated at Rotterdam Cardiology Hospital) Registries. *JACC Cardiovasc Interv.* 2009;2:603–610.

52. Brown RA, et al. Sex-specific outcomes following revascularization with zotarolimus-eluting stents: comparison of angiographic and late-term clinical results. *Catheter Cardiovasc Interv.* 2010;76:804–813.

53. Nakatani D, et al. Sex differences in neointimal hyperplasia following endeavor zotarolimus-eluting stent implantation. *Am J Cardiol.* 2011;108:912–917.

54. Ng VG, et al. Three-year results of safety and efficacy of the everolimus-eluting coronary stent in women (from the SPIRIT III randomized clinical trial). *Am J Cardiol.* 2011;107:841–848.

55. Lansky AJ, et al. Gender-based evaluation of the XIENCE V everolimus-eluting coronary stent system: clinical and angiographic results from the SPIRIT III randomized trial. *Catheter Cardiovasc Interv.* 2009;74:719–727.

56. Fengler K, et al. Gender differences in patients with cardiogenic shock complicating myocardial infarction: a substudy of the IABP-SHOCK II-trial. *Clin Res Cardiol.* 2015;104:71–78.

57. Joseph SM, et al. Women with cardiogenic shock derive greater benefit from early mechanical circulatory support: an update from the cVAD Registry. *J Interv Cardiol.* 2016;29:248–256.

58. Ahmed B, et al. Significantly improved vascular complications among women undergoing percutaneous coronary intervention: a report from the Northern New England percutaneous coronary intervention registry. *Circ Cardiovasc Interv.* 2009;2(5):423–429.

59. Daugherty SL, et al. Patterns of use and comparative effectiveness of bleeding avoidance strategies in men and women following percutaneous coronary interventions: an observational study from the National Cardiovascular Data Registry. *J Am Coll Cardiol.* 2013;61(20):2070–2078.

60. Ng VG, et al. Impact of bleeding and bivalirudin therapy on mortality risk in women undergoing percutaneous coronary intervention (from the REPLACE-2, ACUITY, and HORIZONS-AMI trials). *Am J Cardiol.* 2016;117(2):186–191.

61. Ndrepepa G, et al. Bleeding after percutaneous coronary intervention in women and men matched for age, body mass index, and type of antithrombotic therapy. *Am Heart J.* 2013;166(3):534–540.

62. Argulian E, et al. Gender differences in short-term cardiovascular outcomes after percutaneous coronary interventions. *Am J Cardiol.* 2006;98(1):48–53.

63. Sandgren T, et al. The diameter of the common femoral artery in healthy human: influence of sex, age, and body size. *J Vasc Surg.* 1999;29(3):503–510.

64. Rao SV, et al. A registry-based randomized trial comparing radial and femoral approaches in women undergoing percutaneous coronary intervention. *JACC Cardiovasc Interv.* 2014;7(8):857–867.

65. Steg PG, et al. Women and men with stable coronary artery disease have similar clinical outcomes: insights from the international prospective CLARIFY registry. *Eur Heart J.* 2012;33(22):2831–2840.

66. Daly C, et al. Gender differences in the management and clinical outcome of stable angina. *Circulation.* 2006;113:490–498.

67. Acharjee S, et al. Optimal medical therapy with or without percutaneous coronary intervention in women with stable coronary disease: a pre-specified subset analysis of the Clinical Outcomes Utilizing Revascularization and Aggressive druG Evaluation (COURAGE) trial. *Am Heart J.* 2016;173:108–117.

68. Wallentin L, et al. Outcome at 1 year after an invasive compared with a non-invasive strategy in unstable coronary-artery disease: the FRISC II invasive randomised trial. FRISC II Investigators. Fast Revascularisation during Instability in Coronary artery disease. *Lancet.* 2000;356(9223):9–16.

69. Wallentin L, et al. Early invasive versus non-invasive treatment in patients with non-ST-elevation acute coronary syndrome (FRISC-II): 15

70. Clayton TC, et al. Do men benefit more than women from an interventional strategy in patients with unstable angina or non-ST-elevation myocardial infarction? The impact of gender in the RITA 3 trial. *Eur Heart J.* 2004;25(18):1641–1650.

71. Swahn E, et al. Early invasive compared with a selective invasive strategy in women with non-ST-elevation acute coronary syndromes: a substudy of the OASIS 5 trial and a meta-analysis of previous randomized trials. *Eur Heart J.* 2012;33(1):51–60.

72. Cannon CP, et al. Comparison of early invasive and conservative strategies in patients with unstable coronary syndromes treated with the glycoprotein IIb/IIIa inhibitor tirofiban. *N Engl J Med.* 2001;344(25):1879–1887.

73. O'Donoghue M, et al. Early invasive vs conservative treatment strategies in women and men with unstable angina and non–ST-segment elevation myocardial infarction. *JAMA.* 2008;300(1):71–80.

74. Bucholz EM, et al. Sex differences in long-term mortality after myocardial infarction: a systematic review. *Circulation.* 2014;130(9):757–767.

75. O'Gara PT, et al. 2013 ACCF/AHA guideline for the management of ST-elevation myocardial infarction: executive summary: a report of the American College of Cardiology Foundation/American Heart Association Task Force on Practice Guidelines: developed in collaboration with the American College of Emergency Physicians and Society for Cardiovascular Angiography and Interventions. *Catheter Cardiovasc Interv.* 2013;82(1):E1–E27.

76. Tamis-Holland JE, et al. Benefits of direct angioplasty for women and men with acute myocardial infarction: results of the Global Use of Strategies to Open Occluded Arteries in acute coronary syndromes (GUSTO II-B) angioplasty substudy. *Am Heart J.* 2004;147(1):133–139.

77. Pancholy SB, et al. Sex Differences in short-term and long-term all-cause mortality among patients with ST-segment elevation myocardial infarction treated by primary percutaneous intervention. *JAMA Intern Med.* 2014;174(11):1822–1830.

78. De Luca L, et al. Contemporary trends and age-specific sex differences in management and outcome for patients with ST-segment elevation myocardial infarction. *J Am Heart Assoc.* 2016;5(12). pii: e004202.

79. Khera S, et al. Temporal trends and sex differences in revascularization and outcomes of ST-segment elevation myocardial infarction in younger adults in the United States. *J Am Coll Cardiol.* 2015;66(18):1961–1972.

80. Patti G, et al. Platelet function and long-term antiplatelet therapy in women: is there a gender-specificity? A 'state-of-the-art' paper. *Eur Heart J.* 2014;35(33):2213b–2223b.

81. Stevens RF, Alexander MK. A sex difference in the platelet count. *Br J Haematol.* 1977;37(2):295–300.

82. Wang TY, et al. Platelet biology and response to antiplatelet therapy in women: implications for the development and use of antiplatelet pharmacotherapies for cardiovascular disease. *J Am Coll Cardiol.* 2012;59(10):891–900.

83. Ridker PM, et al. A randomized trial of low-dose aspirin in the primary prevention of cardiovascular disease in women. *N Engl J Med.* 2005;352:1293–1304.

84. Wiviott SD, et al. Prasugrel versus clopidogrel in patients with acute coronary syndromes. *N Engl J Med.* 2007;357(20):2001–2015.

85. Husted S, et al. The efficacy of ticagrelor is maintained in women with acute coronary syndromes participating in the prospective, randomized, PLATelet inhibition and patient Outcomes (PLATO) trial. *Eur Heart J.* 2014;35(23):1541–1550.

86. Boersma E, et al. Platelet glycoprotein IIb/IIIa inhibitors in acute coronary syndromes. *Lancet.* 2002;360:342–343.

87. Subherwal S, et al. Baseline risk of major bleeding in non-ST-segment-elevation myocardial infarction: the CRUSADE (Can Rapid risk stratification of Unstable angina patients Suppress ADverse outcomes with Early implementation of the ACC/AHA guidelines) bleeding score. *Circulation.* 2009;119:1873–1882.

88. Rubanyi GM, Johns A, Kauser K. Effect of estrogen on endothelial function and angiogenesis. *Vasc Pharmacol.* 2002;38:89–98.

89. Alexander KP, et al. Sex differences in major bleeding with glycoprotein IIb/IIIa inhibitors: results from the CRUSADE (Can Rapid risk stratification of Unstable angina patients Suppress ADverse outcomes with Early implementation of the ACC/AHA guidelines) initiative. *Circulation.* 2006;114(13):1380–1387.

90. Lincoff AM, et al. Bivalirudin and provisional glycoprotein IIb/IIIa blockade compared with heparin and planned glycoprotein IIb/IIIa blockade during percutaneous coronary intervention: REPLACE-2 randomized trial. *JAMA.* 2003;289(7):853–863.

91. Chacko M, et al. Ischemic and bleeding outcomes in women treated with bivalirudin during percutaneous coronary intervention: a subgroup analysis of the Randomized Evaluation in PCI Linking Angiomax to Reduced Clinical Events (REPLACE)-2 trial. *Am Heart J.* 2006;151(5):1032. e1–1032.e7.

92. Lansky AJ, et al. Impact of gender and antithrombin strategy on early and late clinical outcomes in patients with non-ST-elevation acute coronary syndromes (from the ACUITY trial). *Am J Cardiol.* 2009;103(9):1196–1203.

93. Nairooz R, et al. Meta-analysis of randomized clinical trials comparing bivalirudin versus heparin plus glycoprotein IIb/IIIa inhibitors in patients undergoing percutaneous coronary intervention and in patients with ST-segment elevation myocardial infarction. *Am J Cardiol.* 2014;114(2):250–259.

94. Schulman KA, et al. The effect of race and sex on physicians' recommendations for cardiac catheterization. *N Engl J Med.* 1999;340:618–626.

95. Poon S, et al. Bridging the gender gap: insights from a contemporary analysis of sex-related differences in the treatment and outcomes of patients with acute coronary syndromes. *Am Heart J.* 2012;163(1):66–73.

96. Kragholm K, et al. Sex-stratified trends in enrollment, patient characteristics, treatment, and outcomes among non-ST-segment elevation acute coronary syndrome patients: insights from clinical trials over 17 years. *Circ Cardiovasc Qual Outcomes.* 2015;8(4):357–367.

97. Fuchs C, et al. Gender differences in clinical presentation and surgical outcome of aortic stenosis. *Heart.* 2010;96(7):539–545.

98. Williams M, et al. Sex-related differences in outcomes after transcatheter or surgical aortic valve replacement in patients with severe aortic stenosis: insights from the PARTNER Trial (Placement of Aortic Transcatheter Valve). *J Am Coll Cardiol.* 2014;63(15):1522–1558.

99. Humphries KH, et al. Sex differences in mortality after transcatheter aortic valve replacement for severe aortic stenosis. *J Am Coll Cardiol.* 2012;60(10):882–886.

100. Buchanan GL, et al. The role of sex on VARC outcomes following transcatheter aortic valve implantation with both Edwards SAPIEN and Medtronic CoreValve ReValving System(R) devices: the Milan registry. *EuroIntervention.* 2011;7:556–563.

101. Hayashida K, et al. Sex-related differences in clinical presentation and outcome of transcatheter aortic valve implantation for severe aortic stenosis. *J Am Coll Cardiol.* 2012;59:566–571.

102. Elhmidi Y, et al. Gender differences in patients undergoing transcatheter aortic valve implantation with the Medtronic CoreValve System [abstract]. *J Am Coll Cardiol.* 2011;58:B204.

103. Tigges E, et al. Transcatheter mitral valve repair in surgical high-risk patients: gender-specific acute and long-term outcomes. *Biomed Res Int.* 2016;2016:3934842.

104. Estévez-Loureiro R, et al. Effect of gender on results of percutaneous edge-to-edge mitral valve repair with MitraClip system. *Am J Cardiol.* 2015;116(2):275–279.

105. Attizzani GF, et al. Gender-related clinical and echocardiographic outcomes at 30-day and 12-month follow up after MitraClip implantation in the GRASP registry. *Catheter Cardiovasc Interv.* 2015;85(5):889–897.

106. Vahanian A, et al. Guidelines on the management of valvular heart disease: the Task Force on the Management of Valvular Heart Disease of the European Society of Cardiology. *Eur Heart J.* 2007;28:230–268.

107. Tomai F, et al. Twenty year follow-up after successful percutaneous balloon mitral valvuloplasty in a large contemporary series of patients with mitral stenosis. *Int J Cardiol.* 2014;177(3):881–885.

108. Seshadri S, et al. The lifetime risk of stroke: estimates from the Framingham study. *Stroke.* 2006;37:345–350.

109. Petrea R, et al. Gender differences in stroke incidence and poststroke disability in the Framingham heart study. *Stroke.* 2009;40(4):1032–1037.

110. Kuy S, et al. Management of carotid stenosis in women. *JAMA Surg.* 2013;148(8):788–790.

111. Howard VJ, et al. Influence of sex on outcomes of stenting versus endarterectomy: a subgroup analysis of the Carotid Revascularization Endarterectomy versus Stenting Trial (CREST). *Lancet Neurol.* 2011;10(6):530–537.

112. Chaikof EL, et al. The care of patients with an abdominal aortic aneurysm: the Society for Vascular Surgery practice guidelines. *J Vasc Surg.* 2009;50(4 suppl):S2–S49.

113. Higgins JP, Higgins JA. Epidemiology of peripheral arterial disease in women. *J Epidemiol.* 2003;13(1):1–14.

114. Hooi JD, et al. Incidence of and risk factors for asymptomatic peripheral arterial occlusive disease: a longitudinal study. *Am J Epidemiol.* 2001;153(7):666–672.

115. Hirsch A, et al. Peripheral arterial disease detection, awareness, and treatment in primary care. *JAMA.* 2001;286:1317–1324.

116. Sigvant B, et al. A population-based study of peripheral arterial disease prevalence with special focus on critical limb ischemia and sex differences. *J Vasc Surg.* 2007;45(6):1185–1191.

117. Sadrzadeh Rafie AH, et al. Sex differences in the prevalence of peripheral artery disease in patients undergoing coronary catheterization. *Vasc Med.* 2010;15(6):443–450.

118. Fowkes FG, et al. Ankle brachial index combined with Framingham Risk Score to predict cardiovascular events and mortality: a meta-analysis. *JAMA.* 2008;300(2):197–208.

119. Hernandez-Vila EA. Peripheral arterial disease in women: the effect of gender on diagnosis and treatment. *Tex Heart Inst J.* 2011;38(2):154–156.

 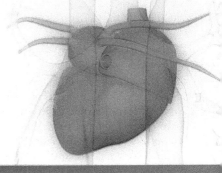

Primary and Secondary Coronary Prevention

Carl J. Lavie, MD, FACC and

Richard V. Milani, MD, FACC

Although the value of preventive cardiology may be emphasized more by the general cardiovascular (CV) community compared to the interventional community, secondary and even primary prevention guidelines are essential in the practice of interventional cardiology. This chapter discusses many aspects of preventive cardiology, including some of the guidelines from the American Heart Association (AHA)/American College of Cardiology (ACC), as well as from many other major organizations.

AHA/ACC Guidelines

During the past decade, major guidelines have emphasized several different classes of medications in addition to therapeutic lifestyle changes (TLCs). Certainly, in interventional cardiology, antiplatelet therapy has been emphasized. In the absence of contraindications, most patients should receive low doses of aspirin (81–325 mg) for life, and dual antiplatelet therapy (clopidogrel, prasugrel, ticagrelor) for at least 3 months, and probably for 12 months, in most patients following acute coronary syndrome (ACS) and percutaneous coronary intervention (PCI). This is discussed in detail elsewhere in this book. Lipid-lowering therapy, generally with statins (discussed in more detail under section Lipid Intervention), is indicated in patients with atherosclerotic cardiovascular disease (ASCVD). Therapy for hypertension (HTN) is indicated to achieve blood pressure (BP) levels of at least <140/90 mm Hg and <150/90 mm Hg in people >60 years of age (lower levels are a consideration for certain patients as discussed under section Hypertension). In patients with diabetes mellitus (DM), hypoglycemic therapy is indicated to achieve near-normal glucose levels (glycosylated hemoglobin or HbA1C <7%). Additionally, for most patients after myocardial infarction (MI) and with coronary heart disease (CHD), angiotensin-converting enzyme inhibitors (ACEIs) and β-blockers (BBs) are indicated. In fact, the AHA developed the Get With The Guidelines (GWTG) campaign during the last decade to increase adherence to many of these and other guidelines.

General CV Risk-Factor Information

Dyslipidemia (DLP) and HTN produce a substantial burden in the United States, and in most of Western civilization (1–3). A substantial number of deaths each year are estimated to be caused by systolic BP (SBP) that is higher than optimal (>115 mm Hg in epidemiologic studies) and by total cholesterol (TC) higher than optimal (estimated to be >150 mg/dL). In fact, almost 60% of the CV disease burden is caused by BP and/or TC higher than optimal. In the US, the combination of HTN and DLP were highly prevalent, with HTN affecting nearly one-quarter of the population, DLP impacting a third of the population, and both HTN and DLP impacting nearly 15%. Almost two-thirds of the patients with HTN also have DLP, and nearly half of those with DLP have HTN. Many studies suggest that most patients with HTN and DLP are not at both goals.

The risk of CHD events and strokes markedly rises with increasing age and increasing SBP. Likewise, there is a strong direct relationship between TC and low-density lipoprotein cholesterol (LDL-C) and major CV and CHD events (1). Although both SBP and TC markedly increase overall risk, as seen with other risk factors, often the individual risk factors are more than additive, and actually potentiate each other in increasing overall risk, emphasizing the importance of multifactorial risk-factor intervention (1).

Hypertension

The lifetime incidence of HTN has been increasing during recent decades and has now reached nearly 90% in the US (1). Approximately 70% of individuals with HTN are aware of their condition, and nearly 60% are receiving treatment. Nevertheless, HTN is controlled in only 30% of patients. Large meta-analyses show nearly 50% increases in the long-term CV mortality for every 20 mm Hg increase in SBP above 115 mm Hg. Lowering elevated BP will decrease the risk of CV events regardless of age, race, gender, or other risk factors.

The recent HTN guidelines are based on the Joint National Commission (JNC) 8 major recommendations (2). Changes in the guidelines since JNC 7 are summarized in Table 30.1. In general, HTN therapy is recommended for BPs >140/90 mm Hg, but the current guidelines indicate treatment in those 60 years of age and older is only definitively needed when BP is >150/90 mm Hg, although this has been questioned (3). Now more intense treatment is not required based on DM or chronic kidney disease (CKD), although a recent major trial (SPRINT) raises the possibility of goal BP being closer to 120/80 mm Hg (or at least <130/80 mm Hg as in the November, 2017 AHA/ACC Updated Guidelines) (4). In the last JNC 7 recommendations, BBs were considered main agents for HTN, along with diuretics, ACEIs, angiotensin receptor blockers (ARBs), and calcium-channel blockers (CCBs). Nevertheless, except for patients with heart failure (HF), post-MI, and also certain

---

TABLE 30.1 JNC 8's New HTN Guidelines

- 60 years and older, cut-point 150/90 mm Hg
- Under 60 years, cut-point 140/90 mm Hg
- 18 and older with DM, cut-point 140/90
- 18 and older with CKD, cut-point 140/90; use ACEI/ARB as first med
- Non-Blacks, use thiazides, CCB, ACEI/ARB; in Blacks, do not use ACEI/ARB (unless CKD)
- Increase dose or add med after 1 month to reach goal
- No ACEI/ARB combination

ACEI, angiotensin-converting enzyme inhibitors; ARB, angiotensin receptor blocker; CCB, calcium-channel blocker; CKD, chronic kidney disease; DM, diabetes mellitus; HTN, hypertension; JNC, Joint National Commission.
Adapted from: James PA, et al. 2014 evidence-based guideline for the management of high blood pressure in adults: report from the panel members appointed to the Eighth Joint National Committee (JNC 8). *JAMA.* 2014;311:507–520.

tachyarrhythmias, considerable evidence has questioned the use of BBs, especially with the older and non-vasodilating BBs early in the course of HTN. Therefore, BBs were taken out of first-line therapy for routine HTN in JNC 8. In African-American patients, ACEIs/ARB are not considered first-line therapy unless there is CKD. In DM, ACEIs/ARBs are given equal status with diuretics and CCBs. Also, ACEIs and ARBs should not generally be combined.

Lipid Intervention

Substantial evidence from epidemiologic and lipid intervention trials demonstrate the importance of TC, LDL-C, high-density lipoprotein cholesterol (HDL-C), and triglycerides (TGs) in the development and progression of atherosclerosis, and especially in the risk of major CV and CHD events (1). Although levels of HDL-C and non-HDL-C actually correlate better with CHD than does LDL-C, the vast majority of the intervention data during the last two decades has focused on the role of LDL-C, especially with statins, which are emphasized in the guidelines.

The National Cholesterol Education Program (NCEP)–ATP III treatment algorithm was based on LDL-C and assessing for CHD, CHD risk equivalents, and common CHD risk factors (by assessing Framingham Risk Score [FRS] in patients with ≥2 risk factors) (5). According to these guidelines, CHD risk equivalents were considered to be DM, as well as other forms of atherothrombotic disease, such as peripheral arterial disease (PAD), abdominal aortic aneurysm, significant carotid disease, or having a FRS that suggests greater than 20% 10-year risk of CAD. Certainly, from a clinical standpoint, many would consider other patients to have a CHD risk equivalent, such as those with a high coronary calcium score, metabolic syndrome (MetS), or symptomatic carotid disease (including those with a carotid bruit or significant stenosis), but these were not official CHD risk equivalents based on the NCEP–ATP III. As discussed with MetS and HTN, TLCs are always recommended for treatment guidelines for lipids. Most of the prior emphasis was placed on the treatment of LDL-C and non-HDL-C (**Table 30.2**). The new ACC/AHA/NCEP IV guidelines (6) now focus on statins, especially in those with ASCVD or who are high risk.

The risk assessment has now changed from the FRS to the Pooled Cohort Equation (7). Also, DM is no longer considered a risk equivalent; risk is now calculated in patients with DM using the Pooled Cohort Equation.

The current AHA/ACC guidelines focus on ASCVD (**Table 30.3**) and four major statin groups (**Table 30.4**). For many groups, intense statin therapy, especially those with ASCVD and ≥LDL-C 190 mg/dL, is defined as 40- and 80-mg doses of atorvastatin and 20 to 40 mg of

TABLE 30.2 ATP III LDL-C and Non–HDL-C Goals

RISK CATEGORY	LDL-C (mg/dL)	NON-HDL-C (mg/dL)
CHD or equivalent (10-year risk >20%)	<100	<130
≥2 Risk factors (10-year risk ≤20%)	<130	<160
0–1 Risk factors	<160	<190

CHD, coronary heart disease; HDL, high-density lipoprotein; LDL, low-density lipoprotein. Adapted from: Expert Panel on Detection, Evaluation, and Treatment of High Blood Cholesterol in Adults. Executive summary of the third report of the National Cholesterol Education Program (NCEP) expert panel on detection, evaluation, and treatment of high blood cholesterol in adults (adult treatment panel III). JAMA. 2001;285:2486–2497.

TABLE 30.3 New ACC/AHA 2013 Cholesterol Guidelines. Emphasis on Clinical ASCVD

- ACS/MI
- Angina, stable or unstable
- Arterial revascularization, coronary and other
- Stroke/TIA
- PAD, presumably atherosclerotic

ACS, acute coronary syndrome; ASCVD, atherosclerotic cardiovascular disease; MI, myocardial infarction; PAD, peripheral arterial disease; TIA, transient ischemic attack. Adapted from: Stone NJ, et al. 2013 ACC/AHA guideline on the treatment of blood cholesterol to reduce atherosclerotic cardiovascular risk in adults: a report of the American College of Cardiology/American Heart Association Task Force on Practice Guidelines. J Am Coll Cardiol. 2014;63:2889–2934.

TABLE 30.4 New ACC/AHA 2013 Cholesterol Guidelines—Four Major Statin Benefit Groups

- ASCVD
- LDL-C 190 mg/dL and higher
- Diabetes, age 40–75
- 10-year risk of major ASCVD of 7.5% and higher, age 40–75

ASCVD, atherosclerotic cardiovascular disease; LDL, low-density lipoprotein. Adapted from: Stone NJ, et al. 2013 ACC/AHA guideline on the treatment of blood cholesterol to reduce atherosclerotic cardiovascular risk in adults: a report of the American College of Cardiology/American Heart Association Task Force on Practice Guidelines. J Am Coll Cardiol. 2014;63:2889–2934.

rosuvastatin. For the elderly (≥75 years), moderate doses of statins are generally recommended, despite data showing the efficacy and safety of higher doses in older patients. Nevertheless, the guidelines do state that clinicians should review and discuss the pros and cons of more aggressive treatments with their elderly patients. The AHA/ACC guidelines do not have definitive recommendations for DM <40 years or ≥75 years, unless LDL-C is ≥190 mg/dL or there is an ASCVD. There are also no goals for LDL-C or non-HDL-C in the ACC/AHA guidelines, although many other groups, such as the National Lipid Association, the American Association of Clinical Endocrinologists, the European Society of Cardiology, the International Atherosclerosis Society, and the European Atherosclerosis Society, and others still have more aggressive goals for LDL-C and non-HDL-C. The current ACC/AHA guidelines have no definitive recommendations for using non-statins, except for patients with severe hypertriglyceridemia with TGs ≥500 mg/dL, with a recommendation similar to previous ones to treat elevated TGs. These prior guidelines recommended treating very high TGs first and then treating LDL-C with statins if required. The ACC now has an Expert Statement for possibly using ezetimibe, bile acid sequestrants, or the new PCSK9 inhibitors (8).

Metabolic Syndrome

During the last decade, the NCEP–ATP III has emphasized the importance of MetS (previously referred to as insulin resistance syndrome or MetS X) in contributing to the overall risk of CHD (5). As demonstrated in **Table 30.5**, the diagnosis depends on the parameters of obesity, TGs, HDL-C, BP, and fasting glucose. The prevalence of MetS markedly increases with age, and current statistics have determined the prevalence of MetS to be nearly one quarter of the adult population, and between 40% and 50% of older patients. Although in the general population the prevalence of MetS markedly

TABLE 30.5 Diagnosis of Metabolic Syndrome (MS)

RISK FACTOR	MEN	WOMEN
Waist circumference (inches)[a]	>40	>35
Triglycerides (mg/dL)	≥150	≥150
HDL-C (mg/dL)	<40	<50
BP (mm/Hg)	≥130/85	≥130/85
FBG (mg/dL)	≥100	≥100

Diagnosis of MS is made when ≥3 risk factors are present.
[a]Current level has been changed and is population/ethnicity specific (37 in. or 94 cm men, and 31.5 in. or 80 cm women in Middle East/Mediterranean).
BP, blood pressure; FBG, fasting blood glucose; HDL, high-density lipoprotein.
Adapted from: Expert Panel on Detection, Evaluation, and Treatment of High Blood Cholesterol in Adults. Executive summary of the third report of the National Cholesterol Education Program (NCEP) expert panel on detection, evaluation, and treatment of high blood cholesterol in adults (adult treatment panel III). JAMA. 2001;285:2486–2497.

increases with age, we have demonstrated that in patients with established CHD, the prevalence of MetS is actually inversely related to age (9). The prevalence of MetS in older CHD patients is similar to the prevalence in the general elderly population. Nevertheless, in younger patients with CHD (e.g., those <60 years of age), the prevalence of MetS is nearly 75%, suggesting that three out of every four younger patients with CHD meets the criteria for MetS.

Although many consider obesity, especially abdominal obesity, to be the major pathologic aspect of MetS, it should be emphasized that 5% of women and nearly 20% of men with MetS do not have a weight circumference that meets the current MetS criteria for abdominal obesity.

Patients with MetS are at markedly increased risk of developing type II DM (T2DM), so a major goal in the management of MetS is to prevent predictable complications, including T2DM, and more importantly, major CV disease events. Therefore, many patients with MetS will require TLCs and pharmacotherapy. The major TLCs in MetS involve dietary restriction of calories, easily digestible and refined carbohydrates, saturated fats, and trans fatty acids. Increases in levels of soluble fiber and "good fats" (omega-9 and omega-3 fatty acids) in a diet is also beneficial. Additionally, achieving and maintaining ideal weight and waist circumference are also very important. Increasing aerobic exercise, which helps with weight reduction and maintenance of weight loss, as well as increasing cardiorespiratory fitness (CRF), which is a major predictor of long-term prognosis and survival, is a mainstay of therapy in patients with MetS. Several studies have demonstrated that TLCs consisting of dietary intervention, a small amount of weight loss, and moderate exercise training produced nearly 60% reductions in the subsequent development of T2DM. On the other hand, pharmacologic therapy, such as metformin or acarbose, reduces the prevalence in developing T2DM by only approximately 30%. Other pharmacologic agents that reduce development of T2DM are ACEIs and ARBs, which were shown to reduce T2DM by nearly 25% (11,12). It should be emphasized that even when pharmacologic therapy is needed in patients with MetS, concomitant TLCs are still important in long-term therapy.

Obesity

Overweight conditions and obesity are strongly correlated with CV disease, because they adversely affect almost all of the major CHD risk factors, including (a) lipids (reducing HDL-C, increasing TGs,

slightly increasing LDL-C but changing LDL to a predominance of small dense particles that are more atherogenic); (b) HTN, by raising BP and promoting left ventricular hypertrophy (LVH), which is a potent independent risk factor for adverse CV events; (c) glucose, thus raising fasting and postprandial glucose levels, which are fundamentally pathophysiologic aspects of MetS and T2DM; (d) fitness, which reduces exercise capacity and CRF (also strongly related to increased CV disease); and (e) systolic and diastolic left ventricular function (obesity worsens both of these parameters) (10). Considering these myriad adverse effects on proven CV risk factors, it is not surprising that obesity is associated with almost all CV diseases, including HTN, CHD, and HF. Nevertheless, despite a strong association with obesity, and with CV risk factors and the development of CV diseases, now numerous studies of cohorts with established CV diseases, including HTN, CHD, HF, atrial fibrillation (AF), and PAD have demonstrated that overweight and obese persons have a better prognosis than do their leaner counterparts, which has been termed the "obesity paradox" (10–13). Although a detailed discussion of the obesity paradox and potential limitations for weight reduction and CV diseases is beyond the scope of this chapter, clearly the overall information available strongly supports efforts to prevent patients from becoming overweight or obese in the first place, something that should go a long way in the prevention of CV disease risk factors and many CV diseases. Additionally, despite the obesity paradox, the "weight" of information still strongly supports efforts at weight loss for most patients with advanced CV diseases, including HTN, CHD, and HF, although clearly better larger-scale outcome studies of significant weight loss is needed for all of these CV diseases.

Diabetes Mellitus

Patients with DM are at a markedly increased risk of CHD, cerebrovascular disease, and PAD (1), yet DM is no longer considered a CHD risk equivalent in the new guidelines. Clearly, CV disease continues to be the leading cause of morbidity and mortality among the DM population, accounting for almost 70% of deaths among patients with T2DM (1). Optimization of the dismal CV prognosis associated with DM requires aggressive, longitudinal, multifactorial CV risk factor treatment, including vigorous efforts at treating and/or preventing HTN, DLP, and obese and overweight conditions. Although detailed discussion of various therapies for T2DM and the potential role of CV risk factor reduction is beyond the scope of this chapter, clearly certain agents for T2DM have been associated with CV risk reduction.

Inflammmation and C-Reactive Protein

Substantial evidence documents the central role of inflammation in the pathogenesis and progression of atherosclerosis and major CV events (14). C-reactive protein (CRP) is a marker of systemic inflammation, and has been implicated in the pathogenesis of many chronic diseases, including CV disease and CHD. There is considerable controversy, however, regarding whether CRP is pathogenic in itself or just a marker of CV disease and CHD, but a detailed discussion of this is beyond the scope of this chapter. Clearly, however, patients with high levels of CRP have an increased risk of major CV events in most studies. In fact, even following CHD events, high CRP predicts further events. As observed in major statin trials following ACS, those patients with both low levels of LDL-C and low CRP have the lowest risk of recurrent CV events.

Although the most recognized CV treatment for lowering levels of CRP is with the statin medications, particularly at higher doses, there is also substantial evidence that cardiac rehabilitation (CR) and exercise training, as well as increased levels of CRF, are associated with marked reductions in the levels of CRP, especially when exercise training is accompanied by significant weight loss (15).

Smoking

The toxic effects of long-term tobacco smoking on CV, CHD, and general health are well recognized, and a graded relationship exists between the number of cigarettes smoked and the risk of MI and ACS. Nevertheless, unlike the impact of smoking to increase the risk of lung cancer, which takes nearly 20 years of smoking cessation to reverse, within 12 to 18 months of successful smoking cessation, most of the increased risk of smoking disappears, with the adverse CV risk of past smoking completely gone within 3 to 5 years after tobacco cessation. Recommendations for smoking cessation are considered a quality measure following ACS, and several medications (nicotine, bupropion, varenicline, and probably clonidine and nortriptyline) are effective in improving the odds of smoking cessation (1).

CR Programs, Exercise, and Fitness

CR programs have been neglected in preventive cardiology, with recent studies of Medicare beneficiaries showing that only 10% to 15% of covered participants actually attend these programs (16). Considerable recent emphasis has been placed in making both the referral and participation in formal CR a performance measure. Clearly, CR programs have been proven to increase exercise capacity and CRF (a potent predictor of prognosis for almost all CV diseases and total mortality), improve CHD risk factors, reduce psychosocial stress (PSS; which also predicts recovery and prognosis) and, most importantly, to reduce major morbidity and mortality (16–18). Considering the importance of physical activity, exercise, and CRF in general health, the national guidelines for physical activity and exercise are approximately 150 min/wk of moderate exercise (e.g., walking) or 75 min/wk of moderate to high-intensity exercise (e.g., running), and these recommendations are typically for both primary and secondary prevention.

Other Preventive Strategies

Long-term prevention also involves anti-platelet therapy in patients with established ASCVD or high risk. Although omega-3 fatty acids and prevention of vitamin D deficiency have potential medical benefits, there are no definitive cardiac guidelines regarding these agents. Small amounts of alcohol protect against most CVD, although any alcohol increases the risk of AF. Nevertheless, high alcohol above two to three drinks per day increases the risk of HTN and hemorrhagic stroke. As mentioned previously, CR is indicated in patients after major CHD events and is now indicated in HF and PAD although the AHA has recently recommended 1 gram of omega-3 after MI and for systolic HF (19).

Key Points

- Current guidelines from JNC-8 recommend pharmacologic BP treatment when BP is >150/90 mm Hg in those age 60 and older, although this has been questioned, especially based on recent evidence.

- β-blockers have been removed as a first-line therapy for HTN, except when needed for HF, CHD, and arrhythmias.

- ACEI/ARBs are not first-line therapy for HTN in African Americans.

- ACEI/ARB, thiazide diuretics, or CCBs are all acceptable first-line anti-hypertensive therapy, even in diabetes.

- The AHA/ACC/NVEP IV has no definitive goals for LDL-C or non-HDL, although many other groups with lipid guidelines differ.

- The AHA/ACC guidelines do not have definitive recommendations for DM or any patients <40 years or ≥75 years, unless LDL-C is ≥190 mg/dL or there is an ASCVD.

- The current ACC/AHA guidelines have no definitive recommendations for using non-statins, except for patients with severe hypertriglyceridemia ≥500 mg/dL.

- For the elderly (≥75 years), moderate doses of statins are generally recommended, despite data showing efficacy and safety of higher doses in older patients.

- Metabolic syndrome is the major component of diabetes associated with increased CHD risk.

References

1. O'Keefe JH, Carter MD, Lavie CJ. Primary and secondary prevention of cardiovascular diseases: a practical evidence-based approach. *Mayo Clin Proc.* 2009;84:741–757.

2. James PA, et al. 2014 evidence-based guideline for the management of high blood pressure in adults: report from the panel members appointed to the Eighth Joint National Committee (JNC 8). *JAMA.* 2014;311:507–520.

3. Bangalore S, et al. 2014 eight Joint National Committee panel recommendations for blood pressure targets revisited: results from the INVEST study. *J Am Coll Cardiol.* 2014;64:784–793.

4. Wright JT Jr, et al. SPRINT Research Group. A randomized trial of intensive versus standard blood-pressure control. *N Engl J Med.* 2015;373:2103–2116.

5. Expert Panel on Detection, Evaluation, and Treatment of High Blood Cholesterol in Adults. Executive summary of the third report of the National Cholesterol Education Program (NCEP) expert panel on detection, evaluation, and treatment of high blood cholesterol in adults (adult treatment panel III). *JAMA.* 2001;285:2486–2497.

6. Stone NJ, et al. 2013 ACC/AHA guideline on the treatment of blood cholesterol to reduce atherosclerotic cardiovascular risk in adults: a report of the American College of Cardiology/American Heart Association Task Force on Practice Guidelines. *J Am Coll Cardiol.* 2014;63:2889–2934.

7. Goff DC Jr, et al. 2013 ACC/AHA guideline on the assessment of cardiovascular risk: a report of the American College of Cardiology/American Heart Association Task Force on Practice Guidelines. *J Am Coll Cardiol.* 2014;63:2935–2959.

8. Lloyd-Jones DM, et al. 2016 ACC expert consensus decision pathway on the role of non-statin therapies for LDL-cholesterol lowering in the management of atherosclerotic cardiovascular disease risk: a report of the American College of Cardiology Task Force on Clinical Expert Consensus Documents. *J Am Coll Cardiol.* 2016;68:92–125.

9. Milani RV, Lavie CJ. Prevalence and profile of metabolic syndrome in patients following acute coronary events and effects of therapeutic lifestyle change with cardiac rehabilitation. *Am J Cardiol.* 2003;92:50–54.

10. Lavie CJ, et al. Obesity and prevalence of cardiovascular diseases and prognosis: the obesity paradox updated. *Prog Cardiovasc Dis.* 2016;58:537–547.

11. O'Keefe JH, et al. Should an angiotensin-converting enzyme inhibitor be standard therapy for patients with atherosclerotic disease? *J Am Coll Cardiol.* 2001;37:1–8.

12. Abuissa H, et al. Angiotensin-converting enzyme inhibitors or angiotensin receptor blockers for prevention of type 2 diabetes: a meta-analysis of randomized clinical trials. *J Am Coll Cardiol.* 2005;46:821–826.

13. Lavie CJ, et al. Update on obesity and obesity paradox in heart failure. *Prog Cardiovasc Dis.* 2016;58:393–400.

14. Lavie CJ, et al. C-reactive protein and cardiovascular diseases: is it ready for primetime? *Am J Med Sci.* 2009;338:486–492.

15. Lavie CJ, et al. Impact of physical activity, cardiorespiratory fitness, and exercise training on markers of inflammation. *J Cardiopulm Rehabil Prev.* 2011;31:137–145.

16. Arena R, et al. Increasing referral and participation rates to outpatient cardiac rehabilitation: the valuable role of healthcare professionals in the inpatient and home health settings: a science advisory from the American Heart Association. *Circulation.* 2012;125:1321–1329.

17. Menezes AR, et al. Cardiac rehabilitation in the United States. *Prog Cardiovasc Dis.* 2014;56:522–529.

18. Lavie CJ, Arena R, Franklin BA. Cardiac rehabilitation and healthy life-style interventions: rectifying program deficiencies to improve patient outcomes. *J Am Coll Cardiol.* 2016;67:13–15.

19. Siscovick DS, et al. Omega-3 Polyunsaturated Fatty Acid (Fish Oil) Supplementation and the Prevention of Clinical Cardiovascular Disease: A Science Advisory From the American Heart Association. *Circulation.* 2017;135:e867–e884.

31 PCI Guidelines for Interventional Cardiology Boards

Zoran Lasic, MD, FSCAI, FACC

In November 2011, the ACCF/AHA/SCAI published guidelines for percutaneous coronary intervention (PCI) (1) with subsequent focused updates on STEMI/NSTEMI (ST-Elevation Myocardial Infarction/non-ST-elevation myocardial infarction), the Clinical Competence Statement, and dual antiplatelet therapy (DAPT) from 2012 to 2016 (2–5). Practice guidelines are the result of a thorough review of evidence with an aim to provide assistance to physicians in selecting the best management strategy for an individual patient. In return, physicians will have to be familiar with the guidelines to optimally manage their patients and to successfully pass the interventional cardiology board exam, given that most questions on the board exam are derived from material contained in the guidelines.

Data on efficacy and outcomes represent the primary basis for the recommendations contained in the guidelines. The Class of Recommendation (COR) is an estimate of the size of the treatment effect, considering risks versus benefits, in addition to evidence and/or agreement that a given treatment or procedure is or is not useful/effective or in some situations may cause harm.

In general, Class I recommendations are for the procedure/treatment that should be performed. Class IIa reflects a recommendation where there is likely benefit from the treatments/procedures to be performed. Class IIb recommendations are made when the benefit-to-risk ratio is less certain. Class III denotes those treatments/procedures where the risks outweigh the benefits and these therapies should not be provided.

The Level of Evidence (LOE) is an estimate of the certainty or precision of the treatment effect, and each recommendation given is associated with the weight of evidence, ranked as LOE A, B, or C according to the number of patients' populations evaluated. When preparing for the interventional cardiology board, one should primarily focus on Class I and III recommendations, and because of this, most of the recommendations listed here will be in Classes I and III. Board questions usually depict a clinical scenario looking for the correct answer that is based on the guidelines. Most of the time, correct answers will be one that is based on Class I (treatment/procedure that should be performed) or Class III (treatment/procedure that should not be performed), regardless of the LOE.

This chapter summarizes many of the recommendations contained within the guideline document, with a focus on Class I and III COR. Most of the basis for specific recommendations are covered in many of the other chapters in this book and therefore not duplicated here.

Heart Team Approach to Revascularization Decisions

Heart Team is composed of an interventional cardiologist, cardiac surgeon, and the patient's general cardiologist. Support for using a multidisciplinary approach is a foundation of a Heart Team approach that originates from reports that patients with complex CAD referred specifically for PCI or coronary artery bypass graft (CABG) in concurrent trial registries have lower mortality rates than those randomly assigned to PCI or CABG in controlled trials. Particularly in patients with stable ischemic heart disease (SIHD) and unprotected left main and/or complex coronary artery disease (CAD) for whom a revascularization strategy is not straightforward, an approach has been endorsed that involves terminating the procedure after diagnostic coronary angiography is completed: This allows a thorough discussion and affords both the interventional cardiologist and cardiac surgeon the opportunity to discuss revascularization options with the patient. Calculation of the Society of Thoracic Surgeons (STS) score and the SYNTAX (6) score is often useful in making revascularization decisions because they have been shown to predict adverse outcomes in patients undergoing CABG and PCI.

Class I

A Heart Team approach to revascularization is recommended in patients with unprotected left main or complex CAD (LOE: C).

Class II

Calculation of the STS and SYNTAX scores is reasonable in patients with unprotected left main and complex CAD (LOE: B).

PCI Outcomes

Three interrelated components define the outcomes of PCI procedures: angiographic, procedural, and clinical success (Table 31.1).

Angiographic Success

Two different sets of criteria characterize the angiographic success of PCI procedures. One is related to a successful balloon angioplasty, defined as the reduction of a minimum stenosis diameter to <50%, and the other for successful deployment of coronary stents where a minimum diameter stenosis of 10% (with the optimal goal of as close to 0% as possible) is a benchmark that defines success. In both procedures, there should be final thrombolysis in myocardial infarction (TIMI) flow grade 3, without occlusion of a significant side branch, flow-limiting dissection, distal embolization, or angiographic thrombus.

TABLE 31.1 PCI Outcomes

Angiographic Success
PTCA: <50% residual stenosis
Stent: <10% residual stenosis
Procedural Success
Angiographic success without MACE
Clinical Success
Angiographic + procedural success + relief of signs and/or symptoms of myocardial ischemia
Short term: <9 months
Long term: >9 months

MACE, major adverse cardiac events; PCI, percutaneous coronary intervention; PTCA, percutaneous transluminal coronary angioplasty.

Procedural Success

Procedural success consists of angiographic success without associated in-hospital major clinical complications (e.g., death, myocardial infarction (MI), stroke, emergency CABG).

Clinical Success

Clinically successful PCI mandates both anatomic and procedural success, along with relief of signs and/or symptoms of myocardial ischemia. Duration of clinical success determines short- and long-term success with the cutoff point of 9 months. The primary driving force behind lack of long-term success is restenosis.

Complications

In spite of the refinement of PCI, in-hospital mortality still occurs in an average of 1.27% of patients undergoing PCI, ranging from 0.65% in elective PCI to 4.81% in STEMI (7). It is more common in patients with risk factors, primarily advanced age, comorbidities (e.g., diabetes, chronic kidney disease [CKD], congestive heart failure), multivessel CAD, high-risk lesions, and the setting of PCI (e.g., STEMI, urgent or emergency procedure, cardiogenic shock).

Procedural and periprocedural MI after PCI occur in 10% to 13% of patients based on the 2012 universal definition of MI which states that, after PCI, elevations of cardiac biomarkers above the 99th percentile upper reference limit indicate periprocedural myocardial necrosis. Increases of biomarkers greater than five times the 99th percentile upper reference limit were designated as defining PCI-related MI when coupled with new ECG changes, angiographic complications, or imaging evidence. Periprocedural MI occur in 1.5% to 2.6% of patients when using the SCAI definition of clinically relevant MI, which require creatine kinase-MB (CK-MB) >10 times, or troponin >70 times the upper limit of normal. Most common causes for MI include acute artery closure, embolization and no-reflow, side-branch occlusion, and acute stent thrombosis. It is critical to differentiate between myonecrosis and a clinical MI. All MIs involve myonecrosis, but not all myonecrosis is a clinical MI.

Incidence of emergency CABG after PCI has dramatically decreased to the current level of 0.4%. In-hospital mortality associated with it remains high, with ranges from 7.8% to 14% of patients. Similarly, the incidence of PCI-related stroke is relatively low—0.22%, but in-hospital mortality in patients with PCI-related stroke is 25% to 30%.

Access-related complications are the most common cause of vascular complications from PCI. With technique refinement, incidence has decreased over time. The most commonly encountered complications are access site hematoma, retroperitoneal hematoma, pseudoaneurysm, arteriovenous fistula, and arterial dissection and/or occlusion. Their incidence varies based on different definitions from 2% to 6%.

Radial artery access and ultrasound guided access could potentially decrease bleeding complications, but vascular closure devices have not been clearly demonstrated to decrease vascular complication rates.

Periprocedural bleeding is associated with subsequent mortality, with higher risk in patients with advanced age, low body mass index, CKD, baseline anemia, vascular access site, and sheath size, as well as the degree of platelet and thrombin inhibition.

Coronary perforation occurs in 0.2% of PCIs, most commonly by wire perforation during PCI for chronic total occlusion (CTO) or by ablative or oversized devices during PCI of heavily diseased or tortuous coronary arteries. Table 31.2 lists the frequency of complications (7–16).

Predictors of Clinical Outcome After PCI

Several models have been developed to predict procedural success and mortality after PCI. For inpatient mortality, the best accepted system is the ACC National Cardiovascular Data Registry (NCDR) CathPCI Risk Score system (7), with C statistic (probability of placing a patient in the right order, giving the higher probability to the one who develops the disease than to the one who does not) of 0.90.

For procedural success, the modified ACC/AHA score (17) and the SCAI score (18) are both in use, with discrimination by the C statistic of 0.70 to 0.82, respectively.

SYNTAX score is based on the location, severity, and extent of coronary stenoses, and is able to predict long-term risk of MACE (defined as a composite of death, stroke, MI, or repeat revascularization) after multivessel intervention (19). A low score indicates less complicated anatomic CAD. In post hoc analyses, a low score was defined as ≤22; intermediate, 23 to 32; and high, ≥33. The occurrence of MACE correlated with the SYNTAX score for drug-eluting stent (DES) patients but not for those undergoing CABG. At 12-month follow-up, the primary endpoint was similar for CABG and DES in those with a low SYNTAX score. In contrast, MACE occurred more often after DES implantation than after CABG in those with an intermediate or high SYNTAX score.

PCI in Hospitals Without On-Site Surgical Backup

Both primary and elective PCI can be performed at hospitals without on-site cardiac surgical backup with a high success rate, a low in-hospital mortality rate, and a low rate for emergency CABG, but only when performed by experienced operators with complication rates and outcomes equivalent or superior to national benchmarks. Hospitals should provide around-the-clock services for STEMI patients so as to achieve the best outcomes in lowering in-hospital mortality and shortening door-to-balloon times (20). Quality control and improvement measures must include comparison of outcomes with regional and national date registries, which include accepted benchmarks.

Specific requirements for PCI programs without on-site surgical backup in regard to strategy for surgical backup based on patient and lesion characteristics are listed in Tables 31.3 and 31.4.

TABLE 31.2 **PCI Complications**					
DEATH (2)		**MI (3,4)**	**CVA (5)**	**EMERGENT CABG (6)**	**VASCULAR (7–10)**
Elective	0.65%	10%–13% or 1.5%	0.22%	0.4%	2%–6%
STEMI	4.81%				

CABG, coronary artery bypass graft; CVA, cerebrovascular accident; MI, myocardial infarction; PCI, percutaneous coronary intervention; STEMI, ST-Elevation Myocardial Infarction.

TABLE 31.3 High-Risk Patient and Lesion Features

High-risk patient features	• Decompensated CHF • LVEF <25% • Left main stenosis (≥50% diameter) or three-vessel disease • Single-target lesion with >50% of myocardium at jeopardy
High-risk lesion features	• Diffuse disease (>2 cm in length) • Excessive tortuosity, calcification, or angulation (>90%) • Inability to protect major side branches • Degenerated SVG • Substantial thrombus formation • Questionable successful stent deployment • CTO intervention

CHF, congestive heart failure; CTO, chronic total occlusion; LVEF, left ventricular ejection fraction; SVG, saphenous vein grafts.

TABLE 31.4 Strategy for Surgical Backup Based on Lesion and Patient Risk

	HIGH-RISK PATIENTS	NON-HIGH-RISK PATIENTS
High-risk lesions	No PCI (transfer)	PCI
Non-high-risk lesions	PCI (discuss backup with CTS)	PCI

CTS, cardiothoracic surgical; PCI, percutaneous coronary intervention.

Class IIa

Primary PCI (PPCI) is reasonable in hospitals without on-site cardiac surgery, provided that appropriate planning for program development has been accomplished (LOE: B).

Class III: Harm

Primary or elective PCI should not be performed in hospitals that do not have on-site cardiac surgery capabilities without a proven plan for rapid transport to a cardiac surgery operating room in a nearby hospital or without appropriate hemodynamic support capability for transfer (LOE: C).

Operator and Institutional Competency and Volume Recommendations

The outcome of PCI is dependent on volume, both on institutional and operator level. Nevertheless, data supporting the evidence are from older observational studies and are increasingly recognized as uncertain, particularly with regard to low-volume institutions and operators. In more recent studies, it appears that operator experience may modify the volume–outcome relationship at the institutional level, so for the quality measures, risk-adjusted outcomes remain preferable to institutional and individual operator volumes (21).

Class I

Elective/urgent PCI should be performed by operators with an acceptable annual volume of 50 PCI procedures per year (averaged over a 2-year period) in centers that perform a minimum of 200 PCI procedures annually.

Elective/urgent PCI should be performed by operators and institutions whose current risk-adjusted outcomes statistics are comparable to those reported in contemporary national data registries.

PPCI for STEMI should be performed by experienced operators who perform more than 11 PCI procedures for STEMI per year. Ideally, these procedures should be performed in institutions that perform more than 200 elective PCIs per year and more than 36 PPCI procedures for STEMI per year.

Class IIa

PPCI is reasonable in hospitals without on-site cardiac surgery, provided that appropriate planning for program development has been accomplished.

Class III: No Benefit

Primary or elective PCI should not be performed in hospitals that do not have onsite cardiac surgery capabilities without a proven plan for rapid transport to a cardiac surgery operating room in a nearby hospital or without hemodynamic support capability for transfer.

Older observational evidence supported a volume–outcome relationship in PCI at both the institutional and operator level. Nevertheless, this relationship is complicated and may be inconsistent across low-volume institutions or operators. More recent data on PPCI suggest that operator experience may modify the volume–outcome relationship at the institutional level. Risk-adjusted outcomes remain preferable to institutional and individual operator volumes as quality measures.

Quality and Performance

PCI quality and performance considerations are defined by attributes related to structure, processes, and risk-adjusted outcomes (Table 31.5). They could be used for internal quality-improvement efforts and public reporting. Public reporting of institutional risk-adjusted outcomes is becoming more common and is more reliable than operator-level outcomes due to lack of statistical power resulting from lower volumes.

Class I

Every PCI program should operate a quality-improvement program that routinely (1) reviews quality and outcomes of the entire program; (2) reviews results of individual operators; (3) includes risk adjustment; (4) provides peer review of difficult or complicated cases; and (5) performs random case reviews (LOE: C).

Every PCI program should participate in a regional or national PCI registry for the purpose of benchmarking its outcomes against current national norms (LOE: C).

CAD Revascularization

The goals of revascularization for patients with CAD are to improve survival and/or relieve symptoms. When one method of revascularization is preferred over the other for improved survival, this consideration, in general, takes precedence over improved symptoms. When discussing options for revascularization with the patient, he or she should understand when the procedure is being performed in an attempt to improve symptoms, survival, or both.

Revascularization recommendations are predominantly based on studies of patients with symptomatic SIHD and should be interpreted in this context. Recommendations on the type of revascularization applicable to patients with unstable angina (UA)/NSTEMI are listed in a separate section Significant Coronary Artery Stenosis.

Angiographic criteria define "significant" coronary artery stenosis of ≥70% (≥50% for left main CAD), and historically, most studies

TABLE 31.5 PCI Quality and Performance Considerations

Structural attributes	Equipment Supplies Staffing Institutional and operator level volumes Availability of electronic medical records
Processes	Strategies for the appropriate patient Protocols for pre- and post-procedural care Appropriate procedural execution and management of complications Participation in databases and registries for benchmarking performance of the program and individual operator
Risk-adjusted outcomes	End result of structural attributes and processes of care

PCI, percutaneous coronary intervention.

of revascularization have been based on and been reported according to those criteria. More recent studies used physiologic criteria (assessment of fractional flow reserve [FFR] with "significant" stenosis defined as FFR ≤80%) to decide when revascularization is indicated.

Revascularization to Improve Survival

Left Main CAD Revascularization

Class I

CABG to improve survival is recommended for patients with significant (≥50% diameter stenosis) left main coronary artery stenosis (level of evidence: B).

Class IIa

PCI to improve survival is reasonable as an alternative to CABG in selected stable patients with significant (≥50% diameter stenosis) unprotected left main CAD with: (1) anatomic conditions associated with a low risk of PCI procedural complications and a high likelihood of good long-term outcome (e.g., a low SYNTAX score [≤22], ostial or trunk left main CAD); and (2) clinical characteristics that predict a significantly increased risk of adverse surgical outcomes (e.g., STS-predicted risk of operative mortality ≥5%) (level of evidence: B).

PCI to improve survival is reasonable in patients with UA/NSTEMI when an unprotected left main coronary artery is the culprit lesion and the patient is not a candidate for CABG (level of evidence: B).

PCI to improve survival is reasonable in patients with acute STEMI when an unprotected left main coronary artery is the culprit lesion, distal coronary flow is less than TIMI (Thrombolysis In Myocardial Infarction) grade 3, and PCI can be performed more rapidly and safely than CABG (level of evidence: C).

Class III Harm

PCI to improve survival should not be performed in stable patients with significant (≥50% diameter stenosis) unprotected left main CAD who have unfavorable anatomy for PCI and who are good candidates for CABG (LOE: B).

Non–Left Main CAD Revascularization

Class I

CABG to improve survival is beneficial in patients with significant (≥70% diameter) stenoses in three major coronary arteries (with or without involvement of the proximal left anterior descending (LAD) or in the proximal LAD plus one other major coronary artery (LOE: B).

CABG or PCI to improve survival is beneficial in survivors of sudden cardiac death with presumed ischemia-mediated ventricular tachycardia caused by significant (≥70% diameter) stenosis in a major coronary artery (CABG LOE: B; PCI LOE: C).

Class III: Harm

CABG or PCI should not be performed with the primary or sole intent to improve survival in patients with SIHD with one or more coronary stenoses that are not anatomically or functionally significant (e.g., <70% diameter non–left main coronary artery stenosis, FFR >0.80, no or only mild ischemia on non-invasive testing), involve only the left circumflex or right coronary artery, or subtend only a small area of viable myocardium (LOE: B).

Revascularization to Improve Symptoms

Revascularization techniques and medical therapy have improved substantially during the last 40 years. The effectiveness in controlling symptoms improved with both modalities. While the gap between revascularization techniques and guideline-directed medical therapy (GDMT) is narrower, the failure of GDMT to provide symptomatic relief justifies the need for elective revascularization.

Class I

CABG or PCI to improve symptoms is beneficial in patients with one or more significant (≥70% diameter) coronary artery stenoses amenable to revascularization and unacceptable angina despite guideline-directed medical therapy (GDMT) (level of evidence: A).

Class III: Harm

CABG or PCI to improve symptoms should not be performed in patients who do not meet anatomic (≥50% diameter left main or ≥70% non–left main stenosis diameter) or physiologic (e.g., abnormal FFR) criteria for revascularization (level of evidence: C).

PCI in Specific Clinical Situations

UA/NSTEMI

In patients with UA/NSTEMI, early risk stratification is essential for selection of ischemia-guided strategy or early invasive strategy to improve symptoms and reduce MI and mortality risk. Invasive strategy is favored in patients with high-risk clinical presentation (Table 31.6).

The choice of revascularization technique is based on the anatomical considerations used for patients with stable CAD, with the caveat that PCI may be initially preferred regardless of anatomical characteristics to stabilize the patient. Early angiography and revascularization (within 24 hours of admission) is favored particularly in patients with high-risk features (22).

Class I

An urgent/immediate invasive strategy—within 2 hours—(i.e., diagnostic angiography with intent to perform revascularization) is indicated in UA/NSTEMI patients who have refractory angina or hemodynamic or electrical instability (without serious comorbidities or contraindications to such procedures) (level of evidence: A).

An early invasive strategy—within 24 hours—(i.e., diagnostic angiography with intent to perform revascularization) is indicated in

TABLE 31.6 High-Risk Features in UA/NSTEMI

- Dynamic EKG changes
- Elevated troponin
- High-risk score (GRACE, TIMI)
- Recurrent symptoms
- Threatened viable myocardium
- CKD
- Large ischemic burden

initially stabilized UA/NSTEMI patients (without serious comorbidities or contraindications to such procedures) who have an elevated risk for clinical events (level of evidence: B).

The selection of PCI or CABG as the means of revascularization in the patient with ACS should generally be based on the same considerations as those without ACS (level of evidence: B).

Class III: No Benefit

An early invasive strategy (i.e., diagnostic angiography with intent to perform revascularization) is not recommended in patients with extensive comorbidities (e.g., liver or pulmonary failure, cancer) in whom: (a) The risks of revascularization and comorbid conditions are likely to outweigh the benefits of revascularization (level of evidence: C); (b) there is a low likelihood of ACS (troponin-negative) despite acute chest pain (level of evidence: C), especially women (level of evidence: B); or (c) consent to revascularization will not be granted regardless of the findings (level of evidence: C).

ST-Elevation Myocardial Infarction

Reperfusion strategies in ST-elevation myocardial infarction include fibrinolytic therapy, primary PCI, and a combination of both. All modalities have evolved over time. The major challenges in primary PCI, which is the preferred modality, remains the achievement of rapid time to treatment and increased patient access to hospitals that provide primary PCI services. All communities should create and maintain a regional system of STEMI care that includes assessment and continuous quality improvement of EMS and hospital-based activities. Performance can be facilitated by participating in programs such as Mission: Lifeline and the D2B Alliance (23–27).

With fibrinolytic therapy, the key decision is for whom and when to perform coronary angiography. Of critical importance is that revascularization, via either modality, be undertaken in a timely fashion. Prolonged delay from medical contact to device (i.e., >120 minutes for transfer patients) suggests lytic therapy is preferred to primary PCI. For unstable patients (e.g., severe heart failure or cardiogenic shock, hemodynamically compromising ventricular arrhythmias) not treated initially with primary PCI, or stable patients treated with fibrinolytic therapy and suspect reperfusion failure, a strategy of immediate coronary angiography followed by PCI improves outcomes. The diagnosis of failed fibrinolysis is best made when there is <50% ST-segment resolution 90 minutes after initiation of therapy in the lead showing the greatest degree of ST-segment elevation at presentation. Given the higher risk of bleeding, patients initially treated with fibrinolytic therapy will attain the greatest benefit from PCI if they belong to a group of moderate and high-risk patients, such as those with anterior MI or inferior MI with right ventricular involvement or precordial ST-segment depression, as well as patients with ongoing pain.

Indications for coronary angiography in STEMI are listed in **Table 31.7**.

TABLE 31.7 Indications for Coronary Angiography in STEMI

	COR	LOE
Immediate Coronary Angiography		
Candidate for primary PCI	I	A
Severe heart failure or cardiogenic shock (if suitable revascularization candidate)	I	B
Moderate to large area of myocardium at risk and evidence of failed fibrinolysis	IIa	B
Coronary Angiography 3–24 Hours after Fibrinolysis		
Hemodynamically stable patients with evidence for successful fibrinolysis	IIa	A
Coronary Angiography before Hospital Discharge		
Stable patients	IIb	C
Coronary Angiography at any Time		
Patients in whom the risks of revascularization are likely to outweigh the benefits, or the patient or designee does not want invasive care	III: no benefit	C

Primary PCI is preferred to fibrinolytic therapy when there is a short first medical contact-to-treatment time in high-volume hospitals with expert operators. Advantages of primary PCI compared to fibrinolytic therapy are listed in **Table 31.8** (28). The greatest mortality benefit of primary PCI is in high-risk patients. For STEMI patients who are undergoing interhospital transfer, the first medical contact–to-device time goal is 120 minutes or less, with emphasis for systems to set the goal for times <90 minutes (29).

PCI of a non-infarct artery may be considered in selected patients with STEMI and multivessel disease who are hemodynamically stable, either at the time of primary PCI or as a planned staged procedure (30–34).

PCI for a hemodynamically significant stenosis in a patent infarct artery >24 hours after STEMI as part of a revascularization strategy improves outcome (35), while PCI of an occluded infarct artery 1 to 28 days after MI in asymptomatic patients without evidence of myocardial ischemia has no incremental benefit beyond optimal medical therapy (36) (**Table 31.9**).

Cardiogenic Shock

Class I

PCI is recommended for patients with STEMI who develop cardiogenic shock and are suitable candidates irrespective of the time delay from MI onset (37) (level of evidence: B).

TABLE 31.8 Advantages of Primary PCI versus Fibrinolytic Therapy

Rates for infarct artery patency	Higher
TIMI flow grade 3	Higher
Recurrent ischemia	Lower
Reinfarction	Lower
Emergency repeat revascularization procedures	Lower
Intracranial hemorrhage	Lower
Death	Lower

TABLE 31.9 Indications for PCI in STEMI

	COR	LOE
Primary PCI[a]		
STEMI symptoms within 12 hours	I	A
Severe heart failure or cardiogenic shock	I	B
Contraindications to fibrinolytic therapy with ischemic symptoms <12 hours	I	B
Clinical and/or electrocardiographic evidence of ongoing ischemia between 12 and 24 hours after symptom onset	IIa	B
Asymptomatic patients presenting between 12 and 24 hours after symptom onset and higher risk	IIb	C
PCI of a non-infarct artery may be considered in selected patients with STEMI and multivessel disease who are hemodynamically stable, either at the time of primary PCI or as a planned staged procedure	IIb	B
Delayed or Elective PCI in Patients with STEMI		
Clinical evidence for fibrinolytic failure or infarct artery reocclusion	IIa	B
Stable patient after successful fibrinolysis before discharge and ideally between 3 and 24 hours	IIa	B
Ischemia on non-invasive testing	IIa	B
Delayed PCI of a significant stenosis in a patent infarct artery >24 hours after STEMI as a part of invasive strategy	IIb	B
Totally occluded infarct artery >24 hours after STEMI in a hemodynamically stable asymptomatic patient without evidence of severe ischemia	III: no benefit	B

[a]Contact to balloon time <90 minutes in primary PCI hospitals, <120 minutes in non-primary PCI hospitals.

Class IIa

The use of intra-aortic balloon pump (IABP) counterpulsation can be useful for patients with cardiogenic shock after STEMI who do not quickly stabilize with pharmacologic therapy (level of evidence: B).

Class IIb

LV assist devices may provide superior hemodynamic support compared to IABP and serve as more effective bridges to recovery or transplantation, although experience with their use in this setting is limited (38) (level of evidence: C).

A leading cause of in-hospital mortality in STEMI is cardiogenic shock, and the only treatment proven to decrease mortality is revascularization, predominately through PCI, but also in selected patients with left main or three-vessel disease with CABG. Patients who present to hospitals without primary PCI capabilities should be transferred to a PCI center to improve their chances for survival (39).

Aspiration Thrombectomy

Routine aspiration thrombectomy before primary PCI is not recommended (Class III). Nevertheless, the strategy of selective or bailout aspiration thrombectomy, defined as thrombectomy that was initially unplanned but was later used during the procedure because of an unsatisfactory initial result or procedural complication, might be considered (Class IIb).

For rheolytic thrombectomy, no clinical benefit has been demonstrated in patients with STEMI undergoing primary PCI (40–43).

Coronary Stents

In primary PCI, BMS implantation is superior to balloon angioplasty because it decreases the risk for target vessel revascularization and possibly reduces MI rates, but does not reduce mortality rates (44). Compared to elective PCI, stent thrombosis is higher in STEMI patients, but there is no difference between DESs and BMSs. Nevertheless, DESs have demonstrated lower restenosis rates compared to BMSs. More recent primary PCI studies and meta-analyses have demonstrated lower restenosis rates without an increased risk of adverse stent outcome with DESs compared with BMSs (45–47). The greatest challenge in deciding the approach at the time of primary PCI is determining emergently whether the patient is a candidate for a prolonged (1-year) course of DAPT.

Class I

DESs are useful as an alternative to BMSs to reduce the risk of restenosis in cases in which the risk of restenosis is increased and the patient is likely to be able to tolerate and comply with prolonged dual antiplatelet therapy (DAPT) (level of evidence: A).

BMS should be used in patients with high bleeding risk, an inability to comply with 1 year of dual antiplatelet therapy (DAPT), or anticipated invasive or surgical procedures in the next year (level of evidence: C).

PCI in Specific Anatomic Situations

PCI in SVGs

Embolic protection devices in SVG intervention demonstrated a reduction of 30-day composite outcomes of death, MI, emergency CABG, or target-lesion revascularization (9.6% vs. 16.5%), in RCT comparing distal balloon occlusion embolic protection with no embolic protection (48), and reduction in periprocedural MI in non-inferiority trials evaluating proximal occlusion and distal filter embolic protection devices (EPDs) versus distal protection and occlusion balloons, respectively (49,50).

PCI in chronic SVG occlusion is not indicated because it is associated with low success rates, high complication rates, and poor long-term patency rates. Similarly, routine use of GP IIb/IIIa inhibitor therapy has not been shown to be helpful (51).

DESs compared with BMSs have a lower rate of restenosis, and target-vessel revascularization rates are lower with similar mortality and stent thrombosis rates (52).

Class I

EPDs should be used during SVG PCI when technically feasible (level of evidence: B).

Class III: No Benefit

Platelet GP IIb/IIIa inhibitors are not beneficial as adjunctive therapy during SVG PCI (level of evidence: B).

Class III: Harm

PCI is not recommended for chronic SVG occlusions (level of evidence: C).

Oral Antiplatelet Therapy

Aspirin (325 mg) should be given before PCI, at least 2 and preferably 24 hours before the procedure to reduce the frequency of ischemic complications (53,54). The optimal aspirin dose in patients treated with DAPT that provides maximal protection from ischemic events and minimizes bleeding risk is 81 mg (range 75–100 mg) (5). Following PCI, aspirin (81 mg daily) should be continued indefinitely (**Table 31.10**).

Clopidogrel loading dose of 600 mg achieves a greater degree of platelet inhibition compared to a 300-mg loading dose (55) and has similar benefits to a 900-mg loading dose.

Duration of DAPT in PATIENT with SIHD Treated with PCI

Class I

After BMS implantation in patients with SIHD treated with PCI, clopidogrel 75 mg should be given for a minimum of 1 month. For DESs, preferred duration of clopidogrel therapy after PCI is at least 6 months.

Class IIb

In patients with SIHD treated with DAPT after BMS or DES implantation who have tolerated DAPT without a bleeding complication and who are not at high bleeding risk (e.g., prior bleeding on DAPT, coagulopathy, oral anticoagulant use), continuation of DAPT with clopidogrel for longer than 1 month in patients treated with BMSs or longer than 6 months in patients treated with DES may be reasonable.

In patients with SIHD treated with DAPT after DES implantation who develop a high risk of bleeding (e.g., treatment with oral anticoagulant therapy) and are at high risk of severe bleeding complications (e.g., major intracranial surgery), or develop significant overt bleeding, discontinuation of P2Y12 inhibitor therapy after 3 months may be reasonable.

Duration of DAPT in PATIENT with ACS Treated with PCI

Class I

In patients with ACS (NSTE-ACS or STEMI) treated with DAPT after BMS or DES implantation, P2Y12 inhibitor therapy (clopidogrel, prasugrel, or ticagrelor) should be given for at least 12 months with aspirin in a daily dose of 81 mg (range, 75–100 mg).

Class IIa

In patients with ACS (NSTE-ACS or STEMI) treated with DAPT after coronary stent implantation, it is reasonable to use ticagrelor in preference to clopidogrel for maintenance P2Y12 inhibitor therapy.

In patients with ACS (NSTE-ACS or STEMI) treated with DAPT after coronary stent implantation who are not at high risk for bleeding complications and who do not have a history of stroke or TIA, it is reasonable to choose prasugrel over clopidogrel for maintenance P2Y12 inhibitor therapy.

TABLE 31.10 Oral Antiplatelet Agents for PCI: Indication Class (COR), Level of Evidence (LOE), and Comments for Practice

	COR	LOE	RELEVANT CAVEATS/COMMENTS
Before PCI			
Aspirin	I	B	81–325 mg before PCI if already on aspirin 325 mg non-enteric before PCI if not on aspirin
P2Y12 inhibitors	I	A	A loading dose of a P2Y12 inhibitor should be given to patients undergoing PCI with stenting.
Clopidogrel	I	B	– 600-mg loading dose (ACS and SIHD) – 300-mg loading dose up to 24 hours after fibrinolysis – 600-mg loading dose >24 hours after fibrinolysis
Prasugrel	I	B	– 60-mg loading dose in ACS – Contraindicated in patients with prior TIA/CVA (Class III: harm; LOE: B) – Generally not recommended in patients >75 years of age – Consideration of using a lower maintenance dose for patients weighing <60 kg
Ticagrelor	I	B	– 180-mg loading dose in ACS – Issues of patient compliance may be important
After PCI			
Aspirin	I	B	– 81 mg, continue indefinitely
P2Y12 Inhibitors PCI with Stenting			
Clopidogrel	I	B	– 75 mg for minimum of 1 month BMS in SIHD – 75 mg for at least 6 months after DES in SIHD – 75 mg for at least 1 year after ACS with BMS or DES
Prasugrel	I	B	– 10 mg for at least 1 year after ACS with BMS or ACS
Ticagrelor	I	B	– 90 mg twice daily for at least 1 year after ACS with BMS or DES
P2Y12 inhibitors after stenting	IIb	C	– In SIHD after DES implantation—if bleeding or high bleeding risk—3 months may be reasonable
Prasugrel	III	B	Prasugrel should not be administered to patients with a prior history of stroke or TIA

Class III

Prasugrel should not be administered to patients with a prior history of stroke or TIA.

Recommendation for Antiplatelet Agent in SIHD and ACS

ACS patients in TRITON–TIMI 38 (Trial to Assess Improvement in Therapeutic Outcomes by Optimizing Platelet Inhibition with Prasugrel–Thrombolysis In Myocardial Infarction) treated with prasugrel had a significant 2.2% reduction in absolute risk and a 19% reduction in relative risk in the composite endpoint of cardiovascular death, nonfatal MI, or nonfatal stroke. Somewhat offsetting this was a significant increase in the rate of TIMI major bleeding (1.8% vs. 2.4%) when compared with patients who received clopidogrel (56). Prasugrel is contraindicated in patients with a history of transient ischemic attack or stroke and is not recommended for patients older than 75 years and in patients weighing less than 60 kg because of an increased risk of bleeding on the 10-mg daily maintenance dose.

Ticagrelor, unlike clopidogrel or prasugrel, is not a thienopyridine and it also does not require metabolic conversion to an active metabolite. In ACS patients enrolled in the PLATO (Platelet Inhibition and Patient Outcomes) trial, ticagrelor was associated with a significant 1.9% reduction in absolute risk and a 16% reduction in relative risk in the primary composite endpoint of vascular death, nonfatal MI, or nonfatal stroke compared to clopidogrel (57). Importantly, a significant reduction in vascular mortality and all-cause mortality was observed. Aspirin above 100-mg doses reduces the effectiveness of ticagrelor and should not be used (58). Maintenance doses of 90 mg twice-daily could be important for patient compliance and should be discussed and emphasized to the patient. Ticagrelor and prasugrel have not been studied in elective PCI, thus no recommendation can be made regarding its use in this clinical setting.

Summary

This chapter represents a summary of interventional cardiology guidelines published in 2011 with subsequent focused updates on STEMI/NSTEMI, Clinical Competence Statement, and dual antiplatelet therapy (DAPT) from 2012 to 2016 (2–5). The material covered here and in other chapters will be the foundation for a majority of interventional cardiology board questions, usually in the form of case scenarios. Special attention is warranted for Class I and III recommendation for a particular topic (unless only IIa/IIb are available) because most of the questions will test candidates' ability to identify "the most appropriate treatment" (Class I) or one that is harmful or not useful (Class III).

Key Points

- For the interventional cardiology board, focus on Class I and III recommendations.
- In unprotected left main and complex CAD, the Heart Team approach and calculation of SYNTAX and STS scores is recommended.
- PCI outcome is defined by angiographic, procedural, and clinical success.

- The most common complications are death, MI, emergent CABG, CVA, and access site complications.
- Models that predict outcomes post-PCI are ACC NCDR, ACC/AHA, SCAI, and SYNTAX scores.
- PCI without on-site surgical backup is feasible if performed in accordance to guidelines.
- Operators should perform ≥50 procedures (averaged over a 2-year period) and at least 11 STEMI PCIs annually.
- PCI programs should have a quality-improvement program and participate in national and regional registry.
- Goals of PCI in patients with CAD are to improve survival and/or symptoms.
- Early invasive strategy is favored in high-risk patients with UA/NSTEMI.
- PCI is the preferred strategy in STEMI, with the goal of first medical contact to balloon time <90 minutes.
- Embolic protection is the preferred strategy in SVG PCI.
- DAPT should continue for 1 month following BMS and at least 6 months after DES in SIHD.
- DAPT should continue for 12 months following BMS or DES in ACS.

References

1. Levine GN, et al. 2011 ACCF/AHA/SCAI guideline for percutaneous coronary intervention. *J Am Coll Cardiol.* 2011;58:44–122. doi:10.1016/j.jacc.2011.08.007.
2. American College of Emergency Physicians, et al. 2013 ACCF/AHA guideline for the management of ST-elevation myocardial infarction. *J Am Coll Cardiol.* 2013;61(4):e78–e140.
3. Amsterdam EA, et al. 2014 AHA/ACC guideline for the management of patients with non–ST-elevation acute coronary syndromes. *J Am Coll Cardiol.* 2014;64(24):e139–e228.
4. Levine GN, et al. 2015 ACC/AHA/SCAI focused update on primary percutaneous coronary intervention for patients with ST-elevation myocardial infarction. *J Am Coll Cardiol.* 2016;67(10):1235–1250.
5. Levine GN, et al. 2016 ACC/AHA guideline focused update on duration of dual antiplatelet therapy in patients with coronary artery disease. *J Am Coll Cardiol.* 2016;68(10):1082–1115.
6. Sianos G, et al. The SYNTAX score: an angiographic tool grading the complexity of coronary artery disease. *EuroIntervention.* 2005;1:219–227.
7. Peterson ED, et al. Contemporary mortality risk prediction for percutaneous coronary intervention: results from 588,398 procedures in the National Cardiovascular Data Registry. *J Am Coll Cardiol.* 2010;55:1923–1932.
8. Alcock RF, et al. Incidence and determinants of myocardial infarction following percutaneous coronary interventions according to the revised Joint Task Force definition of troponin T elevation. *Int J Cardiol.* 2010;140:66–72.
9. Testa L, et al. Myocardial infarction after percutaneous coronary intervention: a meta-analysis of troponin elevation applying the new universal definition. *QJM.* 2009;102:369–378.
10. Aggarwal A, et al. Incidence and predictors of stroke associated with percutaneous coronary intervention. *Am J Cardiol.* 2009;104:349–353.
11. Kutcher MA, et al. Percutaneous coronary interventions in facilities without cardiac surgery on site: a report from the National Cardiovascular Data Registry (NCDR). *J Am Coll Cardiol.* 2009;54:16–24.

12. Ahmed B, et al. Significantly improved vascular complications among women undergoing percutaneous coronary intervention: a report from the Northern New England percutaneous coronary intervention registry. *Circ Cardiovasc Interv.* 2009;2:423–429.

13. Applegate RJ, et al. Trends in vascular complications after diagnostic cardiac catheterization and percutaneous coronary intervention via the femoral artery, 1998 to 2007. *JACC Cardiovasc Interv.* 2008;1:317–326.

14. Jolly SS, et al. Radial versus femoral access for coronary angiography or intervention and the impact on major bleeding and ischemic events: a systematic review and meta-analysis of randomized trials. *Am Heart J.* 2009;157:132–140.

15. Nikolsky E, et al. Vascular complications associated with arteriotomy closure devices in patients undergoing percutaneous coronary procedures: a meta-analysis. *J Am Coll Cardiol.* 2004;44:1200–1209.

16. Patel MR, et al. Arteriotomy closure devices for cardiovascular procedures: a scientific statement from the American Heart Association. *Circulation.* 2010;122:1882–1893.

17. Ellis SG, et al. Coronary morphologic and clinical determinants of procedural outcome with angioplasty for multivessel coronary disease. Implications for patient selection. Multivessel Angioplasty Prognosis Study Group. *Circulation.* 1990;82:1193–1202.

18. Kimmel SE, et al. Development and validation of simplified predictive index for major complications in contemporary percutaneous transluminal coronary angioplasty practice. The Registry Committee of the Society for Cardiac Angiography and Interventions. *J Am Coll Cardiol.* 1995;26:931–938.

19. Serruys PW, et al. Percutaneous coronary intervention versus coronary-artery bypass grafting for severe coronary artery disease. *N Engl J Med.* 2009;360:961–972.

20. Nallamothu BK, et al. Relation between hospital specialization with primary percutaneous coronary intervention and clinical outcomes in ST-segment elevation myocardial infarction: National Registry of Myocardial Infarction-4 analysis. *Circulation.* 2006;113:222–229.

21. Harold JG, et al. ACCF/AHA/SCAI 2013 update of the clinical competence statement on coronary artery interventional procedures: a report of the American College of Cardiology Foundation/American Heart Association/American College of Physicians Task Force on Clinical Competence and Training (Writing Committee to revise the 2007 clinical competence statement on cardiac interventional procedures). *J Am Coll Cardiol.* 2013;62(4):357–396.

22. Damman P, et al. 5-year clinical outcomes in the ICTUS (Invasive versus Conservative Treatment in Unstable coronary Syndromes) trial a randomized comparison of an early invasive versus selective invasive management in patients with non-ST-segment elevation acute coronary syndrome. *J Am Coll Cardiol.* 2010;55:858–864.

23. Le May et al. A citywide protocol for primary PCI in ST-segment elevation myocardial infarction. *N Engl J Med.* 2008;358:231–240.

24. Aguirre FV, et al. Rural interhospital transfer of ST-elevation myocardial infarction patients for percutaneous coronary revascularization: the Stat Heart Program. *Circulation.* 2008;117:1145–1152.

25. Henry TD, et al. A regional system to provide timely access to percutaneous coronary intervention for ST-elevation myocardial infarction. *Circulation.* 2007;116:721–728.

26. Jollis JG, et al. Implementation of a statewide system for coronary reperfusion for ST-segment elevation myocardial infarction. *JAMA.* 2007;298:2371–2380.

27. Nielsen PH, et al. System delay and timing of intervention in acute myocardial infarction (from the Danish Acute Myocardial Infarction-2 [DANAMI-2] trial). *Am J Cardiol.* 2011;108:776–781.

28. Keeley EC, Boura JA, Grines CL. Primary angioplasty versus intravenous thrombolytic therapy for acute myocardial infarction: a quantitative review of 23 randomised trials. *Lancet.* 2003;361:13–20.

29. Andersen HR, et al. Danish multicenter randomized study on fibrinolytic therapy versus acute coronary angioplasty in acute myocardial infarction: rationale and design of the DANish trial in Acute Myocardial Infarction-2 (DANAMI-2). *Am Heart J.* 2003;146:234–241.

30. Engström T, et al. Complete revascularisation versus treatment of the culprit lesion only in patients with ST-segment elevation myocardial infarction and multivessel disease (DANAMI 3-PRIMULTI): an open-label, randomised controlled trial. *Lancet.* 2015;386:665–671.

31. Gershlick AH, et al. Randomized trial of complete versus lesion-only revascularization in patients undergoing primary percutaneous coronary intervention for STEMI and multivessel disease: the CvLPRIT trial. *J Am Coll Cardiol.* 2015;65:963–972.

32. Wald DS, et al. Randomized trial of preventive angioplasty in myocardial infarction. *N Engl J Med.* 2013;369:1115–1123.

33. Hlinomaz O, et al. Multivessel coronary disease diagnosed at the time of primary PCI for STEMI: complete revascularization versus conservative strategy. PRAGUE 13 trial. Presented at: euroPCR. http://sbhci.org.br/wp-content/uploads/2015/05/PRAGUE-13-Trial.pdf. Accessed September 10, 2015.

34. Hannan EL, et al. Culprit vessel percutaneous coronary intervention versus multivessel and staged percutaneous coronary intervention for ST-segment elevation myocardial infarction patients with multivessel disease. *JACC Cardiovasc Interv.* 2010;3:22–31.

35. Erne P, et al. Effects of percutaneous coronary interventions in silent ischemia after myocardial infarction: the SWISSI II randomized controlled trial. *JAMA.* 2007;297:1985–1991.

36. Hochman JS, et al. Coronary intervention for persistent occlusion after myocardial infarction. *N Engl J Med.* 2006;355:2395–2407.

37. Hochman JS, et al. Early revascularization in acute myocardial infarction complicated by cardiogenic shock. *N Engl J Med.* 1999;341:625–634.

38. Kar B, et al. The percutaneous ventricular assist device in severe refractory cardiogenic shock. *J Am Coll Cardiol.* 2011;57:688–696.

39. Babaev A, et al. Trends in management and outcomes of patients with acute myocardial infarction complicated by cardiogenic shock. *JAMA.* 2005;294:448–454.

40. Elgendy IY, et al. Is aspiration thrombectomy beneficial in patients undergoing primary percutaneous coronary intervention? Meta-analysis of randomized trials. *Circ Cardiovasc Interv.* 2015;8:e002258.

41. Fröbert O, et al. Thrombus aspiration during ST-segment elevation myocardial infarction. *N Engl J Med.* 2013;369:1587–1597.

42. Jolly SS, et al. Randomized trial of primary PCI with or without routine manual thrombectomy. *N Engl J Med.* 2015;372:1389–1398.

43. Lagerqvist B, et al. Outcomes 1 year after thrombus aspiration for myocardial infarction. *N Engl J Med.* 2014;371:1111–1120.

44. Nordmann AJ, et al. Clinical outcomes of primary stenting versus balloon angioplasty in patients with myocardial infarction: a meta-analysis of randomized controlled trials. *Am J Med.* 2004;116:253–262.

45. Mauri L, et al. Drug-eluting or bare-metal stents for acute myocardial infarction. *N Engl J Med.* 2008;359:1330–1342.

46. Stone GW, et al. Paclitaxel-eluting stents versus bare-metal stents in acute myocardial infarction. *N Engl J Med.* 2009;360:1946–1959.

47. Suh HS, et al. Drug-eluting stents versus bare-metal stents in acute myocardial infarction: a systematic review and meta-analysis. *Int J Technol Assess Health Care.* 2011;27:11–22.

48. Baim DS, et al. Randomized trial of a distal embolic protection device during percutaneous intervention of saphenous vein aorto-coronary bypass grafts. *Circulation.* 2002;105:1285–1290.

49. Mauri L, et al. THE PROXIMAL trial: proximal protection during saphenous vein graft intervention using the Proxis Embolic Protection System: a randomized, prospective, multicenter clinical trial. *J Am Coll Cardiol.* 2007;50:1442–1449.

50. Stone GW, et al. Randomized comparison of distal protection with a filter-based catheter and a balloon occlusion and aspiration system during percutaneous intervention of diseased saphenous vein aorto-coronary bypass grafts. *Circulation.* 2003;108:548–553.

51. Roffi M, et al. Lack of benefit from intravenous platelet glycoprotein IIb/IIIa receptor inhibition as adjunctive treatment for percutaneous interventions of aortocoronary bypass grafts: a pooled analysis of five randomized clinical trials. *Circulation.* 2002;106:3063–3067.

52. Lee MS, et al. Comparison by meta-analysis of drug-eluting stents and bare metal stents for saphenous vein graft intervention. *Am J Cardiol.* 2010;105:1076–1082.

53. Jolly SS, et al. Effects of aspirin dose on ischaemic events and bleeding after percutaneous coronary intervention: insights from the PCI-CURE study. *Eur Heart J.* 2009;30:900–907.

54. Popma JJ, et al. Antithrombotic therapy during percutaneous coronary intervention: the Seventh ACCP Conference on antithrombotic and thrombolytic therapy. *Chest.* 2004;126:576S–599S.

55. von Beckerath N, et al. Absorption, metabolization, and antiplatelet effects of 300-, 600-, and 900-mg loading doses of clopidogrel: results of the ISAR-CHOICE (Intracoronary Stenting and Antithrombotic Regimen: Choose Between 3 High Oral Doses for Immediate Clopidogrel Effect) trial. *Circulation.* 2005;112:2946–2950.

56. Wiviott SD, et al. Prasugrel versus clopidogrel in patients with acute coronary syndromes. *N Engl J Med.* 2007;357:2001–2015.

57. Wallentin L, et al. Ticagrelor versus clopidogrel in patients with acute coronary syndromes. *N Engl J Med.* 2009;361:1045–1057.

58. AstraZeneca [package insert]. *Brilinta REMS Document.* NDA 22-433. Reference ID: 2976456. http://www.fda.gov/downloads/Drugs/DrugSafety/PostmarketDrugSafetyInformationforPatientsandProviders/UCM264004.pdf. Accessed September 9, 2011.

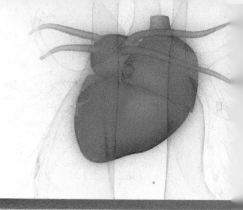

32

Thoracic Aortic, Abdominal Aortic, and Lower Extremity Interventions

Ehrin J. Armstrong, MD, MSc, MAS, FACC, FSCAI, FSVM and Douglas E. Drachman, MD, FACC, FSCAI

Interventional cardiovascular specialists encounter peripheral artery disease (PAD) in all aspects of routine clinical practice. Even the most skilled operators will occasionally cause peripheral vascular complications that require interventional therapy. As such, an understanding of the basic principles and indications for peripheral revascularization is critical for all interventionalists, including those who do not routinely perform non-coronary interventions. Interventionalists are also increasingly involved in the treatment of all manifestations of PAD. This chapter succinctly summarizes thoracic, aortic, and lower extremity interventions, with an emphasis on what should be anticipated on the interventional cardiology board examination.

Thoracic Aorta

Subclavian and Brachiocephalic Intervention

Obstructive disease of the major aortic arch vessels supplying the upper extremities is a common condition affecting up to 7% of individuals in select populations (1). When atherosclerotic in nature, subclavian and brachiocephalic disease is predominantly ostial or proximal in location, but other conditions—such as fibromuscular dysplasia, medium- and large-vessel vasculitides (e.g., Takayasu arteritis, giant cell arteritis), thoracic outlet syndrome, or radiation-induced disease—may cause lesions in more distal locations (2).

Symptoms of subclavian obstruction include arm claudication that manifests as fatigue, paresthesias, or pain during exertion. Proximal left subclavian artery stenosis may also impede antegrade flow through the left vertebral or internal mammary (LIMA) arteries, resulting in symptoms of vertebrobasilar insufficiency or angina when the LIMA has been used for coronary artery bypass grafting (CABG).

Revascularization of the brachiocephalic or subclavian arteries is indicated in the presence of significant symptoms such as arm claudication, vertebrobasilar insufficiency, or angina. Additionally, when the LIMA is required as a conduit for CABG surgery, empiric revascularization of left subclavian artery stenosis is appropriate, even in the absence of symptoms (2). Importantly, isolated identification of flow reversal in the vertebral artery—a common finding on Doppler ultrasound examinations—should not prompt revascularization in asymptomatic patients unless the internal mammary is needed for arterial bypass.

Technically, percutaneous revascularization of the subclavian and brachiocephalic arteries is successful in >95% of cases (3). No randomized data exist comparing open surgical revascularization with stenting. The femoral approach is most often utilized, although brachial or radial access may facilitate treatment of chronic total occlusions, where it may be difficult to localize the vessel's origin from the aortic arch or to maintain adequate catheter support to cross the occlusion (4). Ostial and proximal lesions are generally treated with balloon-expandable stents because radial force is desirable and this region is not exposed to extrinsic compression. For lesions located in the more distal portions of these vessels, self-expanding stents may be preferred to accommodate for the increased mobility of the vessels in these regions. If, however, the lesion is just distal to the origin of the mammary or vertebral arteries, brachial or radial access should be considered to ensure that self-expanding stent deployment does not inadvertently cover the origins of these vessels. Atheroembolization, while uncommon, represents a devastating potential complication, and can occur due to the direct route to the cerebral circulation through the vertebral artery. Some operators advocate the use of cerebral embolic protection at the time of treatment of bulky or angiographically "worrisome" subclavian or brachiocephalic lesions (5), but no convincing data are available to validate this strategy. Figure 32.1 shows stenting of a symptomatic left subclavian artery stenosis.

Coarctation

Aortic coarctation is a discrete narrowing of the thoracic aorta that preferentially occurs in proximity to the ligamentum arteriosum. It is the sixth most common form of congenital heart disease, and commonly occurs with other congenital lesions, classically in association with bicuspid aortic valves. Coarctation in children and adults is most commonly manifested as hypertension, and should be suspected in the presence of a brachial–femoral artery pulse delay (6). Individuals with unrepaired coarctation are at an increased risk of cardiovascular events, including stroke, heart failure, and death.

Endovascular or surgical repair is recommended in individuals with a gradient of >20 mm Hg across the segment of coarctation. Because collateralization may reduce the detectable gradient across the coarcted segment, intervention should also be considered in lower gradient states if diagnostic imaging demonstrates significant collateral flow. Surgical repair and endovascular angioplasty are both acceptable modes of therapy. In general, surgical repair is reserved for those with compelling anatomical indications such as branch artery involvement or associated large aneurysmal dilatation. Angioplasty is associated with significant recurrence rates; primary stenting is therefore generally preferred. The risk of aneurysm formation following surgical or endovascular treatment of coarctation is significant, and patients with a history of coarctation repair should receive annual follow-up with thoracic aortic imaging at regular intervals (7).

Acute Aortic Syndromes

Acute aortic syndromes include aortic dissection, intramural hematoma, aortic pseudoaneurysm, and penetrating aortic ulcer (8). Aortic dissections are classified as Type A (occurring with the proximal tear in the ascending aorta or arch) or Type B (occurring distal to the left subclavian artery). Intramural hematoma represents the presence of an aortic wall hematoma in the absence of an intimal tear. Aortic pseudoaneurysms and penetrating aortic ulcers represent an important subset of acute aortic pathologies. Most

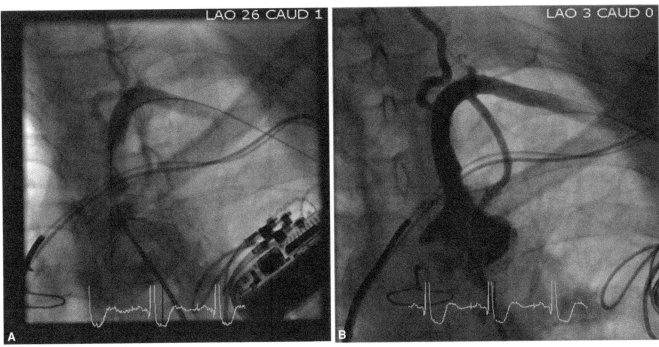

FIGURE 32.1 Subclavian intervention in a 65-year-old male with angina secondary to subclavian-coronary steal. **A:** A severe, ulcerated plaque is demonstrated in the proximal left subclavian artery. A 60-mm Hg gradient was present across this lesion. **B:** Following predilation, an 8 × 29 balloon-expandable stent was deployed with excellent angiographic results. Postdeployment hemodynamic assessment demonstrated no residual translesional pressure gradient.

pseudoaneurysms occur as a result of blunt trauma (e.g. following motor vehicle accident), whereas penetrating aortic ulcers tend to occur among patients with advanced atherosclerotic disease. The presence of a Type A aortic dissection represents a surgical emergency; in contrast, the management of a Type B dissection depends on the presence of distal organ malperfusion, such as renal dysfunction, mesenteric ischemia, or limb ischemia. In the absence of end organ malperfusion, most cases of descending thoracic acute aortic syndromes are managed medically, with a focus on meticulous control of blood pressure to minimize subsequent extension of the dissection flap (9). In the case of Type B aortic dissection with malperfusion, thoracic endovascular aortic repair (TEVAR) with a covered stent graft may be considered to cover the site of the tear. Among patients with Type B aortic dissection who are initially managed conservatively, approximately 25% to 30% develop aneurysmal degeneration of the aorta or extension of the dissection during the ensuing 5 years, and consequently require endovascular repair.

Thoracic Aortic Aneurysm

Thoracic aortic aneurysms (TAAs) comprise approximately one-third of all aortic aneurysms. There are multiple etiologies of TAA, including atherosclerotic disease, aneurysmal progression at a site of prior dissection, and predisposing genetic disease states, such as Marfan's syndrome. The majority of TAAs are asymptomatic and are detected on ultrasound or by CT scan. The indications for repair include a symptomatic TAA, an asymptomatic ascending TAA of 5 to 6 cm, or an asymptomatic descending TAA of 6 to 7 cm diameter (10). These thresholds for repair are a general guide for therapy, because patients with genetic etiologies may benefit from earlier repair, due to the natural history of continued progression, while patients with significant comorbidities may be more favorably managed with

continued monitoring until a higher threshold for repair is reached. The majority of ascending TAA are repaired surgically, although branched and fenestrated stent graft devices are being developed to promote future endovascular approaches. The majority of descending TAA may be repaired with TEVAR stent grafts.

Abdominal Aorta

Abdominal aortic aneurysm (AAA) remains a prevalent condition that poses a significant risk of death from rupture. Tobacco use, Caucasian race, and male gender are the classic associated risk factors, while, interestingly, diabetes is associated with a reduced rate of AAA (11). Current recommendations support a one-time ultrasound screening for AAA in males aged 65 to 74 with a history of smoking (12). Other societal guidelines also suggest screening among patients with a family history of AAA, regardless of gender or smoking history.

Open surgical repair was historically considered the standard of care, but more recently endovascular aneurysm repair (EVAR) has been utilized in the majority of cases owing to its lower periprocedural risk (13). Repair should be considered for the treatment of AAA larger than 5.5 cm, AAA that are expanding rapidly (>0.5 cm over 6 months), or for those of any size that are symptomatic. Current guidelines support open surgical repair for acceptable operative candidates. EVAR is a reasonable option for those at high risk for open repair with suitable anatomy (Class IIA indication). The utility of EVAR for those at low or moderate surgical risk is uncertain (Class IIB indication) (14). Notably, these guidelines were developed prior to the publication of three major randomized trials summarized in **Table 32.1**. Overall, these trials indicate that EVAR is associated with lower short-term mortality than surgical revascularization, but long-term mortality is similar between

TABLE 32.1 Randomized Trials of EVAR versus Open Surgical Repair

TRIAL	PATIENTS	COMPARISON	FOLLOW-UP DURATION	PRIMARY ENDPOINT	SECONDARY ENDPOINTS
DREAM	351	EVAR vs. open repair in surgically eligible patients	6 years	Cumulative survival, 69.9% vs. 68.9%, p = NS	Freedom from re-intervention, 81.9% vs. 70.4% favoring open repair, p = 0.03
EVAR-1	1,252	EVAR vs. open repair in surgically eligible patients	6 years	Death, 7.5 vs. 7.7 deaths per 100 patient-years, p = NS	Re-intervention 5.1 vs. 1.7 per 100 patient-years favoring open repair, p <0.001
EVAR-2	404	EVAR vs. no repair in surgically ineligible patients	6.1 years	Death, 21.0 vs. 22.1 deaths per 100 patient-years, p = NS	Aneurysm-related mortality 3.6 vs.7.3 deaths per 1,000 patient-years, p = 0.02

EVAR, endovascular aneurysm repair; NS, not significant.

treatment groups (15–17). EVAR is associated with a higher rate of re-intervention, approaching 25% at 5-year follow-up. These trials utilized older stent graft devices; newer-generation devices may improve technical success, and are likely associated with lower rates of long-term re-intervention.

Currently, the majority (approximately 80%) of patients with AAA in the US are treated with EVAR. Factors that may favor open surgery include complex anatomy not amenable to endovascular repair, young age, and patients less willing to maintain close follow-up for surveillance and possible re-intervention. There is a growing range of commercially available devices designed for the endovascular treatment of AAA. In general, these devices are comprised of self-expanding stents with interwoven fabric to exclude the aneurysmal segment, and suprarenal fixation to prevent device migration. The sheath sizes of these devices have also decreased over time, and the majority of patients may now be treated using a fully percutaneous approach, including "preclosure" with a large, suture-mediated closure device technique for management of the arteriotomy.

Importantly, patients who undergo EVAR require long-term surveillance with annual CT scans in order to monitor for device failure, while such surveillance is generally not necessary for patients who undergo surgical repair. The major long-term complications associated with EVAR include the following: lack of an effective seal between the endograft and the aorta with consequent "type 1" endoleak and aneurysm expansion; or the persistent communication of collateral arteries and the aneurysm sac, resulting in "type II" endoleak and aneurysm expansion.

Lower Extremity

General Overview

While lower-extremity PAD is a highly prevalent condition affecting 14.5% of the population older than 70 years (18), the majority of patients with PAD are asymptomatic, and most will not develop limb-threatening ischemia over time. Additionally, in symptomatic individuals, natural history studies suggest that most (70%–80%) will have stable claudication symptoms and that, fortunately, <4% will require amputation during long-term follow-up (19). In light of these principles, percutaneous revascularization of the lower extremities is commonly reserved for treatment of lifestyle-limiting symptoms that have persisted despite conservative measures, or for limb-threatening ischemia, namely rest pain or tissue loss (20). Conservative management includes hygienic and supportive measures to prevent skin breakdown and infection, exercise conditioning, pharmacotherapy for claudication, and—most importantly—modification of risk factors to reduce the profound associated cardiovascular

morbidity: smoking cessation, cholesterol reduction, treatment of diabetes, antihypertensive therapy, and antiplatelet therapy (21).

Lower-extremity PAD commonly involves multiple vascular segments. As a general principle, inflow disease (i.e., the more proximal segments) should be treated first for patients with claudication. In cases of critical limb ischemia (CLI), multilevel intervention is often necessary to establish straight-line flow to the affected limb (22).

Iliac Interventions

The TransAtlantic Inter-Society Consensus (TASC) document classification was developed to categorize aortoiliac lesions and guide therapy (Table 32.2) (23). In the TASC document, endovascular therapy was recommended for TASC A and B lesions, surgery was recommended for TASC D lesions, and individually tailored decisions were considered for TASC C lesions. While the TASC classification system provided a useful schema to categorize lesion complexity, the evolution of endovascular technology and techniques have permitted access to increasingly complex patients and lesions, and have rendered the guidelines expressed in this landmark document less relevant to contemporary clinical practice. In the current era, endovascular approaches are considered for most lesion subsets in most patients, because iliac artery stenting is associated with patency rates similar to that of surgery.

In the CLEVER trial, 111 patients with symptomatic aortoiliac stenosis were randomized to treatment with a supervised exercise program, stenting, or optimal medical therapy. The primary endpoint, improvement in peak walking time at 6 months, was highest in those who underwent a supervised exercise program (5.8 ± 4.6 minutes greater than baseline), slightly lower for those treated with stenting (3.7 ± 4.9), and lowest for those randomized to treatment with optimal medical care (1.2 ± 2.6). Of interest, a secondary endpoint, including improvement in quality of life, was achieved in a greater number of patients treated with stenting than with those who underwent an exercise program, calling into question the generalizability and application to clinical practice of the study's primary finding (24). In comparison, the recently published ERASE trial randomized 212 patients with aortoiliac or femoropopliteal disease and symptomatic claudication to exercise therapy alone or exercise therapy plus endovascular revascularization (25). Patients randomized to combination therapy had a significantly improved maximum walking distance compared to supervised exercise therapy alone (264–1,501 m vs. 285–1,240 m) and in pain-free walking distance. These results suggest that revascularization and supervised exercise therapy are complementary among patients with lifestyle-limiting claudication.

The optimal strategy for arterial access in patients undergoing intervention for aortoiliac disease depends on the characteristics and

TABLE 32.2 TASC Lesion Classification

TASC CATEGORY	LESION CHARACTERISTICS
Aortoiliac	
A	Unilateral or bilateral stenosis of CIA, unilateral or bilateral stenoses of EIA (≤3 cm)
B	Stenosis of infrarenal aorta (≤3 cm), unilateral CIA occlusion, stenoses of EIA 3–10 cm in length not involving CFA, unilateral EIA occlusion not involving IIA or CFA
C	Bilateral CIA occlusions, bilateral EIA stenoses 3–10 cm in length, unilateral EIA stenosis extending into CFA, unilateral EIA occlusion involving IIA or CFA, heavily calcified unilateral EIA occlusion
D	Infrarenal aortoiliac occlusion, diffuse aortic and bilateral CIA disease requiring treatment, multiple stenoses involving CIA, EIA, and CFA, unilateral occlusion of CIA and EIA, bilateral EIA occlusions, iliac stenoses with AAA that are not amenable to endograft placement
Femoropopliteal	
A	Single stenosis ≤10 cm, occlusion ≤5 cm
B	Multiple stenoses each <5 cm, stenosis or occlusion ≤15 cm not involving infrageniculate popliteal artery, single or multiple lesions in absence of continuous tibial vessel to improve distal bypass inflow, heavily calcified occlusion ≤5 cm, single popliteal stenosis
C	Multiple stenoses or occlusions >15 cm, recurrent disease needing treatment
D	Occlusions ≥20 cm of CFA or SFA involving popliteal artery, occlusion of popliteal and proximal trifurcation vessels
Infrapopliteal	
A	Single stenosis ≤5 cm in the target tibial artery
B	Multiple stenoses, each ≤5 cm in length, or total length ≤10 cm or single occlusion ≤3 cm in length in the target tibial artery
C	Multiple stenoses in the target tibial artery and/or single occlusion with total lesion length >10 cm
D	Multiple occlusions involving the target tibial artery with total lesion length >10 cm or dense lesion calcification or non-visualization of collaterals. The other tibial arteries are occluded or have dense calcification.

AAA, abdominal aortic aneurysm; CFA, common femoral artery; CIA, common iliac artery; EIA, external iliac artery; IIA, internal iliac artery; SFA, superficial femoral artery; TASC, TransAtlantic Inter-Society Consensus Document.
Adapted from: Jaff M, et al. An update on methods for revascularization and expansion of the TASC lesion classification to include below-the-knee arteries. *J Endovasc Ther.* 2015;22:663–677, with permission.

location of the lesion to be addressed. If entire reconstruction of the aortoiliac bifurcation is required, bilateral femoral access is employed to permit simultaneous bilateral iliac stent placement and "kissing" balloon postdilatations. When treating unilateral disease within the proximal iliac system (e.g., common iliac), ipsilateral access is desired to permit retrograde delivery of balloon and stent. In such cases, the contralateral approach may be more difficult because of the acute bend of the aortoiliac bifurcation and the associated challenges in establishing adequate coaxial support to deliver balloon and stent to a lesion that is proximal in the common iliac artery. In contrast, if the target lesion is in the distal common or external iliac artery, contralateral access may be preferred, particularly in situations where the external iliac disease extends distally to the common femoral region, compromising ipsilateral sheath placement.

The majority of iliac lesions are treated with stent placement, although shorter and anatomically simple lesions may be treated with balloon angioplasty alone (26–28). In the treatment of common iliac and proximal external iliac lesions, balloon-expandable stents are preferred, owing to their superior radial strength and more predictable delivery (29). In vascular segments near the femoral region, which are inherently prone to flexion and extrinsic compression, the superior flexibility of self-expanding stents may outweigh the slightly inferior radial strength compared with balloon-expandable stents. Balloon-expandable covered stents may also be favored for the treatment of anatomically complex (TASC C or D) aortoiliac lesions. In a randomized trial that compared covered balloon-expandable stents to non-covered stents, covered stents were associated with improved long-term patency and a decreased need for re-interventions during long-term follow-up (30).

Femoropopliteal Interventions

The femoropopliteal arterial segment is long and relatively straight, but is subjected to extrinsic compression from the thigh musculature, and to flexion and torsion because of movement at the hip and knee joints. Disease within this segment is often calcific, diffuse, and frequently occlusive; endovascular interventions must be designed to confront these unique and formidable technical challenges. Similar to the schema developed to categorize iliac arterial disease, the TASC classification system describes femoropopliteal lesions as type A, B, C, or D, corresponding to increasing anatomic complexity on the basis of length, presence of occlusion, and territory involved (**Table 32.2**) (23). Virtually all categories may be considered for an endovascular approach, although TASC C and D lesions have historically been regarded as "surgical disease" because the technical approach to complex stenoses and occlusions may be demanding.

Atherosclerotic disease in the common femoral artery represents a unique situation where endovascular therapy is most commonly avoided. Because the common femoral artery represents a valuable target for future peripheral bypass surgery, placing a stent in the vessel could potentially "burn a bridge" to important subsequent revascularization efforts. Moreover, the proximity of the hip joint and constant exposure to flexion increase the risk of stent fracture, and there is a paucity of data supporting balloon angioplasty for the treatment of common femoral disease.

In contrast, endovascular therapy of the femoropopliteal segment is generally the preferred first-line approach, because surgical bypass in this segment is associated with marginally better durability, but poses a much higher risk of global cardiovascular and local (wound-associated) adverse events (23). Restenosis remains the major limitation of endovascular treatment of the femoropopliteal segment. With balloon angioplasty alone, restenosis rates as high as 63% at 1 year have been reported (31,32). Similarly poor outcomes were noted with the use of balloon-expandable stents in this territory, likely due to profound compressive forces that characterize this arterial distribution (33). Advances in stent technology have led to the development of nitinol-based self-expanding stents that better resist the external forces generated by limb movement and muscle compression. For nonfocal disease (i.e., longer than 40 mm), multiple randomized trials have now demonstrated the superiority of nitinol-based self-expanding stents compared with balloon angioplasty with provisional stenting (34).

Newer devices have recently been developed to improve the long-term patency of endovascular interventions. Paclitaxel-eluting nitinol stents have demonstrated superior patency to balloon angioplasty or older-generation bare nitinol stents, with a long-term reduction in the need for re-intervention (35). Newer-generation nitinol stents are also associated with superior patency, due to engineering designs that have increased stent flexibility and resistance to compression (36). More recently, drug-coated balloons (DCB) have demonstrated patency rates similar to those historically garnered by nitinol self-expanding stents. Currently available DCBs deliver paclitaxel to the vessel wall during balloon inflation, where the lipophilic nature of paclitaxel enables it to partition into the vessel wall, upon which it exerts its anti-restenotic effect. In one randomized trial, DCBs were superior to standard balloon angioplasty, with improved primary patency and freedom from repeat re-intervention at 2 years (37). After DCB angioplasty, focal stent placement may be necessary in cases of significant flow-limiting dissection or recoil; real-world studies suggest that the rates of bailout stenting are 10% to 20% and depend on the length of the lesion being treated (38).

Although no randomized data are available, niche devices may also play a role for specific femoropopliteal interventions. Recanalization of long superficial femoral occlusions often requires subintimal tracking with distal reentry (**Fig. 32.2**). In cases of difficult reentry, specialized reentry devices may be utilized to regain access to the true lumen to facilitate angioplasty and stenting (39). Atherectomy using laser, orbital, rotational, or excisional means, may be useful for debulking plaque in regions where stent placement is undesirable, such as at the origin of the superficial femoral artery, within the popliteal artery, or in lesions with high calcific burden.

Infrapopliteal Interventions

The popliteal artery bifurcates below the knee into the anterior tibial (AT) and tibioperoneal trunk; the tibioperoneal trunk gives rise to the posterior tibial (PT) and peroneal arteries. The AT, PT, and peroneal arteries form the major blood supply to the foot and, when diseased, may require endovascular therapy.

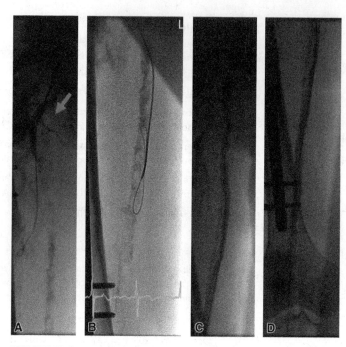

FIGURE 32.2 A 78-year-old male presented with critical limb ischemia. **A:** Angiography demonstrated a long (>20 cm) occlusion originating at the origin of the superficial femoral artery (*red arrow*) with reconstitution at the adductor canal. **B:** Subintimal tracking was used to cross the occlusion, and the native vessel was successfully reentered at the popliteal level. Successful recanalization was achieved with angioplasty and self-expanding stent deployment (**C** and **D**).

In contrast to iliac and femoropopliteal disease, where the majority of interventions are performed for claudication, infrapopliteal revascularization is typically reserved for cases of CLI. This is an important distinction because perfusion requirements for wound healing are much greater than those necessary to maintain tissue integrity. As a result, long-term tibial vessel patency following intervention is less important so long as patency has been durable enough to allow for ischemic ulcerations to heal.

Patients with CLI may be treated with surgical bypass or endovascular techniques. The individual patient approach is based on a number of factors, including anatomic feasibility of revascularization, presence of adequate vein for bypass, and patient comorbidities. The BASIL trial represents a randomized study of surgical bypass versus balloon angioplasty for patients with CLI and femoropopliteal disease; the overall results of this study were negative based on an intention-to-treat analysis and are not generalizable to current endovascular techniques (32). The ongoing BEST-CLI trial is a randomized study of surgical bypass versus endovascular therapy among patients with CLI (40). The trial design includes the use of all available surgical or endovascular strategies. When completed, this study will provide a wealth of data regarding treatment strategies for patients with CLI.

Given the comparable size of the infrapopliteal arteries to the coronaries, the majority of these interventions are performed utilizing equivalent, narrow-caliber equipment compared to those used in coronary interventions, including 0.014-inch wires, angioplasty balloons, and stent systems. A central principle in the treatment of CLI is to reestablish a patent, straight line of blood flow from the heart to the foot, including at least one of the infrapopliteal vessels (**Fig. 32.3**). A more contemporary concept correlates the area of tissue loss with the infrapopliteal artery that subtends the territory

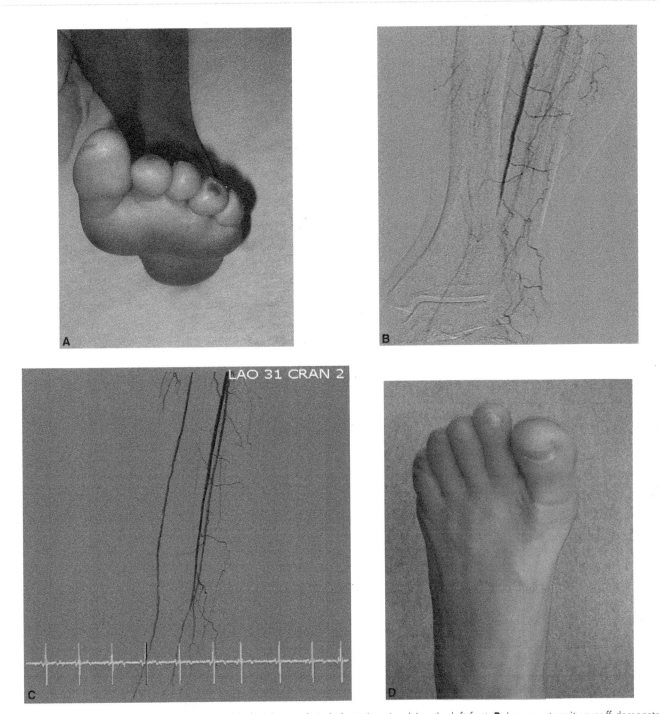

FIGURE 32.3   A: A 60-year-old male presented with ischemic digital ulcerations involving the left foot. **B:** Lower extremity runoff demonstrated occluded anterior (AT) and posterior tibial (PT) arteries, and a patent peroneal artery providing one-vessel runoff to the foot. **C:** Angioplasty of the AT and PT arteries was performed with excellent angiographic results. **D:** Tissue healing occurred, and the patient remains clinically well and has not required repeat revascularization during 6 years of follow-up.

or "angiosome." A revascularization strategy that favors the infrapopliteal artery correlated with the angiosome of tissue loss may enhance wound healing (41). In infrapopliteal intervention, the use of stents is generally reserved for rare cases of severely suboptimal angioplasty results or flow-limiting dissections.

For infrapopliteal intervention, ipsilateral antegrade common femoral arterial access is often preferred. The relatively short distance and the straight access from groin to knee (and below) offer significant technical advantages for wire and catheter manipulation.

Increasingly, arterial access from the "pedal" vessels (dorsalis pedis or PT) is now being considered for treatment of femoropopliteal or proximal infrapopliteal total occlusions. Such "ipsilateral retrograde" access may offer an advantage to cross recalcitrant occlusions where it is difficult to penetrate the proximal segments of occlusion using antegrade technique. Pedal access is often obtained using narrow-caliber needle and wire systems (e.g., micropuncture), in conjunction with an antegrade femoral sheath to permit wire snaring and exteriorization, followed by an antegrade approach to the

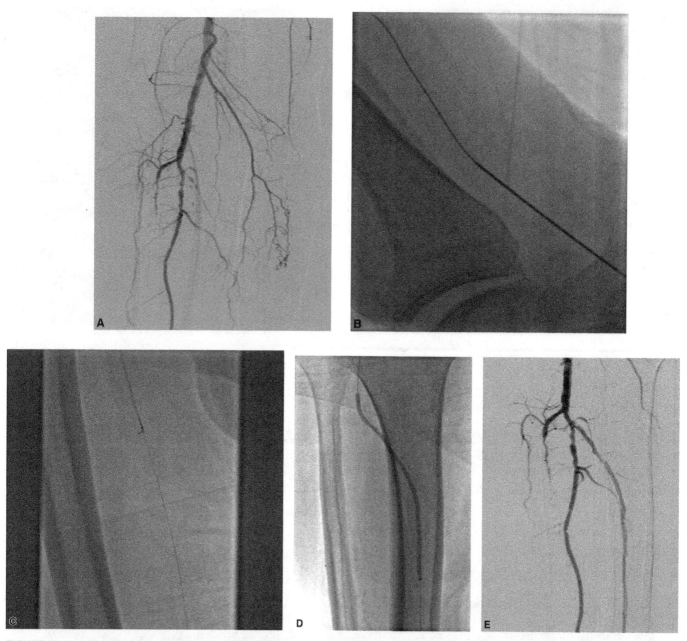

FIGURE 32.4 A 57-year-old male presented with critical limb ischemia. **A:** Runoff showed a diseased peroneal and occlusions of the anterior (AT) and posterior tibial (PT) vessels. Attempts to recanalize the AT and PT through an ipsilateral antegrade approach were unsuccessful. **B:** Antegrade angiography was used to guide access to the PT artery using a micropuncture needle and a 0.018-inch V-18 wire. **C:** The PT occlusion was crossed retrograde using the pedal access, and the wire was exteriorized through the ipsilateral, antegrade common femoral sheath. **D:** Angioplasty of the PT was performed. **E:** The final angiographic result was excellent.

lesion without the use of a large-caliber sheath in the pedal vessel (Fig. 32.4). Pedal access carries a risk of compromising flow in the accessed vessel, which may represent the only outflow to the foot, although recent multicenter data have supported the overall safety of this approach (42).

Endovascular therapy for CLI results in limb salvage for the majority of patients. In a study of 235 sequential patients undergoing angioplasty treatment for tibioperoneal stenosis in the context of CLI, 95% of patients were treated successfully, with a limb salvage rate of 91% among survivors at mean follow-up of 34 months (43). Treatment of infrapopliteal chronic occlusions in patients with minimal runoff is associated with reduced rates of major amputation in patients with successful versus unsuccessful revascularization (44). Although

randomized results are lacking, recent observational analyses suggest that infrapopliteal balloon angioplasty is associated with improved patency compared to tibial bypass among patients with CLI (45).

New technologies are being studied to improve the patency of infrapopliteal interventions. Multiple studies have demonstrated improved lesion patency with coronary drug-eluting stents (DESs), and potentially decreased rates of amputation (46). Nevertheless, these results are based on treatment of short lesions (typically <50 mm) and are not generalizable to the larger population of infrapopliteal interventions, where the treated lesion segments are frequently 100 mm or greater in length. Somewhat surprisingly, a randomized trial of DCB angioplasty versus standard balloon angioplasty failed to find a benefit of DCB, with a trend toward higher amputation rates (47).

It is unclear whether this outcome was related to the specific device or was a possible effect of paclitaxel on wound healing. Ongoing studies are investigating newer generations of DCBs, novel DESs, and other mechanisms for limiting restenosis after infrapopliteal balloon angioplasty (48).

Conclusion

Endovascular therapy has emerged as a safe, less invasive alternative to surgery in most major peripheral vascular beds. Appropriate patient selection coupled with sound procedural technique offers many patients with PAD substantial benefit. With future research, we may refine our clinical insights, applying new technology to deliver optimal patient-centered, lesion-specific care.

Key Points

Thoracic Aorta

- Arm claudication and symptomatic steal syndromes are indications for subclavian revascularization.

- Subclavian revascularization is indicated even in asymptomatic individuals if the disease subtends the internal mammary artery takeoff and the vessel is a required conduit for bypass surgery.

- Steal physiology detected on non-invasive testing should not be treated in asymptomatic patients.

- Patients with Type A aortic dissection are usually treated with emergency surgery. Patients with uncomplicated Type B aortic dissections may often be managed medically, although an increasing percentage are treated with TEVAR.

Abdominal Aorta

- Multiple trials have demonstrated similar long-term mortality with EVAR relative to open surgical repair.

- Re-intervention rates are higher with EVAR, which also makes this a more expensive therapy that requires long-term surveillance.

- In patients with prohibitive surgical risk, EVAR does not appear to reduce all-cause mortality compared with no repair.

Lower Extremity

- Endovascular interventions for claudication should be performed only in individuals with lifestyle-limiting symptoms who have failed conservative measures, including risk-factor modification and exercise.

- Avoid angioplasty of the common femoral artery; disease in this segment should in most cases be reserved for surgery.

- Newer-generation nitinol stents and DCB are each associated with improved patency in the superficial femoral artery.

- Infrapopliteal interventions are primarily reserved for patients with CLI (e.g., rest pain, tissue loss) with the therapeutic goal of restoring straight-line blood flow from the heart to the foot.

References

1. Shadman R, et al. Subclavian artery stenosis: prevalence, risk factors, and association with cardiovascular diseases. *J Am Coll Cardiol*. 2004;44:618–623.
2. Brott TG, et al. 2011 ASA/ACCF/AHA/AANN/AANS/ACR/ASNR/CNS/SAIP/SCAI/SIR/SNIS/SVM/SVS guideline on the management of patients with extracranial carotid and vertebral artery disease: executive summary: a report of the American College of Cardiology Foundation/American Heart Association task force on practice guidelines, and the American Stroke Association, American Association of Neuroscience Nurses, American Association of Neurological Surgeons, American College of Radiology, American Society of Neuroradiology, Congress of Neurological Surgeons, Society of Atherosclerosis Imaging and Prevention, Society for Cardiovascular Angiography and Interventions, Society of Interventional Radiology, Society of NeuroInterventional Surgery, Society for Vascular Medicine, and Society for Vascular Surgery Developed in Collaboration with the American Academy of Neurology and Society of Cardiovascular Computed Tomography. *J Am Coll Cardiol*. 2011;57:1002–1044.
3. Patel SN, et al. Catheter-based treatment of the subclavian and innominate arteries. *Catheter Cardiovasc Interv*. 2008;71:963–968.
4. Yu J, et al. Transradial approach to subclavian artery stenting. *J Invasive Cardiol*. 2010;22:204–206.
5. Michael TT, Banerjee S, Brilakis E. Subclavian artery intervention with vertebral embolic protection. *Catheter Cardiovasc Interv*. 2009;74:22–25.
6. Tanous D, Benson LN, Horlick EM. Coarctation of the aorta: evaluation and management. *Curr Opin Cardiol*. 2009;24:509–515.
7. Warnes CA, et al. ACC/AHA 2008 guidelines for the management of adults with congenital heart disease: a report of the American College of Cardiology/American Heart Association task force on practice guidelines (Writing Committee to develop guidelines on the management of adults with congenital heart disease). Developed in collaboration with the American Society of Echocardiography, Heart Rhythm Society, International Society for Adult Congenital Heart Disease, Society for Cardiovascular Angiography and Interventions, and Society of Thoracic Surgeons. *J Am Coll Cardiol*. 2008:52:e143–e263.
8. Mussa FF, et al. Acute aortic dissection and intramural hematoma: a systematic review. *JAMA*. 2016;316:754–763.
9. Cooper M, et al. Diagnosis and treatment of uncomplicated type B aortic dissection. *Vasc Med*. 2016;21:547–552.
10. Hiratzka LF, et al. 2010 ACCF/AHA/AATS/ACR/ASA/SCA/SCAI/SIR/STS/SVM guidelines for the diagnosis and management of patients with Thoracic aortic disease: a report of the American College of Cardiology Foundation/American Heart Association Task Force on Practice Guidelines, American Association for Thoracic Surgery, American College of Radiology, American Stroke Association, Society of Cardiovascular Anesthesiologists, Society for Cardiovascular Angiography and Interventions, Society of Interventional Radiology, Society of Thoracic Surgeons, and Society for Vascular Medicine. *Circulation*. 2010;121:e266.
11. Lederle FA, et al. The aneurysm detection and management study screening program: validation cohort and final results. Aneurysm Detection and Management Veterans Affairs Cooperative Study investigators. *Arch Intern Med*. 2000;160:1425–1430.
12. Fleming C, et al. Screening for abdominal aortic aneurysm: a best-evidence systematic review for the U.S. Preventive Services task force. *Ann Intern Med*. 2005;142:203–211.
13. Ng TT, et al. Variations in the utilization of endovascular aneurysm repair reflect population risk factors and disease prevalence. *J Vasc Surg*. 2010;51:801–809, 809.e1.
14. Kent KC. Abdominal aortic aneurysms. *N Engl J Med*. 2014;371:2101–2108.
15. De Bruin JL, et al. Long-term outcome of open or endovascular repair of abdominal aortic aneurysm. *N Engl J Med*. 2010;362:1881–1889.
16. United Kingdom EVAR Trial Investigators, et al. Endovascular versus open repair of abdominal aortic aneurysm. *N Engl J Med*. 2010;362:1863–1871.
17. United Kingdom EVAR Trial Investigators, et al. Endovascular repair of aortic aneurysm in patients physically ineligible for open repair. *N Engl J Med*. 2010;362:1872–1880.

18. Selvin E, Erlinger TP. Prevalence of and risk factors for peripheral arterial disease in the United States: results from the National Health and Nutrition Examination Survey, 1999–2000. *Circulation*. 2004;110:738–743.

19. Weitz JI, et al. Diagnosis and treatment of chronic arterial insufficiency of the lower extremities: a critical review. *Circulation*. 1996;94:3026–3049.

20. Gerhard-Herman MD, et al. 2016 AHA/ACC guideline on the management of patients with lower extremity peripheral artery disease: a report of the American College of Cardiology/American Heart Association Task Force on Clinical Practice Guidelines. *J Am Coll Cardiol*. 2017;69(11):e71–e126.

21. Armstrong EJ, et al. Adherence to guideline-recommended therapy is associated with decreased major adverse cardiovascular events and major adverse limb events among patients with peripheral arterial disease. *J Am Heart Assoc*. 2014;3:e000697.

22. Brewster DC. Clinical and anatomical considerations for surgery in aortoiliac disease and results of surgical treatment. *Circulation*. 1991;83:I42–I52.

23. Norgren L, et al. Inter-society consensus for the management of peripheral arterial disease (TASC II). *J Vasc Surg*. 2007;45(suppl S):S5–S67.

24. Murphy TP, et al. Supervised exercise versus primary stenting for claudication resulting from aortoiliac peripheral artery disease: six-month outcomes from the claudication: exercise versus endoluminal revascularization (CLEVER) study. *Circulation*. 2012;125:130–139.

25. Fakhry F, et al. Endovascular revascularization and supervised exercise for peripheral artery disease and intermittent claudication: a randomized clinical trial. *JAMA*. 2015;314:1936–1944.

26. Bosch JL, Hunink MG. Meta-analysis of the results of percutaneous transluminal angioplasty and stent placement for aortoiliac occlusive disease. *Radiology*. 1997;204:87–96.

27. Tetteroo E, et al. Randomised comparison of primary stent placement versus primary angioplasty followed by selective stent placement in patients with iliac-artery occlusive disease. Dutch Iliac Stent Trial Study Group. *Lancet*. 1998;351:1153–1159.

28. AbuRahma AF, et al. Primary iliac stenting versus transluminal angioplasty with selective stenting. *J Vasc Surg*. 2007;46:965–970.

29. Aggarwal V, Waldo SW, Armstrong EJ. Endovascular revascularization for aortoiliac atherosclerotic disease. *Vasc Health Risk Manag*. 2016;12:117–127.

30. Mwipatayi BP, et al. Durability of the balloon-expandable versus bare-metal stents in the Covered versus Balloon Expandable Stent Trial (COBEST) for the treatment of aortoiliac occlusive disease. *J Vasc Surg*. 2016;64:83–94.

31. Ihnat DM, et al. Contemporary outcomes after superficial femoral artery angioplasty and stenting: the influence of TASC classification and runoff score. *J Vasc Surg*. 2008;47:967–974.

32. Adam DJ, et al. Bypass versus angioplasty in severe ischaemia of the leg (BASIL): multicentre, randomised controlled trial. *Lancet*. 2005;366:1925–1934.

33. Surowiec SM, et al. Percutaneous angioplasty and stenting of the superficial femoral artery. *J Vasc Surg*. 2005;41:269–278.

34. Schillinger M, et al. Balloon angioplasty versus implantation of nitinol stents in the superficial femoral artery. *N Engl J Med*. 2006;354:1879–1888.

35. Dake MD, et al. Durable clinical effectiveness with paclitaxel-eluting stents in the femoropopliteal artery: 5 year results of the Zilver PTX randomized trial. *Circulation*. 2016;133:1472–1483.

36. Garcia L, et al. Wire-interwoven nitinol stent outcome in the superficial femoral and proximal popliteal arteries: twelve month results of the SUPERB trial. *Circ Cardiovasc Interv*. 2015;8:e000937.

37. Laird JR, et al. Durability of treatment effect using a drug-coated balloon for femoropopliteal lesions: 24-month results of the IN.PACT SFA trial. *J Am Coll Cardiol*. 2015;66:2329–2338.

38. Micari A, et al. One year results of paclitaxel-coated balloons for long femoropopliteal disease: evidence from the SFA-long study. *JACC Cardiovasc Interv*. 2016;9:950–956.

39. Kitrou P, et al. Targeted true lumen re-entry with the Outback catheter: accuracy, success, and complications in 100 peripheral chronic total occlusions and systematic review of the literature. *J Endovasc Ther*. 2015;22:538–545.

40. Menard MT, et al. Design and rationale of the best endovascular versus best surgical therapy for patients with critical limb ischemia (BEST-CLI) trial. *J Am Heart Assoc*. 2016;5:e003219.

41. Iida O, et al. Long-term results of direct and indirect endovascular revascularization based on the angiosome concept in patients with critical limb ischemia presenting with isolated below-the-knee lesions. *J Vasc Surg*. 2012;55:363.e5–370.e5.

42. Walker CM, et al. Tibiopedal access for crossing of infrainguinal artery occlusions: a prospective multicenter observational study. *J Endovasc Ther*. 2016;23:839–846.

43. Dorros G, et al. Tibioperoneal (outflow lesion) angioplasty can be used as primary treatment in 235 patients with critical limb ischemia: five-year follow-up. *Circulation*. 2001;104:2057–2062.

44. Singh GD, et al. Endovascular recanalization of infrapopliteal occlusions in patients with critical limb ischemia. *J Vasc Surg*. 2014;59:1300–1307.

45. Hicks CW, et al. Below-knee endovascular interventions have better outcomes compared to open bypass for patients with critical limb ischemia. *Vasc Med*. 2017;22(1):28–34.

46. Katsanos K, et al. Comparative effectiveness of plain balloon angioplasty, bare metal stents, drug-coated balloons, and drug-eluting stents for the treatment of infrapopliteal peripheral artery disease: systematic review and Bayesian network meta-analysis of randomized controlled trials. *J Endovasc Ther*. 2016;23:851–863.

47. Zeller T, et al. IN.PACT DEEP trial investigators. Drug-eluting balloon versus standard balloon angioplasty for infrapopliteal revascularization in critical limb ischemia: 12-month results from the IN.PACT DEEP randomized trial. *J Am Coll Cardiol*. 2014;64:1568–1576.

48. Varcoe RL, et al. Experience with the Absorb everolimus-eluting bioresorbable vascular scaffold below the knee: six-month clinical and imaging outcomes. *J Endovasc Ther*. 2015;22:226–232.

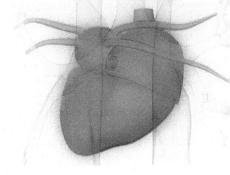

33

Carotid and Cerebrovascular/Acute Stroke Intervention

Jose D. Tafur Soto, MD, Sartaj Hans, MD, FACC, and

Christopher J. White, MD, MSCAI, FACC

Extracranial Carotid Interventions

Epidemiology and Natural History of Carotid Stenosis

Nearly 800,000 strokes occur each year in the United States, and over 120,000 Americans die annually from stroke (1). The estimated direct and indirect cost of stroke for 2012 was $33 billion, and it is expected that, between 2012 and 2030, total direct medical stroke-related costs will triple, from $71.6 billion to $184.1 billion (2). Stroke is the fifth-leading cause of mortality in the US, and among survivors, 30% are permanently disabled (mean Rankin score ≥4) (3). Atherosclerotic carotid artery disease is the leading cause of non-cardioembolic ischemic strokes (4). Carotid plaque most often causes cerebrovascular events due to plaque rupture with atheroembolization, rather than carotid artery occlusion (<20% of ischemic strokes) with thrombosis (5).

The natural history of carotid artery stenosis depends on the presence of symptoms (transient ischaemic attack [TIA], stroke, amaurosis fugax). Symptomatic patients have a 5- to 10-fold risk of stroke compared to asymptomatic patients. In a Medicare registry of patients who underwent carotid revascularization, asymptomatic patients with carotid artery stenosis outnumbered symptomatic patients 2.5:1 (6). Approximately 5% to 10% of patients over age 65 have a carotid stenosis >50%, with 1% having a stenosis ≥75%. Because the majority (≥80%) of ischemic strokes have no warning symptoms, the management of asymptomatic carotid atherosclerosis with either revascularization or medical therapy is important (7).

Transient focal neurologic symptoms are associated with a 30% risk of stroke within 6 months. TIA is currently defined as a transient episode of neurologic dysfunction caused by focal brain, spinal cord, or retinal ischemia, without acute infarction, based on pathologic, imaging, other objective evidence, and/or clinical evidence (8). Stroke, central nervous system (CNS) infarction, is defined by neuropathologic, neuroimaging, and/or clinical evidence of permanent injury. Nevertheless, many of the initial studies that illustrated the natural history of this disease, as well as our current standards of practice, pre-dated this updated definition and included only a clinical definition of infarction.

Asymptomatic Patients: In the 1990s, two large randomized controlled trials (Asymptomatic Carotid Atherosclerosis Study (ACAS) and the Asymptomatic Carotid Surgery Trial (ACST)) showed that carotid endarterectomy (CEA) reduced the incidence of ipsilateral stroke in patients with asymptomatic carotid artery stenosis ≥60% when compared to medical therapy (e.g., aspirin) by 50%. Nevertheless, CEA did not reduce overall stroke and death, and did not show any benefit in women or in patients older than 75 years of age. It is important to note the medical therapy provided in these trials (aspirin) has significantly improved. Currently, the risk of progression of an asymptomatic carotid artery stenosis to occlusion with modern medical therapy is very low. In a cohort of 3,681 patients with yearly duplex follow-up, 316 (8.6%) asymptomatic patients had occlusions that occurred during observation. Of these, 80% (254) of the occlusions occurred before the initiation of modern intensive medical therapy (9) (Fig. 33.1).

Symptomatic Patients: Symptomatic carotid disease is defined as focal neurologic symptoms of sudden onset, in the appropriate carotid artery distribution, within the previous 6 months. The natural history of symptomatic carotid artery stenosis was reflected in the

Percentage of Patients in the Clinic with New Index Occlusion by Year

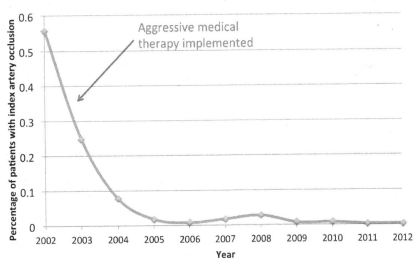

FIGURE 33.1   Percentage of patients with index carotid artery occlusion in a 10-year cohort. (From Yang C, Bogiatzi C, Spence JD. Risk of stroke at the time of carotid occlusion. *JAMA Neurol.* 2015;72:1261–1267.)

373

medical arm of the randomized the North American Symptomatic Carotid Endarterectomy Trial (NASCET). The 5-year risk of ipsilateral stroke in those medically managed was 18.7% among those with lesions <50% in severity. In those with 50% to 69% stenosis, the risk over the same time period was 22.2%. In those with a 70% to 99% stenosis, the 2-year risk of ipsilateral stroke was 26% (10). Results were similar in the European Carotid Surgery Trial (ECST). The incidence of stroke increased with the severity of stenosis, and the 3-year risk of ipsilateral stroke in symptomatic patients with stenosis greater than 80% was 26.5%. Nevertheless, as the stenosis approaches total occlusion (95%–99%), the risk of ipsilateral stroke goes down to 17.2% (11).

Clinical Presentation

Symptoms of carotid artery stenosis include the following: ipsilateral transient visual defects (amaurosis fugax) from retinal emboli; contralateral weakness or numbness of an extremity or of the face, or a combination of these; visual field defect; dysarthria; and, in the case of dominant hemisphere involvement, aphasia. The National Institutes of Health Stroke Scale (NIHSS) should be performed in all symptomatic patients to quantify the neurologic deficit, which correlates with outcome (12).

Anatomic Imaging

Digital subtraction angiography (DSA) is the gold standard for defining carotid anatomy, with the NASCET method of stenosis measurement the most widely accepted methodology (**Fig. 33.2**). Invasive cerebral catheter-based angiography carries a risk of cerebral infarction of 0.5% to 1.2%; therefore, non-invasive imaging should be the initial strategy for evaluation. Carotid duplex imaging, transcranial Doppler imaging, computed tomography angiography (CTA), and magnetic

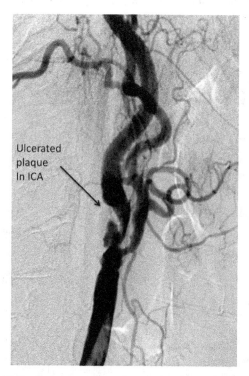

FIGURE 33.2 Catheter angiography of right carotid artery in a patient with recent transient ischemic attack. There is ulcerated plaque at the origin of the internal carotid artery.

resonance angiography (MRA) are the non-invasive methods of assessment. Duplex imaging is the best initial choice given its safety profile, low cost, and wide availability. Cerebral and cervical imaging should define the aortic arch and the Circle of Willis (**Fig. 33.3**).

Medical Therapy

Current anti-atherosclerotic medical therapy has advanced significantly with the development of angiotensin converting enzyme-inhibitors (ACE-I), angiotensin receptor blockers (ARB), statin drugs, and newer antiplatelet agents. Medical therapy for carotid atherosclerosis should focus on preventing stroke and stabilizing atherosclerotic lesions to prevent plaque rupture and atheroembolization. Blood pressure control is of paramount importance because it is a primary risk factor for stroke; it is also a risk factor for atrial fibrillation and myocardial infarction (MI), which both increase the likelihood of stroke. ACE-I and ARB seem to be of particular benefit in stroke prevention, particularly in those at higher risk for cardiovascular disease (13).

Cholesterol lowering with statin drugs in patients treated for cardiovascular disease prevention demonstrated a lower risk of stroke (14). It is possible that statins prevent strokes through pleiotropic effects on endothelial function and plaque stabilization, in addition to their lipid-lowering properties. Current American Heart Association/American Stroke Association (AHA/ASA) Stroke guidelines (7) endorse the ACC/AHA recommendations for the use of statins, which recommend that high-intensity statin therapy be initiated or continued as first-line therapy in patients ≤75 years of age that have clinical atherosclerotic cardiovascular disease unless contraindicated (Class I, Level of evidence (LOE) A), and it should be considered in those >75 years of age if the benefit outweighs the risk (Class IIa, LOE B) (15) (**Table 33.1**).

The guidelines also recognize the FDAs approval of statins for stroke prevention in patients with cardiovascular disease and in high-risk hypertensive patients. The Stroke Prevention by Aggressive Reduction in Cholesterol Levels (SPARCL) trial demonstrated that high-dose atorvastatin is effective for secondary stroke prevention in patients with an ischemic stroke or TIA but no coronary heart disease (16). The Justification for the Use of Statins in Prevention: an Intervention Trial Evaluating Rosuvastatin (JUPITER) study showed that rosuvastatin treatment in patients with normal cholesterol levels but elevated levels of c-reactive protein is effective in reducing the rate of stroke (17). Therefore, statins are an important component of stroke treatment and prevention and are indicated for patients with carotid artery disease.

Antiplatelet medications are a critical component of primary stroke prevention. In the Antithrombotic Trialists' Collaboration meta-analysis of high-risk patients, antiplatelet therapy reduced the occurrence of any vascular event by roughly 25%, non-fatal stroke by about 25%, and death due to vascular cause by about 15%. Aspirin was the most widely used drug with doses of 75 to 150 mg being as beneficial as higher doses. The Women's Health Study found that 100 mg of aspirin every other day resulted in a significant 17% reduction in the risk of stroke over 10 years. In secondary prevention, aspirin reduces the risk of future strokes by 15% to 25%. High-dose aspirin (160–325 mg daily) provided no more benefit than lower doses but was associated with more side effects. Among patients with symptomatic vascular disease, including stroke, the Clopidogrel versus Aspirin in Patients at Risk of Ischemic Events (CAPRIE) trial demonstrated that clopidogrel 75 mg daily was associated with an 8.7% relative risk reduction in ischemic stroke, MI, or vascular death versus aspirin 325 mg daily (5.32% vs. 5.83% p = 0.043). For the patients who presented with stroke, however, the benefit was not significant. Clopidogrel 75 mg daily plus aspirin 75 mg daily was

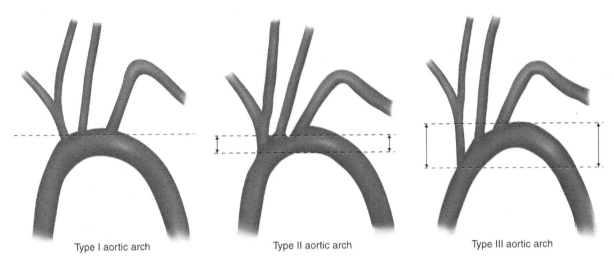

Type I aortic arch   Type II aortic arch   Type III aortic arch

FIGURE 33.3   Types of aortic arch.

TABLE 33.1 AHA/ASA Guidelines for the Primary Prevention of Stroke (7)

Endorsed statin use per 2013 ACC/AHA (62) cholesterol guidelines	ASCVD	Age ≤75—high-intensity statin Age >75—moderate-intensity statin	Class I LOE A
	LDL ≥190	High-intensity statin	
	Age 40–75 with diabetes LDL 70–189	10-year risk ≥7.5%: high-intensity statin 10-year risk <7.5%: moderate-intensity statin	
	Age 40–75 without ASCVD or diabetes 10-year risk ≥7.5%	Moderate- to high-intensity statin	
Niacin[a] may be considered for • Low HDL, or • Elevated lipoprotein(a)			Class IIb LOE B
Fibric acid derivatives[a] may be considered for • Hypertriglyceridemia			Class IIb LOE C
Non-statin lipid-lowering therapies[a], such as fibric acid derivatives, bile acid sequestrants, niacin, and ezetimibe may be considered in patients who cannot tolerate statins			Class IIb LOE C

[a]Efficacy in preventing ischemic stroke in patients with these conditions is not established.
ASCVD, atherosclerotic cardiovascular disease; HDL, high-density lipoprotein; LDL, low-density lipoprotein; LOE, level of evidence.

compared to clopidogrel alone in the Management of Atherothrombosis with Clopidogrel in High-risk Patients (MATCH) trial. This study found that, among stroke patients, the combination regimen did not improve vascular outcomes but significantly increased the number of major and life-threatening bleeding complications. The Clopidogrel for High Atherothrombotic Risk and Ischemic Stabilization, Management, and Avoidance (CHARISMA) trial included over 4,300 patients with a prior TIA or stroke and found that aspirin (75 to 162 mg daily) was as effective as aspirin plus clopidogrel in preventing future MI, stroke, or cardiovascular death in patients with multiple-risk factors or with clinically evident cardiovascular disease. This study also found that 81 mg of aspirin is the optimal dose for safety and efficacy for prevention.

The American Heart Association and the American Stroke Association (AHA/ASA) guidelines recommend that all patients with carotid atherosclerosis be placed on antiplatelet medications (7). Aspirin (81 or 100 mg daily) or clopidogrel alone in patients who cannot tolerate aspirin should be initiated for secondary prevention of stroke.

There is uncertainty regarding the best therapy for asymptomatic carotid artery disease. The CREST-2 trial is currently enrolling patients and features two parallel arms (Fig. 33.4): one compares CEA with best medical management versus best medical management alone, and the other arm compares CAS and best medical management versus best medical management alone. CREST-2 does not compare CEA to CAS (carotid artery stenting), but recognizes the equipoise for these two treatments. CREST-2 medical management goals include systolic blood pressure (SBP) <140 mm Hg (<130 mm Hg for diabetes mellitus [DM]), low-density lipoprotein (LDL) <70 mg/dL, hemoglobin A1c <7.0%, smoking cessation, targeted weight management, and more than 30 minutes of moderate exercise three times per week.

Surgical Therapy to Prevent Stroke

Asymptomatic Patients: The purpose of carotid revascularization is to prevent ischemic stroke. There have been three large randomized studies comparing CEA to antiplatelet (aspirin) therapy in the

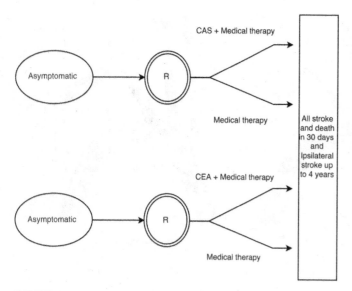

FIGURE 33.4 CREST-2 trial design. CAS, carotid artery stenting; CEA, carotid endarterectomy; CREST, carotid revascularization endarterectomy versus stenting trial.

treatment of moderate (≥50%–60%) carotid stenosis in patients without focal neurologic symptoms, which are all made less relevant by modern medical therapy. The Veterans Affairs Cooperative Study (VACS) (18) randomized 444 men with asymptomatic carotid stenosis of ≥50% by angiography to medical therapy plus CEA or medical therapy alone. All patients were assigned aspirin 650 mg twice daily, although many did not tolerate that dose. The 30-day risk of stroke or death in the CEA group was 4.7%. At nearly 4 years of follow-up, the ipsilateral neurologic event rate (including TIA, transient monocular blindness, and fatal and nonfatal stroke), was 8% in the surgical arm and 20.6% in the medical arm (p < 0.001). The risk of ipsilateral stroke alone was reduced from 9.4% with medical treatment to 4.7% (p < 0.06) with CEA. Notably, there was no difference between surgery and medical therapy for combined stroke or death.

ACAS randomized 1,662 asymptomatic patients with carotid stenosis ≥60% to medical therapy or medical therapy with CEA (19). All patients received aspirin 325 mg daily. Angiography was performed only in the CEA group and was associated with a 1.2% risk of stroke. The 30-day risk of stroke or death in the surgical group, including the risk associated with angiography, was 2.7%. The projected 5-year risk of ipsilateral stroke and any perioperative stroke or death was reduced from 11% in the medical arm to 5.1% with CEA. The number of patients needed to treat (NNT) with surgery to prevent one ipsilateral stroke at 5 years was 19. The benefit for women (17% reduction in events) was less than for men (66% reduction).

ACST evaluated 3,120 asymptomatic patients with ≥60% carotid stenosis by ultrasound. Patients were randomized to CEA with medical management or medical management alone. Drug treatment was left to the discretion of the patients' primary physicians—this usually included antiplatelet medications, antihypertensive therapy, and, in the later years of the study, lipid-lowering agents. The 30-day perioperative risk of stroke or death was 3.1%. The 5-year risk of perioperative death or total stroke was reduced from 11.8% to 6.4% with CEA; roughly half the strokes were disabling. The benefit of surgery was significant across varying degrees of stenosis (60%–90% stenosis). Nevertheless, CEA did not reduce overall stroke and death,

and did not show any benefit in women or in patients older than 75 years of age (20).

Symptomatic Patients: Three large randomized controlled studies have evaluated the benefit of CEA compared to medical therapy (i.e., aspirin) in symptomatic patients with moderate to severe carotid artery disease that are also compromised by outdated and less effective medical than is available today. The Veterans Administration 309 trial (21) screened 5,000 men who presented within 4 months of a small stroke, TIA, or transient monocular blindness and randomized 189 to either CEA with "best medical therapy" or best medical therapy alone. The patients had angiographically defined internal carotid stenosis >50%. The trial was ended prematurely when early results from NASCET and ECST confirmed the significant benefit of CEA. At a mean follow-up of almost 1 year, there was a reduction in ipsilateral stroke or TIA from 19.4% in the medical treatment arm to 7.7% in the surgical arm, an absolute reduction in risk of 11.7%. The benefit of surgery was most profound in patients with stenosis >70% (an absolute risk reduction of 17.7%).

The NASCET investigators randomized patients with a TIA or non-disabling stroke within 180 days to CEA with medical therapy (including aspirin) or medical therapy alone. Patients were originally stratified into three groups according to the degree of carotid stenosis: Group 1 with <50%; Group 2 with 50% to 69%; and Group 3 with 70% to 99%. A total of 659 patients with ≥70% stenosis were randomized with CEA, demonstrating an absolute risk reduction of 17% (26% CEA vs. 9% medical therapy) in the rate of ipsilateral stroke at 2 years (10). CEA lowered the 2-year risk of major or fatal stroke from 13.1% to 2.5%. In patients with <50% stenosis, there was no benefit for stroke prevention with CEA and medical therapy compared to medical therapy alone. Among patients with a 50% to 69% stenosis, the 30-day perioperative stroke or death rate was 6.7% in those treated with CEA (10). The 5-year rate of ipsilateral stroke was 22.2% in those treated medically and 15.7% in those treated with CEA for an absolute risk reduction of 6.5% for those treated with CEA.

ECST studied 3,024 symptomatic patients with carotid stenosis; 60% of patients were randomized to CEA and 40% to medical therapy. All patients received optimal medical therapy that consisted of anti-hypertensive medications, antiplatelet agents, and anti-smoking counseling. The 30-day perioperative risk of major stroke or death with surgery was 7%. While there was no benefit to surgery for stenosis below the 70% to 80% range, among patients with a stenosis ≥80%, the rate of major stroke or death at 3 years was 26.5% in the medical therapy group and 14.9% in the CEA group, an absolute reduction of 11.6% favoring surgery. There was no benefit for patients who had near occlusion of the carotid artery. Of note, ECST defined the degree of stenosis differently than NASCET (**Fig. 33.5**) (22) resulting in an 80% stenosis in ECST being similar to a 60% stenosis in NASCET.

A meta-analysis of these three studies found that for lesions <30% as measured by NASCET criteria, surgery increased the 5-year risk of ipsilateral stroke. CEA provided a marginal benefit in patients with 50% to 69% stenosis (absolute risk reduction of 4.6%) and was highly beneficial for patients who had ≥70% stenosis (16% absolute risk reduction, p < 0.001). In patients with near-occlusion, defined as a stenosis causing reduced flow to the distal internal carotid artery (ICA) and narrowing of the post-stenotic ICA, there was no benefit for CEA (22).

Current AHA/ASA guidelines recommend CEA in symptomatic patients with stenosis of 50% to 99% if the risk of perioperative stroke or death is <6% (23). In asymptomatic patients, guidelines recommend CEA for stenosis of 60% to 99% if the perioperative risk

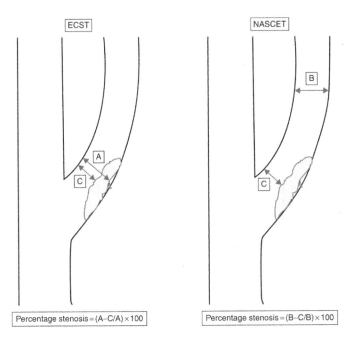

FIGURE 33.5 Angiographic methods for determining carotid stenosis severity. ECST, European carotid surgery trial; NASCET, North American symptomatic carotid endarterectomy trial.

of stroke is <3% and life expectancy is at least 5 years (7). Some have recommended delaying revascularization in asymptomatic patients until the stenosis has reached 80%, but the evidence from ACST demonstrated an equal event rate for asymptomatic patients with moderate compared to severe stenoses.

Carotid Artery Stenting

Clinical Evidence: For CAS to become a routine and commonly used procedure, clinical outcomes must not be inferior to the standard revascularization procedure, CEA. When interpreting data on carotid stenting, it is important to realize that a patient who is at high-risk for surgery is not necessarily at increased risk for stenting (and vice

versa). Features that place a patient at increased risk for complications from CEA and CAS are summarized in Table 33.2.

High-Surgical-Risk (HSR) Patients: The Stenting and Angioplasty with Protection in Patients at High Risk for Endarterectomy (SAPPHIRE) trial is the only randomized trial comparing HSR patients treated with CEA to those treated with CAS (24). Sapphire randomized 334 patients with a symptomatic stenosis of ≥50% or an asymptomatic stenosis ≥80% (~30% were symptomatic) to either CEA or CAS. The primary endpoint of death, stroke, or MI at 30 days plus ipsilateral stroke or death from neurologic cause between day 31 and 1 year occurred in 12.2% of patients in the stenting group and 20.1% in the CEA group (p = 0.004 for non-inferiority). The 30-day stroke and death rate among the asymptomatic patients was 4.6% for the CAS group and 5.4% for the CEA group. At 3 years, there were no differences between the CEA or CAS.

Most of the contemporary registry data focuses on HSR patients, and data from over 10,000 HSR patients have been published. These registries generally include symptomatic patients with ≥50% stenosis and asymptomatic patients with ≥70% to 80% stenosis. Data from many of these studies are summarized in Figure 33.6. It is apparent that in HSR patients who require revascularization for stroke prevention CAS is the preferred procedure in patients who (1) can be treated by an experienced operator and (2) have suitable anatomy for CAS. The current AHA/ASA stroke prevention guidelines regarding carotid revascularization are summarized in Table 33.3.

Average- or Low-Surgical-Risk Patients: Five large randomized studies in average- or low-surgical-risk patients have compared CAS to CEA (25–29). Three of these trials were conducted in Europe, and their results were compromised by allowing very inexperienced CAS operators to participate in the trials and not requiring embolic protection devices (EPDs) to be used. The Endarterectomy Versus Angioplasty in Patients with Symptomatic Severe Carotid Stenosis (EVA-3S) trial randomized symptomatic patients with carotid stenosis of ≥60% to either CEA or CAS. All patients had to be "suitable candidates" for both procedures and had ipsilateral neurologic symptoms within 120 days of enrollment. The use of EPDs was optional and many of the investigators were tutored while treating patients. The study was terminated early. The 30-day incidence of

TABLE 33.2 High-Risk Features of Carotid Artery Stenting (CAS) and Carotid Endarterectomy (CEA)

HIGH-RISK FEATURES FOR CAS		HIGH-RISK FEATURES FOR CEA	
CLINICAL FEATURES	**ANGIOGRAPHIC FEATURES**	**COMORBIDITIES**	**ANATOMIC FEATURES**
Age ≥75/80	Severe tandem lesions	Age ≥80	Lesion C2 or higher
Renal failure	≥2 acute (90° bends)	Class III/IV CHF or angina	Lesion below clavicle
Multiple lacunar strokes	Circumferential calcification	LM ≥ 2-vessel CAD	Prior neck surgery (including ipsilateral CEA)
Dementia	Evidence of thrombus	LVEF ≤30%	Contralateral carotid occlusion
Bleeding disorder	Poor vascular access	Recent MI (>1 but <30 days)	Contralateral laryngeal nerve palsy
		Severe chronic lung disease	Neck radiation
		Renal failure	Tracheostomy

CAD, coronary artery disease; CHF, congestive heart failure; LM, left main; LVEF, left ventricular ejection fraction; MI, myocardial infarction.

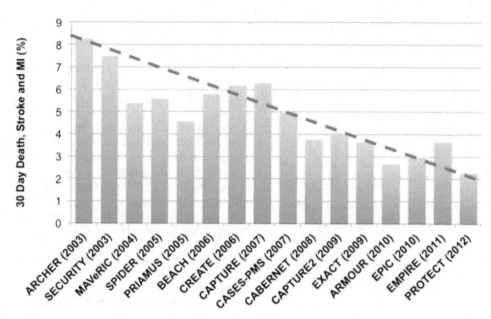

FIGURE 33.6 Trials comparing CAS to CEA in high-surgical-risk patients. CAS, carotid artery stenting; CEA, carotid endarterectomy; MI, myocardial infarction.

TABLE 33.3 Guidelines for Carotid Revascularization (7,63)

	SYMPTOMATIC PATIENTS				ASYMPTOMATIC PATIENTS	
	ESC		AHA/ACCF/SCAI		ESC	AHA/ACCF/SCAI
	50%–69% STENOSIS[a]	70%–99% STENOSIS[a]	50%–69% STENOSIS[b]	70%–99% STENOSIS[b]	≥60% STENOSIS[a]	70%–99% STENOSIS[b]
Carotid endarterectomy	Class IIa LOE—A	Class I LOE—A	Class I LOE—B	Class I LOE—A	Class IIa[c] LOE—A	Class IIa LOE—A
Carotid artery stenting	Class IIa[e] Class IIb[f] LOE—B		Class I LOE—B	Class I LOE—B	Class IIb[d] LOE—B	Class IIb LOE—B

[a]The severity of stenosis is calculated by duplex ultrasound, CTA, and/or MRA.
[b]The severity of stenosis is defined according to the angiographic criteria by the method used in NASCET but generally corresponds as well to assessment by sonography and other accepted methods of measurement.
[c]Perioperative stroke and death rate <3% and life expectancy >5 years.
[d]In high-volume centers with documented death or stroke rate <3%.
[e]In symptomatic patients at high surgical risk, CAS should be considered an alternative to CEA.
[f]CAS may be considered an alternative to CEA in high-volume centers with a documented death or stroke rate <6%.
ACCF, American College of Cardiology Foundation; AHA, American Heart Association; CTA, computed tomography angiography; ESC, European Society of cardiology; MRA, magnetic resonance angiography; LOE, level of evidence; SCAI, The Society for Cardiovascular Angiography and Interventions.

stroke or death was 9.6% in the CAS group and 3.9% (p = 0.004) in the CEA group (28).

The Stent-Supported Percutaneous Angioplasty of the Carotid Artery versus Endarterectomy (SPACE) trial randomized 1,214 symptomatic, average-surgical-risk patients to either CEA or CAS (26). The use of EPDs was optional, and inexperienced operators were tutored during patient enrollment. The 30-day rate of ipsilateral stroke or death was not different between the two groups (6.8% in the CAS group and 6.3% in the CEA group, p = 0.09 for non-inferiority). Nevertheless, the 2-year outcomes for this trial demonstrated a statistically significant benefit for CAS over CEA in patients <68 years of age.

The International Carotid Stenting Study (ICSS) enrolled over 1,700 symptomatic patients and randomized them to either CAS or CEA. Use of EPDs was optional. To qualify as an experienced center, a center had to have a surgeon who had performed 50 CEA procedures and an interventionalist who had performed 10 CAS procedures. If the center was less experienced, they were tutored

until considered proficient by their proctor. The center was upgraded to experienced after randomizing 20 patients and if their outcomes were considered acceptable. The patients were assigned to CAS or CEA in a 1:1 fashion and followed up for a median of 4.2 years. The number of fatal or disabling strokes and cumulative 5-year risk did not differ between the CAS and CEA groups (6.4% vs. 6.5%; hazard ratio [HR] 1.06, 95% CI 0.72–1.57, p = 0.77). The distribution of modified Rankin scale scores at 1 year, 5 years, or final follow-up did not differ between treatment groups (25).

The Carotid Revascularization Endarterectomy versus Stenting Trial (CREST) (27) is the largest (n = 2,502) randomized trial published comparing CAS with EPD to CEA in patients at average risk for surgery and including both symptomatic (n = 1,321) and asymptomatic (n = 1,181) patients. The primary outcome of periprocedural stroke, death, or MI or follow-up ipsilateral stroke was not significantly different between the two groups (7.2% for CAS and 6.8% for CEA). The 30-day risk of all stroke was higher for CAS (4.1% vs. 2.3%, p = 0.01), whereas CEA was associated with a higher 30-day risk of MI (2.3% vs. 1.1%, p = 0.03). The rate of ipsilateral stroke over a mean follow-up of 4 years was similar between groups. CAS appeared safer than CEA for patients ≤69 years of age, while CEA yielded better outcomes in those >70 years of age (Fig. 33.7).

CREST differed from the previous three trials in three significant ways. Most importantly, the European trials, EVA-3S, SPACE, and ICSS, allowed inexperienced operators to treat patients. All allowed stent operators, but not surgery operators, to be "tutored" during the randomized trial. CREST requirements were more stringent. In fact, many of the "experienced" CAS operators in the first three trials were not very experienced (EVA-3S required that operators perform at least five CAS procedures, ICSS required 10 CAS procedures, and SPACE had no minimum number of carotid stents required). The fact that so many neurologic events involve the non-culprit carotid

circulation is testament to the importance of catheter skills, and the value of experience cannot be overstated. Second, CREST mandated the use of EPDs, whereas the other trials did not. Lastly, just over 50% of the patients in CREST were symptomatic, whereas the other trials were entirely for symptomatic patients.

Asymptomatic average surgical risk carotid stenosis patients were enrolled in the Asymptomatic Carotid Trial (ACT-1). CAS was non-inferior to CEA with regard to death, stroke, or MI within 30 days after the procedure, or ipsilateral stroke within 1 year (3.8% vs. 3.4%). There was no difference for CAS versus CEA for rates of stroke or death within 30 days (2.9% and 1.7% [p = 0.33]). Freedom from ipsilateral stroke from 30 days to 5 years was 97.8% in the CAS group and 97.3% in the CEA group (p = 0.51) (29) (Fig. 33.8).

When taken together, the message from these five large randomized controlled trials is that CAS with or without an EPD is a reasonable

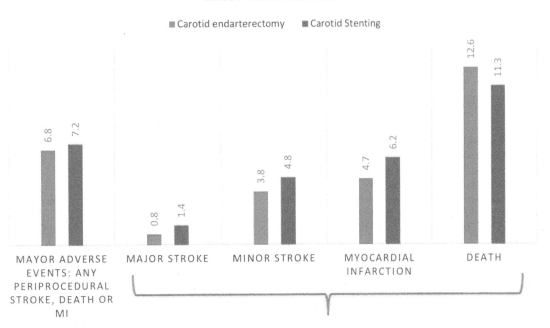

FIGURE 33.7   Results of the Carotid Revascularization Endarterectomy versus Stenting Trial (CREST).

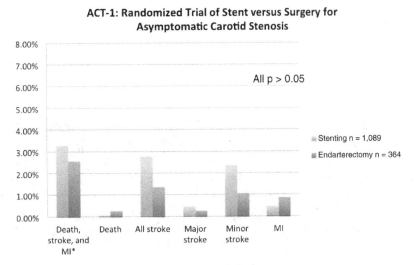

FIGURE 33.8   Results of the asymptomatic carotid trial (ACT-1). MI, myocardial infarction.

alternative to CEA in selected average surgical risk patients, when performed by experienced operators.

Technical Aspects

Baseline Aortography and Cerebral Angiography: An arch aortogram is performed in the 30° to 45° left anterior oblique (LAO) projection. Once the morphology of the aortic arch is determined, catheters are chosen for selective angiography of the cervical arteries supplying the brain (right and left carotid and vertebral arteries) and the cerebral vasculature. For a type I arch, Berenstein or Judkins Right (JR) catheters are often used. For type II or III arch morphologies, shepherd's crook-shaped catheters (i.e., Simmons or Vitek catheters) may be best (**Fig. 33.9**).

Because of the very low incidence of stroke complicating CAS, demonstrating clinical benefit for any EPD in a randomized clinical trial has been difficult. Two meta-analyses support the use of EPDs (30,31); nevertheless, others have failed to demonstrate benefit. Anecdotally, one simply has to retrieve a filter full of debris to realize the empirical benefits relative to the rare complications associated with an EPD. At the present time, optimal practice should include the use of an EPD, one that the operator is most comfortable using.

An alternative to distal embolic protection is proximal protection. Two devices are available: the Gore flow reversal system (W L Gore, Flagstaff, AZ) and the Mo.Ma system (Medtronic, Minneapolis, MN). Both are positioned in a similar fashion. With the Gore device, the external carotid artery is accessed as mentioned earlier and a balloon-tipped sheath is advanced over the 0.035-inch stiff wire into the common carotid artery. This sheath has a port for an occlusion balloon to be placed in the external carotid artery. The external and common carotid balloons are inflated arresting antegrade flow. The Mo.Ma system is similar but consists of a single sheath with two balloons: a proximal balloon in the common carotid artery and a distal balloon in the external carotid artery. When the balloons are inflated, blood flow is arrested. In both systems, once patient tolerance of balloon occlusion is confirmed, the internal carotid lesion is crossed with a 0.014-inch wire, dilated, and stented as described earlier. With the Mo.Ma system, blood is manually aspirated after the stenting procedure to clear the debris distal to the common carotid balloon. The Gore system, however, provides continuous flow reversal by having the arterial sheath connected to a venous sheath. While experience with these devices is limited, data indicate that they can provide excellent results. A 1,300-patient single-center prospective registry reported 99.7% procedural success with the Mo.Ma device and a 30-day death and stroke rate of 1.38% (32).

EPDs are standard of care in the US, and several types exist (**Fig. 33.10**). If the EPD will not cross the lesion, the stenosis may be crossed with a conventional 0.014-inch guide wire and subsequently predilated with a small (2.5 mm) balloon. Then, the EPD

may be placed. After distal EPD deployment, the lesion is often predilated with an undersized coronary balloon, typically 3 to 4 mm in diameter. A self-expanding stent is then placed across the lesion. The stent covering the origin of the ICA is typically sized to fit the common carotid artery. There is no demonstrated benefit for using tapered stents. It is common practice, when treating an internal carotid bifurcation lesion, to place the stent across the ostium of the external carotid artery.

There are two types of self-expanding stents: closed-cell and open-cell. Open-cell stents are more flexible and may better navigate tortuous vessels. Closed-cell stents are more rigid but offer better "coverage"

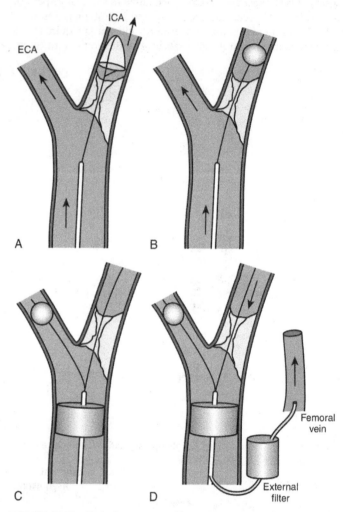

FIGURE 33.10 Embolic protection devices (EPDs). **A**, Filter-type device. **B**, Balloon occlusion of internal carotid artery (ICA). **C,D**, Proximal protection with flow reversal. See text. ECA, external carotid artery.

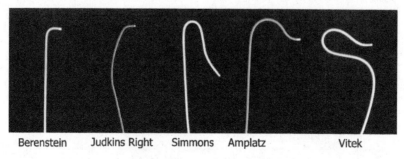

Berenstein   Judkins Right   Simmons   Amplatz   Vitek

FIGURE 33.9 Catheter shapes most used for engagement of great vessels.

of atherosclerotic plaque. While some evidence suggests that the frequency of embolic complications in symptomatic patients is lower with closed-cell stents, others have found no significant correlation between stent design and outcomes. Typical stent sizes are 6 to 10 mm in diameter and 2 to 4 cm in length. Gentle postdilation with a ≤5-mm balloon is often performed to improve stent apposition with the vessel wall. There is no benefit to aggressive postdilation because restenosis and late loss are very low in the carotid artery. Balloons are conservatively sized (≤1:1) to minimize vessel trauma/dissection, plaque embolization, and stimulation of the carotid sinus. A post-stent carotid diameter stenosis of ≤50% is an acceptable result.

Following the procedure, if a filter-type EPD is used, the EPD is retrieved, and final carotid and cerebral angiography is performed. If a proximal protection device is used, the balloons are deflated and final angiography is performed (Fig. 33.11). It is important to confirm that the carotid artery is free of dissection and that the cerebral vasculature is intact. Prior to removal of equipment, a neurologic exam assessing speech, movement, and mental status

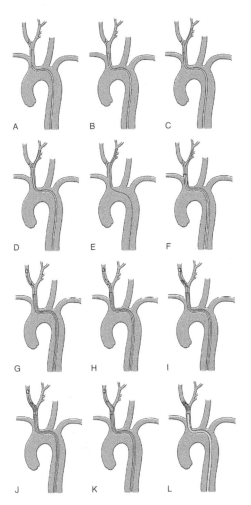

FIGURE 33.11 Stenting of the internal carotid artery (ICA). **A**, The common carotid artery (CCA) is accessed with a diagnostic catheter and standard 0.035-inch J wire. **B**, The catheter is advanced over the J wire but remains in the CCA. **C**, The J wire is exchanged for a hydrophilic stiff-angled 0.035" wire. **D**, The catheter is advanced to the ECA and the hydrophilic wire is removed. **E**, A stiff Amplatz wire is advanced to the ECA and the catheter is removed. **F**, A long 6F sheath is advanced over a dilator to the CCA. **G**, After removing the Amplatz wire and dilator, the lesion is crossed with a wire/filter device. **H**, Predilation. **I**, Stent placement. **J**, Stent deployment. The ostium of the ECA is often "jailed". **K**, postdilation. **L**, Final result..

should be performed. If a neurologic deficit is found, a culprit lesion is sought and neurovascular rescue attempted.

Aorto-Ostial and Common Carotid Interventions: Femoral access is obtained with a 6- to 9-Fr sheath, depending on the diameter of the balloon and stent that will be used.

After anticoagulation (ACT ≥250 seconds) and appropriate diagnostic imaging of the target lesion, a 5-Fr diagnostic catheter is advanced through a guide catheter (i.e., a JR 4 or multipurpose guide) to the ostium of the target common carotid artery. The ostial lesion is crossed with a steerable 0.035-inch hydrophilic glidewire. The diagnostic catheter is then advanced across the lesion into the distal vessel. The glidewire is exchanged for a stiff 0.035-inch Amplatz wire, and the guide catheter is carefully advanced over the diagnostic catheter until it engages the ostium of the common carotid artery. The diagnostic catheter is then slowly removed.

The lesion is predilated with a balloon sized 1:1 with the common carotid artery. As the balloon deflates, the guide is gently advanced or "telescoped" over the balloon and across the lesion. This will facilitate placing the stent across the lesion. The predilation balloon is removed, and a balloon-expandable stent is placed. (In arteries protected by the axial skeleton, balloon-expandable stents are more often used.) After positioning the stent at the target lesion, the guide catheter is withdrawn, uncovering the stent and placing it in contact with the target lesion. The proximal stent should protrude very slightly into the aorta (≤1 mm) to ensure lesion coverage. After verifying adequate placement with contrast injections through the guide catheter, the stent is deployed at nominal pressure. As the balloon deflates, the guide is again gently telescoped over the balloon to allow further stents to be delivered distally if needed. A larger semi-compliant balloon may be used to flare the protruding portion of the stent in order to facilitate future angiography. Final angiography and neurologic assessment are performed (Fig. 33.12).

The access site is managed similarly to other interventional procedures. Sheath removal is performed when the ACT is ≤170 seconds if a closure device is not used.

Complications and Troubleshooting

Stroke: In a review of over 54,000 patients, the 30-day risk of stroke during or after CAS was 3.9% (31). Symptomatic patients were twice as likely to have an adverse event as asymptomatic patients. Most events occur within 24 hours of the procedure. If the patient develops a focal neurologic deficit *during* the procedure, an embolic event is assumed. Immediate cerebral angiography should be performed, and rescue intervention should be attempted. Typically, these emboli are plaque elements and not amenable to thrombolytic agents. Attempts at revascularization with angioplasty and stenting and/or thrombectomy are recommended. Mental status changes *after* the procedure warrant CT evaluation to rule out intracranial bleeding or hyperperfusion syndrome (see the following text).

Hemodynamic Instability: Stimulation of the carotid sinus baroreceptor is common during carotid interventions and can cause hypotension and bradycardia. Typically, patients who are most sensitive will react negatively to predilation of their lesion. Acute hypotension can lead to brain hypoperfusion and neurologic symptoms due to impaired cerebral autoregulation.

Atropine (0.4–1 mg) may be used to treat acute bradycardia. A prophylactic dose may be considered before stent deployment if the patient was sensitive to predilation, but there is a risk of urinary retention in men. The dose may be repeated if necessary.

Aggressive fluid administration is important in treating hypotension, but vasopressor medications may be needed to maintain a

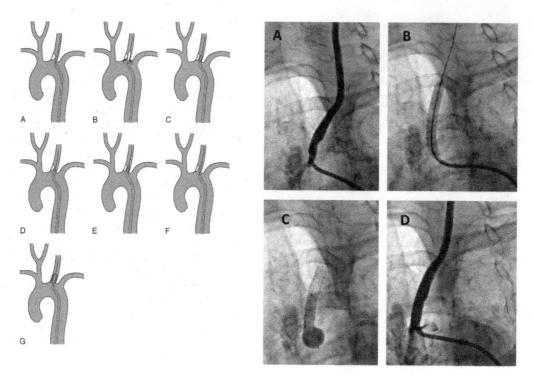

FIGURE 33.12   Dilating and stenting aorto-ostial lesions. Left Panel: **A**, The lesion is crossed with a 0.035-inch wire and pre-dilation balloon is placed. **B**, The lesion is predilated and as the balloon deflates, the guide catheter is advanced, thus "swallowing" the balloon. **C**, The guide is now distal to the lesion. **D**, The balloon is removed. **E**, a balloon-expandable stent is placed, although a portion of it remains within the guide. **F**, The guide is withdrawn, uncovering the stent and leaving it in contact with the lesion. **G**, The stent is deployed. If a stent is required distally, the stent balloon is "swallowed". Right Panel: **A**, Aorto-ostial common carotid stenosis. **B**, Sent inflation with stent partially protruding into the aorta. **C**, Post-dilation with Ostial flash balloon. **D**, Final result.

SBP of $\geq$100 mm Hg. We use repeated boluses, as needed, of 25 to 50 μg of phenylephrine. A continuous infusion may be required if hypotension persists. In most patients, however, phenylephrine can be weaned within several hours of the procedure, and the patient can ambulate in preparation for discharge the next day. Midodrine 2.5 to 10 mg three times daily (and then titrated downward as tolerated) can be useful to support blood pressure in the setting of prolonged hypotension. Adjusting the patient's antihypertensive regimen will be necessary over the short-term. Keep in mind that access site bleeding is a common cause of hypotension and should be ruled out in these patients.

Hyperperfusion Syndrome and Intracranial Hemorrhage: The opening of a stenotic carotid artery can lead to significant increases in cerebral blood flow, sometimes to levels more than twice the pre-procedure flow. Hyperperfusion syndrome occurs in <1% of carotid stent patients and is defined clinically by the presence of an ipsilateral throbbing headache, a seizure, or a focal neurologic deficit. A chronically stenotic carotid artery can cause the cerebral vasculature to remain in a state of constant, maximal vasodilation. When the stenosis is suddenly alleviated, cerebral autoregulatory mechanisms fail to control blood flow, a problem exacerbated by hypertension. The resulting elevated cerebral perfusion pressure can lead to cerebral edema or, worse, intracranial hemorrhage (33).

Neurologic symptoms from cerebral edema are usually transient but must be addressed. A neurology consultation and head CT should be obtained if this diagnosis is entertained. When diagnosed, strict control of blood pressure is critical, and consideration of mannitol, diuretics, or anti-epileptic medications (depending on presentation) is warranted. Medications that cause cerebral arterial vasodilation (i.e., hydralazine) should theoretically be avoided. Intracranial bleeding

is life-threatening. If it occurs, anti-platelet medications should be stopped and a neurosurgical team consulted. Strict blood pressure control (goal systolic pressure of 120–140 mm Hg) may decrease the risk of hyperperfusion syndrome and intracranial bleeding.

Follow-up

Following intervention, patients should be followed to ensure continued continuation of best medical therapy, monitoring patency of the stent with Doppler ultrasound surveillance (DUS) and for the development of focal neurologic symptoms. After carotid artery revascularization, it is recommended to obtain DUS studies at baseline (within 1 month of intervention), at 6, 12 months, and yearly thereafter (34). It is important to remember that carotid DUS velocities are altered after stenting, and that over-estimation of stenosis is very common (35).

Vertebral Artery Interventions

Approximately 80% of strokes are ischemic in etiology, and a minority (one-quarter) are located in the posterior circulation (36). The natural history of symptomatic vertebral artery stenosis (VAS) is a 5% to 11% incidence of stroke or death at 1 year (37). Reversible neurologic deficits caused by extracranial VAS carry a 5-year stroke risk of 30% (38). Symptomatic posterior circulation stenoses that are refractory to medical therapy carry a 5% to 11% incidence of stroke or death at 1 year (39).

Patients with persistent symptoms and anatomically suitable lesions despite optimal anti-atherosclerotic medical therapy should be considered for endovascular revascularization. Classical symptoms of posterior circulation ischemia include dizziness, drop attacks, diplopia, gait disturbance, dysphasia, and bilateral hemianopia. Less frequent symptoms include confusion, global amnesia, syncope, occipital headaches, nausea, vomiting, nystagmus, bilateral facial numbness, cortical blindness, and altered mental status (40).

Reasonable candidates for revascularization include patients with symptomatic vertebrobasilar insufficiency (VBI) and bilateral VAS ≥70% or unilateral vertebral stenosis ≥70% in the presence of an occluded or hypoplastic contralateral vertebral artery (VA) (41,42). VA revascularization may be considered if vertebral perfusion through the Circle of Willis would increase total cerebral blood flow enough to improve symptomatic patients with diffuse atherosclerotic disease and occlusions of both carotid arteries. VA occlusions should not be revascularized. Distal embolic debris to V4 and basilar artery perforators supplying the anterior spinal cord and brain stem could potentially be clinically devastating. Reperfusion of vertebral artery chronic total occlusions is contraindicated to prevent cerebellar, midbrain, pons, medullary, and brainstem infarctions.

Atherosclerotic disease of the VA is most commonly located at the ostium (V0) and proximal segment of the vessel (V1) and typically represents extension of plaque from the subclavian artery. The primary mechanism of stroke in 9% of the cases is artery-to-artery embolism to the distal circulation.

Surgical revascularization of proximal VA disease involves transposition of the VA to the ipsilateral common carotid artery or ICA, VA endarterectomy, and vein patch angioplasty. Given the lack of data regarding the natural history of asymptomatic patients with proximal VA disease, revascularization should be restricted to symptomatic patients, especially those for whom medical therapy has failed and an endovascular approach is preferred. Most proximal VA interventions are performed using femoral artery access. A 6-Fr guide or 8-Fr sheath is delivered to the proximal subclavian artery, and the lesion is crossed using a 0.014-inch coronary wire. Predilation with a coronary balloon is routinely performed to facilitate stent delivery. Stenting with a balloon-expandable stent is preferred to provide radial strength and reduce restenosis. EPDs are used if the distal vessel is large enough to accommodate the device (41).

With the use of contemporary stenting techniques, procedural success approaches 100% and periprocedural neurologic complications are rare. Angioplasty alone carries out high rates of restenosis; however, after stenting, the rate of restenosis is 10% or fewer of patients. Lesion length is an independent predictor of restenosis, and this may be considered for the selection of drug-eluting over bare-metal stents for longer lesions.

A 2011, meta-analysis of 27 articles and 980 patients undergoing VA stenting reported 1.1% stroke rate (11 patients) and 0.8% TIA (8 patients) at 30 days.

Vertebrobasilar infarction (1.3%) and recurrent symptoms (6.5%) remained low at mean follow-up of 21 months (43). In 2014, a meta-analysis of nine retrospective studies examined 480 lesions treated with 309 bare-metal stents and 175 drug-eluting stents. Drug-eluting stents significantly decreased both angiographic and symptomatic restenosis compared to bare-metal stents: 8.2% versus 23.7% and 4.7% versus 11.7%, respectively (44).

The Vertebral Artery Stenting Trial (VAST) enrolled 115 patients with symptomatic VA stenosis and randomized medical therapy versus stenting plus medical therapy. Unfortunately, the trial was prematurely discontinued due to regulatory and funding deficiencies after enrollment of 57 patients in the endovascular arm and 58 patients in the medical therapy arm. There were three strokes and one death (5%) in the stent arm compared to one stroke (2%) in the medical therapy arm at 30 days. At 3-year follow-up, there were more vertebrobasilar strokes with stent therapy compared to

medical therapy, 12% (n = 7) versus 7% (n = 4), respectively, but the trial did not show a significant difference in a composite outcome of death, stroke, and MI between the two groups (45).

Acute Stroke Interventions

For the treatment of acute cerebrovascular syndromes, prior trials of endovascular therapy included the intracranial administration of thrombolysis and the use of early-generation mechanical thrombectomy devices (Merci and Penumbra devices). The initial trials did not demonstrate conclusive benefit for endovascular therapy, although there were promising signals. There seemed to be a balance between early and effective mechanical reperfusion, balanced against the risk of intracranial hemorrhage that was perhaps related to reperfusion of non-viable brain. The newer trials have focused on delivering safe, and effective reperfusion therapy in stroke patients with viable brain tissue at risk (penumbra), determined by pre-treatment brain imaging (Fig. 33.13).

The treatment paradigm for acute stroke has shifted in the last few years. The two main aspects driving this change have been the introduction of new catheter technologies (stent retrievers), and a better pre-intervention patient selection based on the radiologic and clinical data available.

Results of Recent Randomized Clinical Trials

Several prospective trials studying mechanical thrombectomy for acute ischemic stroke—trials that predate "stent-retriever" devices—have been negative or inconclusive. The results of the Interventional Management of Stroke III (IMS-III) trial, published in 2013, showed no benefit of endovascular therapy following the use of intravenous (IV) thrombolysis over IV thrombolysis alone in the treatment of moderate to severe acute ischemic stroke. Nevertheless, in this study, CT-angiography was not required for enrollment, which allowed the inclusion of patients that did not have intracranial large-vessel occlusion. Secondly, the new technologies—stent-retrievers—were used only in five patients.

Between December 2014 and April 2015, five multicenter randomized clinical trials were published with positive results for endovascular therapy (23,46–49). The major differences between these positive endovascular trials and past trials were the use of CTA to select patients with proximal intracranial occlusion and the use of stent-retrievers for thrombectomy in the majority of cases.

The Multicenter Randomized Clinical Trial of Endovascular Treatment for Acute Ischemic Stroke in the Netherlands (MR CLEAN) (47), Endovascular Treatment for Small Core and Anterior Circulation Proximal Occlusion With Emphasis on Minimizing CT to Recanalization Times (ESCAPE) (46), Extending the Time for Thrombolysis in Emergency Neurological Deficits-Intra-Arterial (EXTEND-IA) (48), Solitaire With the Intention for Thrombectomy as Primary Endovascular Treatment (SWIFT PRIME) (49), and thrombectomy within 8 hours after Symptom Onset in Ischemic Stroke (REVASCAT) (23) have demonstrated the efficacy of endovascular therapy versus IV r-tPA (intra-arterial recombinant tissue plasminogen activator) alone in treating patients with acute anterior circulation ischemic stroke. The last three studies were stopped early by their Data Safety Monitoring Boards after the MR CLEAN results were published.

Inclusion Criteria and Time Window: All five trials used CT imaging to select patients. In MR CLEAN, patients were selected based upon plain CT imaging using the Alberta Stroke Program Early CT Score (ASPECTS). In other trials, patients were selected for having

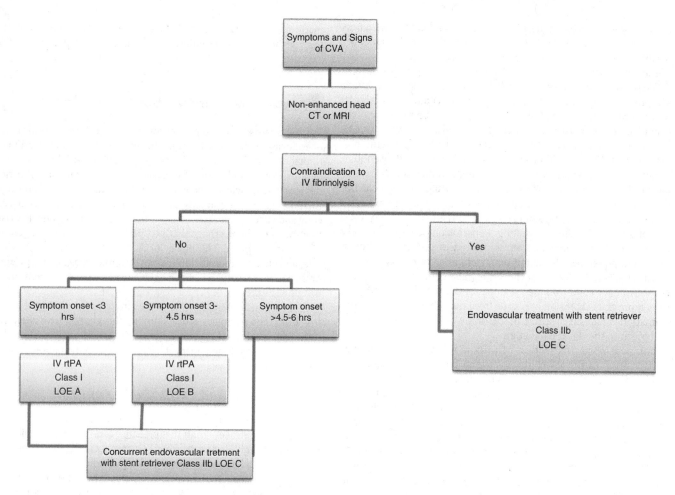

FIGURE 33.13 Algorithm for acute ischemic stroke imaging and treatment. Patients eligible for IV r-tPA should receive IV r-tPA even if endovascular treatments are being considered (Class I: LOE A). Observing patients after IV r-tPA to assess for clinical response before pursuing endovascular therapy is not required to achieve beneficial outcomes and is not recommended (Class III: LOE B-R). CT, computed tomography; CVA, cerebral vascular accident; IV rtPA, intra-arterial recombinant tissue plasminogen activator; LOE, level of evidence; MRI, magnetic resonance imaging.

a small ischemic core at baseline and either adequate collaterals (using CTA in ESCAPE) or a salvageable brain (using CT perfusion) in EXTEND-IA and SWIFT PRIME. The documentation of a proximal anterior circulation intracranial occlusion with CTA was required in all trials, which is a major difference from the negative endovascular reperfusion trials in the past (**Table 33.4**).

The baseline age and gender characteristics were comparable in all trials. The baseline NIHSS stroke scale was high at about 16. In the EXTEND-IA study, the NIHSS was lower in the conservative group compared to the intervention group (13 vs. 16). Patients older than 80 years of age were included in all but SWIFT PRIME.

SWIFT PRIME treated patients up to 4.5 hours from the onset of stroke, while MR CLEAN and EXTEND-IA included those up to 6 hours after onset, REVASCAT up to 8 hours, and ESCAPE up to 12 hours. In practice, however, only a few patients who could not have groin puncture by 6 hours were actually included. Therefore, the positive results of the trials mainly apply to patients treated within 6 hours from symptom onset. A combined approach with IV thrombolysis and thrombectomy was required in SWIFT PRIME and was used in the majority of patients within the other studies. Most patients in the control groups received IV thrombolysis if they presented within the 4.5-hour time window.

Favorable Clinical Outcome: All five recent randomized control trials showed a benefit for endovascular treatment compared to IV

tPA alone with regard to functional outcomes. The percentage of patients achieving a favorable clinical outcome with intra-arterial thrombectomy (IAT) varied between 33% and 71%. There was a consistent positive difference across all studies with a favorable clinical outcome (defined as a modified Rankin Score [mRS] of 0–2 at 90 days) between interventional and control arms, favoring IAT by 14% to 31%. The difference between the groups was more pronounced in the trials in which penumbral imaging with CT-perfusion was used. Nevertheless, even without imaging selection beyond the unenhanced CT, such as the MR CLEAN study, there was a clear benefit favoring IAT. Importantly, IAT was consistently effective overall among the important pre-specified patient subgroups of sex, age, stroke severity, and time of presentation.

Complication and Mortality Rates: In all of the studies, IAT added no additional risk of bleeding over standard management with IV tPA. The intracerebral hemorrhage risk in both interventional and control arms ranged from 0% to 7%. The fact that, in all trials, IAT carried no higher bleeding risk compared to IV tPA demonstrates that thrombectomy is safe, and any bleeding risk is caused mainly by thrombolysis. There was an overall trend toward a reduction in mortality with IAT.

Recanalization Rates: Successful recanalization was defined as a thrombolysis in cerebral infarction (TICI)-score 2b or 3. The use of stent-retrievers in the trials led to recanalization rates of between 59%

TABLE 33.4 Summary of Contemporary Trials in Acute Stroke Intervention

PRE-STENT RETRIEVER	PATIENTS	STENT RETRIEVER USE (% AGE)	VASCULAR IMAGING	DEVICE DEPLOYMENT AND/OR IA tPA (TREATMENT ARM)	RECANALIZATION TICI 2b/3 FLOW	PRIMARY ENDPOINT TREATMENT CONTROL COMPARISON
IMS III	656	1.5	No	77%; IA rtPA 41% IA rtPA + device 38% Device only 21% Stent retriever 1.5%	41%	mRS 0–2 at 90 days 40.8% 38.7% 1.5% (−6 to 9)[a]
MR RESCUE	118	0	CTA, MRA	95% MERCI 58% Penumbra 22% Both 16%	25%	Mean mRS 3.9 3.9 → p = 0.99
SYNTHESIS expansion	362	14	No	91% IA rtPA alone 66% + device 34%	–	mRS 0–1 at 3 months → 30.4% 34.8% → 0.71 (0.44–1.14)[b]
Stent Retriever Era						
MR CLEAN	500	81.5	CTA, MRA, DSA	83.7% Stent retriever 81.5% IAT 21%	58%	Improvement in mRS 1.67 (1.21–2.3)[a] at 90 days
ESCAPE	316	86.1	CTA	91.5% Stent retriever 86.1%	72.4%	Improvement in mRS 3.1 (2.0–4.7)[a] at 90 days
EXTEND-IA	70	100	CTA, MRA	77% Stent retriever 100%	86%	Median Reperfusion 100% 37% 4.7 (2.5–9.0)[a] at 24 hours ↓ in NIHSS 8 or 80% 37% 6.0 (2.0–18.0)[a] NIHSS 0, 1 at 3 days
SWIFT PRIME	196	100	CTA, MRA	88.8% Stent retriever 100%	88%	Rankin shift p <0.001 5 and 6 combined
REVASCAT	206	100	CTA, MRA, DSA	95% Stent retriever 100%	66%	Improvement in mRS 1.7 (1.05–2.8)[a] at 90 days

[a]95% confidence interval
CTA, computed tomography angiography; DSA, digital subtraction angiography; IA rtPA, intra-arterial recombinant tissue plasminogen activator; MRA, magnetic resonance angiography; mRS, modified Rankin Scale; NIHSS, National Institutes of Health Stroke Scale; TICI, thrombolysis in cerebral infarction.

and 88%. The trials also showed that the likelihood of good outcome increased with better recanalization. The highest recanalization rates were achieved in SWIFT PRIME (88%) and EXTEND-IA (86%), correlating with the high rates of good clinical outcomes seen in these trials (60% and 71%). The lowest recanalization rate was in MR CLEAN at 59% with a favorable clinical outcome occurring in only 33% of the patients.

Endovascular Technique/Thrombectomy Devices: The major difference between these randomized trials and the mechanical thrombectomy trials in the past was the use of stent retrievers in the majority of the patients (Table 33.4). Retrievable stents are self-expandable stent-like devices that are fully retrievable. Therefore, these devices combine the advantages of prompt flow restoration and mechanical thrombectomy (Fig. 33.14). The excellent recanalization results

with low complication rates of the stent-retriever devices in registries suggested a high rate of favorable clinical outcome (50,51). This was confirmed in all five randomized trials.

Indications and Patient Selection for Endovascular Treatment

Clinical Status: The NIHSS, a quantitative measure of the severity of a stroke, should be performed at the initial examination in all stroke patients, but especially in patients being considered for IV tPA. Patients with significant deficits manifesting as scores between 8 and 20 are more likely to benefit from reperfusion, making them better candidates for treatment (52). Patients with minor to mild

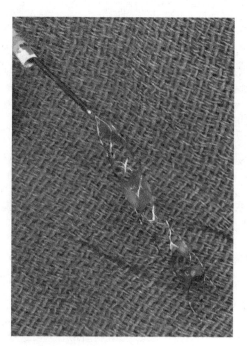

FIGURE 33.14 Stent retriever device.

symptoms (NIHSS score <8) and an existing intracranial large-vessel occlusion were not included in the trials. In these patients, the decision to perform additional IAT is based on the operator's experience and the estimated risk of the procedure.

Time of Presentation: IV tPA and IAT reperfusion therapies have both been shown to improve patient outcome. The time window for treatment of both approaches is limited, however. IV thrombolysis can be given up to 4.5 hours after stroke onset, additional or primary IA therapies can be used up to 12 hours after stroke onset. In anterior circulation strokes, the impact of successful thrombectomy is greater in the first 3 to 4.5 hours after stroke compared to late recanalization after 5 to 8 hours.

Imaging of Acute Stroke: Imaging helps identify target intracranial thrombi and measures the extent of salvageable brain tissue. Imaging the brain and the vasculature that supplies it is a vital first step in evaluating patients with acute ischemic stroke. A comprehensive evaluation may be performed with CTA or magnetic resonance imaging (MRI) techniques. The major advantages of CTA compared to MRI are that CTA is widely available, and a stroke imaging protocol that consists of unenhanced CT, CTA, and CT-perfusion imaging can be executed in 5 minutes for the comprehensive evaluation of the extra and intracranial circulation, the amount of infarcted brain tissue, and the penumbra.

Computed Tomography: With its widespread availability, short scan time, non-invasiveness nature, and safety, CT has been the traditional first-line imaging modality for the evaluation of acute ischemic stroke. Multi-modal CT includes unenhanced CT, CTA, and CT-perfusion. Non-contrast CT can identify intracranial hemorrhage and detect early signs of acute ischemic stroke. CTA can identify the occlusion site, detect arterial dissection, and grade collateral blood flow, whereas CT-perfusion can differentiate between "tissue-at-risk" (the so-called "penumbra") and irreversibly damaged brain tissue (52). Multimodal CT offers rapid data acquisition and can be performed with modern CT equipment.

Non-contrast CT: In the acute ischemic stroke setting, non-contrast CT has been used to rule out intracranial hemorrhage (a contraindication to thrombolysis), or other stroke mimics (e.g., tumor, infection,

etc.), which preclude the use of thrombolytic therapy, and is also used to measure the extent of early ischemic changes within an ischemic brain. The Alberta Stroke Program Early CT Score (ASPECTS) is a simple and systematic approach evaluating stroke patients (53). Patients with a high ASPECTS (8–10) seem to benefit more from IAT. MR CLEAN, which included patients with ASPECTS of 5 to 7, had an odds ratio of 1.97 for benefit, while those with ASPECTS of 8 to 10 had a beneficial odds ratio of 1.61. Those with ASPECTS of 0 to 4 had no benefit (OR 1.09), suggesting that mechanical thrombectomy has less efficacy in patients with a large ischemic core (47).

CT-Angiography: CTA is widely available, with fast, thin-section, volumetric spiral CT images acquired during the injection of a time-optimized bolus of contrast material for vessel opacification. The entire region from the aortic arch to the circle of Willis can be covered in a single image acquisition. CTA allows a detailed evaluation of the intra- and extracranial vasculature. Its utility in acute stroke lies in its ability to detect large-vessel occlusion within intracranial vessels and to evaluate the carotid and vertebral arteries in the neck. CTA can also depict the leptomeningeal collaterals and can identify large vessel occlusions with "good" and "poor" collaterals (54). Good collateral circulation improves the chance of a good neurologic outcome by limiting the extent of brain infarction. The ESCAPE trial used collateral assessment to select patients; the exclusion of participants with a large infarct core and poor collateral circulation was one of the reasons for the high rate of favorable clinical outcome (53%) (46).

CT-Perfusion: CT-perfusion allows rapid, non-invasive, quantitative evaluation of cerebral perfusion. CT-perfusion differentiation of the infarct core from the penumbra is based on the concept of cerebral vascular autoregulation. In the penumbra, autoregulation is preserved, mean transit time (MTT) is prolonged, but cerebral blood volume (CBV) is preserved because of vasodilatation and collateral recruitment as part of the autoregulation process. In the infarct core, autoregulation of blood flow is lost, MTT is prolonged and CBV is reduced. Thus, using appropriate MTT and CBV thresholds, the infarct core and penumbra can be distinguished on CT-perfusion maps (30). Direct assessment of an individual patient's ischemic penumbra may allow more personalized, appropriate selection of candidates for intervention than generalized time criteria because individuals may have different timelines for conversion of penumbra into infarct tissue. CT-perfusion was used to select patients for the EXTEND-IA trial, which achieved an impressive rate of good clinical outcome at 71%.

Pre-procedure Planning

Despite the fact that the efficacy of IV thrombolysis decreases with duration from the onset of symptoms, less than one-third of the patients meet the goal of a "door-to-needle time" of 60 minutes or less due to in-hospital delays (55). Improvements in pre-hospital and in-hospital stroke management can translate into faster treatment (56). Every stroke center should have an optimized stroke management protocol to reduce the "door-to-treatment" time with an on-demand, 24-7-365, stroke reperfusion service. When neuro-interventional providers are not able to provided 24-7-365 interventional stroke coverage, interventional cardiologists with carotid stenting experience can achieve comparable outcomes (57).

Optimized Stroke Management

Emergency services are instructed to bring patients with a suspected stroke directly to the stroke treatment room, which should be located in proximity to the CT scanner. After the neurologic examination, the unenhanced CT scan is acquired. If an intracerebral hemorrhage (ICH) can be ruled out, CT angiography and CT-perfusion are performed. Within the 4.5-hour time window, patients are treated with IV tPA immediately after exclusion of clinical and neuroradiologic contraindications.

If an occlusion of a large proximal intracranial vessel is found, the decision to perform endovascular therapy is based on the clinical condition of the patient, the time window (up to 6 hours after stroke onset), as well as the imaging criteria of the CTA and CT-perfusion (presence of leptomeningeal collaterals and the presence of ischemic penumbra). If the decision to proceed with endovascular therapy is made, the patient is transferred immediately to the angiography suite.

At this point, the decision regarding the need for general anesthesia and ventilation is made, depending on the patient's clinical condition. A subgroup analysis from MR CLEAN indicated that the advantage of IAT may disappear with general anesthesia. One advantage of conscious sedation, compared to general anesthesia, is timesaving, which allows the procedure to start more quickly. Another major advantage of conscious sedation is being able to assess the clinical status of the patient during the procedure and to evaluate the success of treatment. Disadvantages of conscious sedation are the patient's movements, which require experienced operators for a safe and successful procedure.

Using an optimized stroke protocol, with a door-to-device (D2D) time (the time from arrival at the hospital until the thrombectomy device is placed in the target lesion), a D2D time of <100 minutes had a favorable outcome in 66% of patients, compared with 44% of patients with a D2D time of more than 100 minutes (50). By analogy, the D2D time should play an important role in the outcome of these patients, as it does for the door-to-balloon time in the outcome of patients with ST-segment elevation myocardial infarction.

Description of Procedure

From First-Generation Devices to the Flow Restoration Devices (Stent-Retriever): In the last decade, mechanical recanalization devices have been developed to achieve better results than IA thrombolysis. The Merci-device and the Penumbra aspiration system were the first devices for which large clinical experiences have been reported (58,59). Nevertheless, the breakthrough in interventional treatment of acute stroke was achieved by the use of stent-like thrombectomy devices (stent-retriever; see Fig. 33.14) (60,61). The stent-retriever devices allow high recanalization rates, with a reduction in the recanalization time and low complication rates (50,51). In cases with a large thrombus burden, a combination of aspiration through a large lumen reperfusion catheter may be used. In the special groups of patients with extracranial carotid occlusion, arterial dissection and intracranial stenosis, carotid stenting will be necessary.

Stent-Retriever Technique: Stent-retrievers are self-expandable stent-like devices that are fully retrievable. Therefore, these devices combine the advantages of prompt flow restoration and mechanical thrombectomy. The improved clinical outcome with flow restoration devices is due to fast and effective clot removal, and the possibility of temporarily restoring flow. Recanalization rates of TICI 2a/b or 3 flow are high, up to 90%. The results of prospective studies showed high rates of favorable clinical outcomes at 3 months, a low rate of symptomatic ICH, and a low mortality rate. The low mortality rate reflects the low rate of symptomatic ICH and shows the safety of flow-restoration devices compared with reperfusion devices in the past.

Technique Thrombus Aspiration

Despite the impressive results of the stent-retriever devices with successful recanalization results of up to 95%, there are some vessel occlusions and thrombi that are resistant to this technique, even after repeated recanalization attempts. These vessel occlusions include cases

of terminal ICA occlusions. Moreover, "hard" or organized thrombi in other locations, like the MCA, can be resistant to the stent-retriever technique. For these cases, the direct aspiration of the thrombus has been used as an alternative technique. For direct thrombus aspiration, the most common aspiration catheters used for these purposes are 5F systems (e.g., the Penumbra reperfusion catheter), ACE 64 (Penumbra, USA), which has a 0.64-inch inner lumen that is significantly larger than the prior generation of aspiration catheters.

Post-Procedure Management

The use of vascular closure devices can be routinely used with low complication rates, especially in patients that received IV thrombolysis. During intervention, there is no need for any antiplatelet medication. In cases with emergency stent implantation (52) of occlusions at the origin of ICA, antiplatelet therapy is necessary to prevent acute stent thrombosis. In these cases, administration of IV aspirin would be possible. In post-procedure, guidelines recommend aspirin, 325 mg orally, within 24 to 48 hours of ischemic stroke onset.

Although hypertension is common in acute ischemic stroke and is associated with poor outcomes, studies of antihypertensive treatment in this setting have produced conflicting results. A theoretical drawback of blood pressure reduction is that elevated blood pressure may counteract dysfunctional cerebral autoregulation from stroke, but limited evidence suggests that antihypertensive treatment in acute stroke does not change cerebral perfusion. Once intravenous tPA or thrombectomy are performed, the blood pressure must be maintained below 180/105 mm Hg to limit the risk of ICH.

Potential Complications

Complications that can occur during or after the procedure include distal embolization to the same or other vessel territories, dissection of the arteries, and subarachnoid or intracerebral hemorrhage. MR CLEAN reported 5.6% incidence of new symptomatic embolism. With distal embolization, the management depends on how relevant the occluded branch is. If the patient is not intubated, a clinical examination can show if the persistent occlusion is relevant or not. If the occluded branch is a relevant one, a stent-retriever can be used even in M3 branches of the MCA or in A2-segments of the ACA.

Dissections of the vessels mostly occur in the ICA when a distal access catheter is used.

Dissections without flow restriction do not require any therapy. In cases of a flow limiting dissection, stenting of the affected vessel can be performed.

Small subarachnoid hemorrhages are often seen on the control CT and do not require specific therapy. Intracerebral hemorrhage can occur during the procedure due to the intervention or even within 48 hours after the procedure as a result of reperfusion injury. Therefore, blood pressure control is a critical element of post-procedure management.

The occurrence of any worsening of neurologic status should be considered a possible sign of ICH, warranting immediate clinical evaluation and an emergency CT scan of the brain. Should ICH be found, reversal of all antithrombotic agents should be carried out.

Based on the positive outcomes in the five randomized trials comparing endovascular treatments in suitable patients in conjunction with IV thrombolysis or in patients in whom IV thrombolysis was contraindicated, the AHA/ASA published a Focused Update in 2015 for the early management of patients with acute ischemic stroke regarding endovascular treatment (52). Patients should receive endovascular therapy with a stent retriever if they meet the criteria shown in **Table 33.5.**

TABLE 33.5 AHA/ASA (52) Criteria for Endovascular Therapy in Acute Stroke Patients

Criteria for Endovascular Therapy after Acute Ischemic Stroke (Class I; Level of Evidence A)
Pre-stroke mRS score 0–1
Acute ischemic stroke receiving intravenous r-tPA within 4.5 hours of onset according to guidelines from professional medical societies
Causative occlusion of the internal carotid artery or proximal MCA (M1),
Age ≥18 years,
NIHSS score of ≥6,
ASPECTS of ≥6, and
Treatment can be initiated (groin puncture) within 6 hours of symptom onset

MCA, middle cerebral artery; mRS, modified Rankin Scale; NIHSS, National Institutes of Health Stroke Scale; r-tPA, recombinant tissue plasminogen activator.

Conclusion

Recently completed randomized controlled trials have established mechanical thrombectomy for acute ischemic stroke in patients with large-vessel occlusions and appropriate imaging for brain viability. The current endovascular reperfusion therapies allow high recanalization rates, high rates of favorable clinical outcomes, and low complication rates. Nevertheless, to optimize clinical results, image-guided patient selection and the use of an optimized stroke management protocol are required.

Key Points

■ ACCF/ASA/AHA Class I Recommendations for Diagnostic Testing in Patients with Symptoms or Signs of Extracranial Carotid Artery Disease:

1. Initial evaluation of patients with transient retinal or hemispheric neurologic symptoms of possible ischemic origin should include non-invasive imaging for the detection of ECVD (LOE: C).
2. Duplex ultrasonography is recommended to detect carotid stenosis in patients who develop focal neurologic symptoms corresponding to the territory supplied by the left or right ICA (LOE: C).
3. In patients with acute, focal ischemic neurologic symptoms corresponding to the territory supplied by the left or right ICA, MRA or CTA is indicated to detect carotid stenosis when sonography either cannot be obtained or yields equivocal or otherwise nondiagnostic results (LOE: C).
4. When extracranial or intracranial cerebrovascular disease is not severe enough to account for neurologic symptoms of suspected ischemic origin, echocardiography should be performed to search for a source of cardiogenic embolism (LOE: C).

■ Antihypertensive treatment is recommended for patients with hypertension and asymptomatic extracranial carotid or vertebral atherosclerosis to maintain blood pressure below 140/90 mm Hg (Class I, LOE: A).

■ Patients with extracranial carotid or vertebral atherosclerosis who smoke cigarettes should be advised to quit smoking and be offered smoking cessation interventions to reduce the risks of atherosclerosis progression and stroke (Class I, LOE: B).

■ Treatment with a statin medication is recommended for all patients with extracranial carotid or vertebral atherosclerosis to reduce LDL cholesterol below 100 mg/dL (Class I, LOE: B).

■ ACCF/ASA/AHA Class I Recommendations for Antiplatelet Therapy in ECVD:

1. Antiplatelet therapy with aspirin, 75 to 325 mg daily, is recommended for patients with obstructive or non-obstructive atherosclerosis that involves the extracranial carotid and/or vertebral arteries for prevention of MI and other ischemic cardiovascular events. This benefit has not been established for prevention of stroke in asymptomatic patients (Class I, LOE: A).
2. In patients with obstructive or non-obstructive extracranial carotid or vertebral atherosclerosis who have sustained ischemic stroke or TIA, antiplatelet therapy with aspirin alone (75–325 mg daily), clopidogrel alone (75 mg daily), or the combination of aspirin plus extended-release dipyridamole (25 and 200 mg twice daily, respectively) is recommended (Class I, LOE: B) and preferred over the combination of aspirin with clopidogrel (Class I, LOE: B). Selection of an antiplatelet regimen should be individualized on the basis of patient risk-factor profiles, cost, tolerance, and other clinical characteristics, as well as guidance from regulatory agencies.
3. Antiplatelet agents are recommended, rather than oral anticoagulation for patients with atherosclerosis of the extracranial carotid or vertebral arteries with (LOE: B) or without (LOE: C) ischemic symptoms.

■ ACCF/ASA/AHA Class I Recommendations for Vascular Imaging in Patients With Vertebral Artery Disease:

1. CTA or MRA for detection of VA disease should be part of the initial evaluation of patients with neurologic symptoms referable to the posterior circulation and those with subclavian steal syndrome (LOE: C).
2. Patients with asymptomatic bilateral carotid occlusions or unilateral carotid artery occlusion and incomplete circle of Willis should undergo non-invasive imaging for detection of VA obstructive disease (LOE: C).
3. In patients whose symptoms suggest posterior cerebral or cerebellar ischemia, MRA or CTA is recommended rather than ultrasound imaging for evaluation of the vertebral arteries (LOE: C).

■ ACCF/ASA/AHA Recommendations for Management of Atherosclerotic Risk Factors in Patients With Vertebral Artery Disease:

1. Medical therapy and lifestyle modification to reduce atherosclerotic risk are recommended in patients with vertebral atherosclerosis according to the standards recommended for those with extracranial carotid atherosclerosis (LOE: B).
2. In the absence of contraindications, these patients should also receive antiplatelet therapy with aspirin (75–325 mg daily) to prevent MI and other ischemic events (LOE: B).

3. Antiplatelet drug therapy is recommended as part of the initial management for patients who sustain ischemic stroke or TIA associated with extracranial vertebral atherosclerosis. Aspirin (81–325 mg daily), the combination of aspirin plus extended-release dipyridamole (25 and 200 mg twice daily, respectively), and clopidogrel (75 mg daily) are acceptable options. Selection of an antiplatelet regimen should be individualized (LOE: B).

References

1. Writing Group Members, et al. Heart disease and stroke statistics-2016 update: a report from the American Heart Association. *Circulation.* 2016;133:e38–e360.
2. Ovbiagele B, et al. Forecasting the future of stroke in the United States: a policy statement from the American Heart Association and American Stroke Association. *Stroke.* 2013;44:2361–2375.
3. Gargano JW, Reeves MJ, Paul Coverdell National Acute Stroke Registry Michigan Prototype Investigators. Sex differences in stroke recovery and stroke-specific quality of life: results from a statewide stroke registry. *Stroke.* 2007;38:2541–2548.
4. Amarenco P, Steering Committee Investigators of the TIAregistry.org. Risk of stroke after transient ischemic attack or minor stroke. *N Engl J Med.* 2016;375:387.
5. Markus HS, et al. Asymptomatic embolisation for prediction of stroke in the Asymptomatic Carotid Emboli Study (ACES): a prospective observational study. *Lancet Neurol.* 2010;9:663–671.
6. Jalbert JJ, et al. Comparative effectiveness of carotid artery stenting versus carotid endarterectomy among Medicare beneficiaries. *Circ Cardiovasc Qual Outcomes.* 2016;9:275–285.
7. Meschia JF, et al. Guidelines for the primary prevention of stroke: a statement for healthcare professionals from the American Heart Association/American Stroke Association. *Stroke.* 2014;45:3754–3832.
8. Sacco RL, et al. An updated definition of stroke for the 21st century: a statement for healthcare professionals from the American Heart Association/American Stroke Association. *Stroke.* 2013;44:2064–2089.
9. Yang C, Bogiatzi C, Spence JD. Risk of stroke at the time of carotid occlusion. *JAMA Neurol.* 2015;72:1261–1267.
10. Barnett HJ, et al. Benefit of carotid endarterectomy in patients with symptomatic moderate or severe stenosis. North American Symptomatic Carotid Endarterectomy Trial Collaborators. *N Engl J Med.* 1998;339:1415–1425.
11. Inzitari D, et al. Risk factors and outcome of patients with carotid artery stenosis presenting with lacunar stroke. North American Symptomatic Carotid Endarterectomy Trial Group. *Neurology.* 2000;54:660–666.
12. Bates ER, et al. ACCF/SCAI/SVMB/SIR/ASITN 2007 Clinical Expert Consensus Document on carotid stenting. *Vasc Med.* 2007;12:35–83.
13. Constantinou J, Jayia P, Hamilton G. Best evidence for medical therapy for carotid artery stenosis. *J Vasc Surg.* 2013;58:1129–1139.
14. Chou R, et al. Statin use for the prevention of cardiovascular disease in adults: a systematic review for the US Preventive Services Task Force. *JAMA.* 2016;316(19):2008–2024.
15. Stone NJ, et al. 2013 ACC/AHA guideline on the treatment of blood cholesterol to reduce atherosclerotic cardiovascular risk in adults: a report of the American College of Cardiology/American Heart Association Task Force on Practice Guidelines. *Circulation.* 2014;129:S1–S45.
16. Amarenco P, et al. Coronary heart disease risk in patients with stroke or transient ischemic attack and no known coronary heart disease: findings from the Stroke Prevention by Aggressive Reduction in Cholesterol Levels (SPARCL) trial. *Stroke.* 2010;41:426–430.
17. Everett BM, et al. Rosuvastatin in the prevention of stroke among men and women with elevated levels of C-reactive protein: Justification for the Use of statins in Prevention: an Intervention Trial Evaluating Rosuvastatin (JUPITER). *Circulation.* 2010;121:143–150.
18. Hobson RW 2nd, et al. Efficacy of carotid endarterectomy for asymptomatic carotid stenosis. The Veterans Affairs Cooperative Study Group. *N Engl J Med.* 1993;328:221–227.
19. Endarterectomy for asymptomatic carotid artery stenosis. Executive Committee for the Asymptomatic Carotid Atherosclerosis Study. *JAMA.* 1995;273:1421–1428.
20. Halliday A, et al. Prevention of disabling and fatal strokes by successful carotid endarterectomy in patients without recent neurological symptoms: randomised controlled trial. *Lancet.* 2004;363:1491–1502.
21. Mayberg MR, et al. Carotid endarterectomy and prevention of cerebral ischemia in symptomatic carotid stenosis. Veterans Affairs Cooperative Studies Program 309 Trialist Group. *JAMA.* 1991;266:3289–3294.
22. Rothwell PM, et al. Analysis of pooled data from the randomised controlled trials of endarterectomy for symptomatic carotid stenosis. *Lancet.* 2003;361:107–116.
23. Molina CA, et al. REVASCAT: a randomized trial of revascularization with SOLITAIRE FR device vs. best medical therapy in the treatment of acute stroke due to anterior circulation large vessel occlusion presenting within eight-hours of symptom onset. *Int J Stroke.* 2015;10:619–626.
24. Yadav JS. Carotid stenting in high-risk patients: design and rationale of the SAPPHIRE trial. *Cleve Clin J Med.* 2004;71(suppl 1):S45–S46.
25. Bonati LH, et al. Long-term outcomes after stenting versus endarterectomy for treatment of symptomatic carotid stenosis: the International Carotid Stenting Study (ICSS) randomised trial. *Lancet.* 2015;385:529–538.
26. SPACE Collaborative Group, et al. 30 day results from the SPACE trial of stent-protected angioplasty versus carotid endarterectomy in symptomatic patients: a randomised non-inferiority trial. *Lancet.* 2006;368:1239–1247.
27. Mantese VA, et al. The Carotid Revascularization Endarterectomy versus Stenting Trial (CREST): stenting versus carotid endarterectomy for carotid disease. *Stroke.* 2010;41:S31–S34.
28. Mas JL, et al. Endarterectomy Versus Angioplasty in Patients with Symptomatic Severe Carotid Stenosis (EVA-3S) trial: results up to 4 years from a randomised, multicentre trial. *Lancet Neurol.* 2008;7:885–892.
29. Rosenfield K, et al. Randomized trial of stent versus surgery for asymptomatic carotid stenosis. *N Engl J Med.* 2016;374:1011–1020.
30. Garg N, et al. Cerebral protection devices reduce periprocedural strokes during carotid angioplasty and stenting: a systematic review of the current literature. *J Endovasc Ther.* 2009;16:412–427.
31. Touze E, et al. Systematic review of the perioperative risks of stroke or death after carotid angioplasty and stenting. *Stroke.* 2009;40:e683–e693.
32. Stabile E, et al. Cerebral embolic lesions detected with diffusion-weighted magnetic resonance imaging following carotid artery stenting: a meta-analysis of 8 studies comparing filter cerebral protection and proximal balloon occlusion. *JACC Cardiovasc Interv.* 2014;7:1177–1183.
33. Moulakakis KG, et al. Hyperperfusion syndrome after carotid revascularization. *J Vasc Surg.* 2009;49:1060–1068.
34. American College of Cardiology Foundation, et al. ACCF/ACR/AIUM/ASE/ASN/ICAVL/SCAI/SCCT/SIR/SVM/SVS/SVU [corrected] 2012 appropriate use criteria for peripheral vascular ultrasound and physiological testing part 1: arterial ultrasound and physiological testing: a report of the American College of Cardiology Foundation appropriate use criteria task force, American College of Radiology, American Institute of Ultrasound in Medicine, American Society of Echocardiography, American Society of Nephrology, Intersocietal Commission for the Accreditation of Vascular Laboratories, Society for Cardiovascular Angiography and Interventions, Society of Cardiovascular Computed Tomography, Society for Interventional Radiology, Society for Vascular Medicine, Society for Vascular Surgery, [corrected] and Society for Vascular Ultrasound [corrected]. *J Am Coll Cardiol.* 2012;60:242–276.
35. Chi YW, et al. Ultrasound velocity criteria for carotid in-stent restenosis. *Catheter Cardiovasc Interv.* 2007;69:349–354.
36. Savitz SI, Caplan LR. Vertebrobasilar disease. *N Engl J Med.* 2005;352:2618–2626.
37. Turan TN, et al. Risk factors associated with severity and location of intracranial arterial stenosis. *Stroke.* 2010;41:1636–1640.
38. Crawley F, Brown MM. Percutaneous transluminal angioplasty and stenting for vertebral artery stenosis. *Cochrane Database Syst Rev.* 2000:CD000516.
39. Ausman JI, et al. Intracranial vertebral endarterectomy. *Neurosurgery.* 1990;26:465–471.

40. Jenkins JS, et al. Vertebral artery stenting. *Catheter Cardiovasc Interv.* 2001;54:1–5.

41. Jenkins JS, et al. Endovascular stenting for vertebral artery stenosis. *J Am Coll Cardiol.* 2010;55:538–542.

42. Henry M, et al. Angioplasty and stenting of extracranial vertebral artery stenosis. *Int Angiol.* 2005;24:311–324.

43. Stayman AN, Nogueira RG, Gupta R. A systematic review of stenting and angioplasty of symptomatic extracranial vertebral artery stenosis. *Stroke.* 2011;42:2212–2216.

44. Langwieser N, et al. Safety and efficacy of different stent types for the endovascular therapy of extracranial vertebral artery disease. *Clin Res Cardiol.* 2014;103:353–362.

45. Compter A, et al. Stenting versus medical treatment in patients with symptomatic vertebral artery stenosis: a randomised open-label phase 2 trial. *Lancet Neurol.* 2015;14:606–614.

46. Demchuk AM, et al. Endovascular treatment for Small Core and Anterior circulation Proximal occlusion with Emphasis on minimizing CT to recanalization times (ESCAPE) trial: methodology. *Int J Stroke.* 2015;10:429–438.

47. Fransen PS, et al. MR CLEAN, a multicenter randomized clinical trial of endovascular treatment for acute ischemic stroke in the Netherlands: study protocol for a randomized controlled trial. *Trials.* 2014;15:343.

48. Campbell BC, et al. A multicenter, randomized, controlled study to investigate EXtending the time for Thrombolysis in Emergency Neurological Deficits with Intra-Arterial therapy (EXTEND-IA). *Int J Stroke.* 2014;9:126–132.

49. Saver JL, et al. Solitaire with the Intention for Thrombectomy as Primary Endovascular Treatment for Acute Ischemic Stroke (SWIFT PRIME) trial: protocol for a randomized, controlled, multicenter study comparing the Solitaire revascularization device with IV tPA with IV tPA alone in acute ischemic stroke. *Int J Stroke.* 2015;10:439–448.

50. Roth C, et al. Mechanical recanalization with flow restoration in acute ischemic stroke: the ReFlow (mechanical recanalization with flow restoration in acute ischemic stroke) study. *JACC Cardiovasc Interv.* 2013;6:386–391.

51. Roth C, et al. Stent-assisted mechanical recanalization for treatment of acute intracerebral artery occlusions. *Stroke.* 2010;41:2559–2567.

52. Powers WJ, et al. 2015 American Heart Association/American Stroke Association focused update of the 2013 guidelines for the early management of patients with acute ischemic stroke regarding endovascular treatment: a guideline for healthcare professionals from the American Heart Association/American Stroke Association. *Stroke.* 2015;46:3020–3035.

53. Barber PA, et al. Validity and reliability of a quantitative computed tomography score in predicting outcome of hyperacute stroke before thrombolytic therapy. ASPECTS Study Group. Alberta Stroke Programme early CT score. *Lancet.* 2000;355:1670–1674.

54. Lima FO, et al. The pattern of leptomeningeal collaterals on CT angiography is a strong predictor of long-term functional outcome in stroke patients with large vessel intracranial occlusion. *Stroke.* 2010;41:2316–2322.

55. Fonarow GC, et al. Timeliness of tissue-type plasminogen activator therapy in acute ischemic stroke: patient characteristics, hospital factors, and outcomes associated with door-to-needle times within 60 minutes. *Circulation.* 2011;123:750–758.

56. Fonarow GC, et al. Improving door-to-needle times in acute ischemic stroke: the design and rationale for the American Heart Association/American Stroke Association's Target: stroke initiative. *Stroke.* 2011;42:2983–2989.

57. Htyte N, et al. Predictors of outcomes following catheter-based therapy for acute stroke. *Catheter Cardiovasc Interv.* 2015;85:1043–1050.

58. Grunwald IQ, et al. Revascularization in acute ischaemic stroke using the penumbra system: the first single center experience. *Eur J Neurol.* 2009;16:1210–1216.

59. Smith WS, et al. Mechanical thrombectomy for acute ischemic stroke: final results of the Multi MERCI trial. *Stroke.* 2008;39:1205–1212.

60. Papanagiotou P, et al. Treatment of acute cerebral artery occlusion with a fully recoverable intracranial stent: a new technique. *Circulation.* 2010;121:2605–2606.

61. Perez MA, et al. Intracranial thrombectomy using the Solitaire stent: a historical vignette. *J Neurointerv Surg.* 2012;4:e32.

34 Atherosclerotic Renal Artery Disease

Pranav M. Patel, MD, FSCAI, FACC

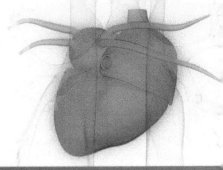

Prevalence and Natural History

Atherosclerotic renal artery stenosis (RAS) is the most common primary disease of the renal arteries, and it is associated with clinical syndromes such as ischemic renal disease and hypertension. It is a common cause of secondary hypertension and is found in 0.5% to 5% of all hypertensive patients (1,2). Renovascular hypertension, ischemic nephropathy, and end-stage renal disease (ESRD) are the potential consequences of atherosclerotic RAS.

The prevalence of RAS has been well documented in patients, affecting ~7% of the population aged >65 years (1). In patients with atherosclerotic coronary and peripheral artery disease (PAD), renal-arterial disease has been documented to be present in 30% of patients undergoing screening renal artery angiography at the time of cardiac catheterization. In these populations, significant obstructive RAS (>50%) has been reported in 11% to 19% of patients (2–4). Prevalence studies have also demonstrated significant RAS in 22% to 59% of patients with PAD (5–9), and bilateral RAS involvement is found in ~44% with RAS (10).

Atherosclerosis accounts for ~90% of cases of stenosis within the renal arterial bed (11). Causes of RAS are listed in **Table 34.1**.

TABLE 34.1 Causes of Renal Artery Stenosis

- Atherosclerotic renal artery stenosis; most common
- Fibromuscular dysplasia
- Renal artery vasculitis
- Diabetic nephropathy
- Scleroderma
- Trauma
- Neurofibromatosis
- Thromboangiitis obliterans
- Nephroangiosclerosis
- Dissection of aorta or renal arteries

Atherosclerotic lesions usually involve the origin and proximal third of the main renal artery and also the perirenal aorta.

Fibromuscular dysplasia (FMD) accounts for <10% of cases of RAS, and usually involves the distal two-thirds of the main renal artery or its branches. Medial fibroplasia, a subtype of medial FMD, is the histologic finding in 75% to 80% of all cases of FMD. Microscopically, there are alternating areas of thinned media and thickened fibromuscular ridges containing collagen. Some areas of the internal elastic membrane are lost (12–14). A "string of beads" is used to describe its angiographic appearance, where the "bead" diameter is larger than the proximal vessel. The classification of FMD is demonstrated in **Table 34.2**. Atherosclerosis and FMD are the most common causes of RAS.

Pathophysiology of RAS

RAS gives rise to renovascular hypertension via the activation of the renin–angiotensin–aldosterone pathway. RAS and subsequent ischemia triggers the release of renin. Renin leads to the conversion of angiotensin I to angiotensin II. Angiotensin II causes vasoconstriction, which leads to hypertension and enhances the adrenal synthesis of aldosterone. Aldosterone causes sodium and fluid retention, which also promotes the development of hypertension. Together with aldosterone release, the sympathetic nervous system is activated and also plays a role in the development of renovascular hypertension. Early revascularization of atherosclerotic RAS will improve hypertension in these patients. Nevertheless, this improvement may not be seen in kidneys that have already experienced damage from sustained hypertension.

Clinical Endpoints and Physical Examination

Atherosclerotic RAS is a progressive disease. Progression to occlusion is more common in renal arteries with more severe stenosis. Over a

TABLE 34.2 Classification of Fibromuscular Dysplasia

TYPE	FREQUENCY	PATHOLOGY
Medial dysplasia		
Medial fibroplasias	80%	Alternating areas of thinned media and thickened fibromuscular ridges containing collagen. Internal elastic membrane may be lost in some areas
Perimedial fibroplasias	10%–15%	Extensive collagen deposition in the outer half of the media
Medial hyperplasia	1%–2%	True smooth muscle cell hyperplasia without fibrosis
Intimal fibroplasias	<10%	Circumferential or eccentric deposition of collagen in the intima. No lipid or inflammatory component. Internal elastic lamina fragmented or duplicated
Adventitial (periarterial) fibroplasias	<1%	Dense collagen replaces the fibrous tissue of the adventitia and may extend into surrounding tissue

3-year period, Zierler and associates found that 48% of patients had progression of RAS from <60% to ≥60% stenosis. The renal arteries that progressed to occlusion were each characterized by a stenosis ≥60% at baseline. Progression of RAS occurred at an average rate of ~7% per year (15). Patients with atherosclerotic RAS who progress to dialysis-dependent ESRD have high mortality rates (16). This may be because of systemic atherosclerotic disease and higher rates of cardiovascular ischemic events in these individuals. Although several retrospective studies have indicated that percutaneous renal artery revascularization improves blood pressure, and stabilizes or retards the deterioration in renal function, recent randomized prospective trials have not indicated the usefulness of such revascularization procedures. As a result, management of such patients is still not completely clear, and the relationship between RAS severity and the impact on renal function remains poorly understood.

Patients with atherosclerotic RAS who progress to ESRD and require dialysis have high mortality rates. The mean life expectancy of individuals older than 65 years with RAS who had ESRD is only ~3 years (16). This is thought to be because of the systemic atherosclerosis and higher rates of cardiovascular events in individuals with atherosclerotic RAS. The severity of renal impairment has been associated with reduced survival in patients with RAS. In patients with serum creatinine levels <1.4 mg/dL, 3-year survival was 92% (±4%). For serum creatinine levels of between 1.5 and 1.9 mg/dL, 3-year survival was 74% (±8%), and for creatinine ≥2.0 mg/dL, it was only 51% (±8%) (17).

Several clinical features provide relative indications for application of more specific diagnostic testing strategies for RAS (**Table 34.3**). One such indication is the presence of an atrophic kidney

---

TABLE 34.3 Clinical Clues to the Diagnosis of Renal Artery Stenosis

- Patients with the onset of hypertension before the age of 30 years.
- Patients with the onset of severe hypertension after the age of 55 years.
- Patients with the following characteristics: (a) accelerated hypertension (sudden and persistent worsening of previously controlled hypertension); (b) resistant hypertension (defined as the failure to achieve goal blood pressure in patients who are adhering to full doses of an appropriate three-drug regimen that includes a diuretic); or (c) malignant hypertension (hypertension with coexistent evidence of acute end-organ damage, i.e., acute renal failure, acutely decompensated congestive heart failure, new visual or neurologic disturbance, and/or advanced [grade III to IV] retinopathy).
- Patients with new azotemia or worsening renal function after the administration of an ACE inhibitor or an angiotensin receptor blocking agent.
- Patients with an unexplained atrophic kidney or a discrepancy in size between the two kidneys of greater than 1.5 cm.
- Patients with sudden, unexplained pulmonary edema (especially in azotemic patients).
- Patients with unexplained renal failure, including individuals starting renal replacement therapy (dialysis or renal transplantation).
- Patients with multivessel coronary artery disease and none of the clinical clues or PAD at the time of arteriography.
- Patients with unexplained congestive heart failure or refractory angina.

ACE, angiotensin converting enzyme; PAD, peripheral artery disease.

(≤7–8 cm) or discrepancy in renal sizes (>1.5 cm) (18,19). If the renal atrophy is unexplained by a prior history of pyelonephritis, reflux nephropathy, or trauma, then this is an indication for additional renal diagnostic tests to define RAS.

The physical examination of patients with RAS should focus on the assessment of blood pressure because RAS may be associated with sustained or labile hypertension. Assessment for fluid retention and history of flash pulmonary edema, unexplained congestive heart failure, and refractory angina are also useful. The patient should also have an evaluation for evidence of atherosclerosis in other vascular territories. The physical exam should include evaluation for a renal abdominal bruit. Epigastric renal bruits that are high-pitched with a diastolic component tend to be more hemodynamically significant.

Diagnostic Testing

Patients at high risk for RAS should undergo a non-invasive screening test to rule out this condition. Various screening tests are available to investigate for RAS (**Table 34.4**).

RAS is best diagnosed with an imaging modality (18). Both the main and the accessory renal arteries should be assessed to identify the hemodynamic significance of lesions, the site and severity of the stenosis, and associated pathology, including the presence of an abdominal aortic aneurysm (AAA) or renal or adrenal masses. Imaging modalities such as duplex ultrasound, magnetic resonance angiography (MRA) and computed tomographic angiography (CTA) are the most effective diagnostic screening methods (**Table 34.5**). The choice of imaging procedure will depend on patient characteristics, renal function, contrast allergy, and presence of prior stents or metallic objects (may be contraindications to MRA or CTA techniques). Renal artery duplex ultrasound is a very sensitive and specific diagnostic tool for diagnosing RAS. CTA and MRA are also very sensitive and specific. CTA may cause contrast-induced nephropathy while gadolinium-enhanced MRA has been associated with nephrogenic systemic fibrosis.

The American College of Cardiology (ACC) and American Heart Association (AHA) have given various recommendations as to diagnostic modalities that can be used to identify RAS. Captopril renal artery scintigraphy is a relatively specific but insensitive test to demonstrate unilateral RAS; however, the incidence of false negatives is substantial. Measurement of plasma renin levels is discouraged because it is neither a specific nor a sensitive indicator of renovascular hypertension.

Renal Artery Angiography in the Cath Lab

Catheter-based renal angiography remains the gold standard for imaging renal arteries, although the non-invasive testing methods mentioned earlier have superseded it as a screening exam. Angiography is required to establish the diagnosis of RAS in the case of ambiguous non-invasive imaging. It is also indicated in individuals in whom concomitant peripheral angiography or coronary angiography is to be performed (and who have consented and have prespecified clinical indications).

Angiographic stenosis severity can be simply categorized as:

- mild (<50%),
- moderate/intermediate (50%–70%), and
- severe (>70%).

TABLE 34.4 Screening Tests for Renal Artery Stenosis

TEST	ADVANTAGE(S)	DISADVANTAGE(S)
Duplex ultrasound	High sensitivity	Difficult specificity in obese patients
	Operator/experience-dependent	
Magnetic resonance angiogram	Good sensitivity and specificity	Increased false positives
	Operator/experience-dependent	Not useful if stents are present
Computed tomographic angiography	Good sensitivity and specificity	Ionizing radiation
	Useful to visualize stents	Iodinated contrast
Captopril renal artery scintigraphy	Good specificity	Poor sensitivity (~10%–25% false negative)
Renal vein renin	Lateralizing renin predicts treatment response	Poor sensitivity/specificity Invasive
Renal catheter-based angiography	High sensitivity and specificity	Invasive

TABLE 34.5 ACC/AHA Recommendations for Diagnostic Methods (18)

Class I

1. Duplex ultrasonography is recommended as a screening test to establish the diagnosis of RAS (level of evidence: B).
2. CTA (in individuals with normal renal function) is recommended as a screening test to establish the diagnosis of RAS (level of evidence: B).
3. MRA is recommended as a screening test to establish the diagnosis of RAS (level of evidence: B).
4. When the clinical index of suspicion is high and the results of non-invasive tests are inconclusive, catheter angiography is recommended as a diagnostic test to establish the diagnosis of RAS (level of evidence: B)

Class III

1. Captopril renal scintigraphy is not recommended as a screening test to establish the diagnosis of RAS (level of evidence: C).
2. Selective renal vein renin measurements are not recommended as a useful screening test to establish the diagnosis of RAS (level of evidence: B).
3. Plasma renin activity is not recommended as a useful screening test to establish the diagnosis of RAS (level of evidence: B).
4. The captopril test (measurement of plasma renin activity after captopril administration) is not recommended as a useful screening test to establish the diagnosis of RAS (level of evidence: B).

CTA, computed tomographic angiography; MRA, magnetic resonance angiography; RAS, renal artery stenosis.

TABLE 34.6 Angiographic and Hemodynamic Significance of RAS (32)

<50% mild stenosis per angiography
50%–70% indeterminate stenosis per angiography
50%–70% severe/significant when resting mean pressure gradient >10 mm Hg
50%–70% severe when systolic hyperemic pressure gradient >20 mm Hg
50%–70% severe when renal P_d/P_a ≤0.80
>70% severe/significant

Nevertheless, such values may not imply the presence of hemodynamically significant stenosis. Angiographic stenoses that are classified as mild (<50%) are not considered hemodynamically significant. Angiographic lesions of >70% are considered to be severe lesions and hemodynamically significant. Moderate angiographic stenosis between 50% and 70% may or may not be hemodynamically significant, but data suggests that significant hemodynamic severity is present when there is a resting mean translesional pressure gradient of >10 mm Hg, a peak systolic translesional pressure gradient of >20 mm Hg (with hyperemia) or renal fractional flow reserve (rFFR) of 0.8 or less. Translesional gradients are measured with nonobstructive catheters such as a 4-French or one with a 0.014-in. pressure wire (P_d/P_a). Hyperemia for measuring FFR can be induced with an intrarenal bolus of papaverine of 30 mg or dopamine at 50 mcg/kg. Adenosine causes vasoconstriction in the renal artery and will not induce renal hyperemia.

Intravascular ultrasound (IVUS) may provide information regarding minimal luminal area and plaque volume. IVUS is also useful in documenting stent apposition. Nonetheless, use of IVUS has not demonstrated any improvement on patient outcomes after renal artery stenting.

Catheter-based angiography has a low rate of complications; nevertheless, care must be taken to reduce the risks of atheroembolization, contrast-related nephropathy, vascular complications/damage, bleeding, and contrast allergy. To avoid these complications, the following is recommended:

- Pre-hydrate with intravenous fluids (normal saline) prior to the administration of contrast.
- Use iso-osmolar, non-ionic contrast agents.
- Obtain as much information from non-invasive studies prior to performing the catheter-based study.

After vascular access is obtained, intravenous heparin or (other intravenous anticoagulation) is administered. Nonselective angiography using a pigtail or universal catheter is performed. Careful catheter manipulation is used to define the status of the aorta and exact locations of the renal ostia in order to facilitate selective cannulation. To reduce contrast volume, aortography can also be performed with diluted contrast and digital subtraction angiography. Alternative angiographic techniques include the use of carbon dioxide angiography or gadolinium as the contrast agent. It is important to make certain that there are no anomalous renal arteries, and that the arterial supply to all portions of the nephrogram is visualized.

Selective renal arteriography is used to evaluate the origin of the renal arteries. Selective renal arterial injections provide the most detail and are easily obtained after initially performing screening aortography. When performing aortography, it should be noted that the renal artery origin usually arises at the level of the first lumbar vertebrae (L1). L1 is found just below the T12 ribs. The anteroposterior (AP) or ipsilateral (up to 30°) angulations provide the best view of the renal artery ostia in most patients. Acutely angled takeoff of the renal artery may require specially shaped catheters, or an arm approach, to achieve vessel cannulation.

Although in the majority of cases retrograde femoral access is used (when the takeoff of the renal artery is horizontal, caudal, or mildly cephalad), in some cases the brachial or radial access is necessary (when the takeoff of the renal artery is downward angulated) to ensure a successful procedure. The choice of access is important, owing to the high rate of PAD in these patients. Downward angulations of the renal arteries may be more readily approached from the left arm. Access from the right arm is sometimes avoided to minimize complications arising from crossing the origin of the great vessels in the neck.

The choice of catheters for selective renal artery angiography is dependent on the anatomy of the renal artery. It is recommended that soft-tipped atraumatic catheters and guide wires be used for these procedures. Commonly used catheters include the internal mammary (IMA), JR4, cobra, renal double curve, hockey stick, multipurpose, or SOS Omni. When brachial access is used for a downward angulated renal artery, a 6F to 7F, 90-cm-long vascular sheath (Shuttle, Raabe, Balkan or Ansel sheath, Cook Inc, Bloomington, IN) is advanced over the guide wire and positioned in the suprarenal abdominal aorta. A 4-F to 6-F IMA catheter, multipurpose, or JR4 is then advanced through the long sheath and is used to engage the renal artery with a telescoping technique. Sometimes a catheter is held away from the aorta-renal ostium with a wire in the aorta (0.018–0.035-inch) while another (0.014–0.018-inch) wire is manipulated into the renal arterial bed using a "no-touch" technique. Using such "no-touch" or telescoping techniques will minimize trauma to the peri-renal aorta and help prevent disruption and embolus of lipid plaque into the distal renal arterial supply.

Treatment

The goals for medical therapy or revascularization of RAS are as follows:

1. Improve blood pressure control with concomitant reduction in the need for antihypertensive medications.
2. Preserve renal function or delay and prevent the need for renal replacement therapy.
3. Reduce the risk of future cardiovascular events and mortality.

Any intervention, whether medical, endovascular, or surgical, should aim to achieve the relevant clinical goals without significant morbidity or mortality from the intervention.

Angiotensin converting enzyme (ACE) inhibitors and calcium-channel blockers are effective in the treatment of hypertension in the presence of RAS. They effectively treat hypertension, and also reduce the progression of renal disease. Treatment with chlorothiazide, hydralazine, and β-blockers is also effective in controlling hypertension in individuals with RAS. In addition, angiotensin II receptor blockers have also shown evidence for controlling blood pressure in individuals with RAS. The use of both ACE inhibitor

TABLE 34.7 ACC/AHA Guidelines for Medical Treatment for RAS (18)

Class I
1. ACE inhibitors are effective medications for treatment of hypertension associated with unilateral RAS (level of evidence: A).
2. Angiotensin receptor blockers are effective medications for treatment of hypertension associated with unilateral RAS (level of evidence: B).
3. Calcium-channel blockers are effective medications for treatment of hypertension associated with unilateral RAS (level of evidence: A).
4. β-blockers are effective medications for treatment of hypertension associated with RAS (level of evidence: A).

ACE, angiotensin converting enzyme; RAS, renal artery stenosis.

and angiotensin receptor blocker (ARB) for the management of hypertension is safe, and is proven to reduce cardiovascular events and slow the progression of renal disease.

Indications for Revascularization

The AHA/ACC/SIR/SCAI/SVMB/SVS 2005 and 2011 guidelines (18) suggest that hemodynamically significant asymptomatic (incidental) renal artery stenosis is defined as RAS in the absence of end-organ dysfunction (e.g., idiopathic pulmonary edema, stroke, visual loss, hypertension, or refractory angina), but in the presence of the following:

1. Greater than or equal to 50% to 70% diameter stenosis by visual estimation with a peak translesional gradient (measured with a ≤5F catheter or pressure wire) of ≥20 mm Hg or a mean gradient ≥10 mm Hg;
2. Any stenosis ≥70% diameter stenosis, or
3. Greater than or equal to 70% diameter stenosis by IVUS measurement.

Initial interventional treatment for RAS involved percutaneous transluminal renal angioplasty (PTRA). The Dutch RAS Intervention Cooperative (DRASTIC) study, in which patients were randomly assigned to treatment by PTRA or medical therapy, demonstrated that patients in the PTRA group were less likely to have deterioration of their blood pressure control or exhibit renal artery occlusion during 12 months of follow-up (20). With use of stent technology and the current use of thienopyridine antiplatelet agents, PTRA with

TABLE 34.8 Indications for Revascularization for Hemodynamically Significant RAS (18)

1. Asymptomatic stenosis where percutaneous revascularization may be considered for treatment of bilateral or solitary viable kidney with a hemodynamically significant RAS.
2. Hypertension in patients with hemodynamically significant RAS and accelerated hypertension, resistant hypertension, malignant hypertension, hypertension with an unexplained unilateral small kidney, and hypertension with intolerance to medication.
3. Preservation of renal function in progressive chronic kidney disease with significant bilateral RAS or a RAS to a solitary functioning kidney.
4. Treatment-significant RAS in patients with unexplained congestive heart failure or sudden, unexplained pulmonary edema, or unstable angina.

RAS, renal artery stenosis.

stent deployment has become the gold standard for endovascular RAS intervention. Additionally, renal artery stenting overcomes the major complication of PTRA, which is elastic recoil. This recoil can lead to a restenosis rate in vessels of 25% or more.

A number of clinical presentations are indications to consider renal artery intervention. These include individuals with hypertension who cannot tolerate medications, or have a unilateral small kidney, or have resistant (more than three antihypertensive medications at maximum dose) or accelerated hypertension with a significant stenosis. In all of these clinical scenarios, consideration should be given to intervention. Similarly, intervention can be considered in individuals with a unilateral kidney and chronic renal failure, or a bilateral or solitary kidney with significant disease and progressive renal failure. In addition, in individuals with unexplained pulmonary edema or heart failure with known significant renal stenosis, intervention could be performed to prevent these cardiac destabilization syndromes. In patients with no clinical symptoms, revascularization may be considered for a hemodynamically significant lesion in a solitary kidney or bilateral significant disease.

Individuals with RAS may also experience "flash" pulmonary edema or may manifest a volume-overload state because they lack normal renal function to respond to pressure natriuresis. Unilateral RAS may play some role in the development of unstable coronary syndromes. It is believed that this may be from increases in myocardial oxygen demand in patients with coronary disease secondary to peripheral vasoconstriction.

Percutaneous Renal Artery Stenting

Percutaneous transluminal renal balloon angioplasty is the treatment of choice for symptomatic RAS caused by FMD (12–14). Nevertheless, atherosclerotic aorto-ostial renal artery stenotic lesions are generally not suitable for treatment by balloon angioplasty alone, owing to a higher restenosis rate. Renal artery stent placement has been shown to be superior to balloon angioplasty in the treatment of renal artery atherosclerotic lesions. It has also been shown that larger-diameter renal arteries (and therefore stents) have lower restenosis rates than smaller-diameter vessels.

The potential benefits of renal stent placement also include reperfusion of the ischemic kidneys. Randomized controlled trials have demonstrated the superiority of renal stents over balloon angioplasty in hypertensive patients with atherosclerotic RAS for procedure success, late patency, and cost-effectiveness (18,21,22).

Patients with a rapid deterioration in renal function derive greater benefit in renal function with stenting than those with stable chronic renal impairment. The lack of any potential benefit in certain patients (and possible deterioration) of renal function may be secondary to hyperperfusion injury, contrast nephropathy, progression of nephrosclerosis, and distal embolization of atherosclerotic material. This potential for embolization of atherothrombotic debris during renal stenting has raised concern that procedure-related renal damage could offset any benefits from improved renal artery blood flow.

Embolic protection devices (EPDs) used during saphenous vein graft angioplasty have been reported to reduce procedural complications and subsequently lead to reduced cardiac events. The use of distal EPDs in renal artery interventions has been advocated as a means of potentially preserving renal function (23,24). Limited data suggest the use of EPDs to prevent embolization of atheromatous material may be improving renal function.

Other data combining EDP with abciximab was noted to cause small significant changes in glomerular filtration rate, but no overall improvement in renal function over that existing at baseline prior to renal artery stenting (25). The evidence supporting the use of EPDs and glycoprotein IIb/IIIa inhibitors has thus far remained unconvincing. The CORAL trial first mandated the use of EPDs for all randomized to stent treatment; however, soon after trial initiation, this requirement was removed. It was felt that only selective use of EPDs was deemed to be appropriate in patients who were at increased risk for renal dysfunction from potential atheromatous embolization.

Technique for RA Revascularization

After vascular access is obtained, nonselective angiography using a pigtail or universal catheter (eg, Omni Flush catheter) is performed. The choice of catheters for selective renal artery angiography is dependent on the anatomy of the renal artery. It is recommended that soft-tipped atraumatic catheters and guide wires be used for these procedures. Commonly used catheters include the IMA, JR4, cobra, renal double curve, hockey stick, multipurpose, or SOS Omni.

When the brachial access is used for a downward angulated renal artery, a 6-F to 7-F, 90-cm-long vascular sheath (Shuttle, Raabe, Balkan or Ansel sheath, Cook Inc., Bloomington, IN) is advanced over the guide wire and positioned in the suprarenal abdominal aorta. A 5-F to 6-F IMA, JR4, or multipurpose catheter is then advanced through the long sheath and is used to engage the renal artery. A 0.014-inch or 0.018-inch wire is then advanced into the renal artery. Alternatively, a soft-tip exchanged-length 0.035-inch steerable guide wire (Wholey wire, Mallinckrodt, St. Louis, MO) is advanced into the renal artery. Keeping the diagnostic catheter engaged in the renal artery and the guide wire in a distal branch of the renal artery, the sheath is advanced over the multipurpose catheter and positioned in contact with the ostium of the renal artery. The diagnostic catheter is then removed, leaving the guide wire in the renal artery, and the sheath in contact with the ostium of the renal artery.

When retrograde Common Femoral Artery (CFA) access is chosen, a short 7-F or 8-F sheath is inserted into the CFA. Otherwise, a 6-F to 7-F, 55-cm sheath (Ansel, Rabbe or Shuttle) can be used. Next, a 5-F to 6-F diagnostic catheter (IMA, cobra, or Judkins right configuration) is advanced to engage the ostium of the renal artery. It is recommended that these diagnostic catheters be inserted through a 7-F to 8-F guiding catheter or 55-cm sheath prior to vessel engagement. This will enable easy exchange and manipulation of the catheters once the wires are in place. Then, a 0.014-inch or 0.018-inch wire or a soft-tip exchange-length 0.035-inch soft-tipped Wholey guide wire is used to cross the lesion, and is positioned in a renal artery branch. The guiding catheter or 55-cm sheath is then positioned in contact with the renal artery ostium. In this way, the diagnostic catheter can then be removed without losing access to the renal vessel.

It is recommended to avoid the use of a Glidewire, because this may cause inadvertent vessel perforation and/or dissection. The use of 5-F or 6-F diagnostic catheters is recommended to locate the ostium of the renal arteries to avoid trauma and potential cholesterol embolization from scraping the aorta, which may occur with larger angioplasty guiding catheters. Using the "no-touch" technique also prevents cholesterol embolization. Using this technique, a 0.035-inch J-tipped guide wire is manipulated to hold the distal tip of the guide catheter away from the wall of the aorta, and a 0.014-inch coronary wire was advanced across the lesion into the distal renal artery. In this way, we minimize the unnecessary scraping of the luminal atherosclerotic aortic plaque from guiding catheter manipulations during cannulation of the renal artery ostium.

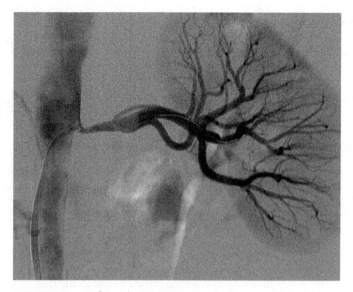

FIGURE 34.1 Left renal artery stenosis.

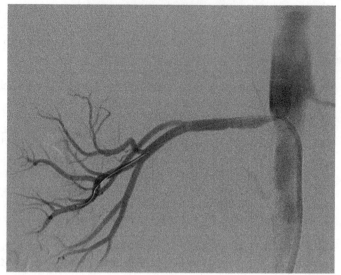

FIGURE 34.3 Right renal artery stenosis.

After the reference vessel diameter (RVD) is measured with quantitative angiography, a peripheral angioplasty balloon (4–8 mm in diameter) is advanced over the guide wire and positioned at the lesion. The lesion is then dilated with a balloon sized 1:1 with the RVD, using the lowest pressure that will fully expand the balloon. Before removal, the balloon is reinflated at a low pressure (1–2 atm) and, while the balloon is deflating, the catheter is advanced across the lesion over the balloon. This maneuver enables the stent to be positioned at the lesion site (within the sheath) without risking its edges catching on the plaque and reducing the risk of stent embolization. The use of distal vessel protection devices during balloon angioplasty and stenting can reduce and prevent the chance of distal vessel atheroembolism in selected patients.

Balloon-expandable stents are used to scaffold the lesion and maximize the angiographic result. The stent is advanced over the guide wire to the lesion site. With contrast injections through the sheath or the guiding catheter, the stent is positioned at the lesion site. When treating ostial lesions, it is important to allow ~1 mm

of the stent to protrude into the aorta to ensure complete coverage of the ostium of the artery. The stent is deployed at 6 to 8 atm, and then the balloon is withdrawn into the sheath or the guiding catheter. Angiography is then performed and, if inadequate expansion of the stent is observed, the operator should repeat dilation of the stent at a higher inflation pressure or with a larger balloon. The goal is to safely reduce the RAS to 30% (or less) angiographic stenosis and abolish the translesional pressure gradient to zero. During angioplasty and stenting, patients will experience discomfort. This may signify stretching of the adventitia and possible vascular rupture. When pain occurs, the balloon should be immediately deflated (**Figs. 34.1–34.4**).

The Szabo technique is another safe and reproducible technique to exactly deploy stents at the aortorenal artery junction (26). This technique was initially used in coronary artery ostial lesions and can also be used in guiding and deploying renal stents into position at the aortorenal junction. Here, for the exact deployment, two 0.014-inch wires (with the second wire inserted through the last cell of a stent) are used for stent deployment. This stent tail wire or anchor

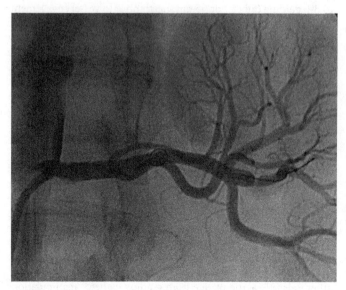

FIGURE 34.2 Angiogram of left renal artery after stenting.

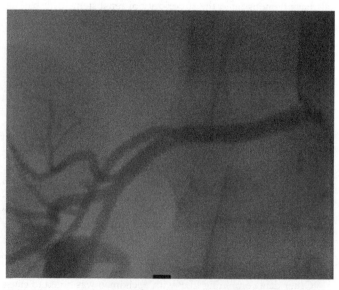

FIGURE 34.4 Angiogram of right renal artery after stenting.

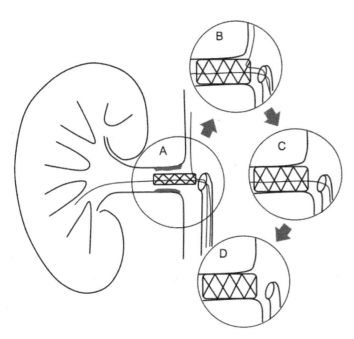

FIGURE 34.5 Szabo technique applied to exact stent deployment in renal artery stenosis. The stent is guided to the lesion with the aid of two wires **(A)**. The aortic wire properly engages the stent at the ostial renal–aorta junction and the stent is partial deployed **(B)**. The aortic wire is then removed and the stent is fully deployed **(C)**. Finally, the guide (renal) wire is removed and the stent remains in the optimal position **(D)**.

technique facilitates precise aorto-ostial stent deployment in cases of atherosclerotic RAS. It also helps to eliminate errors of improper stent positioning at this aortorenal junction, and may possibly minimize patient exposure to ionizing radiation and contrast dye (**Fig. 34.5**).

Surgery for arteriosclerotic renovascular disease must first consider the status of the aorta. When surgery was compared with balloon angioplasty for renal artery revascularization in a randomized clinical trial in hypertensive patients with atherosclerotic RAS, the surgery group had a higher primary patency rate than the balloon angioplasty group. Nevertheless, there was no difference in the secondary patency rate between the groups. The clinical endpoints

TABLE 34.9 ACC/AHA Guidelines for Surgical Correction for RAS (18)

Class I

1. Vascular surgical reconstruction is indicated for patients with fibromuscular dysplastic RAS with clinical indications for interventions (same as for percutaneous transluminal angioplasty), especially those exhibiting complex disease that extends into the segmental arteries and those having macroaneurysms (level of evidence: B).
2. Vascular surgical reconstruction is indicated for patients with atherosclerotic RAS and clinical indications for intervention, especially those with multiple small renal arteries or early primary branching of the main renal artery (level of evidence: B).
3. Vascular surgical reconstruction is indicated for patients with atherosclerotic RAS in combination with pararenal aortic reconstructions (in treatment of aortic aneurysms or severe aortoiliac occlusive disease) (level of evidence: C).

RAS, renal artery stenosis.

of hypertension control and renal function preservation were not different for angioplasty and surgery. Major complications occur more in surgical patients than balloon angioplasty patients. It is therefore suggested that in patients with RAS who are candidates for either surgery or balloon angioplasty, balloon angioplasty should be the first choice of therapy.

Identification of Patients Who May Benefit from Revascularization

B-type natriuretic peptide (BNP) has been studied as a predictor of clinical benefit following renal artery intervention. Unfortunately, the current data supporting BNP as a possible predictor have been conflicting. Results from the HERCULES trial in 2011 demonstrated significant reductions in systolic blood pressure following stenting. Nevertheless, in patients with elevated BNP levels, pre-treatment did not predict a reduction in blood pressure in follow-up (27).

When trying to assess renal artery diameter stenosis angiographically, measurement of translesional pressure gradients can be performed (28). This involves advancing a 4-F or 5-F catheter through a larger caliber guiding catheter distal to the stenosis and measuring distal pressure versus guiding catheter pressure. Using this method, a peak gradient of 20 mm Hg and a mean gradient of 10 mm Hg or cut-off values has been used to diagnose significant RAS. This technique, however, can result in error, as an end-hole 4-F or 5-F catheter is often occlusive and may thereby artificially raise the gradient.

Other trials have looked at the ability of a pressure guide wire to more accurately measure translesional peak systolic gradients than a simple catheter. Use of a 0.014-inch pressure wire to measure translesional pressures, however, has not demonstrated any correlation to the percent diameter stenosis within atherosclerotic renal arteries.

The use of hyperemic translesional pressure gradient assessment via use of intra-arterial papaverine to induce renal hyperemia has been shown to identify patients who will develop an improvement in hypertension following revascularization. The lack of a hyperemic response in the kidney may identify patients with intrinsic microvascular disease who will not respond to revascularization. Another trial suggested that a dopamine-induced mean gradient >20 mm Hg was the optimal cut-off point to predict a favorable response of hypertension after renal artery stenting.

Trials investigating resting renal fractional flow reserve (rFFR), which is the ratio of distal renal pressure to aortic pressure, have suggested that a resting rFFR <0.9 produced significant elevation in bilateral renal vein renin levels. This suggested that lesions which demonstrated an rFFR <0.9 may provide reasonable predictive accuracy for blood pressure improvement in patients who have revascularization of their RAS. As mentioned previously, another study suggested an FFR value of <0.8 under hyperemic conditions improved blood pressure control patients (28). Additionally, significant RAS and subsequent hemodynamic severity is present when there is a resting mean translesional pressure gradient of >10 mm Hg, a peak systolic translesional pressure gradient of >20 mm Hg (with hyperemia) or a renal fractional flow reserve (rFFR) of 0.8 or less. Translesional gradients are measured with non-obstructive catheters, such as a 4-French, or with a 0.014-inch pressure wire (P_d/P_a). Hyperemia for measuring FFR can be induced with an intrarenal bolus of papaverine of 30 mg or dopamine at 50 mcg/kg.

Clinical Conclusion

Current randomized controlled trials of atherosclerotic renal artery disease comparing renal angioplasty and stenting with the best medical therapy have been very conclusive about renal artery stenting. Results from the Cardiovascular Outcomes in Renal Atherosclerotic Lesions (CORAL) trial (29), confirmed that effective medical therapy should be the first line of treatment in patients with presumed renovascular hypertension. For patients who fail medical therapy or are unable to tolerate medical therapy, stenting remains a reasonable option. CORAL also showed that the benefit of medical therapy alone lessened over time. At 3 to 5 years post-enrollment, event-free survival declined in this patient group. This was seen in the treatment of patients with hemodynamically severe lesions and those who failed medical therapy. Continued study of renal stenting is needed to ensure patients have alternatives when medical therapy in not a viable option.

Currently, aggressive risk factor modification, medical therapy, and blood pressure control remain the mainstay of therapy. Renal artery stenting has been shown to improve functional class in patients with unstable angina and congestive heart failure. This probably occurs through a mechanism of improved blood pressure control and by favorably affecting the renin–angiotensin system. One of the most important indications for revascularization of the renal arteries is to improve blood pressure control. The ability to perform physiologic lesion assessment using translesional hyperemic pressure gradient measurement and renal "fractional flow reserve" (FFR) calculation may aid in identifying patients who will benefit from revascularization. Renal artery stenting is superior to balloon angioplasty; nevertheless, balloon angioplasty remains the treatment of choice for FMD.

The Angioplasty and STenting for Renal Artery Lesions (ASTRAL) trial has suggested that revascularization for RAS produces no benefit over medical therapy (30). Unfortunately, the main limitation of this study was that it excluded people who may have benefitted from revascularization. This included patients with flash pulmonary edema or acute renal injury (or rapidly progressing disease) that was thought to be caused by RAS. Whether such patients benefit from revascularization is still unknown. Therefore, further prospective randomized studies are still needed to investigate the role of endovascular therapy in such patients.

Key Points (31)

- ◼ ACC/AHA Class I Diagnostic Methods for RAS.
  - Duplex ultrasonography is recommended as a screening test to establish the diagnosis of RAS (level of evidence: B).
  - CTA (in individuals with normal renal function) is recommended as a screening test to establish the diagnosis of RAS (level of evidence: B).
  - MRA is recommended as a screening test to establish the diagnosis of RAS (level of evidence: B).
  - When the clinical index of suspicion is high and the results of non-invasive tests are inconclusive, catheter angiography is recommended as a diagnostic test to establish the diagnosis of RAS (level of evidence: B).

- ◼ ACC/AHA Class III Diagnostic Methods for RAS (not recommended)
  - Captopril renal scintigraphy is not recommended as a screening test to establish the diagnosis of RAS (level of evidence: C).

- Selective renal vein renin measurements are not recommended as a useful screening test to establish the diagnosis of RAS (level of evidence: B).
- Plasma renin activity is not recommended as a useful screening test to establish the diagnosis of RAS (level of evidence: B).
- The captopril test (measurement of plasma renin activity after captopril administration) is not recommended as a useful screening test to establish the diagnosis of RAS (level of evidence: B).

◼ ACC/AHA Indications for Revascularization.

Asymptomatic Stenosis

Class IIb

1. Percutaneous revascularization may be considered for treatment of an asymptomatic bilateral or solitary viable kidney with a hemodynamically significant RAS (level of evidence: C).
2. The usefulness of percutaneous revascularization of an asymptomatic unilateral hemodynamically significant RAS in a viable kidney is not well established and is presently clinically unproven (level of evidence: C).

Hypertension

Class IIa

1. Percutaneous revascularization is reasonable for patients with hemodynamically significant RAS and accelerated hypertension, resistant hypertension, malignant hypertension, hypertension with an unexplained unilateral small kidney, and hypertension with intolerance to medication (level of evidence: B).

Preservation of Renal Function

Class IIa

1. Percutaneous revascularization is reasonable for patients with RAS and progressive chronic kidney disease with bilateral RAS or a RAS to a solitary functioning kidney (level of evidence: B).

Class IIb

1. Percutaneous revascularization may be considered for patients with RAS and chronic renal insufficiency with unilateral RAS (level of evidence: C).

Impact of RAS on Congestive Heart Failure and Unstable Angina

Class IIa

1. Percutaneous revascularization is reasonable for patients with hemodynamically significant RAS and unstable angina (level of evidence: B).

◼ ACC/AHA Recommendations: Revascularization for RAS (stenting and PTRA)

Class I

1. Renal stent placement is indicated for ostial atherosclerotic RAS lesions that meet the clinical criteria for intervention (level of evidence: B).
2. Balloon angioplasty with bailout stent placement if necessary is recommended for FMD lesions (level of evidence: B).

References

1. Hansen KJ, et al. Prevalence of renovascular disease in the elderly: a population-based study. *J Vasc Surg.* 2002;36:443–451.
2. Harding MB, et al. Renal artery stenosis: prevalence and associated risk factors in patients undergoing routine cardiac catheterization. *J Am Soc Nephrol.* 1992;2:1608–1616.
3. Weber-Mzell D, et al. Coronary anatomy predicts presence or absence of renal artery stenosis: a prospective study in patients undergoing cardiac catheterization for suspected coronary artery disease. *Eur Heart J.* 2002;23:1684–1691.
4. Jean WJ, et al. High incidence of renal artery stenosis in patients with coronary artery disease. *Cathet Cardiovasc Diagn.* 1994;32:8–10.
5. Missouris CG, et al. Renal artery stenosis: a common and important problem in patients with peripheral vascular disease. *Am J Med.* 1994;96:10–14.
6. Olin JW, et al. Prevalence of atherosclerotic renal artery stenosis in patients with atherosclerosis elsewhere. *Am J Med.* 1990;88(1N):46N–51N.
7. Rossi GP, et al. Excess prevalence of extracranial carotid artery lesions in renovascular hypertension. *Am J Hypertens.* 1992;5:8–15.
8. Metcalfe W, Reid AW, Geddes CC. Prevalence of angiographic atherosclerotic renal artery disease and its relationship to the anatomical extent of peripheral vascular atherosclerosis. *Nephrol Dial Transplant.* 1999;14:105–108.
9. Missouris CG, et al. High prevalence of carotid artery disease in patients with atheromatous renal artery stenosis. *Nephrol Dial Transplant.* 1998;13:945–948.
10. Rimmer JM, Gennari FJ. Atherosclerotic renovascular disease and progressive renal failure. *Ann Intern Med.* 1993;118:712–719.
11. Safian RD, Textor SC. Renal artery stenosis. *N Engl J Med.* 2001;344:431–442.
12. Stanley JC, Wakefield TW. Arterial fibrodysplasia. In: Rutherford RB, ed. *Vascular Surgery.* 6th ed. Philadelphia, PA: Saunders; 2004:387–408.
13. Messina LM, Stanley JC. Renal artery fibrodysplasia and renovascular hypertension. In: Rutherford RB, ed. *Vascular Surgery.* 6th ed. Philadelphia, PA: Saunders; 2004:1650–1664.
14. Mounier-Vehier C, et al. Renal atrophy outcome after revascularization in fibromuscular dysplasia disease. *J Endovasc Ther.* 2002;9:605–613.
15. Zierler RE, et al. A prospective study of disease progression in patients with atherosclerotic renal artery stenosis. *Am J Hypertens.* 1996;9:1055–1061.
16. Eggers PW, Connerton R, McMullan M. The Medicare experience with end-stage renal disease: trends in incidence, prevalence, and survival. *Health Care Financ Rev.*1984;5:69–88.
17. Wright JR, et al. A prospective study of the determinants of renal functional outcome and mortality in atherosclerotic renovascular disease. *Am J Kidney Dis.* 2002;39:1153–1161.
18. Hirsch AT, et al. ACC/AHA 2005 guidelines for the management of patients with peripheral arterial disease: executive summary. A collaborative report from the American Association for Vascular Surgery/Society for Vascular Surgery, Society for Cardiovascular Angiography and Interventions, Society for Vascular Medicine and Biology, Society for Interventional Radiology, and the ACC/AHA taskforce on practice guidelines. *J Am Coll Cardiol.* 2006;47(6):1239–1312.
19. Gifford RW Jr, McCormack LJ, Poutasse EF. The atrophic kidney: its role in hypertension. *Mayo Clin Proc.* 1965;40:834–852.
20. van Jaarsveld BC, et al. The effect of balloon angioplasty on hypertension in atherosclerotic renal-artery stenosis. Dutch Renal Artery Stenosis Intervention Cooperative Study Group. *N Engl J Med.* 2000;342:1007–1014.
21. van de Ven PJ, et al. Arterial stenting and balloon angioplasty in ostial atherosclerotic renovascular disease: a randomised trial. *Lancet.* 1999;353:282–286.
22. Dorros G, Prince C, Mathiak L. Stenting of a renal artery stenosis achieves better relief of the obstructive lesion than balloon angioplasty. *Cathet Cardiovasc Diagn.* 1993;29:191–198.
23. Henry M, et al. Protected renal stenting with the PercuSurge GuardWire device: a pilot study. *J Endovasc Ther.* 2001;8(3):227–237.
24. Holden A, Hill A. Renal angioplasty and stenting with distal protection of the main renal artery in ischemic nephropathy: early experience. *J Vasc Surg.* 2003;38(5):962–968.
25. Cooper CJ, et al. Embolic protection and platelet inhibition during renal artery stenting. *Circulation.* 2003;117(21):2752–2760.
26. Salazar M, Kern MJ, Patel PM. Exact deployment of stents in ostial renal artery stenosis using the stent tail wire or Szabo technique. *Catheter Cardiovasc Interv.* 2009;74(6):946–950.
27. Jaff MR, et al. Significant reduction in systolic blood pressure following renal artery stenting in patients with uncontrolled hypertension: results of the HERCULES trial. *Catheter Cardiovasc Interv.* 2012;80(3):343–350.
28. Leesar MA, et al. Prediction of hypertension improvement after stenting of renal artery stenosis: comparative accuracy of translesional pressure gradients, intravascular ultrasound, and angiography. *J Am Coll Cardiol.* 2009;53(250):2263–2271.
29. Cooper CJ, et al. Stenting and medical therapy for atherosclerotid renal artery disease. *N Engl J Med.* 2014;370(1):13–22. doi:10.1056/NEJMoa1210753.
30. The ASTRAL Investigators. Revascularization versus medical therapy for renal artery stenosis. *N Engl J Med.* 2009;361:1953–1962.
31. Anderson JL, et al. Management of patients with peripheral artery disease (compilation of 2005 and 2011 ACCF/AHA guideline recommendations): a report of the American College of Cardiology Foundation/American Heart Association Task Force on Practice Guidelines. *Circulation.* 2013;127:1425–1443.
32. Parikh SA, et al. SCAI expert consensus statement for renal artery stenting appropriate use. *Cathet Cardiovasc Intervent.* 2014;84:1163–1171.

35

Deep Venous Thrombosis

Jayendrakumar S. Patel, MD and Mehdi H. Shishehbor,

DO, MPH, PhD, FSCAI

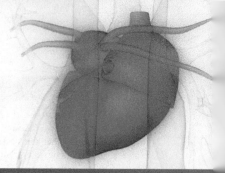

Epidemiology and Diagnosis

With approximately 900,000 new cases diagnosed annually, venous thromboembolism (VTE) represents a source of significant morbidity and mortality and is the third leading cause of cardiovascular death (1–4). Although most cases are preventable with appropriate pharmacologic and nonpharmacologic prophylaxis, the incidence of VTE appears to be on the rise and is estimated to be 1 to 3 cases per 1,000 person-years (2,5). Sequelae are common, expensive, and burdensome in terms of reduced quality of life (6–8). For example, 20% to 50% of patients with proximal deep venous thrombosis (DVT) may go on to develop some degree of post-thrombotic syndrome (PTS) due to valve damage and persistent outflow obstruction despite appropriate anticoagulation (9,10). Some risk factors for the development of PTS include extensive clot burden, severe symptoms, sub-therapeutic anticoagulation, recurrent ipsilateral DVT, obesity, and advanced age (9,11,12). Interestingly, the total duration of anticoagulation, inherited or acquired thrombophilia, sex, or the circumstances of DVT (provoked, malignancy, unprovoked) do not seem to influence the risk of developing PTS. Massive pulmonary embolism (PE), secondary to DVT, causes nearly 300,000 deaths annually in the United States (13). In addition, 1% to 5% of those who experience

an acute PE may develop chronic thromboembolic pulmonary hypertension (CTEPH), which can lead to considerable disability and right heart failure. For all of these reasons, prevention and early diagnosis with appropriate management are key.

Diagnosis of acute VTE can be challenging because not all proximal DVTs are clinically apparent. Physical examination can be helpful, but is neither sensitive nor specific (14). Clinical suspicion should therefore be high. Risk factors for the development of VTE are presented in **Table 35.1** and can be categorized into acquired (some of which may be transient) and genetic factors (5,15). The diagnostic workup of patients with suspected DVT depends upon the estimated pretest probability (**Fig. 35.1**) (16–18). Importantly, the D-dimer test is highly sensitive but cannot rule out VTE in those with high pretest probability. Those patients should proceed to imaging without D-dimer testing (i.e., whole leg compression duplex ultrasonography for suspected DVT, and computed tomography angiography or ventilation–perfusion scan for suspected PE) (17).

It is important to assess the severity of illness, identify important co-morbid conditions (e.g., pregnancy, cancer), and recognize contraindications to anticoagulation at the time of diagnosis, because this will often alter management. For patients with DVT, signs of blanching, cyanosis, edema, compartment syndrome, or even venous gangrene are suggestive of phlegmasia cerulea dolens, which is associated with significantly higher morbidity and mortality (19–21). Furthermore, all proximal DVTs are not equal. Those with iliofemoral DVT have low rates of recanalization and higher rates of recurrent thrombosis (22). For those with PE, risk stratification should be performed using a validated prognostic model such as the PE severity index (PESI) (**Table 35.2**) (23–26).

TABLE 35.1 Risk Factors for the Development of VTE

Acquired
- Acute medical illness
- Inflammatory bowel disease
- Nephrotic syndrome
- Age >60 years
- Previous VTE
- Cancer or chemotherapy
- Surgery
- Trauma
- Immobility
- Pregnancy
- Estrogen therapy
- Obesity
- Antiphospholipid antibody syndrome
- May–Thurner syndrome

Genetic
- Antithrombin deficiency
- Protein C deficiency
- Protein S deficiency
- Hyperhomocysteinemia
- Prothrombin gene mutation
- Factor V Leiden mutation
- Elevated Factor VIII levels

VTE, venous thromboembolism.

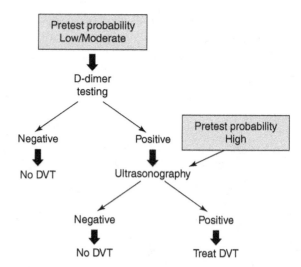

FIGURE 35.1 Diagnostic algorithm for suspected deep venous thrombosis (DVT).

TABLE 35.2 Simplified Pulmonary Embolism Severity Index Score

PREDICTOR	POINTS
Age >80 years	1
History of cancer	1
COPD	1
Pulse ≥100 bpm	1
SBP <100 mm Hg	1
SaO$_2$ <90%	1
Score ≥1 = high risk	

COPD, chronic obstructive pulmonary disease; SBP, systolic blood pressure.

Medical Management

Prompt initiation of therapeutic anticoagulation remains the cornerstone of treatment for patients with suspected and confirmed VTE. Treatment should not be delayed for imaging results, especially if the pretest probability is high. Anticoagulation prevents thrombus propagation, recurrence, and the development of new thrombi, but does not dissolve thrombi that already exist. Current available direct-acting oral anticoagulant (DOAC) options are shown in Table 35.3, and recent guidelines give a weak recommendation for their use as first-line treatment for patients without cancer (27). For those with cancer, low-molecular-weight heparin (LMWH) is the preferred agent (27). DOACs and LMWH offer fairly predictable pharmacomechanics when compared with unfractionated heparin, with a rapid onset of action and short time to achieving therapeutic anticoagulation. Rivaroxaban and apixaban can be given as monotherapy without parenteral anticoagulation. Dabigatran and edoxaban were studied in patients who initially received 5 to 10 days of parenteral anticoagulation. Routine use of compression stockings during the acute phase to prevent PTS is not recommended based on the negative randomized controlled SOX (Compression Stockings to Prevent the Post-Thrombotic Syndrome) trial (27,28).

A minimum of 3 months of therapeutic anticoagulation should be administered to all patients with acute VTE regardless of whether reversible or transient risk factors are identified (27). Anticoagulation may be discontinued in patients with transient risk factors, but should be continued indefinitely in unprovoked cases or in patients with cancer. If anticoagulation needs to be discontinued for patients with unprovoked cases due to intolerance, then aspirin should be prescribed indefinitely (29,30).

Catheter-Directed Management of Acute DVT

As discussed previously, the purpose of conventional therapy with anticoagulation for DVT is to prevent propagation of the clot and the development of new clots and to reduce the risk for PE. Anticoagulation does not resolve the existing clot, reduce the risk of developing venous valvular damage, prevent venous hypertension, or rapidly resolve symptoms, thus it leaves patients with proximal iliofemoral DVT with large thrombus burden vulnerable to the development of venous stasis ulcers, PTS, and perhaps even PE. In such patients, early catheter-directed therapy may prevent PTS and provide faster symptom relief compared with anticoagulation alone (31–38). In the National Venous Thrombolysis Registry, 66% of patients had acute DVT, and 19% had acute on chronic DVT, most (75%) of which involved the iliofemoral system (35). This study reported a success rate of 65% with a 1-year patency rate of 96% in those who had initial procedural success (35,39). Importantly, incomplete clot lysis was associated with venous valvular incompetence, whereas optimal clot lysis was associated with improved valvular function. The rate of bleeding associated with catheter-directed thrombolysis appears to be low (<10%) and most bleeding is related to the access site with intracranial events limited to <1% (34,35,40). More definitive evidence will come from the multicenter randomized ATTRACT (Acute Venous Thrombosis: Thrombus Removal with Adjunctive Catheter-Directed Thrombolysis) trial, which aims to determine whether pharmacomechanical catheter-directed thrombolysis (PMCT) prevents PTS (41).

While routine use of catheter-directed treatment is not encouraged by current guidelines, young patients with acute symptomatic phlegmasia cerulea dolens (especially with a threatened limb), large thrombus burden within the inferior vena cava, or symptomatic massive iliofemoral and femoral vein thrombosis should be considered for catheter-based treatment as an adjunct to oral anticoagulation, because these are the patients at highest risk for PTS (10,27). Until further data is available from randomized trials, isolated femoropopliteal DVT should most likely be treated with medical therapy alone; however, this decision should be personalized. In all cases, the risk of bleeding must be relatively low, and the thrombus must be fairly acute (within 2–4 weeks) in order to have the highest chance

TABLE 35.3 Direct-Acting Oral Anticoagulant Options

	DABIGATRAN	RIVAROXABAN	APIXABAN	EDOXABAN
Target	Thrombin (IIa)	Xa	Xa	Xa
Time to peak (hours)	1.5–3	2–3	3–4	1–2
Half-life (hours)	14–17	5–9	8–15	10–14
Renal excretion %	>80	66	25	50
Antidote	Idarucizumab	None	None	None
Dosing	Oral, once or twice daily	Oral, once or twice daily	Oral, twice daily	Oral, once daily
FDA-labeled indications	• NVAF • VTE ppx THA • VTE tx	• NVAF • VTE ppx THA, TKA • VTE tx	• NVAF • VTE ppx THA, TKA • VTE tx	• NVAF • VTE tx

NVAF, non-valvular atrial fibrillation; THA, total hip arthroplasty; TKA, total knee arthroplasty; VTE, venous thromboembolism.

of clot dissolution (42). Additional contraindications include recent stroke, GI bleed, surgery, or trauma, and presence of malignancy or pregnancy.

Catheter-based therapies can be divided into three major categories: catheter-based lysis alone, mechanical thrombectomy without lysis, and pharmacomechanical thrombolysis plus/minus thrombectomy. Nevertheless, frequently a combination of the preceding types listed is needed. Options for catheter-based lysis include administration of a thrombolytic agent directly into the thrombus for 48 to 72 hours via an infusion catheter with multiple side-holes. Mechanically enhanced thrombolysis can be achieved by rheolytic thrombectomy. Pharmacomechanical thrombolysis can be achieved by pulse spray via AngioJet device

or by ultrasound-based methods such as EKOS. Any combination of these modalities can be employed, and our general approach is shown in **Figure 35.2**. The latter two strategies are preferred and referred to as PMCT and have been shown to reduce the total thrombolytic dose, the duration of exposure to thrombolytic drugs, cost, and hospital days, and may result in more effective clot dissolution (43–48).

For iliofemoral DVT, the ipsilateral popliteal vein is typically accessed ideally with a single puncture using ultrasound guidance. The thrombus is crossed with a 0.035-inch hydrophilic guide wire, and the thrombolytic delivery system is advanced over the wire into position. With the 5.2-French ultrasound-enhanced system (EkoSonic Endovascular System, **Fig. 35.3**), the thrombolytic

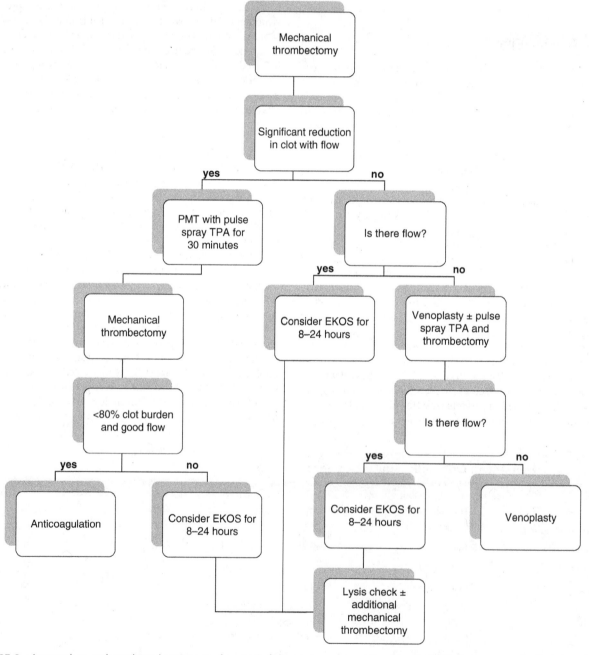

FIGURE 35.2 Approach to catheter-based treatment of acute iliofemoral deep venous thrombosis. PMT, pharmacomechanical thrombectomy; TPA, tissue plasminogen activator.

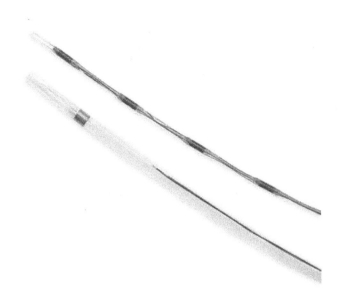

FIGURE 35.3 EkoSonic endovascular system.

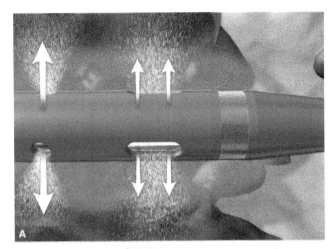

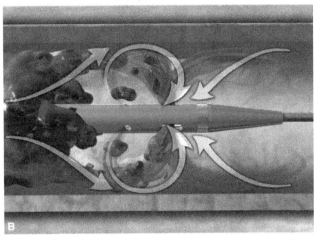

FIGURE 35.4 AngioJet rheolytic thrombectomy system. **A:** Top panel demonstrates power pulse feature where tPA is sprayed into the thrombus. **B:** Bottom panel demonstrates the mechanism of thrombus removal, where high-velocity flow creates a low-pressure zone within and surrounding the catheter tip. The thrombus is subsequently pulled into the catheter. tPA, tissue plasminogen activator.

agent is continuously infused into the catheter, and ultrasound waves accelerate thrombolysis by mechanically disturbing the fibrin matrix and exposing more binding sites for the agent to work. The ultrasound waves also serve to push the thrombolytic drug deeper into the clot. After 12 to 24 hours, repeat venography is performed to assess the clot burden and determine the need for further treatment with either additional thrombolytic infusion or percutaneous thrombectomy. Close monitoring in an intensive care unit for complications such as bleeding or PE is required. Partial thromboplastin time and fibrinogen levels are obtained every 4 to 6 hours. If the fibrinogen level drops to <100 mg/dL, the thrombolytic infusion is reduced or stopped. Intravenous fluids should be administered if possible, because hemolysis may result in renal insufficiency. The 8-French Trellis system (temporarily off the market) isolates the thrombus between two occluding balloons and utilizes a vibrating catheter to facilitate lytic penetration. With the AngioJet rheolytic thrombectomy system (Fig. 35.4), thrombolytic agent is sprayed directly into the thrombus and allowed to percolate for 15 to 30 minutes. During thrombectomy, high-pressure pulsatile saline jets macerate and fragment the thrombus. For large thrombus burden in the inferior vena cava, suction thrombectomy using the AngioVac veno-venous bypass system can be considered. A 22-French central venous cannula is used to suction the thrombus using a centrifugal pump. Blood and clot then pass through an external filtering system, and the filtered blood is then reinfused via a 17-French central venous cannula.

Residual stenosis due to a fibrotic organized thrombus or webs may be present after PMCT and is associated with recurrent thrombosis and PTS (49–51). Balloon angioplasty with or without stenting is commonly performed in such cases to relieve outflow obstruction and has been shown to reduce recurrent thrombosis, improve quality of life, and reduce PTS (52,53). Wallstents are typically used for inferior vena cava (IVC) stenosis, and they are usually safe to balloon across an IVC filter (54). Intravascular ultrasound can assist with accurate placement. For infra-inguinal stenoses, self-expanding stents are preferred, given their resistance to extrinsic compression. Postprocedural duplex ultrasonography is typically performed at 6 to 12 months intervals to assess for patency or restenosis.

Key Points

1. Risk factors for VTE can be categorized into acquired and genetic factors.
2. The diagnostic workup of suspected DVT depends upon the estimated pretest probability.
3. The D-dimer test is highly sensitive but cannot rule out VTE in those with high pretest probability. High-probability patients should proceed to imaging without D-dimer testing (i.e., whole leg compression duplex ultrasonography for suspected DVT, and computed tomography angiography or ventilation-perfusion scan for suspected PE).
4. A minimum of 3 months of therapeutic anticoagulation should be administered to all patients with acute VTE regardless of whether reversible or transient risk factors are identified.
5. PMCT has been shown to reduce the total thrombolytic dose, the duration of exposure to thrombolytic drugs, cost, and hospital days, and may result in more effective clot dissolution.

References

1. Heit JA. The epidemiology of venous thromboembolism in the community. *Arterioscler Thromb Vasc Biol.* 2008;28:370–372.
2. Huang W, et al. Secular trends in occurrence of acute venous thromboembolism: the Worcester VTE study (1985–2009). *Am J Med.* 2014;127:829.e5–839.e5.
3. Kahn SR, et al. Prevention of VTE in nonsurgical patients: antithrombotic therapy and prevention of thrombosis, 9th ed: American College of Chest Physicians Evidence-Based Clinical Practice Guidelines. *Chest.* 2012;141:e195S–e226S.
4. Lindblad B, Sternby NH, Bergqvist D. Incidence of venous thromboembolism verified by necropsy over 30 years. *BMJ.* 1991;302:709–711.
5. Dobromirski M, Cohen AT. How I manage venous thromboembolism risk in hospitalized medical patients. *Blood.* 2012;120:1562–1569.
6. Guanella R, et al. Economic burden and cost determinants of deep vein thrombosis during 2 years following diagnosis: a prospective evaluation. *J Thromb Haemost.* 2011;9:2397–2405.
7. Kahn SR, et al. Determinants of health-related quality of life during the 2 years following deep vein thrombosis. *J Thromb Haemost.* 2008;6:1105–1112.
8. Page RL 2nd, et al. Hidden costs associated with venous thromboembolism: impact of lost productivity on employers and employees. *J Occup Environ Med.* 2014;56:979–985.
9. van Dongen CJ, et al. Relation between quality of anticoagulant treatment and the development of the postthrombotic syndrome. *J Thromb Haemost.* 2005;3:939–942.
10. Kahn SR, et al. The postthrombotic syndrome: evidence-based prevention, diagnosis, and treatment strategies: a scientific statement from the American Heart Association. *Circulation.* 2014;130:1636–1661.
11. Ageno W, et al. Body mass index is associated with the development of the post-thrombotic syndrome. *Thromb Haemost.* 2003;89:305–309.
12. Chitsike RS, et al. Risk of post-thrombotic syndrome after subtherapeutic warfarin anticoagulation for a first unprovoked deep vein thrombosis: results from the REVERSE study. *J Thromb Haemost.* 2012;10:2039–2044.
13. Tapson VF. Acute pulmonary embolism. *N Engl J Med.* 2008;358:1037–1052.
14. Goodacre S, Sutton AJ, Sampson FC. Meta-analysis: the value of clinical assessment in the diagnosis of deep venous thrombosis. *Ann Intern Med.* 2005;143:129–139.
15. Bauer KA. The thrombophilias: well-defined risk factors with uncertain therapeutic implications. *Ann Intern Med.* 2001;135:367–373.
16. Wells PS, et al. Value of assessment of pretest probability of deep-vein thrombosis in clinical management. *Lancet.* 1997;350:1795–1798.
17. Bates SM, et al. Diagnosis of DVT: antithrombotic therapy and prevention of thrombosis, 9th ed: American College of Chest Physicians Evidence-Based Clinical Practice Guidelines. *Chest.* 2012;141:e351S–e418S.
18. Wells PS, et al. Derivation of a simple clinical model to categorize patients probability of pulmonary embolism: increasing the models utility with the SimpliRED D-dimer. *Thromb Haemost.* 2000;83:416–420.
19. Sarwar S, Narra S, Munir A. Phlegmasia cerulea dolens. *Tex Heart Inst J.* 2009;36:76–77.
20. Haimovici H. The ischemic forms of venous thrombosis. 1. Phlegmasia cerulea dolens. 2. Venous gangrene. *J Cardiovasc Surg (Torino).* 1965;5(suppl):164–173.
21. Jaff MR, et al. Management of massive and submassive pulmonary embolism, iliofemoral deep vein thrombosis, and chronic thromboembolic pulmonary hypertension: a scientific statement from the American Heart Association. *Circulation.* 2011;123:1788–1830.
22. Douketis JD, et al. Does the location of thrombosis determine the risk of disease recurrence in patients with proximal deep vein thrombosis? *Am J Med.* 2001;110:515–519.
23. Jimenez D, et al. Effectiveness of prognosticating pulmonary embolism using the ESC algorithm and the Bova score. *Thromb Haemost.* 2016;115:827–834.
24. Jimenez D, et al. Derivation and validation of multimarker prognostication for normotensive patients with acute symptomatic pulmonary embolism. *Am J Respir Crit Care Med.* 2014;189:718–726.
25. Wicki J, et al. Predicting adverse outcome in patients with acute pulmonary embolism: a risk score. *Thromb Haemost.* 2000;84:548–552.
26. Aujesky D, et al. Derivation and validation of a prognostic model for pulmonary embolism. *Am J Respir Crit Care Med.* 2005;172:1041–1046.
27. Kearon C, et al. Antithrombotic therapy for VTE disease: CHEST Guideline and Expert Panel Report. *Chest.* 2016;149:315–352.
28. Kahn SR, et al. Compression stockings to prevent post-thrombotic syndrome: a randomised placebo-controlled trial. *Lancet.* 2014;383:880–888.
29. Becattini C, et al. Aspirin for preventing the recurrence of venous thromboembolism. *N Engl J Med.* 2012;366:1959–1967.
30. Brighton TA, et al. Low-dose aspirin for preventing recurrent venous thromboembolism. *N Engl J Med.* 2012;367:1979–1987.
31. Comerota AJ, et al. Catheter-directed thrombolysis for iliofemoral deep venous thrombosis improves health-related quality of life. *J Vasc Surg.* 2000;32:130–137.
32. Elsharawy M, Elzayat E. Early results of thrombolysis vs anticoagulation in iliofemoral venous thrombosis. A randomised clinical trial. *Eur J Vasc Endovasc Surg.* 2002;24:209–214.
33. AbuRahma AF, et al. Iliofemoral deep vein thrombosis: conventional therapy versus lysis and percutaneous transluminal angioplasty and stenting. *Ann Surg.* 2001;233:752–760.
34. Vedantham S, et al. Quality improvement guidelines for the treatment of lower extremity deep vein thrombosis with use of endovascular thrombus removal. *J Vasc Interv Radiol.* 2006;17:435–447; quiz 48.
35. Mewissen MW, et al. Catheter-directed thrombolysis for lower extremity deep venous thrombosis: report of a national multicenter registry. *Radiology.* 1999;211:39–49.
36. Meissner MH, et al. Deep venous insufficiency: the relationship between lysis and subsequent reflux. *J Vasc Surg.* 1993;18:596–605; discussion 6–8.
37. Watson L, Broderick C, Armon MP. Thrombolysis for acute deep vein thrombosis. *Cochrane Database Syst Rev.* 2016;11:CD002783.
38. Enden T, et al. Long-term outcome after additional catheter-directed thrombolysis versus standard treatment for acute iliofemoral deep vein thrombosis (the CaVenT study): a randomised controlled trial. *Lancet.* 2012;379:31–38.
39. Bjarnason H, et al. Iliofemoral deep venous thrombosis: safety and efficacy outcome during 5 years of catheter-directed thrombolytic therapy. *J Vasc Interv Radiol.* 1997;8:405–418.
40. Patel N, et al. SIR reporting standards for the treatment of acute limb ischemia with use of transluminal removal of arterial thrombus. *J Vasc Interv Radiol.* 2003;14:S453–S465.
41. Vedantham S, et al. Rationale and design of the ATTRACT Study: a multicenter randomized trial to evaluate pharmacomechanical catheter-directed thrombolysis for the prevention of postthrombotic syndrome in patients with proximal deep vein thrombosis. *Am Heart J.* 2013;165:523.e3–530.e3.
42. Theiss W, et al. The success rate of fibrinolytic therapy in fresh and old thrombosis of the iliac and femoral veins. *Angiology.* 1983;34:61–69.
43. Martinez Trabal JL, et al. The quantitative benefit of isolated, segmental, pharmacomechanical thrombolysis (ISPMT) for iliofemoral venous thrombosis. *J Vasc Surg.* 2008;48:1532–1537.
44. Parikh S, et al. Ultrasound-accelerated thrombolysis for the treatment of deep vein thrombosis: initial clinical experience. *J Vasc Interv Radiol.* 2008;19:521–528.
45. O'Sullivan GJ, et al. Pharmacomechanical thrombectomy of acute deep vein thrombosis with the Trellis-8 isolated thrombolysis catheter. *J Vasc Interv Radiol.* 2007;18:715–724.
46. Hartung O, et al. Endovascular management of chronic disabling ilio-caval obstructive lesions: long-term results. *Eur J Vasc Endovasc Surg.* 2009;38:118–124.
47. Latchana N, et al. Ultrasound-accelerated, catheter-directed thrombolysis for inferior vena cava thrombosis after an orthotopic liver transplant. *Exp Clin Transplant.* 2015;13:96–99.
48. Lin PH, et al. Catheter-direct thrombolysis versus pharmacomechanical thrombectomy for treatment of symptomatic lower extremity deep venous thrombosis. *Am J Surg.* 2006;192:782–788.
49. Hartung O, et al. Late results of surgical venous thrombectomy with iliocaval stenting. *J Vasc Surg.* 2008;47:381–387.
50. Neglen P. Stenting is the "Method-of-Choice" to treat iliofemoral venous outflow obstruction. *J Endovasc Ther.* 2009;16:492–493.

51. George R, et al. The effect of deep venous stenting on healing of lower limb venous ulcers. *Eur J Vasc Endovasc Surg.* 2014;48:330–336.

52. Alkhouli M, et al. Comparative outcomes of catheter-directed thrombolysis plus anticoagulation versus anticoagulation alone in the treatment of inferior vena caval thrombosis. *Circ Cardiovasc Interv.* 2015;8:e001882.

53. Delis KT, Bountouroglou D, Mansfield AO. Venous claudication in iliofemoral thrombosis: long-term effects on venous hemodynamics, clinical status, and quality of life. *Ann Surg.* 2004;239:118–126.

54. Neglen P, et al. Stenting of chronically obstructed inferior vena cava filters. *J Vasc Surg.* 2011;54:153–161.

36

Imaging for Structural Heart Disease

Mazen Abu-Fadel, MD, FACC, FSCAI

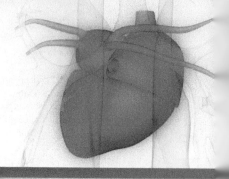

Catheter-based cardiac interventions for structural heart disease (SHD) has emerged as its own specialty within the field of interventional cardiology. While this specialty has existed for over a century, recent technologic advances and a cascade of procedural techniques and devices contributed to a surge in the number and type of performed procedures. SHD interventions range from well-established procedures such as atrial septal defect (ASD) closure and balloon valvuloplasty, to investigational techniques such as mitral valve (MV) replacement and tricuspid annuloplasty. The number of catheter-based corrective procedures is growing rapidly, mainly due to the aging population and the positive outcomes of recent and ongoing clinical trials investigating endovascular treatments of patients with SHD (1). Parallel to the development of these procedures and techniques, the role of imaging in the cardiac catheterization laboratory has become an integral and vital part of such interventions. Different imaging modalities, especially 3D echocardiography and computed tomography, are crucial to help plan, guide, and optimize procedural success and to detect and treat complications when needed.

The first part of this chapter is geared toward briefly understanding the rationale and use of different imaging modalities as an integral part of SHD interventions, while the second part will discuss a general overview of the use of imaging in specific cardiac structural interventions.

Imaging Modalities for SHD

Fluoroscopy

Despite the growth and development of multiple non-invasive imaging techniques, fluoroscopy remains an integral part of any catheterization laboratory interventional procedure. While simple procedures such as patent foramen ovale (PFO) and small ASD closure have been done under echocardiographic guidance only (especially in pregnant females), fluoroscopy remains needed, at this time, for catheter-based interventions. Both fluoroscopy and angiography have an inherent limitation in the accurate diagnosis of SHD. X-ray equipment provides a two dimensional (2D) representation of a three-dimensional (3D) structure. Even with dual plane catheterization laboratories, special information may still be lacking and cardiac soft tissues and defects such as an ASD cannot be identified. Moreover, ionizing radiation use increases the risk of injury to the patient and the operator, especially in long complex cases.

Due to the limitations of fluoroscopy and the development of other reliable and less risky imaging modalities with superior soft tissue images and better special resolution, SHD interventions are currently being performed with much less need for live fluoroscopy. Nevertheless, the overlay of 3D-CT data onto the real-time procedural fluoroscopy, as well as real-time, three-dimensional transesophageal echocardiography (RT 3D TEE), is now used routinely in conjunction with x-ray fluoroscopy to guide percutaneous SHD interventions. Unlike fluoroscopy alone, these two modalities provide excellent details of 3D anatomy and soft tissue structures, and provide "live" intraprocedure guidance (2,3).

Echocardiography

Echocardiography plays an essential role in SHD interventions. It is crucial in identifying patients suitable for the procedure, provides intraprocedural guidance and remains the primary modality for post-procedure follow-up. The demands on the echocardiographer to interpret and guide catheter-based interventions for SHD are much more complex than interpreting a routine echocardiogram. Consequently, interventional cardiologists—if not well trained—will require the assistance of a skilled echocardiographer as part of the interventional SHD team. The major advantage of echocardiography over other imaging modalities, such as computed tomography (CT) and magnetic resonance imaging (MRI), is its mobility and ease of use. In addition, it does not require any contrast agent and does not emit ionizing radiations. It can produce real-time 2D and 3D images and has the ability to detect and diagnose complications in real time during the procedure, which helps for early correction and treatment. Transthoracic echocardiography (TTE), TEE, and intracardiac echocardiography (ICE) are the three modalities widely used for SHD interventions. The advantages and limitations of each are listed in **Table 36.1**.

TRANSTHORACIC ECHOCARDIOGRAPHY

TTE is non-invasive and widely available. It does not require patient sedation or general anesthesia. Newer systems are small, portable, and provide adequate 2D imaging and Doppler capabilities to assist in a number of procedures, including mitral balloon valvuloplasty, alcohol septal ablation (ASA), atrial septostomy, and others (4). TTE images may be challenging to acquire with the patient supine on the catheterization table, while usually the probe and the operator's arm lie in the fluoroscopic field, thus simultaneous images may not be obtainable and so TTE's use is very limited in the cardiac cath lab for SHD interventions (5).

TRANSESOPHAGEAL ECHOCARDIOGRAPHY

Currently, TEE is the standard imaging technique in many centers that perform catheter-based interventions (5). TEE offers superior imaging quality compared to TTE. It provides direct assessment of intraprocedural anatomy and physiology, shows the relationship between catheters/devices and cardiac structures, helps guide interventions and diagnose complications. TEE imaging does not interfere with the operative field and rarely with the fluoroscopic field. One of the most important limitations of TEE includes the need for deep sedation or general anesthesia with endotracheal intubation. In addition, long cases may predispose the TEE probe to overheating and possibly cause burns to the esophagus (4).

On the other hand, TEE has the capability to provide RT 3D imaging. This capability has overcome the limitations of other

TABLE 36.1 Advantages and Limitations of Echocardiographic Imaging Techniques

	ADVANTAGES	LIMITATIONS	USE FOR GUIDANCE
TTE	Easy and rapid access ++ Good image quality (harmonic imaging) Doppler capabilities RT 3D capabilities	Limited acoustic windows ++ Interaction with the sterile field Not usable simultaneously with fluoroscopy	TAVI +
TOE	High-resolution imaging +++ Doppler capabilities Multiplane imaging Accurate assessment of posteriorly situated cardiac structures (interarterial septum, LAA, mitral and aortic valve) Absence of interference with the operative field RT 3D capabilities +++	Semi-invasive Discomfort and aspiration risk in conscious patients Usually requires general anaesthesia and endotracheal intubation ++	Transseptal puncture +++ BMV +++ TAVI ++ Other complex percutaneous procedures +++
ICE	High-resolution imaging +++ Doppler capabilities and four-way steerability (phased array ICE) Accurate assessment of interatrial septum, left atrium, pulmonary veins No need for general anaesthesia Reduced length of procedure and fluoroscopy time 3D (not real-time)	Far field imaging Rare vascular complications (hematomas, venous thrombosis) Arrhythmias Learning curve Additional cost ++	Transseptal puncture +++ BMV++ Percutaneous ASD and PFO closure +++ TAVI +

ASD, atrial septal defect; BMV, balloon mitral valvuloplasty; ICE, intra cardiac echocardiography; LAA, left atrial appendage; PFO, patent foramen ovale; RT 3D, real-time three-dimensional; TAVI, transcatheter aortic valve implantation; TOE, transoesophageal echocardiography; TTE, transthoracic echocardiography.
From: Brochet E, Vahanian A. Echocardiography in the catheterization laboratory. *Heart.* 2010;96(17):1409–1417, with permission.

3D imaging modalities, such as CT and MRI, that have to acquire images prior to the procedure and process them offline to obtain 3D reconstructions. RT 3D TEE has gone from experimental to currently essential for SHD interventions. It has a superior ability to image and navigate open cardiac spaces and show the precise interactions between the 3D structures/defects and the 3D devices being used (**Fig. 36.1**). RT 3D TEE can provide immediate and online textbook-like images of cardiac structure, including mobile structures. It offers superior spatial and temporal resolutions that help with the alignment of catheters and devices with cardiac defects. These defects often have a complex morphology that is sub-optimally visualized by 2D imaging, including for TEE (6). In addition, 3D TEE provides *en face* views of cardiac structures, valves, and surrounding tissues, which has proved to be of great value in some procedures,

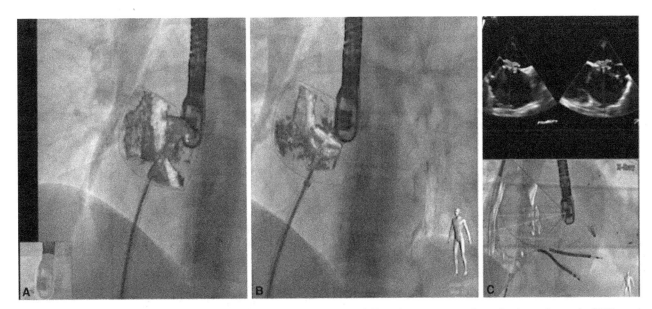

FIGURE 36.1   Fusion imaging guided atrial septal defect (ASD) closure: 2D and 3D real-time transesophageal echocardiography (TEE) overlay on fluoroscopy. Using fusion imaging, the location of the sheet orifice is constantly visualized and the left atrial disc is released under direct vision (**A**). The right atrial disc is opened under echo-guidance (**B**). Color Doppler echocardiography overlay helps to determine correct development, localization, and function of the device without the use of contrast agent (**C**, different patient than **A** and **B**). (From: Biaggi P, et al. Hybrid imaging during transcatheter structural heart interventions. *Curr Cardiovasc Imaging Rep.* 2015;8(9):33, permission not obtained.)

such as the repair of paravalvular leaks (7). RT 3D TEE has a steep learning curve and requires effective communication between the echocardiographer and the interventionalist (1).

Real-time fusion of two or more cardiac imaging modalities, such as fluoroscopy and 3D TEE of the beating heart, is a complex task. The most important step to enable correct real-time fusion is co-registration of the TEE probe position with the cath lab table and the angulation of the C-arm fluoroscope. Special software is needed to recognize the TEE probe within the field of fluoroscopy view and to align its position with that of the C-arm. Once this is done, the TEE probe and the fluoroscopy arm can be moved while image fusion is maintained. In addition, the ability to overlay color Doppler images facilitates the identification of specific targets, improving the rapid and accurate identification of structural defects and landmarks. Fusion imaging potentially increases procedural success, while reducing radiation dose, procedure time, and contrast use. Nevertheless, to date, there is only limited evidence that fusion imaging improves the safety and outcomes of SHD interventions (8).

INTRACARDIAC ECHOCARDIOGRAPHY

ICE has demonstrated excellent potential in guiding and monitoring catheter-based interventions. The image quality of ICE is comparable, or at times superior, to TEE. This technology is widely used for a broad variety of SHD and electrophysiologic procedures. Even though ICE is an invasive procedure, one of its major advantages is the elimination of the need for general anesthesia and endotracheal intubation as in TEE (4).

The most commonly used ICE catheters come in 8-F and 10-F shafts, with a transducer frequency that ranges from about 5 to 10 MHz and has Doppler and color flow capabilities. The catheter is attached to a control handle that helps steer it in four different directions (anterior–posterior and left–right) using two different knobs. The third knob locks the position of the catheter in place once the desired image is displayed (9). The probe is advanced through a separate sheath in the ipsilateral or contralateral femoral vein into the right atrium. Generally, a long sheath from the femoral vein is advanced into the inferior vena cava, followed by the ICE catheter, done under fluoroscopic guidance due to its rigidity and its blunt tip, the latter of which may get wedged in venous branches and possibly harm vital organs and cause bleeding (10). When the catheter reaches the right atrium, the standard starting view is the "home view" that shows the right atrium, right ventricle, tricuspid valve, anterior part of the anterior septum and the right ventricular inflow, and outflow tracks. Depending on the procedure being performed, the ICE catheter can be navigated and its position adjusted to give standardized views that help guide interventions on the atrial septum, ventricular septum, MV, pulmonic valve, left atrial appendage (LAA), and even the descending aorta.

There is a substantial learning curve associated with the use of ICE. This is mainly related to the understanding of the unique images obtained by ICE compared to the standard echocardiographic images. Nevertheless, studies have shown that with the repeated use of ICE, the operator becomes significantly less dependent on fluoroscopy to identify cardiac structures, guide interventions, and diagnose complications (6). This reduction in fluoroscopy times is a potential benefit for both the patient and high-volume operators. Other advantages of ICE include use of only the required minimal additional staff and no additional space for the echocardiography and anesthesia teams, the fact that the patient may be awake for interaction during the procedure, and that the catheter does not interfere with the fluoroscopic field. Some of the disadvantages of this imaging modality include the additional cost of the single-use

TABLE 36.2 Potential Risks of ICE

Vascular
  Trauma at catheterization site
  Bleeding
  Hematoma
  Retroperitoneal bleed
  Perforation of venous structures
Cardiac perforation
  Pericardial effusion
  Tamponade
Arrhythmia
  Atrial premature beats
  AF
  Ventricular ectopy and tachycardia
  Heart block
Thromboembolism
  Venous
  Arterial
Cutaneous nerve palsy

From: Silvestry FE, et al. Echocardiography-guided interventions. *J Am Soc Echocardiogr.* 2009;22(3):213–231, with permission.

AF, atrial fibrillation; ICE, intracardiac Echocardiography.

catheter, the invasive nature of the procedure, and the limited availability and use of 3D ICE imaging. Complications associated with ICE use are mainly due to its invasive nature and the need for maneuvering and manipulation of the stiff catheter in vascular and cardiac structures, which can occur in 1% to 3% of cases (Table 36.2). Reported complications include, but are not limited to, vascular access site complications, venous and cardiac perforation, arrhythmias, thromboembolism, and cutaneous nerve palsy (11).

CT and MRI

CT and MRI 3D images are obtained prior to the procedure, and the images are processed and segmented to include the anatomical area of interest. The data is then transferred to a workstation in the catheterization lab where the images are scaled and overlaid onto the fluoroscopy image in 3D space using anatomical landmarks such as the vertebral bodies or cardiac boarders. This allows the interventional cardiologist to maintain alignment of the two images when the fluoroscopy detector is rotated. The 3D image will maintain the alignment and project a 3D image of the cardiac structures and soft tissues (Fig. 36.2) (12). This can help reduce fluoroscopy time and contrast usage in some cases.

Multi-detector computed tomography (MDCT) has emerged as a key imaging modality in the periprocedural assessment of patients undergoing a variety of SHD interventions (Fig. 36.3). Different imaging protocols to evaluate the cardiac as well as the vascular bed and the aorta are crucial in some cases to decide on the rout of access and plan for the cardiac intervention. The ability of MDCT to provide 3D volumetric data of the entire heart and its surrounding structures has enabled it to become a key imaging modality in the procedural planning and follow-up of the increasing patient population undergoing structural heart interventions. In addition, MDCT allows the operator to identify factors that can affect procedural safety and efficacy (13). CT systems with at least 64-detector technology are recommended. This will give sufficient spatial resolution of cardiac and vascular structures; nevertheless, the temporal resolution

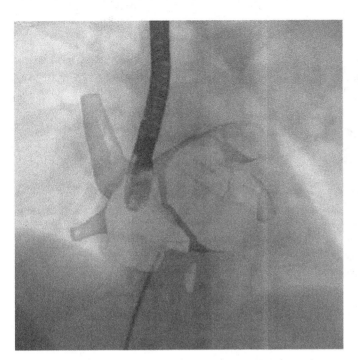

FIGURE 36.2 An image from the workstation is shown here, demonstrating the combining of pre-procedure CTA data with live fluoroscopy during an ASD closure procedure. The delivery cable is seen attached to a partially deployed device in the real-time x-ray image. The CTA contains the soft tissue data that helps identify the location of the ASD, right atrium (*yellow*) and left atrium with pulmonary veins (*blue-green*). The CTA data are first segmented to isolate these important structures, transferred into the workstation in the procedure room, registered with the fluoroscopy, and then actively used during the SHD intervention. ASD, atrial septal defect; CTA, computed tomographic angiography; SHD, structural heart disease.

remains inferior to echocardiography. Some of the disadvantages of CT imaging are related to the use of iodinated contrast and the exposure to ionizing radiation. Using ECG synchronization, advanced scanner technology and imaging protocols can reduce the radiation exposure significantly (Table 36.3) (14).

Cardiovascular MRI has the advantage of visualizing the cardiac and vascular structures without exogenous contrast. Other advantages of MRI include high spatial resolution and excellent soft-tissue characterization. The main drawback of using real-time MRI for catheter-based interventions is due to the compatibility of procedural hardware and catheters with the magnet and the limitation due to respiratory and cardiac motion with the need for rapid image reconstruction and display. The same mechanism that provides unique image quality also makes polymer-only catheters invisible and metal-braded catheters to cause artifact and obscure an entire organ. Most of the equipment used in the catheterization laboratory is not MRI safe, and hybrid MRI/Fluoroscopy suites require dedicated equipment, trained personnel, and additional space and cost. Real-time MRI is available in hybrid suites, but it is mainly used for investigational therapeutic procedures (15).

Use of Imaging to Guide Selected Cardiac Procedures

In this section, a brief review of imaging modalities for specific catheter-based interventions for SHD is discussed. Specific protocols

and step-by-step directions for use is beyond the scope of this review. Irrespective of the imaging modality used to guide all SHD interventions, review of prior diagnostic images (TTE, TEE, CT, MRI, or others) is crucial, especially in patients in whom other associated anomalies are suspected.

Atrial Transseptal Puncture

Access to the left atrium (LA) is required for multiple cardiac interventions. Among the four cardiac chambers, the LA is the most challenging to access. The classic fluoroscopy guided transseptal puncture remains in use by trained and skilled operators. Nevertheless, this technique is less reliable in patients with dilated LA or altered cardiac anatomy. In addition, new interventional procedures such as MV clipping have required the need for a target-specific atrial crossing that is usually at a higher level. This helps the devices cross the MV at a better angle to attain a successful outcome (16). ICE has emerged as the most widely used imaging tool to help operators, especially new ones, achieve a safe and direct visualization of the tenting of the atrial septum by the transseptal sheath prior to needle puncture (Fig. 36.4). This helps increase safety and lowers the risk of canalizing other spaces adjacent to the fossa ovalis, decreases fluoroscopy time, and eliminates the need for sedation and general anesthesia with TEE guidance (4). TTE may be used for this procedure successfully, specifically using 3D TEE to obtain a target-specific crossing (Fig. 36.5).

PFO and ASD Closure

ASD and PFO closure are the most common SHD interventions performed by interventional cardiologists. The majority of these patients will have fluoroscopic imaging as one tool to guide the intervention. Even though fluoroscopy may decrease cost and procedural time, there may be an increase in adverse events such as residual leak, and device malposition if this modality is used alone (17). Two-dimensional TEE without fluoroscopy has been used for successful transcatheter closure of ASD and PFO, but the patients required general anesthetic and higher doses of sedation (18). There are reports in the literature on the use of ICE without fluoroscopy in selected patients that cannot receive sedation or ionizing radiation such as symptomatic pregnant females (19).

Using ICE or TEE, a complete evaluation of the defect and surrounding structures should be performed at the beginning of every case. For patients with ASD, sizing should be done using 2D imaging, and the measurement of surrounding rims should be obtained. Then, the stop-flow diameter of the defect is measured. In patients with PFO, agitated saline contrast images before and after device release should be obtained to document any residual shunting (20).

Advantages of ICE over TEE in performing PFO/ASD closure include shorter procedure and fluoroscopy time, improved imaging, and the addition of supplementary additional diagnostic information. In addition, ICE offers comparable cost when compared to TEE with general anesthesia. As such, ICE is currently the standard imaging modality for these procedures (4). On the other hand, RT 3D TEE provides *en face* views of the intra-atrial septum and can show the exact shape and morphology of the defect, the surrounding rims, and structures that cannot be achieved by any other echocardiographic modality (7).

Valvular Heart Interventions

Valvular heart disease occurs in 2% to 3% of the general population with an increase in prevalence with advancing age. Historically,

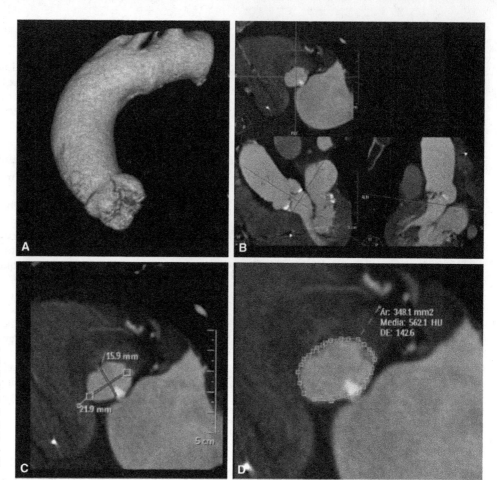

FIGURE 36.3 Multi-slice detector computed tomography reconstruction of the aortic root and ascending aorta **(A)**; 3D orientation for aortic annulus measurement **(B)**; aortic annulus diameters **(C)**; and area and planimetry **(D)** measurement. (From: Zamorano J, et al. The use of imaging in new transcatheter interventions: an EACVI review paper. *Eur Heart J Cardiovasc Imaging.* 2016;17:835, permission being obtained from Elsevier.)

TABLE 36.3 Comparison of Imaging Modalities for Real-Time Procedural Guidance

	REAL-TIME CMR	X-RAY	ECHOCARDIOGRAPHY (SURFACE OR INTRACAVITARY)	COMPUTED TOMOGRAPHY
Ionizing radiation	No	Yes	No	Yes
Structures depicted	Hydrogen- (or other magnetic nuclei) containing tissues	X-ray attenuating (iodinated contrast-filled structures, bone)	Echo dense and echo reflective	Bone and soft tissue
Typical spatial resolution	$1.5 \times 2 \times 5$ mm[a]	<0.4 mm	0.6–1 mm	1–2 mm isotropic
Typical frame rate	5–10 frames/s[a]	15–30 frames/s	20–30 frames/s	2–4 frames/s
Advantages	No ionizing radiation	Widely deployed	Portable	Multislice
	Multiplanar views	Numerous devices available	Lower cost	
	Soft-tissue contrast	High temporal and spatial resolution	High SNR	
	Novel contrast mechanisms		Flow and motion measurements	
Disadvantages	High magnetic field limits devices	Radiation exposure	Limited acoustic windows	Excessive radiation doses
	Low SNR	Limited soft-tissue discrimination	Air and device shadowing	Iodinated contrast
	Potential RF heating	Projection-only (2D) views	Limited "context" (field of view)	
	Gadolinium contrast	Iodinated radiocontrast		

[a]Note the frame rate and spatial resolution given for CMR are arbitrary and represent a typical compromise between spatial and temporal resolution at 1.5-T using parallel imaging with an acceleration factor of 2.
CMR, cardiovascular magnetic resonance; RF, radiofrequency; SNR, signal-to-noise ratio.
From: Saikus CE, Lederman RJ. Interventional cardiovascular magnetic resonance imaging: a new opportunity for image-guided interventions. *JACC Cardiovasc Imaging.* 2009;2(11):1321–1331, with permission.

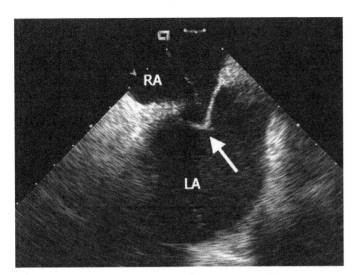

FIGURE 36.4 Phased-array intracardiac echocardiography ICE from the right atrium (RA), demonstrating the tenting of the fossa ovalis *(arrow)* toward the left atrium (LA) before transseptal catheterization. The length of the catheter is seen in the RA.

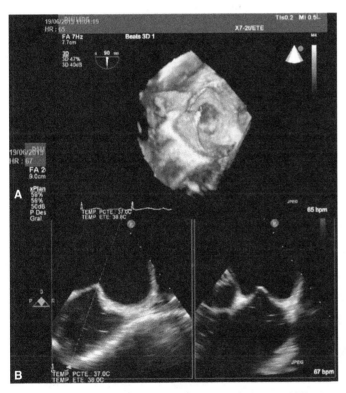

FIGURE 36.5 Three-dimensional **(A)** and two-dimensional **(B)** transesophageal echocardiography to monitor the transseptal puncture in the inferior–posterior portion of the fossa ovalis. (From: Rodríguez Fernandez A, Bethencourt González A. Imaging Techniques in percutaneous cardiac structural interventions: atrial septal defect closure and left atrial appendage occlusion. *Rev Esp Cardiol (Engl Ed).* 2016;69(8):766–777, permission is being obtained from Elsevier.)

percutaneous catheter-based therapy for valvular heart disease was limited to balloon valvuloplasty for aortic, mitral, or pulmonic stenosis. A wide variety of new advances to percutaneous valve therapy is now developing rapidly, including methods for catheter-based valve replacement and repair. All the percutaneous approaches are based on existing surgical techniques and offer less invasive alternatives.

As such, advances in percutaneous interventional approaches have the potential to further improve outcomes for selected patients with valvular heart disease (21).

PERCUTANEOUS BALLOON MITRAL VALVULOPLASTY

Percutaneous balloon mitral valvuloplasty (PBMV) is the treatment of choice for patients with rheumatic mitral stenosis (MS). Many high-volume centers across the world continue to use fluoroscopy guidance and invasive hemodynamics alone to perform this procedure. Two-dimensional TTE in the apical four-chamber, parasternal short axis, and subcostal view is a very helpful addition to fluoroscopy-guided PBMV. Nevertheless, as discussed previously, TTE may interfere with and interrupt the procedure and may prove difficult to help guide the procedure in patients with poor windows. The role of TEE before and during the PBMV is well-established and documented. It is superior to TTE throughout the planning phase and guidance during the intervention. It is crucial in excluding LAA thrombus and assessing the MV and its apparatus for the appropriateness of PBMV. In addition, it can help assess the outcomes of the procedure by measuring transvalvular gradients and ruling out complications, especially worsening mitral regurgitation (MR) (4). ICE can perform all the described steps during the procedure as TEE. It may be superior or inferior to other echocardiographic imaging modalities in visualizing left-sided structures, especially LAA. This depends on the chamber the ICE catheter is imaging from the right versus the LA. In contrast, ICE visualizes the MV structures and apparatus with superior spatial resolution compared to TTE and TEE. Both ICE and TEE can determine the adequacy of valvulotomy, new or worsening MR, and can detect other complications early (4). RT 3D TEE provides additional *en face* views of the MV from both the left ventricular and the left atrial aspects (7).

MITRAL LEAFLET REPAIR

Selected patients suffering from MV regurgitation may benefit from non-surgical catheter-based repair with the MitraClip. This procedure can result in the reduction of the severity of MR. The "clip" grasps the anterior and posterior leaflets of the MV together, in a similar fashion to the Alfieri surgical suture. The biggest challenge of this procedure is to position the device perpendicularly to the coaptation line of the A₂ and P₂ scallops of the MV leaflets to produce two equal mitral orifices (7,22). The anatomic eligibility and patient selection for this procedure is based on a detailed pre-procedural TTE and TEE imaging. The MitraClip is easily imaged using TEE, permitting step-by-step procedural guidance. Once transseptal puncture is obtained under TEE guidance, the device is steered and advanced across the MV under fluoroscopy and TEE guidance. RT 3D TEE greatly facilitates this part of the procedure and is currently the most widely used imaging modality to provide an *en face* view of the MV leaflets and the approaching clip (7,23). Moreover, RT 3D TEE facilitates the perpendicular orientation of the clip to the commissures (Fig. 36.6). Once the leaflets have been clipped, residual MR is assessed with color Doppler in multiple views, and MS should be excluded especially if more than one clip is used. TEE is also crucial to exclude complications and may be used in addition to TTE if needed for outpatient follow-up after the procedure (22,23).

TRANSCATHETER AORTIC VALVE REPLACEMENT

The development of transcatheter aortic valve replacement (TAVR) has provided a viable alternative therapy for patients with severe symptomatic aortic stenosis (AS), which represents high-risk surgical repair. Most commonly, TAVR is performed either through

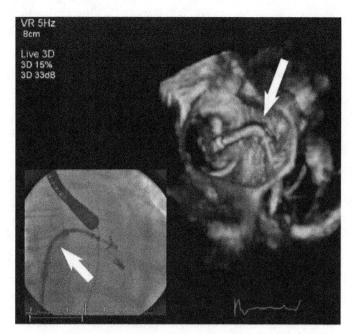

FIGURE 36.6 One of the more challenging investigative structural heart disease (SHD) interventions is the placement of a clip that fastens the mid-portion of the anterior and posterior leaflets of the mitral valve together, in order to reduce the severity of mitral regurgitation. Three-dimensional transesophageal echocardiography (TEE), as shown here, is making a major difference in facilitating the procedure by simultaneously showing the entire guiding catheter and clip delivery system, along with the mitral valve and surrounding structures, in 3D during manipulation of the equipment. This allows easier alignment with the mitral valve orifice, which is challenging in 2D slice images. The insert image is the x-ray image showing a deployed clip and a second clip attached to the delivery system. The *white arrows* point to the delivery catheter in each image.

a retrograde transarterial approach or a transapical approach. Two different types of implants are available: a balloon-expandable valve and a self-expanding prosthesis (24). Due to the technical challenges of TAVR and the lack of direct surgical exposure and visualization of the AV, TAVR relies heavily on imaging for patient selection, pre-procedural planning, intraprocedural decision-making, and post-procedural follow-up. Anatomic information about the aortic annulus, root, valve, coronaries, and aorta and vascular beds for access are critically important (14).

Multidetector CT (MDCT) has emerged as an important imaging modality before and after TAVR. Routine screening with MDCT prior to the procedure has additive information to echocardiographic and angiographic images. ECG synchronized imaging of the aortic root is recommended to avoid image degradation due to motion artifact. Premedication with β-blockers and nitrates should be avoided in this patient population with severe AS (14). Both contrast and non-contrast CT are valuable to obtain. If contrast administration is not possible, a non-contrast scan may provide assessment of aortic and vessel size, tortuosity, and calcification. CT protocols are important to predict access-site complications, aortic narrowing or aneurysms, and protruding aortic arch atheromas that may increase the risk of neurologic complications (**Fig. 36.7**). In such cases, the team may change the strategy to the transapical approach or another type. In addition, pre-procedural CT imaging of the aortic root allows for the prediction of x-ray angiographic planes needed during valve implantation, which in turn help reduce fluoroscopy time and contrast use (25).

MRI and CT have been shown to be more accurate than TEE to assesvs the size of the AV annulus. Three-dimensional TEE, however, has an excellent correlation with CT annular measurement; 2D measurement underestimates the size (23). Complete coronary evaluation with CT is limited in this patient population due to the

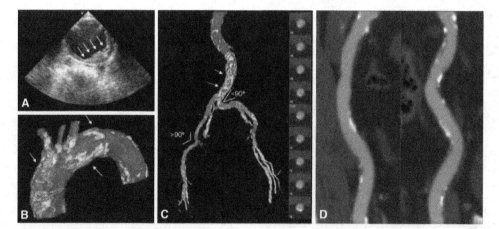

FIGURE 36.7 Aortic atherosclerosis and calcification extent. The presence of extensive atherosclerosis and calcification of the peripheral arteries or thoracic aorta may indicate a transapical approach rather than transfemoral. **A:** An extensive atherosclerotic plaque in the thoracic aortic wall as evaluated with transesophageal echocardiography. **B:** An extensively calcified aortic arch (*arrows*) as assessed with multidetector row–computed tomography. In addition, the presence of the unfavorable anatomy of the iliofemoral arteries can be accurately assessed with multidetector row–computed tomography, by using three-dimensional reconstructions of the arteries (**C**) or multiplanar reformatting views (**D**) showing the cross-sectional area of the arterial lumen and the longitudinal views of the arterial wall. The presence of a minimal luminal diameter of the common iliac, external iliac, or common femoral arteries, 8 mm, more than 60% circumferential calcification at the external–internal iliac bifurcation (*arrows*), and severe angulation between the common and the external iliac arteries define an unfavorable arterial anatomy for the transfemoral approach.

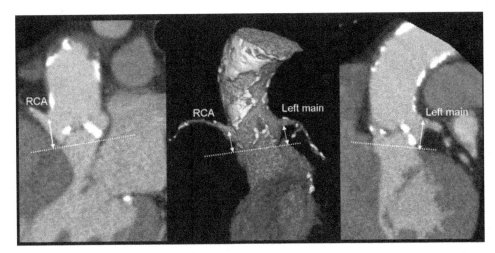

FIGURE 36.8 Assessment of coronary artery ostia height relative to the aortic valve annular plane. RCA, right coronary artery.

universal presence of calcification in the coronary tree. Nevertheless, CT provides the most comprehensive assessment of the relationship between leaflet height and the distance between the annulus and coronary ostia. This helps identify the risk of coronary ostial occlusion by a bulky, long, calcified aortic leaflet after valve prosthesis deployment (Fig. 36.8).

During TAVR, fluoroscopy and TEE play a central role to guide the intervention. The role of ICE is quite limited due to the optimal images that can be obtained by TEE. Exact positioning and deployment of the valve after valvuloplasty is crucial to decrease potential complications. While this is best achieved with a combination of fluoroscopy and TEE, the development of fusion imaging with fluoroscopy and 3D MDCT data help optimize valve plane orientation and visualization of the aorta and aortic valve during the procedure (24). The resulting post-deployment is evaluated by TEE and angiography to rule out complications and post-procedural aortic insufficiency.

LAA Occlusion

In patients with non-valvular AF, embolic stroke is thought to occur from thrombi forming mainly in the LAA, making interventions targeted at the LAA an appealing concept to decrease the risk of stroke especially for patients with contraindications for oral anticoagulation. A number of devices, both endovascular (WATCHMAN, AMPLATZER) and extravascular (LARIAT), have been used to exclude blood flow from the LAA, thereby reducing thrombus formation and CVA risk. The LAA has a highly variable anatomical structure and may be difficult to describe—nevertheless, it is important to correctly evaluate the LAA anatomy in order to optimize procedural success. The best way to determine the configuration and orientation of the LAA lobes is by CT and/or angiography; the LAA orifice and neck can also readily be examined by TEE and 3D TEE (26). From an interventional perspective, understanding the different configurations of the LAA ostium and neck is vital, because the occluder is anchored at the neck and must cover the ostium. TEE and 3D TEE are essential tools at all stages of a percutaneous LAA occlusion procedure: (1) preprocedural TEE is used for LAA examination in multiple planes to exclude the presence of left atrial thrombus, which is a contraindication for device placement. The anatomy of the LAA is highly variable among patients. Therefore, measuring the width of the appendage neck and the length of the appendage is important so that an appropriately sized device can be selected; (2) periprocedural TEE has a major role in guiding delivery and deployment of the device, including transseptal puncture. Placement of this device is performed under fluoroscopy and TEE or RT 3D TEE. After the device is released, TEE imaging is used to examine device stability. Color-flow Doppler is performed to check for leakage. In addition, TEE is used for assessing procedural complications; and (3) postprocedural TEE is important in the surveillance and monitoring of long-term outcomes (27).

A recent study aimed to examine the impact of 3D CT–guided procedural planning for implantation of the WATCHMAN device concluded that 3D CT provides a comprehensive and customized patient-specific LAA assessment that appears to be accurate and may possibly facilitate reducing the early WATCHMAN implantation learning curve (28).

Paravalvular Leaks

Valve replacement surgery is the second most common cardiac surgery after coronary artery bypass grafting. Consequently, the development of a paravalvular leak due to incomplete apposition of the sewing ring and the native tissue is not uncommon. TEE has increased the detection of these defects and allows visualization of the site and the severity of the problem. Paravalvular leaks are most commonly encountered with MV prosthesis but happen with other valves as well. Transcatheter closure of paravalvular leaks was first reported in 2003, and since then various devices have been used with varying degree of success (23). The defects may be multiple, and most of them have a complex 3D anatomy, thus creating a major limitation for device closure and for imaging. TTE plays a limited role in paravalvular leaks, especially in the mitral position, due to extensive acoustic shadowing from the valve rings and leaflets, as well as annular calcification. Both TEE and ICE have been used very successfully for this procedure; however, 3D TEE is currently the preferred imaging modality because it is unique in its capability to show the irregular complex anatomy of the defect and provide accurate sizing. During the procedure, RT 3D TEE guidance plays a major role in confirming the location and the severity of the leak, excluding thrombi and vegetations, facilitating wire and catheter placement, monitoring device deployment, ensuring proper functioning of the valve after device deployment, assessing any residual leaks, and detecting complications if any (23,29). In addition, CT angiography is proving be to a helpful tool and offers incremental value in the periprocedural management of these patients to minimize inaccuracies in the diagnosis and enhance procedural success (30).

Alcohol Septal Ablation

Catheter-based alcohol (ethanol) septal ablation (ASA) was introduced in the early 1990s as a treatment modality for symptomatic hypertrophic obstructive cardiomyopathy. The procedure results in the reduction of the left ventricular outflow track gradient and MR due to systolic anterior motion (SAM) of the MV (31). The septum is perfused by a number of perforators with a significant overlap and variation in the distribution of the myocardial tissue they supply. Contrast echocardiography has been shown to be of great value to guide the selection process of the correct septal perforator to inject with ethanol (4).

After one of the proximal septal perforator arteries is wired and an over-the-wire balloon is inflated in its proximal portion, dye is injected into the balloon catheter lumen to rule out reflux of contrast into the left anterior descending artery. This is followed by injection of 1 to 2 mL of diluted contrast, followed by 1 to 2 mL of saline flushed slowly through the balloon central lumen under continuous TTE or TEE scanning. The target territory of contrast opacification should include the area of maximal flow acceleration seen by color Doppler and the area of SAM, without opacification of any other cardiac structures. Only then should ethanol be administered to ablate the myocardial tissue causing the obstruction (4). If contrast injection opacifies any other right or left ventricular structures, ethanol injection may lead to necrosis of these areas with possible devastating complications (**Fig. 36.9**). Echocardiographic guidance

had a cumulative impact on the interventional strategy in up to 20% of cases (31). Moreover, in 6% of patients, the procedure was aborted because septal perforator injection caused opacification of other cardiac tissues (in addition to the septum) that was not correctable by a target vessel change. These patients are not considered candidates for ASA, and thus need to be referred for myectomy (31).

If TTE is being used to guide the procedure and look for contrast opacification, apical four- and three-chamber views should be obtained. Additional views include the parasternal short and long axis views. Some operators prefer to use TEE for guidance, and in these cases an apical four-chamber view (0°) and a longitudinal view (usually 120°–130°) should be used and supplemented by a transgastric short-axis view to evaluate possible opacification of the papillary muscle (4). An echocardiogram can also be used to measure the drop in the gradient after ethanol injection, to assess if SAM improved, and to detect any complications.

Conclusion

Percutaneous catheter-based intervention for SHD continues to grow as a field of complex interventions, and the number of procedures done annually continues to rise as more patients are considered candidates for these procedures. Unlike surgeons, interventional cardiologists do not have direct visualization of cardiac structures

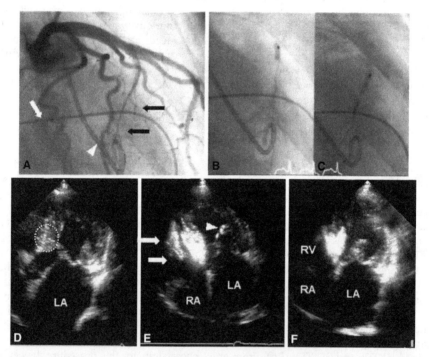

FIGURE 36.9 Interventional and echocardiographic sequence of a (super-selective) septal ablation procedure for symptomatic HOCM. Angio sequence: first major septal perforator artery with two sub-branches (*black arrows*) as the presumed target vessel (**A**, *white arrow*: lead of the temporary pacemaker, *white arrowhead*: pigtail catheter in the left ventricle), balloon within the proximal part of the septal perforator, (**B**) distal vessel bed with two sub-branches contrasted angiographically, (**C**) balloon advanced super-selectively into the left/basal sub-branch. Corresponding echo sequence: subaortic septum as target region in typical SAM-associated, subaortic obstruction (**D**, *dotted line*), (**E**) test injection of the echo contrast agent in balloon position of (**B**) highlighting the basal half of the septum plus a right ventricular papillary muscle (*white arrows*), (**F**) after the super-selective balloon position of (**C**), correct opacification of the target region is achieved. HOCM, hypertrophic obstructive cardiomyopathy; LA, left atrium; RA, right atrium; RV, right ventricle; SAM, systolic anterior motion.

and anatomic relations. Recent advances in cardiac imaging help the accurate visualization of different cardiac structures and thus help in patient selection and guidance of the interventions. Even though all imaging modalities are important and complementary, the combination of fluoroscopy and echocardiography yields an accurate procedural guidance that help attain the highest success with the lowest complication rate. Catheterization laboratories are transforming into hybrid rooms that include CT scans, MRIs, and other modalities to make catheter-based interventions for SHD more efficient and safer.

Key Points

- The number of cardiac catheter-based corrective procedures is on the rise.

- Imaging for SHD interventions assist in diagnosing, planning, guiding, and optimizing these procedures.

- Fluoroscopy remains an integral part of SHD interventions.

- Fluoroscopy is limited by its 2D representations of a 3D structure and its inability to image soft tissues and cardiac structures.

- Ionizing radiation poses a risk for the patient and operator.

- Simultaneous RT 3D TEE and fluoroscopy provides interactive imaging in two modalities that are specifically used for the guidance of SHD interventions.

- Echocardiography is the most available and widely used imaging modality in catheter-based SHD intervention.

- Advanced skills in interpreting echocardiographic images are needed to assist in SHD interventions.

- TTE is widely available, easy to use, and non-invasive.

- Simultaneous fluoroscopy may not be possible with this modality.

- TEE provides superior image quality and does not interfere with the operative field.

- TEE usually requires anesthesia and endotracheal intubation.

- RT 3D TEE provides real-time en face images of complex cardiac structures and defects to facilitate the intervention.

- The combination of TEE with fluoroscopy allows real-time image fusion during SHD interventions, potentially improving procedural success and decreasing radiation dose, contrast use, and procedural time.

- ICE has excellent image quality and eliminates the need for general anesthesia and endotracheal intubation.

- ICE catheters should be advanced to the right atrium under fluoroscopic guidance to decrease complications.

- There is a substantial learning curve to interpret ICE images.

- CT and MRI images are obtained prior to the procedure, and 3D reconstructed images can be overlaid on the fluoroscopic screen.

- These modalities can help evaluate not only cardiac structures but also vascular beds and the aorta for access-related information and procedure planning.

- MDCT has emerged as a key imaging modality in the peri-procedural assessment of patients undergoing a variety of SHD interventions and helps identify factors that can affect procedural safety and efficacy.

- The use of echocardiography is highly recommended for improved safety in performing transseptal punctures.

- ICE has emerged as the leading modality for this procedure because it does not require echocardiographic support and helps in target-specific septal crossing.

- Fluoroscopy combined with another echocardiographic modality remains the standard of care to guide PFO/ASD closure.

- ICE is the current standard imaging modality for this procedure and should be considered when suitable expertise is available.

- Echocardiography is recommended in PBMV for MS and offers significant advantages over sole fluoroscopic guidance.

- TEE or ICE is recommended for procedural guidance, monitoring for complications, and assessment of adequacy of results. The type of imaging used depends on local expertise and the availability of equipment and support staff.

- Mitral leaflet repair with the MitraClip is an alternative procedure for carefully selected patients with MR and high surgical risk.

- RT 3D TEE is the imaging modality of choice to guide this complex procedure.

- Pre-procedural assessment with high-quality CT is crucial for patients undergoing TAVR. This is done to evaluate the aortic root, valve, annulus, aortic arch, descending aorta, iliofemoral arteries, and the relationship of the coronary ostia to the annulus.

- During the procedure, a combination of fluoroscopy and TEE remains the standard of care and provides adequate guidance and evaluation of outcomes and complications.

- 2D TEE imaging is currently the gold standard and recommended imaging modality for LAA occlusion, especially with the WATCHMAN device.

- During the procedure, a combination of fluoroscopy and TEE remains the standard of care and provides adequate guidance and evaluation of outcomes and complications.

- Application of 3D CT imaging allows a comprehensive analysis of LAA anatomy, more appropriate device size selection, and in new implanting sites may reduce the duration of procedures and reduce complications.

- Paravalvular leaks especially in the mitral position are common and present a challenge for treatment.

- Catheter-based closure is possible and RT 3D TEE in addition to fluoroscopy imaging modality to help achieve this complex intervention.

- TTE or TEE is recommended in selecting the appropriate septal perforator to inject with ethanol during ASA.

- Up to 6% of patients will not be considered for ASA due to opacification of cardiac structures other than the desired hypertrophied septum, even when all possible septal perforators are tested.

References

1. Carrol JD, et al. Structural heart disease interventions: rapid clinical growth and challenges in image guidance. *Medicamundi*. 2008;52(2):43–50.
2. Krishnaswamy A, Tuzcu EM, Kapadia SR. Integration of MDCT and fluoroscopy using c-arm computed tomography to guide structural cardiac interventions in the cardiac catheterization laboratory. *Catheter Cardiovasc Interv*. 2015;85:139–147.
3. Clegg SD, et al. Integrated 3D echo-x ray to optimize image guidance for structural heart intervention. *JACC Cardiovasc Imaging*. 2015;8(3):371–374.
4. Silvestry FE, et al. Echocardiography-guided interventions. *J Am Soc Echocardiogr*. 2009;22(3):213–231.
5. Brochet E, Vahanian A. Echocardiography in the catheterisation laboratory. *Heart*. 2010;96(17):1409–1417.
6. Hudson PA, et al. A comparison of echocardiographic modalities to guide structural heart disease interventions. *J Interv Cardiol*. 2008;21(6):535–546.
7. Wunderlich N, et al. 3D echo guidance for structural heart interventions. *Interv Cardiology Rev*. 2009;4(1):16–32.
8. Biaggi P, et al. Hybrid imaging during transcatheter structural heart interventions. *Curr Cardiovasc Imaging Rep*. 2015;8(9):33.
9. Saikus CE, Lederman RJ. Interventional cardiovascular magnetic resonance imaging: a new opportunity for image-guided interventions. *JACC Cardiovasc Imaging*. 2009;2(11):1321–1331.
10. Amin Z, Cao QL, Hijazi ZM. Intracardiac echocardiography for structural heart defects a review of ICE innovations, devices, and techniques. *Cardiac Interventions Today*. April/May 2009:43–50.
11. Bortnick AE, Silvestry FE. In: Gillam LD, Otto CM, ed. *Advanced Approaches in Echocardiography*. 1st ed. Philadelphia, PA: Elsevier Saunders; 2012:73–83.
12. Carroll JD. Dynamic imaging for structural heart disease interventions. *Cardiac Interventions Today*. 2008:65–68.
13. Bo Xu, et al. Clinical utility of multi-detector cardiac computed tomography in structural heart interventions. *J Med Imaging Radiat Oncol*. 2016;60:299–305
14. Schoenhagen P, et al. Computed tomography in the evaluation for Transcatheter Aortic Valve Implantation (TAVI). *Cardiovasc Diagn Ther*. 2011;1(1):44–56. doi:10.3978/j.issn.2223-3652.2011.08.01.
15. Ratnayaka K, et al. Interventional cardiovascular magnetic resonance: still tantalizing. *J Cardiovasc Magn Reson*. 2008;10:62.
16. Shaw TR. Atrial transseptal puncture techniques. *Cardiac Interventions Today*. 2008:69–73.
17. Rhodes JF. Imaging for ASD and PFO closure. *Cardiac Interventions Today*. 2009:24–28.
18. Ewert P, et al. Transcatheter closure of atrial septal defects without fluoroscopy: feasibility of a new method. *Circulation*. 2000;101:847–849.
19. Balzer J, et al. Feasibility, safety, and efficacy of real-time three-dimensional transesophageal echocardiography for guiding device closure of interatrial communications: initial clinical experience and impact on radiation exposure. *Eur J Echocardiogr*. 2010;11(1):1–8.
20. Hijazi ZM, Shivkumar K, Sahn DJ. Intracardiac echocardiography during interventional and electrophysiological cardiac catheterization. *Circulation*. 2009;119:587–596.
21. Feldman T, Herrmann HC, St Goar F. Percutaneous treatment of valvular heart disease: catheter-based aortic valve replacement and mitral valve repair therapies. *Am J Geriatr Cardiol*. 2006;15(5):291–301.
22. Cilingiroglu M, et al. Step-by-step guide for percutaneous mitral leaflet repair. *Cardiac Interventions Today*. 2010:69–76.
23. Zamorano JL, et al. EAE/ASE recommendations for the use of echocardiography in new transcatheter interventions for valvular heart disease. *Eur Heart J*. 2011;32(17):2189–2214.
24. Delgado V, et al. Optimal imaging for planning and guiding interventions in structural heart disease: a multi-modality imaging approach. *Eur Heart J Suppl*. 2010;12(suppl E):E10–E23.
25. Ben-Dor I, et al. Clinical and imaging requirements for TAVI. *Cardiac Interventions Today*. 2010:52–58.
26. Yu CM, et al. Mechanical antithrombotic intervention by LAA occlusion in atrial fibrillation. *Nat Rev Cardiol*. 2013;10:707–722.
27. Nucifora G, et al. Evaluation of the left atrial appendage with real-time 3-dimensional transesophageal echocardiography. Implications for catheter-based left atrial appendage closure. *Circ Cardiovasc Imaging*. 2011;4(5):514–523.
28. Wang DD, et al. Application of 3-dimensional computed tomographic image guidance to WATCHMAN implantation and impact on early operator learning curve. *JACC Cardiovasc Interv*. 2016;9:2329–2340.
29. Booker JD, Rihal CS. Management of paravalvular regurgitation. *Cardiac Interventions Today*. 2009:38–42.
30. Lesser JR, et al. Use of cardiac CT angiography to assist in the diagnosis and treatment of aortic prosthetic paravalvular leak: a practical guide. *J Cardiovasc Comput Tomogr*. 2015;9(3):159–164.
31. Fabera L, et al. Echo-guided percutaneous septal ablation for symptomatic hypertrophic obstructive cardiomyopathy: 7 years of experience. *Eur J Echocardiogr*. 2004;5(5): 347–355.

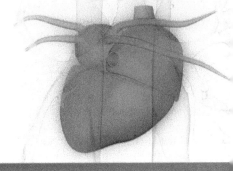

Atrial Septal Defect and Patent Foramen Ovale

Dominik M. Wiktor, MD and

John D. Carroll, MD, FSCAI, FACC

Atrial Septal Defects and Closure

Atrial Septal Anatomy/Embryology

SEPTUM PRIMUM AND SECUNDUM/FORAMEN OVALE AND FOSSA OVALIS

The interatrial septum is composed of the septum primum and the septum secundum. In the first developmental stage of the interatrial septum, the septum primum grows from the roof of the atrium toward the endocardial cushions (1,2), thereby forming the initial separation of the rudimentary right and left atria. As the primum grows, the leading edge is concave (or crescent-shaped), resulting in an interatrial communication referred to as the ostium primum, allowing for right-to-left shunting of blood and bypassing of the fetal pulmonary circulation that is obligatory for fetal development. As the ostium primum ultimately closes, fenestrations develop in the superior aspect of the septum and ultimately coalesce to develop into a new interatrial communication referred to as the ostium secundum, allowing for continued right-to-left shunting of blood during fetal gestation.

The septum primum is leftward and posterior to the septum secundum, which is formed by an infolding of the atria directed rightward and anterior to the septum primum. As the septum secundum grows, its leading edge forms the foramen ovale, which lies in continuity with the ostium secundum and allows for continuous right-to-left shunting of blood. As the septum secundum continues to grow, the septum primum continues to thin and regress, ultimately forming a thin flap of tissue covering the left side of the foramen ovale.

With parturition, left atrial pressure exceeds right atrial pressure, thereby forcing the septum primum against the interatrial septum and terminating right-to-left flow through the foramen ovale. Over time, in normal infant development, the foramen ovale fuses, resulting in an intact anatomical structure known as the fossa ovalis. Nevertheless, in ~25% of the general population, a small channel—a patent foramen ovale (PFO)—persists (3). The relationship of the septum primum to the secundum results in a flap valve mechanism, wherein the superior and leftward aspect of the septum primum (i.e., the "flap") can open toward the left atrium in physiologic scenarios where right atrial pressure exceeds that of left atrial pressure (e.g., Valsalva, cough, mechanical ventilation, etc.), allowing for transient right-to-left inter-atrial shunting and leading to the potential for paradoxical emboli.

Atrial Septal Defect

SECUNDUM ATRIAL SEPTAL DEFECT

The most common atrial septal defect (ASD) is a secundum ASD (Fig. 37.1B), accounting for ~75% of all ASDs (4). The secundum-type defect results from either deficient growth of the septum secundum or excessive resorption of the septum primum (5). Both scenarios result in a centrally located septal defect (near the area of the fossa ovalis in normal hearts) of varying size, shape, and degree of shunting.

With the exception of very large secundum ASDs (>35 mm), and those defects with insufficient rim tissue to accommodate a closure

device, catheter-based closure techniques are recommended over surgery as first-line therapy for ASD repair/closure.

PRIMUM ASD

Primum ASDs (Fig. 37.1D) (also referred to as atrioventricular [AV] septal defects, AV canal defects, and endocardial cushion defects) are less common than the secundum type, on the order of 15% to 20% of all ASDs (4). Partial primum ASDs consist of an absence of the inferior portion of the interatrial septum and frequently a cleft mitral valve, whereas complete primum ASDs are marked by an inlet ventricular septal defect (VSD) and a single AV valve (5). The nature and anatomy of primum ASDs are not amenable to catheter-based closure (partly because of their spatial relationship to the AV valves), so surgical patch repair is the recommended therapy for such defects.

SINUS VENOSUS ASD AND UNROOFED CORONARY SINUS

Occurring in significantly lower frequency are sinus venosus (~5%) and unroofed coronary sinus (<1%) defects. Sinus venosus defects most commonly result from deficiency of the common wall

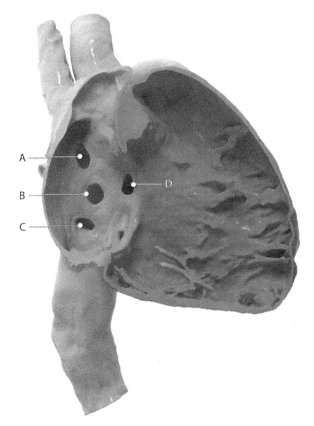

FIGURE 37.1 Atrial septal defect morphologies: superior sinus venosus (A), secundum (B), inferior sinus venosus (C), primum (D). (Courtesy of Adam Hansgen.)

417

between the superior vena cava (SVC) and left atrium (**Fig. 37.1A**), involving the superior, posterior portion of the septum, and are invariably associated with an anomalous right upper pulmonary vein draining into the right atrium (5). Less frequently, the defect is of the inferior, posterior septum, associated with the inferior vena cava (IVC) and an anomalous right lower pulmonary vein draining into the right atrium (**Fig. 37.1C**). The unroofed coronary sinus is an open communication between the left atrium and the coronary sinus, allowing for left-to-right shunting through the intact coronary sinus inlet into the right atrium. Neither sinus venosus nor unroofed coronary sinus defects are amenable to catheter-based closure and therefore must be surgically repaired.

INDICATIONS FOR ASD REPAIR/CLOSURE

Recommendations from the ACC/AHA 2008 Guidelines for the Management of Adults with Congenital Heart Disease (4) are listed in **Table 37.1**.

TABLE 37.1 ACC/AHA Guideline Recommendations for ASD Closure

RECOMMENDATION	CLASS	LEVEL
A sinus venosus, coronary sinus, or primum ASD should be repaired surgically rather than by percutaneous closure.	I	B
Surgeons with training and expertise in CHD should perform operations for various ASD closures (level of evidence: C).	I	C
Surgical closure of secundum ASD is reasonable when concomitant surgical repair/replacement of a tricuspid valve is considered or when the anatomy of the defect precludes the use of a percutaneous device.	IIa	C
Closure of an ASD either percutaneously or surgically is indicated for:		
Right atrial and/or right ventricular enlargement, whether or not the patient is symptomatic	I	B
Paradoxical embolism	IIa	C
Orthodeoxia-platypnea	IIa	B
Presence of net left-to-right shunting, pulmonary artery pressure less than two-thirds systemic levels, PVR less than two-thirds systemic vascular resistance, or when responsive to either pulmonary vasodilator therapy or test occlusion of the defect (patients should be treated in conjunction with providers who have expertise in the management of pulmonary hypertensive syndromes)	IIb	C
Patients with severe irreversible PAH and no evidence of a left-to-right shunt should not undergo ASD closure	III	B

ASD, atrial septal defect; CHD, coronary heart disease; PAH, pulmonary arterial hypertension; PVR, pulmonary vascular resistance.
From: Warnes CA, et al. ACC/AHA 2008 guidelines for the management of adults with congenital heart disease: executive summary: a report of the American College of Cardiology/American Heart Association Task Force on Practice Guidelines (writing committee to develop guidelines for the management of adults with congenital heart disease). *Circulation.* 2008;118:2395–2451, with permission.

ASD Closure Devices

Four devices are currently Food and Drug Administration (FDA)-approved for the closure of ASDs, of which three are currently available for clinical use: the AMPLATZER Septal Occluder (ASO) (St. Jude Medical, St. Paul, MN), the AMPLATZER Multi-Fenestrated (Cribriform) Septal Occluder (St. Jude Medical, St. Paul, MN), the Gore Helex/Cardioform Occluders (Gore Medical, Newark, DE) device. A fourth device, the CardioSEAL STARFlex Septal Occluder (from the now-defunct NMT Medical Inc., Boston, MA) is no longer available.

The ASO device is approved for the closure of secundum-type ASDs and closure of Fontan fenestrations (**Fig. 37.2**). It is composed of a nitinol (nickel/titanium alloy) mesh with left and right atrial discs and a central waist. The size of the device should match the size of the secundum defect measured with a balloon-sizing technique. In the United States, the ASO comes in sizes ranging from 4 to 38 mm (the diameter of the device waist). The left atrial disc is 12 to 16 mm wider in diameter than the waist (depending on waist size), and 4 mm wider than the right atrial disc. Because of its design, the ASO is considered a "self-centering" device.

The AMPLATZER Multi-Fenestrated Septal Occluder (aka, the Cribriform Occluder) device is approved for closure of multi-fenestrated secundum-type ASDs. The device is similar in design to the ASO, but differs in that the left and right atrial discs are of the same size with a small central waist. Sizing of the device is according to disc size, and comes in 18-mm, 25-mm, 30-mm, and 35-mm sizes.

The Gore Helex/Cardioform Occluder consists of a nitinol wire frame covered with polytetrafluoroethylene (PTFE) (**Fig. 37.3**). The original Helex is no longer available, having been replaced by the CardioForm. The Gore Helex/Cardioform Occluder is approved for closure of secundum-type ASDs up to 18 mm in diameter and less than 8 mm in thickness. The recommended size of the device is twice the diameter of the defect (2:1 ratio). Available device sizes are 15 mm, 20 mm, 25 mm, 30 mm, and 35 mm. In contradistinction to the AMPLATZER ASO devices, the Helex/Cardioform device will tend to "ride up" and splay against the retroaortic septum secundum (i.e., non-self-centering).

The CardioSEAL device was approved by the FDA for closure of secundum-type ASDs, but after two negative studies of the related CardioSEAL STARFlex closure device (CLOSURE I [6] and Migraine Intervention with STARFlex Trial [MIST] [7]), the device manufacturer (NMT Medical, Inc.) ceased operations.

Percutaneous Closure Technique

While the specifics of each device's implantation technique are beyond the scope of this review, some important general considerations that apply to transcatheter ASD closure are worth noting.

Sizing of the defect is a critical component, not only for technical success but also for minimizing complications while maximizing long-term outcomes. While each device is sized based on its unique design, they all have the capacity to embolize or erode into surrounding structures. As a rule, ASDs should be measured using a compliant sizing balloon, accompanied by invasive (intracardiac or transesophageal) echocardiography (**Fig. 37.4**). This allows the operator to determine the defect size with a high degree of accuracy. The sizing balloon is advanced across the defect and inflated with low pressure until color-flow Doppler across the defect stops. Importantly, the balloon should not be overinflated because this will lead to larger devices being chosen for closure with increasing risk of device erosion. The defect diameter is then measured in its "stretched" form, and an appropriately sized device is selected for closure.

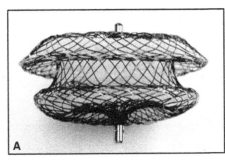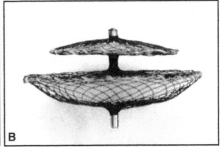

FIGURE 37.2   **A:** Amplatz Atrial Septal Defect Occluder. **B:** Cribriform Occluder (also used for Patent Foramen Ovale Occlusion). (From: Alkashkari W, et al. In: Kern MJ, ed. *The Interventional Cardiac Catheterization Handbook.* Philadelphia, PA: Elsevier pub; 2012, with permission.)

Understanding of the adequacy of the "rim" tissue to allow for device capture is equally important in determining both feasibility of catheter-based closure and ultimate device stability. While retroaortic rim deficiencies are the most common, all rim quadrants of the defect should be carefully examined with echocardiography. In situations where <75% of the defect is accompanied by sufficient rim tissue to safely accommodate a device, surgical defect closure should be strongly considered.

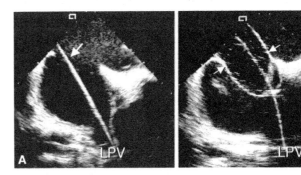

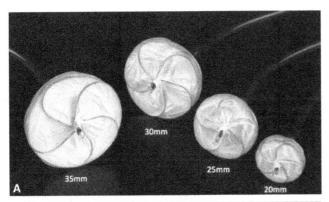

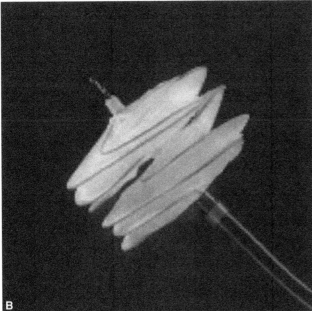

FIGURE 37.3   **A:** Gore CARDIOFORM ASD closure devices of various sizes. **B:** Close-up of CARDIOFORM device attached to delivery cable. ASD, atrial septal defect. (From: W.L. Gore & Associates.)

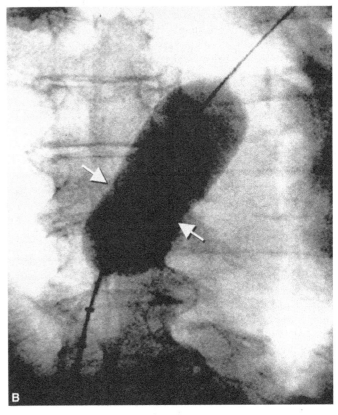

FIGURE 37.4   Intracardiac echocardiographic images showing defect sizing. **A:** The exchange wire *(arrow)* across the defect into the left upper pulmonary vein (LPV). Sizing balloon occluding the defect is noted. This is the stretched diameter *(arrows in the right)* of the defect. **B:** Cineangiographic image during balloon sizing of the defect, demonstrating the stretched diameter *(arrows)* of the defect. (From: Alkashkari W, et al. In: Kern MJ, ed. *The Interventional Cardiac Catheterization Handbook.* Philadelphia, PA: Elsevier pub; 2012, with permission.)

TABLE 37.2 Intention-to-Treat Results of the CLOSURE I Trial

ENDPOINT	CLOSURE (N = 447)	MEDICAL THERAPY (N = 462)	HAZARD RATIO (95% CI)	p VALUE
Composite end point[a]—no. (%)	23 (5.5)	29 (6.8)	0.78 (0.45–1.35)	0.37
Stroke—no. (%)	12 (2.9)	13 (3.1)	0.90 (0.41–1.98)	0.79
TIA—no. (%)	13 (3.1)	17 (4.1)	0.75 (0.36–1.55)	0.44

[a]Defined as stroke or TIA during 2 years of follow-up, death from any cause during the first 30 days, and death from neurologic causes between 31 days and 2 years.
TIA, transient ischemic attack.
From: Furlan AJ, et al. Closure or medical therapy for cryptogenic stroke with patent foramen ovale. *N Engl J Med.* 2012;366:991–999, with permission.

Postclosure Management

Patients are frequently admitted overnight for monitoring, although same-day discharge may be considered in certain subsets of patients. Routine care includes post-procedure monitoring of the access site for hematoma formation, a complete blood count (CBC) for new onset or worsening anemia, electrocardiograms (ECGs) for signs of pericarditis or arrhythmia, and non-invasive hemodynamics for pericardial effusion.

A chest x-ray is recommended within the first 24 hours to check for device positioning and evidence of cardiomegaly suggestive of a large pericardial effusion. More commonly, a transthoracic echo is used to confirm device positioning, rule out pericardial effusion, and ascertain the degree of residual shunt in both the first 24 hours and then at 6 months. It is also typically recommended that patients take aspirin (ASA) (81 to 325 mg daily) for the first 6 months, and clopidogrel (75 mg daily) for the first 2 to 3 months after device implantation (8). Bacterial endocarditis prophylaxis is recommended for the first 6 months post-implantation. It is important to note that many of these post-procedure practices are empirical in nature because there are few data on which to base these recommendations.

Complications

Early potential complications of device implantation include the induction of arrhythmias (~5%), air embolisms (<1%), vascular access complications (<1%), pericardial effusion as a result of perforation of the atrial wall (<1%), and device embolizations (1%–2%) (9–11). Routine screening with chest x-rays, transthoracic echocardiography (TTE), and hemodynamic monitoring should alert the clinician to these rare but serious events.

Device embolization can occur in a delayed fashion as well, but this is much less common. Other rare but potentially significant delayed clinical sequelae include an allergic reaction either to nickel (12,13) or to the device itself (11) and thrombus formation on the device (most commonly associated with the now unavailable CardioSEAL device) (14). More recently, the risk of device erosion (~0.1%, but difficult to truly estimate) has garnered significant interest in national monitoring bodies (e.g., FDA), wherein the implanted device erodes through the atrial wall or into the aorta, most commonly associated with the ASO device (15). While no absolute conclusions can be drawn at this time as to the cause of such erosions, device oversizing, the presence of a deficient retroaortic rim, and repetitive motion have been implicated (15).

Patent Foramen Ovale

Indications for PFO Closure

The recent FDA approval of the AMPLATZER PFO occluder for prevention of recurrent cryptogenic stroke has the potential to markedly alter the landscape of PFO closure in cryptogenic stroke. The most studied indications for PFO closure are cryptogenic stroke (CLOSURE I—**Table 37.2** [6], RESPECT—**Table 37.3** [16], RESPECT extended follow-up **Table 37.4** [18] and PC Trial—**Table 37.5** [17]) and migraine with aura (MIST, **Table 37.6**) (7). The extended results of the RESPECT trial (Table 37.4) served as the impetus for FDA approval of the AMPLATZER PFO occluder and provide the strongest evidence of benefit for PFO closure in highly select patients with cryptogenic stroke to reduce the rise of recurrent stroke as compared with medical therapy alone. The recently published CLOSE and Gore REDUCE trials have strengthened the evidence base for selective closure of PFO in cryptogenic stroke. Both trials demonstrated significant reduction in the rates of recurrent stroke in highly selected patients undergoing percutaneous PFO closure for cryptogenic stroke versus medical therapy alone (19,20). The recently completed PREMIUM trial showed no statistically significant benefit of PFO closure with the AMPLATZER PFO Occluder for the reduction of migraine with aura. PFO closure has also been performed in the treatment of other clinical syndromes, including orthodeoxia-platypnea, systemic hypoxemia, decompression illness, and prior to solid organ transplant. None of these indications, however, have been well studied.

Closure Devices

The recent FDA approval of the AMPLATZER PFO occluder for closure of PFO in cryptogenic stroke marks the first approved device for percutaneous closure of PFO in the United States. The AMPLATZER PFO occluder is most similar to the AMPLATZER Cribriform Occluder. The device consists of a left and right atrial disc joined by a short connecting waist that allows the two discs to move independently. The device comes in four sizes: the 18-mm and 30-mm sizes have equal disc sizes, whereas the 25-mm and 35-mm devices feature left atrial discs that are smaller in diameter than the right atrial discs. The method of closure is shown in **Figures 37.5** and **37.6**.

TABLE 37.3 Primary and Subgroup Analyses of the Primary Endpoint of the RESPECT Trial (16)

	HAZARD RATIO (95% CI)	p VALUE
Intention-to-Treat	0.49 (0.22–1.11)	0.08
Per-protocol	0.37 (0.14–0.96)	0.03
As treated	0.27 (0.10–0.75)	0.007
Substantial right-to-left shunt	0.18 (0.04–0.81)	0.01
Atrial septal aneurysm	0.19 (0.04–0.87)	0.02

TABLE 37.4 Long-Term Efficacy Outcomes of the RESPECT Trial (18)

OUTCOME[a]	CLOSURE GROUP (N = 499)		MEDICAL GROUP (N = 481)		HAZARD RATIO (95% CI)	p VALUE
	PATIENTS WITH EVENTS	EVENT RATE PER 100 PT-YEARS	PATIENTS WITH EVENTS	EVENT RATE PER 100 PT-YEARS		
Recurrent ischemic stroke	18 (3.6%)	0.58	28 (5.8%)	1.07	0.55 (0.31–0.999)	0.046
Recurrent ischemic stroke of undetermined cause (ASCOD)	10 (2.0%)	0.32	23 (4.8%)	0.86	0.38 (0.18–0.79)	0.007
Recurrent cryptogenic ischemic stroke (TOAST)	1 (0.2%)	0.03	11 (2.3%)	0.41	0.08 (0.01–0.58)	0.01
Transient ischemic attack	17 (3.4%)	0.54	23 (4.8%)	0.86	0.64 (0.34–1.20)	0.16

[a]Outcomes shown are first such recurrent event in a patient, not second or later recurrences.
ASCOD, A: atherosclerosis, S: small-vessel disease, C: cardiac pathology, O: other causes; TOAST, Trial of ORG 10172 in Acute Stroke Treatment.

TABLE 37.5 Primary and Secondary Outcomes of the PC Trial

	PFO CLOSURE N (%)	MEDICAL THERAPY N (%)	HAZARD RATIO/RELATIVE RISK (95% CI)	p VALUE
Death, stroke, TIA, or peripheral embolism	7 (3.4)	11 (5.2)	0.63 (0.24–1.62)	0.34
Death	2 (1.0)	0	5.20 (0.25–107.61)	0.24
Cardiovascular	0	0	N/A	
Noncardiovascular	2 (1.0)	0	5.20 (0.25–107.61)	0.24
Thromboembolic Event				
Stroke	1 (0.5)	5 (2.4)	0.20 (0.02–1.72)	0.14
TIA	5 (2.5)	7 (3.3)	0.71 (0.23–2.24)	0.56
Peripheral embolism	0	0	N/A	
Stroke, TIA, or peripheral embolism	5 (2.5)	11 (5.2)	0.45 (0.16–1.29)	0.14

PC, percutaneous closure; PFO, patent foramen ovale; TIA, transient ischemic attack.
Adapted from: Meier B, et al. Percutaneous closure of patent foramen ovale in cryptogenic embolism. *N Engl J Med.* 2013;368:1083–1091.

TABLE 37.6 Intention-to-Treat Results of the MIST Trial

ENDPOINT	IMPLANT (N = 74)		SHAM PROCEDURE (N = 73)		STATISTICAL ANALYSES	
	BASELINE	ANALYSIS PHASE	BASELINE	ANALYSIS PHASE	DIFFERENCE BETWEEN IMPLANT AND SHAM ARMS (95% CI)	p VALUE
Patients with no migraine attacks, N	0	3	1	3	−0.06% (−6.45 to 6.34)	1.0
Frequency of migraine attacks/month, mean ± SD	4.82 ± 2.44	3.23 ± 1.80	4.51 ± 2.17	3.53 ± 2.13	0.45 (−0.16 to 1.05)	0.14
Total MIDAS score, median (range)	36 (3–108)	17 (0–270)	34 (2–189)	18 (0–240)	1 (−11 to 10)	0.88
Headache days/3 months (MIDAS), median (range)	27 (0–70)	18 (0–90)	30 (5–80)	21 (0–80)	1 (−5 to 6)	0.79
HIT-6 total score, mean_SD	67.2 ± 4.7	59.5 ± 9.3	66.2 ± 5.1	58.5 ± 8.6	0 (−3 to 2)	0.77

MIDAS, migraine disability assessment; MIST, Migraine Intervention with STARFlex Trial; SD, standard deviation.
From: Dowson A, et al. Migraine Intervention with STARFlex Technology (MIST) trial: a prospective, multicenter, double-blind, sham-controlled trial to evaluate the effectiveness of patent foramen ovale closure with STARFlex septal repair implant to resolve refractory migraine headache. *Circulation.* 2008;117:1397–1404, with permission.

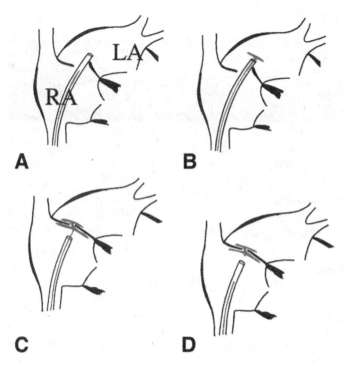

FIGURE 37.5 Schematic demonstration of patent foramen ovale closure using the AMPLATZER PFO Occluder. **A:** Sheath in mid left atrium (LA). **B:** Deployment of left atrial disc. **C:** Deployment of connecting waist and right atrial disc. **D:** Device released. PFO, patent foramen ovale. (From: Alkashkari W, et al. In: Kern MJ, ed. *The Interventional Cardiac Catheterization Handbook.* Philadelphia, PA: Elsevier pub; 2012, with permission.)

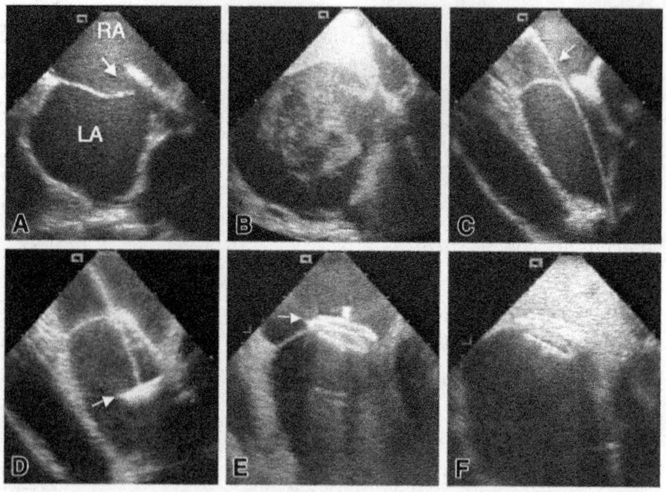

FIGURE 37.6 Intracardiac echocardiographic images in a young patient who has a patent foramen ovale (PFO), demonstrating the steps of closure. **A:** Septal view demonstrating the PFO *(arrow)* and the thin septum primum. **B:** Contrast bubble study demonstrating significant right-to-left shunt. **C:** Guide wire *(arrow)* positioned through the defect into the left pulmonary vein. **D:** Deployment of the left atrial disc *(arrow)*. **E:** Deployment of the right atrial disc *(arrow)*; release of the device. **F:** Contrast bubble study repeated after the device has been released, demonstrating successful closure. (From: Alkashkari W, et al. In: Kern MJ, ed. *The Interventional Cardiac Catheterization Handbook.* Philadelphia, PA: Elsevier pub; 2012, with permission.)

Clinical Trial Data

The CLOSURE I trial was a prospective, randomized, open label trial of the STARFlex closure device compared with medical therapy for the prevention of recurrent cryptogenic stroke (6). A total of 909 patients with a cerebrovascular accident (CVA) or transient ischemic attack (TIA) within the previous 6 months, demonstrated PFO with right-to-left shunting; no other obvious cause of CVA was included. No difference in recurrent ischemic events was found, although the rate of adverse events in the closure group was higher.

The RESPECT trial was a randomized, controlled, multicenter, open-label trial conducted in the United States comparing the AMPLATZER PFO Occluder to medical therapy for prevention of recurrent cryptogenic stroke (16). It enrolled 980 patients. Compared to the CLOSURE I study, the rate of successful device implantation was higher, and the rate of adverse events was lower. A non-significant trend toward lower event rates was seen in the initial intention-to-treat analysis (p = 0.08), while the per-protocol (p = 0.03) and as-treated (p = 0.007) analyses suggested benefit to closure. Recently, the extended follow-up results of RESPECT have been published, demonstrating the benefit of PFO closure in this selected population versus medical therapy alone (p = 0.046) for prevention of recurrent stroke (18). Subpopulation analyses suggested benefit in patients with "substantial" right-to-left shunts and atrial septal aneurysms.

The PC Trial also used the AMPLATZER PFO Occluder, and enrolled 414 patients in Europe, Canada, Brazil, and Australia (29). No benefit to closure was seen either in the intention-to-treat analysis

(p = 0.34), or the per-protocol analysis (p = 0.48). This trial was notable for both slow enrollment and a lower-than-anticipated event rate in the medical therapy group.

The CLOSE trial was a multicenter, prospective, randomized, open label trial in 663 patients who had a recent stroke attributed to PFO with associated atrial septal aneurysm or large interatrial shunt in which patients were assigned in a 1:1:1 ratio to transcatheter PFO closure plus long-term antiplatelet therapy, antiplatelet therapy alone, or oral anticoagulation. Among these patients, the rate of recurrent stroke was lower in the PFO closure arm than in the antiplatelet therapy alone arm (0 vs 14 events, p<0.001). The antiplatelet therapy alone versus oral anticoagulation subgroup of the study was underpowered and thus no conclusions could be drawn regarding the optimal medical therapy for reducing recurrent stroke in this patient population (19).

The Gore REDUCE trial was a multicenter, prospective, randomized trial in 664 patients with PFO and cryptogenic stroke who were assigned in a 2:1 ratio to either PFO closure with Gore Helex/Cardioform plus antiplatelet therapy or antiplatelet therapy alone. The rate of recurrent stroke was lower in the PFO closure arm than in the antiplatelet therapy alone arm (1.4 vs 5.4%, p=0.002) (20).

The MIST trial was a prospective, randomized, double-blind, sham-controlled trial comparing the STARFlex closure device with medical therapy in 147 patients with moderate to large right-to-left shunts (7). No difference in migraine cessation was seen between the two groups, although the implanted group demonstrated a higher rate of serious adverse events.

Key Points

- Primum and sinus venosus ASDs and unroofed coronary sinuses must be repaired surgically.

- Secundum-type ASDs are the most common form of ASD, are generally amenable to catheter-based closure, and carry a Class I recommendation for closure in the setting of RA/RV enlargement.

- Currently approved ASD closure devices are the AMPLATZER Septal and Cribriform Occluders and the Gore Cardioform Occluder.

- The AMPLATZER PFO occluder has recently been approved by the FDA for closure of PFO in select patients with recurrent cryptogenic stroke.

- The MIST trial failed to show benefit of PFO closure for migraine reduction using the CardioSEAL STARflex device, while the PREMIUM trial studying the AMPLATZER PFO occluder for this same indication is ongoing.

References

1. Anderson RH, Webb S, Brown NA. Clinical anatomy of the atrial septum with reference to its developmental components. *Clin Anat.* 1999;12:362–374.
2. Anderson RH, Brown NA, Webb S. Development and structure of the atrial septum. *Heart.* 2002;88:104–110.
3. Hagen PT, Scholz DG, Edwards WD. Incidence and size of patent foramen ovale during the first 10 decades of life: an autopsy study of 965 normal hearts. *Mayo Clin Proc.* 1984;59:17–20.
4. Warnes CA, et al. ACC/AHA 2008 guidelines for the management of adults with congenital heart disease: executive summary: a report of the American College of Cardiology/American Heart Association Task Force on Practice Guidelines (writing committee to develop guidelines for the management of adults with congenital heart disease). *Circulation.* 2008;118:2395–2451.
5. Bonow RO, Zipes DP, Libby P, ed. *Braunwald's Heart Disease: A Textbook of Cardiovascular Medicine.* 9th ed. Philadelphia, PA: Elsevier; 2011.
6. Furlan AJ, et al. Closure or medical therapy for cryptogenic stroke with patent foramen ovale. *N Engl J Med.* 2012;366:991–999.
7. Dowson A, et al. Migraine Intervention with STARFlex Technology (MIST) trial: a prospective, multicenter, double-blind, sham-controlled trial to evaluate the effectiveness of patent foramen ovale closure with STARFlex septal repair implant to resolve refractory migraine headache. *Circulation.* 2008;117:1397–1404.
8. Franke A, Kuhl HP. The role of antiplatelet agents in the management of patients receiving intracardiac closure devices. *Curr Pharm Des.* 2006;12:1287–1291.
9. Du ZD, et al. Comparison between transcatheter and surgical closure of secundum atrial septal defect in children and adults: results of a multicenter nonrandomized trial. *J Am Coll Cardiol.* 2002;39:1836–1844.
10. Everett AD, et al. Community use of the Amplatzer™ atrial septal defect occluder: results of the multicenter MAGIC atrial septal defect study. *Pediatr Cardiol.* 2009;30:240–247.
11. Jones TK, et al. Results of the U.S. multicenter pivotal study of the HELEX® septal occluder for percutaneous closure of secundum atrial septal defects. *J Am Coll Cardiol.* 2007;49:2215–2221.
12. Khodaverdian RA, Jones KW. Metal allergy to Amplatzer™ occluder device presented as severe bronchospasm. *Ann Thorac Surg.* 2009;88:2021–2022.
13. Wertman B, et al. Adverse events associated with nickel allergy in patients undergoing percutaneous atrial septal defect or patent foramen ovale closure. *J Am Coll Cardiol.* 2006;47:1226–1227.
14. Krumsdorf U, et al. Incidence and clinical course of thrombus formation on atrial septal defect and patient foramen ovale closure devices in 1,000 consecutive patients. *J Am Coll Cardiol.* 2004;43:302–309.
15. Crawford GB, et al. Percutaneous atrial septal occluder devices and cardiac erosion: a review of the literature. *Catheter Cardiovasc Interv.* 2012;80:157–167.
16. Carroll JD, et al. Closure of patent foramen ovale versus medical therapy after cryptogenic stroke. *N Engl J Med.* 2013;368:1092–1100.
17. Meier B, et al. Percutaneous closure of patent foramen ovale in cryptogenic embolism. *N Engl J Med.* 2013;368:1083–1091.
18. Saver JL, et al. Long-term outcomes of PFO closure of medical therapy in cryptogenic stroke. *N Engl J Med.* 2017;377:1022–1032.
19. Søndergaard L, et al. Patent foramen ovale closure or antiplatelet therapy for cryptogenic stroke. *N Engl J Med* 2017; 377: 1033–42.
20. Mas J-L, vet al. Patent foramen ovale closure or anticoagulation vs. antiplatelets after stroke. *N Engl J Med* 2017; 377: 1011–21.

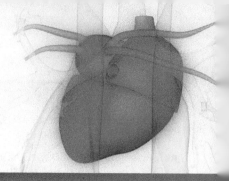

38

Left Atrial Appendage Closure

Matthew J. Price, MD, FSCAI, FACC

Atrial fibrillation (AF) is the most common sustained arrhythmia. Increasing age is a major risk factor for onset of AF, and therefore the global burden of AF is growing substantially as the population ages. Overall, the presence of AF increases stroke risk approximately 5-fold, and paroxysmal, persistent, and permanent AF appear to increase thromboembolic risk to a similar degree. AF-related ischemic strokes are more likely to be fatal than strokes not related to AF, and among survivors, AF-related strokes are great in severity and recur more frequently than non-AF-related strokes. The prevalence of AF-related strokes is particularly pronounced in the very elderly: AF accounts for approximately one in four strokes among octogenarians (1). Treatment with oral anticoagulants (OACs) is the traditional approach to reducing thromboembolic risk in AF patients. Nevertheless, treatment with vitamin K–dependent OACs (e.g., warfarin) is challenging due to warfarin's narrow therapeutic window, the need for drug monitoring, and numerous drug–drug and food–drug interactions (2). Large randomized trials have demonstrated the safety and efficacy of non-vitamin K-dependent OACs (NOACs), but these agents are still associated with a significant hazard for bleeding and have substantial cost. AF patients at thromboembolic risk are undertreated despite the availability of NOACs (3). The left atrial appendage (LAA) appears to be the dominant source of thromboembolism in AF (4). LAA closure, by eliminating the nidus for thrombus formation, may reduce the thromboembolic risk in AF while abrogating the need for long-term anticoagulation and thereby eliminating the long-term bleeding risk observed with medical therapy. Therefore, transcatheter closure of the LAA represents a local, non-pharmacologic approach to stroke prevention in AF patients.

LAA Anatomy

The LAA is a multi-lobed, trabeculated, broad-shaped structure with a narrow neck, predisposing to stagnation and thrombosis. The LAA is an anterior and superior structure arising from the left atrium. The ostium is formed *superiorly* by the limbus of the left upper pulmonary vein (LUPV) and *inferiorly* by the area adjacent to the mitral valve annulus and above the left atrioventricular groove, which contains the left circumflex artery (Fig. 38.1). The morphology of the LAA is variable, and can be generally classified into one of the following categories: windsock, cactus, cauliflower, and chicken wing (Fig. 38.2). The chicken-wing-type anatomy may be particularly challenging for successful transcatheter closure. Transthoracic echocardiography (TTE) is insufficient to evaluate LAA anatomy. A thorough evaluation of the LAA by transesophageal echocardiography (TEE) includes an assessment for LAA thrombus, the presence of baseline pericardial effusion, and the interrogation of the appendage from the mid-esophageal view in four planes (0°, 45°, 90°, and 135°) to determine the overall shape, depth, and number of lobes and the maximal width and depth of the LAA ostium. For the purpose of LAA closure with the WATCHMAN occluder, the

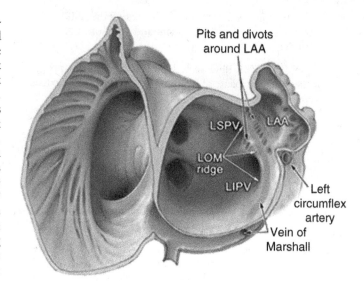

FIGURE 38.1 Anatomy of the left atrial appendage and its surrounding structures. LAA, left atrial appendage; LIPV, left inferior pulmonary vein; LOM, ligament of Marshall; LSPV, left superior pulmonary vein. (Adapted from: DeSimone CV, et al. A review of the relevant embryology, pathohistology, and anatomy of the left atrial appendage for the invasive cardiac electrophysiologist. *J Atr Fibrillation*. 2015;8(2):81–87.)

ostial diameter is defined as the distance from a point just distal to the left circumflex artery to approximately 1 to 2 cm from the tip of the LUPV limbus. Cardiac computed tomography (CT) may be useful in cases where the LAA anatomy is unclear or of borderline feasibility according to TEE; nevertheless, the data for the safety and efficacy of LAA closure did not incorporate routine CT scanning.

Thromboembolic and Bleeding Risk Scores

The assessment of thromboembolic and bleeding risks are essential components for patient selection for LAA closure, because the procedure is indicated only in patients who are at high stroke risk and who have a rationale to seek a non-pharmacologic approach to stroke reduction. The $CHADS_2$ and CHA_2DS_2VASc scores are well-validated risk schemes based on a particular individual's co-morbidities that can estimate a yearly risk of thromboembolic events and identify patients who may derive clinical benefit from OAC (Tables 38.1 and 38.2) (5–7).

LAA Occluders

Several devices can be used for the purpose of LAA closure (2). At present, only the WATCHMAN occluder (Boston Scientific, Natick, MA) has been evaluated in randomized clinical trials, and is the only

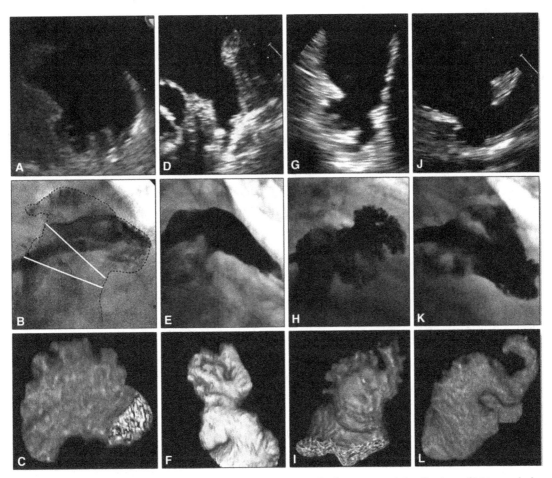

FIGURE 38.2 Various morphologies of the left atrial appendage. The four proposed classifications of LAA morphologies as shown by transesophageal echocardiography (**top**), cineangiography (**middle**), and 3D-computed tomography (**bottom**). (**A–C**): Cauliflower; (**D–F**): windsock; (**G–I**): cactus; (**J–L**): chicken wing. (Adapted from: Biegel R, et al. The left atrial appendage: anatomy, function, and noninvasive evaluation. *J Am Coll Cardiol Img.* 2014;7(12):1251–1265.)

device that has been approved by the Food and Drug Administration (FDA) for clinical use (Fig. 38.3). The device is introduced into the LAA through a 14-Fr sheath delivered from the right femoral vein via an infero-posterior transseptal puncture. The device is made of a self-expanding nitinol frame with a polyethylene terephthalate (PET) fabric 160-μm mesh cap. Distal fixation anchors secure the device within the LAA trabeculae. It attaches to a delivery cable at a central threaded insert, and is advanced through a delivery sheath that is placed deep within the LAA. In combination with radial force at the device shoulders, distal fixation anchors secure the device within the LAA trabeculae. The device size corresponds to the width of the device at its proximal shoulders. The length of the device is approximately equal to its diameter.

Randomized Clinical Trial Data for LAA Closure

The safety and clinical efficacy of WATCHMAN LAA closure have been evaluated in two Bayesian, randomized, clinical trials that tested whether LAA occlusion was non-inferior to warfarin therapy for the primary efficacy endpoint of stroke, systemic embolism, and cardiovascular/unexplained death in AF patients who were eligible for long-term OAC. In these trials, patients who received the WATCHMAN device were continued on warfarin therapy for

approximately 6 weeks post-procedure, at which time they were transitioned to dual antiplatelet therapy with aspirin and clopidogrel for 6 months, followed by indefinite aspirin monotherapy if LAA seal was confirmed by TEE (Fig. 38.4). The PROTECT-AF (WATCHMAN Left Atrial Appendage System for Embolic Protection in Patients with Atrial Fibrillation) trial randomly assigned 707 AF patients with a CHADS$_2$ score $\geq$1 who were eligible for long-term OAC to either WATCHMAN LAA closure or warfarin in a 2:1 ratio (8). LAA closure was both non-inferior and superior to warfarin for the primary efficacy endpoint at a mean follow-up of 3.8 $\pm$ 1.7 years (2,625 patient-years) (rate ratio, 0.60 [95% credible interval (CrI), 0.41–1.05], posterior probability of non-inferiority >99.9%, posterior probability for superiority = 96%) (Fig. 38.5). Cardiovascular and all-cause mortality were reduced with LAA closure (HR 0.40 [95% CI, 0.21–0.75], p = 0.005 and HR 0.66 [95% CI, 0.45–0.98], p = 0.04, respectively). Safety events were initially greater in the device group, driven by procedural complications, although by the end of the follow-up the overall rate of safety events in both arms were similar due to bleeding events in the warfarin group (Fig. 38.5) (9). Peri-device flow on follow-up TEE was frequent (41% and 32% of patients at 6 weeks and 1-year post-procedure, respectively), was mostly <3 mm in diameter, and did not appear to be associated with thromboembolic events (10).

TABLE 38.1 Thromboembolic Risk Scores for Patients with Atrial Fibrillation

CHADS₂	
CHARACTERISTIC	**POINTS**
Congestive heart failure	1
Hypertension	1
Age ≥ 75 years	1
Diabetes mellitus	1
Stroke, transient ischemic attack, or thromboembolism	2
Maximum score	6

CHA₂DS₂VASC	
CHARACTERISTIC	**POINTS**
Congestive heart failure	1
Hypertension	1
Age ≥75 years	2
Diabetes mellitus	1
Stroke, transient ischemic attack, or thromboembolism	2
Vascular disease (prior MI, PAD, or aortic plaque)	1
Age 65–74 years	1
Sex category = female	1
Maximum score	9

MI, myocardial infarction; PAD, peripheral arterial disease.
Adapted from: January CT, et al. 2014 AHA/ACC/HRS guideline for the management of patients with atrial fibrillation: a report of the American College of Cardiology/ American Heart Association Task Force on Practice Guidelines and the Heart Rhythm Society. *J Am Coll Cardiol.* 2014;64:e1–e76.

TABLE 38.2 HAS-BLED Bleeding Risk Score

CHARACTERISTIC	POINTS
Hypertension (uncontrolled systolic blood pressure >160 mm Hg)	1
Abnormal liver or renal function[a]	1 each, maximum 2
Stroke (previous history)	1
Bleeding history or disposition (e.g., anemia)	1
Labile INR (i.e., time in therapeutic range <60%)	1
Elderly age (>65 years)	1
Drugs that promote bleeding or excess alcohol consumption (>7 units/week)	1 each, maximum 2
Maximum score	9

INR, internationalnormalized ratio.
[a]Abnormal liver function was defined as cirrhosis or biochemical evidence of significant hepatic derangement; abnormal renal function was defined as serum creatinine >200 μmol/L (2.26 mg/dL).
Adapted from: Pisters R, et al. A novel user-friendly score (HAS-BLED) to assess 1-year risk of major bleeding in patients with atrial fibrillation: the Euro Heart Survey. *Chest.* 2010;138:1093–1100.

The aim of the smaller PREVAIL (Prospective Randomized Evaluation of the WATCHMAN Left Atrial Appendage Closure Device In Patients with Atrial Fibrillation Versus Long Term Warfarin Therapy) trial was to confirm procedural safety, particularly among newer operators, and to further explore clinical efficacy of LAA closure compared with warfarin (11). A total of 407 AF patients with CHADS₂ ≥2 were randomly assigned to either WATCHMAN LAA closure or warfarin in a 2:1 ratio. The WATCHMAN device met the performance goal for procedural and device safety prespecified by the sponsor and the FDA, with safety events occurring in 2.2% of patients. Implantation by new operators was not associated with reduced rates of implant success or an increased risk of major adverse events. The rate of procedural complications, including stroke and serious pericardial effusions, were significantly reduced in PREVAIL compared to PROTECT-AF. At a mean follow-up of 11.8 ± 5.8 months, the primary efficacy endpoint of stroke, systemic embolism, or cardiovascular death was similar between study arms, but LAA closure did not achieve non-inferiority (device event rate, 0.064 vs. warfarin event rate, 0.064; rate ratio, 1.07 [95% CrI, 0.57–1.89] rate ratio for non-inferiority criterion: upper bound of 95% CrI <1.75).

A pooled, patient-level meta-analysis of these two randomized trials demonstrated that the rate of the primary efficacy endpoint was similar with device closure compared with chronic warfarin therapy (HR 0.79, 95%CI: 0.53-1.2, P=0.22) (12). All-cause stroke and systemic embolism were similar between LAAC and warfarin; there was numerically more ischemic strokes in the device group, significantly more hemorrhagic strokes in the warfarin group, and

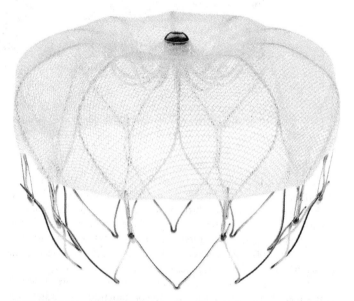

FIGURE 38.3 WATCHMAN device. The device is comprised of a self-expanding nitinol frame with a polyethylene terephthalate fabric cap. Distal tines secure the device within the LAA trabeculae. The device is fully retrievable prior to release from the delivery cable. Device length is approximately equal to its diameter. Device size is selected based upon the largest diameter of the LAA ostium, which is measured by drawing a line from the mitral valve annulus across to the ridge of the left upper pulmonary vein, perpendicular to the planned axis of the delivery sheath. Alternatively, the LAA ostium can be measured from the mitral valve annulus to a point approximately 2 cm distal from the tip of the left upper pulmonary vein ridge. The device is delivered through a 14-Fr delivery sheath introduced into the LAA through an infero-posterior transseptal puncture. According to the device's instructions for use, the device should only be released after deployment if the criteria for its adequate position (i.e., not too distal or proximal), anchoring (good tug test), size (device compression 8%–20%), and seal (no peridevice flow by TEE or fluoroscopy) are achieved. LAA, left atrial appendage; TEE, transesophageal echocardiography.

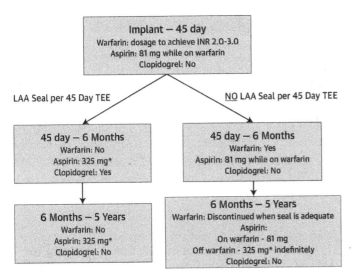

significantly fewer cardiovascular deaths in the device group. Another pooled analysis demonstrated a significant reduction in major bleeding with LAA closure once the 6-month period of post-procedure pharmacotherapy was completed (Fig. 38.6) (13).

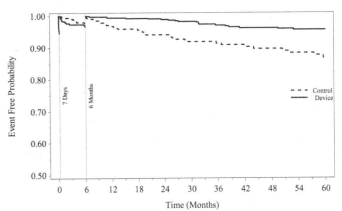

FIGURE 38.4 Anticoagulant and antiplatelet management strategy in patients receiving device therapy in the randomized clinical trials of the WATCHMAN LAA occluder. After device implantation, patients were treated with a combination of warfarin and aspirin for approximately 6 weeks, at which time TEE was performed. If the LAA was sealed (defined as a residual leak <5 mm in width without evidence of thrombus), warfarin was discontinued and the patient was treated with aspirin and clopidogrel until 6 months post-procedure, at which time the clopidogrel was discontinued and the patient continued on aspirin monotherapy. *Asterisk*: recommended dosage. INR, international normalized ratio; LAA, left atrial appendage; TEE, transesophageal echocardiography. (Adapted from: Holmes DR, et al. Prospective randomized evaluation of the WATCHMAN left atrial appendage closure device in patients with atrial fibrillation versus long-term warfarin therapy: the PREVAIL trial. *J Am Coll Cardiol.* 2014;64:1–12.)

FIGURE 38.6 Landmark analysis of the freedom from major bleeding after transcatheter LAA closure over three intervals of follow-up in a pooled, patient level analysis of the PROTECT-AF and PREVAIL trials. Landmarks are from randomization to day 7, representing the periprocedural period for patients randomly assigned to LAA closure; 8 days to 6 months post-randomization, during which device-treated patients received warfarin and aspirin followed by dual antiplatelet therapy; and beyond 6 months, when device-treated patients were eligible to receive aspirin alone. Major bleeding after 6 months post-procedure was significantly lower with LAA closure compared with ongoing warfarin (HR 0.28; 95% CI: 0.23–0.35, p < 0.001). LAA, left atrial appendage; PREVAIL, Prospective Randomized Evaluation of the WATCHMAN Left Atrial Appendage Closure Device In Patients with Atrial Fibrillation Versus Long Term Warfarin Therapy; PROTECT-AF, WATCHMAN Left Atrial Appendage System for Embolic Protection in Patients with Atrial Fibrillation. (Adapted from: Price MJ, et al. Bleeding outcomes after left atrial appendage closure compared with long-term warfarin: a pooled, patient-level analysis of the WATCHMAN randomized trial experience. *JACC Cardiovasc Interv.* 2015;8:1925–1932.)

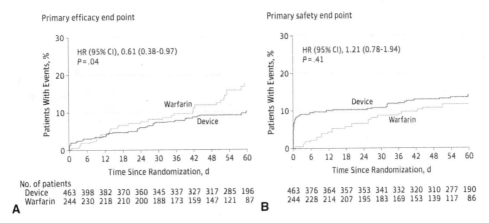

FIGURE 38.5 Long-term clinical and safety outcomes in the PROTECT-AF randomized trial of WATCHMAN LAA closure compared with warfarin therapy. **A:** Primary efficacy outcome of cardiovascular death, stroke, or systemic embolism. At a mean of 3.8 years (2,621 patient-years) of follow-up, transcatheter LAA occlusion with the WATCHMAN met pre-specified criteria for non-inferiority and superiority compared with warfarin. **B:** Primary safety outcomes, a composite of major bleeding events and procedure-related complications. While an early hazard was apparent around the periprocedural period with device therapy, the overall rate of safety events was similar in both groups, primarily due to ongoing bleeding events in the warfarin group. LAA, left atrial appendage; PROTECT-AF, WATCHMAN Left Atrial Appendage System for Embolic Protection in Patients with Atrial Fibrillation. (Adapted from: Reddy VY, et al. Percutaneous left atrial appendage closure vs warfarin for atrial fibrillation: a randomized clinical trial. *JAMA.* 2014;312:1988–1998.)

Procedural Complications with LAA Closure

Major complications associated with LAA closure include pericardial effusion and tamponade, procedural stroke, device embolization, and vascular injury or bleeding (14). In PROTECT-AF, serious pericardial effusion (requiring drainage or surgical intervention) occurred in 22 patients (4.8%). Nevertheless, procedural outcomes have improved since this initial experience (Table 38.3), although pericardial effusion remains the most common adverse event. Device thrombus over follow-up has also been observed in approximately 3% to 4% of cases.

FDA Approval of LAA Closure

At present, the WATCHMAN occluder (Boston Scientific, Natick, MA) is the only LAA closure device approved by the FDA for stroke prevention. The indications for use are listed in Box 38.1.

TABLE 38.3 Comparison of Complication Rates in Device Patients in PROTECT-AF and PREVAIL

EVENT	PROTECT-AF (N = 463)	PREVAIL (N = 269)	P VALUE
All 7-day procedural complications	8.7%	4.5%	0.004
Pericardial effusion requiring surgery	1.6%	0.4%	0.03
Pericardial effusion with pericardiocentesis	2.4%	1.5%	0.32
Procedure-related stroke	1.1%	0.7%	0.02
Device embolization	0.4%	0.7%	0.47

PROTECT, WATCHMAN Left Atrial Appendage System for Embolic Protection in Patients with Atrial Fibrillation; PREVAIL, Prospective Randomized Evaluation of the WATCHMAN Left Atrial Appendage Closure Device In Patients with Atrial Fibrillation Versus Long Term Warfarin Therapy.
Adapted from: Holmes DR Jr, et al. Prospective randomized evaluation of the WATCHMAN left atrial appendage closure device in patients with atrial fibrillation versus long-term warfarin therapy: the PREVAIL trial. *J Am Coll Cardiol*. 2014;64:1–12.

BOX 38.1 FDA Indications for Use of the WATCHMAN LAA Occluder

The WATCHMAN is indicated to reduce the risk of thromboembolism from the LAA in patients with non-valvular AF who:

- Are at an increased risk of stroke and systemic embolism based on $CHADS_2$ or CHA_2DS_2VASc scores and are recommended for OAC
- Are deemed by their physicians to be suitable for warfarin; and
- Have an appropriate rationale to seek a non-pharmacologic alternative to warfarin, taking into account the safety and effectiveness of the device compared to warfarin.

Appropriate rationales for seeking an alternative to warfarin include:

- a history of major bleeding while taking therapeutic anticoagulation therapy
- the patient's prior experience with OAC (if applicable),
- a medical condition, occupation, or lifestyle placing the patient at high risk of major bleeding secondary to trauma

AF, atrial fibrillation; FDA, Food and Drug Administration; LAA, left atrial appendage; OAC, oral anticoagulation

Society Guidelines

The 2014 American Heart Association (AHA)/American College of Cardiology (ACC)/Heart Rhythm Society (HRS) Guideline for the Management of Patients with Atrial Fibrillation (15) recommend no antithrombotic therapy or treatment with an oral anticoagulant or aspirin be considered in nonvalvular AF and a CHA_2DS_2-VASc score of 1 (Class IIB, level of evidence: C) and the use of OACs in patients with CHA_2DS_2VASc score ≥ 2 (Class I, level of evidence: A). Society recommendations pertaining to LAA closure are shown in Table 38.4.

TABLE 38.4 Society Recommendations Pertaining to Left Atrial Appendage Closure

CLASSIFICATION	LEVEL OF EVIDENCE	RECOMMENDATION
AMERICAN HEART ASSOCIATION/AMERICAN COLLEGE OF CARDIOLOGY/HEART RHYTHM SOCIETY 2014 GUIDELINE FOR THE MANAGEMENT OF PATIENTS WITH ATRIAL FIBRILLATION (16)		
IIb	C	Surgical excision of the LAA may be considered in patients undergoing cardiac surgery.
AMERICAN HEART ASSOCIATION/AMERICAN STROKE ASSOCIATION GUIDELINE FOR PRIMARY PREVENTION OF STROKE (17)		
IIB	C	LAA closure may be considered for high-risk patients with AF who are deemed unsuitable for anticoagulation if performed at a center with low rates of periprocedural complications and the patient can tolerate the risk of at least 45 days of post-procedural anticoagulation
EUROPEAN SOCIETY OF CARDIOLOGY 2016 GUIDELINES FOR THE MANAGEMENT OF ATRIAL FIBRILLATION (18)		
CLASSIFICATION	LEVEL OF EVIDENCE	RECOMMENDATION
IIb	B	Surgical occlusion or exclusion of the LAA may be considered in patients with AF undergoing cardiac surgery.
IIb	B	LAA occlusion may be considered in patients with AF and contraindications for long-term anticoagulant treatment (e.g., those with a previous life-threatening bleed without a reversible cause).

Key Points

■ The LAA appears to be a major source of thromboembolism in nonvalvular AF. The randomized clinical trials of LAA closure compared the WATCHMAN device with warfarin in patients with nonvalvular AF who were candidates for long-term warfarin anticoagulation. In these trials, patients assigned to WATCHMAN LAA closure were treated post-procedure with 6 weeks of aspirin and warfarin, 5 months of aspirin and clopidogrel, and then indefinite aspirin maintenance therapy.

■ Pooled analysis of the two randomized trials for LAA closure demonstrated similar rates of all-cause stroke, lower rates of

intracranial hemorrhage, and lower rates of cardiovascular death with LAA closure compared with warfarin.

■ WATCHMAN LAA closure is indicated to reduce the risk of thromboembolism from the LAA in patients with nonvalvular AF who are at an increased risk of stroke and systemic embolism based on CHADS$_2$ or CHA$_2$DS$_2$VASc scores and are recommended for OAC, are deemed by their physicians to be suitable for warfarin, and have an appropriate rationale to seek a non-pharmacologic alternative to warfarin.

■ The most common complication of transcatheter LAA closure is pericardial effusion and tamponade.

References

1. Mozaffarian D, et al. Heart disease and stroke statistics-2016 update: a report from the American Heart Association. *Circulation.* 2016;133:e38–e360.
2. Price MJ, Valderrabano M. Left atrial appendage closure to prevent stroke in patients with atrial fibrillation. *Circulation.* 2014;130:202–212.
3. Marzec LN, et al. Influence of direct oral anticoagulants on rates of oral anticoagulation for atrial fibrillation. *J Am Coll Cardiol.* 2017;69:2475–2484.
4. Blackshear JL, Odell JA. Appendage obliteration to reduce stroke in cardiac surgical patients with atrial fibrillation. *Ann Thorac Surg.* 1996;61:755–759.
5. Gage BF, et al. Validation of clinical classification schemes for predicting stroke: results from the National Registry of Atrial Fibrillation. *JAMA.* 2001;285:2864–2870.
6. Lip GY, et al. Comparative validation of a novel risk score for predicting bleeding risk in anticoagulated patients with atrial fibrillation: the HAS-BLED (Hypertension, Abnormal Renal/Liver Function, Stroke, Bleeding History or Predisposition, Labile INR, Elderly, Drugs/Alcohol Concomitantly) score. *J Am Coll Cardiol.* 2011;57:173–180.
7. Lip GY, et al. Refining clinical risk stratification for predicting stroke and thromboembolism in atrial fibrillation using a novel risk factor-based approach: the Euro Heart Survey on atrial fibrillation. *Chest.* 2010;137:263–272.
8. Holmes DR, et al. Percutaneous closure of the left atrial appendage versus warfarin therapy for prevention of stroke in patients with atrial fibrillation: a randomised non-inferiority trial. *Lancet.* 2009;374:534–542.
9. Reddy VY, et al. Percutaneous left atrial appendage closure vs warfarin for atrial fibrillation: a randomized clinical trial. *JAMA.* 2014;312:1988–1998.
10. Viles-Gonzalez JF, et al. The clinical impact of incomplete left atrial appendage closure with the Watchman Device in patients with atrial fibrillation: a

PROTECT AF (Percutaneous Closure of the Left Atrial Appendage Versus Warfarin Therapy for Prevention of Stroke in Patients With Atrial Fibrillation) substudy. *J Am Coll Cardiol.* 2012;59:923–929.
11. Holmes DR Jr, et al. Prospective randomized evaluation of the Watchman Left Atrial Appendage Closure device in patients with atrial fibrillation versus long-term warfarin therapy: the PREVAIL trial. *J Am Coll Cardiol.* 2014;64:1–12.
12. Holmes DR Jr, et al. Left atrial appendage closure as an alternative to warfarin for stroke prevention in atrial fibrillation: a patient-level meta-analysis. *J Am Coll Cardiol.* 2015;65:2614–2623.
13. Price MJ, et al. Bleeding outcomes after left atrial appendage closure compared with long-term warfarin: a pooled, patient-level analysis of the WATCHMAN randomized trial experience. *JACC Cardiovasc Interv.* 2015;8:1925–1932.
14. Price MJ. Prevention and management of complications of left atrial appendage closure devices. *Interv Cardiol Clin.* 2014;3:301–311.
15. January CT, et al. 2014 AHA/ACC/HRS guideline for the management of patients with atrial fibrillation: executive summary: a report of the American College of Cardiology/American Heart Association Task Force on Practice Guidelines and the Heart Rhythm Society. *J Am Coll Cardiol.* 2014;64:2246–2280.
16. January CT, et al. 2014 AHA/ACC/HRS guideline for the management of patients with atrial fibrillation: a report of the American College of Cardiology/American Heart Association Task Force on Practice Guidelines and the Heart Rhythm Society. *J Am Coll Cardiol.* 2014;64:e1–e76.
17. Meschia JF, et al. Guidelines for the primary prevention of stroke: a statement for healthcare professionals from the American Heart Association/American Stroke Association. *Stroke.* 2014;45:3754–3832.
18. Kirchhof P, et al. 2016 ESC Guidelines for the management of atrial fibrillation developed in collaboration with EACTS. *Eur Heart J.* 2016;37:2893–2962.

39

Mitral Valvuloplasty and Percutaneous Mitral Valve Repair

Ted Feldman, MD, MSCAI, FACC, FESC, Mayra Guerrero, MD, FACC, FSCAI, Michael H. Salinger, MD, FSCAI, FACC, and Justin P. Levisay, MD, FACC, FSCAI

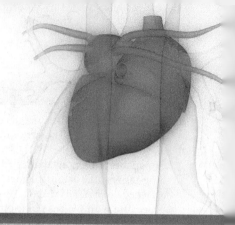

Although percutaneous techniques for the treatment of structural heart disease represent revolutionary technology, the basic principles of these therapies were born from concepts developed several years ago. For example, pulmonic valve stenosis was treated with percutaneous catheter therapy as early as the 1950s. Balloon valvuloplasty was first described in 1982 by Inoue (1), and has subsequently developed into a mature therapy for mitral (2), pulmonic, and aortic stenosis (3). This chapter reviews percutaneous mitral valvuloplasty as it is practiced today and provides an overview of the next horizon in catheter valve therapy, percutaneous mitral valve repair, and replacement.

Balloon Commissurotomy for Mitral Stenosis

Rheumatic heart disease is an infrequent diagnosis in the United States, but remains an important disease process (4). Immigrants have entered the United States from all over the world, importing rheumatic heart disease from Mexico, Asia, and Central and South America. Also, new strains of *Streptococci* have been associated with rheumatic fever in the United States, and streptococcal skin and kidney infections have been implicated in some outbreaks of rheumatic disease (5). There is suboptimal utilization of secondary antibiotic prophylaxis, oral anti-coagulation, and contraception in this population (6).

It is important to recall that initial attacks of rheumatic fever require specific therapy. The rheumatic disease process not only attacks the valves but also produces a pancarditis, which may adversely affect atrial and ventricular function. Atrial fibrillation in association with rheumatic mitral stenosis (MS) is probably caused by both left atrial distention and damage to the atrial tissue at the time of the acute rheumatic infection. MS has historically been synonymous with rheumatic valve disease. Etiologies other than rheumatic are encountered less frequently. Congenital MS, carcinoid drug-induced potentially reversible MS associated with methysergide, and eosinophilic endomyocardial fibroelastosis represent rare causes of MS. Increasingly, calcific MS in association with severe mitral annular calcification associated with our aging population or among patients on chronic hemodialysis is being recognized and associated with our aging population.

It is critically important to recognize the difference between calcific and rheumatic disease. The hallmark of rheumatic MS is commissural fusion, usually in association with subvalvular thickening, and in almost all cases with some involvement of aortic, tricuspid, and/or pulmonic valves. In contrast, the typical chronic calcific patient has calcification extending from the annulus toward the body of the leaflets, with free movement of the leaflet tips, little involvement of the chordae, and no evidence for commissural fusion. Thus, the bases of the leaflets have diminished motion, while the commissures show no signs of fusion. Clinical history is critical for the diagnosis of MS. The sine qua non of the disease is dyspnea on exertion. Patients may be misdiagnosed with a history of asthma or other lung diseases. Some patients have even had lung biopsy for a long-standing diagnosis of interstitial disease until pulmonary congestion from rheumatic MS is diagnosed. Exercise intolerance and dyspnea develop in almost all patients with clinically significant disease. With exercise, cardiac output rises slowly with a disproportionately greater increase in the left atrial and pulmonary artery pressures.

Disease progression can be slow, and many patients with MS adamantly deny any limitation in exercise tolerance. Patients often decrease their activity level to avoid symptoms. Thus, the history requires some effort to elicit. Exercise testing can be helpful when the symptomatic status of a patient is not clear (7). In particular, serial exercise testing over a period of several years is often very helpful when a patient presents with moderate disease initially.

Echocardiographic Evaluation

Transthoracic echocardiography (TTE) is the primary tool for assessment of patients for suitability for balloon mitral commissurotomy (BMC). A scoring system has been described that utilizes four characteristics to characterize the spectrum of mitral valve deformity (Table 39.1) (8). The score combines descriptions of leaflet mobility, leaflet thickening, calcification, and subvalvular involvement on a scale, where 1 is minimal deformity and 4 represents severe deformity. The scoring system is relatively subjective and has a large amount of interobserver variability. Many other scoring systems have been described, but the original Wilkins score remains the simplest and most widely used. Despite the limitations of the Wilkins score, it represents a

TABLE 39.1 Wilkins Score

	MOBILITY	SUBVALVULAR	THICKENING	CALCIUM
1	Tips restricted	Minimal thickening	Normal (4–5 mm)	Single area
2	Mid and base normal	1/3 chordal length	Leaflet margins 5–8 mm	Scattered
3	Valve moves forward	Thick to distal chords	Entire leaflet 5–8 mm	Mid leaflets
4	Barely mobile	Extensive to paps	>8–10 mm thick	Extensive

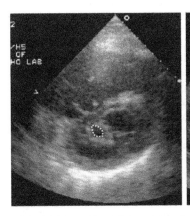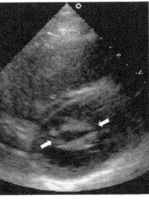

FIGURE 39.1 The left-hand panel shows a short-axis transthoracic echocardiographic image at the level of the mitral valve orifice. Planimetry of the orifice shows the typical fishmouth appearance (*dotted circle*). The interventricular septum is flattened due to chronic pulmonary hypertension. There is dense, symmetrical commissural fusion. On the right, after balloon mitral commissurotomy, there is bilateral commissural splitting, shown by the *white arrows*. The interventricular septum is now more round, consistent with immediate diminution of the pulmonary artery pressure.

common currency for describing the degree of valve deformity and MS. Scores of 8 or less have been associated with excellent long-term results from BMC, while scores >12 have poor long-term outcomes and a high incidence of mitral regurgitation complicating the procedure. Echocardiographic scores between 9 and 12 are associated with intermediate long-term outcomes. Patients with lower echo scores have event-free survival rates over 5 years after BMC exceeding 80%. The event-free rate over 5 years declines to about 60% among those with intermediate scores. Patients with severe valve deformity are usually poor candidates for any form of therapy and may receive BMC as a palliative therapy when the risk of surgery is prohibitive. These patients typically present at a later age in states of advanced disease, and have poor long-term outcomes, and in some cases are currently subjects being evaluated for transcatheter mitral valve replacement (TMVR).

The short axis transthoracic echo view can be used to assess the symmetry of commissural fusion (**Fig. 39.1**). Symmetric commissural fusion and the absence of leaflet calcification are associated with the best balloon dilatation results. Asymmetric fusion and/or calcification of the commissures typically yield less optimal results from balloon dilatation because of the reduced ability of the balloon to split the commissures in a controlled, predictable fashion.

Indications for coronary arteriography were described in detail in older guidelines, but are not addressed specifically in the 2014 valve disease document. Based on older guidelines, coronary angiography prior to BMC should be considered for patients with chest pain or evidence of ischemia, poor left ventricular (LV) function, a history of coronary artery disease, for male and postmenopausal female patients over the age of 35 years, and in premenopausal female patients when risk factors for coronary artery disease are present.

Patient Selection

BMC has become the therapy of choice for the majority of patients with symptomatic MS (**Table 39.2**) (9). BMC is recommended for symptomatic patients with a valve area of <1.5 cm^2 who have favorable valve morphology, no left atrial thrombus, and no severe mitral regurgitation. Treatment decisions for asymptomatic patients are challenging. Those who have no symptoms and a mitral valve

---

TABLE 39.2 AHA/ACC Guideline Recommendations for Mitral Stenosis Intervention

Class I

BMC is recommended for symptomatic patients with severe MS (MVA 1.5 cm^2, stage D) and favorable valve morphology in the absence of contraindications.

Mitral valve surgery is indicated in severely symptomatic patients (NYHA class III/IV) with severe MS (MVA 1.5 cm^2, stage D) who are not high risk for surgery and who are not candidates for or failed previous PMBC.

Concomitant mitral valve surgery is indicated for patients with severe MS (MVA 1.5 cm^2, stage C or D) undergoing other cardiac surgery.

Class IIa

BMC is reasonable for asymptomatic patients with very severe MS (MVA 1.0 cm^2, stage C) and favorable valve morphology in the absence of contraindications.

Mitral valve surgery is reasonable for severely symptomatic patients (NYHA class III/IV) with severe MS (MVA 1.5 cm^2, stage D), provided there are other operative indications.

Class IIb

BMC may be considered for asymptomatic patients with severe MS (MVA 1.5 cm^2, stage C) and favorable valve morphology who have new onset of AF in the absence of contraindications.

BMC may be considered for symptomatic patients with MVA >1.5 cm^2 if there is evidence of hemodynamically significant MS during exercise.

BMC may be considered for severely symptomatic patients (NYHA class III/IV) with severe MS (MVA 1.5 cm^2, stage D) who have suboptimal valve anatomy and are not candidates for surgery or at high risk for surgery.

Concomitant mitral valve surgery may be considered for patients with moderate MS (MVA 1.6–2.0 cm^2) undergoing other cardiac surgery.

Mitral valve surgery and excision of the left atrial appendage may be considered for patients with severe MS (MVA 1.5 cm^2, stages C and D) who have had recurrent embolic events while receiving adequate anticoagulation.

AF, atrial fibrillation; BMC, balloon mitral commissurotomy; MS, mitral stenosis; MVA, mitral valve area; NYHA, New York Heart Association; PMBC, percutaneous mitral balloon commissurotomy.

---

area of <1.5 cm^2 may be considered for catheter commissurotomy if the pulmonary artery systolic pressure is >50 mm Hg at rest or 60 mm Hg after exercise. New atrial fibrillation has also been defined as an indication for BMC in patients without symptoms. Patients with moderate to severe MS and New York Heart Association (NYHA) Class III or IV symptoms, who have restricted, nonpliable calcified leaflets and are at high risk for mitral valve surgery, are also candidates for BMC (Class IIa). There is a common misconception that an echo score >8 is a "contraindication" to BMC. While the long-term outcomes among patients with higher scores is clearly less good, the score must be considered in conjunction with the risks for surgery and the goals of therapy. At the extreme of higher scores, octogenarian patients with no other therapy options may have a year or two of palliation, freedom from heart failure hospitalizations, and improved quality of life from BMC. Some younger female patients may have BMC despite some valve deformity to allow for pregnancy before ultimately having surgical mitral valve replacement.

Acute Results and Complications

The hemodynamic results of BMC have been consistent regardless of the method or type of balloon used for the procedure. The immediate intraprocedure results are dramatic (**Fig. 39.2**). There is a decline of left atrial pressure and transmitral pressure gradient with an associated increase in cardiac output and, consequently, an increase in mitral valve area. In patients with hypertensive heart disease or LV diastolic pressure elevations, the diminution in gradient may be overshadowed by persistently high ventricular diastolic and left atrial pressures. On average, the mitral valve area increases from 1.0 cm^2 to between 1.8 and 2.2 cm^2. Pulmonary hypertension typically decreases by between 10% and 25% as soon as the valve has been successfully dilated. Immediate declines in left atrial and pulmonary artery pressure often lead patients to spontaneously comment on improvement in their sense of breathing while they are still on the cardiac cath lab table (10). Additional decreases in pulmonary pressure usually take place over several weeks or months after the procedure. Despite these improvements, severe pulmonary hypertension usually does not completely resolve. Atrial fibrillation reverts in only 20% to 25% of patients. This is probably because of rheumatic involvement of the atria and the persistent fibrosis of atrial tissue caused by chronic left atrial distension.

The most important complication of BMC is an increase in mitral regurgitation. About 2% to 3% of patients require mitral valve replacement for mitral regurgitation during the hospitalization for the procedure. As many as one-third of patients have an increase in mitral regurgitation associated with a net benefit in clinical outcome. Intraprocedural or hospital death occurs in <1% of patients. In a large cross-sectional study of balloon mitral valvuloplasty in the

United States, trends of decreasing overall utilization and increasing procedural complication rates and cost were noted over a period of 13 years, between 1998 and 2010, corresponding to increasing age and the burden of comorbidities in patients (11).

BMC-related stroke or transient ischemic attack as a consequence of embolization from the left atrial appendage has been virtually eliminated by the routine use of transesophageal echo as a pre-procedure screening tool. The incidences of these complications are similar to other catheterization procedures. Cardiac perforation associated with transseptal puncture occurs in about 1% in most series. Perforation of the ventricle by the balloon is rare with the Inoue Balloon, and is more frequent with the longer, sharper-tipped balloons used for the two-balloon technique.

Most techniques for BMC involve transseptal puncture, with creation of an atrial septal defect (12). Color-flow Doppler demonstrates shunt flow in almost all patients immediately after the procedure, but most atrial septal defects close spontaneously within a few weeks or months. Less than 2% of patients have atrial septal shunting with shunt ratios >1.5. Consequently, the need for septal closure is rare. Persistent shunting is often related to suboptimal left atrial decompression and persistently elevated left atrial pressure, which maintains left-to-right intra-atrial flow.

Outcomes after BMC for calcific MS are not well-characterized. In some cases, there is an excellent acute hemodynamic result, but this seems unpredictable, and catastrophic mitral regurgitation (MR) may just as easily occur.

Long-Term Outcomes

After 5 years, about 70% of patients remain event-free following BMC. Up to 20 years after successful BMC, one-third to half of patients still exhibit a good clinical result defined as freedom from cardiovascular death or the need for mitral surgery or repeat BMC (13). The subgroups of patients with more or less pliable valves have significantly different results. The ideal patient with little valve deformity has a 5-year event-free survival rate that exceeds 80%, while older patients with severe valve and subvalvular deformity may have a 5-year event-free survival closer to 50%. For these older patients, achieving the optimum, durable hemodynamic result is less important, and palliation is the goal of therapy. Re-intervention may be needed in over one-third of patients over the decade following BMC (14). Repeat BMC may be feasible in one out of four of these cases, thereby allowing for postponement of surgery in a substantial number of patients.

An important consideration in assessing the outcomes after BMC is the patient population that is being described. The country from which a report originates is critical to understanding differences in reported procedure outcomes. Patients from the United States undergoing BMC have a mean age of around 55 years. In contrast, reports from Asia describe populations with mean age of 25 to 35 years, and those from India, an even younger population. The course of rheumatic disease differs greatly among these different demographic and age groups. It is critical to understand the differences in specific populations to adequately assess whether surgery or a particular percutaneous approach might be optimal in a given clinical setting. Thus, comparisons among structural heart trials performed in different geographic areas must be made with great caution.

Randomized trials are the ideal manner in which to compare surgical commissurotomy with BMC. Randomized comparisons of balloon and surgical commissurotomy have shown that the two approaches are equivalent. The hemodynamic and valve area results in these trials have been reported with up to a 10-year follow-up (15).

Treatment for patients with significant valve deformity remains an important challenge. Those with echocardiographic scores of <8 can be

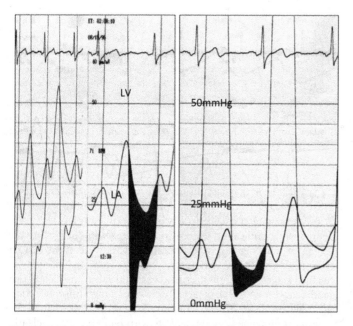

FIGURE 39.2 Simultaneous left atrial (LA) and left ventricular (LV) pressures before and after BMC. On the *left*, the shaded area shows a large transmitral pressure gradient. On the *right*, immediately after BMC, the gradient has been reduced. The left atrial waveform remains unchanged, with no increase in the "V" wave, indicating that this result has been achieved without any significant worsening of mitral regurgitation. BMC, balloon mitral commissurotomy.

expected to have excellent acute and long-term outcomes. Patients with scores >10 have less optimal results, although many are poor candidates for surgery and thus reasonable for BMC as a palliative procedure.

The presence of a left atrial thrombus is a relative contraindication for BMC. Transesophageal echocardiographic screening is a necessary step in preparation for BMC. When left atrial thrombus is found, anticoagulation therapy may be continued for several months with either newly initiated or more aggressive anticoagulant therapy. About 80% of thrombi will resolve after 2 or 3 months. Patients with large mobile thrombi might best be referred for valve replacement surgery to minimize the risk of stroke. Intense left atrial smoke on TTE or transesophageal echocardiography (TEE) is not a contraindication to BMC.

BMC during Pregnancy

Some patients present with MS during pregnancy. Hemodynamic changes in pregnancy provoke dyspnea and sometimes overt heart failure. BMC is the procedure of choice in this setting (16). When clinical circumstances permit, BMC is best performed upon completion of the first trimester, so that fetal organogenesis is relatively complete with lesser risks from radiation exposure for the fetus. Utilization of transthoracic echocardiographic assistance to evaluate improvement in the valve area and the development of mitral regurgitation during the procedure is important to help minimize use of fluoroscopic guidance.

Fluoroscopy times under 4 or 5 minutes should be achievable by experienced operators in pregnant patients. There are reports of successful BMC procedures with echocardiographic guidance without fluoroscopy. The potential for severe mitral regurgitation is no different in a pregnant patient, so a conservative approach to balloon sizing is important. Relief of hemodynamic overload for the short term is the major goal of therapy.

Techniques for BMC

Several techniques have been described to accomplish BMC. Inoue first described the single-balloon antegrade approach in 1984 (Fig. 39.3). Conventional single, double, and monorail balloons have also been utilized (Figs. 39.4 and 39.5). Dilatation is usually performed via an antegrade approach using transseptal puncture. Retrograde access via the aorta with passage of the balloon back into the left atrium is only rarely employed. A catheter metal commissurotomy device, replicating that used in open surgical procedures, has been described, but is no longer manufactured.

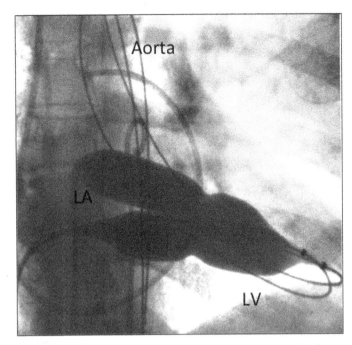

FIGURE 39.4 The double balloon technique. Two conventional balloons have been positioned across the mitral orifice. Double wires can be seen looped in the left ventricle (LV). The course of the wire is from the left atrium (LA), across the mitral valve and through the left ventricle into the aorta. The wires are anchored in the descending aorta.

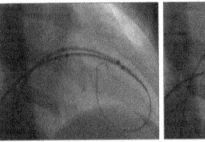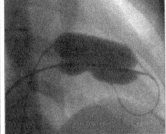

FIGURE 39.5 The multi-track system. On the *left*, a single guide wire can be seen looped in the left ventricular apex. On the *right*, the inflated balloons make it easier to see that the superior of the two balloons is delivered via a short monorail, while an over-the-wire balloon sits below it. This allows a single wire to be utilized for the double balloon approach.

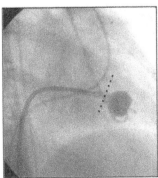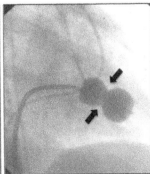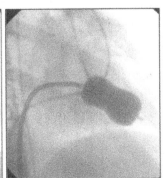

FIGURE 39.3 The Inoue-Balloon Catheter. The left-hand panel shows the partially inflated balloon. It has been pulled back to the plane of the mitral orifice (*dotted line*). This fixes the balloon in the correct position so that with further inflation, shown in the middle panel, the waist of the balloon engages the mitral orifice, shown by the *black arrows*. On the right, the balloon has fully inflated, with relief of the stenosis. From the appearance of the balloon, it is not possible to tell whether one or both commissures have been split.

An adjunct to transseptal procedures is imaging with transesophageal or intracardiac ultrasound (ICE). ICE eliminates the need for general anesthesia during the procedure and involves placement of an 8- or 10-Fr ultrasound catheter in the right atrium. The fossa ovalis can be easily visualized when a transseptal needle is engaged in the fossa, and tenting of the fossa by the transseptal needle toward the left atrium is seen. This imaging modality eliminates some of the risks and difficulties of the transseptal puncture. An additional femoral venous puncture and placement of a 9- or 11-Fr venous sheath is required for ICE. Real-time three-dimensional TEE has recently been introduced. When used in conjunction with BMC, it is associated with expedited transseptal puncture and balloon catheter navigation as reflected in the decreased transseptal-to-balloon time and less reliance on fluoroscopic navigation (17). It comes with the burden of general anesthesia, in comparison to ICE for transseptal puncture, or TTE for procedure monitoring.

The most commonly used device for BMC worldwide is the Inoue-Balloon Catheter (18). The Inoue catheter is introduced into the left atrium, and the partially inflated balloon is passed across the mitral annulus into the left ventricle. Partial inflation of the balloon while it traverses the mitral valve insures that it will be free from chordal entanglement. Once positioned in the left ventricle, the distal end of the balloon is inflated, and the balloon is pulled back until the distal end engages the stenotic mitral orifice (Fig. 39.3). With further inflation, the proximal portion of the balloon inflates, thus straddling the valve. As the balloon is completely inflated, the middle section opens, applying pressure to the commissures and resulting in commissural splitting. The balloon may be inflated with increasing volumes of dilute contrast with resultant sequential or stepwise increases in diameter. After each balloon inflation, the pressure gradient can be measured, and mitral regurgitation assessed either by echocardiographic visualization or by repeat ventriculography. According to the stepwise inflation technique, successive inflations at larger balloon diameters can be performed until either a minimum gradient is achieved or mitral regurgitation begins to increase (19).

BMC may also be accomplished using conventional balloons. Typically, two balloons of 15 to 20 mm in diameter are used together. Two wires must be passed through the transseptal puncture to accomplish this. The wires are looped in the ventricular apex and sometimes passed antegrade into the aorta to provide stability for advancing the balloons into the mitral orifice. The balloon catheters for this approach are longer than the Inoue Balloon, and either the balloon catheter tips or the guide wire may cause perforation of the LV apex. An attractive feature of the Inoue approach is that the balloon is passed or floated into the left ventricle without the use of a guide wire in the left ventricle. Ventricular perforation is thus a rare complication of the Inoue technique.

A double-balloon commissurotomy may also be performed using a single wire across the transseptal access point, with a monorail balloon advanced initially and then a second over-the-wire balloon to follow the first on the same wire. This "multitrack" technique accomplishes the same mechanical effect as double-balloon valvuloplasty, but is simpler and may result in less damage to the atrial septum. The multitrack balloons are not approved for use in the United States.

Finally, it is also possible to accomplish BMC by passing balloons retrograde from the aorta through the left ventricle and across the mitral valve. This approach avoids transseptal puncture, but requires large-caliber bilateral femoral arterial access, and is only rarely employed (20).

Bioprosthetic Stenosis

Porcine or bovine pericardial prosthetic valves all suffer from a limited lifespan due to a process of mineralization and collagen degeneration over time. Cuspal tears, fibrin deposition, disruption of the fibrocollagenous structure, perforation, fibrosis, and calcium infiltration begin to appear after a few years, and by 10 years, tissue valve failure occurs in about 30%. The process then accelerates, and by 15 years, over half of the valves will have failed. Patients on dialysis are particularly susceptible to early prosthetic leaflet failure. Other factors that have been identified include younger age, pregnancy, and hypercalcemia.

Commissural fusion is uncommon in these valves, the major problem being leaflet immobility. At times, these valves become functionally stenotic. From an anatomic standpoint, the use of percutaneous balloon valvuloplasty procedures is problematic given the lack of commissural fusion. There are limited data regarding the use of balloon procedures in prosthetic valve stenosis. It has been reported successfully in isolated cases. Limited follow-up is available and restenosis occurs quickly. There is a strong reporting bias in the case reports that are available, because failures are rarely reported. Bench-top testing in degenerated valves has demonstrated leaflet tearing and fragmentation due to the patchy nature of calcification, with areas of calcium adjacent to areas of thinning, creating interface where tearing may occur. There are no prospective studies that have addressed the safety and efficacy of this procedure, and it is not recommended based on the anecdotal evidence for poor results. The valve-in-valve technique using transcatheter aortic valve replacement (TAVR) devices in the mitral position is emerging as the best transcatheter therapy for bioprosthetic deterioration. This approach has been successful for a wide range of modes of failure of bioprosthetic valves (21).

Percutaneous Mitral Valve Repair

Percutaneous mitral valve repair has developed steadily over the past decade and transcatheter mitral replacement has now emerged in early human clinical trials. Mitral repair in particular has entered practice in many parts of the world and has growing use in the United States. Percutaneous mitral repair in US practice at this point is synonymous with leaflet repair using the MitraClip device. The MitraClip is an implantable device that is delivered transvenously, via a transseptal approach. The clip is used to grasp the anterior and posterior mitral valve leaflets. This leaflet repair therapy is modeled on a surgical method for suturing the free edges of the mitral leaflets together to create a double orifice valve, known as the Alfieri or edge-to-edge repair. It is most applicable to patients with mitral regurgitation that arises from the central parts of the line of mitral leaflet coaptation. A randomized trial comparing surgical repair with MitraClip has been completed, and demonstrates that while the MitraClip device is less effective at reducing mitral regurgitation, the impact on favorable LV remodeling, clinical outcomes measured by quality-of-life questionnaires, and the NYHA Class had similar outcomes compared to surgical valve repair or replacement (22).

Importantly, subgroup analysis of this pivotal randomized trial demonstrated the most favorable outcomes in patients who are over age 70 years, with abnormal LV function, and with functional rather than degenerative mitral regurgitation. Accordingly, a registry of over 350 patients with predominantly functional MR have 1-year outcomes reported, with excellent reductions in mitral regurgitation and improvement in symptoms (23). This high-risk cohort showed a significant decrease in hospitalizations for heart failure following MitraClip therapy, and improved survival compared to a small nonrandomized control group. Importantly, despite advanced age and a high level of comorbidities, the procedural safety and 30-day mortality is low, with a short hospital stay averaging under 3 days, and a rate of discharge to home over 85%.

TABLE 39.3 AHA/ACC Guideline Recommendations for Surgery or Intervention for Chronic Primary MR

Class I

MV surgery is recommended for symptomatic patients with chronic severe primary MR (stage D) and LVEF > 30%.

MV surgery is recommended for asymptomatic patients with chronic severe primary MR and LV dysfunction (LVEF 30%–60% and/or LVESD 40 mm, stage C2).

MV repair is recommended in preference to MVR when surgical treatment is indicated for patients with chronic severe primary MR limited to the posterior leaflet.

MV repair is recommended in preference to MVR when surgical treatment is indicated for patients with chronic severe primary MR involving the anterior leaflet or both leaflets when a successful and durable repair can be accomplished.

Concomitant MV repair or replacement is indicated in patients with chronic severe primary MR undergoing cardiac surgery for other indications.

Class IIa

MV repair is reasonable in asymptomatic patients with chronic severe primary MR (stage C1) with preserved LV function (LVEF >60% and LVESD <40 mm) in whom the likelihood of a successful and durable repair without residual MR is >95% with an expected mortality rate of <1% when performed at a Heart Valve Center of Excellence

MV repair is reasonable for asymptomatic patients with chronic severe nonrheumatic primary MR (stage C1) and preserved LV function in whom there is a high likelihood of a successful and durable repair with (1) new onset of AF or (2) resting pulmonary hypertension (PA systolic arterial pressure >50 mm Hg).

Concomitant MV repair is reasonable in patients with chronic moderate primary MR (stage B) undergoing cardiac surgery for other indications.

Class IIb

MV surgery may be considered in symptomatic patients with chronic severe primary MR and LVEF 30% (stage D).

MV repair may be considered in patients with rheumatic mitral valve disease when surgical treatment is indicated if a durable and successful repair is likely or if the reliability of long-term anticoagulation management is questionable.

Transcatheter MV repair may be considered for severely symptomatic patients (NYHA class III/IV) with chronic severe primary MR (stage D) who have a reasonable life expectancy but a prohibitive surgical risk because of severe comorbidities.

Class III

MVR should not be performed for treatment of isolated severe primary MR limited to less than one half of the posterior leaflet unless MV repair has been attempted and was unsuccessful.

AF, atrial fibrillation; LV, left ventricle; LVEF, left ventricular ejection fraction; LVESD, left ventricular end-systolic diameter; MR, mitral regurgitation; MV, mitral valve; MVR, mitral valve replacement; NYHA, New York Heart Association; PA, pulmonary artery.

A subgroup analysis of patients with degenerative MR from this high-risk group ultimately led to the FDA approval of MitraClip for high-risk degenerative mitral regurgitation (DMR) in the United States (24). MitraClip in these prohibitive surgical risk patients was associated with safety and good clinical outcomes, including decreases in rehospitalization, functional improvements, and favorable ventricular remodeling, at 1 year. The specific language of the approval states that the MitraClip Clip Delivery System is indicated for the percutaneous reduction of significant symptomatic mitral regurgitation (MR ≥ 3+) due to primary abnormality of the mitral apparatus (degenerative MR) in patients who have been determined to be at prohibitive risk for mitral valve surgery by a heart team, which includes a cardiac surgeon experienced in mitral valve surgery and a cardiologist experienced in mitral valve disease, and in whom existing comorbidities would not preclude the expected benefit from reduction of the mitral regurgitation (Table 39.3). The MitraClip Clip Delivery System is contraindicated in DMR patients who cannot tolerate procedural anticoagulation or a post-procedural antiplatelet regimen, have active endocarditis of the mitral valve, rheumatic etiology for mitral valve disease, or evidence of intra-cardiac, inferior vena cava or femoral venous thrombus.

The majority of use for MitraClip in international practice is for high-risk patients with ischemic functional mitral regurgitation (FMR). To date, all of the reported outcomes in this patient group are registries. The results of the registries are all concordant, with procedure results of low early mortality, short hospital stays, and high rates of discharge to home (Table 39.4). The clinical outcomes have similarly been good

TABLE 39.4 Patient Characteristics and Procedure Outcomes in the ACC/STS TVT Valve Registry (29)

N = 564	
Age, years	83 (74–87)
Atrial fibrillation	63%
Prior CABG	33%
STS-PROM score replacement ≥8%	44%
Left ventricular ejection fraction, %	56 (45–63)
Device implant success	94%
Post-implant MR grade >2+	6.9%
Single leaflet device attachment	1.1%
Device embolization	0.4%
Delivery system component embolization	0
Device thrombosis	0
Open heart surgery	0.7%
Median length of hospital stay	3 days
Death 30 days	5.8%
Any stroke 30 days	1.8%

CABG, coronary artery bypass grafting; MR, mitral regurgitation; PROM, predicted risk of mortality; TVT, transcatheter valve therapies.

TABLE 39.5 AHA/ACC Guideline Recommendations for Surgery or Intervention for Chronic Secondary MR

Class IIa

MV surgery is reasonable for patients with chronic severe secondary MR (stages C and D) who are undergoing CABG or AVR.

Class IIb

MV surgery may be considered for severely symptomatic patients (NYHA class III/IV) with chronic severe secondary MR (stage D)

MV repair may be considered for patients with chronic moderate secondary MR (stage B) who are undergoing other cardiac surgery

AVR, aortic valve replacement; CABG, coronary artery bypass grafting; MR, mitral regurgitation; MV, mitral valve; NYHA, New York Heart Association.

with most patients feeling improved, and with decreased rates of heart failure hospitalization (25). There remains uncertainty about the role of mitral repair for functional ischemic MR (**Table 39.5**). What has been missing from this clinical database is a comparison of MitraClip with medical therapy (including cardiac resynchronization therapy), which is necessary for FDA approval in the US. Two randomized

trials to address this open question are underway. Mitra-France is ongoing and is randomizing 288 patients, with a combined 1-year endpoint of death and heart failure hospitalizations. The COAPT trial is randomizing 610 patients, with a 1-year endpoint of heart failure hospitalizations (**Figs. 39.6–39.10**). The results of these trials will define the role of MitraClip in functional ischemic MR.

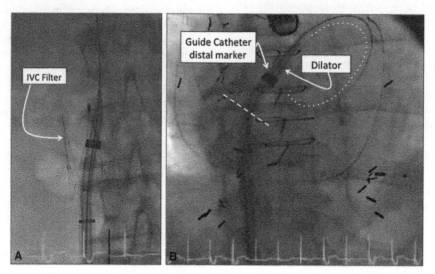

FIGURE 39.6 Figures 39.6–39.9 represent the procedure sequence in a single patient undergoing MitraClip repair for functional mitral regurgitation in the COAPT trial. MitraClip guide catheter insertion. The 24-French guide catheter is inserted into the femoral vein and passed into the left atrium after transseptal puncture. Panel **A** shows the guide catheter traversing an inferior vena cava filter over a guide wire. Panel **B** shows the guide catheter and dilator across the atrial septum (*dashed line*). The guide wire is a pre-curved 0.035-inch wire, denoted by the *dotted line*.

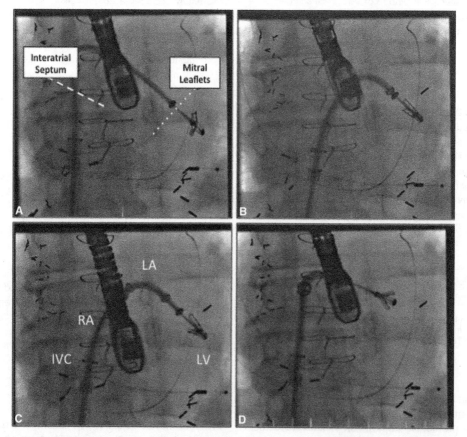

FIGURE 39.7 Panel **A** shows the MitraClip device inserted through the guide catheter and passed across the mitral valve into the left ventricle. A transesophageal echo probe is noted in the picture. Panel **B** shows the clip having been pulled back and closed to capture the mitral leaflets. Panel **C** shows the clip being released due to insufficient reduction in mitral regurgitation. Panel **D** shows the clip everted, so it can be safely pulled back into the left atrium and another grasp attempted. IVC, inferior vena cava; LA, left atrium; LV, left ventricle; RA, right atrium.

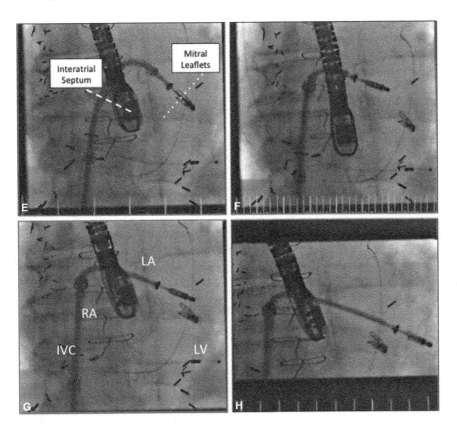

FIGURE 39.8   Panel **E** shows the second grasp attempt with the clip closed on the leaflets. Panel **F** shows the first clip released and in place. A second clip is now being passed through the mitral orifice lateral to the first clip. Panel **G** shows the second clip traversing the mitral leaflets and orifice adjacent to the first clip. Panel **H** shows the second clip in the left ventricle in a closed position. IVC, inferior vena cava; LA, left atrium; LV, left ventricle; RA, right atrium.

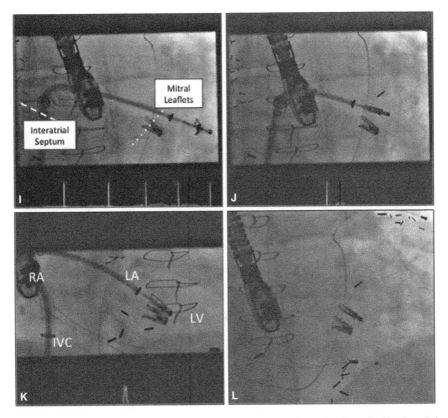

FIGURE 39.9   Panel **I** shows the second clip open in the left ventricle, and Panel **J** shows the clip pulled back and closed on the mitral leaflets. Panel **K** shows the second clip adjacent to the first clip in a closed position. Panel **L** shows both clips after release in their final positions. IVC, inferior vena cava; LA, left atrium; LV, left ventricle; RA, right atrium.

Three other technologies are approved for use outside the United States in Europe and internationally (26). All of them are annuloplasty devices. The Cardiac Dimensions Carillon (Fig. 39.11), Valtech Cardioband (Fig. 39.12), and Mitralign annuloplasty (Fig. 39.13) devices all have CE approval based on small registries. Only the Carillon and Cardioband are being distributed and used. The Carillon is an indirect annuloplasty approach, utilizing a wireform device that is implanted in the coronary sinus. The Cardioband is delivered via transseptal approach to the left atrial side of the mitral annulus. The Cardioband most closely approximates a surgical annuloplasty device. Early results with this group of devices has shown consistent 1 to

2 grade improvements in MR severity, improved exercise capacity, and improved quality of life and NYHA Class. Randomized pivotal US trials are being planned.

Transcatheter Mitral Valve Replacement

TMVR is also under development (27). Proof of concept can be found in some experience using TAVR valves for implantation in prior mitral bioprosthetic vales (Fig. 39.14), annuloplasty rings (Fig. 39.15), or native mitral valves with stenosis due to mitral annular calcification

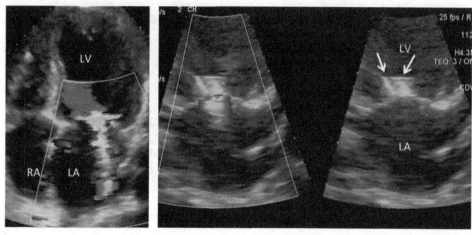

FIGURE 39.10   On the *left* is a transthoracic echocardiogram from the MitraClip patient in Figures 39.7–39.9, taken before the MitraClip procedure. Severe mitral regurgitation is easily seen. On the *right*, two clips can be seen, denoted by the *arrows*. The mitral regurgitation has been reduced to a trivial grade. LA, left atrium; LV, left ventricle.

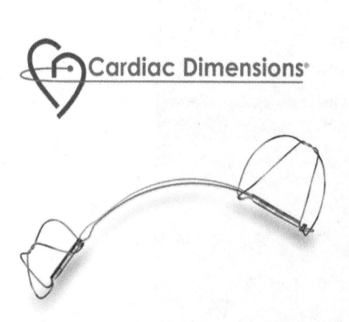

FIGURE 39.11   The Cardiac Dimensions Carillon device. This is a coronary sinus annuloplasty device. A smaller anchor is placed distally in the great cardiac vein, and the larger anchor near the coronary sinus ostium. The device is tensioned to reduce the mitral annular circumference.

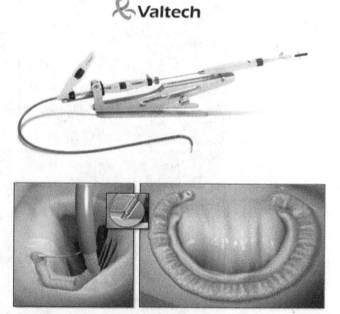

FIGURE 39.12   The Valtech Cardioband. The upper part of the figure shows the delivery system. On the *left*, a transseptal catheter delivers the annuloplasty band in steps. A screw is used to anchor each of the segments of the device. On the *right*, the final incomplete annuloplasty ring can be seen.

(28). There are significant challenges that differentiate native mitral from aortic catheter valve replacement. For transcatheter aortic valve replacement, the aortic stent valve can anchor securely in the deformed and calcified native aortic valve. For the mitral valve, the challenge of anchoring is more complex due to the larger annulus area, asymmetry, and lack of calcification. Several concepts to overcome these limitations are under development, and early human therapy is underway. Ultimately, mitral valve replacements may be a more generally applicable catheter therapy for severe mitral regurgitation than the various repair approaches. Over 30 companies have TMVR device concepts, prototypes, or some level of early human experience. Among the challenges is thrombus formation, due in part to the large bulk of these devices and the low flow or stasis in the left atrium. One trial,

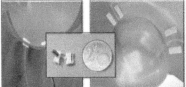

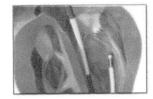

FIGURE 39.13 The Mitralign device. On the *left*, a guide catheter has been passed retrograde across the aortic valve with the distal tip of the guide catheter behind the anterior mitral leaflet. In the center, pledgets are placed through the annulus and then cinched together to reduce the annular circumference as seen on the *right*.

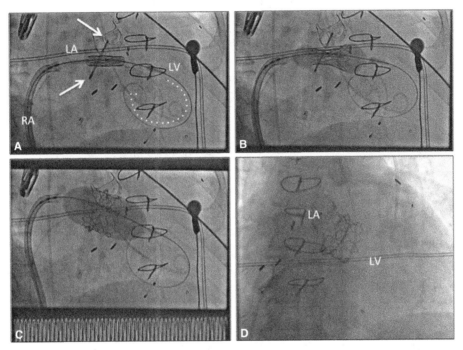

FIGURE 39.14 A transcatheter aortic valve device being placed in a prior mitral annuloplasty ring. Panel **A** has two *arrows* that denote the edges of the ring. The TAVR device delivery system is introduced transseptally and the device is passed from the left atrium to the left ventricle across the ring. The *dotted line* shows a pre-formed curved guide wire in the left ventricular apex. Panel **B** shows balloon inflation of the neo-valve in the mitral annuloplasty ring. Panel **C** shows full inflation of the valve. The electrocardiographic trace at the bottom of the image shows the rapid ventricular pacing used during balloon inflation and valve deployment. Panel **D** shows the final appearance of the fully deployed valve prosthetic. LA, left atrium; LV, left ventricle; TAVR, transcatheter aortic valve replacement.

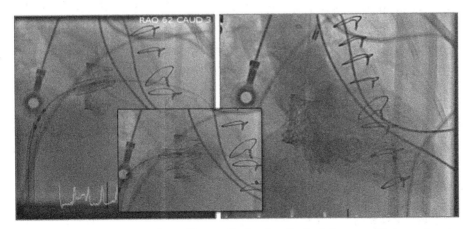

FIGURE 39.15 Aortic valve device and degenerated mitral bioprosthetic valve. On the *left*, a transcatheter aortic valve replacement (TAVR) device can be seen across the bioprosthetic mitral valve. The *middle* in-stent shows balloon inflation. On the *right*, a ventriculogram demonstrates a competent mitral valve-in-valve.

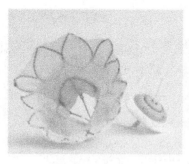
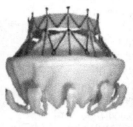
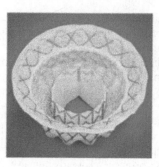

Tendyne-Abbott   CardiAQ-Edwards   TWELVE-Medtronic

FIGURE 39.16 Transcatheter mitral valve replacement devices.

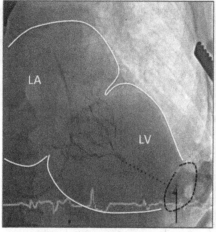
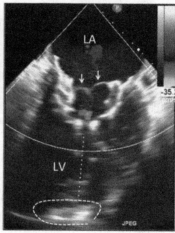

FIGURE 39.17 The Tendyne valve is placed via apical access, using a left ventricular apical anchor (*dashed circle*) and a tether (*dotted line*). The valve prosthesis can be seen in the mitral annulus. On the *right*, an echocardiographic image shows the same features with *arrows* pointing at the neo-leaflets of the prosthetic mitral valve. LA, left atrium; LV, left ventricle.

using the Edwards Fortis valve, was stopped due to device thrombus formation. Despite the complexity inherent in TMVR development, three device companies spent an aggregate of over $1 billion in the second half of 2015 to acquire TMVR startup companies. Edwards, Medtronic, and Abbott purchased CardiAQ, Twelve, and Tendyne Holdings, respectively (**Fig. 39.16**). These TMVR devices are implanted mostly via transapical access (**Fig. 39.17**), with plans to develop antegrade transseptal delivery systems. Another concept for TMVR is to implant a frame or docking device, into which the valve itself is placed. The M-Valve system uses this approach to place a dock, into which a standard TAVR device can be placed. Caisson Interventional has a system that places an atrial frame and then the leaflets from a transseptal approach, and has successfully started early human trials.

Key Points

Percutaneous Transvenous Mitral Commissurotomy

■ Percutaneous transvenous mitral commissurotomy (PTMC) is the therapy of choice for most patients with predominant MS.

■ Randomized comparisons with surgery show no advantages to surgical commissurotomy.

■ Asymptomatic patients with MS should be considered for catheter commissurotomy when the pulmonary artery systolic pressure is >50 mm Hg at rest or 60 mm Hg with exercise.

■ Urgent or emergency surgery is required for the PTMC complication of severe MR in 2% to 3% of cases.

■ PTMC has not had predictable results for non-rheumatic MS, such as due to mitral annular calcification.

Percutaneous Mitral Valve Repair

■ Percutaneous mitral repair in US practice at this point is synonymous with leaflet repair using the MitraClip device.

■ Current FDA approval of MitraClip is for high-risk degenerative MR in the United States.

■ The majority of use for MitraClip in international practice is for high-risk patients with ischemic FMR. Ongoing trials will compare medical therapy with MitraClip for FMR.

■ Three other annuloplasty devices are approved for use internationally and will undergo US trials.

■ TMVR is also under development but is at an early stage.

References

1. Inoue K, et al. Clinical application of transvenous mitral commissurotomy by a new balloon catheter. *J Thorac Cardiovasc Surg.* 1984;87:394–402.

2. Lock JE, et al. Percutaneous catheter commissurotomy in rheumatic mitral stenosis. *N Engl J Med.* 1985;313:1515–1518.

3. Cribier A, et al. Percutaneous transluminal valvuloplasty of acquired aortic stenosis in elderly patients: an alternative to valve replacement? *Lancet.* 1986;1:63–67.

4. Nulu S, Bukhman G, Kwan GF. Rheumatic heart disease: the unfinished global agenda [review]. *Cardiol Clin.* 2017;35(1):165–180. doi:10.1016/j.ccl.2016.08.006.

5. Feldman T. Rheumatic heart disease. *Curr Opin Cardiol.* 1996;11:126–130.

6. Zühlke L, et al. Characteristics, complications, and gaps in evidence-based interventions in rheumatic heart disease: the Global Rheumatic Heart Disease Registry (the REMEDY study). *Eur Heart J.* 2015;36(18):1115a–1122a.

7. Picano E, et al. The emerging role of exercise testing and stress echocardiography in valvular heart disease. *J Am Coll Cardiol.* 2009;54(24):2251–2260.

8. Wilkins GT, et al. Percutaneous balloon dilatation of the mitral valve: an analysis of echocardiographic variables related to outcome and the mechanism of dilatation. *Br Heart J.* 1988;60:299–308.

9. Nishimura RA, et al. 2014 AHA/ACC guideline for the management of patients with valvular heart disease: a report of the American College of Cardiology/American Heart Association Task Force on Practice Guidelines. *J Am Coll Cardiol.* 2014;63:e57–e185.

10. Hart SA, et al. Pulmonary hypertension and elevated transpulmonary gradient in patients with mitral stenosis. *J Heart Valve Dis.* 2010;19(6):708–715.

11. Badheka AO, et al. Balloon mitral valvuloplasty in the United States: a 13-year perspective. *Am J Med.* 2014;127(11):1126.e1–1126.e12. doi:10.1016/j.amjmed.2014.05.015.

12. Manjunath CN, et al. Incidence and predictors of atrial septal defect after percutaneous transvenous mitral commissurotomy—a transesophageal echocardiographic study of 209 cases. *Echocardiography.* 2013;30(2):127–130.

13. Tomai F, et al. Twenty year follow-up after successful percutaneous balloon mitral valvuloplasty in a large contemporary series of patients with mitral stenosis. *Int J Cardiol.* 2014;177(3):881–885. doi:10.1016/j.ijcard.2014.10.040.

14. Bouleti C, et al. Reinterventions after percutaneous mitral commissurotomy during long-term follow-up, up to 20 years: the role of repeat percutaneous mitral commissurotomy. *Eur Heart J.* 2013;34(25):1923–1930.

15. Reyes VP, et al. Percutaneous balloon valvuloplasty compared with open surgical commissurotomy for mitral stenosis. *N Engl J Med.* 1994;331:961–967.

16. Esteves CA, et al. Immediate and long-term follow-up of percutaneous balloon mitral valvuloplasty in pregnant patients with rheumatic mitral stenosis. *Am J Cardiol.* 2006;98(6):812–816.

17. Eng MH, et al. Implementation of real-time three-dimensional transesophageal echocardiography for mitral balloon valvuloplasty. *Catheter Cardiovasc Interv.* 2013;82(6):994–998.

18. Feldman T, Herrmann HC, Inoue K. Technique of percutaneous transvenous mitral commissurotomy using the Inoue balloon catheter. *Cathet Cardiovasc Diagn.* 1994;2(suppl):26–34.

19. Feldman T, et al. Effect of balloon size and stepwise inflation technique on the acute results of Inoue mitral commissurotomy: Inoue balloon catheter investigators. *Cathet Cardiovasc Diagn.* 1993;28:199–205.

20. Nath RK, Soni DK. Retrograde non trans-septal balloon mitral valvotomy in mitral stenosis with interrupted inferior vena cava, left superior vena cava, and hugely dilated coronary sinus. *Catheter Cardiovasc Interv.* 2015;86(7):1289–1293. doi:10.1002/ccd.25973.

21. Codner P, et al. Treatment of aortic, mitral and tricuspid structural bioprosthetic valve deterioration using the valve-in-valve technique. *J Heart Valve Dis.* 2015;24(3):345–352.

22. Feldman T, et al. Percutaneous repair or surgery for mitral regurgitation. *N Engl J Med.* 2011;364:1395–1406.

23. Glower DD, et al. Percutaneous mitral valve repair for mitral regurgitation in high-risk patients: results of the EVEREST II study. *J Am Coll Cardiol.* 2014;64(2):172–181.

24. Lim DS, et al. Improved functional status and quality of life in prohibitive surgical risk patients with degenerative mitral regurgitation after transcatheter mitral valve repair. *J Am Coll Cardiol.* 2014;64(2):182–192.

25. Philip F, et al. MitraClip for severe symptomatic mitral regurgitation in patients at high surgical risk: a comprehensive systematic review. *Catheter Cardiovasc Interv.* 2014;84(4):581–590.

26. Feldman T, Guerrero M, Salinger MH. Emerging technologies for direct and indirect percutaneous mitral annuloplasty. *EuroIntervention.* 2016;12:Y1–Y6.

27. Feldman T, Guerrero M. The future of transcatheter therapy for mitral valve disease. *Cardiovasc Innov Appl.* 2016;1(3):287–299. doi:10.15212/CVIA.2016.0017.

28. Guerrero M, et al. Transcatheter mitral valve replacement in native mitral valve disease with severe mitral annular calcification results from the first multicenter global registry. *JACC Cardiovasc Interv.* 2016;9(13):1361–1371. doi:10.1016/j.jcin.2016.04.022.

29. Sorajja P, et al. Initial experience with commercial transcatheter mitral valve repair in the United States. *J Am Coll Cardiol.* 2016;67(10):1129–1140. doi:10.1016/j.jacc.2015.12.054.

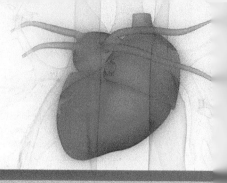

40 Transcatheter Aortic Valve Replacement

William Suh, MD, FSCAI

Age-related calcific aortic stenosis (AS) is the most common form of AS. Approximately 3% of patients over the age of 75 years have severe AS. The presence of symptoms (i.e., angina, syncope, heart failure) in the setting of severe AS is known to portend a dismal prognosis (1). Surgical aortic valve replacement (SAVR) has been proven to improve both survival and quality of life in symptomatic AS patients and remains the standard of care for low-surgical-risk AS patients. Per AHA/ACC guidelines, SAVR is a class I recommendation with level of evidence B in symptomatic AS patients (2). The reason the recommendation does not have a level of evidence A is that no randomized trials have ever been done comparing SAVR to medical therapy. Despite the guideline recommendation, many patients with severe symptomatic AS are not offered surgery. In fact, the Euro Heart Survey on valvular heart disease documented that 33% of patients above the age of 75 years with severe symptomatic AS were denied SAVR (3). The reason for this is believed to be the combination of advanced age and the presence of medical comorbidities.

Before the advent of transcatheter aortic valve replacement (TAVR), the alternative to SAVR in patients deemed too "high risk" for surgery was balloon aortic valvuloplasty (BAV). Introduced in the mid-1980s, BAV as a therapy had been limited by high rates of both early and late restenosis (4). BAV is a procedure in which a stiff 0.035-inch guide wire is placed into the left ventricle in a retrograde fashion and a 20- to 25-mm diameter balloon is inflated multiple times to "crack" the stenotic valve open. In addition to high rates of restenosis, the procedural risks of BAV include embolic stroke, vascular complications, and severe aortic insufficiency. Currently, the AHA/ACC guidelines limit the use of BAV to either cases of palliation or situations "to bridge" unstable patients to a more definitive therapy, such as aortic valve replacement (AVR) (2).

In 2011, the FDA approved the Edwards SAPIEN valve for TAVR in inoperable patients. The following year, the FDA approved the SAPIEN valve for TAVR in high-risk patients (STS predicted risk of mortality 8% or higher). In 2014, the FDA approved the Medtronic CoreValve for TAVR in extreme-risk and high-risk patients. This chapter discusses the TAVR procedure, the data supporting its use, and issues surrounding the procedure.

TAVR Valves

The Edwards SAPIEN 3 valve and the Medtronic CoreValve Evolut R are the only two FDA-approved aortic transcatheter heart valves currently available for commercial use (Fig. 40.1). The SAPIEN family of valves has been studied in the Placement of Aortic Transcatheter Valves (PARTNER) and PARTNER 2 trials (5–7), the latter investigating TAVR in intermediate-risk patients (STS PROM 4%–8%). The SAPIEN 3 valve is a balloon-expandable cobalt chromium frame with bovine pericardial leaflets. It also has a polyethylene terephthalate (PET) outer sealing skirt to reduce paravalvular leak (PVL). The CoreValve family of valves has been studied in the CoreValve US Pivotal Trials (8,9). SURTAVI is the CoreValve intermediate-risk trial. CoreValve

Evolut R is a self-expanding nitinol frame with porcine pericardial leaflets. It has an extended sealing skirt compared to previous CoreValve designs, so as to reduce PVL. Evolut R also is recapturable and repositionable, unlike the balloon-expandable valves.

Preprocedural Evaluation

Paramount to a successful TAVR procedure is the pre-procedural evaluation of the patient and procedural planning. This assessment should provide key information regarding the patient's candidacy for TAVR. STS score and EuroSCORE provide a predicted risk of mortality with SAVR. As of August 2016, patients in the United States with symptomatic AS are eligible for TAVR if they are intermediate risk, high risk, or inoperable. Low-risk patients may be eligible for clinical trial participation. Patients being evaluated for TAVR should be assessed by the Heart Team, a multidisciplinary team that performs a comprehensive evaluation of the patient. An evaluation should include an assessment of the severity of the valve disease, the presence of any coronary artery disease and/or left ventricular dysfunction, the presence of concomitant medical comorbidities (e.g., chronic obstructive pulmonary disease [COPD], peripheral arterial disease, or renal insufficiency), a thorough evaluation of the peripheral arteries for vascular access, and an assessment of the patient's frailty.

The workup entails transthoracic echocardiography (TTE) and/or transesophageal echocardiography (TEE), cardiac catheterization for evaluation of coronary anatomy and hemodynamic parameters, pulmonary function testing, carotid duplex imaging, computed tomography angiography (CTA), and objective testing to measure frailty. The four main components of frailty include independence in activities of daily living, gait speed, grip strength, and nutrition. CTA has emerged as the imaging modality of choice for the preprocedural workup of the TAVR patient. In addition to obtaining accurate and reproducible measurements of the ileofemoral

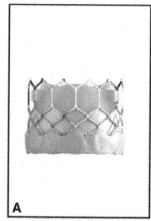
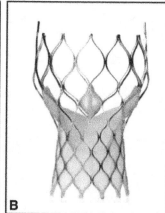

FIGURE 40.1 Panel **A:** Edwards balloon-expandable SAPIEN 3 transcatheter aortic valve. Panel **B:** Medtronic self-expanding CoreValve Evolut R transcatheter aortic valve.

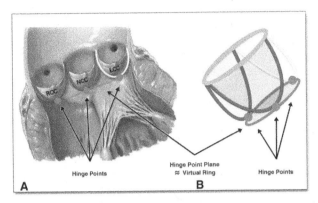

FIGURE 40.2 Normal Anatomy of the Aortic Annulus. The aortic annulus accounts for the tightest part of the aortic root **(A)** and is defined as a virtual ring (green line) with 3 anatomical anchor points at the nadir (green points) of each of the attachments of the 3 aortic leaflets **(B)**. LCC = left coronary cusp; NCC = noncoronary cusp; RCC = right coronary cusp. (From: Kasel AM, et al. Standardized imaging for aortic annular sizing: implications for transcatheter valve selection. *JACC Cardiovasc Imaging*. 2013;6(2):249–262.)

anatomy for access, CTA provides valuable information regarding aortic valve annular dimensions, the presence of ascending aortic calcification (porcelain aorta), and the anatomy of the ascending aorta and related structures.

Accurate measurements of the annular area and perimeter are the most critical aspect of procedural planning because this determines which prosthesis size will be implanted. If the prosthesis is too small, there is increased risk of device embolization and PVL. If the prosthesis is too large, there is increased risk of annular rupture, aortic dissection, and coronary obstruction. The aortic annulus accounts for the narrowest part of the aortic root and is defined as a virtual ring with three anatomical anchor points at the nadir of each coronary cusp (**Fig. 40.2**) (10). Three-dimensional multiplanar reconstruction CTA is considered the gold standard for measuring the aortic annulus, as well as coronary heights, the presence of annular calcification, and Sinuses of Valsalva and sinotubular junction dimensions (**Fig. 40.3**). Three-dimensional TEE is an alternative imaging modality, especially for a patient with chronic kidney disease who is at risk for contrast nephropathy (**Fig. 40.4**).

The presence of medical comorbidities needs to be addressed at the evaluation stage. The presence of any malignancy should be evaluated for short- and long-term prognosis. The benefits of TAVR

in patients with severe dementia or very frail patients may be limited. These patients are sometimes referred to as cohort C patients; they are "too sick" for even TAVR. Decisions should also be made regarding the need for pre-TAVR coronary revascularization procedures.

Preprocedural evaluation of vascular access is another critical aspect to determine suitability for a transfemoral (TF) approach for TAVR. The Edwards SAPIEN valve originally came in two sizes: 23 mm and 26 mm. The 23-mm valve required a minimum ileofemoral diameter (MID) of 7 mm for a 22-F sheath, and the 26-mm valve required a MID of 8 mm for a 24-F sheath. SAPIEN 3 is available in four sizes (20 mm, 23 mm, 26 mm, and 29 mm). The three smaller sizes can be delivered via a 14-F expandable sheath (MID 5.5 mm), whereas the largest 29-mm valve is delivered via a 16-F expandable sheath (MID 6.0 mm). CoreValve was originally available in four sizes (23 mm, 26 mm, 29 mm, and 31 mm). All valve sizes could be delivered via an 18-F sheath. CoreValve Evolut R is available in the same four sizes, but the delivery sheath has been reduced to 14F (MID 5.0 mm). The reduction in delivery sheath diameters has drastically reduced vascular complication rates and the need for alternative access. Nevertheless, if a patient does not have adequate ileofemoral access, alternative access sites can be used. Transapical (TA) access is only feasible with the balloon-expandable valves. Transaortic, subclavian, and carotid access can be considered for both balloon-expandable and self-expanding systems.

A careful assessment needs to be made of the vessel size, angulation, calcification, and tortuosity in planning a strategy for access (**Fig. 40.5**).

Procedural Imaging Modalities

Fluoroscopy/angiography is the mainstay of imaging used for all aspects of the transcatheter valve delivery, positioning, and deployment. It is not used in isolation, but echocardiography and CT are complementary. Fluoroscopy is used to carefully obtain vascular access and position the delivery sheath. In addition, fluoroscopy is used to identify aortic valvular calcification and to establish landmarks for valve positioning prior to deployment.

Selecting the optimal angiographic view is necessary for proper valve positioning. The view must identify the three aortic valve sinuses in a coplanar configuration, with minimal overlap with the spine so that the calcification of the aortic valve/annulus can be clearly visualized. The coplanar alignment of the sinuses allows for proper assessment of valve position prior to deployment. The image detector angulation to give the coplanar view can be predicted by CTA but the coplanar view can also be achieved by using the "follow the right cusp" rule (**Fig. 40.6**) (11).

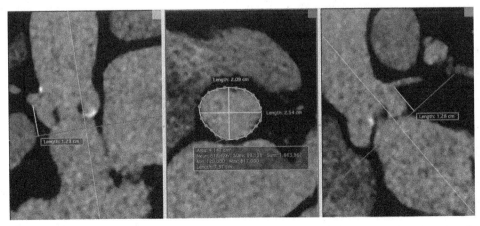

FIGURE 40.3 Multiplanar reconstruction of the aortic annulus from computed tomography angiography (CTA). Annular area, perimeter, and minimum and maximum diameters are all measured. The distance from the annular plane to the left and right coronary arteries are also measured.

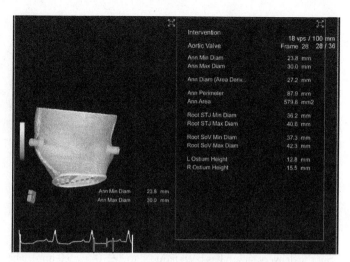

FIGURE 40.4 Automated 3D reconstruction of the aortic valve complex from transesophageal echocardiography (TEE). Annulus, Sinuses of Valsalva, sinotubular junction, and coronary heights are all measured.

Echo (TTE or TEE) during the procedure is important for defining valvular anatomy, annular sizing, and quantifying valvular regurgitation and ventricular function intraprocedurally. After deployment, echo is necessary to accurately assess for either valvular or paravalvular aortic regurgitation (AR), ventricular function, mitral valve function, and pericardial effusion/tamponade. An immediate assessment can be helpful in identifying a potential complication of the valve deployment.

Transcatheter Valve Delivery, Positioning, and Deployment

For the purposes of this chapter, we will focus on the TF approach to TAVR (TF-TAVR) because TF is primarily an interventional cardiology procedure and is feasible in almost 90% of cases.

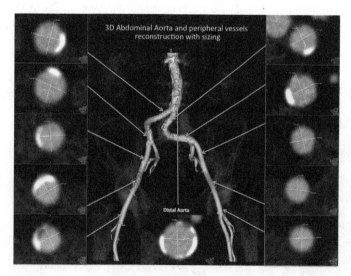

FIGURE 40.5 Three-dimensional reconstruction of the ileofemoral anatomy demonstrating dimensions, calcification, angulation, and tortuosity of the arterial vessels. The axial images also provide the circumferential extent of calcification.

A hybrid operating room/catheterization laboratory that will allow for simultaneous fluoroscopy-guided catheter manipulation and possible conversion to open surgery is necessary for TAVR procedures. It should also be large enough to accommodate a team consisting of cardiac anesthesiologists, echocardiographers, perfusionists, cardiac surgeons, and interventional cardiologists.

In the early experience of TF-TAVR, endovascular access was obtained via surgical cutdown to expose the common femoral artery, given the large sheath diameters. Currently, percutaneous access of the common femoral artery is the preferred mode of vascular access utilizing a suture-based preclose method. Shifting to a totally percutaneous procedure and reduced need for TEE in evaluating PVL with the newer devices has allowed many operators to take a "minimalist" approach to TAVR. TAVR is more commonly being performed without general anesthesia, without invasive hemodynamic monitoring (arterial line and pulmonary artery catheter), or bladder catheterization. Conversion to open heart surgery is so rare that many centers have also removed cardiopulmonary bypass and perfusionist standby from the procedure. Taking a "minimalist" approach can make a substantial impact on recovery time, reduce length of stay, and reduce costs. Elderly patients often are fearful of general anesthesia and its potential complications, and therefore often welcome a conscious sedation approach.

Once percutaneous access is obtained in the common femoral artery and preclosed, the vessel is serially dilated and the valve sheath is carefully inserted under fluoroscopic guidance. Anticoagulation with heparin should be initiated before placement of the large valve sheath. Bivalirudin should not be used because there is no clinical benefit and cannot be reversed in case there is a bleeding complication (12). Venous and arterial access is also obtained on the contralateral side for placement of a temporary transvenous pacemaker and a pigtail catheter, respectively.

Once the desired view has been decided upon for valve positioning, a BAV is routinely performed prior to valve delivery to create space for the transcatheter valve inside the native stenosed aortic valve. It is important to be aware of the degree of aortic insufficiency present prior to BAV, as a sudden worsening of aortic insufficiency can sometimes lead to hemodynamic instability.

The delivery of the valve catheter is generally accomplished under fluoroscopic guidance and positioned across the native aortic valve. An aortogram is performed to identify calcium landmarks and to assess overall valve position prior to deployment (**Fig. 40.7**). Once the optimal position is confirmed, steps for valve implantation are initiated. For balloon-expandable TAVR, rapid pacing is absolutely necessary to halt ventricular ejection during balloon inflation. For self-expanding TAVR, the valve can be deployed without rapid pacing. Nevertheless, rapid pacing will be needed if any postdilations are needed.

In the immediate post-valve-deployment stage, it is imperative to resuscitate the patient following the ventricular pacing run. Valve position, valve function, presence of valvular insufficiency (central or paravalvular), presence of a pericardial effusion/tamponade, and ventricular function must be assessed using a combination of fluoroscopy, angiography, and echo. The information attained acutely after valve deployment will determine the need for further intervention (i.e., postdilation, second valve).

Clinical Data

The first successful TAVR was performed in France by Dr. Cribier and colleagues using an antegrade transseptal technique (13).

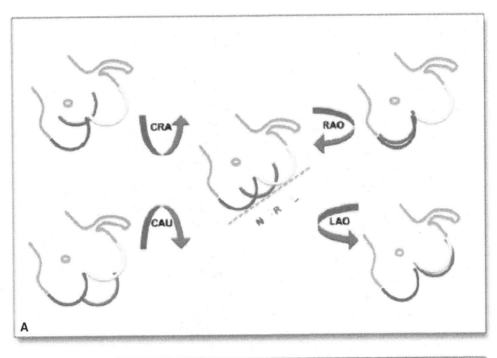

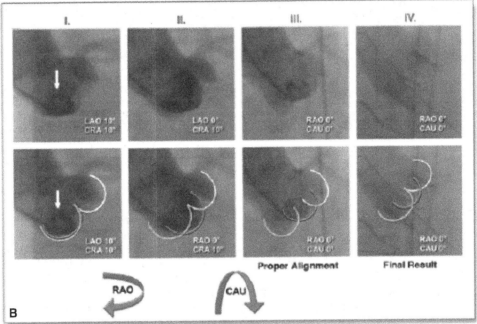

FIGURE 40.6 Follow the right coronary cusp rule to attain the optimal coplanar view for valve deployment. **A:** Diagrams of cusp orientations. **B:** Overlay of positions on the aortograms. (From: Kasel AM, et al. Fluoroscopy-guided aortic root imaging for TAVR: "follow the right cusp" rule. *JACC Cardiovasc Imaging.* 2013;6(2):274–275.)

Following this, the same group reported on their initial feasibility experience in six patients with end-stage AS (14), and then on their midterm follow-up from their initial 36-patient safety and feasibility experience (Registry of Endovascular Critical Aortic Stenosis Treatment, RECAST, trial), demonstrating feasibility and real clinical improvement in inoperable patients (15). Several European and Canadian registries have enrolled patients who have undergone TAVR. These early studies and registries demonstrated reasonable short- and mid-term outcomes with TAVR. Nevertheless, FDA approval for the TAVR valves relied on the outcomes of randomized trials comparing SAVR and TAVR.

Partner Trials

In the United States, the landmark trial that led to FDA approval for TAVR in inoperable patients with severe AS was the PARTNER trial (5,6). There were two cohorts in this study: A and B. Cohort B were patients with severe symptomatic AS who were deemed inoperable by two cardiac surgeons, so enrollment into this part of the trial was completed first (5). Prior chest radiation, porcelain aorta, severe lung disease, and frailty were all reasons for inoperability as determined by the surgeons. These patients were randomized either to TAVR or standard medical therapy. Of note, 83.8% of patients in the standard

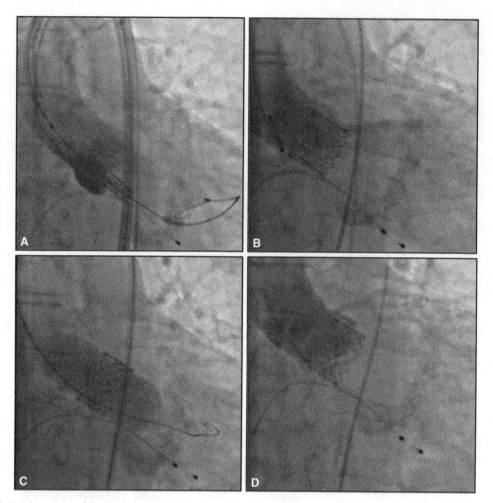

FIGURE 40.7   A: Optimal position of the SAPIEN 3 valve prior to deployment. The bottom of the middle marker band is at the level of the aortic annulus. **B:** Postdeployment angiogram shows moderate-severe PVL. **C:** Postdilatation balloon with 24-mm balloon. **D:** Postdilatation angiogram shows no central regurgitation or residual PVL. PVL, paravalvular leak.

therapy arm underwent BAV. A total of 358 patients were randomized in the PARTNER B cohort. The primary endpoint was superiority of TAVR in all-cause mortality. The 1-year all-cause mortality rate in those undergoing standard therapy was 50.7% versus 30.7% in patients treated with TAVR (p < 0.001). This was an absolute reduction in mortality of 20% and the number needed to treat to prevent one death in 1 year was only five. Despite a large number of patients in the standard therapy arm treated with BAV, it did not alter the dismal prognosis associated with severe inoperable AS.

There was also significant improvement in symptoms and quality of life in those patients having undergone TAVR. At 1 year, 74.8% of those having undergone TAVR had New York Heart Association (NYHA) Class I or II symptoms as compared with 42% in the medical therapy group (p < 0.001). Despite these positive findings, TAVR was noted to have a higher rate (5.0% vs. 1.1%, p = 0.06) of major strokes at 30-days post-procedure. Largely due to the mortality benefit seen with TAVR in the PARTNER trial, the FDA approved the use of the SAPIEN valve for inoperable patients with severe symptomatic AS in November 2011.

PARTNER cohort A examined the role of TAVR in patients with severe symptomatic AS deemed to be surgical candidates, albeit high risk (6). These patients were deemed to be high risk on the basis of a STS PROM of at least 10%. A total of 699 patients were randomized to TAVR (either TF or TA, depending on peripheral arterial size) or SAVR. Of the 348 patients randomized to TAVR,

244 underwent TF-TAVR. The TA TAVR patients had higher rates of peripheral vascular disease and prior coronary bypass surgery.

Unlike PARTNER B, PARTNER A's primary endpoint was non-inferiority in all-cause mortality. At 1 year, there were no significant differences in all-cause mortality between TAVR versus SAVR and non-inferiority was seen out to 3 years. Nevertheless, the major stroke rate in PARTNER A at 1 year was 5.1% in the transcatheter group and 2.4% in the surgical group (p = 0.07).

With regard to symptoms, the transcatheter group had a significant improvement in NYHA symptom class at 30 days versus the open AVR group; nevertheless, by 1 year, there was no difference between the groups. TAVR was also associated with higher rates of vascular complications, permanent pacemakers, and paravalvular regurgitation. On the basis of non-inferiority, in October 2012 the FDA approved the use of the SAPIEN valve for high-risk patients with severe symptomatic AS.

PARTNER 2A study design was similar to PARTNER 1A, but this trial was different in that it was investigating SAPIEN XT (a second-generation valve) in intermediate-risk patients (STS 4%–8%) (7). This study randomized 2,032 patients, and the primary endpoint was all-cause mortality or disabling stroke at 2 years. At 2 years, there were no significant differences in the primary endpoint between the groups; TAVR was non-inferior to SAVR, and stroke rates showed no significant differences.

PARTNER 1A and 2A were both randomized studies. PARTNER 2 S3i was a nonrandomized study of intermediate-risk patients (16). A total of 1,032 patients were enrolled in the study, and all the patients were treated with TAVR using the third-generation SAPIEN 3 valve. This cohort of patients was then compared to the surgical cohort in PARTNER 2A. A propensity score analysis showed that SAPIEN 3 TAVR was superior to SAVR for the primary endpoint of all-cause mortality and all stroke (10.8% vs. 18.8%). Nevertheless, surgery was still superior for patients with moderate or greater AR after TAVR. On the basis of the results from PARTNER 2A and PARTNER S3i, in August 2016 the FDA approved the use of the SAPIEN XT and SAPIEN 3 valves for intermediate-risk patients with severe symptomatic AS.

CoreValve US Pivotal Trials

Unlike PARTNER cohort B, the CoreValve US Pivotal Extreme Risk Trial was not randomized to standard therapy (8). This study enrolled 489 patients and met its primary endpoint of death or major stroke at 1 year with a rate of 25.5%, which was 40.7% lower (p < 0.0001) in patients treated with the CoreValve than was expected (based on a performance goal developed in partnership with the FDA). At 1 year, 75.6% of patients were still alive, and stroke was low at 4.1%. On the basis of these results, in January 2014 the FDA approved the use of CoreValve for extreme-risk patients with severe symptomatic AS.

The CoreValve US Pivotal High Risk Trial was a randomized trial comparing CoreValve TAVR to SAVR, with 795 patients enrolled in the study (9). The high-risk trial showed that CoreValve TAVR was associated with a lower mortality at 1 year compared to SAVR (14.1% vs. 18.9%) and a lower stroke rate (8.7% vs. 12.5%). These benefits were sustained out to 3 years. The need for a permanent pacemaker and significant paravalvular regurgitation were again higher with TAVR. On the basis of these results, in June 2014 the FDA approved the use of CoreValve for high-risk patients with severe symptomatic AS.

Bicuspid Valves

Patients with bicuspid AS were excluded from the randomized clinical trials. Anatomically, the aortic annulus is usually more elliptical in bicuspid AS, and asymmetric expansion of the prosthesis may have adverse effects on PVL and durability. Perlman et al. reported the feasibility of SAPIEN 3 TAVR in 51 patients with bicuspid AS (17). Post-implantation AR was none/trivial in 63% and mild in 37%; there were no cases of moderate or severe AR. At 30-day follow-up, there were two deaths (3.9%), two major vascular complications, and 12 patients (23.5%) required pacemaker implantation. Further studies with longer follow-up are required before TAVR can be routinely recommended for bicuspid AS.

Valve-in-Valve TAVR

The CoreValve US Pivotal Study also had an observational arm, the Expanded Use Study, which enrolled 143 patients who underwent aortic valve-in-valve TAVR for a failing surgical heart valve (27th annual Transcatheter Cardiovascular Therapeutics Scientific Symposium, October 2015, San Francisco, CA). This study showed low rates of both mortality and stroke at 30 days and 6 months, along with significant improvements in valve hemodynamics and patients' quality of life. In March 2015, the FDA approved CoreValve for aortic valve-in-valve TAVR for high- and extreme-risk patients with a failing bioprosthetic valve.

SAPIEN XT was also studied in valve-in-valve procedures as part of the PARTNER 2 Valve-in-Valve Study (27th annual Transcatheter Cardiovascular Therapeutics Scientific Symposium, October 2015, San Francisco, CA). The study enrolled 197 patients and also showed low rates of mortality and stroke at 30 days and 1 year. In October 2015, the FDA approved SAPIEN XT for aortic valve-in-valve TAVR for high-risk patients with a failing bioprosthetic valve.

Dr. Vinayak Bapat developed an iOS app called Valve in Valve, which is available as a free download. The app provides detailed information about a wide variety of surgical heart valves, including prosthesis height and inner diameter. The app then provides suggested TAVR valves with the appropriate size as well as fluoroscopic examples of an actual valve-in-valve procedure (**Fig. 40.8**). There is another version of the app for mitral valve-in-valve. The SAPIEN valve has also been used for valve-in-valve applications in the tricuspid and pulmonic positions.

TAVR Procedural Risks

Stroke

Potential mechanisms for stroke associated with TAVR include embolization of calcific debris from the aortic valve, atheroma in the aorta, or embolism from the TAVR valve. These mechanisms largely account for the strokes seen within the first 30 days after TAVR. In fact, most strokes occur within the first 2 days of TAVR (18). Diffusion-weighted MRI studies have shown multiple embolic lesions in more than 75% of TAVR patients, although the majority of these are clinically silent with no stroke symptoms or cognitive impairment (19). Furthermore, new onset atrial fibrillation after the procedure also leads to increased stroke risk and can partially explain the increased stroke seen beyond 30 days but within the first year of TAVR (20). In PARTNER cohort A, the 30-day major stroke rate was higher in TAVR compared to SAVR (3.8% vs. 2.1%, p = 0.20), as well as for the 1-year major stroke rate (5.1% vs. 2.4%, p = 0.07) (6). With a reduction in delivery system size, the stroke rates have dramatically decreased. In PARTNER S3i, the life-disabling stroke rate was only 1.0% at 30 days and 2.3% at 1 year (16).

Several strategies are being investigated to potentially reduce the risk of cerebral embolization. One such strategy is the use of emboli protection devices during valve positioning and deployment.

To reduce the risk of embolic stroke, patients are typically anticoagulated with dual antiplatelet therapy with aspirin and plavix, lifelong for the former, and 3 to 6 months for the latter. This recommendation was initially based on expert opinion, but the addition of plavix may increase bleeding risk without decreasing thromboembolic events. A randomized trial is ongoing that will help answer the question of whether the addition of plavix has clinical benefit (21). Patients with atrial fibrillation should be anticoagulated with warfarin. In patients treated with warfarin, concomitant antiplatelet therapy does not appear to reduce stroke or major adverse cardiovascular events while increasing the risk of bleeding (22). Further studies are needed to clarify optimal anticoagulation regimens after TAVR.

Vascular Complications

Although delivery sheath sizes are dramatically smaller, the risk for significant vascular complications remains important, and when it occurs, it can lead to major morbidity and even mortality. In the PARTNER trial, major vascular complications were identified as an independent predictor of 1-year mortality (23). Vascular complications such as aortic dissections and root disruptions can also occur with

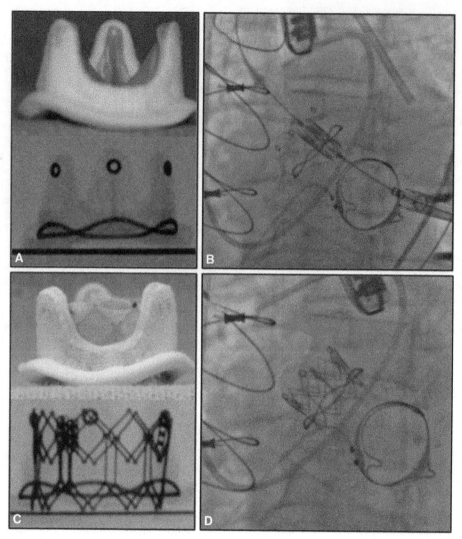

FIGURE 40.8   A: Photograph and radiograph of a Hancock surgical heart valve from the Valve in Valve iOS app. **B:** Positioning of the SAPIEN XT valve within the failing Hancock surgical valve. The top of the transcatheter aortic valve replacement (TAVR) valve is aligned with the three circular markers of the surgical prosthesis. Guiding catheter, coronary guide wire, and balloon are in place to protect the left main. **C:** Photograph and radiograph of valve-in-valve with SAPIEN XT from the iOS app. **D:** Post-valve-in-valve fluoroscopy showing an ideal implant.

device manipulation and oversizing of prosthesis. Familiarity with recognizing and treating vascular complications is an important aspect of the TAVR procedure.

Conduction System Abnormalities

The conduction system (notably, the bundle of His) is located in the membranous septum of the left ventricular outflow tract (LVOT), a location that is highly susceptible to direct trauma, compression, and ischemia during and after valve deployment (24). Following TAVR, varying degrees of heart block and left bundle branch block (LBBB) can occur. While some of these disturbances may be transient, some may require a permanent pacemaker. Prosthesis implantation depth, degree of oversizing, preexisting right bundle branch block, and small LVOT diameter are factors that increase the risk of a pacemaker after TAVR.

Valvular Insufficiency

As reported in the 2-year data of PARTNER A cohort, the presence of even mild aortic paravalvular regurgitation post-TAVR was associated with decreased survival at 2 years (25). Extensive annular and root calcification, improper prosthesis positioning, and undersizing of the valve may predispose to the development of paravalvular regurgitation. The management of this complication includes postdeployment balloon dilatation of the prosthesis, either with additional saline in the delivery balloon or with a larger diameter balloon (Fig. 40.7, Panel C). In some cases, a second valve within the first valve may be required to treat this complication.

Coronary Ostium

One of the most important observations made at the pre-procedural assessment stage is the determination of the coronary ostial anatomy in relationship to the aortic valve annulus, the aortic root, and the height of the sinotubular junction. With proper placement of the valve, there should not be obstruction to the coronary ostia; nevertheless, in situations of high valve placement or a short aortic root, there is the possibility that the valve can obstruct the coronary ostium. The risk of coronary obstruction is markedly higher in valve-in-valve procedures involving stentless surgical valves. When coronary obstruction occurs, urgent percutaneous coronary revascularization will be necessary. If the risk of coronary obstruction is identified during pre-procedural planning, a coronary guide and guide wire can be placed prophylactically into the coronary artery prior to valve deployment to allow easier access to the ostium if necessary (Fig. 40.8, Panel B).

Conclusions

TAVR is one of the most exciting developments in interventional cardiology and has ushered in a new era in the percutaneous management of valvular heart disease. Advances in device design have made TAVR safer and more effective. Initially only an option for inoperable or high-risk patients, TAVR indications have expanded to intermediate-risk patients based on clinical trial data proving non-inferiority of TAVR compared to SAVR in a randomized clinical trial. Although there is eagerness to treat all AS patients with TAVR, SAVR remains the standard of care for low-risk patients pending the results of the low-risk randomized trials.

Patient selection and proper procedural planning are essential for success. This is best done by a multidisciplinary evaluation by the Heart Team. Use of multimodality imaging is critical in preprocedural planning and in the assessment of post-procedural complications.

Although TAVR is associated with decreased mortality and stroke compared to SAVR, TAVR's weaknesses still include higher vascular complications, a permanent pacemaker, and PVL. New technology will hopefully be able to address these issues as the space continues to mature in the years ahead.

Key Points

- Mortality is high in patients with severe symptomatic AS. Aortic valve replacement is an AHA/ACC Class I recommendation (level of evidence: B) in these patients.

- Many patients with symptomatic critical AS are not offered surgical AVR, given advanced age and medical comorbidities. TAVR has been shown to improve survival and symptoms in a patient population that previously had not been treated.

- TAVR is now indicated in inoperable, high-risk, and, more recently, intermediate-risk patients. SAVR is still the standard of care for low-surgical-risk patients.

- TAVR requires a multidisciplinary approach toward treating patients, often involving interventional cardiology, cardiac surgery, cardiac anesthesia, and non-invasive cardiology all working together.

- Preprocedural evaluation of the TAVR patient is often extensive and requires multimodality testing in order to ensure candidacy for TAVR.

- Accurate measurement of the aortic annulus (virtual ring) and aortic root is critical in TAVR planning. Complications such as PVL, annular rupture, and coronary obstruction can be avoided with careful assessment and planning. Three-dimensional imaging with either CTA or TEE is essential. Remember the Marine adage: 7Ps. Proper Prior Planning Prevents Piss Poor Performance.

- Ninety percent of patients can be treated via TF approach. CTA provides essential information about vessel dimensions, calcification, and tortuosity. If femoral access is not feasible, TAVR can be performed via alternate access such as TA, transaortic, subclavian, or carotid access.

- TAVR is associated with higher vascular complications, a permanent pacemaker, and PVL compared to SAVR.

- Implantation depth, degree of oversizing, preexisting right bundle branch block, and small LVOT are factors that increase the need for a permanent pacemaker after TAVR.

- Most strokes occur within the first 2 days of TAVR. New onset atrial fibrillation increases stroke risk after TAVR.

References

1. Varadarajan P, et al. Clinical profile and natural history of 453 nonsurgically managed patients with severe aortic stenosis. *Ann Thorac Surg.* 2006;82(6):2111–2115.
2. Nishimura RA, et al. 2014 AHA/ACC guideline for the management of patients with valvular heart disease: a report of the American College of Cardiology/American Heart Association Task Force on Practice Guidelines. *J Thorac Cardiovasc Surg.* 2014;148(1):e1–e132.
3. Iung B, et al. Valvular heart disease in the community: a European experience. *Curr Probl Cardiol.* 2007;32(11):609–611.
4. Otto CM, et al. Three-year outcome after balloon aortic valvuloplasty: insights into prognosis of valvular aortic stenosis. *Circulation.* 1994;89(2):642–650.
5. Leon MB, et al. Transcatheter aortic-valve implantation for aortic stenosis in patients who cannot undergo surgery. *N Engl J Med.* 2010;363(17):1597–1607.
6. Smith CR, et al. Transcatheter versus surgical aortic valve replacement in high-risk patients. *N Engl J Med.* 2011;364(23):2187–2198.
7. Leon MB, et al. Transcatheter or surgical aortic-valve replacement in intermediate-risk patients. *N Engl J Med.* 2016;374(17):1609–1620.
8. Popma JJ, et al. Transcatheter aortic valve replacement using a self-expanding bioprosthesis in patients with severe aortic stenosis at extreme risk for surgery. *J Am Coll Cardiol.* 2014;63(19):1972–1981.
9. Adams DH, et al. Transcatheter aortic-valve replacement with a self-expanding prosthesis. *N Engl J Med.* 2014;370(19):1790–1798.
10. Kasel AM, et al. Standardized imaging for aortic annular sizing: implications for transcatheter valve selection. *JACC Cardiovasc Imaging.* 2013;6(2):249–262.
11. Kasel AM, et al. Fluoroscopy-guided aortic root imaging for TAVR: "follow the right cusp" rule. *JACC Cardiovasc Imaging.* 2013;6(2):274–275.
12. Dangas GD, et al. Bivalirudin versus heparin anticoagulation in transcatheter aortic valve replacement: the randomized BRAVO-3 Trial. *J Am Coll Cardiol.* 2015;66(25):2860–2868.
13. Cribier A, et al. Percutaneous transcatheter implantation of an aortic valve for calcific aortic stenosis: first human case description. *Circulation.* 2002;106(24):3006–3008.
14. Cribier A, et al. Early experience with percutaneous transcatheter implantation of heart valve prosthesis for the treatment of end-stage inoperable patients with calcific aortic stenosis. *J Am Coll Cardiol.* 2004;43(4):698–703.
15. Cribier A, et al. Treatment of calcific aortic stenosis with the percutaneous heart valve: mid-term follow-up from the initial feasibility studies: the French experience. *J Am Coll Cardiol.* 2006;47(6):1214–1223.
16. Thourani VH, et al. Transcatheter aortic valve replacement versus surgical valve replacement in intermediate-risk patients: a propensity score analysis. *Lancet.* 2016;387(10034):2218–2225.
17. Perlman GY, et al. Bicuspid aortic valve stenosis: favorable early outcomes with a next-generation transcatheter heart valve in a multicenter study. *JACC Cardiovasc Interv.* 2016;9:817–824.
18. Kapadia S, et al. Insights into timing, risk factors, and outcomes of stroke and transient ischemic attack after transcatheter aortic valve replacement in

the PARTNER trial (placement of aortic transcatheter valves). *Circ Cardiovasc Interv.* 2016;9(9). pii: e002981.

19. Kahlert P, et al. Silent and apparent cerebral ischemia after percutaneous transfemoral aortic valve implantation: a diffusion-weighted magnetic resonance imaging study. *Circulation.* 2010;121:870–878.

20. Auffret V, et al. Predictors of early cerebrovascular events in patients with aortic stenosis undergoing transcatheter aortic valve replacement. *J Am Coll Cardiol.* 2016;68(7):673–684.

21. Nijenhuis VJ, et al. Rationale and design of POPular-TAVI: antiPlatelet therapy fOr Patients undergoing Transcatheter Aortic Valve Implantation. *Am Heart J.* 2016;173:77–85.

22. Abdul-Jawad Altisent O, et al. Warfarin and antiplatelet therapy versus warfarin alone for treating patients with atrial fibrillation undergoing transcatheter aortic valve replacement. *JACC Cardiovasc Interv.* 2016;9(16):1706–1717.

23. Genereux P, et al. Vascular complications after transcatheter aortic valve replacement: insights from the PARTNER (Placement of AoRTic TraNscath-etER Valve) trial. *J Am Coll Cardiol.* 2012;60(12):1043–1052.

24. Moreno R, et al. Cause of complete atrioventricular block after percutaneous aortic valve implantation: insights from a necropsy study. *Circulation.* 2009;120(5):e29–e30.

25. Kodali SK, et al. Two-year outcomes after transcatheter or surgical aortic-valve replacement. *N Engl J Med.* 2012;366(18):1686–1695.

41

Hypertrophic Cardiomyopathy

Paul Sorajja, MD, FSCAI, FACC, FAHA

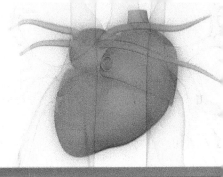

Hypertrophic cardiomyopathy (HCM) is a common, inheritable cardiac disorder with a prevalence of 1 in 500 persons in the general population. Clinically, HCM is defined as the presence of severe myocardial hypertrophy in the absence of a known local or systemic etiology (1). For patients with coexistent diseases that also may cause myocardial hypertrophy (e.g., hypertension or aortic stenosis), the degree of hypertrophy must be out of proportion to the hemodynamic burden imposed by that disease in order to meet diagnostic criteria for HCM. Mutations in sarcomeric genes cause HCM, with thousands of such mutations in >14 different genes identified in these patients thus far.

The clinical diagnosis of HCM is typically made by detection of severe myocardial hypertrophy using two-dimensional echocardiography and, in some cases, cardiac magnetic resonance imaging (MRI). Doppler echocardiography can accurately diagnose and quantify left ventricular outflow tract (LVOT) obstruction using the modified Bernoulli equation (gradient = $4 \times$ velocity^2) in most instances. During cardiac catheterization, the operator should suspect HCM when there is a hypertrophied left ventricle with a small cavity and normal or hyperdynamic systolic function on ventriculography. Regional hypertrophy, such as basal septal or apical hypertrophy, may be present (Fig. 41.1). Left ventricular diastolic pressures may be elevated, reflecting diastolic dysfunction. Dynamic LVOT obstruction should be suspected if there is a gradient between the left ventricular apex and base or if there is a "spike and dome" pattern on the aortic pressure trace (Fig. 41.2). Of note, the presence of dynamic LVOT obstruction is highly dependent on ventricular loading conditions and the contractile state, and may be evident only with physical maneuvers or drug provocation.

Pathophysiology

Diastolic dysfunction with elevated ventricular filling pressures is the major pathophysiologic mechanism contributing to signs and symptoms for patients with HCM. Abnormalities of diastolic dysfunction arise due to abnormal relaxation and poor compliance in the presence of altered loading conditions, myocardial ischemia, ventricular non-uniformity, and severe hypertrophy. The end result of diastolic dysfunction is an increase in left ventricular filling pressures that causes the typical symptoms of dyspnea and angina. For patients with HCM, there may be a significant discrepancy between the mean left atrial pressure and left ventricular end diastolic pressure. Therefore, both measurements should be made when possible.

Dynamic LVOT obstruction is present in 75% of patients with HCM (2). Determining the presence and severity of the LVOT obstruction is essential because this then provides the basis for therapy. Two

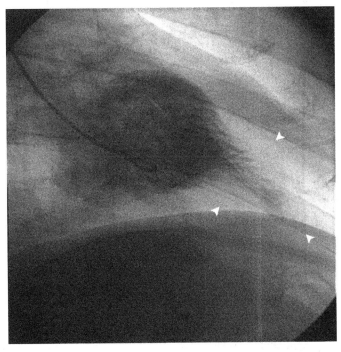

FIGURE 41.1 Left ventriculography of a patient with apical hypertrophic cardiomyopathy. This is an end-diastolic angiographic frame showing severe apical hypertrophy (*arrowheads*).

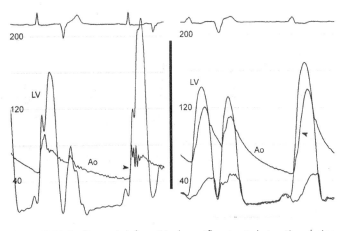

FIGURE 41.2 Dynamic left ventricular outflow tract obstruction during cardiac catheterization in a patient with hypertrophic cardiomyopathy versus aortic valvular stenosis. **Left:** In a patient with obstructive hypertrophic cardiomyopathy, there is a left ventricular outflow tract gradient with a "spike-and-dome" configuration in the aortic pressure. On the post-ectopic beat, there is a decrease in stroke volume and consequently a decrease in the aortic pulse pressure (*arrowhead*), with further exaggeration of the spike-and-dome contour. **Right:** In a patient with aortic stenosis, increased contractility on the postectopic beat leads to an increase in stroke volume and an increase in the aortic pulse pressure (*arrowhead*). Ao, ascending aorta; LV, left ventricle.

mechanisms underlie the development of dynamic LVOT obstruction: (a) septal hypertrophy and narrowing of the LVOT, which lead to Venturi forces that accelerate during ventricular emptying and pull the mitral apparatus anteriorly; and (b) anterior papillary muscle displacement, which subjects the mitral leaflets to intraventricular currents during systole that drag the apparatus anteriorly. Decreased mitral leaflet coaptation occurs due to systolic anterior motion of the mitral valve, leading to secondary mitral regurgitation in patients with LVOT obstruction.

It is important to note the dynamic nature of LVOT obstruction and secondary mitral regurgitation. LVOT obstruction is exacerbated by increases in inotropy and decreases in either ventricular afterload (e.g., vasodilators) or preload (e.g., dehydration, diuretic therapy). The severity of LVOT obstruction is highly sensitive to ventricular load and contractility, with changes in the gradient even observed during quiet respiration (Fig. 41.3). Although the clinical significance of LVOT obstruction in HCM historically has been debated, modern studies have demonstrated its relation to heart failure and poor survival when severe.

Medical Therapy

Negative inotropic agents, such as β-receptor antagonists, disopyramide, and calcium-channel blockers (i.e., verapamil, diltiazem) are the cornerstone of drug therapy for symptomatic LVOT obstruction. By depressing contractility, these agents increase diastolic filling time, improve myocardial relaxation, reduce the imbalance of myocardial oxygen supply and demand, and ameliorate the propensity toward LVOT obstruction by reducing the intraventricular flow velocities that aggravate the development of systolic anterior motion of the mitral valve. It is important to note that large doses of these medications are frequently required (e.g., 480 mg verapamil or 200 mg metoprolol) to completely suppress LVOT obstruction. Verapamil should be used only with caution, if at all, in patients with advanced heart failure, high LVOT gradients, and bradycardia. Furthermore, disopyramide should be prescribed with a concomitant atrioventricular (AV) node

blocker in patients with atrial fibrillation, as disopyramide may accelerate AV conduction.

Peripheral vasodilators, inotropic agents (e.g., digoxin, β-receptor agonists), and high-dose diuretics should be avoided as they will aggravate the development of LVOT obstruction. Patients should also be counseled on the need to maintain hydration and general avoidance of circumstances that precipitate vasodilatation (e.g., saunas). When severe symptoms persist despite optimal drug therapy, definitive septal reduction therapy should be considered in patients with obstructive HCM.

Surgical Myectomy

The time-honored standard for septal reduction therapy is surgical myectomy (3–5). In this procedure, a surgeon uses a transaortic approach to widen the LVOT through direct resection of the hypertrophied ventricular septum. Not uncommonly, the myectomy is extended to the base of the papillary muscles, leading to full reconstruction of the LVOT. While early historical series raised concern about the safety of the procedure, surgical myectomy now has an operative mortality of <1% with a success rate of >90% when performed in experienced centers. Complications, such as aortic regurgitation, ventricular septal defect, and pacemaker dependency are infrequent (<5%). Importantly, long-term studies (10-year follow-up) have demonstrated no impairment of survival after surgical myectomy. In national practice guidelines on HCM, surgical myectomy is the preferred mode of therapy for septal reduction in highly symptomatic patients and is utilized in HCM patients of all ages (1). Myectomy should be performed in only experienced surgical centers.

Alcohol Septal Ablation

Percutaneous alcohol septal ablation is an alternative to surgical myectomy for the relief of LVOT obstruction in patients with HCM. The aim of alcohol septal ablation is to induce a localized myocardial infarction and thinning of the basal ventricular septum, thereby leading to a reduction in septal thickening and systolic excursion into the LVOT.

Patient Selection

Proper patient selection is critical to the success of septal ablation. A comprehensive clinical evaluation and echocardiogram should be performed in all candidates, ideally in a center with expertise in the care of HCM patients. Criteria for septal ablation include the following: (a) severe, drug-refractory cardiac symptoms (New York Heart Association functional class III/IV dyspnea or Canadian Cardiac Society angina class III/IV) due to obstructive HCM; (b) dynamic LVOT obstruction (gradient ≥30 mm Hg at rest or ≥50 mm Hg with provocation) that is due to septal hypertrophy and systolic anterior motion of the mitral valve; (c) ventricular septal thickness ≥15 mm; (d) absence of significant intrinsic mitral valve disease; (e) absence of need for concomitant cardiac surgical procedure (e.g., bypass grafting, valve replacement); and (f) informed patient consent. A comprehensive two-dimensional and Doppler echocardiogram is elementary to proper patient selection. This evaluation should document the dynamic nature of the LVOT obstruction and exclude anatomic findings that would impede the clinical efficacy of the procedure (Figs. 41.4 and 41.5).

Informed patient consent requires full understanding of the limited data on long-term survival after the procedure, risk of pacemaker dependency, the relatively lower success rate due to its dependence

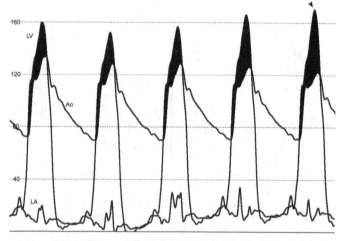

FIGURE 41.3 Dynamic changes in left ventricular outflow tract obstruction. The left ventricular outflow tract gradient (*shaded*) is highly sensitive to ventricular loading conditions and the contractile state, with effects seen even during quiet respiration. During expiration, an increase in thoracic pressure leads to lower afterload, and consequently an increase in the left ventricular outflow tract gradient. Reciprocal changes occur during inspiration. *Arrowhead* indicates peak end-expiration. Ao, ascending aorta; LA, left atrium; LV, left ventricle.

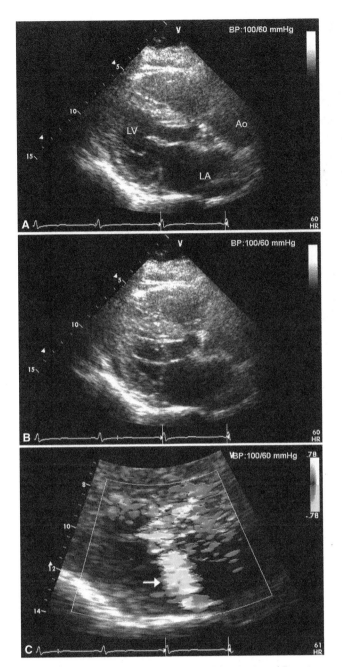

FIGURE 41.4 Patient selection for septal ablation. **A** and **B** are parasternal long axis views and **C** is color doppler showing point of gradient. This patient has appropriate anatomy for consideration of septal ablation. There is ventricular septal hypertrophy, systolic anterior motion of the mitral valve, and posteriorly directed mitral regurgitation that is secondary to the outflow obstruction (*arrow*). Ao, ascending aorta; LA, left atrium; LV, left ventricle.

on coronary anatomy, and potential complications related to cardiac catheterization and instrumentation of the coronary arteries. It is advised that decision making regarding surgical myectomy or alcohol septal ablation be undertaken in the context of a longitudinal, multidisciplinary program with expertise in the care of HCM patients, with experienced operators performing these procedures (1).

Although younger age is not an absolute contraindication to the procedure, septal ablation has generally been reserved for older adult patients due to the limited data on long-term survival of the procedure. In the 2011 ACCF/AHA practice guidelines on HCM, septal ablation is a class III recommendation for patients under the

age of 21 years, and the procedure is also strongly discouraged in those aged <40 years if surgical myectomy is a viable option (1).

Hemodynamic Evaluation

Proper performance of septal ablation requires a complete and accurate evaluation of the severity of LVOT obstruction due to HCM. Characteristically, LVOT obstruction in HCM is dynamic and exquisitely sensitive to ventricular loading conditions and contractility. The operator should be cognizant of this sensitivity when examining hemodynamic data from both the echocardiogram and invasive catheterization. Careful attention must be given not only to the initial LVOT gradient observed at rest, but all dynamic and provocable gradients (e.g., variation with respiration, post-PVC accentuation) observed during the procedure.

The most accurate method for the invasive evaluation of LVOT obstruction in HCM entails a transseptal approach with positioning of a balloon-tipped catheter (e.g., 7-F Berman catheter, Arrow International Inc., Reading, PA) at the left ventricular inflow region, and a pigtail catheter placed retrograde in the ascending aorta for simultaneous measurement of the LVOT gradient. The transseptal approach helps to avoid catheter entrapment, which can be difficult to distinguish from changes in left ventricular pressure that occur due to the dynamic nature of LVOT obstruction (**Fig. 41.6**). Use of an 8-F Mullins sheath for transseptal access also enables recording of left atrial pressure via the sidearm for assessment for concomitant diastolic dysfunction.

Alternatively, left ventricular pressure can be assessed with a 5-F or 6-F catheter placed retrograde across the aortic valve. In this technique, a catheter with shaft side holes should not be used because some or all of the holes will be positioned above the level of subaortic obstruction, leading to erroneous measurements of left ventricular pressure and the LVOT gradient. Catheters that may be used for this purpose are a multipurpose or a Halo pigtail catheter. Absence of catheter entrapment should be confirmed with hand contrast injections or demonstration of pulsatile flow from the catheter with disconnection from the extenders used for pressure transduction.

Temporary Pacemaker Placement

The risk of pacemaker dependency from septal ablation varies according to the baseline electrocardiographic abnormalities. Septal ablation results in right bundle branch block in approximately 50% of cases. Thus, for those patients with left bundle branch block, severe left axis deviation, or a very wide QRS interval, the rate of pacemaker dependency approaches 50%. In patients with a normal electrocardiogram, permanent pacemaker dependency from complete AV block occurs in 10% to 15% (6). Thus, for patients without a permanent pacemaker, a temporary device is placed at the right ventricular septum via the right internal jugular vein prior to septal ablation. Conventional 5-F or 6-F temporary pacemakers can be utilized. Of note, these devices have been associated with cardiac perforation, at least partly because of their long dwelling time while patients are observed in the intensive care unit after the procedure. A more preferable approach is placement of active fixation leads connected to a temporary generator. In all cases, the temporary pacemaker should be placed away from the target site of ablation to ensure continuous capture following induction of the septal infarction.

Procedure

Coronary angiography is performed to determine the most appropriate septal artery for the procedure. Both arteries should be evaluated, as basal septal branches occasionally arise from the proximal right coronary artery. With a right anterior oblique angulation of the

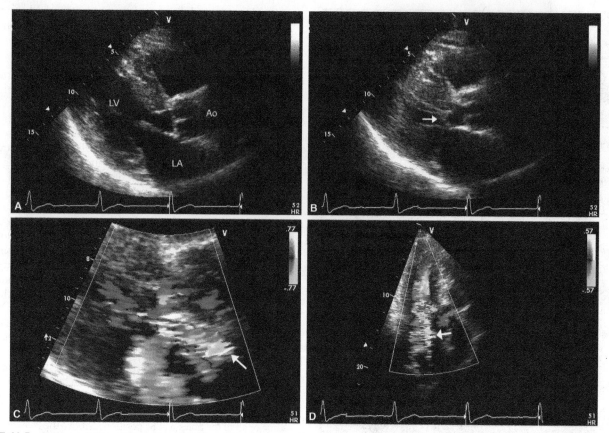

FIGURE 41.5 Patient selection. This patient has obstructive hypertrophic cardiomyopathy and was referred for alcohol septal ablation. Although there is systolic anterior motion of the mitral valve (part **B**, *arrow*), there is also mitral regurgitation secondary to a flail mitral leaflet. Note the anterior course of the mitral regurgitant jet (parts **C** and **D**, *arrows*), which is not typical for that owing to outflow obstruction. Ao, ascending aorta; LA, left atrium; LV, left ventricle.

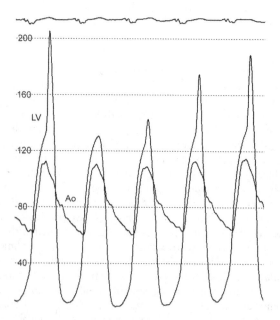

FIGURE 41.6 Catheter entrapment. Although there appears to be a significant variable gradient between the ascending aorta (Ao) and the left ventricle (LV), this appearance is an artifact due to catheter entrapment. The distinguishing features of entrapment in this figure are the absence of variation in the ascending aortic pressure with a corresponding change in the LV pressure, and significant damping of the pressure tracings. This artifact easily occurs during retrograde assessment of left ventricular outflow tract obstruction in hypertrophic cardiomyopathy.

left coronary artery, straight and caudal views help to examine the angulation of the origin of the septal artery, while cranial projections can assist with the length of the vessel. Left anterior oblique projections should be used to demonstrate the course of the artery in the ventricular septum.

Conventional 6-F or 7-F guide catheters are used to engage the left coronary artery with standard procedural anticoagulation (e.g., heparin 70–100 units/kg). A stable, relatively large guide is preferred because complete contrast opacification of the left coronary artery with minimization of movement of the balloon catheter is needed during the procedure. Both a primary and a large secondary bend should be placed on the tip of a 0.014-inch guide wire to facilitate entry into the candidate septal artery. A slightly oversized, short-length, over-the-wire balloon is placed *entirely* (i.e., at least one balloon length) into the septal artery using standard catheter techniques. Oversizing of the balloon allows occlusion of the artery at low pressures (3–4 atm), which permits relatively easier injection of material through the wire lumen of the catheter.

Following inflation of the balloon catheter, the guide wire is withdrawn. Angiography of the left coronary artery is then performed to demonstrate balloon occlusion and no communication between the septal artery and left anterior descending artery, and also to confirm the course of the target vessel through the ventricular septum on fluoroscopy (**Fig. 41.7**). Next, using full-strength contrast, angiography of the septal artery through the balloon catheter confirms patency of the vessel for ablation and localization (i.e., no untoward collateralization). Both angiographic and echocardiographic contrast are injected to identify the perfusion bed of the septal perforator

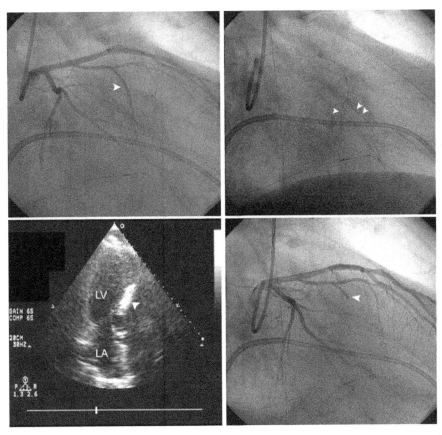

FIGURE 41.7 Percutaneous septal alcohol ablation. **Top left:** Baseline angiogram of the left coronary artery showing the septal perforator artery (*arrowhead*) to be used for ablation. **Top right:** An over-the-wire balloon is inflated in the perforator artery followed by contrast injection through the balloon for septal angiography (*arrowheads*). **Bottom left:** Echocardiographic contrast is injected through the balloon and visualized with simultaneous echocardiography. **Bottom right:** Following injection of alcohol, the septal artery (*arrowhead*) is obliterated. LA, left atrium; LV, left ventricle.

artery with simultaneous two-dimensional echocardiography. The injection of contrast should be done gently to avoid dissection of the vessel, and to minimize opening of distal septal collaterals. Multiple echocardiographic views are used to confirm enhancement of the septal hypertrophy intimately related to LVOT obstruction, but with no targeting of undesirable locations, such as the right ventricle, free walls, or papillary muscles.

After delineation of the targeted myocardium, 1 to 3 mL of desiccated ethanol is infused slowly over a period of 3 to 5 minutes, followed by a slow normal saline flush. The use of alcohol is preferred because this agent immediately results in a discrete myocardial infarction. In other percutaneous methods (e.g., vascular coiling, covered stent placement), septal infarction may not result, owing to septal collateralization that is either preexisting or that develops during follow-up.

The balloon should be left inflated following the saline flush for 5 to 10 minutes to reduce the likelihood of alcohol extravasation. For patient comfort, intravenous analgesia (e.g., fentanyl 25 mg) is frequently given prophylactically or intermittently as needed. For patients without significant reduction of either the resting or provoked LVOT gradient, other septal perforator arteries can be targeted and treated in similar fashion.

Acute Procedural Success

In published series, the magnitude of LVOT gradient reduction with septal ablation has ranged from 55% to 75% (7,8). Acute procedural success, when defined as a ≥50% reduction in the peak resting or provoked LVOT gradient with a final residual resting gradient of <20 mm Hg, occurs in 80% to 85% of patients (Fig. 41.8). In addition to proper patient selection, factors associated with higher likelihood of acute hemodynamic success include relatively less septal hypertrophy, lower LVOT gradients, and operator experience. It is important to note that myocardial edema from the infarction can lead to recurrent LVOT obstruction during hospitalization and typically subsides in follow-up. Further reduction in the LVOT gradient over 3 to 6 months after the procedure also occurs due to ventricular remodeling and basal septal thinning. Regression of myocardial hypertrophy both at the site of LVOT obstruction and remote from the ventricular septum has been demonstrated using cardiac MRI. Overall, alcohol septal ablation results in a transmural infarction that typically quantitates as ~10% of the left ventricular mass.

The major limitation to higher success is the lack of an appropriate septal artery, which may be absent in up to 20% of patients. The most common complication of septal ablation is temporary or complete AV block. Other potential complications are cardiac tamponade, dissection of the left anterior descending artery, ventricular tachycardia or fibrillation, and free wall myocardial infarction. For these reasons, patients are observed in an intensive care setting for at least 3 days after the procedure (6). Overall, the published periprocedural mortality rates are 1% to 2%.

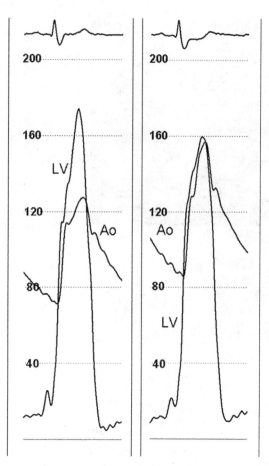

FIGURE 41.8 Hemodynamic effects of septal alcohol ablation. **Left:** Baseline hemodynamic study demonstrating a 48-mm Hg gradient across the left ventricular outflow tract. **Right:** Following successful septal ablation, the left ventricular outflow tract gradient is <5 mm Hg. Ao, ascending aorta; LV, left ventricle.

Symptom Improvement

Septal ablation leads to significant clinical improvement, as measured by both subjective functional class and objective testing, such as treadmill exercise time and peak myocardial oxygen consumption. The clinical efficacy of septal ablation is related to the degree of reduction in severity of the LVOT gradient. Overall, septal ablation typically results in a 20% to 30% increase in objective measures of functional capacity (7,8). These clinical improvements are sustained in follow-up, with several reports showing effects comparable to that of surgical myectomy (**Fig. 41.9**) (7–12). Nonetheless, in younger patients (age <65 years), symptom relief may be greater with surgical myectomy (**Fig. 41.10**) (12). The reasons for this observation are not clear, but may be related to the residual gradients present after ablation (typically, 10–20 mm Hg) that are higher than those after surgical myectomy (typically, <10 mm Hg). These relatively higher residual gradients may be less tolerated by younger, more active individuals.

Survival

Most studies that have compared septal ablation to surgical myectomy have been limited to a mid-term follow-up of 4 years. Overall survival has been comparable to that of myectomy, although the total number of ablation patients examined remains relatively small. Meta-analyses of alcohol septal ablation and surgical myectomy

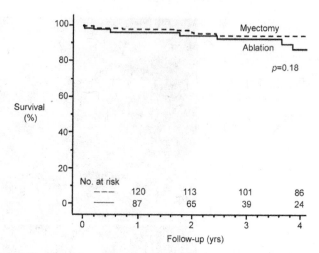

FIGURE 41.9 Comparison of survival after septal ablation to a matched cohort of surgical myectomy patients. The 4-year survival free of all mortality (including defibrillator discharge for lethal arrhythmia) among septal ablation patients was similar to that observed among age and sex-matched patients who underwent isolated surgical myectomy. (Reprinted from: Sorajja P, et al. Outcome of alcohol septal ablation for obstructive hypertrophic cardiomyopathy. *Circulation.* 2008;118:131–139, by permission from Lippincott Wilkins.)

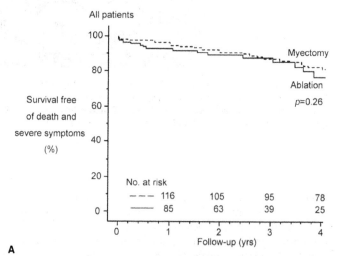

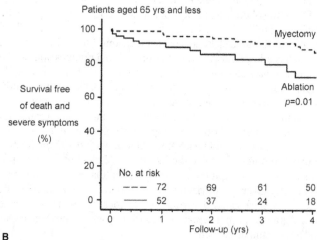

FIGURE 41.10 Symptom-free survival for septal ablation patients in comparison with surgical myectomy. Survival free of severe symptoms and death was comparable in the overall population (**A**), but was inferior among patients aged <65 years (**B**). (Reprinted from: Sorajja P, et al. *Circulation.* 2008;118:131–139, with permission from Lippincott Wilkins.)

have also demonstrated no difference in sudden death or all-cause mortality with medium-term follow-up (10).

Although the current studies suggest that there is no impairment of early to mid-term survival after septal ablation, the long-term effects and risk of sudden death remain debatable owing to limited data on extensive follow-up. In the Mayo Clinic experience (n = 177), survival at 8 years was comparable to that of myectomy patients, and to the expected survival for the US general population (12). In another report of 55 ablation patients with a mean follow-up of 8 ± 1 years, survival was comparable to matched myectomy patients. For a separate study of 629 patients with a mean follow-up of 4.6 ± 2.5 years, sudden cardiac death occurred in only 7 patients, although 24 patients were either lost to follow-up or succumbed to an unknown cause of death (13). Conversely, in a single-center experience of 91 patients who had alcohol septal ablation, 21% experienced sudden cardiac death, aborted sudden death, or appropriate discharge of a defibrillator with an annual event rate of 4.4% (14). Moreover, a multicenter HCM implantable cardioverter-defibrillator registry reported that defibrillator discharge rates were markedly higher in ablation patients (10.3% per year) than in other patients (2.6% per year). Further study regarding the long-term effects of alcohol septal ablation, including an examination of the effects on younger patients, is still required (15,16).

Key Points

- LVOT obstruction in patients with HCM is highly dependent on ventricular load and the contractile state. Increases in contractility and decreases in either preload or afterload will lead to worsening of LVOT obstruction in these patients.

- Dynamic LVOT obstruction is characterized by a "spike-and-dome" configuration in the aortic pressure contour, with a decrease in the aortic pulse pressure and exaggeration of this contour on the postectopic ventricular beat.

- Negative inotropic agents, such as β-receptor antagonists, disopyramide, and non-dihydropyridine calcium-channel blockers (i.e., verapamil, diltiazem), are the cornerstone of drug therapy for symptomatic LVOT obstruction. Peripheral vasodilators, intropes, and high-dose diuretics should be avoided.

- Surgical myectomy is currently the standard therapy for symptomatic obstructive HCM, with success rates of >90%, operative mortality of <1%, and no impairment of long-term survival when performed in experienced centers.

- Patient selection is essential to the acute and long-term outcome of alcohol septal ablation. In particular, operators should be wary of intrinsic mitral valve disease that requires open surgical repair.

- The outcomes of alcohol septal ablation approach that of surgical myectomy in selected patients and when performed in experienced centers, although the relative lack of long-term data with ablation remains a concern. The rate of pacemaker dependency after ablation is highly dependent on the baseline conduction abnormalities.

References

1. Gersh BJ, Maron BJ, Bonow RO. 2011 ACCF/AHA guideline for the diagnosis and treatment of hypertrophic cardiomyopathy: a report of the American College of Cardiology Foundation/American Heart Association Task Force on Practice Guidelines. *J Am Coll Cardiol.* 2011;58:e212–e260.
2. Maron MS, et al. Effect of left ventricular outflow tract obstruction on clinical outcome in hypertrophic cardiomyopathy. *N Engl J Med.* 2003;348:295–303.
3. Ommen SR, et al. Long-term effects of surgical septal myectomy on survival in patients with obstructive hypertrophic cardiomyopathy. *J Am Coll Cardiol.* 2005;46:470–476.
4. Maron BJ, et al. The case for surgery in obstructive hypertrophic cardiomyopathy. *J Am Coll Cardiol.* 2004;44:2044–2053.
5. Olivotto I, et al. Surgical myectomy versus alcohol septal ablation for obstructive hypertrophic cardiomyopathy. *J Am Coll Cardiol.* 2007;50:831–834.
6. Kern MJ, et al. Delayed occurrence of complete heart block without warning after alcohol septal ablation for hypertrophic obstructive cardiomyopathy. *Catheter Cardiovasc Interv.* 2002;56:503–507.
7. Nagueh SF, et al. Comparison of ethanol septal reduction therapy with surgical myectomy for the treatment of hypertrophic obstructive cardiomyopathy. *J Am Coll Cardiol.* 2001;38:1701–1706.
8. Qin JX, et al. Outcome of patients with hypertrophic obstructive cardiomyopathy after percutaneous transluminal septal myocardial ablation and septal myectomy surgery. *J Am Coll Cardiol.* 2001;38:1994–2000.
9. Kwon DH, et al. Long-term outcomes in high-risk symptomatic patients with hypertrophic cardiomyopathy undergoing alcohol septal ablation. *JACC Cardiovasc Interv.* 2008;1:432–438.
10. Agarwal S, et al. Updated meta-analysis of septal alcohol ablation versus myectomy for hypertrophic cardiomyopathy. *J Am Coll Cardiol.* 2010;55:823–834.
11. Ralph-Edwards A, et al. Hypertrophic obstructive cardiomyopathy: comparison of outcomes after myectomy or alcohol ablation adjusted by propensity score. *J Thorac Cardiovasc Surg.* 2005;129:351–358.
12. Sorajja P, et al. Survival after alcohol septal ablation for obstructive hypertrophic cardiomyopathy. *Circulation.* 2012;126:2374–2380.
13. Cuoco FA, et al. Implantable cardioverter-defibrillator therapy for primary prevention of sudden death after alcohol septal ablation of hypertrophic cardiomyopathy. *J Am Coll Cardiol.* 2008;52:1718–1723.
14. Ten Cate FJ, et al. Long-term outcome of alcohol septal ablation in patients with obstructive hypertrophic cardiomyopathy: a word of caution. *Circ Heart Fail.* 2010;3:362–369.
15. Kim LK, et al. Hospital volume outcomes after septal myectomy and alcohol septal ablation for treatment of obstructive hypertrophic cardiomyopathy: US nationwide inpatient database, 2003–2011. *JAMA Cardiol.* 2016;1:324–332.
16. Liebregts M, et al. Long-term outcome of alcohol septal ablation for obstructive hypertrophic cardiomyopathy in the young and the elderly. *JACC Cardiovasc Interv.* 2016;9:463–469.

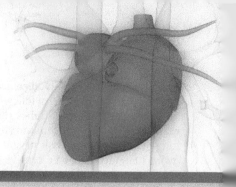

42 Paravalvular Leaks

Adnan K. Chhatriwalla, MD, FACC, FSCAI and

Paul Sorajja, MD, FSCAI, FACC, FAHA

Paravalvular regurgitation (PVR) after surgical valve replacement is relatively common, occurring in 5% to 17% of patients, and it has been even more common with early-generation transcatheter valves (1–5). Common etiologies for PVR include tissue friability, annular calcification and infection, and an early occurrence of PVR typically relates to technical aspects of the surgery. Both bioprosthetic and mechanical valves can be affected, and clinically significant PVR more commonly occurs with mitral prostheses, less commonly with aortic prostheses, and rarely with tricuspid or pulmonary prostheses. Patients may be asymptomatic, or may present with symptoms of heart failure, hemolytic anemia, or both. Additionally, significant PVR after transcatheter valve replacement has been associated with increased mortality (6). Medical therapy may be helpful in terms of management of congestive heart failure (CHF) symptoms; however, medical therapy alone may not prevent the progression of symptoms or the need for transfusion. While reoperation has historically been the standard of care for management of refractory symptoms, it is associated with more morbidity and mortality than the index procedure. Furthermore, reoperation may not be successful due to the underlying annular pathology predisposing to PVR (7). For these reasons, transcatheter paravalvular leak (PVL) closure has become the preferred therapy for many symptomatic patients at experienced centers. Importantly, catheter-based techniques permit a subsequent surgical attempt in the event of an unsuccessful outcome, if desired. Thus, transcatheter PVL closure is inherently attractive as a relatively less invasive option for many patients.

In the 2014 AHA/ACC guideline for the management of patients with valvular heart disease, transcatheter PVL closure is recommended as reasonable for high-risk surgical patients with severe CHF symptoms or refractory hemolysis and suitable anatomy, when performed at centers with expertise (class IIa recommendation) (8).

Clinical Evaluation and Patient Selection

Patients considered for transcatheter PVL closure require a comprehensive, multidisciplinary evaluation with a Heart Team approach, where there is close collaboration between the cardiologist, interventionalist, cardiac surgeon, and imaging specialists. Surgical consultation should be considered and the assessment of surgical risk by objective measures, such as the STS risk calculator, may be beneficial. Although patients' reoperative risk will be increased relative to their initial surgery, the risk of reoperation may not be prohibitive in many patients. All patients with PVR should be evaluated for both hemolytic anemia and active endocarditis, even when there are not suspicious clinical findings. If hemolytic anemia is present, it is unlikely to resolve unless the PVL is completely closed, and this should be known when discussing therapeutic options. Active endocarditis is a contraindication to transcatheter PVL closure.

While echocardiography is the primary imaging modality for the evaluation of PVR, cardiac computed tomography (CT) imaging may also be beneficial. Two-dimensional transthoracic echocardiography

(TTE) and transesophageal echocardiography (TEE) may quantify the degree of regurgitation, confirm its paravalvular nature, and rule out endocarditis or annular dehiscence. When transcatheter PVL closure is being considered, 3D echocardiography is essential in providing detailed morphology, including size, shape, and location of the defect(s), as well as the distance of the defect(s) from the prosthetic leaflets (Fig. 42.1) (9). In some patients, acoustic shadowing can pose significant challenges for visualizing PVR. Contrast CT imaging can also provide information regarding the size of defects, their orientation, and the presence of surrounding calcification. Furthermore, CT studies can also provide information regarding camera setup in the catheterization laboratory, which can facilitate transcatheter PVL closure. In properly equipped laboratories, CT "fusion" imaging may also be used to guide the procedure and enhance the success of transcatheter closure.

Of note, while criteria for echocardiographic quantification of valvular regurgitation are well-established, the criteria for quantification of PVR are not as well understood (10–12). Furthermore, patients with PVR can have symptoms out of proportion to the severity of PVR, as assessed by conventional standards. Cardiac magnetic resonance imaging (MRI) can be beneficial in assessing regurgitant volume, particularly for patients with equivocal echocardiographic findings (13). For symptomatic patients with inconclusive noninvasive studies, a detailed invasive hemodynamic assessment and aortography or ventriculography should be considered. Even defects that are not severe can be hemodynamically significant and may benefit

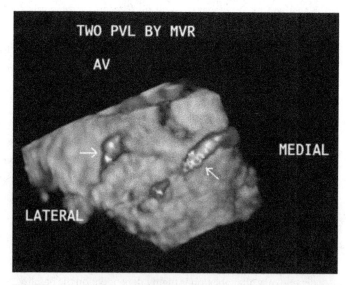

FIGURE 42.1 A three-dimensional transesophageal echocardiography (TEE) image depicting two paravalvular defects around a mechanical mitral prosthesis. This is the so-called "surgeons' view," with the aortic valve above (anterior to) the mitral valve, the atrial septum to the right (medial to) the valve, and the left atrial appendage to the left (lateral to) the valve. AV, aortic valve; MVR, mitral valve replacement; PVL, paravalvular leak.

from therapy; thus, direct measurement of filling pressures may be beneficial. In each case, clinical judgment must be exercised regarding the severity of PVR and the likelihood of associated symptoms, with the decision to pursue treatment individualized for all patients.

Despite the increasing use of transcatheter PVL closure for the treatment of PVR in symptomatic patients, some strict contraindications remain. Patients with active endocarditis, intracardiac thrombus, annular dehiscence (a rocking prosthesis), significant valvular regurgitation, or a paravalvular defect comprising >1/3 of the annular circumference should not be treated with transcatheter repair (14,15).

Procedural Techniques

Device Occluders

Transcatheter PVL closure requires off-label use of vascular occluders. The most commonly used devices are the AMPLATZER (Abbott Vascular, Abbott Park, IL) vascular plugs (AVP) and duct occluders (ADO). These devices are made of self-expanding nitinol, deliverable through small-caliber catheters, and have retention disks to help reduce the risk of embolization after deployment. The AVP-2, AVP-4, and ADO II devices are circular in shape, and are available for use in the United States, while the AVP-3, which has an oblong shape, is available only in Europe. Other devices include the AMPLATZER muscular ventricular septal defect occluder, which requires relatively larger sheaths for delivery, and the Occlutech PLD (Helsingborg, Sweden), specifically designed for transcatheter PVL closure, and only available in Europe. Accommodation of occluder devices within delivery catheters with or without wires is not described well in the manufacturers' labeling; however, as transcatheter PVL closure has become more prominent, descriptive tables have been published that may help to facilitate the selection of equipment for the procedure (16).

Aortic PVR

For patients with aortic PVR, the most common approach for transcatheter closure is retrograde via the femoral artery (Fig. 42.2). The echocardiographic imaging modality may be selected based on the location of the defect and the need to minimize acoustic shadowing of the regurgitant jet (TEE for posterior defects; TTE for anterior defects). Intracardiac echocardiography can also be performed from the right atrium, and manipulation of the catheter into the right ventricular outflow tract may provide additional imaging details.

Imaging angles in the catheterization laboratory should be obtained such that no overlap is observed between the defect and the aortic prosthesis, to ensure that the guide wire is being passed into the defect external to the prosthesis. This positioning can be approximated (e.g., left anterior oblique [LAO] cranial for posterior defects; right anterior oblique [RAO] caudal for anterior defects) or accurately determined from CT imaging. In biplane laboratories, the additional camera can be positioned *en face* to help with external placement of the wire, although this view is not required.

The defect is approached with a steerable coronary catheter, and an angled-tip, exchange-length hydrophilic wire is placed through the defect and can be passed antegrade through the aortic valve in the event that a guide-wire rail is desired. A delivery catheter is then advanced over the wire into the left ventricle. Selection of the delivery catheter is dependent on: (1) the size and number of device occluders needed; (2) the difficulty encountered in crossing the defect; and (3) the need for an anchor wire. With the delivery

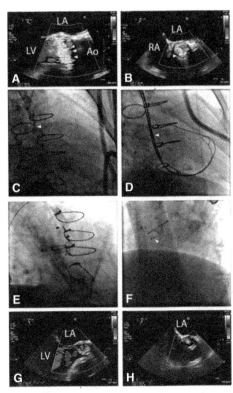

FIGURE 42.2 Transcatheter aortic PVL closure (**A** and **B**) TEE imaging demonstrating PVR (*arrowheads*). **C:** The defect is crossed with a hydrophilic wire (*arrowhead*). **D:** A guide catheter is advanced over the wire to the LV, and the hydrophilic wire is exchanged for two stiff wires. **E:** A delivery catheter is advanced separately over each wire to the LV, and two device occluders are positioned in the defect. **F:** The devices are deployed and released (*arrowhead* marking the ventricular retention disks). **G** and **H:** TEE imaging demonstrates resolution of PVR after PVL closure. Ao, ascending aorta; LA, left atrium; LV, left ventricle; PVL, paravalvular leak; PVR, paravalvular regurgitation; RA, right atrium; TEE, transesophageal echocardiography.

catheter in the left ventricle, the device occluder is extruded with retention disks positioned on the ventricular and aortic sides of the defect or, as frequently with AVP-4 plugs, wholly within the defect. The final assessment must include evaluation for prosthetic leaflet impingement, residual regurgitation, and coronary occlusion. Coronary angiography can be considered to exclude coronary occlusion in patients requiring large device occluders, and those with small aortic sinuses, low coronary height, or defects located near the coronary ostia. Once the final assessment is satisfactory, the device occluders are released.

Mitral PVR

For patients with mitral PVR, transcatheter PVL closure is typically performed with general anesthesia and TEE. The most commonly used approach is femoral venous access with transseptal puncture and antegrade cannulation of the defect from the left atrium. Alternatively, direct transapical puncture or a retrograde approach (via the femoral artery) with retrograde cannulation of the defect from the left ventricle also can be successful (16–18).

For the antegrade approach, standard transseptal technique with guidance from fluoroscopy and echocardiography are used to access the left atrium. A steerable guide catheter is loaded with a telescoped catheter system—e.g., a 6-Fr 100-cm multipurpose guide and a 5-Fr 125-cm multipurpose diagnostic catheter (Fig. 42.3).

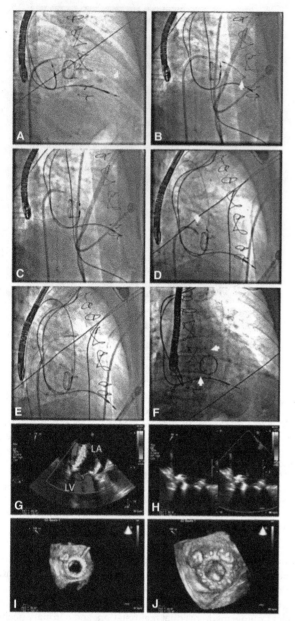

FIGURE 42.3 Transcatheter mitral PVL closure. **A:** A lateral defect is crossed with a hydrophilic wire (*arrow*). **B:** A delivery catheter is advanced over the wire to the LV and a device occluder is advanced to the LV. The *arrow* indicates the distal retention disk in the LV. **C:** The device is positioned across the defect and further unsheathed. **D:** The device is released with the proximal retention disk positioned on the left atrial side of the defect (*arrow*). **E:** A medial defect is crossed in retrograde fashion with a hydrophilic wire from the LV and snared in the LA to form a guide-wire rail. **F:** Two occluder devices are deployed in the medial defect using the guide-wire rail. *Arrows* indicate the lateral and medial devices. **G:** TEE imaging demonstrating medial and lateral jets of PVR prior to PVL closure. **H:** TEE imaging demonstrating trivial residual PVR medially, and no PVR laterally. **I:** Three-dimensional TEE imaging demonstrating the deployed lateral occluder device and a catheter crossing the medial defect. **J:** Three-dimensional TEE imaging demonstrating device deployment in both the lateral and medial defects. LA, left atrium; LV, left ventricle; PVL, paravalvular leak closure; PVR, paravalvular regurgitation; TEE, transesophageal echocardiography.

A steerable guide with a small-sized curve may be particularly helpful for medial defects. This system is steered toward the defect, which is crossed with a hydrophilic wire. Fluoroscopy should demonstrate positioning of the steerable guide and the guide wires external to

the prosthesis ring. The telescoped catheters are placed sequentially into the left ventricle, followed by removal of the diagnostic catheter. A device occluder can be passed through the guide catheter, or exchanged over a stiff wire for a larger sheath, depending on the size and number of device occluders needed and the need for an anchor wire. Similar to treatment of aortic defects, the distal retention disk of the occluder is extruded from the guide into the left ventricle, followed by straddling of the defect with the retention disks on both sides. Once leaflet impingement has been excluded on both echocardiography and fluoroscopy, the device occluder is released.

In the retrograde approach from the femoral artery, a coronary catheter is placed into the left ventricle and oriented posteriorly toward the defect. This technique can be used when the transseptal approach is not successful, especially if the defect is located medially. The defect can be crossed with relatively softer wires, such as 0.014-inch or 0.018-inch coronary guide wires, if needed. In the transapical technique, defect cannulation and device placement is similar to the antegrade approach.

Transcatheter Rails

Placement of guide catheters can be challenging due to the serpiginous and often calcific nature of paravalvular defects. In these instances, transcatheter rails can be utilized for greater support for catheter passage.

Originally described for the treatment of congenital heart lesions, transcatheter rails are created by snaring of a guide wire that has been placed across the paravalvular defect, followed by exteriorization to provide the operator with both ends of the wire. For mitral paravalvular defects, a transcatheter rail can be placed left atrial–ventricular–aortic or left atrial–ventricular–apical. For aortic paravalvular defects, the rail can be placed aortic–ventricular–aortic, aortic–ventricular–apical, or left atrial–ventricular–aortic. Once the rail has been created, the operator can advance a guide catheter with support from an assistant who provides tension on both ends of the wire.

It is important to note that guide-wire tension from transcatheter rails can result in injury to the surrounding structures, and damage to the prosthetic or native leaflets, as well as cause myocardial injury, atrioventricular node injury and resultant bradycardia, or disrupt the mitral valve apparatus from chordal entanglement. Therefore, transcatheter heart rails should only be utilized by experienced operators and with careful hemodynamic monitoring and simultaneous echocardiography.

Multiple Device Placement and Anchor Wiring

Paravalvular defects frequently are eccentric and in close proximity to the surgical sewing ring. As a result, successful closure can be challenging with the use of large occluders, because device overhang can result in leaflet impingement of the valve, particularly with mechanical prostheses, which do not have struts. Alternatively, multiple, smaller-device occluders can be deployed using an anchor wire technique. In these instances, after the defect is crossed with a hydrophilic guide wire, a larger bore sheath is placed into the ventricle. The sheath can accommodate multiple, stiff guide wires that can then be used to place the delivery catheters either simultaneously or sequentially over each wire. The anchor wire technique is also useful for maintaining a position across the paravalvular defect in the event that an occluder needs to be exchanged for different or multiple other devices. If anchor wiring is used, large bore sheaths are required at the arterial or venous access site to accommodate the multiple delivery catheters and wires. The DrySeal sheath (W.L. Gore, Flagstaff, AZ), with its inflatable cuff, is uniquely suitable for maintaining hemostasis for this purpose.

CT Guidance

Cardiac CT can identify paravalvular defects and assist with transcatheter PVL closure. Using information from echocardiography, the CT scan is reconstructed using views of the exit point of the regurgitant jet, whose paravalvular continuity can then be examined (Fig. 42.4). Imaging with CT can help with sizing of the defect and identifying its course, and can provide information on surrounding calcification. The information gained from CT imaging may be of particular clinical benefit when there is significant acoustic shadowing on echocardiography.

Fusion CT imaging can also be used to facilitate transcatheter PVL closure. In this technique, CT data are coregistered to cardiac structures (i.e., chambers, valves, coronary arteries), enabling overlay onto the fluoroscopy screen. Fusion CT imaging is then used to guide access (transseptal antegrade vs. retrograde apical), defect wiring, and device placement (17).

Clinical Outcomes

Transcatheter PVL closure was first described over 25 years ago, and interest in this therapy has greatly increased in the last decade

(18). Procedural success in achieving no more than a mild residual leak with no major adverse events is approximately 80%, and is approximately 90% in achieving moderate residual regurgitation or less (19,20). Complications are relatively infrequent. A series of 115 patients (20) reported the following rate of adverse events at 30 days: stroke (2.6%), emergency surgery (0.9%), sudden or unexplained death (1.7%), and periprocedural bleeding (5.2%). Procedural death is uncommon (~0.5%) and the rate of device embolization is approximately 2.5%. Coronary artery occlusion is another potential concern in aortic PVL closure, and is dependent on the height of the coronary arteries and the location of the defect.

The most common reasons for procedural failure are prosthetic leaflet impingement and the inability to cross the defect with a wire or delivery catheter. The rate of leaflet impingement ranges from 5% to 7% and can occur with any prosthesis, but is more common in mechanical valves due to the absence of valve struts. The circular shape of some AVP occluders and the close proximity of the defect to the surgical annular ring increase the likelihood of impingement, and impingement can be minimized by using multiple, smaller devices if necessary. Prior to device release, careful echo, fluoroscopic, and hemodynamic assessment is required

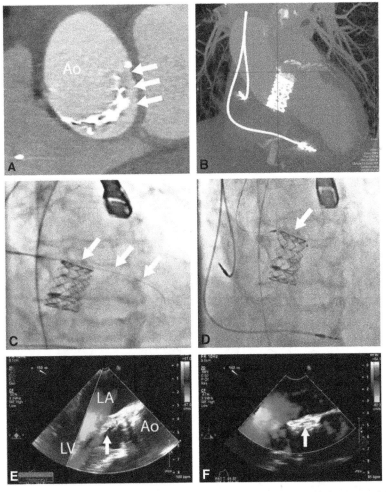

FIGURE 42.4   CT guidance for transcatheter PVL closure. **A:** CT imaging identifies the paravalvular defect (*arrows*). **B:** CT imaging aligns the defect exterior to the prosthesis, providing cath lab camera angles to facilitate the procedure. **C:** Using the camera angle provided by CT, the defect is easily wired (*arrows*). **D:** A device occluder is deployed in the paravalvular defect (*arrow*). **E:** TEE imaging demonstrating severe paravalvular regurgitation prior to transcatheter PVL closure (*arrow*). **F:** TEE imaging demonstrating mild residual paravalvular regurgitation after transcatheter PVL closure (*arrow*). Ao, aorta; CT, computed tomography; LA, left artery; LV, left ventricle; PVL, paravalvular leak; TEE, transesophageal echocardiography.

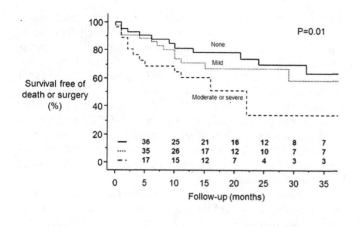

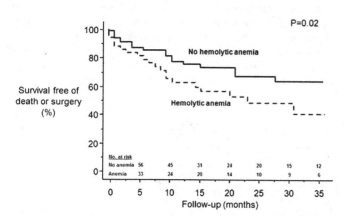

FIGURE 42.5 Survival after transcatheter PVL closure. **Top:** Survival free of death or reoperation according to residual PVL following transcatheter PVL closure. **Bottom:** Survival free of death or reoperation according to the presence or absence of hemolytic anemia. PVL, paravalvular leak. (From: Sorajja P, et al. Long-term follow-up of percutaneous repair of paravalvular regurgitation. *J Am Coll Cardiol.* 2011;58:2218–2224.)

to assess leaflet motion and valve gradient. Because the release of tension on the system after device release can lead to reorientation of the occluder, leaflet impingement should be reassessed after final deployment as well.

In a long-term evaluation of 126 patients who underwent transcatheter PVL closure, the 3-year survival was 64% (**Fig. 42.5**) (21). Cardiac death occurred in 9.5%, while the incidence of noncardiac death was between 7.1% and 12.7%, indicating the high-risk nature of this patient population. Notably, 72% of survivors were free of severe symptoms or the need for surgical reintervention. Clinical success and relief of symptoms have been shown to be related to the degree of residual regurgitation, and are greater for patients with symptoms of congestive heart failure than for those with hemolysis (Fig. 42.5) (21). Importantly, the New York Heart Association (NYHA) functional class has been demonstrated to improve only in those patients with less than or equal to a mild residual leak. On the other hand, successful treatment of hemolysis ideally requires complete closure of the paravalvular defect. In addition, operator experience with advanced closure techniques (e.g., anchor wire, three-dimension imaging, transcatheter rails) is an important predictor of procedural success (**Fig. 42.6**) (22).

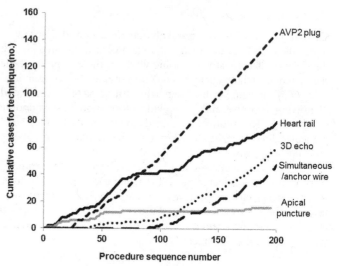

FIGURE 42.6 Adoption of procedural techniques for transcatheter PVL closure at a single center. The graph depicts the cumulative experience with each technique over a series of 200 cases. AVP, AMPLATZER vascular plug; PVL, paravalvular leak closure. (From: Sorajja P, et al. The learning curve in percutaneous repair of paravalvular prosthetic regurgitation: an analysis of 200 cases. *JACC Cardiovasc Interv.* 2014;7:521–529.)

Key Points

- PVR after surgical valve replacement is relatively common, and may be related to tissue friability, annular calcification, or infection.

- Significant PVR may result in hemolysis, congestive heart failure, or both.

- Transcatheter PVL closure is indicated for patients with severe CHF symptoms or refractory hemolysis who are at high-risk for reoperation, if their anatomy is suitable.

- Procedural success of transcatheter PVL closure may be as high as 90% through antegrade and retrograde approaches; however, potential complications include bleeding, stroke, valve leaflet impingement, and device embolization.

- Transcatheter PVL closure should be performed at experienced centers.

References

1. Akins CW, et al. Early and late results of the surgical correction of cardiac prosthetic paravalvular leaks. *J Heart Valve Dis.* 2005;14(6):792–799; discussion 799–800.
2. Davila-Roman VG, et al. Prevalence and severity of paravalvular regurgitation in the Artificial Valve Endocarditis Reduction Trial (AVERT) echocardiography study. *J Am Coll Cardiol.* 2004;44(7):1467–1472.
3. Hwang HY, et al. Paravalvular leak after mitral valve replacement: 20-year follow-up. *Ann Thorac Surg.* 2015;100(4):1347–1352.
4. Miller DL, et al. Reoperation for aortic valve periprosthetic leakage: identification of patients at risk and results of operation. *J Heart Valve Dis.* 1995;4(2):160–165.
5. Genereux P, et al. Paravalvular leak after transcatheter aortic valve replacement: the new Achilles' heel? A comprehensive review of the literature. *J Am Coll Cardiol.* 2013;61(11):1125–1136.

6. Kodali SK, et al. Two-year outcomes after transcatheter or surgical aortic-valve replacement. *N Engl J Med.* 2012;366(18):1686–1695.

7. Orszulak TA, et al. Results of reoperation for periprosthetic leakage. *Ann Thorac Surg.* 1983;35(6):584–589.

8. Nishimura RA, et al. 2014 AHA/ACC guideline for the management of patients with valvular heart disease: executive summary: a report of the American College of Cardiology/American Heart Association Task Force on Practice Guidelines. *J Am Coll Cardiol.* 2014;63(22):2438–2488.

9. Altiok E, et al. Comparison of two- and three-dimensional transthoracic echocardiography to cardiac magnetic resonance imaging for assessment of paravalvular regurgitation after transcatheter aortic valve implantation. *Am J Cardiol.* 2014;113(11):1859–1866.

10. Kappetein AP, et al. Updated standardized endpoint definitions for transcatheter aortic valve implantation: the Valve Academic Research Consortium-2 consensus document. *J Am Coll Cardiol.* 2012;60(15):1438–1454.

11. Zoghbi WA, et al. Recommendations for evaluation of prosthetic valves with echocardiography and doppler ultrasound: a report from the American Society of Echocardiography's Guidelines and Standards Committee and the Task Force on Prosthetic Valves, developed in conjunction with the American College of Cardiology Cardiovascular Imaging Committee, Cardiac Imaging Committee of the American Heart Association, the European Association of Echocardiography, a registered branch of the European Society of Cardiology, the Japanese Society of Echocardiography and the Canadian Society of Echocardiography, endorsed by the American College of Cardiology Foundation, American Heart Association, European Association of Echocardiography, a registered branch of the European Society of Cardiology, the Japanese Society of Echocardiography, and Canadian Society of Echocardiography. *J Am Soc Echocardiogr.* 2009;22(9):975–1014; quiz 1082–1084.

12. Zoghbi WA, et al. Recommendations for evaluation of the severity of native valvular regurgitation with two-dimensional and Doppler echocardiography. *J Am Soc Echocardiogr.* 2003;16(7):777–802.

13. Ribeiro HB, et al. Cardiac magnetic resonance versus transthoracic echocardiography for the assessment and quantification of aortic regurgitation in patients undergoing transcatheter aortic valve implantation. *Heart.* 2014;100(24):1924–1932.

14. Eleid MF, et al. Techniques and outcomes for the treatment of paravalvular leak. *Circ Cardiovasc Interv.* 2015;8(8):e001945.

15. Sorajja P. Mitral paravalvular leak closure. *Interv Cardiol Clin.* 2016;5(1):45–54.

16. Gossl M, Rihal CS. Percutaneous treatment of aortic and mitral valve paravalvular regurgitation. *Curr Cardiol Rep.* 2013;15(8):388.

17. Kliger C, et al. CT angiography-fluoroscopy fusion imaging for percutaneous transapical access. *JACC Cardiovasc Imaging.* 2014;7(2):169–177.

18. Hourihan M, et al. Transcatheter umbrella closure of valvular and paravalvular leaks. *J Am Coll Cardiol.* 1992;20(6):1371–1377.

19. Ruiz CE, et al. Clinical outcomes in patients undergoing percutaneous closure of periprosthetic paravalvular leaks. *J Am Coll Cardiol.* 2011;58(21):2210–2217.

20. Sorajja P, et al. Percutaneous repair of paravalvular prosthetic regurgitation: acute and 30-day outcomes in 115 patients. *Circ Cardiovasc Interv.* 2011;4(4):314–321.

21. Sorajja P, et al. Long-term follow-up of percutaneous repair of paravalvular prosthetic regurgitation. *J Am Coll Cardiol.* 2011;58(21):2218–2224.

22. Sorajja P, et al. The learning curve in percutaneous repair of paravalvular prosthetic regurgitation: an analysis of 200 cases. *JACC Cardiovasc Interv.* 2014;7(5):521–529.

43 Pericardial Disease Interventions

Paul Sorajja, MD, FSCAI, FACC, FAHA

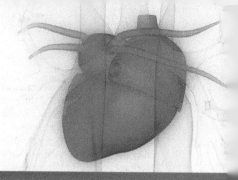

Cardiac tamponade is a life-threatening disorder that can result from any condition that causes a pericardial effusion. Although the most frequent cause is malignancy, tamponade may also occur from pericarditis (e.g., viral, uremic, inflammatory, or idiopathic), aortic dissection from disruption of the aortic annulus, ventricular rupture from myocardial infarction, and virtually any disorder that causes a pericardial effusion (1). In the cardiac catheterization laboratory, tamponade can result from cardiac perforation from a variety of invasive procedures and lead to rapid demise of the patient, owing to the swift accumulation of fluid in a poorly compliant pericardial space. Prompt recognition of the salient hemodynamic features and immediate pericardiocentesis are elementary in the successful treatment of cardiac tamponade.

Diagnosis of Cardiac Tamponade

Cardiac tamponade should be suspected in any patient in the cardiac catheterization laboratory with unexplained hypotension. The hemodynamic effects of a pericardial effusion may be acute or gradual, depending on the amount and rate of fluid accumulation. Localized tamponade can result from loculated pericardial effusions, such as those that may be present adjacent to the atria in the postoperative setting or those due to local injury from invasive cardiology pressures.

Normally, the pericardial space contains 15 to 50 mL of fluid, with an intrapericardial pressure that approximates the intrapleural pressure (-5 to $+5$ cm H_2O). Fluid accumulation and pericardial restraint leads to rises in intrapericardial pressure. Cardiac tamponade occurs when intrapericardial pressure exceeds intracardiac pressure, leading to impaired ventricular filling throughout the entire diastolic period, followed by increases in pulmonary venous and jugular venous pressures, and reduction in forward stroke volume and cardiac output. With inspiration, there is a fall in the driving pressure to fill the left ventricle, subsequently leading to a reduction in ventricular filling and stroke volume. The fall in left ventricular stroke volume during inspiration manifests as a relative decrease in pulse pressure or peak systolic pressure, which is the hallmark finding of *pulsus paradoxus* in patients with cardiac tamponade. Of note, cardiac tamponade also may occur without marked elevation of atrial pressures when the intracardiac filling pressures (i.e., low-pressure tamponade) are relatively low, such as in dehydrated patients (2). This latter scenario is commonly seen following pericardiocentesis with large intravascular volume loss, leading to intracardiac pressures falling lower than pericardial pressures.

Two-dimensional and Doppler echocardiography is commonly used for diagnosing cardiac tamponade (3,4). Specific signs of tamponade include diastolic inversion or collapse of the right atrium and right ventricle, ventricular septal shifting with respiration, and plethora of the inferior vena cava (Fig. 43.1). Respiratory variation in the Doppler mitral inflow is a highly sensitive measure that occurs early in tamponade, and may precede changes in cardiac output, blood pressure, and other echocardiographic findings.

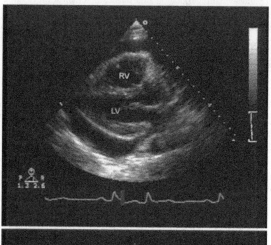

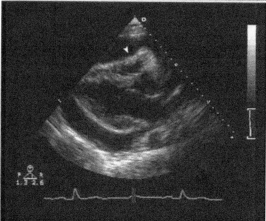

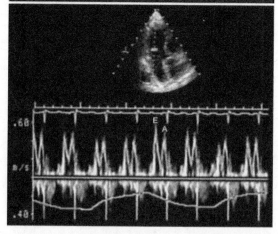

FIGURE 43.1 Echocardiographic findings of cardiac tamponade. **Top:** Parasternal long-axis view showing a circumferential pericardial effusion. **Middle:** Diastolic inversion and collapse of the right ventricle is present. **Bottom:** Doppler echocardiography of the mitral valve flow demonstrates significant respiratory variation in left ventricular filling. LV, left ventricle; RV, right ventricle.

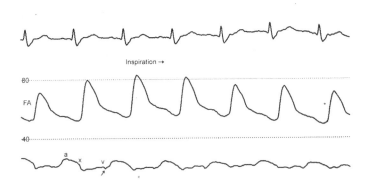

FIGURE 43.2 Invasive hemodynamic findings of cardiac tamponade. On the last beat in the femoral artery (FA) pressure tracing, there is an inspiratory decline in the aortic pulse pressure (*asterisk*), analogous to the bedside finding of pulsus paradoxus. In the right atrial pressure tracing, there is loss of the y descent (*arrow*) that normally follows the V wave.

The invasive hemodynamic hallmark of cardiac tamponade is blunting of the y descent in the atrial pressure tracings, or blunting of the early diastolic filling wave in ventricular pressure contour. The x descent is usually preserved because of the decrease in intracardiac volume during systolic ejection, which leads to a temporary reduction in intrapericardial and right atrial pressures (**Fig. 43.2**). Elevated intrapericardial pressure impairs ventricular filling during the remainder of the cardiac cycle, resulting in blunting of the y descent. These hemodynamic consequences can also manifest in the

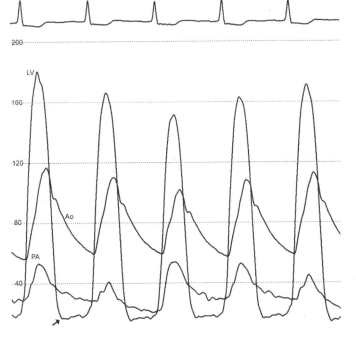

FIGURE 43.3 Change in left ventricular diastolic pressure with cardiac tamponade. This patient underwent retrograde evaluation of her aortic stenosis in the cardiac catheterization laboratory. There is blunting of the left ventricular early diastolic (or minimum) pressure (*arrow*), corresponding to blunting of the y descent that would be seen in the atrial pressure recording. Inspiratory decline in the aortic pulse pressure also is evident on the third beat. Emergent echocardiography confirmed the presence of a pericardial effusion with tamponade physiology. AO, ascending aorta; LV, left ventricle; PA, pulmonary artery.

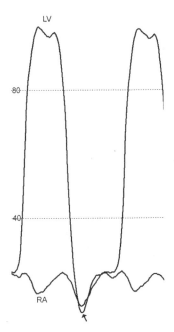

FIGURE 43.4 Early rapid ventricular filling. This figure illustrates the presence of early rapid ventricular filling and prominent y descents (*arrow*), which are a feature of constrictive pericarditis, restrictive cardiomyopathy, and other forms of heart failure. The preservation (or accentuation) of the y descent allows one to distinguish these entities from cardiac tamponade (see Figs. 43.2 and 43.3). LV, left ventricle; RA, right artery.

left ventricular early diastolic (or early minimum) pressure, whose changes may be subtle (**Fig. 43.3**). The blunting or loss of the early rapid ventricular filling wave is the hallmark of cardiac tamponade that distinguishes it from other diastolic filling disorders (**Fig. 43.4**). The reduction in left ventricular filling and stroke volume manifests as a decrease in aortic pulse pressure during inspiration in a manner analogous to the bedside finding of pulsus paradoxus.

Technique for Pericardiocentesis

For most patients, pericardiocentesis is performed with echocardiographic guidance (**Table 43.1**) (5). Certainly, in emergent situations where echocardiography is not immediately available, pericardiocentesis can be performed in a blinded or ECG-guided fashion, usually from the subxyphoid approach (6). However, adjunctive echocardiography plays a significant role in the evaluation of patients with cardiac tamponade and will reduce the incidence of complications related to pericardiocentesis. Of note, pericardiocentesis should not be performed in patients with tamponade and aortic dissection. In such patients, relief of the tamponade will lead to an abrupt increase in systolic blood pressure that may exacerbate the aortic dissection (7). Careful imaging with transthoracic or transesophageal echocardiography is required to determine the presence of these manifestations of tamponade.

For all patients, volume resuscitation can help provide hemodynamic stability and should be performed immediately in patients with cardiac tamponade. Reversal of anticoagulation and antiplatelet therapy should be performed as clinically permitted. Agents that augment ventricular afterload (e.g., phenylephrine) should be avoided, because this increase will further impair forward stroke volume and worsen the hemodynamic effects of cardiac tamponade. During pericardiocentesis, right heart catheterization with simultaneous

TABLE 43.1 Equipment for Pericardiocentesis

Sterile gloves, mask, and gown

Povidone-iodine solution or other skin antiseptic

Sterile transparent plastic drape

20G or 25G needle for local anesthesia administration

Local anesthesia (e.g., 1% lidocaine)

18-gauge polytef-sheathed venous needles of varying lengths (5–8 cm)

Syringes (10, 20, and 50 mL)

0.035" J-tipped guide wire

Scalpel (no. 11 blade)

5-F or 6-F introducer sheath

5-F or 6-F, 65-cm pigtail catheter with multiple side holes

4" × 4" gauze for dressing and ointment

1 L vacuum bottle or comparable fluid receptacle

Labels for specimen collection

Sterile isotonic saline (for catheter flush)

measurement of right atrial and pulmonary capillary wedge pressures assist in the diagnosis and for determining efficacy of the procedure.

Patient Positioning

The patient is usually positioned with head raised ~30° to facilitate inferior and apical pooling of the pericardial effusion.

Site of Entry

Echocardiography helps to determine the most appropriate site of entry and needle direction. Most frequently, the echocardiographic window that is closest to the effusion is selected (Fig. 43.5). Common portals of entry are subxiphoid and apical, but other locations have included axillary, and left or right parasternal. Advantages of the subxiphoid approach are a lower risk of pneumothorax and laceration of internal mammary or intercostal arteries. For the subxiphoid approach, the needle must be angled clear below the bottom rib because it attaches to the inferolateral surface above the xiphoid process (typically one fingerbreadth inferior and lateral to the edge of the xiphoid). Punctures that are too high and near the recess at the xiphoid angle can pose challenges to delivering the needle under the rib. When using a parasternal approach, the needle should pass 1 cm lateral to the sternum to avoid injury to the internal mammary artery; the risk of pneumothorax increases with further lateral positioning. For intercostal approaches, the needle should pass superior to the rib margins to reduce the risk of injury to the neurovascular bundle. The angle of entry and direction should be fixed in the operator's mind. The site of entry can be marked with an indelible pen. The precordium or subxiphoid area is sterilized with antiseptic solution and covered with a sterile drape.

Needle Insertion

Following local anesthesia, an 18-G, thin-walled Polytef-sheathed needle is inserted at the entry site using the predetermined angulation. Some operators, include those in our cardiac catheterization laboratory, prefer use of a micropuncture needle. In all cases, the needle is advanced with gentle aspiration into the pericardial space. Aggressive aspiration may cause tissue occlusion of the needle and inhibit detection of pericardial fluid. Once fluid is obtained, the polytef needle is advanced slightly further (~2 mm) to ensure placement of the sheath into the pericardial space. The polytef sheath is then advanced over the needle, followed by withdrawal of the needle. The needle should not be readvanced once it has been removed from the sheath. For micropuncture needle use, a standard sheath wire can be used followed by placement of the sheath.

Confirmation of Location

Agitated saline is injected into the sheath via a three-way stopcock with echocardiographic imaging (Fig. 43.6). If the agitated saline does not enhance the pericardial space, then repositioning of the needle by either withdrawal or another needle passage is performed. Radiographic contrast can also be administered under fluoroscopy. Small test injections should be given initially to exclude myocardial positioning, which is seen as myocardial staining. Contrast swirling will indicate a ventricular location, while pooling suggests intrapericardial positioning. Alternatively, the needle (before it is withdrawn) or the sheath can be connected to tubing connectors for pressure transduction. Intrapericardial pressure will be similar to the atrial pressure, while ventricular systolic pressure waveforms can immediately alert the operator to inadvertent ventricular perforation. For operators using an ECG-guided approach, the needle is connected to an alligator-tipped electrode. With myocardial contact, ST-segment elevation (i.e., injury current) will be detected that may not appear on other electrocardiographic leads.

Catheter Placement

Following confirmation of the position, a J-tipped guide wire is inserted through the polytef or micropuncture sheath into the pericardial space. A small skin incision with a scalpel is made, followed by exchange for a 5-F or 6-F introducer sheath and removal of the dilator. A multihole pigtail catheter is then inserted, followed by removal of the introducer sheath, leaving only the smooth-walled pigtail catheter in place. Positioning of the pigtail catheter can be reconfirmed using either echocardiography or pressure measurement.

Aspiration

Manual techniques or vacuum bottles can be used to remove the pericardial effusion. For patients with tamponade caused by cardiac perforation, care should be taken to remove as much pericardial fluid as possible because this will facilitate sealing of the perforated site. For patients with other causes of pericardial effusion, complete apposition of the parietal and visceral layers also will reduce the risk of recurrence. The inability to aspirate despite a persistent pericardial effusion on echocardiography should lead to repositioning of the pigtail catheter. Occasionally, puncture of a tense pericardium will lead to discharge of pericardial contents into a pleural space, resulting in less than expected removal via aspiration. Normalization of atrial pressures documented with simultaneous right-heart catheterization helps to ensure successful removal of the pericardial effusion and relief of the cardiac tamponade. For patients with large volume removal because of acute hemorrhage, cell savers are often used to minimize blood loss.

Postpericardiocentesis Management

The pigtail catheter is sutured to the chest wall, connected to a stopcock, and flushed every 4 to 6 hours with heparinized saline to maintain patency. Standard indwelling catheter care with complete dressing changes every 72 hours is recommended. When drainage becomes minimal (<25 mL/day) and echocardiography shows no recurrent effusion, the pigtail catheter can be removed. For completely drained pericardial effusions, the risk of recurrence is low (<10%), with the exception of certain etiologies (e.g., bacterial infection, malignancy).

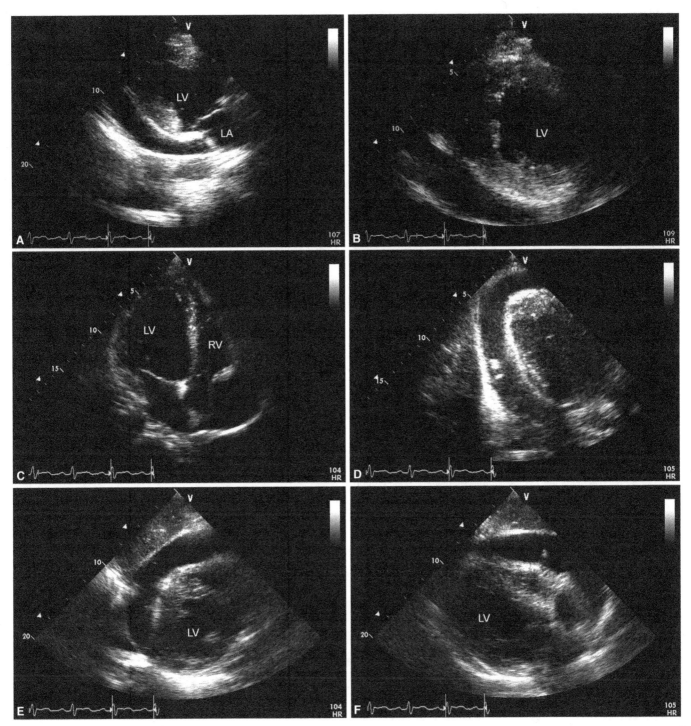

FIGURE 43.5 Echocardiography for site location for pericardiocentesis. Multiple views are required to determine the most appropriate site of pericardiocentesis, with examination of parasternal (**A** and **B**), apical (**C** and **D**), and sub-coastal (**E** and **F**) windows. The apical window in panel **D** was chosen for pericardiocentesis. LA, left artery; LV, left ventricle; RA, right artery; RV, right ventricle.

Complications

When performed by experienced operators, complications of pericardiocentesis are infrequent (<1.5% of patients) (8–12). The most serious complication is laceration of a coronary artery. Perforation of either the right or the left ventricle also may occur, but this is rarely of clinical significance. Bleeding and tamponade from coronary or ventricular perforation can be detected by continuous

monitoring of atrial pressure, which will increase in the event of these complications. Acute left ventricular failure with pulmonary edema has been reported as a complication of pericardiocentesis, but the cause of this phenomenon is not known (13).

·Although most pericardial effusions can be treated percutaneously, a surgical approach may still be required. Loculated effusions, posterior effusions, or pericardial clot formations from a recent hemorrhage may all be difficult to remove percutaneously. Large

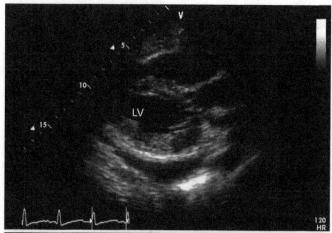

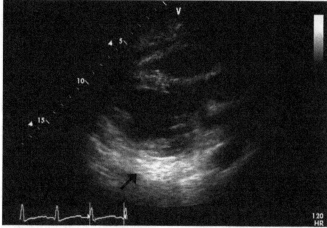

FIGURE 43.6 Use of agitated saline contrast medium for confirmation of sheath position in pericardial space. Pericardial effusion was visualized by imaging remote from entry site on chest wall, before injection of agitated saline contrast medium (**top**). Injection of agitated saline contrast medium provides dense opacification of pericardial space, confirming sheath position (**bottom**, *arrow*). LV, left ventricle.

surgical drainage is often required for effusions caused by bacterial infection. For patients with refractory pericardial effusions (e.g., caused by malignancy), balloon pericardiotomy to allow drainage into the pleural or peritoneal space may be a therapeutic option (14).

Key Points

- The hemodynamic hallmark of cardiac tamponade is blunting of the y descent in the atrial pressure tracing. This finding corresponds to blunting of the early minimum diastolic pressure in the ventricular pressure tracing, and reflects impairment of ventricular filling during the entire diastolic period because of elevated intrapericardial pressure.

- *Pulsus paradoxus* is an inspiratory fall in left ventricular stroke volume, which manifests as a decrease in the systolic pressure or pulse pressure.

- Patients with cardiac tamponade should be treated initially with volume resuscitation, followed by emergent pericardiocentesis under echocardiographic guidance.

References

1. Atar S, et al. Bloody pericardial effusion in patients with cardiac tamponade: is the cause cancerous, tuberculous, or iatrogenic in the 1990s. *Chest*. 1999;116:1564–1569.
2. Walsh BM, Tobias LA. Low-pressure pericardial tamponade: case report and review of the literature. *J Emerg Med*. 2017;52(4):516–522. doi:10.1016/j.jemermed.2016.06.069.
3. Appleton CP, Hatle LK, Popp RL. Cardiac tamponade and pericardial effusion: respiratory variation in transvalvular flow velocities studied by Doppler echocardiography. *J Am Coll Cardiol*. 1988;11:1020–1030.
4. Maisch B, et al. Guidelines on the diagnosis and management of pericardial diseases executive summary; the task force on the diagnosis and management of pericardial diseases of the European Society of Cardiology. *Eur Heart J*. 2004;25:587–610.
5. Tsang SM, et al. Echocardiographically guided pericardiocentesis: evolution and state-of-the-art technique. *Mayo Clin Proc*. 1998;73:647–652.
6. Campbell PT, et al. Subxiphoid pericardiotomy in the diagnosis and management of large pericardial effusions associated with malignancy. *Chest*. 1992;101:938–943.
7. Isselbacher EM, Cigarroa JE, Eagle KA. Cardiac tamponade complicating proximal aortic dissection: is pericardiocentesis harmful? *Circulation*. 1994;90:2375–2378.
8. Duvernoy O, et al. Complications of percutaneous pericardiocentesis under fluoroscopic guidance. *Acta Radiol*. 1992;33:309–313.
9. Galli M, et al. Percutaneous balloon pericardiotomy for malignant pericardial tamponade. *Chest*. 1995;108:1499–1501.
10. Markiewicz W, Borovik R, Ecker S. Cardiac tamponade in medical patients: treatment and prognosis in the echocardiographic era. *Am Heart J*. 1986;111:1138–1142.
11. Tsang TS, et al. Rescue echocardiographically guided pericardiocentesis for cardiac perforation complicating catheter-based procedures. The Mayo Clinic experience. *J Am Coll Cardiol*. 1998;32:1345–1350.
12. Tsang TS, et al. Consecutive 1,127 therapeutic echocardiographically guided pericardiocentesis: clinical profile, practice patterns, and outcomes spanning 21 years. *Mayo Clin Proc*. 2002;77:429–436.
13. Wolfe MW, Edelman ER. Transient systolic dysfunction after relief of cardiac tamponade. *Ann Intern Med*. 1993;119:42–44.
14. Ziskind AA, et al. Percutaneous balloon pericardiotomy for the treatment of cardiac tamponade and large pericardial effusions: description of technique and report of the first 50 cases. *J Am Coll Cardiol*. 1993;21:1–5.

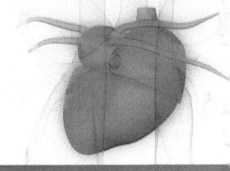

Interventional Procedures in Adult Congenital Heart Disease

Vikas Singh, MD and Ignacio Inglessis, MD

Improved treatment strategies and interventions have increased survival in adult congenital heart disease (ACHD) so much that up to 85% of the children born with cardiac birth defects are expected to live well into adulthood (1–3). Over the last decade, the field of interventional cardiology has also witnessed a dramatic advancement driven by technologic improvement. Percutaneous therapies are now acceptable alternatives, additions, or treatments of choice when surgical or medical interventions are contemplated in ACHD. Interventional cardiology is a well-established component of any center that provides care to this unique patient population. Guidelines recommendations for catheter interventions have also been published in the context of overall care of ACHD in the United States and Europe (1,4).

In this chapter, we review the most commonly performed percutaneous procedures in adults with congenital heart disease (CHD), including valvuloplasty, transcatheter valve replacement, angioplasty/stenting, device closure, and coil embolization. The guidelines recommendations for these procedures, along with their level of evidence, are provided in **Table 44.1**.

Valvuloplasty

Balloon Pulmonary Valvuloplasty

Pulmonary valve stenosis (PS) is almost always congenital in origin and usually results from commissural fusion of thin and pliable leaflets. The majority of the cases are characterized by a narrow central opening with preserved valve motion (i.e., dome-type PS). Less frequently, the pulmonary valve is dysplastic, with thickened valve leaflets and a relatively immobile valve. The 2008 ACC/AHA guidelines for management of adults with congenital heart disease classify the severity of PS into mild, moderate, and severe, based on the peak Doppler gradient of <30 mm Hg, 30 to 50 mm Hg, and >50 mm Hg, respectively (1).

Balloon pulmonary valvuloplasty (BVP) is the treatment of choice for isolated PS, with high technical success and excellent short- and long-term results. Most patients are free of events in the long term after a single procedure.

Further reduction in residual gradients may be seen over time because of resolution of residual hypertrophic subvalvular stenosis (5,6). The use of an oversized balloon (1.2–1.25 times the annulus) has been advocated to achieve a successful result, which is defined by a peak valve gradient of <20 mm Hg. More aggressive balloon sizing (>1.4 times the annulus) has been associated with development of moderate to severe pulmonary regurgitation (PR) in 11% of the cases (7). An undersized balloon (<1.2 times the annulus) is a predictor for restenosis, which is reported in 10% of the patients (5). Transient severe right ventricular outflow tract obstruction ("suicide" right ventricle [RV]) has been reported after BPV, particularly in the pediatric population; however, this may be treated by volume expansion and β-blocker therapy (5). BPV has also been attempted in subvalvular PS and in adults with dysplastic pulmonary valves, but results are typically suboptimal and surgical valvotomy is usually

indicated for these patients. The impact of associated aneurysmal dilation of the main pulmonary (and potentially aortic) trunk in patients (and their relatives) with PS remains unclear.

Balloon Aortic Valvuloplasty

Obstructive lesions of the left ventricular outflow tract comprise nearly 6% of the congenital heart diseases in children, of which valvular aortic stenosis (AS) is the most common. Bicuspid aortic valve accounts for the majority of the cases, and in contrast to PS, AS secondary to bicuspid aortic valve disease is a progressive disorder in the adult. Those affected are at risk for sudden death, particularly undiagnosed young adults exposed to strenuous exercise.

The standard approach for balloon aortic valvuloplasty (BAV) in adults is a retrograde transfemoral arterial approach; however, it has been suggested that the antegrade venous transseptal technique may be associated with fewer vascular complications and reduce the risk of aortic leaflet perforation, despite increased risk of damage to the mitral valve (8). Outcomes following BAV vary according to age. The aortic valve leaflets in children are typically pliable and usually easy to dilate. This is in contrast to adult patients with AS in whom the aortic valve becomes thickened and calcified by the fourth decade of life, making them less suitable to effective balloon dilation. The standard approach to BAV results in more than a 50% reduction in gradients in the majority of patients; however, 15% to 30% of the cases develop moderate to severe aortic regurgitation (AR) and 15% require repeat BAV (9). Serial graded inflations starting with undersized balloons to the annulus diameter and real-time echocardiographic assessment (via transthoracic echocardiography [TTE] or intracardiac echocardiography [ICE]) is advised to avoid severe aortic insufficiency. Repeat intervention is required more often in newborns, while older patients are more likely to develop AR following BAV (9). Long-term follow-up data suggest up to 88% survival and just fewer than 50% of the patients requiring aortic valve replacement at 20 years (10).

In contrast to valvar AS, subvalvar AS does not respond well to balloon dilation. Thus, the appropriate intervention for patients with significant obstruction is surgical resection of the subvalvar membrane. Nevertheless, BAV has been offered as a short-term alternative. Long-term outcomes of patients with discrete subaortic stenosis who underwent balloon dilation suggest a restenosis rate of 15% (11). Larger annulus diameter and thinner membranes are known to yield better results. Balloon dilation has also been used for congenital supravalvar AS, but this approach has failed to become mainstream therapy.

Balloon Mitral Valvuloplasty

While balloon mitral valvuloplasty (BMV) is frequently performed in the treatment of patients with rheumatic mitral stenosis (MS), there is limited experience with BMV in congenital MS. Surgery is the preferred treatment for adults with congenital MS, in view of their complex anatomy, the significant stenosis of the subvalvular apparatus, and the potential risk for severe residual mitral insufficiency postdilation.

TABLE 44.1 Most Commonly Performed Catheter-Based Interventions in Adults with Congenital Heart Diseases: Indications and Guidelines Recommendations (Level of Evidence)

INTERVENTION	INDICATION	RECOMMENDATION (LEVEL OF EVIDENCE)

Balloon aortic valvuloplasty	I. In young adults and others without significantly calcified aortic valves and no AR
	  a. Symptomatic on exertion, and peak-to-peak gradients >50 mm Hg.
	  b. Asymptomatic young adults who demonstrate ST or T-wave abnormalities in the left precordial leads on ECG at rest or with exercise and a peak-to-peak >60 mm Hg.
		I (C)

	II. Asymptomatic young adult with AS and a peak-to-peak gradient >50 mm Hg when the patient is interested in playing competitive sports or becoming pregnant.	IIa (C)
	III. Bridge to surgery in hemodynamically unstable adults with AS, adults at high risk for AVR, or when AVR cannot be performed secondary to significant comorbidities.	IIb (C)
Balloon pulmonary valvuloplasty	a. Asymptomatic patients with a domed pulmonary valve and a peak Doppler gradient >60 mm Hg or a mean gradient >40 mm Hg (in association with less than moderate pulmonic valve regurgitation).	I (B)
	b. Asymptomatic patients with a dysplastic pulmonary valve and a peak Doppler gradient >60 mm Hg or a mean Doppler gradient >40 mm Hg.	IIb (C)
	c. Symptomatic patients with a domed pulmonary valve and a peak Doppler gradient >50 mm Hg or a mean Doppler gradient >30 mm Hg (in association with less than moderate pulmonic regurgitation).	I (C)
	d. Symptomatic patients with a dysplastic pulmonary valve and peak Doppler gradient >50 mm Hg or a mean Doppler gradient >30 mm Hg.	IIb (C)
Tricuspid valvuloplasty	a. Isolated, symptomatic severe tricuspid stenosis without TR.	IIb (C)
VSD closure	a. Muscular VSD, especially if remote from the tricuspid valve and the aorta, if the VSD is associated with severe left-sided heart chamber enlargement, or if there is PAH. b. Restrictive VSDs with a significant left-to-right shunt (Qp/Qs >1.5:1), or history of bacterial endocarditis c. Residual defects after prior attempts at surgical closure d. Trauma or iatrogenic artifacts after surgical replacement of the aortic valve.	IIb (C)
PDA closure	a. Left atrial and/or LV enlargement or if PAH is present, or in the presence of net left-to-right shunting. b. Prior endarteritis.	I (C)
Pulmonary artery dilation	a. Focal branch and/or peripheral pulmonary artery stenosis with >50% diameter narrowing, an elevated RVSP >50 mm Hg, and/or symptoms.	I (B)
Coarctation of aorta dilation	a. Peak-to-peak coarctation gradient ≥20 mm Hg.	I (C)
	b. Peak-to-peak coarctation gradient <20 mm Hg in the presence of anatomic evidence of significant coarctation with radiologic evidence of significant collateral flow.	I (B)
	c. Recurrent, discrete coarctation and a peak-to-peak gradient of at least 20 mm Hg.	IIb (C)
	d. Stent placement for long-segment coarctation.	
RVOT stenting	a. Symptomatic patients with discrete RV–pulmonary artery conduit obstructive lesions with >50% diameter narrowing or when a bioprosthetic pulmonary valve has a peak Doppler gradient >50 mm Hg or a mean gradient >30 mm Hg.	IIa (C)
	b. Asymptomatic patients when a pulmonary bioprosthetic valve has a peak Doppler gradient greater than 50 mm Hg	IIa (C)
Aortopulmonary collateral closure	a. Unexplained LV or RV dysfunction, fluid retention, chest pain, or cyanosis	IIb (C)
Coronary artery fistula closure	a. A large fistula, regardless of symptomatology, should be closed via either a transcatheter or surgical route	I (C)
	b. A small to moderate fistula in the presence of myocardial ischemia, arrhythmia, otherwise unexplained ventricular systolic or diastolic dysfunction or enlargement, or endarteritis should be closed via either a transcatheter or surgical approach	I (C)
Misc	Baffle leak closure Stenting of superior vena cava or inferior vena cava Stenting of pulmonary venous pathway obstruction.	I (B)

AR, aortic regurgitation; AS, aortic stenosis; AVR, aortic valve replacement; ECG, electrocardiography; LV, left ventricle; PAH, pulmonary arterial hypertension; PDA, patent ductus arteriosus; RV, right ventricle; RVOT, right ventricular outflow tract; RVSP, right ventricular systolic pressure; TR, tricuspid regurgitation; VSD, ventricular septal defect.

Transcatheter Valve Replacement and Repair

Transcatheter Pulmonary Valve Replacement

Transcatheter pulmonary valve replacement (TPVR) is a less invasive alternative to surgical conduit replacement and is now available for patients with right ventricular outflow dysfunction (stenosis or regurgitation). The initial experience involved dysfunctional right ventricular to PA conduits; however, the indications have expanded to native right ventricular outflow tracks and dysfunctional pulmonary bioprosthesis.

Two types of valves are commercially available: the Medtronic Melody pulmonary valve (18 mm, 20 mm, and 22 mm) and the Edwards SAPIEN pulmonary valve (23 mm, 26 mm, and 29 mm). Short- and medium-term results of TPVR are available for both Melody and SAPIEN valves; however, more data are available for the Melody valve (up to 7 years of follow-up). The data for the Melody valve suggest that the gradient over right ventricular outflow tract (RVOT) falls significantly from a median of 35 to 40 mm Hg to 10 to 20 mm Hg, instability of the device is reported in 1% of patients, there is compression of coronary arteries in 1%, endocarditis in 1% to 3%, stent fractures in 20%—which reduces to 5% with aggressive presenting and freedom from reintervention in 95% of the patients (12,13). For the SAPIEN valve, the limited available data suggest a decrease in peak-to-peak gradients from 27 to 12 mm Hg. PR was moderate or less in 97% (14,15).

The implantation technique is similar for the two valves via venous access in the femoral or jugular vein. Because coronary compromise is a life-threatening complication, a balloon test is performed to exclude potential coronary artery compression. This is performed by inflation of a high-pressure balloon equal to the size of the intended diameter of the landing zone for the pulmonary valve in the RVOT conduit, with a simultaneous aortogram to visualize coronary arteries. Impairment of coronary blood flow is a contraindication for TPVR. Presenting of the conduit, usually with a covered stent, is another important measure taken during the procedure to minimize the risk of transcatheter valve fracture or conduit rupture. A valve-in-valve procedure can also be performed in cases of primary device failure.

Transcatheter Tricuspid Valve Replacement

In general, tricuspid repair is preferred to replacement; however, the risk of recurrent regurgitation is high and many patients will eventually receive a bioprosthetic tricuspid valve. Over the years, these valves may fail, resulting in stenosis or regurgitation. Transcatheter tricuspid valve replacement (TTVR) may thus help in this patient population, representing a lower-risk alternative than redo surgery (16). This approach was described in 15 patients with a 100% procedural success with the use of the Melody percutaneous pulmonary valve (Medtronic, Inc., Minneapolis, MN) (17). The mean gradient in stenotic valves reduced from 12.9 to 3.9 mm Hg, whereas the degree of TR in regurgitant valves reduced from severe to mild or none to mild to none (17). One patient developed complete heart block and one developed endocarditis after 2 months (17). Larger series, and ultimately prospective studies, will determine the safety and efficacy of these techniques and help identify the ideal patients for each approach.

Transcatheter tricuspid valve (systemic AV valve) repair with MitraClip (Abbott, USA) has also been described in high-surgical-risk patients with congenitally corrected transposition of the great arteries who present with severe tricuspid regurgitation (18). In contrast to treatment of the mitral valve, the use of MitraClip on the tricuspid valve aims to clip together two of the three leaflets to create a double orifice tricuspid valve. The choice of leaflets depends on the location of the regurgitant jet and ease of imaging (19).

Angioplasty/Stenting

Coarctation of the Aorta

Coarctation of the aorta accounts for 4% to 6% of all congenital heart defects. In adults, it is typically located just distal to the origin of the left subclavian artery. The presence of cystic medial necrosis in the aortic wall adjacent to the coarctation site predisposes the patients to aortic wall rupture and aneurysm formation with percutaneous or surgical interventions. When left untreated, coarctation is associated with a mean survival rate of 35 years, with 75% mortality at 46 years of age (1). This is due to uncontrolled systemic hypertension, accelerated coronary artery disease, stroke, aortic dissection, and heart failure.

Studies suggest that balloon angioplasty and surgical correction are equally effective in reducing the peak systolic pressure gradient early after intervention; however, the surgical approach is associated with higher immediate procedural complications and longer hospital stays, whereas balloon angioplasty is associated with a higher incidence of recoarctation (up to 25%) and aneurysm (7%) formation at follow-up (20,21). Therefore, stent placement with the advantage of sustained hemodynamic benefit is now considered the treatment of choice for older children and adults with native coarctation. Balloon angioplasty is still performed in patients with isolated recoarctation regardless of age.

Retrospective data from over 500 patients demonstrate the efficacy and relative safety of stent placement, with a success rate of 98% and an acute complications rate of 14% (22). The rates of stent restenosis or aneurysms on follow-up imaging are very low (<1%) (22). In the Coarctation of the Aorta Stent Trial (COAST) trial, a prospective, multicenter, single-arm clinical trial of 105 patients (median age 16 years), Cheatham Platinum stent implantation was successful in 99% (23). At 2-years follow-up, 10% of the patients required reinterventions for stent redilation (either as part of an intentionally staged approach or to compensate for somatic growth) or to address aneurysms (23).

It has been suggested that the use of covered stents, which consist of a bare-metal stent with a polytetrafluoroethylene sleeve, may reduce the risk of aneurysms; however, a randomized study of 120 patients with a mean age of 23.60 ± 10.99 years comparing the two strategies showed that patients who underwent covered stent implantation experienced a nonsignificantly lower recoarctation rate and a higher occurrence of pseudoaneurysm formation compared to bare-metal stent placement (24). More recently, the COAST II trial (Covered Cheatham-Platinum Stents for Prevention or Treatment of Aortic Wall Injury Associated with Coarctation of the Aorta Trial) included 158 patients and demonstrated that placement of covered stents can effectively treat and potentially prevent arterial wall injury associated with coarctation of the aorta (25). Long-term results of this study are awaited. Commercially made covered stents are now currently available in the United States and in Europe. Further data are awaited to determine if there is a subset of patients who benefit from covered stents.

Pulmonary Artery Stenosis

Pulmonary artery stenosis (PAS) in patients with congenital heart disease may occur anywhere in the pulmonary vascular tree. PAS is typically associated with other congenital defects or syndromes, such as tetralogy of Fallot, ventricular septal defect (VSD), or Alagille syndrome. Additionally, PAS may result as sequelae of surgical interventions (including systemic-pulmonary shunts, homograft or conduit implantation, pulmonary artery (PA) banding, pulmonary arterioplasty or after arterial switch operation) or may be a residue of acquired diseases (including chronic thromboembolic disease) (6).

In persons with abnormal pulmonary resistance, isolated branch obstruction can result in pulmonary hypertension, increased subpulmonary ventricular afterload, pulmonary valve insufficiency, or a sufficient perfusion–ventilation imbalance that may lead to symptoms.

Quantitative radiographic assessment of lung perfusion and ventilation should be part of the diagnostic algorithm and should be used as a tool to evaluate the results of dilation procedures in such patients. Surgical access and correction of PAS may be cumbersome and limited. Consequently, percutaneous therapy is the preferred treatment method to restore pulmonary blood flow and balance and to decrease resistance for patients with PAS. PA (Pulmonary Arterial) procedures such as balloon angioplasty and/or stenting (PA rehabilitation) may account for up to 20% of all catheter-based interventions in this population (26).

Data from multicenter registries (NCDR and Congenital Cardiac Catheterization Project on Outcomes) suggest major adverse events in up to 10% of patients (26,27). While vascular/cardiac tear is the most common adverse event, balloon rupture (5%) and stent embolization/malposition (6%) have also been reported (27). PA stenting provides an effective relief for PAS in adults with congenital heart disease; however, multiple and bilateral stents may be required. The presence of significant PR predisposes to stent embolization (28). Certain lesions remain problematic for stent therapy, such as proximal main pulmonary stenosis close to the pulmonary valve and bifurcation stenoses.

PA stenting provides effective relief of narrowing in adults with congenital heart disease. Bilateral and/or multiple stenting are often required. Stent embolization may occur particularly in patients with associated significant PR.

RVOT Stenting

The standard treatment for many congenital heart defects includes placement of a conduit from the RV to the PA. The lifespan of RV–PA conduits is limited because of progressive obstruction and regurgitation secondary to severe angulation, calcification, sternal compression, or tissue proliferation, most notably at anastomotic sites. This may lead to right ventricular pressure and volume overloading. Stenting obstructed RV–PA conduits with bare-metal stents prolongs the conduit lifespan and reduces the number of open heart surgeries by acutely reducing the peak pressure gradient across the conduit, RV systolic pressure, and the RV:aortic pressure ratio. Older patients achieve a longer median freedom from conduit surgery (29). Follow-up data suggest that the majority of these patients require additional stents or redilations. Stent fractures (16%), associated with stent compression and substernal location, usually do not cause any acute hemodynamic compromise (29). Finally, the potential for coronary compression (coursing of a coronary artery sufficiently adjacent to the conduit) by stent implantation has been reported, with catastrophic potential, and must be assessed before intervention.

Baffle Stenosis

Conduit stenosis can be observed after Glenn or Fontan operations. Similarly, systemic baffle obstruction is observed in up to 15% of patients undergoing atrial switch (Mustard or Senning) procedures. Balloon angioplasty occasionally results in long-term relief; however, stent deployment has been highly successful in relieving obstruction, with low complication rates and superior results, especially when performed in the superior portion of the systemic venous baffle after atrial switch operations (6).

Device Closure

Ventricular Septal Defects

VSD is the most common CHD, which presents in 3 to 3.5 infants per 1,000 live births. This incidence is much less in adults because of the high incidence of spontaneous closure, especially of small VSDs, and surgical closure of hemodynamically significant defects in childhood. VSDs are classified as outflow/supracristal, perimembranous/infracristal (most common; 80% of all VSDs), muscular, or inflow based on their location in the septum (4). VSD closure in the adult is usually recommended either when left ventricular volume overload, unexplained by any alternative mechanism, is present, correlating with Qp/Qs >1.5, in the presence of multiple recurrences of otherwise unexplained bacterial endocarditis or when accompanied by progressive AR (1).

Percutaneous closure of VSD offers an attractive alternative to surgical management in selected patients with isolated uncomplicated defects, increased surgical risk, multiple previous cardiac surgical interventions, or with poorly accessible muscular VSDs. Transcatheter VSD closure is generally technically more challenging than atrial septal defect closure, with intravascular passage through the VSD with the use of a balloon-tipped catheter (to ensure passage via the largest lumen) from the left ventricular side, snaring a guide wire in the PA, formation and externalization of a venous–arterial–venous vascular loop, and subsequent device deployment based on a pathway allowing maximal device arm–septal apposition, without interference from adjacent intracardiac structures.

Several reports of transcatheter closure of VSDs have been published with high procedural success rates (95%), with major complication rates up to 12%, and the need for permanent pacemaker implantation in up to 6% of patients (30–32). The AMPLATZER Muscular and Membranous VSD device, AMPLATZER Septal Occluder, and the AMPLATZER Duct Occluder and the Duct Occluder II (St. Jude Medical, Inc. St. Paul, Minnesota, USA) are available in the US. Currently in the United States, the only FDA-approved available device that is specifically designed to close VSDs is the AMPLATZER Muscular VSD device. The AMPLATZER Perimembranous VSD device underwent a clinical trial in the US; however, concerns regarding the development of complete heart block prevented the device from ever receiving FDA approval (33). The other devices listed earlier are either not available in the US or must be used off label. Newer devices are in development, with the aim of reducing the radial force on the conduction tissue and thus reducing the incidence of heart blocks. More recent studies on transcatheter closure of membranous VSDs show a similar procedural success rate, without an increased risk of significant valvular regurgitation or heart block when compared with surgical closure (34,35).

Transcatheter closure of acquired VSD secondary to myocardial infarction (MI) is associated with significant morbidity and mortality (up to 50%), similar to surgical closure. This is more due to the underlying critical condition of the patients with heart failure and cardiogenic shock during acute MI than direct outcome of the percutaneous procedure, which has been described with high rates of success (90%) (36).

Patent Ductus Arteriosus

Patent ductus arteriosus (PDA) is an abnormally persistent arterial connection after birth between the descending aorta and the PA, most commonly to the junction of the main and left PA branches. Similar to VSD, patients with large PDA may develop left-sided volume overload and pulmonary hypertension at younger ages, leading to diagnosis early in life. It is not uncommon that the diagnosis of PDA is made in adulthood by means of physical examination and the presence of the continuous murmur typical of PDA, or as an incidental finding on echocardiography (6). Additional problems associated with PDA include infectious endarteritis, aneurysm formation, calcification, and rare rupture. Large PDA with a significant left-to-right shunt should be closed to reduce occurrence of the sequelae of subaortic ventricular failure or pulmonary arterial hypertension. There are adult-specific closure issues, such as calcification of ductal tissue, change in orientation of the duct with age, leading to a more horizontal entry into the PA and a higher incidence of pulmonary hypertension.

First introduced in 1967, percutaneous closure of PDA has been performed for over four decades with several generations of devices and is the preferred mode of therapy worldwide given increasing surgical risk with age because of PDA calcification and the potential for intraoperative recurrent laryngeal nerve damage. If the PDA is associated with other conditions that require surgical correction, the ductus may be closed during the same operation, although percutaneous closure of the PDA before other cardiac surgery may decrease the risk of cardiopulmonary bypass (1). Currently, in adults with PDA, the AMPLATZER ductal occluder (ADO) is the most commonly used device typically implanted during an outpatient procedure, with MRI-compatible coil embolization reserved for PDA measuring <2 to 3 mm or for residual leaks. Complete closure has been reported in >95% of patients at 6 months with both techniques, with device embolization being rarely encountered (37,38). The current FDA-approved occluder devices are ADO, ADO II, and PFM Nit-Occlud; all are MRI-safe. Contrary to PDA closure in children, left PA obstruction is not a concern in adults. The postimplantation antiplatelet regimen remains unsubstantiated, although it is typically recommended for 3 to 4 months, and patients continue to receive antibiotic prophylaxis against subacute bacterial endocarditis for 6 months after device implantation.

Fontan Fenestrations and Atrial Switch Baffle Leaks

Following Fontan operations, patients may have spontaneous or surgically created residual fenestrations that may lead to a right-to-left shunt and consequent systemic oxygen desaturation, systemic emboli, and exercise incapacity. These fenestrations can be closed with the use of the AMPLATZER or Gore CardioForm septal occluder devices. Patients typically receive long-term anticoagulation and prophylaxis against subacute bacterial endocarditis. Recent studies have suggested that closure of fenestrations may contribute to late tachyarrhythmias in this patient population (39).

Up to 25% of patients undergoing Mustard or Senning operations will demonstrate late baffle leaks, likely as the result of suture dehiscence. Although many of these shunts are hemodynamically unapparent and do not require therapy, closure is indicated for large defects, resulting in significant intracardiac shunting. Percutaneous closure has been reported with the AMPLATZER devices as alternatives to surgery.

Ruptured Sinus of Valsalva Aneurysm

The weakness at the junction of the aortic media and annulus fibrosis can lead to formation of a sinus of Valsalva aneurysm (SVA). Aneurysms are asymptomatic in the majority of the cases; however, a rupture may cause significant hemodynamic change. The rupture usually occurs into the Right atrium (RA) or RV Right ventricle causing a significant left-to-right shunt and heart failure. Surgical repair remains the treatment of choice; however, transcatheter closure of a ruptured SVA has been successfully performed since 1994, with success rates of 91%, thus

avoiding sternotomy and cardiopulmonary bypass in critically ill patients. The AMPLATZER duct occluder remains the most commonly used device, with some cases using the muscular VSD occluder (40). Rare procedure-related aortic valve regurgitation, as well as severe procedure-related complications, should be considered in the risk assessment.

Coil Embolization

Aortopulmonary Arterial Collaterals

Aortopulmonary collaterals may be observed in patients with congenital malformations associated with decreased pulmonary flow, including pulmonary atresia, as well as variations of single-ventricle physiology, or after a Glenn shunt or Fontan palliation. These collaterals can arise from any systemic artery and connect directly to the pulmonary arteries at the lung hilum or at the periphery (6). Resulting left-to-left systemic arterial to pulmonary arterial shunting may cause pulmonary vascular disease, elevation of systemic ventricular filling pressure, systemic ventricular volume loading, and ultimate failure. Residual surgically created systemic to pulmonary arterial shunts share the same pathophysiologic sequelae. In addition to the aforementioned factors, aortopulmonary collateral embolization is indicated before the final stage of surgical subpulmonary ventricle to PA connection because the left-to-right shunt directly into the pulmonary arteries complicates cardiopulmonary bypass, and the dual supply to the vascular branches leads to over-circulation and development of pulmonary arterial hypertension. Embolization is typically performed in those collaterals that share significant flow from the main or additional unifocal pulmonary arteries to avoid lung infarction. Embolization is typically performed with coils; however, use of AMPLATZER vascular plugs, microspheres, and copolymers of ethylene vinyl alcohol has also been reported with similar success.

Coronary Artery Fistulae

Coronary fistulae can originate from all major epicardial coronary arteries (55% from Right coronary artery), and drainage usually occurs to the RV (40%), RA (25%), coronary sinus, or PA. These collaterals can become markedly enlarged and can lead to significant left-to-right shunting with right-sided volume overload and effective coronary arterial steal leading to ischemia. Surgical correction is associated with low mortality and morbidity; nevertheless, percutaneous catheter techniques have become the method of choice. Embolization has been reported predominantly with coils (Gianturco coils; interlocking detachable coils); however, other devices such as AMPLATZER duct occluders and AMPLATZER vascular plugs have been used successfully as well (41,42). Risks include MI (15%) and the migration of coils or discs to extracoronary vascular structures or within the coronary artery branches. Long-term follow-up suggests that patients with distal type, large fistulae, and older age at presentation may be at highest risk for coronary thrombosis (41,42).

Other Forms of Collaterals

Collaterals from the systemic to the pulmonary veins (venous–venous collaterals) can occur in patients with single ventricle physiology, especially after Glenn or Fontan operations, in part because of chronically elevated systemic venous pressures. Pulmonary arteriovenous fistulae may also present late after Glenn anastomosis, as well as in patients with chronic liver failure or with hereditary hemorrhagic telangiectasia (Osler–Weber–Rendu syndrome). In both instances, there is a right-to-left shunt, with various degrees of cyanosis. Both types of abnormal connections can be treated successfully with coil embolization or AMPLATZER vascular plugs; however, this is rarely indicated (43). In addition, the recurrence of collaterals is not uncommon unless the underlying physiology driving their development is modified significantly.

Interventions in patients with ACHD presents unique challenges to caregivers. Decreased exercise capacity, altered anatomy in combination with potential for extracardiac comorbidities contribute to physiologic occurrences, risks, and complications encountered less frequently in typical pediatric or adult transcatheter interventions. It is important that these patients are treated in centers of excellence equipped with appropriately trained and experienced operators. There is a critical need for centralized data collection to determine prevalence, demographics, and long-term outcomes in patients with ACHD. This will advance the field with the goal of providing evidence-based care for this unique population.

Key Points

- BPV is the treatment of choice for isolated PS. The use of oversized balloon (1.2–1.25 times the annulus) has been advocated to achieve a successful result, which is defined by a peak valve gradient of <20 mm Hg.

- In contrast to valvar AS, subvalvar AS does not respond well to balloon dilation.

- TPVR is a less invasive alternative to surgical conduit replacement and is now available for patients with right ventricular outflow dysfunction (stenosis or regurgitation).

- Stent placement is the treatment of choice for older children and adults with native coarctation of aorta. Balloon angioplasty is still performed in patients with isolated recoarctation regardless of age.

- Commercially made covered stents (bare metal stents with a polytetrafluoroethylene sleeve) are now available in the United States for coarctation. These may reduce the risk of aneurysms.

- Quantitative radiographic assessment of lung perfusion and ventilation should be part of the diagnostic algorithm and should be used as a tool to evaluate the results of dilation procedures in patients with PAS.

- PA stenting provides an effective relief for PAS in adults with congenital heart disease; however, multiple and bilateral stents may be required.

- Stenting obstructed RV–PA conduits with bare-metal stents prolongs the conduit lifespan and reduces the number of open-heart surgeries by acutely reducing the peak pressure gradient across the conduit, the RV systolic pressure, and the RV:aortic pressure ratio.

- Percutaneous closure of VSD is an attractive alternative to surgical management in selected patients with isolated uncomplicated defects, increased surgical risk, multiple previous cardiac surgical interventions, or with poorly accessible muscular VSDs.

- In adults with PDA, the ADO is the most commonly used device with MRI-compatible coil embolization reserved for PDA measuring <2 to 3 mm or for residual leaks.

References

1. Warnes CA, et al. ACC/AHA 2008 guidelines for the management of adults with congenital heart disease: a report of the American College of Cardiology/American Heart Association Task Force on Practice Guidelines (writing committee to develop guidelines on the management of adults with congenital heart disease). *Circulation.* 2008;118:e714–e833.
2. Gurvitz M, et al. Emerging research directions in adult congenital heart disease: a report from an NHLBI/ACHA Working Group. *J Am Coll Cardiol.* 2016;67:1956–1964.
3. Marelli AJ, et al. Congenital heart disease in the general population: changing prevalence and age distribution. *Circulation.* 2007;115:163–172.
4. Baumgartner H, et al. ESC guidelines for the management of grown-up congenital heart disease (new version 2010). *Eur Heart J.* 2010;31:2915–2957.
5. Rao PS. Percutaneous balloon pulmonary valvuloplasty: state of the art. *Catheter Cardiovasc Interv.* 2007;69:747–763.
6. Inglessis I, Landzberg MJ. Interventional catheterization in adult congenital heart disease. *Circulation.* 2007;115:1622–1633.
7. Harrild DM, et al. Long-term pulmonary regurgitation following balloon valvuloplasty for pulmonary stenosis risk factors and relationship to exercise capacity and ventricular volume and function. *J Am Coll Cardiol.* 2010;55:1041–1047.
8. Cubeddu RJ, et al. Retrograde versus antegrade percutaneous aortic balloon valvuloplasty: immediate, short- and long-term outcome at 2 years. *Catheter Cardiovasc Interv.* 2009;74:225–231.
9. Brown DW, et al. Aortic valve reinterventions after balloon aortic valvuloplasty for congenital aortic stenosis intermediate and late follow-up. *J Am Coll Cardiol.* 2010;56:1740–1749.
10. Maskatia SA, et al. Twenty-five year experience with balloon aortic valvuloplasty for congenital aortic stenosis. *Am J Cardiol.* 2011;108:1024–1028.
11. de Lezo JS, et al. Long-term outcome of patients with isolated thin discrete subaortic stenosis treated by balloon dilation: a 25-year study. *Circulation.* 2011;124:1461–1468.
12. Cheatham JP, et al. Clinical and hemodynamic outcomes up to 7 years after transcatheter pulmonary valve replacement in the US melody valve investigational device exemption trial. *Circulation.* 2015;131:1960–1970.
13. McElhinney DB, et al. Short- and medium-term outcomes after transcatheter pulmonary valve placement in the expanded multicenter US melody valve trial. *Circulation.* 2010;122:507–516.
14. Kenny D, et al. Percutaneous implantation of the Edwards SAPIEN transcatheter heart valve for conduit failure in the pulmonary position: early phase 1 results from an international multicenter clinical trial. *J Am Coll Cardiol.* 2011;58:2248–2256.
15. Boone RH, et al. Transcatheter pulmonary valve implantation using the Edwards SAPIEN transcatheter heart valve. *Catheter Cardiovasc Interv.* 2010;75:286–294.
16. Patel JS, et al. Transcatheter advances in the treatment of adult and congenital valvular heart disease. *Curr Treat Options Cardiovasc Med.* 2015;17:52.
17. Roberts PA, et al. Percutaneous tricuspid valve replacement in congenital and acquired heart disease. *J Am Coll Cardiol.* 2011;58:117–122.
18. Picard F, Tadros VX, Asgar AW. From tricuspid to double orifice morphology: percutaneous tricuspid regurgitation repair with the MitraClip device in congenitally corrected-transposition of great arteries. *Catheter Cardiovasc Interv.* 2017;90(3):432–436.
19. van Melle JP, et al. Percutaneous tricuspid valve repair using MitraClip® for the treatment of severe tricuspid valve regurgitation in a patient with congenitally corrected transposition of the great arteries. *Neth Heart J.* 2016;24:696–697.
20. Rodes-Cabau J, et al. Comparison of surgical and transcatheter treatment for native coarctation of the aorta in patients ≥1 year old. The Quebec Native Coarctation of the Aorta study. *Am Heart J.* 2007;154:186–192.
21. Fawzy ME, et al. Twenty-two years of follow-up results of balloon angioplasty for discreet native coarctation of the aorta in adolescents and adults. *Am Heart J.* 2008;156:910–917.
22. Forbes TJ, et al. Intermediate follow-up following intravascular stenting for treatment of coarctation of the aorta. *Catheter Cardiovasc Interv.* 2007;70:569–577.

23. Meadows J, et al. Intermediate outcomes in the prospective, multicenter Coarctation of the Aorta Stent Trial (COAST). *Circulation*. 2015;131:1656–1664.

24. Sohrabi B, et al. Comparison between covered and bare Cheatham-Platinum stents for endovascular treatment of patients with native post-ductal aortic coarctation: immediate and intermediate-term results. *JACC Cardiovasc Interv*. 2014;7:416–423.

25. Taggart NW, et al. Immediate outcomes of covered stent placement for treatment or prevention of aortic wall injury associated with Coarctation of the Aorta (COAST II). *JACC Cardiovasc Interv*. 2016;9:484–493.

26. Lewis MJ, et al. Procedural success and adverse events in pulmonary artery stenting: insights from the NCDR. *J Am Coll Cardiol*. 2016;67:1327–1335.

27. Holzer RJ, et al. Balloon angioplasty and stenting of branch pulmonary arteries: adverse events and procedural characteristics: results of a multi-institutional registry. *Circ Cardiovasc Interv*. 2011;4:287–296.

28. Kenny D, et al. Medium-term outcomes for peripheral pulmonary artery stenting in adults with congenital heart disease. *J Interv Cardiol*. 2011;24:373–377.

29. Peng LF, et al. Endovascular stenting of obstructed right ventricle-to-pulmonary artery conduits: a 15-year experience. *Circulation*. 2006;113:2598–2605.

30. Dua JS, et al. Transcatheter closure of postsurgical residual ventricular septal defects: early and mid-term results. *Catheter Cardiovasc Interv*. 2010;75:246–255.

31. Chessa M, et al. Transcatheter closure of congenital ventricular septal defects in adult: mid-term results and complications. *Int J Cardiol*. 2009;133:70–73.

32. Carminati M, et al. Transcatheter closure of congenital ventricular septal defects: results of the European Registry. *Eur Heart J*. 2007;28:2361–2368.

33. Fu YC, et al. Transcatheter closure of perimembranous ventricular septal defects using the new Amplatzer membranous VSD occluder: results of the U.S. phase I trial. *J Am Coll Cardiol*. 2006;47:319–325.

34. Saurav A, et al. Comparison of percutaneous device closure versus surgical closure of peri-membranous ventricular septal defects: a systematic review and meta-analysis. *Catheter Cardiovasc Interv*. 2015;86:1048–1056.

35. Yang J, et al. Transcatheter versus surgical closure of perimembranous ventricular septal defects in children: a randomized controlled trial. *J Am Coll Cardiol*. 2014;63:1159–1168.

36. Singh V, et al. Ventricular septal defect complicating ST-elevation myocardial infarctions: a call for action. *Am J Med*. 2017;130(7):863.e1:863.e12.

37. Pass RH, et al. Multicenter USA Amplatzer patent ductus arteriosus occlusion device trial: initial and one-year results. *J Am Coll Cardiol*. 2004;44:513–519.

38. Yan C, et al. Transcatheter closure of patent ductus arteriosus with severe pulmonary arterial hypertension in adults. *Heart*. 2007;93:514–518.

39. Ono M, et al. Clinical outcome of patients 20 years after Fontan operation—effect of fenestration on late morbidity. *Eur J Cardiothorac Surg*. 2006;30:923–929.

40. Zhong L, et al. Clinical efficacy and safety of transcatheter closure of ruptured sinus of valsalva aneurysm. *Catheter Cardiovasc Interv*. 2014;84:1184–1189.

41. Gowda ST, et al. Intermediate to long-term outcome following congenital coronary artery fistulae closure with focus on thrombus formation. *Am J Cardiol*. 2011;107:302–308.

42. Valente AM, et al. Predictors of long-term adverse outcomes in patients with congenital coronary artery fistulae. *Circ Cardiovasc Interv*. 2010;3:134–139.

43. Wiegand G, et al. Transcatheter closure of abnormal vessels and arteriovenous fistulas with the Amplatzer vascular plug 4 in patients with congenital heart disease. *Pediatr Cardiol*. 2013;34:1668–1673.

INDEX

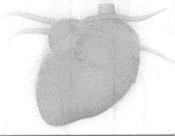

Note: Page numbers followed by *f* indicate figures; page numbers followed by *t* indicate tables; page numbers followed by *b* indicate boxes.

A

AAA. *See* Abdominal aortic aneurysm (AAA)
Abciximab, 220
  biologic half-life, 36
  indications, 36
  mechanisms of action, 35–36
  pharmacologic properties and dosing, 35*t*
  restenosis, 19
  side effects, 36
Abdominal aortic aneurysm (AAA)
  endovascular aneurysm repair, 365–366, 366*t*
  in women, 345
ABI. *See* Ankle Brachial Index (ABI)
ABSORB III trial, 285
Absorb Bioresorbable Vascular Scaffold System
  (BVS-EES), 193
Absorbed dose, 64
Academic Research Consortium (ARC), 190*t*
ACAS (Asymptomatic Carotid Atherosclerosis
  Study), 373
ACCOAST trial, 220
ACEI (Angiotensin converting enzyme inhibitor),
  350
Acetylcholine, 6–8, 55
ACHD. *See* Adult congenital heart disease
  (ACHD)
ACS. *See* Acute coronary syndrome (ACS)
ACST. *See* Asymptomatic Carotid Surgery Trial
  (ACST)
Active approximation devices, 331, 332*t*,
  333*f*
ACUITY trial, 222, 344
Acute coronary syndrome (ACS)
  anti-ischemic therapies, 217, 217*t*
  antiplatelet therapies
    ADP receptor antagonists, 219–220
    aspirin, 219
    clopidogrel, 220
    prasugrel, 220
    ticagrelor, 220
  antithrombotic therapies
    bivalirudin, 221–222
    fondaparinux, 221
    low molecular weight heparins, 221
    unfractionated heparin, 221
  clinical presentation, 216
  coronary artery bypass surgery, 219
  diagnosis, 216
  early invasive *vs.* conservative approach, 218,
    219*f*
  epidemiology, 215
  fractional flow reserve, 88
  glycoprotein IIb/IIIa inhibitors, 220–221
  multivessel PCI, 266–267
  pathology, 215–216
  percutaneous coronary intervention, timing
    of, 219

Acute Venous Thrombosis: Thrombus
  Removal with Adjunctive Catheter-Directed
  Thrombolysis (ATTRACT) trial, 401
Adenosine, 8, 59
  agonists, 54
Adenosine diphosphate (ADP) receptor
  antagonists, 219–220
Adenosine-induced hyperemia, 84, 84*f*
ADO (AMPLATZER duct occluder), 459, 473
Adult Cardiovascular Life Support (ACLS)
  protocols, 308
Adult congenital heart disease (ACHD)
  angioplasty/stenting, 471–472
  coil embolization, 473–474
  device closure, 472–473
  transcatheter valve replacement and repair, 471
  valvuloplasty, 469, 470*t*
AF. *See* Atrial fibrillation (AF)
AGILITY trial, 182
Air embolism, 308
Air kerma, 64
ALARA (As Low As Reasonably Achievable), 64
Alberta Stroke Program Early CT Score
  (ASPECTS), 383, 386
Alcohol septal ablation (ASA)
  acute procedural success, 455, 456*f*
  echocardiographic guidance, 414, 414*f*
  hemodynamic evaluation, 453, 454*f*
  patient selection, 452–453, 453*f*, 454*f*
  procedure, 453–455
  survival, 456–457
  symptom improvement, 456, 456*f*
  temporary pacemaker placement, 453
American Heart Association (AHA)/American
  College of Cardiology (ACC) guidelines, 147*t*
  anticoagulation therapy for STEMI, 242*t*
  atherosclerotic cardiovascular disease, 350
  lipid intervention, 350, 350*t*
  surgical correction of RAS, 397*t*
American Heart Association and the American
  Stroke Association (AHA/ASA) guidelines
  carotid atherosclerosis, 375
  carotid endarterectomy for stenosis, 376
  endovascular treatment, 388*t*
  stroke prevention, 374, 375*t*
Amiodarone, 59
Amplatz atrial septal defect occluder, 418, 419*f*
Amplatz Left curve guides, 179
AMPLATZER duct occluder (ADO), 459, 473
AMPLATZER Perimembranous VSD device, 472
AMPLATZER PFO Occluder, 420, 422*f*
AMPLATZER vascular plugs (AVP), 459
AMRO trial, 184
Anaphylactoid reactions
  delayed anaphylactoid reactions, 73
  immediate anaphylactoid reactions, 72–73,
    72*t*, 73*t*
  recommendations, 308

Angina, 4
  nitroglycerin's anti-ischemic effect, 53
  stable chronic
    CABG *vs.* PCI, 202–208, 204–207*t*
    coronary revascularization, 201
    diagnosis, 196
    life style goals, 200*t*
    management, 198, 199*t*, 200*t*
    optimal medical therapy, 199, 201
    optimal revascularization PCI technique,
      208–209
    pathophysiology, 198
  unstable angina
    acute coronary syndrome, 4
    anti-ischemic therapies, 217, 217*t*
    epidemiology, 215
    pathology, 216
    risk stratification, 217–218, 218*f*
Angiography
  chronic total occlusions PCI, 318–319
  coronary artery disease, 431
  LVOT obstruction, 453
  percutaneous coronary intervention
    anteroposterior imaging, 143, 144*f*
    collateral flow, 145
    coronary lesion characteristics, 145, 147*t*,
      148
    coronary stenosis assessment, 145, 146*f*
    left anterior oblique imaging, 143, 144*f*
    peripheral vascular angiography, 148–153,
      151*f*, 152*f*, 152*t*, 154*f*
    quantitative coronary angiography, 145
    radiographic contrast media, 148
    right anterior oblique imaging, 143
    saphenous vein grafts, 143–144, 145*t*
    SYNTAX score, 148, 149–151*f*
    TIMI flow grades, 144, 146*t*
  ST-elevation myocardial infarction, 227, 227*t*,
    358, 358*t*
  ULMCA PCI, 292, 292*f*, 294, 296*f*
  vulnerable plaques, 105
AngioJet device, 402
AngioJet rheolytic thrombectomy system, 403,
  403*f*
Angioplasty. *See* Balloon angioplasty; Laser
  angioplasty; Stents
Angioscopy, 111
AngioSculpt scoring balloon, 182–183
Angio-Seal device, 331–332, 332*t*, 333*f*
Angiotensin converting enzyme inhibitor (ACEI),
  350
Angiotensin receptor blockers (ARBs), 350
Ankle Brachial Index (ABI), 345
Anomalous origin
  of circumflex coronary artery, 152, 154*f*
  of left main coronary artery, 151–152, 152*f*,
    153*t*
  of right coronary artery, 152–153

Anteroposterior imaging, 143, 144f
Antiarrhythmic drugs
  adenosine, 59
  amiodarone, 59
  β blockers, 59
  calcium channel blockers, 59
  classification and properties, 57–58t
  lidocaine, 58–59
  procainamide, 57H
Anticoagulant therapy
  non-ST segment acute coronary syndromes,
    43–44
    ACC/AHA guideline recommendations, 38
    anticoagulant dosing, 39t
    apixaban, 47
    coagulation cascade inhibition, 38
    direct thrombin inhibitors, 43–44
    early invasive management strategy, 38–39
    fondaparinux, 45–46
    ischemia-guided management strategy, 39
    low-molecular-weight heparins, 42–43
    PCI, 39–40
    rivaroxaban, 46–47
    unfractionated heparin, 40–42
    warfarin, 46
  radial artery occlusion, 325
  restenosis, 19
  ST-elevation myocardial infarction (STEMI)
    ACC/AHA guidelines, 48, 218
    with delayed PCI, 50
    dosing, 49t
    with fibrinolytic therapy, 49–50
    intervention, 241–243, 241f
    with primary PCI, 48–49
Anti-ischemic therapies, 217, 217t
Antiplatelet therapy, 352
  ADP receptor antagonists, 219–220
  aspirin, 219
  clopidogrel, 220
  prasugrel, 220
  ST-elevation myocardial infarction, 243–245
  stroke prevention, 374
  ticagrelor, 220
  trials of, 6
  vorapaxar, 28
  in women, 344
Antiplatelet Trialist Collaboration, 19
Antithrombotic therapy
  bivalirudin, 221–222
  fondaparinux, 221
  low molecular weight heparins, 221
  unfractionated heparin, 221
Aortic annulus, 443, 443f
Aortic arch, 374, 375f
Aortic coarctation, 364
Aortic regurgitation, hemodynamics, 126,
  127–130f
Aortic stenosis, hemodynamics
  femoral artery, 123–124
  low gradient and ejection fraction, 126, 128,
    131f, 132f
  LV-Ao pressure tracings, 124, 126f
  pathophysiology, 124, 125f
aortic syndrome, acute, aortic dissection, 364–365
Aorto-ostial lesions, 381, 382f
Aortopulmonary arterial collaterals, 473
Apixaban, 47, 401
Apoptosis, 3

ARBs (angiotensin receptor blockers), 350
Arrhythmia, 308–309
Arterial dissection, 307–308, 308t
Arterial grafts, 303
Artery fistulae, coronary, 473
As Low As Reasonably Achievable (ALARA), 64
ASA. See Alcohol septal ablation (ASA)
ASCEND-HF Trial, 161t
ASD. See Atrial septal defect (ASD)
ASPECTS. See Alberta Stroke Program Early CT
  Score (ASPECTS)
Aspiration thrombectomy, 239, 359
Aspirin, 219, 359–360
  indications, 28–29
  mechanisms of action, 28, 28f
  restenosis, 19
  side effects, 29
  stroke prevention, 374
Asymptomatic Cardiac Ischemia Pilot (ACIP)
  Study, 197
Asymptomatic Carotid Atherosclerosis Study
  (ACAS), 373
Asymptomatic Carotid Surgery Trial (ACST), 373,
  376
Atherectomy
  orbital atherectomy, 179–180
  rotational atherectomy, 175–179
Atheroembolism, 307
Atherosclerosis
  clinical sequelae of, 4–6, 4–7f
  endothelial dysfunction, 6–9, 8t
  epidemiology, 1, 1t
  immune response in, 2–3
  inflammation and, 1
  injury causing, 1, 1t
  leukocyte recruitment, 1–2
  lipid accumulation, 1
  mature atherosclerotic plaque, 3
  medical therapy, 8–9
  plaque angiogenesis, 3
  smooth muscle cells and mineralization, 3
  vascular remodeling, 3–4
Atorvastatin Versus Revascularization Treatment
  (AVERT) trial, 202
Atrial fibrillation (AF)
  left atrial appendage closure. See WATCHMAN
    LAA occluder
  oral anticoagulants, 424
  stroke risk, 424
  thromboembolic and bleeding risk scores,
    424, 426t
Atrial septal anatomy/embryology, 417
Atrial septal defect (ASD)
  closure
    device implantation complications, 420
    devices, 418
    percutaneous closure technique, 418–419,
      419f
    postclosure management, 420
    recommendations, 417, 418t
  primum, 417, 417f
  secundum, 417, 417f
  sinus venosus, 417–418, 417f
  unroofed coronary sinus ASD, 418
Atrial switch baffle leaks, 473
Atrial transseptal puncture, 409, 411f
ATTRACT trial. See Acute Venous Thrombosis:
  Thrombus Removal with Adjunctive

Catheter-Directed Thrombolysis (ATTRACT)
  trial
AVP (AMPLATZER vascular plugs), 459
Axxess stent, 277

B
Baffle stenosis, 472
Balloon angioplasty
  vs. bare-metal stent, 188–189, 234, 235–236f,
    236, 282t
  coarctation of the aorta, 471
  cutting, 180–182
  pulmonary artery stenosis, 472
  restenosis, 12, 14, 15
  scoring, 182–183
  venous thromboembolism, 403
Balloon aortic valvuloplasty (BAV), 469
Balloon catheters
  compliant and noncompliant, 169
  monorail catheters, 169
  OTW balloon catheter, 168
Balloon injury vs. stent-induced injury, 15–16
Balloon mitral commissurotomy (BMC)
  complications, 432
  double balloon approach, 433, 433f, 434
  echocardiographic evaluation, 430–431, 430t
  5-year event-free survival, 432
  hemodynamic results, 432, 432f
  long-term outcomes, 432–433
  multi-track system, 433, 433f, 434
  patient selection, 431–432
  during pregnancy, 433
  pulmonary hypertension, 432
  single-balloon antegrade approach, 433, 433f
  transseptal puncture, 434
Balloon mitral valvuloplasty (BMV), 469
Balloon pericardiotomy, 468
Balloon pulmonary valvuloplasty (BPV), 469, 470t
Bare-metal stent (BMS)
  vs. balloon angioplasty, 188–189
  diffuse disease, 287
  restenosis, 18
    rate, 272
    reduction, 359
  SV PCI
    vs. balloon angioplasty, 282t
    and cilostazol, 282
    cutting balloon, 283
    heparin stent coating, 282
    intravascular ultrasound, 282–283
    restenosis rate, 281–282
    stent thrombosis, 283
    and strut thickness, 282
BARI (Bypass Angioplasty Revascularization
  Investigation), 258
Basel Kosten Effektivitäts Trial—SAphenous
  Venous Graft Angioplasty Using GP IIa/IIIb
  Receptor Inhibitors and Drug-Eluting Stents
  (BASKET-SAVAGE) trial, 300
BEIR VII model, 66
BENESTENT study, 18, 188
BES (biolimus A9-eluting stents), 191–192
β blockers, 59
  chronic stable angina, 199
  spontaneous coronary artery dissection, 342
  UA/NSTEMI, 217
Bicuspid valves, 447

Bifurcation Optimization Stent System (BIOSS), 277

Bifurcation lesions
    Bifurcations Bad Krozingen 2008, 277
    bio-resorbable scaffold, 277
    British Bifurcation Coronary Study, 278
    CACTUS 2009, 277–278
    classification, 273, 273f, 274f
    DK CRUSH II 2011, 278
    drug-eluting balloons, 276
    EBC TWO trial, 279
    elastic recoil, 272
    hemodynamic significance, 272
    intravascular imaging techniques, 277
    neointimal formation, 272
    Nordic Baltic Bifurcation Study III 2010, 278
    NORDIC Bifurcation Study 2006, 277
    NORDIC IV study, 278–279
    nosologic approach, 273
    pathophysiologic considerations, 272
    quantitative coronary angiography, 273
    stenting guidelines, 279
    stenting strategies
        crush technique, 275, 276f
        culottes stenting, 275, 276f
        Double Kiss Crush II, 276
        new-generation DES, 274
        open-celled stent, 276
        provisional stenting, 274
        randomized trials, 274
        simultaneous kissing stents, 274, 275f
        skirt stent technique, 276
        T and Protrusion, 275–276
        T stent, 275, 275f
        V stenting, 274, 274f
        Y stent technique, 276

Bifurcations Bad Krozingen 2008, 277

Bioabsorbable stents
    diffuse disease, 289
    drug-eluting stents, 193

BioFreedom drug-coated stent, 192

BioLinx tripolymer coating, 191

BioMatrix stent, 192

Bioprosthetic stenosis, 434

Bioresorbable scaffold (BRS), 102, 277

Biplane coronary angiography, 75

Bivalirudin, 221–222
    heparin-induced thrombocytopenia, 325
    ST-elevation myocardial infarction, 241
    STEMI, 48
    for women, 344

BMC. *See* Balloon mitral commissurotomy (BMC)

BMS. *See* Bare-metal stent (BMS)

BMV (balloon mitral valvuloplasty), 469

BPV (balloon pulmonary valvuloplasty), 469, 470t

Brachial artery, 323

Brachytherapy, 22

Bradycardia
    orbital atherectomy, 180
    rotational atherectomy, 178

British Bifurcation Coronary Study, 278

BRS (bioresorbable scaffold), 102, 277

B-type natriuretic peptide (BNP), 216

Burr selection
    orbital atherectomy, 179
    rotational atherectomy, 176

BVS-EES (Absorb Bioresorbable Vascular Scaffold System), 193

Bypass Angioplasty Revascularization Investigation (BARI), 258

Bypass Angioplasty Revascularization Investigation 2 Diabetes (BARI 2D) trial, 203

C

CABG surgery. *See* Coronary artery bypass graft (CABG) surgery

CACTUS 2009, 277–278

Calcification, intravascular ultrasound, 94

Calcium channel blockers, 54, 59, 217

Calcium-channel antagonists, 199

CAMs (cell adhesion molecules), 1

Canadian Cardiovascular Society (CCS) Class, 202

Cangrelor, 31, 221

Cangrelor *versus* Standard Therapy to Achieve Optimal Management of Platelet Inhibition (CHAMPION) PCI study, 161

CAPAS trial, 181

Caravel catheter, 172, 173f

Cardiac allograft disease
    chronic total occlusion lesions, 101
    near-infrared spectroscopy, 102
    optical coherence tomography, 101–102

Cardiac catheterization
    hypertrophic cardiomyopathy, 451, 451f
    left ventricular outflow tract obstruction during, 451f
    radiation safety for, 69

Cardiac cycle, 116, 116f

Cardiac Dimensions Carillon device, 438, 438f

Cardiac tamponade
    diagnosis, 464–465, 464–465f
    hemodynamics, 140, 141f
    pericardial pressure, 140
    pericardiocentesis. *See* Pericardiocentesis

Cardiogenic shock (CS), 216
    causes, 250–251
    circulatory support devices, 253–256
    diagnosis, 252
    hemodynamic criteria, 250
    hemodynamics, 251–252, 252f
    percutaneous coronary intervention, 358–359
    pharmacologic therapy, 253, 253t
    revascularization, 253
    tissue hypoperfusion, 249

CardioSEAL device, 418

Cardiovascular effects, use of contrast media, 71

Cardiovascular Inflammation Reduction Trial, 8

Cardiovascular Outcomes in Renal Atherosclerotic Lesions (CORAL) trial, 398

Carotid artery stenting (CAS), 345
    Asymptomatic Carotid Trial, 379
    clinical evidence, 377
    complications, 381
    CREST, 378–379
    high-surgical-risk patients, 377
    International Carotid Stenting Study, 378
    low-surgical-risk patients, 377–378
    SPACE trial, 378

Carotid endarterectomy (CEA), 375–377

Carotid Revascularization Endarterectomy *versus* Stenting Trial (CREST), 345, 378–379

Carotid stenosis
    anatomic imaging, 374, 374f
    aorto-ostial lesions, 381, 382f
    asymptomatic patients, 373

    baseline aortography, 380
    carotid artery stenting, 377–380
    carotid endarterectomy, 375–377
    cerebral angiography, 380
    clinical presentation, 374
    Doppler ultrasound surveillance, 382
    embolic protection devices, 380–381
    medical therapy, 374–375
    natural history, 373
    symptomatic patients, 373–374

CART (controlled antegrade and retrograde tracking), 319

CAS. *See* Carotid artery stenting (CAS)

Case–control study, 156–157, 157f, 157t

Catheter-related dissection, 308

CEA (carotid endarterectomy), 375–377

Ceiling-mounted shields, 69

Cell adhesion molecules (CAMs), 1

Cerebral vascular accident (CVA), 307

CFA. *See* Common femoral artery (CFA)

CFR. *See* Coronary flow reserve (CFR)

CHAMPION-PHOENIX trial, 221

Cheatham Platinum stent implantation, 471

Chemokines, 2

Chest pain
    initial diagnosis, 216
    in women, 339

Chronic thromboembolic pulmonary hypertension (CTEPH), 400

Chronic total occlusion (CTO)
    arrhythmia prevention, 313, 315
    complications, 319–320, 320f
    coronary artery bypass graft surgery, 313
    definition, 313
    estimated likelihood of success, 315
    estimated risk, 315, 317
    hybrid approach
        algorithm, 319f
        angiogram, 318–319
        antegrade dissection/reentry, 318f, 319
        antegrade wire escalation, 318f, 319
        retrograde approach, 318f, 319
    improve myocardial function, 313
    improve quality of life, 313
    lesion, 101
    long-term survival, 313
    medical therapy, 313
    percutaneous coronary intervention, 355
    procedural planning and equipment selection, 317–318, 317t
    recanalization, shorter guide catheter, 168
    revascularization options, 314f
    saphenous vein grafts PCI, 303
    tolerance of subsequent coronary events, 313
    in women, 342

CI-AKI. *See* Contrast-induced acute kidney injury (CI-AKI)

Cilostazol for Restenosis (CREST) trial, 19

Circumflex coronary artery, anomalous origin, 152, 154f

Clinical Outcomes Utilizing Revascularization and Aggressive Drug Evaluation (COURAGE) trial, 201

Clinical research statistics
    analysis method, considerations, 161–162
    case–control study, 156–157, 157f, 157t
    cohort study design, 157–158, 157f
    evidence-based medicine, 156, 156t

Clinical research statistics (*continued*)
    experimental studies, 158, 158f, 158t
    interpretation, 162, 162t
    sample size, 159–161, 159t, 160f
    study endpoints, 158–159
Clopidogrel, 220, 360
    mechanisms of action, 30–31, 32f
    pharmacologic properties, 29, 29t
    stroke prevention, 374–375
Clopidogrel for High Atherothrombotic Risk
    and Ischemic Stabilization, Management, and
    Avoidance (CHARISMA) trial, 375
Clopidogrel *versus* Aspirin in Patients at Risk of
    Ischemic Events (CAPRIE) trial, 374
CLOSE trial, 422
CLOSURE I trial, 420, 420t, 422
Coagulation issues, contrast media, 71
COAPT trial, 436
Coarctation of the Aorta Stent Trial (COAST) trial,
    471
Coated balloon drug delivery, 22
Coated coronary guide wires, 171
Cohort study design, 157–158, 157f
Coil embolization, 473–474
Collateral circulation, 145
Collateral flow, angiographic classification of, 145
COLOR registry, 102
Common femoral artery (CFA)
    access site, 326, 326f
    bifurcation, 326, 326f
    considerations, 326
    fluoroscopy guided access, 326–327, 327f,
      328f
    sedation, 326
COMPARE trial, 191, 288
Compliant *vs.* noncompliant balloons, 169
Composite endpoints, 158–159
Computed tomography angiography (CTA)
    acute ischemic stroke, 386
    aortic annulus reconstruction, 443, 443f
    atherosclerotic renal artery stenosis (RAS), 392
Computed tomography (CT) imaging
    acute ischemic stroke, 386
    paravalvular regurgitation, 458
    transcatheter paravalvular leak closure, 461,
      461f
Conduction system abnormalities, transcatheter
    aortic valve replacement, 448
Confianza Pro 12, 318
Confidence intervals, 162, 162f
Congenital Cardiac Catheterization Project on
    Outcomes, 472
Constrictive and restrictive cardiac
    hemodynamics, 134, 137, 138–140f, 138t
Continuous data, 161
Continuous veno-venous hemofiltration (CVVH),
    75
Contrast media
    allergic reactions, 72
    coagulation issues, 71
    complications, 308
    contrast-induced acute kidney injury, 73–75,
      73t, 74f
    delayed anaphylactoid reactions, 73
    direct cardiovascular effects, 71
    hyperthyroidism, 72
    immediate anaphylactoid reactions, 72–73,
      72t, 73t
    ionic, 70, 70f

non-ionic, 70, 71f, 71t
    for PCI, 148
    percutaneous coronary intervention, 148
    structure and properties, 70–71, 71f
Contrast-induced acute kidney injury (CI-AKI)
    cause of, 73
    chronic kidney disease, 73
    clinical course, 73
    definition, 73
    metformin-associated lactic acidosis, 75
    preventive strategies, 73t, 74–75, 74f
    risk factors, 73–74
Contrast-induced nephropathy (CIN). *See*
    Contrast-induced acute kidney injury (CI-AKI)
Controlled antegrade and retrograde tracking
    (CART), 319
Controlled clinical trials, 158
CORAL (Cardiovascular Outcomes in Renal
    Atherosclerotic Lesions) trial, 398
CoreValve US Pivotal trial, 442, 447
Coronary Angioplasty Study Amlodipine
    Restenosis (CAPARES), 19
Coronary artery bypass graft (CABG) surgery, 219
    angioplasty *vs.*, 258
    bare-metal stents *vs.*, 258, 259t, 260
    DESs *vs.*, 260
    guidelines, 260–261, 262t
    Heart Team approach, 354
    ST-elevation myocardial infarction, 232–233
Coronary artery disease (CAD). *See also*
    Multivessel coronary artery disease
    angiography, 431
    DES, 342
    revascularization
      angiographic criteria, 356
      fractional flow reserve, 357
      guideline-directed medical therapy, 357
      left main CAD revascularization, 357
      recommendations, 356
      survival improvement, 357
Coronary flow reserve (CFR), 7–8
    coronary Doppler flow velocity, 84, 84f
    coronary stenosis severity, 79
    coronary thermodilution technique, 84, 85f
    experimental dog model, 79, 80f
    factors affecting, 79, 80t
    normal coronary flow and velocity reserve, 84
Coronary lesion characteristics, PCI, 145, 147t,
    148
Coronary ostium, transcatheter aortic valve
    replacement, 448–449
Corrected TIMI frame count (CTFC), 144
Corsair catheter, 172, 173f
Corsair Pro catheter, 172, 173f
Counterpulsation to Reduce Infarct Size Pre-PCI
    Acute MI (CRISP-AMI) trial, 254
COURAGE trial, 215, 343
Covered Cheatham-Platinum Stents for Prevention
    or Treatment of Aortic Wall Injury Associated
    with Coarctation of the Aorta Trial, 471
Covered stents, 299–300
C-reactive protein (CRP), 13, 351–352
Creatine kinase-MB (CK-MB), 216
CREST trial, 282
CREST-2 trial, 375, 376f
Cribriform occluder, 418, 419f
CRP (C-reactive protein), 13, 351–352
Crush stenting, 275, 276f
CS. *See* Cardiogenic shock (CS)

CTEPH (chronic thromboembolic pulmonary
    hypertension), 400
CTO. *See* Chronic total occlusion (CTO)
Culottes stenting, 275, 276f
CURE trial, 220
Cutting balloon angioplasty
    complications, 181–182
    device, 180, 181f
    indications and contraindications, 180–181,
      181t
    outcomes, 181, 182t
    procedure, 180
CVA (cerebral vascular accident), 307
CVVH (continuous veno-venous hemofiltration),
    75
Cyclic adenosine monophosphate (cAMP)
    pathway, 16
CYP2C19 enzyme, 30
Cypher stent, 190
Cytokines, 2, 3

D

Dabigatran, 401
DAPT. *See* Dual antiplatelet therapy (DAPT)
DART trial, 283
D-dimer test, 400
De novo coronary artery lesions, 184
DEA (desethylamiodarone), 59
DECLARE-DIABETES trial, 285
Deep venous thrombosis (DVT). *See* Venous
    thromboembolism
DEFER study, 209
DES. *See* Drug-eluting stents (DES)
Desethylamiodarone (DEA), 59
Diabetes mellitus
    BARI trial, 264
    FREEDOM trial, 264
    prevention, 351
    restenosis, 12
    SYNTAX trial, 264
Diastolic dysfunction, 451
Diffuse coronary narrowing, 55
Diffuse disease
    and bare-metal stents, 287
    bioabsorbable stents, 289
    definition, 287
    drug-eluting stents
      first-generation, 287–288
      full-metal jacket strategy, 288
      IVUS and OCT, 288
      second- and third-generation, 288
      stent overlap, 288
      stent thrombosis, 288–289
Diffuse intrastent, in-stent restenosis, 14
Diffuse proliferative, in-stent restenosis, 14
Digital communication in medicine (DICOM), 64
Digital imaging system, 62, 63f
Digital subtraction angiography (DSA), 374
Digoxin, 59
Dihydropyridines, 54
Diltiazem, 54, 452
Dipyridamole, 19, 28
Direct ionization, 65
Direct-acting oral anticoagulant (DOAC), 401,
    401t
Dissection
    coronary, 307–308, 308t
    reentry, antegrade, 318f, 319

Distal angiographic contrast runoff, classification of, 144
Distal bifurcation lesions, 294
DK CRUSH II 2011, 278
Dobutamine, 56
Dopamine, 56
Doppler echocardiography, 464, 464f
Dose–area product (DAP), 65
Double balloon commissurotomy, 433, 433f, 434
Double Kiss Crush II, 276
Drug-eluting balloons, 276
Drug-Eluting stent Implantation versus optimal Medical Treatment in patients with Chronic Total Occlusion (DECISION-CTO), 313
Drug-eluting stents (DES)
    anti-restenotic agents, 190
    bioabsorbable, 193
    biolimus A9-eluting stents, 191–192
    vs. BMS, 236–237, 237–238t, 238–239f
    components, 189, 190f
    coronary artery disease, 342
    diffuse disease
        first-generation, 287–288
        full-metal jacket strategy, 288
        IVUS and OCT, 288
        second- and third-generation, 288
        stent overlap, 288
        stent thrombosis, 288–289
    drug carriers, 190
    everolimus-eluting stents, 21, 191
    fracture, 13
    hybrid sirolimus eluting stents, 192
    paclitaxel-eluting stents, 20, 190
    restenosis rate, 188t, 272
    restenosis reduction, 359
    saphenous vein grafts, 300
    sirolimus vs. paclitaxel, 20–21
    sirolimus-eluting stents, 20, 190
    SV PCI
        bioabsorbable polymer, 284–285
        and cilostazol, 285
        contemporary United States practice, 285
        different polymers, 284
        first-generation, 283
        in-stent late loss, 285, 286f
        IVUS and OCT in, 286
        major adverse cardiac events, 287f
        second- and third-generation, 283–284
        stent thrombosis, 285
        strut thickness and metallurgy, 284
    thrombosis, 190, 191t
    zotarolimus-eluting stents, 21–22, 191
Drug-Eluting Stents vs. Bare Metal Stents In Saphenous Vein Graft Angioplasty (DIVA) trial, 300
DrySeal sheath, 460
Dual antiplatelet therapy (DAPT), 359–361
    acute coronary syndrome, 219–220
    spontaneous coronary artery dissection, 342
    ULMCA PCI, 294
    in women, 344
Dynaglide mode, 175
Dyspnea, 216, 430

E

EBC TWO trial. See European Bifurcation Club 2 (EBC TWO) trial
ECG. See Electrocardiography (ECG)

ECMO (extracorporeal membrane oxygenation), 255–256
ECST (European Carotid Surgery Trial), 374, 376
EDHFs (endothelium-derived hyperpolarizing factors), 7
Edoxaban, 401
Edwards SAPIEN 3 valve, 442, 442f
Edwards SAPIEN pulmonary valve, 471
EES (everolimus-eluting stent), 21, 191, 284
Effective dose, 65
8-Fr guiding catheters, 166
8-French Trellis system, 403
EkoSonic endovascular system, 403f
Elastic recoil, 14
ELCA. See Excimer laser coronary atherectomy (ELCA)
Electrocardiography (ECG). See also Transesophageal echocardiography (TEE); Transthoracic echocardiography (TTE)
    acute coronary syndrome, 216
    advantage of, 406
    Doppler, 451
    paravalvular regurgitation, 458
    for ST-elevation myocardial infarction, 228
    structural heart disease, 406, 407t
Element stent, 190
Ellis classification of coronary perforations, 309, 309t
Ellis lesion-specific classification, 147t
Embolic protection devices (EPDs)
    carotid stenosis, 380–381
    ST-elevation myocardial infarction, 240
Endeavor stent, 191
Endothelial cells, 7
Endothelial dysfunction
    acetylcholine in, 6–7
    coronary blood flow, 7–8
    coronary flow reserve, 7–8
    Framingham risk score, 8
    microvascular dysfunction, 8
    treatment, 8
    vascular tone changes, 7
Endothelin 1, 7
Endothelium, 7
Endothelium-derived hyperpolarizing factors (EDHFs), 7
Endovascular Treatment for Small Core and Anterior Circulation Proximal Occlusion With Emphasis on Minimizing CT to Recanalization Times (ESCAPE), 383
End-systolic pressure-volume point (ESPV), 121, 121f
Enoxaparin, 48, 221
EPDs. See Embolic protection devices (EPDs)
Epicardial vessel resistance, 79
Epinephrine, 56, 56t
Eptifibatide, 220
    indications, 36
    mechanisms of action, 36
    pharmacologic properties and dosing, 35t
Equivalence trial, 159, 160f
Equivalent dose, 65
Ergonovine, 55
E-selectin, 1
Esmolol, 59
ESPV (end-systolic pressure-volume point), 121, 121f
ESSENCE-DIABETES trial, 191

European Bifurcation Club 2 (EBC TWO) trial, 274, 279
European Carotid Surgery Trial (ECST), 374, 376
European System for Cardiac Operative Risk Evaluation (euroSCORE), 262, 442
euroSCORE (European System for Cardiac Operative Risk Evaluation), 262, 442
Evaluate the Safety and Efficacy of OAS in Treating Severely Calcified Coronary Lesions (ORBIT II) study, 342
Evaluating XIENCE and Left Ventricular Function in Percutaneous Coronary Intervention on Occlusions After ST-Elevation Myocardial Infarction (EXPLORE) trial, 313
Everolimus-eluting stent (EES), 21, 191, 284
Everolimus-Eluting Stents or Bypass Surgery for Left Main Coronary Artery Disease (EXCEL) trial, 294
Evidence-based medicine, 156, 156t
EVOLVE trial, 191
Excimer laser coronary atherectomy (ELCA), 183, 183f
Exertional angina, 4
EXOSEAL device, 332, 332t, 333f, 334
Experimental studies, 158, 158f, 158t
Exposure, 64
Express open-cell slotted-tube stainless-steel stent platform (PES[E]), 190
Extending the Time for Thrombolysis in Emergency Neurological Deficits-Intra-Arterial (EXTEND-IA), 383
Extracellular matrix, 5
Extracorporeal membrane oxygenation (ECMO), 255–256

F

Facilitated angioplasty, 230
Femoral artery access
    common femoral artery
        access site, 326, 326f
        bifurcation, 326
        considerations, 326
        fluoroscopy guided access, 326–327, 327f, 328f
        sedation, 326
    inferior epigastric artery, 326
    micropuncture technique, 325
    posterior wall approach, 325
FemoSeal vascular closure device, 334
Fentanyl, 455
FFR. See Fractional flow reserve (FFR)
Fibrinogen, 6, 19
Fibrinolysis, 229–230
Fibrinolytic therapy, 49–50, 224, 224t, 358, 358t
Fibromuscular dysplasia (FMD), 391, 391t
Fielder FC, 318
Fielder XT, 318
Fighter, 318
FineCross catheter, 172, 173f
First-generation drug-eluting stenting
    comparison among, 190, 190t
    paclitaxel-eluting stents, 190
    vs. second-generation DES, 190
    sirolimus-eluting stents, 190
First-in-man (FIM) study, 190
FISH device, 332, 332t, 333f
FK-binding protein 12 (FKBP-12), 12
Flat panel system, 62–63, 63f

Flextome Cutting balloon angioplasty, 180
Fluoroscopic beam, 62
Fluoroscopic time (FT), 65
Fluoroscopy
    common femoral artery access, 326–327,
        327f, 328f
    pregnancy, 433
    structural heart disease, 406, 413
    transesophageal echocardiography, 443
FMD (fibromuscular dysplasia), 391, 391t
Foam cells, 1–3, 2f
Fondaparinux, 221
    adverse events, 46
    dosing strategies, 45–46
    elective PCI, 45
    NSTE-ACS, 45
Fontan fenestrations, 473
Foramen ovale, 417
Fossa ovalis, 417, 434
Fractional flow reserve (FFR), 357
    acute coronary syndrome, 88
    collateral supply, 81
    of coronary artery, 81
    coronary side-branch bifurcation lesion, 272
    ischemic stress testing, 85
    left main CAD lesions, 87–88
    multivessel CAD, 86–87
    myocardium, 81
    in non-ST segment myocardial infarction,
        90–91
    pressure–flow velocity measurements, 85, 86t
    serial epicardial lesions, 88
    small vessel PCI, 286
    in STEMI, 89
    ULMCA PCI, 294, 296t
Fractional Flow Reserve and Intravascular
    Ultrasound Relationship (FIRST) study, 95
Fractional Flow Reserve versus Angiography for
    Multivessel Evaluation (FAME) trial, 209
Framingham Risk Score (FRS), 8, 350
Framingham study, 158
Free radicals, 65
FRISC2 trial, 218
FRS. See Framingham Risk Score (FRS)
Full-metal jacket stenting, 288
Fusion imaging guided atrial septal defect closure,
    407f

G

Gaia second, 318
GDMT (guideline-directed medical therapy), 357
Global Registry of Acute Coronary Events
    (GRACE) risk score, 217, 218t
Global restenosis trial (GST), 181
Global Utilization of Streptokinase to Open
    occluded arteries study (GUSTO-I), 253
Glycoprotein IIb/IIIa inhibitors, 220–221
    adverse effect, 36
    indications, 36
    mechanisms of action, 35–36
    pharmacologic properties and dosing, 35t
    saphenous vein grafts PCI, 299
Gore CardioForm septal occluder device, 473
Gore Helex/Cardioform ASD closure devices, 418,
    419f
Gore REDUCE trial, 422
Gorlin equation, 125
GuardWire, 302, 302f

Guide catheters
    active support, 165
    vs. diagnostic catheters, 164
    factors affecting, 165t
    length, 168
    for LIMA-LAD anastomosis, 168
    passive support, 165
    for radial access, 168, 168f
    for saphenous vein bypass grafts, 168
    shapes, 166, 167f, 168
    sheath sizes, 164f
    side holes for, 168
    sizes, 165–166, 166t
    styles and lengths, 165, 165t
    traditional guide catheter, 164
Guideline-directed medical therapy (GDMT), 357
Guideliner, 165, 171f, 172
Guide wires
    coronary
        buddy wire, 170
        chronic total occlusions PCI, 318
        complications, 171–172
        construction, 169, 170f
        extra-long guide wires, 170
        hydrophilic coating, 170
        selection, 170
        shaping ribbon, 170
        specialty wire, 171
        support wires, 170–171
        workhorse wires, 170, 170f
    fracture, 310
    thermodilution blood flow technique, 84, 85f
Guidezilla devices, 165

H

Hakke formula, 125
Hard clinical endpoints, 158
HCM. See Hypertrophic cardiomyopathy (HCM)
Heart Team approach, 263, 354
Hematoma, 337
Hemodynamic instability, 381–382
Hemodynamics
    aortic regurgitation, 126, 127–130f
    aortic stenosis
        femoral artery, 123–124
        low gradient and ejection fraction, 126,
            128, 131f, 132f
        LV-Ao pressure tracings, 124, 126f
        pathophysiology, 124, 125f
    cardiac tamponade, 140, 141f
    constrictive and restrictive cardiac physiology,
        134, 137, 138–140f, 138t
    hypertrophic obstructive cardiomyopathy,
        128–129, 132f, 133f
    intracardiac shunts, 122–123
    left atrial pressure waveform, 117–118, 119f
    mitral regurgitation, 131, 136–137f
    MV stenosis
        cusps thickening, 134f
        LV and PCW tracings, 130, 134f
        percutaneous balloon mitral valvuloplasty,
            130, 135f
        subvalvular apparatus retraction, 129, 134f
    pressure volume relationships, 120–122, 121f,
        122f
    right atrial pressure, 116, 117f, 118f
    right atrial waveform
        dyspnea, 118, 119f

    tricuspid regurgitation, 118, 120f
    transcatheter aortic valve replacement, 126,
        127f
    valve area calculations, 124–126
Heparin
    low-molecular-weight heparin. See Low-
        molecular-weight heparin (LWMH)
    restenosis, 15
    unfractionated heparin. See Unfractionated
        heparin (UFH)
High-definition IVUS, 100f
High-osmolar contrast media (HOCM), 71
Hirudin, 19
HMR (hyperemic microvascular resistance), 85
HORIZONS-AMI trial, 48, 241
HSGs (hyperemic renal artery systolic gradients),
    55
HSR (hyperemic stenosis resistance), 85
Hybrid CTO crossing
    algorithm, 319f
    angiogram, 318–319
    antegrade dissection/reentry, 318f, 319
    antegrade wire escalation, 318f, 319
    retrograde approach, 318f, 319
Hybrid sirolimus eluting stents, 192
Hyperemic microvascular resistance (HMR), 85
Hyperemic renal artery systolic gradients (HSGs),
    55
Hyperemic stenosis resistance (HSR), 85
Hyperglycemia, 1
Hyperhomocysteinemia, 1
Hyperlipidemia, 1
Hyperperfusion syndrome, 382
Hypersensitivity reactions, 72
Hypertension (HTN)
    coronary prevention, 349–350, 349t
    JNC recommendations, 349–350, 349t
    lifetime incidence, 349
Hyperthyroidism, 72
Hypertrophic cardiomyopathy (HCM)
    clinical diagnosis, 451
    gene mutation, 451
    left ventriculography, 451f
    LVOT obstruction. See Left ventricular outflow
        tract (LVOT) obstruction
    prevalence, 451
Hypertrophic obstructive cardiomyopathy
    (HOCM), 128–129, 132f, 133f

I

Ibuprofen, 219
ICAM-1. See Intracellular cell adhesion molecules
    (ICAM-1)
ICE. See Intracardiac echocardiography (ICE)
Image intensifier, 62, 63f, 144f
Immunity, adaptive, 2
Impella device, 254–255
Index of microcirculatory resistance (IMR), 85
Inflammation
    and atherosclerosis, 1
    and in-stent restenosis, 12–13
    of leukocyte recruitment and infiltration, 15
    prevention, 351–352
    and restenosis, 15
    in women, 341
Infra-inguinal stenoses, 403
In-hospital mortality, 306
Innate immunity

vs. adaptive immunity, 2
in atherosclerosis, 2–3
Inner Coil technology of coronary guide wire construction, 170, 170f
Inotropes, 55–57, 56t, 253. *See also* Vasopressors and inotropes
Inoue-balloon catheter, 433f
In-stent restenosis (ISR)
  inflammatory response, 14
  intravascular ultrasound, 100–101, 101f
  laser angioplasty, 184
  neointimal formation, 14
  patterns of, 13–14, 13f
  vs. plain balloon angioplasty, 14, 14f
Intention to treat (ITT), 161
Interagency Registry for Mechanically Assisted Circulatory Support (INTERMACS), 251
Interatrial septum, 417
Interferon (IFN)-γ, 3, 5
Interleukin-8 (IL-8), 2
International Carotid Stenting Study (ICSS), 378
International Study of Comparative Health Effectiveness with Medical and Invasive Approaches (ISCHEMIA) trial, 208
Interventional reference point (IRP), 65
Intra-aortic balloon pump (IABP), 254
Intracardiac echocardiography (ICE)
  advantages, 407t, 408
  ASD closure, 419f
  atrial transseptal puncture, 409, 411f
  catheters, 408
  disadvantages, 407t, 408, 408t
  image quality, 408
  patent foramen ovale closure, 422f
  percutaneous balloon mitral valvuloplasty, 411
  PFO/ASD closure, 409
  transcatheter aortic valve replacement, 413
Intracardiac shunts, 122–123
Intracellular cell adhesion molecules (ICAM-1), 2
Intracranial hemorrhage, 382
Intravascular brachytherapy, 22
Intravascular ultrasound (IVUS)
  angiographically unrecognized disease, 94
  artifacts and limitations, 93
  bifurcation lesion stent, 277
  calcification, 94
  calcium assessment, 143
  cardiac allograft disease, 101–102
  devices, 93
  in-stent restenosis, 100–101, 101f
  left main lesions, 95
  lesions of uncertain severity, 94–95
  quantitative luminal measurements, 93–94, 94f
  safety, 93
  stent deployment, 95, 95f, 96–98f
  ULMCA PCI, 294, 296t
  vulnerable plaques
    clinical outcome studies, 108
    conventional grayscale IVUS, 106
    fibrous cap thickness, 107
    plaque burden, 106
    plaque compositional features, 108
    plaque rupture and thrombosis, 107, 108f
    while grayscale IVUS, 107
Inverse square law, 69, 143
Iodine, 70
  allergy, 72
Iodixanol (visipaque), 71

Ionic contrast media, 70, 70f
Ionization
  direct, 65
  indirect, 65
  patient exposure to, 67, 67t
Ioxaglate, 71
"Is Drug-Eluting-Stenting Associated with Improved Results in Coronary Artery Bypass Grafts?" (ISAR-CABG) study, 300
ISAR CLOSURE study, 334
ISAR-COOL trial, 219
ISAR-DESIRE 4 trial, 182
ISAR-REACT 4 trial, 222
ISAR-STEREO trial, 189
ISAR-STEREO-2 trial, 282
Ischemia without obstructive CAD, 342
Iso-osmolar contrast agents (IOCM), 71
Isoproterenol, 56
IVUS. *See* Intravascular ultrasound (IVUS)

J

Japanese Stable Angina Pectoris (JSAP) trial, 203
J-CTO score, 315, 315f
Joint National Commission (JNC) 8 major recommendations, 349–350, 349t
Judkins left guide catheters (JLs), 166, 167f
JUPITER trial, 8
Justification for the Use of Statins in Prevention: an Intervention Trial Evaluating Rosuvastatin (JUPITER) study, 374

K

Kerma, 64
Kidney Disease Improving Global Outcomes (KDIGO), 73

L

LAA. *See* Left atrial appendage (LAA)
Laser angioplasty
  chronic total occlusion, 184
  complications, 184
  contraindications, 184
  de novo coronary artery lesions, 184
  device, 183, 183f
  indications, 183–184
  in-stent restenosis, 184
  principles, 183
  recommendations, 184t
  technique, 183
  thrombus rich lesion, 184
  undilatable stents, 184
Late lumen loss (LLL), 11
LAVA trial, 184
LCBI (lipid core burden index), 102
LEADERS trial, 281
Left anterior descending coronary arteries, 153, 178
Left anterior oblique (LAO) imaging, 143, 144f
Left atrial appendage (LAA)
  anatomy, 424, 424f
  morphologies, 425f
  WATCHMAN occluder
    distal fixation anchors, 425
    indications, 428b
    procedural complications, 428, 428t

randomized clinical trial data, 425–427, 427f
  society recommendations, 428, 428t
Left internal mammary artery (LIMA) graft, 258
Left internanal mammary artery-left anterior descending (LIMA-LAD) interventions
  guide catheters, 168
Left main CAD lesions
  fractional flow reserve, 87–88
  revascularization, 357
Left main coronary artery (LMCA)
  anterior free wall course, 151
  anteroposterior view, 143
  interarterial course, 152
  retroaortic course, 151
  septal course, 151
Left ventricular dysfunction, 216
Left ventricular end-diastole (LVED), 121
Left ventricular hypertrophy (LVH), 351
Left ventricular outflow tract (LVOT) obstruction
  alcohol septal ablation
    acute procedural success, 455, 456f
    hemodynamic evaluation, 453, 454f
    patient selection, 452–453, 453f, 454f
    procedure, 453–455
    survival, 456–457
    symptom improvement, 456, 456f
    temporary pacemaker placement, 453
  cardiac catheterization, 451f
  medical therapy, 452
  pathophysiology, 451–452, 452f
  surgical myectomy, 452
LEONARDO trial, 183
Leukocyte recruitment and infiltration, 1–2, 15
Liberte stent, 190
Lidocaine, 58–59
Limbus of the left upper pulmonary vein (LUPV), 424
Lipid accumulation, 1
Lipid core burden index (LCBI), 102
Lipid Research Clinic Primary Prevention Trial (LRCPPT), 197
LMCA. *See* Left main coronary artery (LMCA)
LOCM. *See* Low-osmolar contrast media (LOCM)
Low density lipoprotein (LDL), 1
Lower extremity
  angiography, 150, 151f
  peripheral artery disease
    femoropopliteal interventions, 367–368
    iliac interventions, 366–367
    infrapopliteal interventions, 368–371, 369f, 370f
Low-molecular-weight heparin (LWMH), 221, 401
  adverse consequences, 43
  comparisons, 42
  dosing strategies, 42–43
  elective PCI, 42
  NSTE-ACS, 42
  vs. UFH, 42
Low-osmolar contrast media (LOCM), 71
LRCPPT (Lipid Research Clinic Primary Prevention Trial), 197
LVED (left ventricular end-diastole), 121
LVH (left ventricular hypertrophy), 351
LVOT obstruction. *See* Left ventricular outflow tract (LVOT) obstruction
LWMH. *See* Low-molecular-weight heparin (LWMH)

M

MACE. *See* Major adverse cardiac events (MACE)
Macrophages, 1–3
Magnetic resonance imaging (MRI)
    acute ischemic stroke, 386
    paravalvular regurgitation, 458
Main, Across, Distal, Side (MADS) classification, 276
Major adverse cardiac events (MACE), 187
    chronic total occlusions PCI, 315
    endothelial dysfunction, 341
    ULMCA PCI, 294
Major adverse vascular events (MAVE), 335t
Management of Atherothrombosis with
    Clopidogrel in High-risk Patients (MATCH)
    trial, 375
Matrix metalloproteinases (MMPs), 3, 13
MATRIX trial, 222, 242
MAVE (major adverse vascular events), 335t
Maximal radiographic contrast dose (MCRD), 74
Mechanically rotated imaging devices, 93
Medicine, Angioplasty or Surgery Study (MASS), 203
Medina classification system, 273, 273f, 274f
Medtronic Melody pulmonary valve, 471
Medtronic self-expanding CoreValve Evolut R, 442, 442f
Melody percutaneous pulmonary valve, 471
Metabolic syndrome, 350–351, 351t
Metformin-associated lactic acidosis, 75
Microcirculatory resistance, 79
Microvascular catheters, 172, 173f
Migraine Intervention with STARFlex Trial
    (MIST), 418
Milrinone, 56–57
Minimal lumen diameter (MLD), 11
Minimal stent area (MSA), 100
Minimally important difference (MID), 159, 160
MIST trial, 420, 421t, 422
MitraClip, 411, 471
Mitral leaflet repair, 411
Mitral regurgitation
    balloon mitral commissurotomy, 432
    hemodynamics, 131, 136–137f
Mitral stenosis
    atrial fibrillation, 430
    balloon commissurotomy. *See* Balloon mitral
        commissurotomy (BMC)
Mitral valve stenosis
    hemodynamics
        cusps thickening, 134f
        LV and PCW tracings, 130, 134f
        percutaneous balloon mitral valvuloplasty, 130, 135f
        subvalvular apparatus retraction, 129, 134f
Mitral valvuloplasty. *See* Balloon mitral
    commissurotomy (BMC)
Mitralign annuloplasty, 438, 439f
MMPs. *See* Matrix metalloproteinases (MMPs)
Monocyte chemoattractant protein-1 (MCP-1), 2, 13
Monocytes, 2
Monorail balloon catheters, 169
Morphine, UA/NSTEMI, 217
Mortality rate, PCI, 306–307
Mother-daughter extension catheters, 165

Multicenter Randomized Clinical Trial of
    Endovascular Treatment for Acute Ischemic
    Stroke in the Netherlands (MR CLEAN), 383
Multi-detector computed tomography (MDCT)
    3D volumetric data, 408
    transcatheter aortic valve replacement, 412, 412f
Multi-element electronic phased-array device, 93
Multi-Link Duet stent, 189
Multiple Risk Factor Intervention Trial (MRFIT), 197
Multivessel coronary artery disease (CAD)
    acute coronary syndromes, 266–267
    advanced age, 263
    bifurcation lesions, 267
    coronary anatomy, 267
    coronary artery bypass graft surgery
        vs. angioplasty, 258
        vs. bare-metal stents, 258, 259t, 260
        vs. DESs, 260
        guidelines, 260–261, 262t
    diabetes, 264
    fractional flow reserve, 86–87
    functional stress testing, 264–265
    Heart Team approach, 263
    hybrid coronary revascularization, 262
    LV dysfunction and viability, 263–264
    patient comorbidities, 262
    revascularization, 265–266
MYNX, 332t, 333f, 334
Myocardial Blush Grades (MBG), 144
Myocardial flow, 79f
Myocardial infarction (MI), 216, 217t
    non ST-segment elevation MI. *See* Non-ST
        segment elevation myocardial infarction
        (NSTEMI)
    ST-elevation myocardial infarction. *See* ST-
        elevation myocardial infarction (STEMI)

N

N-acetyl procainamide (NAPA), 57
N-acetylcysteine (NAC), 75
National Cardiovascular Data Registry (NCDR), 226, 315, 355
National Cholesterol Education Program (NCEP)–
    ATP III treatment algorithm, 350
National Council on Radiation Protection (NCRP), 67, 67t
National Heart Lung and Blood Institute (NHLBI)
    classifications of coronary dissection, 307–308, 308t
National Institutes of Health Stroke Scale
    (NIHSS), 374
Near-infrared spectroscopy (NIRS)
    cardiac allograft disease, 102
    with IVUS, lipid-rich plaque detection, 101f
    vulnerable plaques, 110–111, 111f
Negative remodeling, 16
Neoatherosclerosis, 16–17, 17f
Neointimal hyperplasia (NIH), 13
Neointimal proliferation, 14
Neosynephrine, 55
Neutrophils, 15
New York Heart Association (NYHA) Class III or
    IV symptoms, 431
NEXT trial, 192
Nicardipine, 54
Niche devices

atherectomy
    orbital atherectomy, 179–180
    rotational atherectomy, 175–179
balloon angioplasty
    cutting, 180–182
    scoring, 182–183
NIRS. *See* Near-infrared spectroscopy (NIRS)
Nitroglycerin, 53, 217
Nitroprusside, 53–54
Nobori DES stent, 192
Nominal data, 161
Noncompliant balloons, 169
Non-inferiority trial, 159–160, 160f
Non-ionic contrast agents, 70, 71, 71f, 71t
Non-left main CAD revascularization, 357
Nonrandomized clinical trial, 158
Non-ST segment elevation myocardial infarction
    (NSTEMI)
    anticoagulants
        ACC/AHA guideline recommendations, 38
        anticoagulant dosing, 39t
        apixaban, 47
        coagulation cascade inhibition, 38
        direct thrombin inhibitors, 43–44
        early invasive management strategy, 38–39
        fondaparinux, 45–46
        ischemia-guided management strategy, 39
        low-molecular-weight heparins, 42–43
        PCI, 39–40
        rivaroxaban, 46–47
        unfractionated heparin, 40–42
        warfarin, 46
    epidemiology, 215
    fractional flow reserve, 90–91
    pathology, 216
    risk stratification, 217–218, 218f
    in women and percutaneous interventions, 343
Non-ST-elevation ACS (NSTE-ACS)
    electrocardiography, 216
    epidemiology, 215
Non-uniform rotational distortion (NURD), 93
Non-vitamin K-dependent OACs (NOACs), 424
Nordic Baltic Bifurcation Study III 2010, 278
NORDIC Bifurcation Study 2006, 277
NORDIC IV study, 278–279
No-reflow phenomenon, 309
Norepinephrine (Levophed), 55–56
Normal pressure wave forms, 116
North American Symptomatic Carotid
    Endarterectomy Trial (NASCET), 374, 376
NSTEMI. *See* Non-ST segment elevation
    myocardial infarction (NSTEMI)
Number needed to treat (NNT) principle, 161
NURD (non-uniform rotational distortion), 93

O

OAS. *See* Orbital atherectomy system (OAS)
Obesity, 351
Observational studies, 156–158
Occluder devices, 459
Occlutech PLD, 459
Occupational radiation dose limits, 67–68
OCT. *See* Optical coherence tomography (OCT)
Oculostenotic reflex, 191
Odds ratios, 161t
Optical coherence tomography (OCT)
    bifurcation lesion stent, 277

cardiac allograft disease, 101–102
vulnerable plaques, 100–110
Optical Coherence Tomography Assessment
  of Gender Diversity In Primary Angioplasty
  (OCTAVIA) study, 340
Optically simulated luminescent (OSL) badge, 68
OPTIMIZE PCI trial, 102
Oral anticoagulants (OACs), 424
Orbital atherectomy system (OAS)
  adjunctive techniques, 180
  burr selection, 179
  complications, 180
  components, 179
  device, 179
  guide catheter, 179
  indications and contraindications, 180t
  outcomes, 180
  principles, 179
  procedural technique, 179–180
Ordinal data, 161
Orsiro (Biotronik) stent, 192
Osmolality, contrast media, 70–71
Ostium secundum, 417
Over-the-wire (OTW) balloon catheter, 166, 168

P

P wave, 116
P2Y12 inhibitors
  clopidogrel, 29
  indications, 31, 33–34t
  mechanisms of action, 30–31, 32f
  side effects, 34–35
  ticlopidine, 29
Paclitaxel, 20
Paclitaxel In-Stent Controlled Elution Study
  (PISCES) trial, 20
Paclitaxel-eluting stents (PESs), 190, 283
Palmaz-Schatz stent, 188–189
Papaverine, 54–55
Papillary muscle displacement, anterior, 452
Paravalvular leaks
  closure. See Transcatheter paravalvular leak
    (PVL) closure
  CT angiography, 413
  transesophageal echocardiography, 413
  transthoracic echocardiography, 413
Paravalvular regurgitation (PVR)
  computed tomography, 458
  echocardiographic quantification, 458
  magnetic resonance imaging, 458
  paravalvular leak closure
    anchor wiring, 460
    aortic PVR, 459, 459f
    clinical outcomes, 461–462, 462f
    CT guidance, 461, 461f
    device occluders, 459
    mitral PVR, 459–460, 460f
    multiple device placement, 460
    patient selection, 458–459
    transcatheter rails, 460
Passive approximation devices, 331, 332t, 333f
Patent ductus arteriosus (PDA), 472–473
Patent foramen ovale (PFO), 409
  anatomy/embryology, 417
  closure
    AMPLATZER PFO Occluder, 420, 422f
    clinical trial data, 422
    CLOSE trial, 422

CLOSURE I trial, 420, 420t, 422
    Gore REDUCE trial, 422
    indications, 420
    intracardiac echocardiographic images,
      422f
    MIST trial, 420, 421t, 422
    PC trial, 420, 420t, 422
    RESPECT trial, 420, 421t, 422
Patent hemostasis, 325
PBMV (percutaneous balloon mitral
  valvuloplasty), 130, 135f, 345, 411
PDA (patent ductus arteriosus), 472–473
Peak skin dose (PSD), 65
Perclose devices, 332, 332t, 333f
Percutaneous Access Versus Open Femoral
  Exposure for Endovascular Aortic Aneurysm
  Repair (PEVAR) trial, 337
Percutaneous balloon mitral valvuloplasty
  (PBMV), 130, 135f, 345, 411
Percutaneous coronary intervention (PCI)
  adjunctive equipment, 172–174
  angiographic success, 354, 354t
  aspiration thrombectomy, 359
  balloon catheters, 168–169
  cardiogenic shock, 358–359
  chronic total vessel occlusion, 143
  clinically successful PCI, 354t, 355
  complications, 306, 306t, 355, 355t
    air embolism, 308
    arrhythmia, 308–309
    arterial dissection, 307–308
    atheroembolism, 307
    contrast media reactions, 308
    coronary perforation, 309, 309t
    mortality, 306–307
    no-reflow phenomenon, 309
    retained PCI equipment components,
      310
    stent thrombosis, 310–311
    vascular access/bleeding, 307
  coronary angiography
    anteroposterior imaging, 143, 144f
    collateral flow, 145
    coronary lesion characteristics, 145, 147t,
      148
    coronary stenosis assessment, 145, 146f
    left anterior oblique imaging, 143, 144f
    peripheral vascular angiography, 148–153,
      151f, 152f, 152t, 154f
    quantitative coronary angiography, 145
    radiographic contrast media, 148
    right anterior oblique imaging, 143
    saphenous vein grafts, 143–144, 145t
    SYNTAX score, 148, 149–151f
    TIMI flow grades, 144, 146t
  coronary guide wires, 169–172
  coronary stents, 359
  dual antiplatelet therapy, 360–361
  guide catheters, 164–168
  Heart Team approach, 354
  high-risk, 249, 250f
  operator and institutional competency, 356
  oral antiplatelet therapy, 359–360, 360t
  predictors of clinical outcome, 355
  procedural success, 354t, 355
  quality and performance considerations, 356,
    357t
  radiation exposure, 143
  recommendations, 354

saphenous vein grafts. See Saphenous vein
    grafts (SVGs)
  ST-elevation myocardial infarction, 358, 358t
    antiplatelet agents, 243–245
    balloon angioplasty vs. BMS, 234, 235–
      236f, 236
    drug-eluting stents vs. BMS, 236–237,
      237–238t, 238–239f
    emergency CABG surgery, 232–233
    fibrinolysis, 229–230, 245
    hospitals without, 227–228
    indications, 228, 228t
    late-arriving STEMI patients, 231–232
    non-infarct vessel, 233–234
    with or without on-site surgery, 229t
    parenteral anticoagulants, 241–243
    pharmacoinvasive approach, 231
    spontaneous reperfusion, 232
    surgical and nonsurgical hospitals, 228
    thrombus management, 237, 239–240
  SVG occlusion, 359
  timing of, 219
  UA/NSTEMI, 357–358, 358t
  volume recommendations, 356
  without on-site surgical backup, 355–356,
    356t
Percutaneous mitral valve repair
  Cardiac Dimensions Carillon device, 438, 438f
  MitraClip device, 434–436, 436–438f
  Mitralign annuloplasty, 438, 439f
  Valtech Cardioband, 438, 438f
Percutaneous renal artery stenting, 395
Percutaneous transluminal coronary angioplasty
  (PTCA), 13, 177, 258
Perforation, coronary, 309, 309t, 355
Pericardial effusions, 467–468
Pericardiocentesis
  aspiration, 466
  catheter placement, 466
  complications, 467–468
  equipment for, 465, 466t
  management, 466
  needle insertion, 466
  patient positioning, 466
  sheath position confirmation, 466, 468f
  site of entry, 466, 467f
  subxyphoid approach, 465
Periprocedural MI, 307
PERSEUS SV trial, 284
PESI (pulmonary Embolism severity index), 400,
  400t
PESs (paclitaxel-eluting stents), 190, 283
PFO. See Patent foramen ovale (PFO)
Phased array IVUS, 100f
Phenylephrine, 55
Phosphodiesterase 3 (PDE3), 19
Phosphodiesterase inhibitors, 56–57
Pilot 200, 318
Placement of Aortic Transcatheter Valves
  (PARTNER) trial, 442
Plaque. See also Vulnerable plaques
  angiogenesis of, 3
  atherosclerotic, 3
  fibrous cap over, 5
  and hypoxia, 3
  mineralization of, 3
  rupture of, 4–5
  vulnerability of, 3
Plaque-associated macrophages (PAMs), 3

Plasminogen activator inhibitor-1 (PAI-1), 6
Platelet Inhibition and Patient Outcomes (PLATO) trial, 361
PLATO trial, 220
Poly-l-lactic acid [PLLA], 192
Polymer release kinetics, 20
Post-thrombotic syndrome (PTS), 400
Prasugrel, 30, 220, 361
Precapillary arterioles, 79
Premier of Randomized Comparison of Bypass Surgery Versus Angioplasty Using Sirolimus-Eluting Stent in Patients With Left Main Coronary Artery Disease (PRECOMBAT) trial, 294
Pressure and flow measurements, coronary
    coronary flow reserve, 83–85
    epicardial resistance, 79
    fractional flow reserve, 81, 81f, 86
        acute coronary syndrome, 88
        ischemic stress testing, 85
        left main CAD lesions, 87–88
        multivessel CAD, 86–87
        in non-ST segment myocardial infarction, 90–91
        pressure–flow velocity measurements, 85, 86t
        serial epicardial lesions, 88
        in STEMI, 89
    microcirculatory resistance, 79
    precapillary arterioles, 79
    stenosis
        angioplasty sensor-guide wire, 81
        coronary hyperemia, 82
        coronary pulse-wave analysis, 82–83, 83f
        pressure loss, 79, 80f, 81
PREVAIL trial, 428, 428t
Primary and secondary coronary prevention
    AHA/ACC guidelines, 349
    anti-platelet therapy, 352
    CR programs, 352
    diabetes mellitus, 351
    hypertension, 349–350, 349t
    inflammmation and C-reactive protein, 351–352
    lipid intervention, 350, 350t
    metabolic syndrome, 350–351, 351t
    obesity, 351
    smoking, 352
Primum atrial septal defect, 417, 417f
Procainamide, 57
ProGlides, 336, 337
Progress-CTO Complications score, 315, 316f
Progressive lumen encroachment, 4
Prophylactic intracoronary nitroglycerin, 53
Prospective Global Registry for the Study of Chronic Total Occlusion Intervention (PROGRESS CTO), 315
Prospective Natural-History Study of Coronary Atherosclerosis Trial (PROSPECT), 94, 108, 191
ProspeCtive observational LongitudinAl RegIstry oF patients with stable coronarY artery disease (CLARIFY) registry, 197, 343
ProStar, 336, 337
PROTECT-AF trial, 425, 427f, 428, 428t
Provisional stenting, 274
PTCA. See Percutaneous transluminal coronary angioplasty (PTCA)
PTS. See Post-thrombotic syndrome (PTS)

Pulmonary artery stenosis (PAS)
    balloon angioplasty, 472
    congenital defects, 471
    stenting, 472
    surgical interventions, 471
Pulmonary capillary wedge (PCW), 116, 117f
Pulmonary Embolism severity index (PESI), 400, 400t
Pulse-wave analysis, coronary, 82–83, 83f
Pulsus paradoxus, 464
p-values, 161–162
PVR. See Paravalvular regurgitation (PVR)

Q

Quantitative coronary angiography, 145

R

RA. See Rotational atherectomy (RA)
Rabbit model, 15
Radial artery, 323
Radial artery access
    case selection, 323, 325t
    complications, 323–325, 325t
    Seldinger technique, 323
    ultrasound-guided, 323
Radial Artery Access with Ultrasound trial (RAUST), 323
Radial artery occlusion (RAO), 323, 325
Radial artery spasm (RAS), 323–325
RADIAL Versus Femoral Access for Coronary Artery Bypass Graft Angiography and Intervention (RADIAL CABG) trial, 299
Radiation
    absorbed dose, 64–65
    ALARA principle, 64
    assessment in fluoroscopic procedures, 65
    deterministic effects of, 65
    effective dose, 65
    equivalent dose, 65
    exposure, 64
        maternal and fetal risks, 68
        operator and staff exposure, 67–68, 67t
        patient exposure and risk, 67, 67t
        patient lifetime exposure, 68
        personnel dosimetry, 68
    kerma, 64
    procedural radiation awareness, 65
    radiation protection units, 64
    safety program
        dose optimization, 68
        optimal procedural dose management, 69–70, 69t
        post-procedure, 69
        pre-procedure planning, 68
        procedure justification, 68
        training, 68
Radiation absorbed dose (rad), 64
Radiation caps, 69–70
Randomized clinical trial, 158, 158f
Randomized Intervention Treatment of Angina (RITA) trial, 202
Randomized Study with the Sirolimus-Eluting Velocity Balloon-Expandable Stent (RAVEL), 20, 190
Rapid-exchange (RX) balloon catheters, 169
RAS (radial artery spasm), 323–325
Ratio plots, 162

REALITY trial, 21
REDUCE I trial, 181
Reduction of Restenosis In Saphenous vein grafts with Cypher sirolimus-eluting stent trial (RRISC), 300
Regadenoson, 54
Register of Information and Knowledge about Swedish Heart Intensive Care Admissions (RIKS-HIA), 342
Registry of Endovascular Critical Aortic Stenosis Treatment (RECAST) trial, 445
Rems, 64
Renal arteriography, 148, 150
Renal artery stenosis (RAS)
    catheter-based renal angiography, 392–394
    clinical endpoints and physical examination, 391–392
    diagnostic testing, 392, 392t
    pathophysiology, 391
    percutaneous renal artery stenting, 395
    prevalence and natural history, 391, 391t
    revascularization
        identification of patients, 397
        indications, 394–395, 394t
        technique, 395–397
    screening test, 393t
    treatment, 394
Rescue angioplasty, 230
RESCUT trial, 181
Resolute Integrity platform, 191
RESOLUTE-US trial, 284
RESPECT trial, 420, 421t, 422
Restenosis
    balloon angioplasty, 12, 14
    bare-metal ISR, 12
    coated balloon drug delivery, 22
    definition, 11
    drug-eluting stents, 20–22
    Gaussian distribution, 11, 11f
    and inflammation, 15
    inflammation and cell proliferation, 19
    in-stent
        intravascular ultrasound and, 100–101
        restenosis, 11, 14
    late loss and binary restenosis, 11, 12f
    left main stenting, 12
    leukocyte recruitment and infiltration inflammation mechanism, 15
    mechanical strategies, 17–18
    negative remodeling, 16
    neoatherosclerosis, 16–17, 17f
    pathogenesis, 14
    pathophysiology, 16
    pharmacologic therapies, 18
    risk factors, 12–13
    stent-induced injury vs. balloon, 15–16
    vascular recoil and remodeling, prevention, 19–20
    VSMC, intracellular molecular basis of, 16
Reverse crush technique, 275
RG3 guide wire, 318
Rheolytic thrombectomy, 240
Rheumatic heart disease, 430
RIDDLE-NSTEMI trial, 219
Right anterior oblique (RAO) imaging, 143
Right coronary artery, anomalous origin, 152–153
Right ventricular (RV) myocardial infarction (RVMI), 251
Risk ratios, 161t

RITA-3 trial, 218
Rivaroxaban, 401
    non-ST segment acute coronary syndromes, 46–47
Rivaroxaban Once Daily Oral Direct Factor Xa Inhibition Compared with Vitamin K Antagonism for Prevention of Stroke and Embolism (ROCKET), 159
ROCKET. See Rivaroxaban Once Daily Oral Direct Factor Xa Inhibition Compared with Vitamin K Antagonism for Prevention of Stroke and Embolism (ROCKET)
Roentgen (R), 64
Rotablator, 175, 175f
Rotational atherectomy (RA)
    adjunctive techniques, 176–177
    burr selection, 176
    complications, 178–179
    device, 175f, 175
    guide catheter selection, 176
    indications and contraindications, 177, 177t
    outcomes, 177–178, 177t, 178t
    principles, 175–176
    procedural technique, 176, 176t
Rotational IVUS, 100f
ROTAXUS trial, 178
RVOT stenting, 472

S

Sample size calculation
    equivalence trial, 159, 160f
    non-inferiority trial, 159–160, 160f
    superiority trial, 159, 160f
    type I error, 159, 159t
    type II error, 159, 159t
Saphenous vein bypass grafts, 168
Saphenous VEin De novo (SAVED) trial, 299
Saphenous vein graft Angioplasty Free of Emboli Randomized (SAFER) trial, 301
Saphenous vein grafts (SVGs)
    angulations for, 143–144, 145t
    percutaneous coronary intervention
        acute occlusion, 303
        adjunctive pharmacotherapy, 299
        BASKET-SAVAGE trial, 300
        chronic total occlusions, 303
        covered stents, 299–300
        DIVA trial, 300
        drug-eluting stents, 300
        embolic protection devices, 301–302, 301–303f
        intermediate lesions, 303
        ISAR-CABG study, 300
        multipurpose guide, 299
        radial approach, 299
        RRISC study, 300
        Stenting Of Saphenous Vein Grafts trial, 300
SAVR (surgical aortic valve replacement), 442
SCAAR (Swedish Coronary Angiography and Angioplasty Registry), 12, 342
SCAD. See Spontaneous coronary artery dissection (SCAD)
SCAI lesion-specific characteristics, 147t
Scoring balloon angioplasty
    complications, 183
    device, 182
    indications and contraindications, 182, 182t

outcomes, 182
    procedure, 182
Second-generation drug-eluting stents
    bioabsorbable drug-eluting stents, 193
    biolimus A9-eluting stents, 191–192
    everolimus-eluting stents, 191
    vs. first-generation DES, 190
    hybrid sirolimus eluting stents, 192
    zotarolimus-eluting stents, 191
Secundum atrial septal defect, 417, 417f
Seldinger technique, 323
Septal hypertrophy, 452
Septum primum, 417
Septum secundum, 417
SES. See Sirolimus-eluting stent (SES)
SES-SMART trial, 283
SHD. See Structural heart disease (SHD)
SHOCK trial, 253
Silent (asymptomatic) myocardial ischemia (SMI)
    ambulatory EKG monitoring, 197–198
    asymptomatic ischemia, 197
    coronary revascularization, 201
    definition, 197
    iceberg effect, 197f
    pathophysiology, 198
Simultaneous kissing stents (SKSs), 274, 275f
Single-balloon antegrade approach, 433, 433f
Single-operator balloon catheters, 169
Sinus venosus atrial septal defect, 417–418, 417f
Sion, 318
SIRIUS 2.25 trial, 283
SIRIUS trial, 190
Sirolimus-eluting stent (SES), 190
    vs. paclitaxel-eluting stent trials, 20–21
    small vessel PCI, 283
SIRTAX trial, 283
6-Fr guiding catheters, 165–166
Skin injury, radiation exposure, 65
Skirt stent technique, 276
Small vessel (SV), late loss on diameter stenosis in, 281
Small vessel percutaneous coronary intervention (SV PCI)
    bare-metal stenting
        vs. balloon angioplasty, 282t
        and cilostazol, 282
        cutting balloon, 283
        heparin stent coating, 282
        intravascular ultrasound, 282–283
        restenosis rate, 281–282
        stent thrombosis, 283
        and strut thickness, 282
    BVS, 285–286
    clinical trials, 281
    DESs
        bioabsorbable polymer, 284–285
        and cilostazol, 285
        contemporary United States practice, 285
        different polymers, 284
        first-generation, 283
        in-stent late loss, 285, 286f
        IVUS and OCT in, 286
        major adverse cardiac events, 287f
        second- and third-generation, 283–284
        stent thrombosis, 285
        strut thickness and metallurgy, 284
    fractional flow reserve, 286
    rotational atherectomy, 283
    thin-strut DESs, 281

SMI. See Silent (asymptomatic) myocardial ischemia (SMI)
Smoking prevention, 352
Smooth muscle dysfunction, in women, 341
Society of Thoracic Surgeons (STS) score, 262, 354
Sodium bicarbonate, 75
"Soft" balloons, 169
Soft clinical endpoints, 158
Solitaire With the Intention for Thrombectomy as Primary Endovascular Treatment (SWIFT PRIME), 383, 384
Specialty wire, 171
SPIRIT trial, 191, 284, 288
Spontaneous coronary artery dissection (SCAD)
    classification, 341–342
    management strategies, 342
SPORT trial, 178
St. Jude Medical pressure-wire system, 84, 85f
Stable coronary artery disease (CAD)
    CABG vs. PCI, 202–208, 204–207t
    coronary revascularization, 201
    diagnosis, 196
    life style goals, 200t
    management, 198, 199t, 200t
    optimal medical therapy, 199, 201
    optimal revascularization PCI technique, 208–209
    pathophysiology, 198
Staphylococcus aureus
    stent thrombosis, 311
    VCD infection, 337
StarClose device, 331, 331f, 332t, 333f
Statins, stroke prevention, 374
STEEPLE trial, 42
ST-elevation myocardial infarction (STEMI)
    anticoagulants
        ACC/AHA guideline, 48
        with delayed PCI, 50
        dosing, 49t
        with fibrinolytic therapy, 49–50
        with primary PCI, 48–49
    balloon angioplasty, 224, 226
    coronary angiography, 227, 227t, 358, 358t
    ECG criteria for, 228
    electrocardiography, 216
    epidemiology, 215
    fibrinolytic therapy, 47–48, 48t, 224, 224t, 358, 358t
    fractional flow reserve, 89
    ITT analysis, 161
    percutaneous coronary intervention, 358–359, 359t
        antiplatelet agents, 243–245
        balloon angioplasty vs. BMS, 234, 235–236f, 236
        drug-eluting stents vs. BMS, 236–237, 237–238t, 238–239f
        emergency CABG surgery, 232–233
        fibrinolysis, 229–230, 245
        hospitals without, 227–228
        indications, 228, 228t
        late-arriving STEMI patients, 231–232
        non-infarct vessel, 233–234
        with or without on-site surgery, 229t
        parenteral anticoagulants, 241–243
        pharmacoinvasive approach, 231
        spontaneous reperfusion, 232
        surgical and nonsurgical hospitals, 228

ST-elevation myocardial infarction (STEMI) (*continued*)
    thrombus management, 237, 239–240
    reperfusion approach, 224, 227f
    thrombolytic therapy, 224, 225t
    triage and transfer for PCI in, 226, 227f
    in women and percutaneous interventions, 343–344
STEMI. *See* ST-elevation myocardial infarction (STEMI)
Stenosis assessment, coronary, 145, 146f
Stent underexpansion and malapposition, 13
Stenting and Angioplasty with Protection in Patients at High Risk for Endarterectomy (SAPPHIRE) trial, 377
Stenting Of Saphenous Vein Grafts trial (SOS), 300
Stents. *See also* Bare-metal stent (BMS); Drug-eluting stents (DES)
    bifurcation lesions
        crush technique, 275, 276f
        culottes stenting, 275, 276f
        Double Kiss Crush II, 276
        new-generation DES, 274
        open-celled stent, 276
        provisional stenting, 274
        randomized trials, 274
        simultaneous kissing stents, 274, 275f
        skirt stent technique, 276
        T and Protrusion, 275–276
        T stent, 275, 275f
        V stenting, 274, 274f
        Y stent technique, 276
    coronary
        angiographic outcomes, 187, 187f
        bare-metal stent *vs.* balloon angioplasty, 188–189
        clinical outcomes, 187
        coatings, 188, 188t
        device and procedural success, 187
        drug-eluting stents. *See* Drug-eluting stents (DES)
        material composition, 187
        mode of implantation, 187
        scaffold configuration, 187
    dislodgement and embolization, 310
    fracture, 13
    induced injury *vs.* balloon injury, 15–16
    malapposition
        intravascular ultrasound, 99f
        optical coherence tomography, 100f
    retriever device, 385, 386f
    thrombosis, 191t
        Academic Research Consortium Criteria for, 310t
        mortality rates, 310
        risk factors, 310, 311t
        ST-elevation myocardial infarction, 237
        stent infection, 310–311, 311t
    underexpansion, 99f
Stent-Supported Percutaneous Angioplasty of the Carotid Artery *versus* endarterectomy (SPACE) trial, 378
Stentys, 277
Step crush technique, 275
STICH. *See* Surgical Treatment of Ischemic Heart Failure (STICH)
"Stiff" balloons, 169
Stiff guide wires, 171

Stingray system, 318, 319
Stochastic effects of radiation, 65–66
STRESS study, 188
Stroke
    acute ischemic stroke
        algorithm, 384f
        endovascular treatment, 385–388
        optimized stroke management, 386–387
        post-procedure management, 387
        pre-procedure planning, 386
        randomized clinical trials, 383–385
        stent-retriever technique, 387
        thrombus aspiration technique, 387
    after CAS, 381
    balloon mitral commissurotomy, 432
    medical therapy, 374–375
    percutaneous coronary intervention, 307
    surgical therapy, 375–377
    transcatheter aortic valve replacement, 447
    in women, 345
    volume, 121
Stroke Prevention by Aggressive Reduction in Cholesterol Levels (SPARCL) trial, 374
Structural heart disease (SHD)
    alcohol septal ablation, 414
    atrial transseptal puncture, 409, 411f
    cardiovascular MRI, 410
    CT imaging, 408–409, 410f
    echocardiography, 406–408
    fluoroscopy, 406
    LAA occlusion, 413
    mitral leaflet repair, 411, 412f
    paravalvular leaks, 413
    percutaneous balloon mitral valvuloplasty, 411
    PFO/ASD closure, 409
    transcatheter aortic valve replacement, 411–413, 412f, 413f
    valvular heart interventions, 409, 411
Study design
    case–control study, 156–157, 157f, 157t
    cohort study design, 157–158, 157f
    experimental studies, 158, 158f, 158t
Study of Access Site for Enhancement of PCI for Women (SAFE-PCI), 343
Sublingual nitroglycerin, 53
Substantial Radiation Dose Level (SRDL), 66t
SuperCross microcatheters, 173–174
Superior Yield of the New strategy of Enoxaparin, Revascularization and GlYcoprotein IIb/IIIa inhibitors (SYNERGY), 159
Superiority trial, 159, 160f
Support wires, 170–171
Surgical aortic valve replacement (SAVR), 442
Surgical Treatment of Ischemic Heart Failure (STICH), 202
SURTAVI, 442
SV PCI. *See* Small vessel percutaneous coronary intervention (SV PCI)
SVG occlusion, percutaneous coronary intervention, 359
Swedish Coronary Angiography and Angioplasty Registry (SCAAR), 12, 342
Swiss Interventional Study on Silent Ischemia Type II (SWISSI II) trial, 201
Synergy between Percutaneous Coronary Intervention with Taxus and Cardiac Surgery (SYNTAX) trial, 148, 149–151f, 219, 260, 265f, 287, 293, 354, 355

Synergy stent, 191
Systolic ejection period (SEP), 125

T

T and Protrusion (TAP), 275–276
T stent, 275, 275f
"T" wave, 116
Table-mounted shields, 69
TACTICS-TIMI 18 trial, 218
TandemHeart, 255
Target lesion revascularization (TLR), 12, 187
Target vessel failure (TVF), 187
Target vessel revascularization (TVR), 187
Target-lesion failure (TLF), 285
TAVR. *See* Transcatheter aortic valve replacement (TAVR)
TAXi trial, 20
TAXUS ATLAS LL trial, 288
TAXUS ATLAS SV trial, 284
TAXUS stent, 190
TAXUS V trial, 283, 284
TEE. *See* Transesophageal echocardiography (TEE)
Tendyne valve, 440, 440f
Thermionic emission, 62
Thermistors, 84
Thermodilution coronary flow reserve, 84, 85f
Thermoluminescent dosimeter (TLD) badge, 68
Thin-strut 316L stainless-steel bare-metal stents, 189
Thoracic aorta
    abdominal aortic aneurysm, 365–366, 366t
    acute aortic syndrome, 364–365
    coarctation, 364
    subclavian and brachiocephalic intervention, 364, 365f
    thoracic aortic aneurysm, 365
Thoracic aortic aneurysm (TAA), 365
Thrombin inhibitors, direct
    adverse events, 45
    elective PCI, 44, 45
    NSTE-ACS, 43–44
    for women, 344
Thrombocytopenia, 36
Thrombolysis in cerebral infarction (TICI)-score, 384
Thrombolysis in myocardial infarction (TIMI)
    flow grades
        distal runoff, 144
        Grade and Blush Scores, 146t
        Myocardial Blush Grades, 144
        TIMI frame count, 144
    risk score, 217, 218f, 218t
Thrombolytic therapy
    acute coronary syndrome, 4
    ST-elevation myocardial infarction, 224, 225t
Thrombosis
    coronary, 215–216
    plaque rupture, 4–6
    stents, 191t
        Academic Research Consortium Criteria for, 310t
        mortality rates, 310
        risk factors, 310, 311t
        ST-elevation myocardial infarction, 237
        stent infection, 310–311, 311t
Thromboxane, 216
Thrombus aspiration technique, 387

Ticagrelor, 30–31, 220, 361
Ticlopidine, 29, 220
TIMACS trial, 219
TIMI. *See* Thrombolysis in myocardial infarction (TIMI)
TIMI frame count (TFC), 144
Tirofiban, 220
    indications, 36
    mechanisms of action, 36
    pharmacologic properties and dosing, 35*t*
TLF (target-lesion failure), 285
TMVR. *See* Transcatheter mitral valve replacement (TMVR)
Tortuous vessels, venture catheter for, 174
TPVR (transcatheter pulmonary valve replacement), 471
TransAtlantic Inter-Society Consensus (TASC), 366, 367*t*
Transcatheter aortic valve replacement (TAVR)
    angiographic view, 443, 445*f*
    balloon-expandable, 444
    bicuspid valves, 447
    bioprosthetic deterioration, 434
    clinical data, 444–445
    conduction system abnormalities, 448
    CoreValve Evolut R, 442, 442*f*
    CoreValve US Pivotal trials, 447
    coronary ostium, 448–449
    Edwards SAPIEN 3 valve, 442, 442*f*
    fluoroscopy, 413, 443
    hemodynamics, 126, 127*f*
    implants, 412
    multi-detector computed tomography, 412, 412*f*
    partner trials, 445–447
    post-valve-deployment stage, 444
    preprocedural evaluation, 442–443, 443*f*
    stroke, 447
    three-dimensional TEE, 412–413
    transapical access, 443
    transfemoral approach, 443, 444, 446*f*
    valve-in-valve TAVR, 447
    valvular insufficiency, 448
    vascular complications, 447–448
    in women, 344–345
Transcatheter mitral valve replacement (TMVR)
    degenerated mitral bioprosthetic valve, 438, 439*f*
    devices, 440
    mitral annuloplasty ring, 438, 439*f*
    Tendyne valve, 440, 440*f*
Transcatheter paravalvular leak (PVL) closure
    anchor wiring, 460
    aortic PVR, 459, 459*f*
    clinical outcomes, 461–462, 462*f*
    CT guidance, 461, 461*f*
    device occluders, 459
    mitral PVR, 459–460, 460*f*
    multiple device placement, 460
    patient selection, 458–459
    transcatheter rails, 460
Transcatheter pulmonary valve replacement (TPVR), 471
Transcatheter rails, 460
Transcatheter tricuspid valve replacement (TTVR), 471
Transducer design, intravascular ultrasound, 93
Transesophageal echocardiography (TEE)
    3D imaging modalities, 406–407

    advantages and limitations, 407*t*
    alcohol septal ablation, 414
    aortic annulus reconstruction, 443, 444*f*
    balloon mitral commissurotomy, 433
    fluoroscopy, 443
    left atrial appendage, 424
    paravalvular leaks, 413
    paravalvular regurgitation, 458, 458*f*
    percutaneous balloon mitral valvuloplasty, 411
    PFO/ASD closure, 409
    real-time fusion imaging, 408
    three-dimensional TEE
        atrial transseptal puncture, 409, 411*f*
        mitral leaflet repair, 411
        paravalvular leaks, 413
        percutaneous LAA occlusion procedure, 413
        transcatheter aortic valve replacement, 412
        transcatheter aortic PVL closure, 459*f*
Transient focal neurologic symptoms, 373
Transient ischemic attack (TIA), 307, 432
Transit catheter, 172
Transseptal approach, 453
Transthoracic echocardiography (TTE)
    advantages and limitations, 407*t*
    alcohol septal ablation, 414
    balloon mitral commissurotomy, 430–431, 431*f*
    left atrial appendage, 424
    paravalvular leaks, 413
    paravalvular regurgitation, 458
    percutaneous balloon mitral valvuloplasty, 411
TrapLiner, 172, 172*f*
Trial to Assess Improvement in Therapeutic Outcomes by Optimizing Platelet Inhibition with Prasugrel–Thrombolysis In Myocardial Infarction (TRITON–TIMI), 220, 361
Tricuspid valvuloplasty, 470*t*
Troponin assay, acute coronary syndrome, 216
Tryton stent, 277
TTVR (transcatheter tricuspid valve replacement), 471
Turnpike catheter, 172, 173*f*
TVF (target vessel failure), 187
TVR (target vessel revascularization), 187
TWENTE trial, 21
Type II DM (T2DM), 351
Tyrosine kinase cascade, 16

U

Unfractionated heparin (UFH), 221
    adverse consequences, 41–42
    bioavailability, 40
    dosing strategies and therapeutics, 40–41
    elective PCI, 40
    NSTE-ACS, 40
    ST-elevation myocardial infarction, 241
    STEMI, 48
United Nations Scientific Committee on the Effects of Atomic Radiation (UNSCEAR), 68
Unprotected left main coronary artery (ULMCA) PCI
    coronary angiography, 292, 292*f*, 294, 296*f*
    distal bifurcation lesions, 294
    dual antiplatelet therapy, 294
    fractional flow reserve, 294, 296*t*
    IVUS, 294, 296*t*

    post-revascularization issues and follow-up, 294
    pre-procedural considerations
        anatomical predictors, 293
        distal bifurcation lesions, 293, 293*f*
        EXCEL trial, 294
        low-risk clinical predictors, 293
        PRECOMBAT trial, 294
        predictive models, 293–294
        SYNTAX trial, 293
Unroofed coronary sinus atrial septal defect, 418
Unstable angina (UA)
    acute coronary syndrome, 4
    anti-ischemic therapies, 217, 217*t*
    epidemiology, 215
    pathology, 216
    Percutaneous coronary intervention, 357–358, 358*t*
    risk stratification, 217–218, 218*f*
Upper extremity arterial circulation, 324*f*

V

V stenting, 274, 274*f*
VACSS. *See* Veterans Administration Cooperative Study of Surgery (VACSS)
VALIDATE-SWEDEHEART trial, 49
Valsalva aneurysm (SVA), ruptured sinus of, 473
Valtech Cardioband, 438, 438*f*
Valve-in-valve TAVR, 447
Valvular insufficiency, 448
Valvuloplasty
    balloon aortic valvuloplasty, 469
    balloon mitral valvuloplasty, 469
    balloon pulmonary, 469, 470*t*
VAS (vertebral artery stenosis), 382–383
Vascade vascular closure system, 332*t*, 333*f*, 334
Vascular access
    femoral artery access
        common femoral artery, 326–327, 327*f*, 328*f*
        inferior epigastric artery, 326
        micropuncture technique, 325
        posterior wall approach, 325
    percutaneous coronary intervention, 307
    radial artery access
        case selection, 323, 325*t*
        complications, 323–325, 325*t*
        Seldinger technique, 323
        ultrasound-guided, 323
    radial *vs.* femoral access, 328
Vascular angiography, peripheral
    anomalous origin
        circumflex coronary artery, 152, 154*f*
        left main coronary artery, 151–152, 152*f*, 153*t*
        right coronary artery, 152–153
    circumflex coronary arteries, 153
    common coronary anomalies, 150–151, 152*f*
    left anterior descending coronary arteries, 153
    lower extremity angiography, 150, 151*f*
    renal arteriography, 148, 150
Vascular closure devices (VCDs)
    ACCF/AHA/SCAI/PCI guidelines, 330, 330*t*
    Angio-Seal device, 331, 332*t*, 333*f*
    classification, 331, 332*t*, 333*f*
    clinical utility, 335–337
    comparisons, 335
    complications, 337, 337*t*

Vascular closure devices (VCDs) (continued)
  EXOSEAL device, 332, 332t, 333f, 334
  FISH device, 332, 332t, 333f
  indications and guidelines, 330–331, 330t
  infection control, 331
  MYNX, 332t, 333f, 334
  proficiency, 331
  randomized clinical trials, 334–335, 334–335t
  re-access after, 331
  registries, 335
  StarClose device, 331, 331f
  vascade vascular closure system, 332t, 333f, 334
Vascular reactivity tests, 7
Vascular remodeling, 3–4, 4f, 19–20
Vascular smooth muscle cells (VSMCs)
  calcium channel on, 54
  hyperpolarization, 7
  intracellular molecular basis, 16
  nitroglycerin metabolism, 53
  and restenosis, 13
Vascular tone regulation, 7
Vasoactive drugs
  adenosine agonists, 54
  calcium channel blockers, 54
  coronary vasoconstrictors, 55
  papaverine, 54–55
  vasodilators, 53–54
  vasopressors and inotropes, 55–57
Vasoconstrictors, coronary, 55
Vasodilators
  nitroglycerin, 53
  nitroprusside, 53–54
Vasopressin, 57
Vasopressors and inotropes
  cardiogenic shock, 253
  dobutamine, 56
  dopamine, 56
  indications and doses, 56t
  isoproterenol, 56
  norepinephrine, 55–56
  phenylephrine, 55
  phosphodiesterase inhibitors, 56–57
  side effects, 57
  vasopressin, 57
VAST (Vertebral Artery Stenting Trial), 383
VCDs. See Vascular closure devices (VCDs)
VEin Graft LEsion Stenting With the Taxus Stent and Intravascular Ultrasound (VELETI) Pilot Trial, 303
Venestent trial, 299
Venous thromboembolism (VTE)
  catheter-directed management
    AngioJet rheolytic thrombectomy system, 403, 403f
    ATTRACT trial, 401
    catheter-based lysis, 402
    EkoSonic endovascular system, 403f
    femoropopliteal DVT, 401
    iliofemoral deep venous thrombosis, 402, 402f

    residual stenosis, 403
  diagnosis, 400, 400f
  incidence, 400
  medical management, 401, 401t
  PE severity index, 400, 400t
  risk factors, 400
Venous–venous collaterals, 473
Ventricular filling wave, 465
Ventricular septal defects (VSDs)
  incidence, 472
  percutaneous closure, 472
  transcatheter closure, 472
Venture catheter, 174
Verapamil, 54, 452
Vertebral artery stenosis (VAS), 382–383
Vertebral Artery Stenting Trial (VAST), 383
Veterans Administration Cooperative Study of Surgery (VACSS), 202
Veterans Affairs Cooperative Study (VACS), 376
ViperSlide, 180
Viscosity, contrast media, 71
Vorapaxar, 28
VSDs. See Ventricular septal defects (VSDs)
VSMCs. See Vascular smooth muscle cells (VSMCs)
VTE. See Venous thromboembolism (VTE)
Vulnerable plaques
  angioscopy, 111
  coronary angiography, 105
  histopathology, 105–106, 106f, 106t
  imaging guidelines, 112, 113–114t
  intravascular ultrasound
    clinical outcome studies, 108
    conventional grayscale IVUS, 106
    fibrous cap thickness, 107
    plaque burden, 106
    plaque compositional features, 108
    plaque rupture and thrombosis, 107, 108f
    while grayscale IVUS, 107
  near-infrared fluorescence molecular imaging, 111–112, 113f
  near-infrared spectroscopy, 110–111, 111f
  optical coherence tomography, 100–110

W

Wallstents, 188, 403
Warfarin, 59
  atrial fibrillation, 424
  non-ST segment acute coronary syndromes, 46
WATCHMAN LAA occluder
  distal fixation anchors, 425
  indications, 428b
  procedural complications, 428, 428t
  randomized clinical trial data
    anticoagulant and antiplatelet management strategy, 425, 427f
    bleeding reduction, 426–427, 427f
    PROTECT-AF trial, 425, 427f
    warfarin therapy, 425

  society recommendations, 428, 428t
Wiggers diagram, 116, 116f
Wiggle wire, 171
Wilkins score, 430, 430t
Wire escalation, antegrade, 318f, 319
Women and percutaneous interventions
  abdominal aortic aneurysms, 345
  coronary artery disease
    anatomical considerations, 342
    bleeding events, 343
    demographics, 340
    hemodynamic support, 343
    ischemia without obstructive CAD, 342
    medical comorbidities, 340
    non ST-segment elevation MI, 343
    pharmacotherapy, 344
    physician awareness and referral, 344
    plaque morphology, 340–341, 341f
    research studies, 344
    spontaneous coronary artery dissection, 341–342
    stable CAD, 343
    stent type, 342–343
    ST-segment elevation MI, 343–344
    symptoms, 339
    vascular function, 341
  peripheral vascular disease, 345
  secondary prevention and guidelines, 345
  stroke, 345
  valvular heart disease, 344–345
Women Ischemic Syndrome Evaluation (WISE) study, 341
Workhorse wires, 170, 170f

X

XIENCE Nano trial, 284
Xience V, 21
X-ray beam focal spot, 62
X-ray imaging
  advancement in, 70
  biologic effects, 65–66, 66t
  cine/fluoroscopic unit, 63–64, 64f
  contrast media. See Contrast media
  image formation, 63–64
  image quality, 62–63
  image storage, 64
  image transfer, 62
  patient exposure and risk, 67, 67t
  physics, 62–63
  radiation. See Radiation
  radiation dose, 64–65
X-ray tube, 62, 62f

Y

Y stent technique, 276

Z

Zotarolimus-eluting stents (ZES), 21–22, 191, 284